D1376845

JAMA and ARCHIVES JOURNALS

Alternative Medicine

An Objective Assessment

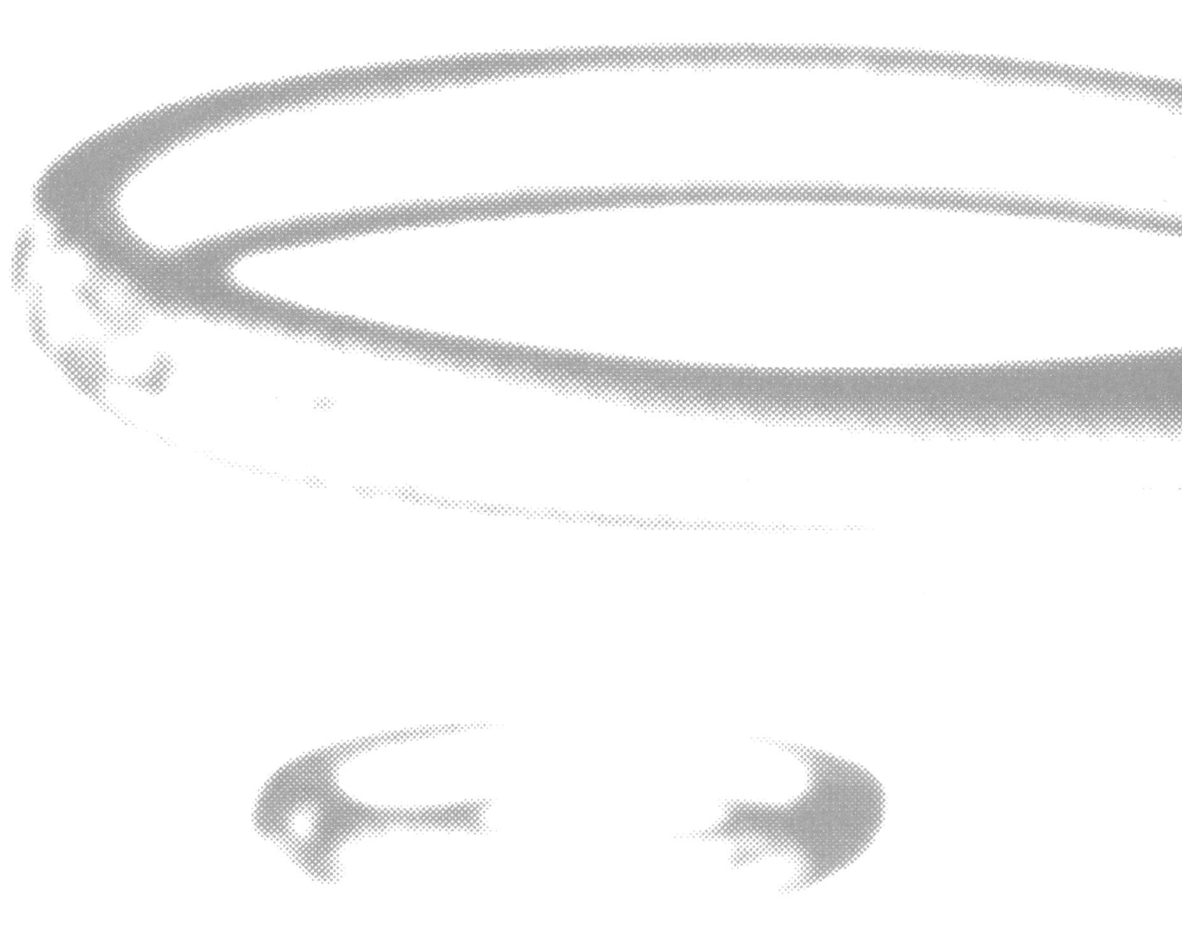

Edited by
Phil B. Fontanarosa, MD

Property of Library
Cape Fear Comm College
Wilmington, N. C.

Publisher: Anthony J. Frankos
Editorial Director: Mary Lou White
Marketing Services Director: Rhonda Taira
Manager, Database and New Media: Mary Ellen Johnston
Senior Acquisitions Editor: Barry Bowlus
Managing Editor: Jean Roberts
Project Manager: Denise M. Bryson
Production Designer: Dawn Goldammer
New Media Specialist: Joel Brammeier
Editorial Assistant: David Arispe

***JAMA* and *Archives* Journals Book Liaisons:** Annette Flanagin, Cheryl Iverson

© 2000 by the American Medical Association.
All rights reserved. Printed in the USA.

Internet address http://www.ama-assn.org

No part of this publication may be reproduced, stored in a retrieval system, or transmitted, in any form or by any means, electronic, mechanical, photocopying, recording, or otherwise, without prior written permission of the publisher.

Additional copies may be ordered from:
Order Department OP210599
ISBN 1-57947-002-5
American Medical Association
For order information, call toll-free 800 621-8335.

BQ64:99-0332:7.2M:1/00

Foreword

From acupuncture to aromatherapy, herbal therapies to homeopathy, and reflexology to relaxation therapy, numerous practices that are termed alternative, complementary, or unconventional medicine have become increasingly prevalent and popular. Even though many of these therapies encompass diverse modalities and philosophies that traditionally are considered outside the realm of mainstream medicine, the use of alternative therapies, visits to alternative medicine practitioners, and expenditures for these therapies are substantial. Yet despite increasing public interest and worldwide use of alternative therapies, high-quality scientific evidence that clearly establishes the safety and effectiveness (or lack thereof) of these interventions is lacking. Consequently, many physicians traditionally have viewed alternative medicine in general, and most practices contained therein, with skepticism and mistrust.

Given the burgeoning interest in alternative therapies among the general public, patients, physicians, other health care professionals, academic medical centers, and health care payers, it is not surprising that a 1997 survey of *JAMA* physician-readers ranked alternative medicine as the seventh most important topic for *The Journal* to address. Moreover, considering that alternative and complementary therapies have the potential to involve patients seen by physicians in virtually all specialties, the *JAMA* Editorial Board and Editorial staff, and the editors of the American Medical Association *Archives* Journals ranked alternative medicine among the top 3 subjects for their journals to address in 1998. Alternative medicine was selected as the subject for theme issues of these scientific journals, which were published concurrently in November of that year.

Alternative Medicine: An Objective Assessment represents the results of this concerted initiative—to provide original research studies and scholarly articles that present new scientific information and critical perspectives on alternative medicine to the medical and scientific communities. Most of the articles in this book were published in the 1998 alternative medicine theme issues of *JAMA* and the *Archives* Journals, or have been published in these journals within the previous or subsequent year. As such, these articles have been subject to the usual exacting editorial evaluation and rigorous peer review characteristic of these scientific publications.

Accordingly, *Alternative Medicine: An Objective Assessment* presents clinically relevant, methodologically reliable, and scientifically valid information. By using this critically evaluated scientific information—rather than relying on anecdotal reports, unproven theories, or unfounded opinions—physicians and other health care professionals should be better prepared to serve as useful sources of information about alternative therapies for patients, should be more comfortable answering their patients' questions appropriately, and should be able to provide evidence-based guidance and advice about the complex and diverse practices known as alternative medicine.

Phil B. Fontanarosa, MD

Phil B. Fontanarosa, MD
Editor, *Alternative Medicine: An Objective Assessment*

(modified from *JAMA;* 1997; 278:2111–2112)

Preface

It is fitting that *Alternative Medicine: An Objective Assessment* tackles perhaps the most controversial arena in medicine—an arena that some purport to be a circus, where fantasy and illusion regularly mingle with reality. Yet where the truth begins and ends is widely debated, and even more widely reported in the popular press. This book answers many of the questions previously unanswered by science.

The authors and editors of *JAMA* and the *Archives* Journals deliver, through the rigors of science, a cogent and well-constructed survey of the evidence-based understanding of alternative medicine. This is a milestone. The authors and editors delineate where the science begins and ends as of today, outlining where further study is needed: all of this, combined with the journalistic excellence we have come to expect from the authors and editors of *JAMA* and the *Archives* Journals.

Physicians, nurses, and other health care professionals seek knowledge from a wide range of sources. The desire for "need-to-know" information about alternative and complementary therapies is strong. It is our duty and responsibility to examine the scientific bases of complementary and alternative medicine. Treatments that initially look "alternative" to Western culture may be part of the medical mainstream in the originating culture. Some estimates suggest that 80% of the world uses "alternative" treatment as their primary means of medical care while struggling to afford Western medicine. In America alone, billions are spent on these "recently discovered" therapies.

As physicians, we are often asked, "Do they work?" As scientists, it is our obligation to ask and to seek the evidence. What works? What doesn't? What is still open to question? What are the limits of our evidence? Where do we direct our future investigations? With this scrutiny, this book creates the milestone.

Thomas R. Reardon, MD

Thomas R. Reardon, MD
President, American Medical Association

Acknowledgments

Sincere appreciation is extended to the many individuals who contributed to *Alternative Medicine: An Objective Assessment,* especially the authors and peer reviewers of the published articles, and the editors of the participating AMA journals (on facing page).

Special thanks is also extended to all members of the editorial staff and publishing staff who served *JAMA* and the *Archives* Journals in 1998 and 1999. This book would not have been possible without their efforts.

Finally, special recognition is given to George D. Lundberg, MD, former Editor-in-Chief (1982–1999) of *JAMA* and AMA Scientific Publications, for having the courage and vision to bring solid scientific information on alternative medicine to physicians through publication in leading conventional medical journals.

Participating Editors, *JAMA* and the *Archives* Journals

Phil B. Fontanarosa, MD
Chicago, Ill
Coeditor, *JAMA*

Richard M. Glass, MD
Chicago, Ill
Coeditor, *JAMA*

Daniel M. Albert, MD, MS
University of Wisconsin, Madison
Editor, *Archives of Ophthalmology*

Kenneth A. Arndt, MD
Beth Israel Deaconess Medical Center
Boston, Mass
Editor, *Archives of Dermatology*

Jack D. Barchas, MD
Cornell Medical Center
New York, NY
Editor, *Archives of General Psychiatry*

Marjorie A. Bowman, MD, MPA
University of Pennsylvania Health System
Philadelphia
Editor, *Archives of Family Medicine*

James E. Dalen, MD, MPH
University of Arizona, Tucson
Editor, *Archives of Internal Medicine*

Catherine D. DeAngelis, MD
Johns Hopkins School of Medicine
Baltimore, Md
Editor, *Archives of Pediatrics & Adolescent Medicine*

Michael E. Johns, MD
Emory University
Atlanta, Ga
Editor, *Archives of Otolaryngology—Head & Neck Surgery*

Claude H. Organ, Jr, MD
University of California–Davis, East Bay
Oakland
Editor, *Archives of Surgery*

Roger N. Rosenberg, MD
University of Texas Southwestern Medical Center
Dallas
Editor, *Archives of Neurology*

Table of Contents

1 Alternative Medicine—Prevalence and Use

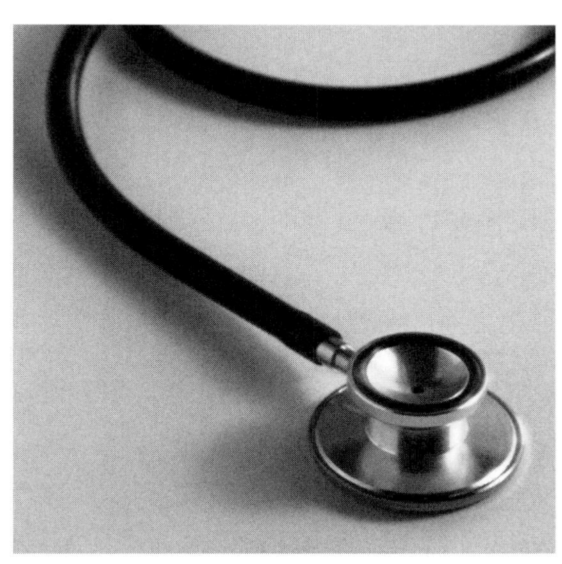

Overview

William R. Harlan, MD
From the National Institutes of Health, Bethesda, Md.

The remarkable growth in the use of complementary and alternative medicine (CAM) in the United States has been likened to a populist movement, one reminiscent and similar to the social movements of 30 years ago. The characteristics include self-determination (or improvement), return to naturalistic foundations and their integration into a technological society, and leadership by educated, affluent segments of the population. The articles in this section document the extent of use, the demographics and characteristics of those using CAM, the attitudes of physicians toward its use, and the implications for practice.

The surveys provide a broad landscape of CAM products and services used by the general public in the United States. The report by Eisenberg et al[1] indicates high use of CAM in 2 cross-sectional surveys and increasing use from 1990 to 1997. Remarkably, 42% of those surveyed had used at least 1 alternative therapy in 1997, and this represented an increase from the earlier survey. The expenditures for these products and services are estimated at $27 billion; more than half were paid out of pocket. The estimate of out-of-pocket payments for CAM equated roughly to similar payments for all services provided for conventional physician services. Given the discretionary nature of payments for these services, it is not surprising that use of CAM was most frequent among middle-income, more highly educated individuals.[2] In the national population survey, over half (58%) of the use was to "prevent future illness from occurring or to maintain health or vitality."[1] This illustrates a limitation of populational surveys of therapeutic products. In surveys of the general population, few persons with serious health problems are likely to be sampled, and the findings would describe patterns of use among generally healthy individuals. Therefore, respondents' emphasis on health maintenance and prevention is not surprising.

However, focusing surveys on patients with serious conditions, such as HIV (Fairfield et al[3]), provides important detail that complements the broad picture. Those with serious conditions report a particularly high use (70% or greater) and even greater expenditures. These patients made almost twice as many visits to CAM providers as to conventional primary care providers. Similar findings might be expected for other serious conditions, such as cancer. The major reason for information requests to the Public Information Clearinghouse at the National Center for Complementary and Alternative Medicine is cancer. For similar reasons, a broad national telephone survey would not provide a clear picture of CAM use by minority or underserved populations, and further work is needed to clarify this picture. Taken as a whole, these surveys should focus the development of studies to validate CAM products and services and to compel conventional practitioners to learn more about the benefits and risks of CAM therapy.

The study by Astin[2] provides an interesting insight into the reasons that people use CAM. His findings suggest that a substantial proportion of those using CAM place considerable value on the holistic aspects of health and did not use CAM because of dissatisfaction with conventional medicine. Rather, its use seemed to complement the use of conventional care and evoke a mind-body holism and a spiritual side of health and healing. This affords insight into the choice of CAM and should provide conventional practitioners with a better understanding of how to relate to patients and understand their interest in these therapies.

A review of 25 national surveys of physician attitudes toward CAM indicates that respondent physicians from industrialized countries use and refer patients for several CAM modalities.[4] The responses reported across surveys and encompassing several countries were characterized by large ranges, and this limits inferences. Chiropractic, acupuncture, massage, herbal medicines, and homeopathy were the modalities most often utilized by conventional physicians in patient management. However, the range of responses by physicians was great and the surveys were limited in sample size. Pediatricians in Michigan were surveyed,[5] and they expressed an open and accepting attitude toward CAM use and referral to CAM practitioners. Despite the variability of response in these surveys, the attitude of conventional physicians who responded could not be characterized as interested in the use of CAM therapies and/or willing to discuss their use with patients. There is greater acceptance of modalities that have been widely used and investigated and are more closely related to approaches that have "stood the test of time" and usage. There is an important caveat that nonrespondents might have different attitudes, and the variability noted in the surveys may reflect differential response rates.

In light of the generally positive attitudes about CAM, the discussion by Studdert et al[6] offers useful information about liability for practice and referral. The claims experience from 1990 to 1996 for nonconventional practitioners was considerably better than for primary care physicians in terms of either rates of claims or average payment per paid claim. Importantly, there is in this chapter a very useful discussion of liability related to referral by conventional practitioners for complementary and alternative therapy. The referring physician should be familiar with the efficacy of CAM treatments and the referring entity—physician or managed care organization or hospital—should exert due diligence to select competent CAM practitioners.

The extent and investment in these complementary and alternative therapies, as well as the growth in use, provide a clarion call to providers to learn about CAM, to researchers to provide the evidence-based approach to generate information about efficacy and adverse effects, and to purveyors of dietary supplements and botanicals that the market deserves investment in research and in manufacturing a good product.

References

1. Eisenberg DM, Davis RB, Ettner SL, et al. Trends in alternative medicine use in the United States, 1990–1997. *JAMA.* 1998;280:1569–1575.

2. Astin JA. Why patients use alternative medicine. *JAMA.* 1998;279:1548–1553.

3. Fairfield KM, Eisenberg DM, Davis RB, Libman H, Phillips RS. Patterns of use, expenditures, and perceived efficacy of complementary and alternative therapies in HIV-infected patients. *Arch Intern Med.* 1998;158:2257–2264.

4. Astin JA, Marie A, Pelletier KR, Hansen E, Haskell WL. A review of the incorporation of complementary and alternative medicine by mainstream physicians. *Arch Intern Med.* 1998;158:2303–2310.

5. Sikand A, Laken M. Pediatricians' experience with and attitudes toward complementary/alternative medicine. *Arch Pediatr Adolesc Med.* 1998;152:1059–1064.

6. Studdert DM, Eisenberg DM, Miller FH, Curto DA, Kaptchuk TJ, Brennan TA. Medical malpractice implications of alternative medicine. *JAMA.* 1998;280:1610–1615.

1 Trends in Alternative Medicine Use in the United States, 1990–1997

Results of a Follow-up National Survey

David M. Eisenberg, MD; Roger B. Davis, ScD; Susan L. Ettner, PhD; Scott Appel, MS; Sonja Wilkey; Maria Van Rompay; Ronald C. Kessler, PhD
From the Center for Alternative Medicine Research and Education, Department of Medicine, Beth Israel Deaconess Medical Center (Drs Eisenberg and Davis, Mr Appel, and Mss Wilkey and Van Rompay), and the Department of Health Care Policy, Harvard Medical School (Drs Ettner and Kessler), Boston, Mass.

Context

A prior national survey documented the high prevalence and costs of alternative medicine use in the United States in 1990.

Objective

To document trends in alternative medicine use in the United States between 1990 and 1997.

Design

Nationally representative random household telephone surveys using comparable key questions were conducted in 1991 and 1997 measuring utilization in 1990 and 1997, respectively.

Participants

A total of 1539 adults in 1991 and 2055 in 1997.

Main Outcomes Measures

Prevalence, estimated costs, and disclosure of alternative therapies to physicians.

Results

Use of at least 1 of 16 alternative therapies during the previous year increased from 33.8% in 1990 to 42.1% in 1997 (*P*≤.001). The therapies increasing the most included herbal medicine, massage, megavitamins, self-help groups, folk remedies, energy healing, and homeopathy. The probability of users visiting an alternative medicine practitioner increased from 36.3% to 46.3% (*P*=.002). In both surveys alternative therapies were used most frequently for chronic conditions, including back problems, anxiety, depression, and headaches. There was no significant change in disclosure rates between the 2 survey years; 39.8% of alternative therapies were disclosed to physicians in 1990 vs 38.5% in 1997. The percentage of users paying entirely out-of-pocket for services provided by alternative medicine practitioners did not change significantly between 1990 (64.0%) and 1997 (58.3%) (*P*=.36). Extrapolations to the US population suggest a 47.3% increase in total visits to alternative medicine practitioners, from 427 million in 1990 to 629 million in 1997, thereby exceeding total

visits to all US primary care physicians. An estimated 15 million adults in 1997 took prescription medications concurrently with herbal remedies and/or high-dose vitamins (18.4% of all prescription users). Estimated expenditures for alternative medicine professional services increased 45.2% between 1990 and 1997 and were conservatively estimated at $21.2 billion in 1997, with at least $12.2 billion paid out-of-pocket. This exceeds the 1997 out-of-pocket expenditures for all US hospitalizations. Total 1997 out-of-pocket expenditures relating to alternative therapies were conservatively estimated at $27.0 billion, which is comparable with the projected 1997 out-of-pocket expenditures for all US physician services.

Conclusions

Alternative medicine use and expenditures increased substantially between 1990 and 1997, attributable primarily to an increase in the proportion of the population seeking alternative therapies, rather than increased visits per patient.

JAMA. 1998;280:1569–1575

Alternative medical therapies, functionally defined as interventions neither taught widely in medical schools nor generally available in US hospitals,[1] have attracted increased national attention from the media, the medical community, governmental agencies, and the public. A 1990 national survey of alternative medicine prevalence, costs, and patterns of use[1] demonstrated that alternative medicine has a substantial presence in the US health care system. Data from a survey in 1994[2] and a public opinion poll in 1997[3] confirmed the extensive use of alternative medical therapies in the United States. An increasing number of US insurers and managed care organizations now offer alternative medicine programs and benefits.[4] The majority of US medical schools now offer courses on alternative medicine.[5]

National surveys performed outside the United States suggest that alternative medicine is popular throughout the industrialized world.[6] The percentage of the population who used alternative therapies during the prior 12 months has been estimated to be 10% in Denmark (1987),[7] 33% in Finland (1982),[8] and 49% in Australia (1993).[9] Public opinion polls and consumers' association surveys suggest high prevalence rates throughout Europe and the United Kingdom.[10–13] The percentage of the Canadian population who saw an alternative therapy practitioner during the previous 12 months has been estimated at 15% (1995).[14] The wide range of utilization rates can be explained, in part, by the disparity in definitions of alternative therapy and the selection of therapies assessed.

The presumption is that alternative medicine use in the United States has increased at a considerable pace in recent years. The purpose of this follow-up national survey was to investigate this presumption and document trends in alternative medicine prevalence, costs, disclosure of use to physicians, and correlates of use since 1990.

Methods

Sample

We conducted parallel nationally representative telephone surveys in 1991 and 1997. Survey methods were approved by the Beth Israel Deaconess Institutional Review Board, Boston, Mass. Both surveys used random-digit dialing to select households and random selection of 1 household resident, aged 18 years or older, as the respondent. Eligibility was limited to English speakers in whom cognitive or physical impairment did not prevent completion of the interview. We asked respondents about their use of alternative therapies during the prior 12 months. We consider the results of the 1991 survey, fielded between January and March of that year, representative of 1990, and the results of the 1997 survey, fielded between November 1997 and February 1998, representative of 1997.

The sampling scheme was designed with a target sample of 1500 in 1990 and 2000 in 1997. The latter sample size was chosen to provide power in excess of 80% to detect an increase from 34% to 39% in the proportion of adults who used at least 1 form of alternative therapy during the prior 12 months. The actual numbers of completed interviews were 1539 in 1990 (67% response rate) and 2055 in 1997 (60% weighted response rate). A secular trend in lower survey response required us to offer a $20 financial incentive for participation in the 1997 survey to maintain a response rate near the one achieved in 1990. No financial incentive was used in the 1990 survey.

The data in each survey were separately weighted to adjust for geographic variation in cooperation (eg, by region of country and urbanicity) and for household variation in probability of selection (ie, the inverse relationship between size of household and probability of selection because only 1 interview was completed in each sample household). The data were then weighted in parallel on sociodemographic variables to adjust for aggregate discrepancies between the sample distributions and population distributions provided by the US Census Bureau. This last stage of weighting was based on the 1997 Current Population Survey data[15] and was done in parallel across the 2 surveys to remove any between-survey discrepancies of weighted sociodemographic distributions.

Of the initial sample of 9750 telephone numbers in 1997, 26% were nonworking, 17% were not assigned to households, and 9% were unavailable (ie, despite 6 attempted follow-up contacts). We declared 481 households ineligible because respondents did not speak English or because of cognitive or physical incapacity. Among the remaining 4167 eligible respondents, 1720 (41.3%) completed the interview on initial request. Attempts were then made to convert a random subsample of 1066 refusers by offering them an increased stipend ($50). A total of 335 (31.4%) of the 1066 contacted were converted in this manner. Extrapolating this conversion rate to all of the refusers and weighting the data for the undersampling of initial refusers, we obtained a 60% (41.3% + [31.4% × (100% − 41.3%)]) weighted overall response rate among eligible respondents.

Interview

In both years, the interview was presented as a survey conducted about the health care practices of Americans by investigators from Harvard Medical School. No mention was made of alternative or complementary therapies. The substantive questions began by asking about perceived health, health worries, days spent in bed, and functional impairment due to health problems. We then asked respondents about their interactions with a *medical doctor,* defined as "a medical doctor (MD) or a doctor of osteopathic medicine (DO), not a chiropractor or other nonmedical doctor." The term *medical doctor* was used throughout the remainder of the interview.

To document trends we explored the following: (1) Respondents in both surveys were presented with a list of common medical conditions and asked if they had experienced each of these conditions during the previous 12 months. (2) Respondents who reported more than 3 conditions were asked to identify their 3 most bothersome or serious medical conditions and were then asked about seeing a medical doctor for these principal medical conditions and about the perceived quality of these interactions. (3) Respondents were asked about their lifetime and past 12-month use of 16 alternative therapies and whether each of these therapies was used for each of the principal medical conditions. The 1997 survey also asked about use for a representative sample of other medical conditions and expanded the list of therapies beyond the original 16 assessed in 1990. (4) We distinguished between use under the supervision of a practitioner of alternative therapy and use without such supervision. Respondents who reported supervised use were asked about their number of visits in the past 12 months to practitioners of each therapy. (5) All users of alternative therapies in 1997 who acknowledged seeing a medical doctor during the past year were then asked if they had discussed their use of each therapy with a medical doctor and, if not, why not.

Prior use of 16 targeted therapies was explored using a computer-assisted interview transcript, which included the following clarifications in both 1990 and 1997: When asking about high-dose vitamin or megavitamin therapies, interviewers made clear that the survey sought information on vitamins not including a daily vitamin or vitamin prescribed by a doctor. Prayer or spiritual healing by others was asked about separately from prayer or spiritual practice for individual health concern. Commercial diet programs were described as "the kind you have to pay for, but not including trying to lose or gain weight on your own." A lifestyle diet included examples like vegetarianism or macrobiotics. Questions regarding energy healing included examples of magnets, energy-emitting machines, or the "laying on of hands," and use of relaxation techniques was explained using the examples of meditation or the relaxation response. The remaining 9 therapies were asked about without interviewer clarification.

The 1997 survey was longer (average, 30 minutes) than the 1990 survey (average, 25 minutes) because we sought to explore a number of areas in more depth. All the important questions in the 1990 survey were repeated in 1997. These replicated questions are the focus of the current report. One major change in the 1997 survey involved replicated questions: respondents who reported using more than 3 alternative therapies were asked in-depth questions (eg, use of a practitioner of alternative therapies, number of visits, out-of-pocket expenses, reasons for use) for all such therapies in 1990 but only for a random sample of 3 such therapies in 1997. This was required because of expansion in both the number of alternative therapies we assessed in 1997 and questions about each therapy. The 1997 data were weighted to adjust for this sampling in making comparisons with the 1990 data.

Insurance Coverage

For each therapy for which respondents said they used services of an alternative medicine practitioner, we asked whether insurance helped pay for any of the costs of the therapy and whether the respondent paid any of the costs out-of-pocket. Based on the answers to these questions, we calculated the proportion of users of each therapy who had complete, partial, or no insurance coverage for that therapy. We also calculated the overall frequency of insurance coverage by weighting the insurance frequencies within each therapy by the proportion of all user therapies accounted for by that therapy.

Construction of Cost Measures

The total cost of visits to alternative medicine practitioners was calculated by multiplying the number of visits for each therapy by a per-visit price and adding the prices of the following therapies: relaxation techniques, herbal medicine, massage therapy, chiropractic care, megavitamins, self-help groups, imagery techniques, commercial diet, folk remedies, lifestyle diet, energy healing, homeopathy, hypnosis, biofeedback, and acupuncture. Out-of-pocket costs were constructed for each therapy by multiplying each user's visits by the full price of the visit if the user had no insurance coverage, by 0.2 if the user had partial insurance coverage, and by zero if insurance paid the full price of the visit. The assumption of a 20% coinsurance rate among users with partial insurance coverage should yield a conservative estimate of out-of-pocket costs, because it ignores deductibles and benefit caps and assumes that insurance benefits for alternative therapy are similar to medical coverage.

We calculated costs based on per-visit prices chosen from typical prices paid for such services by private insurers using a Resource-Based Relative Value Scale (RBRVS)[16] system in selected states. We then recalculated costs using a second set of prices chosen partly to reflect empirical data on the out-of-pocket costs paid by the respondents, but primarily to represent conservative estimates of the per-visit cost of alternative therapies. Total costs based on this second set of prices should represent a lower bound on true expenditures.

Out-of-pocket costs of herbs, megavitamin supplements, and commercial diet products were calculated by multiplying the total population of users by the average out-of-pocket expenditures reported by respondents who used each of these products. In 1997, each respondent who used an alternative therapy was also asked, "Did you spend any additional money on things like books, classes, equipment, or any other items related to [the alternative therapy] in the past 12 months?" Out-of-pocket expenditures on these other items were calculated following the same procedures used for herbs, megavitamins, and commercial diet products. Out-of-pocket expenditures on herbs, megavitamins, commercial diet products, and related items were based on actual dollar amounts reported, so changes between 1990 and 1997 include inflation. To isolate the increase in the cost of practitioner visits between 1990 and 1997 solely because of the increase in the use of alternative therapies, we calculated 1990 practitioner costs using 1997 prices. The differences between the 1990 and 1997 costs of practitioner services reported are understated because they do not take into account inflation, estimated at 44% by the medical component of the Consumer Price Index.[17]

Statistical Analysis

Analyses reported herein consist of computation of prevalence and mean estimates and comparisons of these estimates through the years. As the data in both surveys are weighted, the Taylor series method was used to compute significance tests using SUDAAN software.[18] χ^2 Tests of independence were used for comparing proportions, while *t* tests were used for continuous measures. Extrapolations of survey estimates to the total population were based on the assumption that there were 180 million adults living in the US household population in 1990 and 198 million in 1997.[15]

Results

Characteristics of Respondents

The characteristics of the subjects we interviewed are shown in Table 1. The sociodemographic characteristics of the survey sample are similar to the population distributions published by the US Bureau of the Census.[15]

Patterns of Use

Use of alternative therapies in 1997 was not confined to any narrow segment of society. Rates of use ranged from 32% to 54% in the wide range of sociodemographic groups examined. Use was more common among women (48.9%) than men (37.8%) (P=.001) and less common among African Americans (33.1%) than members of other racial groups (44.5%) (P=.004). People aged 35 to 49 years reported higher rates of use (50.1%) than people either older (39.1%) (P=.001) or younger (41.8%) (P=.003). Use was higher among those who had some college education (50.6%) than with no college education (36.4%) (P=.001)

Table 1. Characteristics of the 1997 (N=2055) and 1990 (N=1539) Subjects Interviewed Compared With the US Population*

Characteristic	1997 Survey, %	1997 US Bureau of the Census,[17] %	1990 Survey, %
Sex			
Female	52	52	48
Male	48	48	52
Age, y			
18-24	10	13	16
25-34	22	20	23
35-49	33	32	27
≥50	35	35	34
Race/ethnicity			
White	77	73	82
African American	8	12	9
Hispanic	10	11	6
Asian	1	4	1
Other	4	1	2
Education			
<High school	14	18	24
High school graduate	37	34	35
College or more	49	48	40
Annual income, $			
<20,000	27	33	30
20,000-49,999	45	41	53
≥50,000	27	26	18
Region			
Northeast	21	19	22
North central	24	24	32
South	35	35	26
West	20	22	19

*Due to rounding, percentages do not always total 100.

and more common among people with annual incomes above $50,000 (48.1%) than with lower incomes (42.6%) (P=.03). Use was more common among those in the West (50.1%) than elsewhere in the United States (42.1%) (P=.004). With the exception of observed sex differences in 1997, these patterns are consistent with those identified in 1990.

Population prevalence estimates of alternative medicine use in 1990 and 1997 are shown in Table 2. The 1990 survey estimated that 33.8% of the US adult population (60 million people) used at least 1 of the 16 alternative therapies listed, while the 1997 survey estimated that this proportion increased significantly to 42.1% (83 million people). A comparison of specific therapies in the first column shows increases in 15 of the 16 therapies; 10 of these were statistically significant ($P \leq .05$). The largest increases were in the use of herbal medicine, massage, megavitamins, self-help groups, folk remedies, energy healing, and homeopathy. Summing Table 2 (first column) data shows a 65% increase in total number of therapies used, from 577 therapies per 1000 population in 1990 to 953 per 1000 in 1997.

Several categories of alternative therapy warrant clarification about the actual modalities used. Three quarters of respondents who acknowledged use of relaxation techniques said they used meditation. Among those who reported using energy healing, the most frequently cited technique involved the use of magnets. Other modalities common to this category included Therapeutic Touch, Reiki, and energy healing by religious groups. The use of self-prayer, in contrast to spiritual or energy healing performed by others, was investigated in terms of prevalence of use but not in terms of costs, referral patterns, or insurance reimbursement. All analyses in this article exclude data involving self-prayer.

Table 2 (second column) shows that a significantly higher proportion of alternative therapy users saw an alternative medicine practitioner in 1997 (46.3%, equivalent to 39 million people) than in 1990 (36.3%, equivalent to 22 million people). Of the 15 therapies for which the question was asked, the proportion of users who saw a practitioner increased for 11. However, even in 1997 there were only 5 therapies in which a majority of users consulted a practitioner: massage, chiropractic, hypnosis, biofeedback, and acupuncture. Unsupervised use (ie, a form of expanded self-care) remains the usual method of use for all other alternative therapies.

Table 2 (third column) reveals no consistent change in the average number of visits among respondents who consulted practitioners of alternative therapy between 1990 (19.2%) and 1997 (16.3%). However, because of the increase in the proportion of people using these therapies, the total number of visits increased substantially from 1990 to 1997. This 47.3% increase in total visits is largely because of increases in visits for relaxation therapy, massage, chiropractic, self-help, and energy healing. The visits to practitioners of alternative therapy in 1997 exceeded the projected number of visits to all primary care physicians in the United States by an estimated 243 million (Figure 1).[19,20] Visits to chiropractors and massage therapists accounted for nearly half of all visits to practitioners of alternative therapies.

Prevalence estimates for selected additional therapies assessed in 1997 but not 1990 include: aromatherapy (5.6%), neural therapy (1.7%), naturopathy (0.7%), and

Table 2. Comparison of Prevalence and Frequency of Use of Alternative Therapies Among Adult Respondents, 1997 vs 1990*

Type of Therapy	Used in Past 12 mo, %		Saw a Practitioner in Past 12 mo, %		Mean No. of Visits per User in Past 12 mo		No. of Visits per 1000 Population		Estimated Total No. of Visits in 1997 (in Thousands)†	Total Visits, %‡§
	1997	1990	1997	1990	1997	1990	1997	1990		
Relaxation techniques	16.3¶	13.1	15.3	9.0	20.9	18.6	521.2	219.3	103,203	16.4
Herbal medicine	12.1**	2.5	15.1	10.2	2.9	8.1	53.0	20.7	10,491	1.7
Massage	11.1**	6.9	61.6#	41.4	8.4	14.8	574.4	422.8	113,723	18.1
Chiropractic	11.0	10.1	89.9**	71.1	9.8	12.6	969.1¶	904.8	191,886	30.5
Spiritual healing by others ‖	7.0#	4.2	...	9.2	...	14.2	...	54.9	...	...
Megavitamins	5.5**	2.4	23.7	11.8	8.6	12.6	112.1	35.7	22,196	3.5
Self-help group	4.8**	2.3	44.4	38.3	18.9	20.5	402.8	180.6	79,754	12.7
Imagery	4.5	4.2	23.1	15.1	11.0	14.2	114.3	90.1	22,640	3.6
Commercial diet	4.4	3.9	43.2	24.0	7.3	20.7	138.8	193.8	27,474	4.4
Folk remedies	4.2**	0.2	6.2	0.0	1.0	...	2.6	...	516	0.1
Lifestyle diet	4.0	3.6	8.0	12.5	2.8	8.1	9.0	36.5	1774	0.3
Energy healing	3.8**	1.3	26.3	32.2	20.2#	8.3	201.9¶	34.7	39,972	6.4
Homeopathy	3.4**	0.7	16.5	31.7	1.6	6.1	9.0	13.5	1777	0.3
Hypnosis	1.2	0.9	62.7	51.8	2.8	2.6	21.1	12.1	4171	0.7
Biofeedback	1.0	1.0	54.3	20.8	3.6	6.4	19.5	13.3	3871	0.6
Acupuncture	1.0¶	0.4	87.6	91.3	3.1	38.4	27.2	140.2	5377	0.9
≥1 of 16 alternative therapies	42.1**	33.8	46.3#	36.3	16.3	19.2	**3176.0**	**2373.0**	**628,825**	...
SE	1.2	1.4	1.9	2.5	1.8	4.5	378.7	599.7	74,997	...
Self-prayer‖	35.1**	25.2	...	...	...	...	...	...	...	...

*Percentages are of those who used that type of therapy. Ellipses indicate data not applicable.
†Estimate based on 1997 population estimate of 198 million.
‡Percentage of total visits of the 16 therapies (ie, excluding self-prayer).
§Because of rounding, percentages do not total 100.
‖Respondents who received spiritual healing by others were not asked for details of visits in 1997, nor were those who used self-prayer in either year.
¶$P \leq .05$; #$P \leq .01$; **$P \leq .001$.

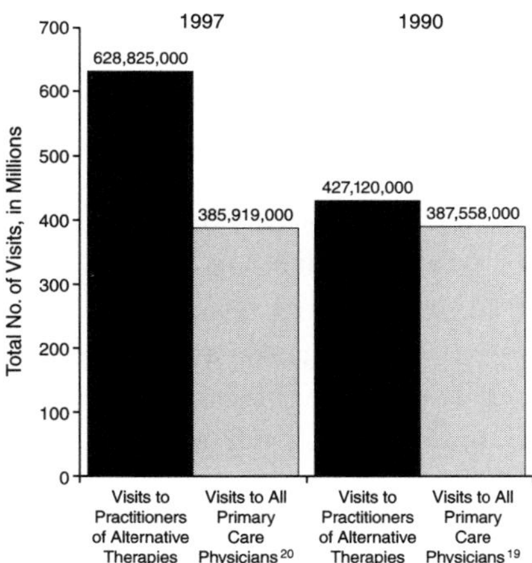

Figure 1. Trends in annual visits to practitioners of alternative therapies vs visits to primary care physicians, United States, 1997 vs 1990. Data are from the National Ambulatory Medical Care Survey from 1996[20] and 1990.[19]

chelation therapy (0.13%) (data not shown). Comparisons of total visits and costs for 1990 and 1997 were performed without inclusion of these data. Prevalence estimates for the simultaneous use of prescription medications with herbs, with high-dose vitamins, or with both were obtained. Among the 44% of adults who said they regularly take prescription medications, nearly 1 (18.4%) in 5 reported the concurrent use of at least 1 herbal product, a high-dose vitamin, or both.

Table 3 summarizes results regarding use of alternative therapies for the most commonly reported principal medical conditions in either survey. In each year, a majority of respondents reported 1 or more principal medical conditions. The list of conditions was expanded in 1997 (37 conditions) compared with 1990 (24 conditions). Significant increases in the proportion using alternative therapies for principal condition(s) (second column) occurred for back problems, allergies, arthritis, and digestive problems. The highest condition-specific rates of alternative therapy use in 1997 were for neck (57.0%) and back (47.6%) problems. The proportion of respondents

Table 3. Comparison of Use of Alternative Therapies for the Most Frequently Reported Principal Medical Conditions, 1997 vs 1990

	Percentage Reporting Condition		Used Alternative Therapy for Condition in Past 12 mo, %		Saw Alternative Practitioner for Condition in Past 12 mo, %		Saw Medical Doctor and Used Alternative Therapy for Condition in Past 12 mo, %		Saw Medical Doctor and Alternative Practitioner for Condition in Past 12 mo, %		
Condition	**1997**	**1990**	**1997**	**1990**	**1997**	**1990**	**1997**	**1990**	**1997**	**1990**	**Therapies Most Commonly Used in 1997**
Back problems	24.0#	19.9	47.6#	35.9	30.1#	19.5	58.8**	36.1	39.1#	23.0	Chiropractic, massage
Allergies	20.7#	16.0	16.6#	8.7	4.2	3.3	28.0¶	15.7	6.4	5.0	Herbal, relaxation
Fatigue*	16.7	. . .	27.0	. . .	6.3	. . .	51.6	. . .	13.1	. . .	Relaxation, massage
Arthritis	16.6	15.9	26.7¶	17.5	10.0	7.6	38.5¶	23.8	15.9	13.8	Relaxation, chiropractic
Headaches	12.9	13.2	32.2	26.5	13.3¶	6.3	42.0	31.8	20.0	12.1	Relaxation, chiropractic
Neck problems*	12.1	. . .	57.0	. . .	37.5	. . .	66.6	. . .	47.5	. . .	Chiropractic, massage
High blood pressure	10.9	11.0	11.7	11.0	0.9	2.9	11.9	11.6	1.1	3.5	Megavitamins, relaxation
Sprains or strains	10.8	13.4	23.6	22.3	10.3	9.6	29.4	24.7	15.9	13.6	Chiropractic, relaxation
Insomnia	9.3#	13.6	26.4	20.4	7.6	4.0	48.4	19.8	13.3	10.9	Relaxation, herbal
Lung problems	8.7	7.3	13.2	8.8	2.5	0.5	17.9	11.1	3.4	0.6	Relaxation, spiritual healing, herbal
Skin problems	8.6	8.0	6.7	6.0	2.2	1.6	6.8	6.9	0.0	2.5	Imagery, energy healing
Digestive problems	8.2	10.1	27.3#	13.2	9.7¶	3.6	34.1¶	15.3	10.7	5.8	Relaxation, herbal
Depression†	5.6	8.4	40.9	20.2	15.6	7.0	40.9	35.2	26.9	14.0	Relaxation, spiritual healing
Anxiety‡	5.5	9.5	42.7	27.9	11.6	6.5	42.7	45.4	21.0	10.4	Relaxation, spiritual healing
Weighted average across all conditions§	. . .	. . .	28.2**	19.1	11.4**	6.8	31.8**	19.9	13.7#	8.3	. . .
People with ≥1 condition‖	77.8¶	81.5	33.7**	22.9	15.3**	6.9	. . .	. . .	. . .	. . .	. . .

*Not included as a separate question in 1990 survey. Ellipses indicate data not applicable.
†The 1997 question asked about severe depression, which is not directly comparable with the 1990 question that asked about depression.
‡The 1997 question asked about anxiety attacks, which is not directly comparable with the 1990 question that asked about anxiety.
§The weighted averages are calculated based on all 37 conditions studied in 1997 and all 24 conditions studied in 1990, ie, condition is unit of analysis.
‖This row shows percentage of respondents who reported 1 or more principal medical conditions, along with the percentage of these respondents who reported use of therapy or practitioners for at least 1 of these conditions, ie, person is the unit of analysis.
¶$P≤.05$; #$P≤.01$; **$P<.001$.

with 1 or more medical conditions who reported use of an alternative therapy for at least 1 of those conditions increased significantly from 22.9% in 1990 to 33.7% in 1997 ($P≤.001$). The weighted condition-specific proportion who saw an alternative medicine practitioner for a given condition also increased significantly from 6.8% in 1990 to 11.4% in 1997 ($P≤.001$).

Table 3 also summarizes the probability that individuals who saw a medical doctor for a particular condition also used an alternative therapy (fourth column) or also saw a practitioner of alternative therapy (fifth column) for that same condition during the same year. A generally increasing pattern of alternative medicine use can be seen across the range of conditions studied. In 1990, an estimated 1 (19.9%) in 5 individuals seeing a medical doctor for a principal condition also used an alternative therapy. This percentage increased to nearly 1 (31.8%) in 3 in 1997 ($P≤.001$). The percentage who saw a medical doctor and also sought the services of an alternative practitioner increased significantly from 8.3% in 1990 to 13.7% in 1997 ($P≤.01$). In both 1990 and 1997, chiropractic, relaxation techniques, and massage therapy were among the alternative therapies used most commonly to treat principal medical conditions.

As in 1990, 96% of 1997 respondents who saw a practitioner of alternative therapy for a principal condition also saw a medical doctor during the prior 12 months, and only a minority of alternative therapies used were discussed with a medical doctor. Among the 618 respondents in 1997 who used 1 or more alternative therapies and had a medical doctor, only 377 (38.5%) of the 979 therapies used were discussed with the respondent's medical doctor. This is not significantly different from the 353 (39.8%) of the 886 therapies discussed by the comparable group of respondents (n=501) in the 1990 survey. Given that most alternative therapy is used without the supervision of an alternative practitioner, a substantial portion of alternative therapy use for principal medical conditions (46.0% in 1997 and 51.3% in 1990) was done without input from either a medical doctor or practitioner of alternative therapy.

Payment for Alternative Therapy

Data on insurance coverage of expenditures for alternative therapy services are shown in Table 4. The majority of people who saw alternative therapy practitioners paid all the costs out-of-pocket in both 1990 (64.0%) and 1997 (58.3%). None of the changes in insurance coverage between 1990 and 1997 were statistically significant, probably due in part to small sample sizes.

Using conservative assumptions about the fees charged by practitioners of alternative therapies and assuming no changes in visit prices, Americans spent an estimated $14.6 billion on visits to these practitioners in 1990 and $21.2 billion in 1997 (Table 5). Using less conservative (RBRVS) price figures, the amount spent on services of practitioners of alternative therapies was estimated at $22.6 billion in 1990 and $32.7 billion in 1997. Regardless of which set of prices is used, total expenditures for practitioners of alternative therapies are estimated to have increased by approximately 45% between 1990 and 1997 exclusive of inflation.

Estimated out-of-pocket expenditures for high-dose vitamins increased from $0.9 billion in 1990 to $3.3 billion in 1997. Smaller increases were observed for commercial diet products ($1.3 billion vs $1.7 billion). Unlike the 1990 survey, the 1997 survey included questions about expenditures for herbal products ($5.1 billion) and respondents' alternative therapy–specific books, classes, or equipment ($4.7 billion).

The estimated total out-of-pocket component of the alternative medicine market in 1997 is shown in Figure 2. Projected out-of-pocket expenditures for all hospitalizations in 1997 in the United States totaled $9.1 billion, while projected out-of-pocket expenses for all US physician services in the same year were $29.3 billion.[21] This compares to a conservatively estimated $12.2 billion in out-of-pocket payments to alternative medicine practitioners for the 15 therapies studied. Adding the estimates of $5.1 billion for herbal therapies, $3.3 billion for megavitamins, $1.7 billion for diet products, and $4.7 billion on alternative therapy–specific books, classes, and equipment, the total out-of-pocket expenditures for

Table 4. Insurance Coverage of Alternative Medicine Services in the United States, 1997 vs 1990*

	Percentage of Users of Services					
	Coverage, 1997			Coverage, 1990		
Type of Therapy	Complete	Partial	None	Complete	Partial	None
Relaxation techniques	28.8	6.6	64.7	5.3	25.9	68.7
Herbal medicine	8.6	11.2	80.2	30.7	15.5	53.8
Massage	11.8	16.7	71.5	19.1	18.3	62.6
Chiropractic	17.6	38.1	44.3	11.5	32.8	55.9
Spiritual healing by others†	...	...	...	0.0	0.0	100.0
Megavitamins	2.7	53.3	44.0	0.0	100.0	0.0
Self-help group	11.7	36.9	51.5	2.8	17.4	79.8
Imagery	51.5	3.5	45.0	16.1	0.0	83.9
Commercial diet	5.0	40.1	54.9	0.0	5.1	94.9
Folk remedies	0.0	0.0	100.0	...	...	...
Lifestyle diet	0.0	44.9	55.1	62.3	0.0	37.7
Energy healing	30.8	8.2	61.1	0.0	19.1	80.9
Homeopathy	0.0	0.0	100.0	0.0	24.7	75.3
Hypnosis	5.1	0.0	94.9	7.0	0.0	93.0
Biofeedback	30.5	43.7	26.0	14.1	19.9	66.0
Acupuncture	0.0	40.7	59.3	21.6	23.0	55.4
Weighted average across all therapies	15.3	26.4	58.3	12.3	23.7	64.0

*Data are percentage of users of alternative therapies provided by practitioners. Ellipses indicate data not applicable.

†Reimbursement patterns not explored in 1997.

Table 5. National Projections of Expenditures for Alternative Therapies in the United States, 1997 vs 1990*

Category of Expenditure	1997 (Billions of Dollars) Conservative (SE)	1997 (Billions of Dollars) RBRVS (SE)	1990 (Billions of Dollars) Conservative (SE)	1990 (Billions of Dollars) RBRVS (SE)	Change (%), 1997 vs 1990 (Billions of Dollars) Conservative	Change (%), 1997 vs 1990 (Billions of Dollars) RBRVS
Total expenditures on professional services for 15 alternative therapies†	21.2 (2.4)	32.7 (3.8)	14.6 (4.0)	22.6 (6.1)	6.6 (45.2)	10.1 (44.7)
Out-of-pocket expenditures						
Professional services, 15 therapies†‡	12.2 (1.7)	19.6 (3.3)	7.2 (1.3)	11.0 (2.1)	5.0 (69.4)§	8.6 (78.2)§
Megavitamins	3.3 (0.4)		0.9 (0.3)		2.4 (266.7)‖	
Commercial diet products	1.7 (0.3)		1.3 (0.3)		0.4 (30.8)	
Subtotal of out-of-pocket expenditures assessed in 1997 and 1990†	17.2	24.6	9.4	13.2	7.8 (83.0)	11.4 (86.4)
Out-of-pocket expenditures assessed only in 1997						
Herbal medicine	5.1 (0.5)		...		...	
Therapy-specific books, classes, and equipment	4.7 (0.8)		...		...	
Total out-of-pocket expenditures for alternative therapies in 1997†	27.0	34.4	...	...	...	...

*The 1990 and 1997 cost measures are based on 1990 and 1997 population estimates, respectively (180 million vs 198 million). Both used 1997 per-visit price estimates as follows (conservative price estimate is followed by Resource-Based Relative Value Scale [RBRVS] estimate for each therapy): relaxation techniques ($20, $50), herbal medicine ($40, $60), massage therapy ($40, $60), chiropractic care ($40, $65), megavitamins ($40, $50), self-help groups ($20, $20), imagery techniques ($45, $50), commercial diet ($20, $20), folk remedies ($20, $50), lifestyle diet ($20, $60), energy healing ($40, $50), homeopathy ($45, $60), hypnosis ($60, $80), biofeedback ($60, $80), and acupuncture ($40, $60). (Price estimates for spiritual healing by others were not included because respondents reporting use were not asked for details of professional visits). Ellipses indicate data not applicable.

†These figures reflect the range in out-of-pocket expenditures for conservative vs RBRVS-derived visit prices.

‡Assumes a 20% copayment for users with partial insurance coverage.

§$P \leq .05$.

‖$P \leq .001$.

alternative medicine are conservatively estimated to be $27.0 billion. Using the average per-visit prices derived from an RBRVS system[16] rather than our conservative estimates (Table 5), the estimated total out-of-pocket expense is approximately $34.4 billion, which is comparable with the projected 1997 out-of-pocket expenditures for all physician services.[21] These estimates exclude out-of-pocket expenditures associated with therapies unique to the 1997 survey (eg, naturopathy, aromatherapy, neural therapy, and chelation therapy).

Comment

The results of our study are limited by the restriction of the sampling frame to people who speak English and have telephones and by the low response rate. The decrease in overall response rate from 67% in 1990 to 60% in 1997 is consistent with secular trends for US telephone interviews in recent years.[22] It is difficult to know what, if any, bias was introduced or whether trend estimates are biased by the fact that financial incentives were used in 1997 but not 1990. Furthermore, we have no data on the accuracy of self-reports concerning recollections of number of visits and amounts spent on books, classes, relevant equipment, herbs, or supplements. To the extent possible, we adjusted by weighting data on sociodemographic variables associated with alternative therapy use (eg, income, education, age, region). It is conceivable that the estimated prevalence and costs of alternative therapy use would have been lower if it were possible to correct for those limitations.

Within the context of these limitations, the results of these 2 surveys suggest that the prevalence and expenditures associated with alternative medical therapies in the United States have increased substantially from 1990 to

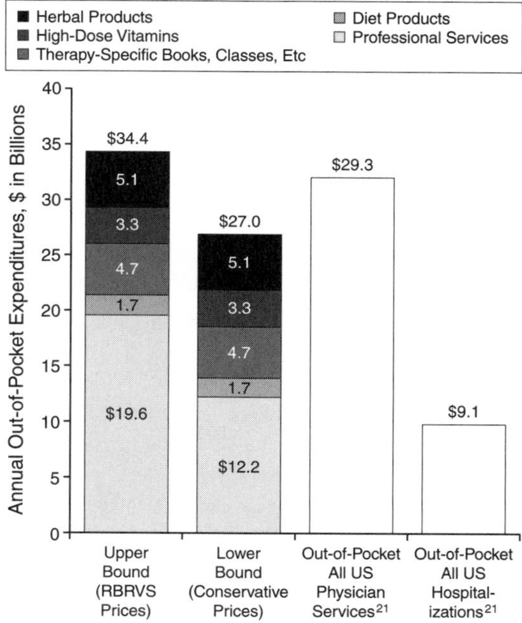

Figure 2. Estimated annual out-of-pocket expenditures for alternative therapies vs conventional medical services, United States, 1997. Data are from the Health Care Financing Administration, United States.[21] RBRVS indicates Resource-Based Relative Value Scale.

1997. This increase appears to be primarily due to increases in the prevalence of use and in the frequency with which users of alternative therapy sought professional services. In 1997, an estimated 4 in 10 Americans used at least 1 alternative therapy as compared with 3 in 10 in 1990. For adults aged 35 to 49 years in 1997, it is estimated that 1 of every 2 persons used at least 1 alternative therapy. Overall prevalence of use increased by 25%, total visits by an estimated 47%, and expenditures on services provided by practitioners of alternative therapies by an estimated 45% exclusive of inflation. Moreover, the use of alternative therapies is distributed widely across all sociodemographic groups.

It is possible to arrange the 16 principal therapies common to the 1990 and 1997 surveys along a spectrum that varies from "more alternative" to "less alternative" in relationship to existing medical school curricula, clinical training, and practice. Arguably, therapies such as biofeedback, hypnosis, guided imagery, relaxation techniques that involve elicitation of the relaxation response (<1% of the sample), lifestyle diet, and (possibly) vitamin therapy can be considered as representative of the more conventional (ie, less alternative) side of the spectrum. Visits associated with these 6 categories accounted for less than 10% of total visits to alternative medicine practitioners; the remainder were associated with the more alternative therapies.

In light of the observed 380% increase in the use of herbal remedies and the 130% increase in high-dose vitamin use, it is not surprising to find that nearly 1 in 5 individuals taking prescription medications also was taking herbs, high-dose vitamin supplements, or both. Extrapolations to the total US population suggest that an estimated 15 million adults are at risk for potential adverse interactions involving prescription medications and herbs or high-dose vitamin supplements. This figure includes nearly 3 million adults aged 65 years or older. Adverse interactions of this nature, including alterations of drug bioavailability or efficacy, are known to occur[23–27] and are more likely among individuals with chronic medical illness, especially those with liver or kidney abnormalities. No adequate mechanism currently is in place to collect relevant surveillance data to document the extent to which the potential for drug-herb and drug-vitamin interaction is real or imaginary.

The magnitude of the demand for alternative therapy is noteworthy, in light of the relatively low rates of insurance coverage for these services. Unlike hospitalizations and physician services, alternative therapies are only infrequently included in insurance benefits. Even when alternative therapies are covered, they tend to have high deductibles and co-payments and tend to be subject to stringent limits on the number of visits or total dollar coverage. Because the demand for health care (and presumably alternative therapies) is sensitive to how much patients must pay out-of-pocket,[28] current use is likely to underrepresent utilization patterns if insurance coverage for alternative therapies increases in the future.

In 1990, a full third of respondents who used alternative therapy did not use it for any principal medical condition.[1] From these data, we inferred that a substantial amount of alternative therapy was used for health promotion or disease prevention. In 1997, 42% of all alternative therapies used were exclusively attributed to treatment of existing illness, whereas 58% were used, at least in part, to "prevent future illness from occurring or to maintain health and vitality."

Despite the dramatic increases in use and expenditures associated with alternative medical care, the extent to which patients disclose their use of alternative therapies to their physicians remains low. Less than 40% of the alternative therapies used were disclosed to a physician in both 1990 and 1997. It would be overly simplistic to blame either the patient or their physician for this inadequacy in patient-physician communication. The current status quo, which can be described as "don't ask and don't tell," needs to be abandoned.[29] Professional strategies for responsible dialogue in this area need to be further developed and refined.

Data from this survey, reflective of the US population, are representative of a predominantly white population. Even if we were to combine data sets from the 1990 and 1997 surveys, we would not have a sufficiently large database to provide precise estimates of the patterns of alternative therapy use among African Americans, Hispanic Americans, Asian Americans, or other minority groups. Parallel surveys, modified to include therapies unique to minority populations and translated when appropriate, should be conducted using necessary sampling strategies. Only then can we compare patterns across ethnic groups and prioritize research agendas for individual populations. As alternative medicine is introduced by third-party payers as an attractive insurance product, it would be unfair for individuals without health insurance and those with less expendable income to be excluded from useful alternative medical services or consultation (eg, professional advice on use or avoidance of alternative therapies).

In conclusion, our survey confirms that alternative medicine use and expenditures have increased dramatically from 1990 to 1997. In light of these observations, we suggest that federal agencies, private corporations, foundations, and academic institutions adopt a more proactive posture concerning the implementation of clinical and basic science research, the development of relevant educational curricula, credentialing and referral guidelines, improved quality control of dietary supplements, and the establishment of postmarket surveillance of drug-herb (and drug-supplement) interactions.

This study was supported in part by National Institutes of Health grant U24 AR43441, Bethesda, Md, the John E. Fetzer Institute, Kalamazoo, Mich, The American Society of Actuaries, Schaumburg, Ill, the Friends of Beth Israel Deaconess Medical Center, and the Kenneth J. Germeshausen Foundation, Boston, Mass, and the J. E. and Z. B. Butler Foundation, New York, NY.

The authors thank the staff of DataStat, Inc, Ann Arbor, Mich, for their assistance with telephone data collection, Linda Bedell-Logan for assistance with RBRVS data analyses, Dan Cherkin, PhD, Murray Mittleman, MD, Ted Kaptchuk, OMD, and Thomas Delbanco, MD, for their review of the manuscript, and Debora Lane, Marcia Rich, and Robb Scholten for their technical assistance.

References

1. Eisenberg DM, Kessler RC, Foster C, et al. Unconventional medicine in the United States. *N Engl J Med.* 1993;328:246–252.

2. Paramore LC. Use of alternative therapies. *J Pain Symptom Manage.* 1997;13:83–89.

3. Landmark Healthcare. *The Landmark Report on Public Perceptions of Alternative Care.* Sacramento, Calif: Landmark Healthcare; 1998.

4. Pelletier KR, Marie A, Krasner M, et al. Current trends in the integration and reimbursement of complementary and alternative medicine by managed care, insurance carriers, and hospital providers. *Am J Health Promot.* 1997; 12:112–122.

5. Wetzel MS, Eisenberg DM, Kaptchuk TJ. Courses involving complementary and alternative medicine at US medical schools. *JAMA.* 1998;280:784–787.

6. Goldbeck-Wood S, Dorozynski A, Lie LG, et al. Complementary medicine is booming worldwide. *BMJ.* 1996;313:131–133.

7. Rasmussen NK, Morgall JM. The use of alternative treatments in the Danish adult population. *Complementary Med Res.* 1990;4:16–22.

8. Vaskilampi T, Meriläinen P, Sinkkonen S, et al. The use of alternative treatments in the Finnish adult population. In: Lewith GT, Aldridge D, eds. *Clinical Research Methodology for Complementary Therapies.* London, England: Hodder & Stoughton; 1993:204–229.

9. MacLennan AH, Wilson DH, Taylor AW. Prevalence and cost of alternative medicine in Australia. *Lancet.* 1996;347:569–573.

10. Fisher P, Ward A. Complementary medicine in Europe. *BMJ.* 1994;309:107–111.

11. Sermeus G. Alternative health care in Belgium. *Complementary Med Res.* 1990;4:9–13.

12. Bouchayer F. Alternative medicines. *Complementary Med Res.* 1990;4:4–8.

13. Piel E. Erfahrungen mit Naturheilmitteln-Umfrageergebnisse aus West- und Ostdeutschland. *Therapeutikon.* 1991; 5:549–551.

14. Millar WJ. Use of alternative health care practitioners by Canadians. *Can J Public Health.* 1997; 88:154–158.

15. US Bureau of the Census. United States population estimates, by age, sex, race, and Hispanic origin, 1990 to 1997. Available at: http://www.census.gov/population/estimates/nation/intfile2-1.txt.

16. Resource-Based Relative Value Scale Converter. *Customized Report for Medical Billing and Collection of All CPT Codes.* Salt Lake City, Utah: Medicode Inc; 1996.

17. US Bureau of Labor Statistics Data. *Consumer Price Index—All Urban Consumers.* US Bureau of Labor Statistics Web site. Available at: http://146.142.4.24/cgi-bin/surveymost?cu. 1998. Series ID: CUUR0000SAM.

18. *SUDAAN: Professional Software for Survey Data Analysis* [computer program]. Version 7.5. Research Triangle Park, NC: Research Triangle Institute; 1997.

19. Schappert SM. *National Ambulatory Medical Care Survey: 1990 Summary.* Hyattsville, Md: National Center for Health Statistics, 1992. Advance Data From Vital and Health Statistics, No. 213:1–11.

20. Woodwell DA. *National Ambulatory Medical Care Survey: 1996 Summary.* Hyattsville, Md: National Center for Health Statistics; 1997. Advance Data From Vital and Health Statistics, No. 295:1–25.

21. Health Care Financing Administration, Office of the Actuary, National Health Statistics Group. National health care expenditure projections tables. Available at: http://www.hcfa.gov/stats/NHE-Proj/tables/.

22. Groves RM, Couper MP. Societal environmental influences on survey participation. In: *Nonresponse in Household Interview Surveys.* New York, NY: John Wiley & Sons Inc; 1998:159.

23. Ernst E. Harmless herbs? *Am J Med.* 1998; 104:170–178.

24. D'Arcy PF. Adverse reactions and interactions with herbal medicines, part 1: adverse reactions. *Adverse Drug React Toxicol Rev.* 1991; 10:189–208.

25. D'Arcy PF. Adverse reactions and interactions with herbal medicines, part 2: drug interactions. *Adverse Drug React Toxicol Rev.* 1993; 12:147–162.

26. De Smet PAGM, D'Arcy PF. Drug interactions with herbal and other non-orthodox remedies. In: D'Arcy PF, McElnay JC, Welling PG, eds. *Mechanisms of Drug Interactions.* New York, NY: Springer Publishing Co Inc; 1996:327–352.

27. De Smet PA. Health risks of herbal remedies. *Drug Saf.* 1995;13:81–93.

28. Shekelle PG, Rogers WH, Newhouse JP. The effect of cost sharing on the use of chiropractic services. *Med Care.* 1996;34:863–872.

29. Eisenberg DM. Advising patients who seek alternative medical therapies. *Ann Intern Med.* 1997;127:61–69.

2 Why Patients Use Alternative Medicine

Results of a National Study

John A. Astin, PhD
From the Stanford Center for Research in Disease Prevention, Stanford University School of Medicine, Palo Alto, Calif.

Context
Research both in the United States and abroad suggests that significant numbers of people are involved with various forms of alternative medicine. However, the reasons for such use are, at present, poorly understood.

Objective
To investigate possible predictors of alternative health care use.

Methods
Three primary hypotheses were tested. People seek out these alternatives because (1) they are dissatisfied in some way with conventional treatment; (2) they see alternative treatments as offering more personal autonomy and control over health care decisions; and (3) the alternatives are seen as more compatible with the patients' values, worldview, or beliefs regarding the nature and meaning of health and illness. Additional predictor variables explored included demographics and health status.

Design
A written survey examining use of alternative health care, health status, values, and attitudes toward conventional medicine. Multiple logistic regression analyses were used in an effort to identify predictors of alternative health care use.

Setting and Participants
A total of 1035 individuals randomly selected from a panel who had agreed to participate in mail surveys and who live throughout the United States.

Main Outcome Measure
Use of alternative medicine within the previous year.

Results
The response rate was 69%.The following variables emerged as predictors of alternative health care use: more education (odds ratio [OR], 1.2; 95% confidence interval [CI], 1.1–1.3); poorer health status (OR, 1.3; 95% CI, 1.1–1.5); a holistic orientation to health (OR, 1.4; 95% CI, 1.1–1.9); having had a

transformational experience that changed the person's worldview (OR, 1.8; 95% CI, 1.3–2.5); any of the following health problems: anxiety (OR, 3.1; 95% CI, 1.6–6.0); back problems (OR, 2.3; 95% CI, 1.7–3.2); chronic pain (OR, 2.0; 95% CI, 1.1–3.5); urinary tract problems (OR, 2.2; 95% CI, 1.3–3.5); and classification in a cultural group identifiable by their commitment to environmentalism, commitment to feminism, and interest in spirituality and personal growth psychology (OR, 2.0; 95% CI, 1.4–2.7). Dissatisfaction with conventional medicine did not predict use of alternative medicine. Only 4.4% of those surveyed reported relying primarily on alternative therapies.

Conclusion

Along with being more educated and reporting poorer health status, the majority of alternative medicine users appear to be doing so not so much as a result of being dissatisfied with conventional medicine but largely because they find these health care alternatives to be more congruent with their own values, beliefs, and philosophical orientations toward health and life.

JAMA. 1998;279:1548–1553

In 1993 Eisenberg and colleagues[1] reported that 34% of adults in the United States used at least 1 unconventional form of health care (defined as those practices "neither taught widely in U.S. medical schools nor generally available in U.S. hospitals") during the previous year. The most frequently used alternatives to conventional medicine were relaxation techniques, chiropractic, and massage. Although educated, middle-class white persons between the ages of 25 and 49 years were the most likely ones to use alternative medicine, use was not confined to any particular segment of the population. These researchers estimated that Americans made 425 million visits to alternative health care providers in 1990, a figure that exceeded the number of visits to allopathic primary care physicians during the same period.

Recent studies in the United States[2] and abroad[3,4] support the prevalent use of alternative health care. For example, a 1994 survey of physicians from a wide array of medical specialties (in Washington State, New Mexico, and Israel) revealed that more than 60% recommended alternative therapies to their patients at least once in the preceding year, while 38% had done so in the previous month.[2] Forty-seven percent of these physicians also reported using alternative therapies themselves, while 23% incorporated them into their practices.

When faced with the apparent popularity of unconventional medical practices and the fact that people seem quite willing to pay out-of-pocket for these services,[1] the question arises: What are the sociocultural and personal factors (health status, beliefs, attitudes, motivations) underlying a person's decision to use alternative therapies?

At present, there is no clear or comprehensive theoretical model to account for the increasing use of alternative forms of health care. Accordingly, the goal of the present study was to develop some tentative explanatory models that might account for this phenomenon.

Three theories that have been proposed to explain the use of alternative medicine were tested:

1. Dissatisfaction: Patients are dissatisfied with conventional treatment because it has been ineffective,[5,6] has produced adverse effects,[6,7] or is seen as impersonal, too technologically oriented, and/or too costly.[6–15]
2. Need for personal control: Patients seek alternative therapies because they see them as less authoritarian[16] and more empowering and as offering them more personal autonomy and control over their health care decisions.[14,16–19]
3. Philosophical congruence: Alternative therapies are attractive because they are seen as more compatible with patients' values, worldview, spiritual/religious philosophy, or beliefs regarding the nature and meaning of health and illness.[19–24]

In addition to testing the validity of these 3 theoretical perspectives, this study also sought to determine on an exploratory basis how the decision to seek alternative therapies is affected by patients' health status and demographic factors.

Methods

Participants completed an extensive mail survey that gathered information on use of alternative health care, perceived benefits and risks of these therapies, health beliefs and attitudes, views toward and experiences with conventional medicine, political beliefs, and worldview. The original survey instrument was developed by Ray,[24] and the survey was conducted through National Family Opinion, Inc, which maintains a panel of persons who have agreed to be participants in mail surveys. This panel constitutes a representative national sample from which subsamples can be drawn. A random sample of 1500 individuals was drawn from this panel, with 1035 people completing the questionnaire (a response rate of 69%).

Dependent Variable

Following Eisenberg et al,[1] the dependent variable, alternative health care use, a dichotomous measure, was operationalized as used within the previous year of any of the following treatments: acupuncture, homeopathy, herbal therapies, chiropractic, massage, exercise/movement, high-dose megavitamins, spiritual healing, lifestyle diet, relaxation, imagery, energy healing, folk remedies, biofeedback, hypnosis, psychotherapy, and art/music therapy. Several of these treatments, however, were deemed not to be alternative or unconventional if they were used to treat particular health-related problems: (1) exercise for lung problems, high blood pressure, heart problems, obesity, muscle strains, or back problems; (2) psychotherapy for depression or anxiety; and (3) self-help groups for depression or anxiety. The category "alternative medicine" was thus delimited to exclude those practices that are already part of standard medical care and recommendations such as exercise to treat hypertension or psychotherapy to treat depression. (The category "lifestyle diet" could include more standard or conventional dietary recommendations such as a low-fat or low-salt regimen for treating cardiovascular disease or hypertension.)

Analyses were repeated using a second dependent variable, primary reliance on alternative medicine, a dichotomous measure defined by those respondents who reported using primarily alternative therapies to treat health-related problems.

Independent Variables

Table 1 lists the independent variables considered possible predictors of alternative health care use. Since constructs like "satisfaction with conventional medicine" are highly generalized, multiple measures of these variables were used. Using principal components analysis with varimax rotation of selected questionnaire items, 4 multi-item factors were identified: satisfaction with conventional practitioners; health status; belief in the power of religious faith to heal; and belief in the efficacy of conventional medicine.

Since the dependent variable was dichotomous, logistic regression analyses were carried out. Demographic variables were entered in a first block with the remaining variables entered in a second block. These variables were entered together in the second block because their precise causal ordering was not readily apparent (ie, there was no clear theoretical rationale for entering them in separate blocks). The variables that then remained significant ($P<.05$) in the logistic regression analyses constituted the final multivariate model.

Hypotheses

The following hypothesized relationships were tested in the multiple logistic regression:

1. Users of alternative health care will be distinguished from nonusers in that they will (*a*) report less satisfaction with conventional medicine; (*b*) demonstrate a greater desire to exercise personal control over health-related matters; and (*c*) subscribe to a holistic philosophical orientation to health.
2. Since the majority of health care alternatives are not covered by insurers, having access to more financial resources will predict use of alternative medicine.[25,26]
3. As suggested by previous research,[1,26–28] higher levels of education will be predictive of alternative medical use.
4. Users of alternative health care will be more likely to be part of a cultural group, described by Ray[24,29] as "cultural creatives," and identifiable by the following values: commitment to environmentalism; commitment to feminism; involvement with esoteric forms of spirituality and personal growth psychology, self-actualization, and self-expression; and love of the foreign and exotic. These individuals tend to be at the leading edge of cultural change and innovation, coming up with the most new ideas in the society, and are therefore hypothesized to be more inclined to use alternative health care.

(Ray developed his value classifications, what he termed "value subcultures," empirically using factor analysis and multidimensional scaling to create orthogonal value dimensions. K-means clustering was then used to cluster respondents into the different value groupings. According to Ray,[24] the cultural creative group has been steadily growing in the culture at large since the late 1960s and now represents approximately 44 million Americans [23.6% of the adult population]. While there is likely some crossover in terms of values and orientation with those identified by the popular media as New Agers, the latter

Table 1. Independent Variables

Satisfaction with conventional medicine

General satisfaction: Thinking about the last time you went to see a medical doctor, how satisfied were you with the care you received? (4-point scale*)

Satisfaction with practitioners†

The last time you had important questions about your health care, and you asked a medical doctor about them, did you understand the answers? (4-point scale)

How much confidence do you have in the medical doctor you see most often for your health care? (4-point scale)

How much trust do you have in the medical doctor you see most often for your health care? (5-point scale)

Lack of trust: I don't trust doctors and hospitals, so I use them as little as possible. (yes/no)

Need for control

What do you prefer for involvement in decisions about your health care? Would you prefer to

__Keep control in your own hands?

__Have an equal partnership with the doctor?

__Leave it in the doctor's hands?

Philosophical/value congruence

Belief in the power of religion†

When I have health problems, I try prayer first, then go to the doctor if I get really sick. (yes/no)

When I have health problems, I depend primarily on prayer and God's help. (yes/no)

Holistic philosophy

The health of my body, mind, and spirit are related, and whoever cares for my health should take that into account. (yes/no)

Classification in the value subculture "cultural creatives,"‡ those who are at the leading edge of cultural change and tend to be interested in psychology, spiritual life, self-actualization, self-expression, like the foreign and exotic, and enjoy mastering new ideas

Experiences of and/or beliefs about religion and spirituality (19 questions: yes/no/not sure)

Participation in a nontraditional religious or spiritual group (yes/no)

Belief in the efficacy of conventional medicine†

I put myself into my doctor's hands, to take care of things for me, and to tell me what's best for my health. (yes/no)

I take my body to the doctor's office, and I expect the doctor to "fix it." (yes/no)

I trust my medical doctor to do the best that Western medicine can do for me regardless of cost. (yes/no)

Health factors

Health problems

26 specific health problems (dichotomous measures: lung; hypertension; heart; diabetes; cancer; digestive; urinary tract; gynecologic; neurological; sprains; dermatological; allergies; dizziness; anxiety; depression; insomnia; acquired immunodeficiency syndrome; addiction; obesity; chronic dental; arthritis; back; headaches; chronic pain; chronic fatigue; other condition)

Health status†

Would you say that your health in general is excellent, very good, good, fair, poor?

During the past 12 months, about how many days did illness or injury keep you in bed more than half the day?

How much bodily pain have you had during the past 4 weeks? (5-point scale)

Demographic factors

Education, sex, income, race, and age

*All such multiple-point questions used standard Likert checkoff scales.
†Multi-item variable derived from factor analysis of selected questionnaire items.
‡Ray[24,29] has identified 3 value subcultures in the US population, termed "the cultural creatives," "the moderns" who represent mainstream popular culture and values, and "the heartlanders," a subculture characterized by fundamentalist and traditional values and beliefs.

term has no operational definition while the categorization of cultural creative is based on empirical research examining specific values held by individuals in the culture at large.)

5. Those who report relying primarily on alternative forms of health care will be more likely to subscribe to a holistic philosophy of health (their greater commitment to these health practices being reflected in a set of health beliefs that are more congruent with many forms of alternative medicine).

Results

Demographic Characteristics

Survey respondents were comparable to census data from the same time period with the exception of a slight underrepresentation of younger, less educated, and poor persons (Table 2).

Health Problems

Respondents were asked whether they had experienced any of a list of 26 health-related problems within the past

Table 2. Demographic Characteristics of Survey Sample (N=1035)

Variables	Sample, %	Users of Alternative Medicine, %
Age, y		
18-24	7.9	35
25-34	21.5	41
35-49	34.8	42
50-64	18.0	44
>64	17.9	35
Race/ethnicity		
White	79.5	41
Black	8.3	29
Hispanic	7.5	40
Asian/Pacific Islander	0.9	44
Native American	0.7	71
Other	3.1	44
Sex		
Male	48.6	39
Female	51.4	41
Education		
High school or less	30.2	31
Some college	26.3	47
Bachelor's degree	15.3	45
Graduate degree	8.7	50
Household income, $		
<12,500	11.9	33
12,500–24,999	15.3	42
25,000–39,999	25.3	36
40,000–59,999	22.9	44
≥60,000	24.7	44

year (Table 1). They were then asked to list the 3 most "bothersome" or "serious" ones. The top 5 problems listed were (1) back problems (19.7%); (2) allergies (16.6%); (3) sprains/muscle strains (15.7%); (4) digestive problems (14.5%); and (5) lung problems, pneumonia, or respiratory infections (13%).

Frequency of Use of Alternative Medicine

Forty percent of respondents reported using some form of alternative health care during the past year. The top 4 treatment categories were chiropractic (15.7%); lifestyle diet (8.0%); exercise/movement (7.2%); and relaxation (6.9%). The most frequently cited health problems treated with alternative therapies were chronic pain (37%); anxiety, chronic fatigue syndrome, and "other health condition" (31% each); sprains/muscle strains (26%); addictive problems and arthritis (both 25%); and headaches (24%).

Analyses were also carried out to determine which specific treatments were being used for which therapeutic modalities. Table 3 lists the top 10 health problems (in terms of percentage who treated them with alternative medicine) and the most frequently used alternative therapies for each.

Table 3. Most Frequently Used Alternative Therapies for Specific Health Problems

Health Problems	Most Frequently Used Alternatives (No.)
Chronic pain	Exercise (12)
	Chiropractic (7)
	Massage (6)
Anxiety	Relaxation (11)
	Exercise (8)
	Herbs (3)
	Art/music therapy (3)
	Massage (3)
Chronic fatigue syndrome	Massage (3)
	Exercise (3)
	Self-help group (2)
	Megavitamins (2)
Sprains/muscle strains	Chiropractic (38)
	Exercise (22)
	Massage (10)
	Relaxation (6)
	Herbs (6)
Addictive problems	Psychotherapy (2)
	Self-help groups (2)
Arthritis or rheumatism	Exercise (17)
	Chiropractic (12)
	Homeopathy (5)
	Herbs (5)
	Other (5)
Severe headaches	Chiropractic (20)
	Massage (5)
	Exercise (5)
	Relaxation (4)
Depression	Relaxation (9)
	Exercise (5)
	Herbs (4)
Digestive problems	Lifestyle diet (7)
	Other (6)
	Relaxation (6)
	Herbs (5)
	Chiropractic (5)
Diabetes	Lifestyle diet (8)
	Exercise (7)
	Other (2)

Although certain alternative therapies tended to be used more frequently, a broad range of alternatives were, in fact, being used for the majority of health problems. For example, although chiropractic care represented close to 50% of all alternative treatments used for headaches, individuals also reported using acupuncture, homeopathy, megavitamins, spiritual healing, lifestyle diets, relaxation, massage, folk medicine, exercise, psychotherapy, and art/music therapy to treat this health problem. A similar pattern is evident across many of the health problems listed on the survey; ie, although particular alternative treatments may predominate, use is by no means confined to any particular therapy or even a few therapies.

Multivariate Statistics

The following variables predicted use of alternative medicine in the multiple logistic regression (criterion for entering was $P<.05$): (1) being more educated; (2) being classified in the value subculture of cultural creatives; (3) having a transformational experience that changed the person's worldview; (4) having poorer overall health; (5) believing in the importance of body, mind, and spirit in treating health problems (holistic health philosophy); and (6) reporting any of the following health problems: anxiety, back problems, chronic pain, or urinary tract problems. Table 4 presents the intercorrelations of all hypothesized predictors and use of alternative medicine. Table 5 presents the adjusted odds ratios and 95% confidence intervals for the independent variables that emerged as significant predictors.

Contrary to a number of previous findings[6–13,27] and the present study's hypothesis, negative attitudes toward or experiences with conventional medicine were not predictive of alternative health care use. Among those who reported being highly satisfied with their conventional practitioners (54%), 39% used alternative therapies, while 40% of those reporting high levels of dissatisfaction (9% of respondents) were users of alternative medicine.

Although there was a trend in the direction of those desiring to keep control in their own hands being more likely to use alternative medicine, this variable was also not a significant predictor of alternative medicine use as hypothesized.

Racial/ethnic differences also did not predict use of alternative medicine. Use was found across all groups (eg, whites, 41%; blacks, 29%; Hispanics, 40%). (Percentages of Asian and Native American respondents who used alternative medicine are not reported here as their overall numbers in the sample are too small. Also, the fact that certain ethnic groups had relatively low representation in the sample may explain why they did not emerge as predictors in the regression.) No significant differences were found with respect to sex with 41% of women and 39% of men reporting use of alternative health care. Finally, neither income nor age predicted use of alternative medicine in the regression.

The results do, however, provide strong support for the philosophical/value congruence theory in several ways. First, as hypothesized, having a holistic philosophy of health ("The health of my body, mind, and spirit are related, and whoever cares for my health should take that into account") was predictive of alternative health care use. Among those subscribing to this philosophy, 46% reported being users of alternative medicine, while only 33% of those not endorsing the item were users. This finding suggests that use of alternative medicine may, in part, reflect shifting cultural paradigms, particularly with respect to recognizing the importance of spiritual factors in health. Second, the statement, "I've had a transformational experience that causes me to see the world differently than before," also emerged as

Table 4. Intercorrelations of Hypothesized Predictor Variables and Use of Alternative Medicine

Variables	1	2	3	4	5	6	7	8	9	10	11	12	13	14
1. Use of alternative medicine	...													
2. Being a "cultural creative"	0.17*	...												
3. Having desire for control over health	0.03	0.04	...											
4. More education	0.13*	0.12*	0.07†	...										
5. Belief in efficacy of conventional care	–0.08†	–0.17*	–0.17*	–0.17*	...									
6. Poorer health status	0.13*	–0.01	–0.11*	–0.14*	0.10‡	...								
7. Higher income	0.06†	0.18*	0.16*	0.41*	–0.16*	–0.19*	...							
8. Dissatisfaction with conventional care	0.01	0.03	0.12*	–0.11‡	–0.14*	0.11‡	–0.05	...						
9. Urinary tract problems	0.07†	0.01	–0.01	–0.03	0.03	0.02	–0.05	–0.01	...					
10. Chronic pain	0.10‡	0.06	0.00	0.01	0.02	0.13*	0.03	0.08‡	–0.01	...				
11. Back problems	0.15*	0.03	0.03	–0.02	–0.03	0.10‡	0.02	0.11‡	–0.08†	0.01	...			
12. Anxiety	0.12*	0.06	0.00	0.03	–0.01	0.02	0.10‡	–0.04	–0.03	–0.04	–0.02	...		
13. Transformational experience	0.12*	0.02	0.04	0.01	–0.02	0.06	–0.05	0.03	–0.02	0.03	–0.01	0.01	...	
14. Holistic philosophy	0.13*	0.18*	0.07†	0.07†	0.04	0.00	0.07†	–0.02	–0.02	0.05	–0.02	0.11*	0.11*	...

*$P<.001$.
†$P<.05$.
‡$P<.01$

Table 5. Significant Predictors in the Multiple Logistic Regression (N=1035)

Variables	Adjusted Odds Ratio (95% Confidence Interval)	*P*
Education*	1.20 (1.10–1.31)	<.001
Health status*	1.32 (1.15–1.52)	<.001
"Cultural creative"	1.95 (1.43–2.67)	<.001
Holistic philosophy	1.42 (1.08–1.86)	<.02
Had transformational experience	1.76 (1.26–2.48)	<.005
Anxiety	3.13 (1.64–5.96)	<.001
Back problems	2.30 (1.66–3.20)	<.001
Urinary tract problems	2.16 (1.32–3.52)	<.005
Chronic pain	1.98 (1.13–3.48)	<.02

*These variables were coded on a 5-point Likert scale (all other independent variables were dichotomous).

a significant predictor. Of those who answered "yes" (18.3%), 53% reported use of alternative health care compared with 37% of those who responded "no" or "not sure." Third, those categorized as cultural creatives were significantly more likely to use alternative health care. Among this subcultural group, 55% reported using alternative health care compared with only 35% of those not in this group.

Education emerged as the 1 sociodemographic variable that predicted use of alternative medicine; individuals with higher educational attainment were more likely to use alternative forms of health care (eg, 31% of those with high school education or less reported use compared with 50% of those with graduate degrees).

The 3-item factor, health status, also emerged as a significant predictor of alternative health care use, with use increasing as health status declined. A number of specific health problems (ie, back problems, chronic pain, anxiety, and urinary tract problems) were also predictive of alternative health care use. These results suggest that experiencing certain health problems increases the likelihood that one will be a user of alternative medicine in a general sense (ie, not simply to treat that particular disorder). For example, those individuals citing anxiety as 1 of their 3 most serious health problems were almost twice as likely as nonanxiety sufferers (67% vs 39%) to be users of alternative health care.

To test the validity of the logistic regression model, 2 techniques were used. First, predicted values from the multivariate equation were divided into quintiles. The percentage of respondents within each quintile who used alternative medicine was then calculated. This analysis is typically used to assess the extent to which there is any clinical or policy relevance to the predictor variables beyond their being statistically significant.[30] Within the quintile of lowest predicted value scores, 17% used alternative medicine; within the highest quintile, 68% were users. These results suggest that the model is fairly strong and has practical (not merely statistical) significance.

To further examine the model's validity, the sample was randomly split into 2 even subsamples, and separate logistic regressions were run for each. These multivariate models were then compared, and there were no significant differences observed in the coefficients of each model. Finally, predicted values were again divided into quintiles in each subsample, and the spread of probabilities across each group was quite consistent between each model and in comparison with the overall regression model.

Primary Reliance on Alternative Medicine

To test whether individuals who report relying primarily on alternative forms of health care show a different profile from those who use alternative medicine more in conjunction with conventional means, separate logistic analyses were carried out. This exploratory analysis suggests that primary reliance on alternative forms of medicine is explained by a considerably different set of variables. The following independent variables were significant predictors in the multiple logistic regression: (1) distrust of conventional physicians and hospitals; (2) desire for control over health matters; (3) dissatisfaction with conventional practitioners; and (4) belief in the importance and value of one's inner life and experiences. The fact that only 4.4% (n=45) of the sample was categorized as relying primarily on alternative forms of health care is consistent with previous findings[1] suggesting that the vast majority of individuals appear to use alternative therapies in conjunction with, rather than instead of, more conventional treatment.

In contrast to individuals who use alternative therapies in conjunction with conventional medicine, for whom dissatisfaction with conventional medicine was not a significant predictor of alternative health care use, 2 of the 4 predictors of primary reliance on alternative medicine reflect a general lack of trust in and satisfaction with conventional medical care. It is also individuals who report a desire to keep control in their own hands who are more likely to report relying primarily on unconventional forms of health care.

Education and health status did not predict primary reliance on alternative medicine. Neither being a cultural creative nor holding a holistic philosophy of health was a significant predictor in this model. These findings suggest that, contrary to my hypothesis, those evidencing a greater commitment to or reliance on alternative health care may be doing so primarily as a result of their dissatisfaction with conventional medicine rather than on ideological or philosophical grounds.

Because of the small sample size in the above analyses and the relatively imprecise measure of the dependent variable (ie, one can only infer that respondents who report relying primarily on these alternatives tend to use them more as a replacement than as a complement to conventional approaches), one must interpret these findings with caution.

Perceived Benefits of Alternative Medicine

Perceived benefits of alternative therapies were considered as potential determinants of use (eg, if someone reports receiving some benefit from a given treatment, this could in turn serve as an important determining factor in future health care decisions). The 2 most frequently endorsed benefits were, "I get relief for my symptoms, the pain or discomfort is less or goes away, I feel better," and "The treatment works better for my particular health problem than standard medicine's." These responses suggest that the most influential or salient factor in people's decision to use alternative health care may be its perceived efficacy. The response, "The treatment promotes health rather than just focusing on illness," was the third most frequently reported benefit and offers further support for the philosophical congruence theory.

Comment

The present study was designed to provide a comprehensive analysis of factors influencing the decision to use various forms of alternative health care. Based on the results from the multiple logistic regression, users of alternative medicine (40% of those surveyed) can generally be characterized as follows: Users tend to be better educated and to hold a philosophical orientation toward health that can be described as holistic (ie, they believe in the importance of body, mind, and spirit in health). They are more likely to have had some type of transformational experience that has changed their worldview in some significant way, and they tend to be classified in a value subculture as cultural creatives. Users of alternative health care are also more likely to report poorer health status than nonusers.

Relief of symptoms is the main benefit reported (the perceived efficacy of alternative medicine being cited nearly twice as often as other reported benefits). A central finding is that users of alternative health care are no more dissatisfied with or distrustful of conventional care than nonusers are.

Among those categorized as primarily reliant on alternative health care—fewer than 5% of the surveyed population—a different pattern emerged. Unlike those who used alternative therapies in conjunction with or as a supplement to conventional forms of medical care, these individuals were more likely to be dissatisfied with and distrustful of standard care as well as desirous of maintaining exclusive control over their health care decisions. They were also more likely to report being interested in their inner life and experiences, suggesting some crossover with the set of spiritually relevant variables that predicted nonexclusive use of alternative health care. These results suggest that future studies examining predictors of alternative health care use need to more carefully measure this phenomenon so that individuals who use these therapies in conjunction with or as a supplement to conventional means can be clearly distinguished from those who use them predominantly or more exclusively.

Several possible interpretations can be offered for certain variables that emerged as predictors of alternative health care use. Education, for example, may increase the likelihood that people will (1) be exposed to various nontraditional forms of health care through their own reading of popular or academic books on the subject; (2) educate themselves about their illnesses and the variety of treatments available to them; and/or (3) question the authority of conventional practitioners (ie, be less inclined simply to accept unquestionably the physician's knowledge and expertise).

There are also at least 2 possible explanations for the finding that poorer health status predicts alternative medical use. First, since those who are in poor health have, by definition, had less success in treating their health problems, their continued suffering may have prompted them to seek out alternatives. Second, a significant number of individuals who report poor health, more pain, disability, and physical symptoms may be somatizers. Somatization has been defined as "the propensity to experience and report somatic symptoms that have no pathophysiological explanation, to misattribute them to disease, and to seek medical attention for them."[31] Since research suggests that somatizers are disproportionately high users of medical services, get more medical tests, and tend to experiment with (shop around for) different health care practitioners, it seems reasonable that they would be more likely to seek out various health care alternatives.[32] It would be useful to design future studies examining predictors of alternative health care use in such a way that somatizers and nonsomatizers can be differentiated more clearly.

There are also several possible explanations for the finding that alternative medicine users are more likely to subscribe to a holistic philosophy of health. People who hold this philosophical orientation may be attracted to alternative forms of health care because they see in these therapeutic systems a greater acknowledgment of the role of nonphysical (mind/spirit) factors in creating health and illness. An alternate explanation (which would reverse the direction of causation) is that people who have been involved with alternative medicine have had their belief systems influenced by these therapeutic modalities and the philosophies underlying them.

That users of alternative health care are more likely to report having had a transformational experience that changed the way they saw the world lends partial support to the hypothesis that involvement with alternative medicine may be reflective of shifting cultural paradigms regarding beliefs about the nature of life, spirituality, and the world in general. As suggested by Charlton,[20] a subset of individuals may be attracted to these nontraditional therapies because they find in them an acknowledgment of the importance of treating illness within a larger context of spirituality and life meaning.

The apparent effect of one's spiritual/philosophical orientation on involvement with alternative health practices is further supported by the finding that being a cultural creative is a significant predictor of use. This suggests that the growing interest in alternative medicine may not simply represent a shift in individual beliefs about the nature of health and illness, but is rather a phenomenon that is transmitted through and influenced by the culture. This interpretation is supported by the finding that the effect of membership in this value subculture is not accounted for simply by holding a holistic philosophy of health; that is, both of these variables contributed independently in the logistic regression equation.

As with other studies that attempt to explain complex human behavioral phenomena, a significant amount of variance is not explained by the regression equation. There are obviously unaccounted for variables such as a general openness to novelty and experimentation, or curiosity, that need to be examined in future studies. Another possibility is measurement error associated with the independent variables; for example, the variable "belief in the importance of body, mind, and spirit" might be interpreted differently depending on one's religious background. Moreover, the decision to use alternative medicine is sufficiently context or situation dependent (eg, influence of significant others who have used or not used various alternatives) to make prediction quite difficult.

Another limitation to this study is its cross-sectional nature, which precludes drawing any definitive conclusions regarding cause-and-effect relationships. For example, it is unclear whether holding a holistic philosophical orientation has led certain individuals to seek out alternative therapies, whether exposure to these therapies has somehow influenced the way they view health and illness, or whether both effects occur. Moreover, the reliance on self-report may weaken the internal validity of the study as retrospective accounts of one's health status, health practices, and reasons for making certain health care decisions may be subject to distortion and inaccuracy.

Since the sample underrepresented the poorer, less educated, and non-English-speaking segments of the population, it is unclear if (and how) the results would be different had these groups been better represented. It is possible that the modest overrepresentation of more educated respondents in the study sample may have slightly inflated the estimates of use of alternative therapies. Finally, since information could not be obtained on nonrespondents, there remains the possibility of some self-selection bias in the study sample.

Despite these limitations, the study results make several contributions to our understanding of alternative health care use. First, the results provide useful information to conventional practitioners about the health beliefs and practices of many of their patients and may suggest areas where practitioners and the present health care system may be failing to meet peoples' health care needs adequately. This seems particularly important given research suggesting that the vast majority of medical symptoms are self-diagnosed and self-treated[33] and that a significant portion of alternative medical use (eg, use of herbal therapies and nutritional supplements) falls into the realm of self-care.[1] Subsequently, if health care professionals are to effectively support individuals in making informed, safe, and appropriate choices, it is critical that they develop greater awareness of the nature of, potential efficacy of, and reasons for patients' use of unconventional self-care approaches.

Second, the results can help identify and clarify prevailing cultural conceptions about and attitudes toward health and illness and examine the degree to which the growing interest in alternative medicine may represent a type of cultural (Kuhnian[34]) paradigm shift regarding health beliefs and practices. Results from the present study lend support to the notion that for many individuals, the use of alternative health care is part of a broader value orientation and set of cultural beliefs, one that embraces a holistic, spiritual orientation to life.

Third, the information derived from this and similar studies can serve as a useful adjunct to data derived from controlled studies of the clinical efficacy of alternative therapies. These combined research efforts not only have the potential to change some of the ways conventional biomedicine is practiced, but can also serve to stimulate further dialogue among the biomedical community, governmental agencies, insurance companies, and managed care organizations regarding the potential value of alternative treatments.

Finally, as policymakers and health care professionals continue to debate reforms of the present health care system, it seems important to understand why a significant portion of the population is going outside mainstream biomedicine to treat a variety of illnesses and to maintain their general health and well-being.

I would like to thank Paul Ray, PhD, for making available the data set that was used in the present study, Helena Kraemer, PhD, for her statistical consultation, and Helen Astin, PhD, and Alexander Astin, PhD, for their very helpful comments and suggestions on earlier drafts of the manuscript.

References

1. Eisenberg DM, Kessler RC, Foster C, Norlock FE, Calkins DR, Delbanco TL. Unconventional medicine in the United States: prevalence, costs, and patterns of use. *N Engl J Med.* 1993; 328:246–252.
2. Borkan J, Neher JO, Anson O, Smoker B. Referrals for alternative therapies. *J Fam Pract.* 1994;39:545–550.
3. Perkin MR, Pearcy RM, Fraser JS. A comparison of the attitudes shown by general practitioners, hospital doctors, and medical students towards alternative medicine. *J R Soc Med.* 1994; 87:523–525.
4. MacLennan AH, Wilson DH, Taylor AW. Prevalence and cost of alternative medicine in Australia. *Lancet.* 1996;347:569–573.
5. Avina RL, Schneiderman LJ. Why patients choose homeopathy. *West Med J.* 1978; 128:366–369.
6. Jensen P. Alternative therapy for atopic dermatitis and psoriasis: patient-reported motivation, information source and effect. *Acta Derm Venereol.* 1990;70:425–428.
7. Cassileth BR, Lusk EJ, Strouse TB, Bodenheimer BJ. Contemporary unorthodox treatments in cancer medicine: a study of patients, treatments, and practitioners. *Ann Intern Med.* 1984;101:105–112.
8. Oths K. Communication in a chiropractic clinic: how a DC treats his patients. *Cult Med Psychiatry.* 1994;18:83–113.
9. Marquis MS, Davies AR, Ware JE. Patient satisfaction and change in medical-care provider: a longitudinal study. *Med Care.* 1983; 21:821–829.
10. Sutherland LR, Verhoef MJ. Why do patients seek a second opinion or alternative medicine? *J Clin Gastroenterol.* 1994;19:194–197.
11. Furnham A, Bhagrath R. A comparison of health beliefs and behaviours of clients of orthodox and complementary medicine. *Br J Clin Psychiatry.* 1993;32:237–246.
12. Furnham A, Smith C. Choosing alternative medicine: a comparison of the beliefs of patients visiting a general practitioner and a homeopath. *Soc Sci Med.* 1988;26:685–689.
13. Furnham A, Forey J. The attitudes, behaviors, and beliefs of patients of conventional vs complementary alternative medicine. *J Clin Psychiatry.* 1994;50:458–469.
14. McGuire MB. *Ritual Healing in Suburban America*. New Brunswick, NJ: Rutgers University Press; 1988.
15. Murray RH, Rubel AJ. Physicians and healers: unwitting partners in health care. *N Engl J Med.* 1992;326:61–64.
16. Riesmann F. Alternative health movements. *Soc Policy*. Spring 1994:53–57.
17. Duggan R. Complementary medicine: transforming influence or footnote to history? *Altern Ther Health Med.* 1995;1:28–33.
18. Kleinman A. Indigenous systems of healing: questions for professional, popular, and folk care. In: Salmon JW, ed. *Alternative Medicines: Popular and Policy Perspectives*. New York, NY: Tavistock Publications; 1984.
19. Vincent C, Furnham A. Why do patients turn to complementary medicine? An empirical study. *Br J Clin Psychol.* 1996;35:37–48.
20. Charlton BG. The doctor's aim in a pluralistic society: A response to "healing and medicine." *J R Soc Med.* 1993;86:125–126.
21. Fuller RC. *Alternative Medicine and American Religious Life.* New York, NY: Oxford University Press; 1989.
22. Levin JS, Coreil J. New-age healing in the US. *Soc Sci Med.* 1986;23:889–897.
23. Salmon JW, ed. *Alternative Medicines: Popular and Policy Perspectives.* New York, NY: Tavistock Publications; 1984.
24. Ray PH. The emerging culture. *American Demographics.* February 1997. Available at: www.demographics.com. Accessed April 10, 1998.
25. Millar WJ. Use of alternative health care practitioners by Canadians. *Can J Public Health.* 1997;88:154–158.
26. Ostrow MJ, Cornelisse PG, Heath KV, et al. Determinants of complementary therapy use in HIV-infected individuals receiving antiretroviral or anti-opportunistic agents. *J Acquir Immune Defic Syndr Hum Retrovirol.* 1997;15:115–120.
27. Dimmock S, Troughton PR, Bird HA. Factors predisposing to the resort of complementary therapies in patients with fibromyalgia. *Clin Rheumatol.* 1996;15:478–482.
28. Bernstein JH, Shuval JT. Nonconventional medicine in Israel: consultation patterns of the Israeli population and attitudes of primary care physicians. *Soc Sci Med.* 1997;44:1341–1348.
29. Ray PH, Anderson SR. *The Cultural Creatives.* In press.
30. Kraemer HC, Kazdin AE, Offord DR, Kessler RC, Jensen PS, Kupfer DJ. Coming to terms with the terms of risk. *Arch Gen Psychiatry.* 1997; 54:337–343.
31. Barsky AJ, Borus JF. Somatization and medicalization in the era of managed care. *JAMA.* 1995;274:1931–1934.
32. Lipowski ZJ. Somatization: the concept and its clinical application. *Am J Psychiatry.* 1988; 145:1358–1368.
33. Dean K. Self-care responses to illness: a selected review. *Soc Sci Med.* 1981;15:673–687.
34. Kuhn T. *The Structure of Scientific Revolutions.* Chicago, Ill: University of Chicago Press; 1970.

3 Pediatricians' Experience With and Attitudes Toward Complementary/Alternative Medicine

Anju Sikand, MD; Marilyn Laken, PhD
From the Division of Adolescent Medicine, Department of Pediatrics, Children's Hospital of Michigan, Wayne State University School of Medicine, Detroit (Dr Sikand); and College of Nursing, Medical University of South Carolina, South Charleston (Dr Laken).

Objective

To assess (1) pediatricians' attitudes toward and practice of complementary and alternative medicine (CAM) for their patients; (2) their knowledge, experience, and referral patterns for selected CAM therapies; and (3) their desire for continuing medical education courses on CAM therapies.

Method

An anonymous, self-report, 25-item questionnaire was mailed to fellows of the Michigan chapter of the American Academy of Pediatrics.

Results

Of 860 pediatricians, 348 (40.5%) responded; their median age ranged from 35 to 45 years, 54.3% were men, 67.6% were white, 67.9% were general pediatricians, and 65.2% were trained in the United States. Of the respondents, 83.5% believed their patients use CAM therapies, but 55.1% believed this constituted less than 10% of patients. Of the pediatricians who talked about CAM (53.8%), 84.7% said the discussion was initiated generally by the patient's family. More than half of the physicians (55.2%) said they would use CAM therapies personally, and 50.3% would refer for CAM therapies. Therapies referred for were biofeedback (23.6%), self-help groups (23.3%), relaxation (14.9%), hypnosis (13.8%), and acupuncture or acupressure (10.9%). Of the physicians who responded, 54.1% were interested in continuing medical education courses on CAM therapies. White respondents, US medical school graduates, and general pediatricians were most likely to believe their patients use CAM and discuss or refer for CAM therapies (*P*<.01). Female pediatricians were most likely to discuss or refer for CAM and to want more continuing medical education on CAM therapies (*P*<.05).

Conclusions

A majority of pediatricians sampled believed a small percentage of their patients were seeking alternatives to conventional medicine. Half would consider referring patients for

CAM, and most were interested in continuing medical education courses on CAM. Larger studies surveying pediatricians, along with more education and research on CAM therapies, need to be considered for the future.

Arch Pediatr Adolesc Med. 1998;152:1059–1064

Complementary/alternative medicine (CAM) refers to a large range of therapies outside the domain of mainstream Western medicine. This covers a vast number of different therapies with different philosophies and practices, ranging from 1000-year-old systems of medicine, such as Ayurvedic[1] medicine and Traditional Chinese Medicine, to homeopathy, prayer, energy healing, massage, chiropractic, and mind-body connections such as biofeedback. Interest in CAM among the public and medical community is rapidly growing in the United States and in Europe. The National Institutes of Health acknowledged this interest in 1992, establishing the Office of Alternative Medicine aimed at facilitating research in these therapies.[2]

In April 1995, a panel of experts from the Office of Alternative Medicine held a conference on research methods to evaluate research needs in the large, diverse, and dynamic field of complementary and alternative medicine. This panel defined CAM as

> a broad domain of healing resources that encompasses all health systems, modalities, and practices and their accompanying theories and beliefs, other than those intrinsic to the politically dominant health system of a particular society or culture in a given historical period. CAM includes all such practices and ideas self-defined by their users as preventing or treating illness or promoting health and well being. Boundaries within CAM and between the CAM domain and the domain of the dominant system are not always sharp or fixed. In the United States the dominant healthcare system is, for want of better term, biomedicine. CAM in the U.S. therefore is that broad domain of all healthcare resources to which people have recourse other than practice models of biomedicine.[3]

Interest in CAM has been heightened by some of the pervasive structural problems of biomedicine, such as high cost, bureaucratization, overspecialization, and limited success in dealing with such problems as chronic illness, mental disorders, and substance abuse. Furthermore, the biomedical model largely concerns itself with physical disease. These limitations of biomedicine may lead many people to seek alternative approaches.[4–6] The advent of antibiotics, immunizations, improved technology, and better sanitation has been associated with lower infant mortality rates, increased life expectancies, and less poverty-related disease in most Western societies. This has shifted focus to issues of improving the quality of our lives. Many CAM therapies focus on improving this quality by means of preventive medicine.

A record number of patients are turning to complementary practitioners in Western countries, including the United States and Canada.[7–11] Eisenberg and colleagues in 1993 indicated that approximately one third of Americans used at least 1 form of alternative therapy. Interestingly enough, only 3 of 10 people in that study informed their physicians of their alternative therapy use. A majority of these patients were well educated and affluent.[12,13]

In 1993, the American Medical Association published information to evaluate health care approaches that are not based on established scientific knowledge and that are commonly referred to as "alternative" therapies. This publication portrays many CAM therapies as being "quackery" or "health frauds." This portrayal by the American Medical Association may influence physicians to perceive CAM in a negative manner, thus negating working toward integrating biomedicine and CAM therapies.[14]

Several studies assessing attitudes, beliefs, and use of CAM by primary care physicians in North America and Europe report that the majority of physicians studied expressed an interest in CAM and would refer patients for CAM.[15–27] A study done in Israel also showed that 54% of family physicians thought CAM may be clinically useful and 42% referred patients.[28]

The use of CAM by parents and children is less well known. A study in Quebec showed that 11% of parents of children seen in an allopathic clinic had consulted 1 or more CAM practitioners for their children.[29] Other studies that assess the use and perceived benefit of nonmedical treatments by patients with cystic fibrosis, juvenile arthritis, and cancer found that 66%, 70%, and 46%, respectively, had used some form of nonconventional treatment in conjunction with their conventional care.[30–32] These findings indicate that CAM is an aspect of pediatrics that we cannot ignore.

This statewide study was conducted to assess (1) pediatricians' beliefs and attitudes toward their patients' use, and use in their personal lives, of CAM therapies; (2) their knowledge, experience, and referral patterns regarding certain CAM therapies; and (3) their desire for continuing medical education (CME) courses on various CAM therapies.

Participants and Methods

An anonymous, self-designed questionnaire assessing attitudes, training, and practices regarding CAM was mailed to fellows of the Michigan chapter of the American Academy of Pediatrics in January 1997. Pediatricians in training were excluded. The questionnaire consisted of 25 questions divided into demographic information, pediatricians' perception of their patients' use of CAM, whether their patients or the parents of their patients discussed their use of CAM, personal and family use of CAM, referral practices, formal training in CAM, whether they practiced any CAM therapies, and attitudes regarding the safety or harmfulness and the effectiveness of 14 complementary/alternative therapies. A table format was used that listed 14 CAM therapies: acupuncture/acupressure, biofeedback, chiropractic, herbs, high-dose antioxidant vitamins, homeopathy, hypnosis, imagery, lifestyle diet, massage therapy, osteopathic manipulation, prayer healing, relaxation, and self-help groups. For each therapy the respondents indicated therapies practiced, personal/family use, and referral for treatment, and rated the therapies as effective, safe, harmful, or didn't know. Finally, the survey asked about the respondent's desire for more training in the form of CME courses in CAM. The survey was pretested on 15 pediatricians. The study was approved by the institutional review board of the Wayne State University School of Medicine, Detroit, Mich, and is available from us.

Statistical analysis was performed by means of SPSS software (SPSS Inc, Chicago, Ill). Frequency distributions were generated for all variables. Six variables representing attitudes and behaviors related to CAM were subjected to factor analysis in an attempt to derive 2 scales to be used as outcome variables for a multiple regression analysis. The 6 variables were (1) personal or family use of CAM, (2) interest in more education in CAM, (3) whether pediatricians refer their patients for CAM, (4) whether they talk to their patients about CAM, (5) the percentage of their patients they believe use CAM, and (6) whether they believe their patients would tell them if they used CAM. A 2-factor principal-components factor analysis followed by varimax rotation was conducted.

Results

A total of 860 questionnaires were mailed; 369 were returned after a second mailing, and only questionnaires that were 75% complete were analyzed. The results of 348 questionnaires are reported in this study, for a 40.5% response rate. The 348 fellows who responded to the questionnaire were compared with all fellows in Michigan for age and sex. No significant differences were noted; the sample was representative of the population. The median age of the sample ranged from 35 to 45 years, median years in practice ranged from 5 to 13, 54.5% were men, 67.6% were white, 67.9% considered themselves to be general pediatricians, and 65.2% had graduated from US medical schools.

Compared with other ethnic groups, more white pediatricians reported that they believe their patients are using CAM and that they talk to their patients about CAM ($P<.001$). More US medical school graduates than non-US medical school graduates reported that they believe their patients are using CAM and talk to their patients about CAM ($P<.001$). More generalists than specialists reported that they believe their patients are using CAM and refer for CAM ($P<.01$).

Perceptions of Personal Use of CAM by Patients and Pediatricians

Of the sample, 83.5% believe some of their patients are using some form of CAM therapies, although most (55.1%) believe that this use constitutes less than 10% of their patients. While 53.5% talk with their patients and the parents of their patients about CAM, the discussion is generally initiated by the patient's family (84.7%). More than three quarters (76.1%) believe their patients or the parents of their patients would tell them if they were using CAM. Whereas 55.2% said they would consider using 1 or more CAM therapies for themselves or their family, half (50.3%) would consider referring their patients to other practitioners for CAM therapies. Table 1 lists medical problems for which respondents either use CAM themselves or refer patients. These were more often for chronic problems (headaches, backaches, pain management, seizures), for which traditional therapies had failed, for behavioral problems, and for psychiatric disorders (anxiety, depression). Less than 20% would use CAM or refer patients for CAM for medical problems such as cancer, chronic diseases for which there are no cures, neurological diseases (demyelinating), and human immunodeficiency virus infection.

Attitudes Toward Specific Therapies

Table 2 summarizes responses to questions about 14 common CAM therapies. Only 37% used any form of CAM in their personal lives (most frequently cited were relaxation, massage, herbs, and prayer healing). Pediatricians stated that they would refer patients for some therapies, especially biofeedback (23.6%), self-help groups (23.3%), relaxation (14.9%), hypnosis (13.8%), and acupuncture/acupressure (10.9%).

Therapies considered to be most effective were relaxation (56.0%), self-help groups (54.3%), acupuncture/acupressure (51.1%), hypnosis (50.3%), biofeedback (49.1%), and massage therapy (46.3%). Therapies considered to be most effective were similar to those considered to be safe, for personal use, or for which they would refer patients. Interestingly, while pediatricians ranked some therapies (such as chiropractic, herbs, high-dose antioxidant vitamins or minerals, homeopathy, lifestyle diet, and osteopathic manipulation) as effective, they were less likely to consider them safe. More than half of the pediatricians (54.1%) were interested in learning about 1 or more CAM therapies, especially biofeedback (41.3%), acupuncture/acupressure (40.1%), relaxation (36.6%), herbs (34.3%), hypnosis (31.4%), and massage therapy (25.0%).

Table 1. Medical Problems for Which 348 Pediatricians Use or Refer for CAM Therapies*

Medical Problems	%
Chronic problems (headaches, backaches, pain management, muscular dystrophy, seizures)	55.9
When traditional therapy fails	45.8
Behavioral problems (eg, ADHD, nightmares)	32.8
Psychiatric disorders (eg, anxiety, depression)	26.7
Cancer	15.9
Other chronic diseases for which there are no cures	14.8
Neurological diseases (eg, demyelinating)	13.0
HIV infection	9.6

*CAM indicates complementary/alternative medicine; ADHD, attention-deficit/hyperactivity disorder; and HIV, human immunodeficiency virus.

Factors Affecting Positive Attitudes Toward CAM and Patient-Physician Relationship

Table 3 presents the derived 2-factor varimax rotated solution (named as follows: factor 1, positive attitudes toward CAM [eigenvalue, 2.3]; and factor 2, physician-patient relationships [eigenvalue, 1.3]) as it relates to CAM therapies. Eigenvalues greater than 1 represent a significant relationship.

Table 4 presents the stepwise linear multiple regression results for the described factor-derived outcome variables, positive attitudes toward CAM and patient-physician relationship. Intercorrelations among 6 demographic variables (US or foreign medical school, age, sex, years in practice, generalist/specialist, and ethnicity) and the 2 outcome variables eliminated ethnicity as a potential predictor. Five demographic predictor variables were entered into the 2 outcome analyses: age, sex, generalist/ specialist, US/foreign medical school, and years in practice.

In the stepwise linear multiple regression analysis for factor 1, positive attitudes toward CAM, 2 significant predictors were found: younger age and female sex, accounting for 7.8% of the variance for more favorable attitudes. In the stepwise linear multiple regression analysis for factor 2, patient-physician relationship, the same 5 variables were entered into the analysis and 3 predictors were found: female sex, US medical school, and fewer years in practice, explaining 12.4% of the variance for more interaction between the pediatrician and the patient and the patient's family regarding CAM.

Table 2. Usage (Personal and Practice), Referral Patterns, Effectiveness, Safety, and Desire for More Continuing Medical Education (CME) on Various Complementary/Alternative Therapies Among 348 Responding Physicians

	% of Respondents						
Therapies	Therapies Practiced	Self/ Family Use	Refer for	May Be Effective	Safe	May Be Harmful	Learn About (More CME)
Acupuncture/acupressure	1.4	7.5	10.9	51.1	30.7	3.4	40.1
Biofeedback	6.6	6.9	23.6	49.1	37.9	0.3	41.3
Chiropractic manipulation	0.0	4.3	7.2	32.5	6.9	40.8	12.8
Herbs	2.3	11.2	4.0	33.3	10.1	29.0	34.3
High-dose antioxdant vitamins/minerals	2.3	7.2	1.7	20.7	5.2	39.9	15.7
Homeopathy	1.1	5.5	4.0	21.0	12.1	13.5	25.0
Hypnosis	2.3	4.6	13.8	50.3	24.4	4.9	31.4
Imagery	4.3	6.9	9.2	31.9	21.8	0.9	15.7
Lifestyle diet	1.4	3.7	4.3	18.4	7.2	17.2	17.4
Massage therapy	4.3	16.1	13.2	46.3	36.8	1.1	25.0
Osteopathic manipulation	2.6	6.3	10.3	35.3	17.0	15.2	14.0
Prayer healing	4.0	11.2	4.6	35.9	31.3	6.0	11.6
Relaxation (yoga, meditation)	8.0	17.8	14.9	56.0	40.2	0.6	36.6
Self-help groups	7.2	8.0	23.3	54.3	37.1	4.9	14.0

Table 3. Two-Factor Varimax Rotated Solution of Attitudes and Patient Relationships as Related to CAM*

Variable	Factor 1, Positive Attitudes Toward CAM	Factor 2, Physician-Patient Relationship
Self or family use CAM	0.86	NA
More CME	0.81	NA
Refers patients for CAM	0.76	NA
Talks to patients about CAM	NA	0.79
Uses CAM in practice	NA	0.79
Patients tell physician they use CAM	NA	0.46

*CAM indicates complementary/alternative medicine; NA, not applicable; and CME, continuing medical education.

Table 4. Stepwise Linear Multiple Regressions (N=348)

Variable	Cumulative R^2	F to Remove	Zero-Order Correlation
	Positive Attitudes Toward CAM*		
Younger age	0.05	10.86	−0.23
Female sex	0.08	7.06	0.20
	Patient-Physician Relationship†		
US medical school	0.07	18.47	0.26
Female sex	0.10	7.39	0.18
Fewer years in practice	0.12	6.22	0.19

*Predictor variables that were not significant ($P<.05$) were years in practice, age, and generalist vs specialist. CAM indicates complementary/alternative medicine.
†Predictor variables that were not significant ($P<.05$) were age and generalist vs specialist.

Comment

The key findings of this study indicate that the majority of pediatricians surveyed in Michigan believe their patients are using some form of CAM (83.5%) and discussions of CAM are generally initiated by parents of the patients or the patients themselves (84.7%). Furthermore, while 50.3% of pediatricians would consider referring patients for CAM, they are most likely to refer patients with chronic diseases, such as headaches, backaches, chronic pain, and seizures (55.9%). Female pediatricians are more likely to discuss CAM with their patients (52.2%), and the majority of pediatricians are interested in CME courses in CAM (54.1%).

Results of this study are similar to those of studies of other primary care physicians. Schachter et al[28] in Israel and Anderson and Anderson[16] in Oxford, England, indicated that 89% of family physicians and 95% of general practitioners believe their patients use "nonconventional" therapies. Verhoef and Sutherland[26] reported that 65% of general practitioners perceive a demand for alternative medicine from their patients. Similarly, other studies report that the majority of physicians surveyed would refer patients for CAM and desire more CME on CAM.[15,19,20,22–25,27]

Greater than 50% (53.8%) of the pediatricians in this study reported that they talk to the parents of the patients or to the patients themselves about CAM, but the majority stated that the discussion was usually initiated by the patient's family. Most believe that the parents of the patients or the patients would tell them if they use CAM. The study by Elder et al[7] supports this belief, as 53% of family practice patients surveyed in Oregon said that they would tell their physician about their use of CAM therapies. This is in contrast to the study by Eisenberg et al[12] that indicates that only one third of the patients surveyed would tell their physicians if they were using CAM therapies.

The majority of the pediatricians in our study would consider using CAM in their personal life, but only a little more than 35% (37.2%) use any of the 14 CAM therapies listed. Relaxation, massage therapy, prayer healing, and herbs were the most commonly used. Studies by Schachter et al[28] and Borkan et al[24] indicate that 27% of family physicians and 55% of primary care physicians, respectively, use CAM personally. A study of general practitioner trainees indicated that 22% of these physicians use CAM therapies.[22] Only 10.3% of the pediatricians in our study practice any form of CAM. This is less than the percentages in other reports of primary care physicians, which range from 13% to 38%.[16,19,20,23,24,28]

A substantial number of pediatricians (26.7%-55.9%) in our study reported that they would use CAM or refer patients for CAM for chronic medical problems (headaches, backaches, pain management, muscular dystrophy, seizures, etc), when traditional therapy fails, for behavioral problems (attention-deficit/hyperactivity disorder, nightmares, etc), and for psychiatric disorders (anxiety, depression, etc). This was similar to other studies.[15,18,26] Conversely, studies of patients with similar health problems found that most of these patients used CAM.[7,12,29,31] Interestingly, less than one fourth of the pediatricians surveyed in our study referred patients for CAM for cancer, human immunodeficiency virus infection, and other medical conditions for which there is no cure.

The most common CAM therapies to which pediatricians in our study refer patients were biofeedback, self-help groups, relaxation, hypnosis, massage therapy, and acupuncture/acupressure. Less than 10% refer for chiropractic manipulation, osteopathic manipulation, homeopathy, herbal medicine, and prayer healing. This is contrary to studies in Europe that indicate that manipulative therapies (chiropractic and osteopathic), acupuncture, and homeopathy were therapies referred to more often.[15,16,19,20,23] This may be because many of these therapies have been accepted by mainstream medicine in Europe more so than in the United States.

More than one fourth of pediatricians in our study consider acupuncture/acupressure, biofeedback, chiropractic or osteopathic manipulation, herbs, hypnosis, imagery, massage therapy, prayer healing, relaxation, and self-help groups to be effective. Even though one third of the physicians reported that they think manipulative therapies may be effective, less than 20% believe they are safe, and less than 10% refer patients for these therapies. One explanation for this discrepancy may be that manipulative therapies for children are often used for nonmusculoskeletal disorders, such as otitis media, respiratory tract disorders, colic, enuresis, etc, often delaying appropriate and effective medical treatment.[33,34] Furthermore, no scientific studies have proved these therapies to be useful for these conditions. In adults, manipulative therapies are most often used for musculosketelal disorders, where they may be effective.

Sex, ethnicity, practice type, and location of medical training all have a significant effect on pediatricians' attitudes toward CAM therapies. This study supports results of other studies that indicate that female sex is a significant positive predictor of favorable attitudes toward CAM and of more interaction between pediatricians and the patients or their parents.[15,23] More female pediatricians refer patients for CAM, and more female pediatricians wanted CME courses on CAM therapies. More whites and more graduates of US medical schools compared with foreign-born or -trained physicians believe their patients use CAM, and they also are more likely to discuss CAM with their patients and the parents of their patients. This may be explained by the fact that non-US medical school graduates may have firm beliefs in biomedicine and may reject CAM so as to be seen as integrated into the US allopathic biomedical model.

Pediatricians in general practice were more likely than specialists to believe their patients use CAM, to refer for CAM, and to want more CME courses in CAM. Our results are similar to those of the study of primary care physicians by Borkan et al,[24] who believe that the physician-patient relationship between physicians in general practice vs subspecialties may be more open, and that physicians in general practice may be more aware of the limitations of biomedicine or deal with less severe, but often chronic, conditions for which CAM may be more appropriate.

This study has implications for clinical practice and for future medical education. It is clear from this and other studies that primary care physicians, including pediatricians, are generally aware that their patients are seeking alternatives to conventional biomedicine. This awareness is associated with an interest in and referral to complementary/alternative therapies despite the lack of substantial scientific basis for some therapies. Many CAM therapies focus on preventive medicine and emphasize a holistic approach to the patient, considering the patient in the context of mind, body, emotions, and environment.[34,35] Patients have a positive attitude toward CAM, and its use is increasing even in children. Pediatricians need to be aware of this and maintain an attitude that is open and nonthreatening. Inquiries about the use of CAM should be a part of the routine pediatric medical history.[33]

This study has several limitations. The survey instrument was administered only to pediatricians in the state of Michigan who were members of the Michigan chapter of the American Academy of Pediatrics, and therefore the results may not be generalizable to all pediatricians. The fact that we had a 40% response rate to our survey raises the possibility of response bias, since many physicians may have strong views for or against CAM, therefore accounting for the large number of nonresponders. Also, although the use of CAM is widespread, it is not widely used in the United States for children; thus, many pediatricians may not be aware of many of these therapies and their use in pediatrics. Finally, many CAM therapies have not been widely studied in children, and even practitioners of CAM may not see a large number of children.

Conclusions

Primary care physicians, including pediatricians surveyed in this and other studies, are interested in CME courses that involve training in CAM. Clearly, there is a need and a demand for more education, along with clinical guidelines for CAM therapies within the context of biomedicine.[36,37] Given the use of CAM by patients and the growing scientific support for some therapies, perhaps some CAM therapies can be integrated as part of both undergraduate and postgraduate medical education. More research in various CAM therapies and larger studies surveying attitudes and referral patterns of pediatricians need to be considered for the future.

We thank Mary Lu Angelilli, MD; Howard Fisher, MD; Paul T. Giblin, PhD; and Howard Schubiner, MD, of Children's Hospital of Michigan, Wayne State University School of Medicine, Detroit, Mich, for their review of the manuscript.

References

1. Micozzi MS, ed. *Fundamentals of Complementary and Alternative Medicine.* New York, NY: Churchill Livingstone; 1996.
2. National Institutes of Health, Office of Alternative Medicine. *Alternative Medicine General Information Package.* Washington, DC: US Government Printing Office; 1996.
3. Panel on Definition and Description, CAM Research Methodology Conference. Defining and describing complementary and alternative medicine. *Altern Ther Health Med.* 1997;3:49–57.
4. Vincent C, Furnham A. Why do patients turn to complementary medicine? an empirical study. *Br J Clin Psychol.*1996;35:37–48.
5. Furnham A, Kirkcaldy B. The health beliefs and behaviors of orthodox and complementary medicine clients. *Br J Clin Psychol.* 1996; 35:49–61.
6. Furnham A, Forey J. The attitudes, behaviors and beliefs of patients of conventional vs complementary (alternative) medicine. *J Clin Psychol.* 1994;50:458–469.
7. Elder NC, Gillcrist A, Minz R. Use of alternative health care by family practice patients. *Arch Fam Med.* 1997;6:181–184.
8. Verhoef MJ, Sutherland LR, Brkich L. Use of alternative medicine by patients attending a gastroenterology clinic. *CMAJ.* 1990;142:121–125.
9. Fisher P, Ward A. Complementary medicine in Europe. *BMJ.* 1994;309:107–111.
10. Thomas KJ, Carr J, Westlake L, et al. Use of non-orthodox and conventional health care in Great Britain. *BMJ.* 1991;302:207–210.
11. Burg MA. Women's use of complementary medicine: combining mainstream medicine with alternative practices. *J Fla Med Assoc.* 1996;83:482–488.
12. Eisenberg DM, Kessler RC, Foster C, et al. Unconventional medicine in the United States: prevalence, costs and patterns of use. *N Engl J Med.* 1993;328:246–252.
13. McGuire MB. *Middle-Class Use of Nonmedical Healing: Ritual Healing in Suburban America.* New Brunswick, NJ: Rutgers University Press; 1988:3–17.
14. Zwicky JF, Hafner AW, Barrett S, et al. *Reader's Guide to Alternative Health Methods: Scientific Perspective.* Chicago, Ill: American Medical Association; 1993:3–13.
15. Marshall RJ, Gee R, Israel M, et al. The use of alternative therapies by Auckland general practitioners. *N Z Med J.* 1990;103:213–215.
16. Anderson E, Anderson P. General practitioners and alternative medicine. *J R Coll Gen Pract.* 1987;37:52–55.
17. Knipschild P, Kleijnen J, Riet GT. Belief in the efficacy of alternative medicine among general practitioners in the Netherlands. *Soc Sci Med.* 1990;31:625–626.
18. Himmel W, Schulte M, Kochen MM. Complementary medicine: are patients' expectations being met by their general practitioners? *Br J Gen Pract.* 1993;43:232–235.
19. Wharton R, Lewith G. Complementary medicine and the general practitioner. *BMJ.* 1986; 101:766–768.
20. Hadley CM. Complementary medicine and the general practitioner: a survey of general practitioners in the Wellington area. *N Z Med J.* 1988; 101:766–768.
21. Visser GJ, Peters L. Alternative medicine and general practitioners in the Netherlands: towards acceptance and integration. *Fam Pract.* 1990;7:227–232.
22. Reilly DT. Young doctors' views on alternative medicine. *BMJ.* 1983;287:337–339.
23. Goldszmidt M, Levitt C, Duarte-Franco E, et al. Complementary health care services: a survey of general practitioners' view. *CMAJ.* 1995; 153:29–35.
24. Borkan J, Neher JO, Anson O, et al. Referrals for alternative therapies. *J Fam Pract.* 1994; 39:545–550.
25. Berman BM, Singh BK, Lao L, et al. Physicians' attitudes toward complementary or alternative medicine: a regional survey. *J Am Board Fam Pract.* 1995;8:361–366.
26. Verhoef MJ, Sutherland LR. General practitioners' assessment of and interest in alternative medicine in Canada. *Soc Sci Med.* 1995; 41:511–515.
27. Ernst E, Resch KL, White AR. Complementary medicine: what physicians think of it: meta-analysis. *Arch Intern Med.* 1995; 155:2405–2408.
28. Schachter L, Weingarten MA, Kahan EE. Attitudes of family physicians to nonconventional therapies: a challenge to science as the basis of therapeutics. *Arch Fam Med.* 1993; 2:1268–1270.
29. Spigelblatt L, Laine-Ammara G, Pless B, et al. The use of alternative medicine by children. *Pediatrics.* 1994;94:811–814.
30. Southwood TR, Nalleson PN, Roberts-Thomson PJ, et al. Unconventional remedies used for patients with juvenile arthritis. *Pediatrics.* 1990; 85:150–154.
31. Stern RC, Canada ER, Doershuk CF. Use of nonmedical treatment by cystic fibrosis patients. *J Adolesc Health.* 1992;13:612–615.
32. Sawyer MG, Gannoni AF, Toogood IR, et al. The use of alternative therapies by children with cancer. *Med J Aust.* 1994;160:320–322.
33. Spigleblatt LS. Alternative medicine: should it be used by children? *Curr Probl Pediatr.* 1995; 25:180–188.
34. Spigleblatt LS. Alternative medicine: a pediatric conundrum. *Contemp Pediatr.* 1997;14:51–64.
35. Kemper KJ. Separation or synthesis: a holistic approach to therapeutics. *Pediatr Rev.* 1996; 17:279–283.
36. LaValley JW, Verhoef MJ. Integrating complementary medicine and health care services into practice. *CMAJ.* 1995;153:45–49.
37. Practice and Policy Guidelines Panel, National Institutes of Health Office of Alternative Medicine. Clinical practice guidelines in complementary and alternative medicine: an analysis of opportunities and obstacles. *Arch Fam Med.* 1997;6:149–154.

4 A Review of the Incorporation of Complementary and Alternative Medicine by Mainstream Physicians

John A. Astin, PhD; Ariane Marie, BA; Kenneth R. Pelletier, PhD; Erik Hansen; William L. Haskell, PhD
From the Stanford Center for Research in Disease Prevention, Stanford University School of Medicine, Stanford, Calif (Drs Astin, Pelletier, and Haskell), University of Southern California School of Medicine, Los Angeles (Ms Marie), and Stanford University (Mr Hansen).

Background
Studies suggest that between 30% and 50% of the adult population in industrialized nations use some form of complementary and/or alternative medicine (CAM) to prevent or treat a variety of health-related problems.

Method
A comprehensive literature search identified 25 surveys conducted between 1982 and 1995 that examined the practices and beliefs of conventional physicians with regard to 5 of the more prominent CAM therapies: acupuncture, chiropractic, homeopathy, herbal medicine, and massage. Six studies were excluded owing to their methodological limitations.

Results
Across surveys, acupuncture had the highest rate of physician referral (43%) among the 5 CAM therapies, followed by chiropractic (40%) and massage (21%). Rates of CAM practice by conventional physicians varied from a low of 9% for homeopathy to a high of 19% for chiropractic and massage therapy. Approximately half of the surveyed physicians believed in the efficacy of acupuncture (51%), chiropractic (53%), and massage (48%), while fewer believed in the value of homeopathy (26%) and herbal approaches (13%).

Conclusions
This review suggests that large numbers of physicians are either referring to or practicing some of the more prominent and well-known forms of CAM and that many physicians believe that these therapies are useful or efficacious. These data vary considerably across surveys, most likely because of regional differences and sampling methods, suggesting the need for more rigorous surveys using national, representative samples. Finally, outcomes studies are needed so that physicians can make decisions about the use of CAM based on scientific evidence of efficacy rather than on regional economics and cultural norms.

Arch Intern Med. 1998;158:2303–2310

Complementary and alternative medicine (CAM), a subject that was covered extensively in the last issue of the *Archives,* includes a variety of medical interventions that are not taught extensively at US medical schools or generally provided at US hospitals.[1] In 1990, an estimated 33% of the general public in the United States reported using[1] or more types of CAM, and the number of visits to CAM providers was greater than the number of visits to all primary care physicians.[1] A national survey conducted in 1994 found 40% of the general public reporting the use of CAM within the previous year.[2] Surveys in Europe and Australia have reported similar uses of CAM (range, 20% to 49%).[3–6] The popularity of particular types of CAM varies geographically, but generally includes chiropractic, relaxation techniques, massage, herbal medicine, and homeopathy.[1–5] The demographic characteristics of frequent CAM users do not vary regionally. Different international surveys consistently report that users of CAM tend to be more educated, have higher incomes, and are more likely to be between the ages of 30 and 49 years.[1,7–9] However, Astin[2] found that among demographic variables only educational level predicted use of CAM.

The most frequently cited reason for consumer use of CAM is dissatisfaction with the ability of conventional medicine to adequately treat chronic illnesses.[1,10,11] However, in a recent multivariate analysis,[2] dissatisfaction failed to predict use of CAM in a national sample. This study found that having more education, poorer health status, and a holistic philosophical orientation to health and life (ie, belief in the importance of mind, body, and spirit) were all predictive of alternative health care use. Use of CAM has been found to be especially high in patients with Alzheimer disease, multiple sclerosis, rheumatic diseases, cancer, acquired immunodeficiency syndrome, back problems, anxiety, headaches, and chronic pain.[1,2,12–17] Use of alternative treatments by both the public and practitioners is likely to escalate with the growing incidence of chronic illnesses as populations age.[18] Additional reasons for consumer use of CAM include (1) a dislike of the reductionist, mechanical model of medicine and/or preference for a holistic, integrative model of medicine[2,10,19,20]; (2) a desire to avoid treatments with adverse effects and to reduce iatrogenic conditions[10,20]; and (3) a greater knowledge of how nutritional, emotional, and lifestyle factors affect health.[11,21–23]

Physicians have had a range of responses to patient interest in CAM. Three of the most common arguments used by opponents are as follows: (1) alternative therapists do not have the extensive knowledge that is required to diagnose an illness properly[24,25]; (2) there is a lack of evidence of the efficacy of CAM[26,27]; and (3) CAM is potentially harmful owing to its adverse effects or indirectly through the failure of patients to seek appropriate medical care.[26,28] By contrast, clinicians have become strong proponents of particular types of CAM, regardless of whether or not there is scientific evidence of efficacy.[29,30] Somewhere between overenthusiastic belief and stubborn disbelief is a balanced perspective that will help patients and advance medical science.[29]

Physicians need to be informed about CAM because their patients are using CAM and will continue to use CAM if they believe that these therapies are helpful to them.[31] Approximately 7 of 10 patients using CAM for a serious health problem do not tell their physicians that they are using unconventional therapy.[1] Hence, physicians need to know enough about CAM to provide information about possible interactions with pharmaceutical prescriptions and to provide reliable information to help patients sort through all the multilevel marketing of CAM products.[32,33] Also, knowledge about CAM may help to expand and improve clinical care, as has been done in the past, such as by incorporating new approaches (eg, nutritional supplements) or by eliminating ineffective approaches (eg, bloodletting).[29,34]

Providing information about the efficacy of CAM is not straightforward, in part because the general area of CAM refers to a variety of methods that may be more or less effective for different medical conditions and individuals. One way to direct future investigation of the efficacy of CAM, particularly given the hundreds of alternative therapies that are being practiced, is to examine which CAM therapies are considered most useful by physicians based on their clinical experience.

Several international surveys have asked about physicians' practices and beliefs with regard to CAM. One meta-analysis published in 1995[6] assessed whether physicians believe that complementary medicine is useful and/or effective based on 12 of these surveys. The authors found that, on average, physicians judged CAM therapies to be moderately effective (the average rating across surveys was 48 on a 100-point scale). However, one of the difficulties in interpreting these data is that across surveys researchers have tended to define CAM quite distinctly. For example, the lists of possible CAM therapies can vary from as few as 3 modalities to as many as 25. Furthermore, numerous surveys examining physicians' attitudes toward CAM have included such categories as diet and exercise and psychotherapy, which most conventional physicians would not consider to be alternative or unconventional. The meta-analysis by Ernst et al[6] also did not include any analyses of physicians' practice of, referrals for, or reasoning behind their use of or belief in such therapies.

The present study addresses the above limitations by (1) focusing on physicians' attitudes toward *specific* CAM therapies rather than toward CAM in general, since it is difficult to interpret the precise meaning or significance of the latter; (2) including an analysis of physicians' practice of, referrals for, and reasoning behind specific CAM use. This review focuses on conventional physicians' attitudes toward the following 5 therapies: acupuncture, chiropractic, herbal medicine, homeopathy, and massage. Research suggests that these therapies are the ones most frequently used by consumers.[1,2] Also, these therapies have tended to receive the most attention by the popular media and are the modalities that insurance companies and health maintenance organizations appear most interested in or willing to offer coverage for. The specific factors that were evaluated in this review include physicians' (1) practice, training, and type of referrals in general, (2) belief in the efficacy or use of CAM, and (3) reasons for practice of, referrals for, and/or interest in CAM. The attitudes of conventional physicians toward these 5 alternative therapies may suggest which types of CAM show clinical potential and would merit further research based on the clinical experience of physicians.

Methods

Literature Review

An international literature search using a multistage process was undertaken in February 1997. In the first stage, systematic searches were undertaken in several databases, including MEDLINE, MED90, MED85, ABI, SOCIOLOGICAL ABSTRACTS (SOCA), PSYCINFO, and BIOSIS. Search terms used were "attitudes, opinions, views" with "physicians, practitioners" and "alternative medicine, alternative therapies." In the second stage, 2 reviewers examined the reference sections of the initial articles in order to identify additional surveys. Additional articles were retrieved, and their reference sections were examined until no more new surveys were identified. In the third stage, directors of the National Institutes of Health's Office of Alternative Medicine national centers as well selected key authors were provided a list of physician surveys and asked to identify any other relevant surveys known to them.

Surveys: Inclusion/Exclusion Criteria

All surveys evaluating physicians' attitudes toward or use of CAM in general were considered. Only surveys of *mainstream physicians* (MDs with no known vested interest in CAM) were included. From these, surveys were excluded if they (1) were not in English, (2) were based on previously published reports of an original survey,[35] (3) were not mail or questionnaire surveys,[36] and (4) did not have a response rate of at least 50%.[35,37–39] Based on these criteria, we identified 19 studies that examined the practices and beliefs of mainstream physicians with regard to CAM. These studies are described in Table 1.

All studies were conducted between 1982 and 1995. Ten studies used a random sampling method; 5 sampled all the physicians in a particular region or regions; 2 distributed surveys at conferences or clinical sites; and 2 combined a random sampling method with a sampling of all the physicians in a particular region. Six of the surveys compared mainstream physicians with other groups, and, when relevant to the purpose of this study, this information is mentioned in the "Results" section. None of the surveys tested the reliability of the survey questions. Nine of the surveys indicated that nonrespondents were demographically similar to respondents, and 1 of these also indicated that nonrespondents were similar in their attitude toward CAM.

Three of 19 surveys did not specify what types of therapies were meant by CAM but asked respondents to specify the types of therapies themselves.[40–42] The other surveys defined the particular types of therapies meant by CAM and asked specific questions related to these therapies.

Two reviewers identified factors to be examined based on the purpose of the study. Both reviewers independently entered the data. Any discrepancies in the data entry were resolved by referring to the original articles. Differences between the 2 reviewers that could not be resolved were decided by a third reviewer.

Results

Methodological Critique

For this analysis, the 19 studies reviewed included 17 heterogeneous surveys. None of the studies tested the reliability of the survey questions. Hence, variation in how individual questions were asked probably confounds the validity of all of the studies reviewed. Samples sizes ranged from 40 to 594 physicians (mean±SD, 201±141). Although a few studies included physicians from different regions within a country, the small sample sizes and the regional specificity of the sampling undermine the generalizability of the results. Furthermore, the limited number of countries and the restriction to English-language publications also limit the generalizability of the findings.

Table 1. Study Characteristics*

Source, Year of Study	Location	Sample Size†	Response Rate, %	Mean Age, y	Sex, % M/F	GP/S, %
Anderson and Anderson,[40] 1986	Oxfordshire, England	222	81	. . .	. . .	100/0
Berman et al,[48] NA	Chesapeake Region, US	180	61	42.8	80/20	82/18
Borkan et al,[53] 1992	Southern Israel and US (Wash, NM)	138	64.7	43.4	. . .	44/56
Cherkin et al,[51] NA	US (Wash)	476	79	43.6	84/16	100 (FPs)/0
Golstein et al,[35] 1984	US (Calif)	142	71.4	44	84.5/16.5	100 (FPs)/0
Goldszmidt et al,[52] 1993	Quebec, Canada	146	73	41	64/36	100/0
Hadley et al,[49] 1986	New Zealand (Wellington, Hutt)	173	77	. . .	75/25	100/0
Himmel et al,[4] NA	Kassel, Germany	40	56.3	. . .	. . .	100/0
King et al,[43] 1990	US (NC, Fla, NY, Ill, Tex, Colo, Calif)	594	59	41	85/15	100 (FPs)/0
Knipschild et al,[54] 1989	The Netherlands	293	74	. . .	. . .	100/0
Lynoe and Svensson,[47] 1990	Sweden	330	81	43	69/31	LPs
Marshall et al,[41] 1989	Auckland, New Zealand	249	67.3	44	82.6/17.4	100/0
Perkin et al,[45] NA	England	168	84	. . .	. . .	51.8/48.2
Reilly,[46] 1982	Scotland	86	86	. . .	52.3/43	100 (Trs)/0
Schacter et al,[42] 1991	Central Israel	89	89	37	54/46	100/0
Verhoef and Sutherland,[44] 1992	Canada (Ontario, Alberta)	200	52	44	76/24	100/0
Visser,[8] NA	The Netherlands	71	70	. . .	29/71	0/100 (Rhs)
Wharton and Lewith,[50] 1985	Avon, England	145	72.5	. . .	. . .	100/0
Zubek,[55] 1993	British Columbia, Canada	79	63.2	40.4	71.4/28.6	100 (FPs)/0

*GP indicates general practitioner; S, specialist; ellipses, information not provided; NA, not available; US, United States; FPs, family practitioners; LPs, licensed physicians; Trs, trainees; and Rhs, rheumatologists.

†Mainstream physicians.

Participation Rates. Response rates ranged from 52% to 89% (mean±SD, 72%±10.4%). In general, surveys with lower response rates are more likely to be influenced by participant self-selection. In evaluating physician practices and beliefs with regard to CAM, it is critical to determine whether nonresponders and responders are similar in their attitude toward CAM. Only 1 of the studies included in this review asked whether nonresponders had a similar attitude toward CAM.[44] Thus, it is possible that many of the surveys with lower response rates are skewed toward participants who were eager to participate because of their either highly favorable or highly unfavorable opinion of CAM. Along these lines, there was a nonsignificant negative association between sample size and belief in efficacy ($r=-0.79$; $P<.07$) and practice of CAM ($r=-0.70$; $P<.40$)

Analysis of Results. A meta-analysis of the studies was not possible because of the heterogeneity of the surveys and the corresponding lack of standardization with respect to methodology, sampling procedures, statistical analyses, and reporting of data. A minority of the studies conducted (7 of 19) did not examine the statistical effects of age and sex on physicians' responses. None of the studies considered differential responses from racial and/or ethnic subpopulations of physicians. Only 1 study compared the responses of physicians based on their specialization.[45]

Along with the 5 CAM therapies we focused on for the present review (acupuncture, chiropractic, homeopathy, herbal therapies, and massage), surveys examined physicians' use of, and attitudes toward, a number of other health care approaches that have been considered alternative or complementary in previous research. Additional CAM therapies included various nutritional approaches, such as use of megavitamin therapy and fasting; mind-body modalities, such as meditation, relaxation, imagery, and hypnosis; spiritual or faith healing; and various body-based techniques, including osteopathy, polarity therapy, electromagnetic healing, chelation therapy, Alexander technique, acupressure, reflexology, and therapeutic touch.

Practice Of CAM

Table 2 summarizes the rates of practice for the 5 specific CAM therapies we reviewed. Across surveys, practice rates varied from a high of 78% for herbal medicine[4] to no reported practice of this modality.[46] Reported rates of practice were quite varied across all CAM modalities. For example, for acupuncture, rates varied from a high of 24%[47] to a low of 1%,[46] while for chiropractic, practice rates varied from a high of 27%[48] to a low of 6%.[40] (The higher practice and

Table 2. Physician Practice of CAM Therapies*

Source, y	Country	Acupuncture	Chiropractic	Homeopathy	Herbal Medicine	Massage
		Type of Therapy, %				
Goldszmidt et al,[52] 1995	Canada	...	...	...	...	...
Verhoef and Sutherland,[44] 1995	Canada	...	...	...	...	...
Perkin et al,[45] 1994	England	8	...	7	...	...
Anderson and Anderson,[40] 1987	England	3	6	1	...	...
Wharton and Lewith,[50] 1986	England	3	24	5	1	...
Himmel et al,[4] 1993	Germany	15	20	45	78	...
Marshall et al,[41] 1990	New Zealand	21	...	4	2	0.04
Hadley,[49] 1988	New Zealand	18	11	4	...	...
Reilly,[46] 1983	Scotland	1	7	2	0	...
Lynoe and Svensson,[47] 1992	Sweden	24	...	1	...	...
Berman et al,[48] 1995	United States	14	27	5	7	35
Borkan et al,[53] 1994	United States and Israel	...	...	...	...	...
Goldstein et al,[35] 1988	United States	51	...	8	9	22
Visser,[8] 1992	The Netherlands	...	51	14	...	...
Knipschild et al,[54] 1990	The Netherlands	...	9	...	...	...
Mean±SD		17±15	19±14	9±13	16±30	19±18
Median		15	18	5	5	22
Range		1–51	6–51	1–45	0–78	0.04–35

*CAM indicates complementary and alternative medicine; ellipses, practice of this modality not assessed.

referral rates reported by Goldstein et al,[35] eg, 51% for acupuncture, are the result, in part, of their having combined practice and referral rates as 1 value.) Across surveys, mean practice rates for physicians varied from a high of 19% for massage and chiropractic to a low of 9% for homeopathy. On average, 17% of physicians reported practicing acupuncture, while 16% reported practicing herbal therapy. Table 2 also lists medians for practice rates, as the mean values in certain instances have been inflated by outlier values, such as the 78% practice rate for herbal medicine reported by Himmel et al[4] (in that study, the mean was 16% and the median was 5%).

The practice of CAM in general is greater among younger physicians according to 1 survey.[44] However, 2 studies found no difference in the practice of CAM by age.[40,41] Two surveys[40,44] found that the practice of CAM is more common among male physicians, and 2 studies found no difference in practice rates by sex.[41,49]

Four surveys also inquired about training in, and practice of, CAM.[40,48–50] Among these surveys, an equal or higher number of physicians reported training in various types of CAM compared with the number of physicians who reported practice of those types of CAM. The only exceptions in which more physicians claimed to practice than claimed training were acupuncture (2 of 4 surveys), chiropractic (3 of 3 surveys), naturopathy (1 of 1 survey), osteopathy (1 of 1 survey), and spiritual or faith healing (2 of 2 surveys).

Referrals for CAM

Table 3 summarizes referral rates for the 5 CAM therapies. As with the practice of CAM, reported referral rates were quite varied, ranging from highs of 83% for chiropractic[44] and 71% for acupuncture,[49] to lows of 2% for chiropractic[41] and 1% for herbal medicine[40] and homeopathy,[47] to no reported referrals for herbal medicine.[46] Mean referral rates ranged from a high of 43% for acupuncture to a low of 4% for herbal medicine. As shown in Table 3, across surveys, the mean rates of referral for chiropractic were 40%, while the rates for homeopathy (15%) and massage (21%) were considerably lower. The highest referral rates reported for homeopathy were 42%[50] and 35%[45] and for massage 35%[48] and 26%.[41] The highest reported referral rates for herbal medicine were 9% (which includes practice as well)[35] and 5%.[41,48]

Three surveys report that referral rates for CAM in general[8,41] and for chiropractic in particular[51] are higher among younger physicians. However, 3 studies found no difference in referral rates for CAM by age.[40,52,53] One survey[42] found that referral rates for CAM are higher among female physicians; however, 3 studies found no difference in referral rates by sex.[40,52,53]

Table 3. Physician Referral for CAM Therapies*

Source, y	Country	Type of Therapy, % Acupuncture	Chiropractic	Homeopathy	Herbal Medicine	Massage
Goldszmidt et al,[52] 1995	Canada	68	58	...	...	...
Verhoef and Sutherland,[44] 1995	Canada	42	83	...	...	...
Perkin et al,[45] 1994	England	62	34	35	...	...
Anderson and Anderson,[40] 1987	England	20	50	18	1	1
Wharton and Lewith,[50] 1986	England	28	51	42	2	...
Himmel et al,[4] 1993	Germany	...	...	...	...	...
Marshall et al,[41] 1990	New Zealand	61	2	21	5	26
Hadley,[49] 1988	New Zealand	71	27	8	...	...
Reilly,[46] 1983	Scotland	8	20	11	0	...
Lynoe and Svensson,[47] 1992	Sweden	24	...	1	...	...
Berman et al,[48] 1995	United States	26	56	6	5	35
Borkan et al,[53] 1994	United States and Israel	11	15	3	...	...
Cherkin et al,[51] 1989	United States	...	57	...	...	...
Goldstein et al,[35] 1988	United States	51	51	8	9	22
Visser,[8] 1992	The Netherlands	...	...	...	...	...
Knipschild et al,[54] 1990	The Netherlands	...	...	...	...	...
Mean±SD		43±22	40±23	15±14	4±3	21±14
Median		47	50	10	4	24
Range		8–71	2–83	1–42	0–9	1–35

*CAM indicates complementary and alternative medicine; ellipses, referrals for this modality not assessed.

Table 4. Physician Belief in the Efficacy of CAM Therapies*

Source, y	Country	Type of Therapy, % Acupuncture	Chiropractic	Homeopathy	Herbal Medicine	Massage
Goldszmidt et al,[52] 1995	Canada	78	70	...	...	...
Verhoef and Sutherland,[44] 1995	Canada	71	59	12	17	...
Perkin et al,[45] 1994	England	...	...	...	...	...
Anderson and Anderson,[40] 1987	England	15	32	7	1	...
Wharton and Lewith,[50] 1986	England	67	89	47	23	...
Himmel et al,[4] 1993	Germany	...	...	...	...	...
Marshall et al,[41] 1990	New Zealand	...	...	...	...	...
Hadley,[49] 1988	New Zealand	67	67	...	...	...
Reilly,[46] 1983	Scotland	88	19	52	15	...
Lynoe and Svensson,[47] 1992	Sweden	43	...	...	...	...
Berman et al,[48] 1995	United States	49	49	27	23	58
Borkan et al,[53] 1994	United States and Israel	...	...	...	...	...
Cherkin et al,[51] 1989	United States	...	91	...	...	...
Goldstein et al,[35] 1988	United States	18	13	1	2	6
Visser,[8] 1992	The Netherlands	37	49	23	9	...
Knipschild et al,[54] 1990	The Netherlands	33	...	40	...	80
Mean±SD		51±26	53±26	26±19	13±9	48±38
Median		49	49	25	15	58
Range		15–88	13–91	1–52	1–23	6–80

*CAM indicates complementary and alternative medicine; ellipses, belief in the efficacy of this modality not assessed.

Belief in the Use or Efficacy of CAM

Once again, the extent to which physicians reported believing in the value or efficacy of CAM therapies varied considerably across both surveys and modalities. As shown in Table 4, belief in the usefulness of CAM ranged from as high as 91% and 89% for chiropractic,[50,51] 88% for acupuncture,[46] and 80% for massage[54] to as low as 1% for homeopathy,[35] 1% to 2% for herbal medicine,[35,40] and 6% for massage.[35] Also, while belief in efficacy tended to be higher for acupuncture and chiropractic, and to a slightly lesser extent massage, several surveys identified fairly high rates of belief for homeopathy and herbal medicine. For example, belief in the value of homeopathy ran as high as 52% and 47%,[46,50] while 2 surveys found 23% of physicians believing in the efficacy or clinical usefulness of herbal medicine.[48,50]

The results of this analysis suggest that, on average, physicians perceive chiropractic to be more useful or effective than acupuncture and acupuncture to be more useful or effective than homeopathy, findings that are consistent with the meta-analysis by Ernst et al.[6]

Belief in CAM is greater among younger physicians according to a survey by Perkin et al[45] and the meta-analysis by Ernst et al.[6] However, 5 studies found no difference in beliefs by age,[40,42,50,53,55] and 1 study found belief in hypnosis to be greater among older physicians.[52] Belief in CAM is greater among female physicians according to 1 survey,[52] although 4 studies found no difference in belief by sex.[40,42,53,55]

Reasons for Practice of, Referrals for, or Interest in CAM

Among the reasons listed by physicians for their practice of, referrals for, or interest in CAM are (in order of frequency) (1) patient's lack of response to conventional treatment, (2) patient's request or preference, (3) belief in efficacy, and (4) fewer adverse effects.[4,41,44,47,53] Less frequently cited reasons include (1) the belief that the scientific world view that is espoused by conventional, academic medicine is limited,[47] (2) the conception that there is a synergy between CAM and patients' cultural beliefs,[53] and (3) the perception that patients' diseases are nonorganic or psychological in nature.[53] Conditions for which physicians use CAM or refer for CAM include psychological problems, pain, back problems, musculoskeletal disorders, chronic illnesses, anxiety, headaches, smoking cessation, and weight problems.[4,40,41,44,46,53]

Comment

Examination of practice of, referrals for, and belief in the efficacy of specific types of CAM revealed a tremendous variation across surveys. However, this variation did not appear to correlate with the year or the country in which the study was conducted. This observation is consistent with that of Ernst et al,[6] who did not identify a change in belief in the efficacy or use of CAM over time or a trend suggesting that 1 country has an increased belief in CAM. It is also consistent with the findings of Borkan et al,[53] who did not identify a significant difference in practice, referrals, or belief in effectiveness among practice locations in the United States and southern Israel. Further corroboration is provided by Schacter et al,[42] who found that a physician's country of origin did not have a significant effect on his or her belief in CAM. However, in some instances, the extent to which certain CAM therapies are accepted and practiced as part of medical care can vary considerably depending on the country or culture one is observing. For example, in a survey of physicians in Kassel, Germany, Himmel et al[4] found that 45% practiced homeopathy, while 78% reported practicing herbal medicine, which likely reflects the greater acceptance of these modalities in this European country.

Other possible explanations for the variation in data for specific types of CAM between surveys could be (1) differences in demographic characteristics of the samples (as well as in how the samples were selected); (2) wording of surveys (including how the various CAM therapies were defined); (3) differences in the ratio of general practitioners to specialists; and/or (4) local/regional differences in the familiarity or availability of particular types of CAM. Demographic variation is a less likely reason, since the mean age and sex ratios were fairly similar among surveys, in addition to the fact that the data are inconclusive with regard to the influence of age or sex on the use of or belief in CAM. One survey found practice of, referrals for, and belief in CAM to be greater among general practitioners than among hospital-based physicians.[45] Unfortunately, too few of the other surveys reported data by specialty for us to be able to evaluate whether general practitioners do indeed use and believe in CAM more than specialists do and therefore to account for the variation in data between survey samples for specific types of CAM use or referral.

Regional differences in familiarity and availability of CAM are the most likely cause of the variation in data for particular types of CAM. For example, Himmel and colleagues[4] examined both patients' use and physicians' practice of CAM and found that herbal medicine, chiropractic, homeopathy, and acupuncture are popular among both patients and physicians. By contrast, relaxation techniques, chiropractic, and massage are most often used by consumers in the United States.[1,2] Studies suggest that physicians in the United States are more similar to consumers in the United States than to physicians in Germany in that relaxation techniques, chiropractic, and massage are more popular than herbal medicine or homeopathy.[35,48] Thus, it appears that the incorporation of particular types of CAM by physicians is influenced by the regional popularity of those therapies. This hypothesis is supported by interviews with hospital CAM program directors, who stated that they most often decided what types of CAM to include in their programs based on the availability of licensed or certified practitioners in their area.[56] It is a matter of concern that scientific evidence of efficacy is not the primary reason for the incorporation of CAM. However, it is not too surprising, since differences in conventional medical practices also correlate more strongly with regional economics, practitioner specialties, and cultural norms than with outcomes.[57]

Despite the variation in data for particular types of CAM, a review of the studies suggests that a number of such interventions may hold clinical promise and merit further research. Conditions for which physicians use or refer to CAM are similar to the conditions for which consumers use these therapies, with the most common being chronic pain, back problems, psychological problems, headaches, and chronic illnesses in general.[1,2] Physician and consumer use of CAM for these health-related problems suggests that conventional medicine may lack satisfactory interventions for the management of these conditions. However, further research is needed to determine whether particular types of CAM provide better outcomes for these conditions than does conventional medicine.

Comparison of information on the training and practice of CAM suggests that few physicians are practicing CAM without training. However, the fact that a few physicians are practicing modalities such as acupuncture and chiropractic (as well as naturopathy, osteopathy, and spiritual healing) without training suggests that physician education about the appropriate use of these therapies is needed.

Conclusions from this study are limited owing to the lack of large, representative national samples of physicians. It is difficult to interpret the variations in findings across surveys, since such differences could be the result of biased samples instead of reflecting true national or regional differences. It is also difficult to draw definitive conclusions from this review of physicians' attitudes toward CAM given (1) the failure to test the reliability of questions, (2) inconsistencies in the definition of CAM, and (3) a bias toward English-language publications. Therefore, future surveys of physicians' practices and beliefs with regard to CAM should consider the following recommendations in order to improve study quality and to allow comparison of different surveys:

- Keep the sample size minimum to 50 practitioners.
- Establish the reliability of questions.
- Use random (representative) samples from a defined region(s).
- Maintain a response rate of at least 75%.

Physicians' practice of and belief in different types of CAM may be influenced by personal experience. Thus, responses should be evaluated by region, sex, age, race and/or ethnic heritage, and medical specialty. Significant differences in responses should be reported (although such analyses will necessitate increasingly larger sample sizes).

Since CAM is largely a political term, the particular types of interventions considered to be alternative are likely to change over time and vary from region to region. Therefore, terms should be defined as precisely as possible, avoiding general terms that incorporate more than 1 intervention, such as *healing, movement,* or *self-care*. In general, data that do not distinguish between types of CAM are less useful. Nonresponders and responders should be similar demographically and have a similar attitude toward CAM.

The impact of physicians incorporating CAM therapies into their practice (or referring patients to CAM providers) may change the delivery of health care in more than one way. For example, the trend toward managed care, standardization of care, and shorter office visits is inconsistent with patients' and physicians' interest in more individualized treatments based on a more extensive understanding of each patient's history and current circumstances. There is also some evidence that incorporating CAM would more than double consultation time.[40] However, a growing body of scientific literature in mind-body medicine suggests that incorporation of some types of CAM, in particular interventions that consider the psychological, social, and environmental aspects of a particular patient, would result in better clinical outcomes.[18] Outcomes studies for both conventional and CAM therapies are needed to determine what diagnostic methods and medical treatments are in the best interests of the patient. Without this information, it is difficult to know how to set limitations on cost, length or number of office visits, and treatments.

Conclusions

This review of 19 international surveys suggests that large numbers of conventional physicians are either referring patients to or practicing some of the more prominent and well-known forms of CAM. Across studies, acupuncture had the highest rate of physician referral (43%) among the 5 CAM therapies we reviewed, followed by chiropractic (40%), and massage (21%). Rates of CAM practice by conventional physicians varied from a low of 9% for homeopathy to a high of 19% for chiropractic and massage therapy. Approximately half of the surveyed physicians believed in the efficacy of acupuncture (51%), chiropractic (53%), and massage (48%), while fewer believed in the value of homeopathy (26%) and herbal approaches (13%). Conditions for which physicians used or made referrals for these and other CAM therapies included chronic pain, back problems, psychological problems, headaches, and chronic illnesses.

These results vary considerably across surveys, most likely because of regional differences and sampling methods, suggesting the need for surveys using more national, representative samples. Finally, outcomes studies are needed so that physicians can make decisions about the use of CAM based on scientific evidence of efficacy rather than on regional economics and cultural norms.

This study was supported by grant AR43558 from the National Institute of Arthritis and Musculoskeletal and Skin Diseases, National Institutes of Health Office of Alternative Medicine, and by the Fetzer Institute, the Nathan Cummings Foundation, and the American Health Association.

We are grateful for the support of the National Institutes of Health Office of Complementary and Alternative Medicine, John W. Farquhar, MD, Cindy Wood, Adeline Hwang, and Ellen DiNucci.

References

1. Eisenberg DM, Kessler RC, Foster C, Norlock FE, Calkins DR, Delbanco TL. Unconventional medicine in the United States: prevalence, costs, and patterns of use. *N Engl J Med.* 1993; 328:246–252.
2. Astin JA. Why patients use alternative medicine: results of a national study. *JAMA.* 1998;279:1548–1553.
3. Risberg T, Lund E, Wist E. Use of non-proven therapies: differences in attitudes between Norwegian patients with non-malignant disease and patients suffering from cancer. *Acta Oncol.* 1995;34:893–898.
4. Himmel W, Schulte M, Kochen MM. Complementary medicine: are patients' expectations being met by their general practitioners? *Br J Gen Pract.* 1993;43:232–235.
5. MacLennan AH, Wilson DH, Taylor AW. Prevalence and cost of alternative medicine in Australia. *Lancet.* 1996;347:569–573.
6. Ernst E, Resch KL, White AR. Complementary medicine: what physicians think of it: a meta-analysis. *Arch Intern Med.*1995; 155:2405–2408.
7. Szanto S. Toward a pluralistic health care: unconventional medicine in Hungary. Paper presented at: Annual Meeting of the American Sociological Association; August 8, 1994; Los Angeles, Calif.
8. Visser J. Alternative medicine in the Netherlands. *Comp Med Res.* 1990;4:28–31.
9. Lloyd P, Lupton D, Wiesner D, Hasleton S. Choosing alternative therapy: an exploratory study of sociodemographic characteristics and motives of patients resident in Sydney. *Aust J Pub Health.*1993;17:135–144.
10. Mitchell S. Healing without doctors. *Am Demogr.* 1993;15:46–49.
11. Perelson GH. Alternative medicine: what role in managed care? *FHPJ Clin Res.* 1996;5:32–38.
12. Clinical Oncology Group. New Zealand cancer patients and alternative medicine. *N Z Med J.* 1987;100:110–113.
13. Fawcett J, Sidney JS, Hanson MJ, Riley-Lawless K. Use of alternative health therapies by people with multiple sclerosis: an exploratory study. *Holistic Nurs Pract.* 1994;8:36–42.
14. Vecchio PC. Attitudes to alternative medicine by rheumatology outpatient attenders. *J Rheumatol.* 1994;21:145–147.
15. Boisset M, Fitzcharles MA. Alternative medicine use by rheumatology patients in a universal healthcare setting. *J Rheumatol.*1994; 21:148–152.
16. Coleman LM, Fowler LL, Williams ME. Use of unproven therapies by people with Alzheimer's disease. *J Am Geriatr Soc.* 1995;43:747–750.
17. Singh N, Squier C, Sivek C, Nguyen MH, Wagener M, Yu VL. Determinants of nontraditional therapy use in patients with HIV infection: a prospective study. *Arch Intern Med.* 1996;156:197–201.
18. Gordon JS. *Manifesto for a New Medicine: Your Guide to Healing Partnerships and the Wise Use of Alternative Therapies.* New York, NY: Addison-Wesley Publishing Co Inc; 1996.
19. Ullman D. The mainstreaming of alternative medicine. *Healthcare Forum J.* 1993;3:24–30.
20. Featherstone C, Forsyth L. *Medical Marriage: The New Partnership Between Orthodox and Complementary Medicine.* Forres, Scotland: Findhorn Press; 1997.
21. Sabatino F. Mind and body medicine: a new paradigm? *Hospitals.* 1993;67:66–72.
22. Furnham A, Smith C. Choosing alternative medicine: a comparison of the beliefs of patients visiting a general practitioner and a homeopath. *Soc Sci Med.* 1988;26:685–689.
23. Furnham A, Forey J. The attitudes, behaviors and beliefs of patients of conventional vs. complementary (alternative) medicine. *J Clin Psychol.* 1994;50:458–469.
24. Weber DO. The mainstreaming of alternative medicine. *Healthcare Forum J.* November/ December 1996;39:16–27.
25. Mandelbaum-Schmid J. Blazing trails: an innovative insurer embraces alternative medicine. *Self.* 1997;19:62.
26. Levin S. Alternative medicine: a doctor's perspective. *S Afr Med J.* 1996;86:183–184.
27. Rees MK. Alternative medicine: down the slippery slope. *ModMed.* 1997;65:67–68.
28. Plaut GS. A comparison of the attitudes shown by general practitioners, hospital doctors, and medical students toward alternative medicine. *J R Soc Med.* 1995;88:238.
29. Ernst E. Complementary medicine: common misconceptions. *J R Soc Med.* 1995; 88:244–247.

30. Brown E. Alternative medicine converts its skeptics. *Managed Healthcare.* 1996;6:24–27.

31. Edelson M. Can the new medicine cure you? *Washingtonian.* 1996;31:68–85.

32. Blair L. Opening Pandora's box: family physicians and alternative medicine. *Can Fam Physician.* 1995;41:1807–1810.

33. Lehrman S. Alternative medicine: insurers cover new ground. *Harv Health Lett.* 1996;2:1–3.

34. Padgug RA. Alternative medicine and health insurance. *Mt Sinai J Med.* 1995;62:152–162.

35. Goldstein MS, Sutherland C, Jaffe DT, Wilson J. Holistic physicians and family practitioners: similarities, differences and implications for health policy. *Soc Sci Med.* 1988;26:853–862.

36. Bourgeault IL. Physicians' attitudes toward patients' use of alternative cancer therapies. *CMAJ.* 1996;155:1679–1685.

37. Blumberg D, Grant WD, Hendricks SR, Kamps CA, Dewan MJ. The physician and unconventional medicine. *Altern Ther Health Med.* 1995; 1:31–35.

38. White AR, Resch KL, Ernst E. Complementary medicine: use and attitudes among GPs. *Fam Pract.* 1997;14:302–306.

39. Cameron-Blackie G, Mouncer Y. *Complementary Therapies in the NHS.* Yorkshire, England: National Association for Health Authorities and Trusts; 1993.

40. Anderson E, Anderson P. General practitioners and alternative medicine. *J R Coll Gen Pract.* 1987;37:52–55.

41. Marshall RJ, Gee R, Israel M, Neave D, et al. The use of alternative therapies by Auckland general practitioners. *N Z Med J.* 1990; 103:213–215.

42. Schachter L, Weingarten MA, Kahan EE. Attitudes of family physicians to nonconventional therapies: a challenge to science as the basis of therapeutics. *Arch Fam Med.* 1993; 2:1268–1270.

43. King DE, Sobal J, Haggerty J, Dent M, Patton D. Experiences and attitudes about faith healing among family physicians. *J Fam Pract.* 1992; 35:158–162.

44. Verhoef MJ, Sutherland LR. Alternative medicine and general practitioners: opinions and behaviour. *Can Fam Physician.* 1995;41:1005–1011.

45. Perkin MR, Pearcy RM, Fraser JS. A comparison of the attitudes shown by general practitioners, hospital doctors and medical students towards alternative medicine. *J R Soc Med.* 1994; 87:523–525.

46. Reilly DT. Young doctors' views on alternative medicine. *BMJ.* 1983;287:337–339.

47. Lynoe N, Svensson T. Physicians and alternative medicine: an investigation of attitudes and practice. *Scand J Soc Med.* 1992;20:55–60.

48. Berman BM, Singh BK, Lao L, Singh BB, Ferentz KS, Hartnoll SM. Physicians' attitudes toward complementary or alternative medicine: a regional survey. *J Am Board Fam Pract.* 1995; 8:361–366.

49. Hadley CM. Complementary medicine and the general practitioner: a survey of general practitioners in the Wellington area. *N Z Med J.* 1988;101:766–768.

50. Wharton R, Lewith G. Complementary medicine and the general practitioner. *BMJ.* 1986;292:1498–1500.

51. Cherkin D, MacCornack FA, Berg AO. Managing of back pain: a comparison of the beliefs and behaviors of family physicians and chiropractors. *West J Med.* 1988;149:475–480.

52. Goldszmidt M, Levitt C, Duarte-Franco E, Kaczorowski J. Complementary health care services: a survey of general practitioners' views. *CMAJ.* 1995;153:29–35.

53. Borkan J, Neher J, Anson O, Smoker B. Referrals for alternative therapies. *J Fam Pract.* 1994; 39:545–550.

54. Knipschild P, Kleijnen J, Riet GT. Belief in the efficacy of alternative medicine among general practitioners in the Netherlands. *Soc Sci Med.* 1990;31:625–626.

55. Zubek EM. Traditional native healing: alternative or adjunct to modern medicine? *Can Fam Physician.* 1994;40:1923–1931.

56. Pelletier KR, Marie A, Krasner MA, Haskell WL. Current trends in the integration and reimbursement of complementary and alternative medicine by managed care, insurance carriers, and hospital providers. *Am J Health Promotion.* 1997;12:112–122.

57. Wennberg J. *The Dartmouth Atlas of Health Care in the United States.* Chicago, Ill: American Hospital Publications Inc; 1996.

5 Patterns of Use, Expenditures, and Perceived Efficacy of Complementary and Alternative Therapies in HIV-Infected Patients

Kathleen M. Fairfield, MD; David M. Eisenberg, MD; Roger B. Davis, ScD; Howard Libman, MD; Russell S. Phillips, MD

From the Division of General Medicine and Primary Care (Drs Fairfield, Eisenberg, Davis, Libman, and Phillips) and the Center for Alternative Medicine Research (Dr Eisenberg), Department of Medicine, Beth Israel Deaconess Medical Center, and Harvard Medical School, Boston, Mass.

Background

Complementary and alternative medicine (CAM) use is common in the general population, accounting for substantial expenditures. Among patients with human immunodeficiency virus (HIV) infection, few data are available on the prevalence, costs, and patterns of alternative therapy use.

Methods

We carried out detailed telephone surveys and medical chart reviews for 289 active patients with HIV in a general medicine practice at a university-based teaching hospital in Boston, Mass. Data were collected on prevalence and patterns of CAM use, out-of-pocket expenditures, associated outcomes, and correlates of CAM use.

Results

Of 180 patients who agreed to be interviewed, 122 (67.8%) used herbs, vitamins, or dietary supplements, 81 (45.0%) visited a CAM provider, and 43 (23.9%) reported using marijuana for medicinal purposes in the previous year. Patients who saw CAM providers made a median of 12 visits per year to these providers compared with 7 visits per year to their primary care physician and nurse practitioner. Mean yearly out-of-pocket expenditures for CAM users totaled $938 for all therapies. For the main reason CAM was used, respondents found therapies "extremely" or "quite a bit" helpful in 81 (81.0%) of 100 reports of supplement use, in 76 (65.5%) of 116 reports of CAM provider use, and in 27 (87%) of 31 reports of marijuana use. In multivariable models, college education (odds ratio [OR]=3.7, 95% confidence interval [CI]=1.9–7.1) and fatigue (OR=2.7, 95% CI=1.4–5.2) were associated with CAM provider use; memory loss (OR=2.3, 95% CI=1.1–4.8) and fatigue (OR=0.4, 95% CI=0.2–0.9) were associated with supplement use; and weight loss (OR=2.6, 95% CI=1.2–5.6) was associated with marijuana use.

Conclusions

Patients with HIV infection use CAM, including marijuana, at a high rate; make frequent visits to CAM providers; incur substantial expenditures; and report considerable improvement with these treatments. Clinical trials of frequently used CAMs are needed to inform physicians and patients about therapies that may have measurable benefit or measurable risk.

Arch Intern Med. 1998;158:2257–2264

Complementary or alternative medical therapies, defined as those treatments that have not generally been promoted and taught in Western medical schools and that have not generally been available at Western hospitals and clinics,[1–4] have been the focus of increasing interest by patients, clinicians, and researchers. A nationwide telephone survey in 1990 found that 34% of those surveyed used at least 1 complementary or alternative medical therapy to treat a serious or bothersome problem within the previous year. Based on data collected in that survey, the authors estimated that in 1990, 60 million US citizens used these therapies and spent an estimated $14 billion, of which $10.5 billion was spent "out-of-pocket."[1]

Use of complementary or alternative medicine (CAM) may be substantially more prevalent among patients with human immunodeficiency virus (HIV) than among the general population. A small study[5] of 2 groups of HIV-infected patients in northern California from 1988 to 1990 found that 70% had used CAM at some point. According to results from a Boston, Mass, survey, Cohen et al[6] reported in 1990 that 73% of patients used CAM. This study showed that those patients with higher education levels and lower helper T cells were more likely to use CAM. These studies were performed before the availability of protease inhibitors, which may have affected CAM use. In addition, few data are available on the specific therapeutic goals or symptoms that patients with HIV may attempt to treat with CAM, their associated outcomes, and expenditures for CAM by HIV-infected patients.

Among patients cared for in a primary care practice, we sought to determine patterns of use, associated expenditures, and perceived efficacy of CAM use among patients with HIV. We hypothesized that prevalence and expenditures for CAM would be high in this population, that patients with more advanced disease would use CAM to a greater degree, and that patients would generally perceive CAM to be efficacious.

Patients and Methods

Study Population

The study included a telephone survey and detailed medical chart review of all known HIV-infected patients at a primary care internal medicine practice at Beth Israel Deaconess Medical Center, Boston. This practice includes approximately 30 faculty, 100 house officers, and 10 nurse practitioners. The medical records for the practice are completely computerized, including all notes, medications, and problem lists.7 The practice provides more than 50,000 patient visits annually. Approximately 30% of patients are covered by Medicaid or by a hospital system of free care.

In December 1996, we identified all known HIV-positive patients in our practice. We contacted the primary care physician for each patient by mail in January 1997 and asked for permission to include their patients in a study of CAM use. If permission was given, we contacted patients by mail with a letter sent jointly by their primary care physician and the study's principal investigator. Patients had the opportunity to request that they not be contacted for interview either by sending back a refusal card included with the letter or by calling within 2 weeks. To preserve patient confidentiality, neither the initial letter nor the card included any mention of HIV infection as a criterion for study eligibility. Also, the letter did not specifically mention CAM in an attempt to avoid enriching our sample for patients interested in describing CAM use. After 2 weeks, we attempted to contact by telephone those patients who had not refused to participate. We obtained informed consent verbally at the beginning of the telephone survey after informing patients that they were confidentially identified as HIV positive for research purposes. We informed patients that researchers at Beth Israel Deaconess Medical Center were carrying out the study to investigate types of therapies people may use for health problems. At no point during the interview did we use the term "alternative therapy" or an equivalent term to avoid value judgments about what therapies might be "alternative." The

Beth Israel Deaconess Medical Center Committee on Clinical Investigations approved the consent process and study design.

As of December 1996, there were 289 active patients with HIV who received primary care in the practice. We excluded 14 hospital employees, 4 non–English-speaking or deaf patients, 3 patients with no working telephone, and 23 patients whose households were never reached by telephone despite numerous attempts during the study. Primary care physicians excluded 7 patients for reasons including severe psychiatric disease, difficult social situations, and extreme physical illness. Of 238 patients who remained eligible, 59 refused the telephone interview. We completed 180 interviews, yielding a response rate of 75.6%.

Data Collection

Telephone Survey. We interviewed all patients by telephone between April 22 and June 30, 1997, using professional interviewers. The interviews averaged 22 minutes. We asked patients whether they had experienced specific symptoms in the past year that were bothersome enough to keep them from their usual activities. These symptoms included pain, fatigue, weight loss and anorexia, and memory impairment or difficulty concentrating. Within each of these symptom categories, patients were queried about conventional therapies a physician may have prescribed for each problem and the perceived efficacy of those therapies. We then asked about the use of vitamins, herbal therapies, dietary supplements, marijuana for medicinal purposes, off-label prescription medications, and any other supplements in the past year using open-ended questions. Off-label prescription medications were described as medications that were generally available only by prescription but that the patient was able to obtain in another manner. We asked patients specifically if they had visited an acupuncturist, chiropractor, herbalist, homeopath, massage therapist, or other provider in the past year. We then asked open-ended questions about use of other therapies not already discussed or visits to other practitioners not specifically queried earlier. For those who use CAM providers or dietary supplements such as herbs or vitamins, we asked the respondent to identify the 3 most helpful therapies they used and then asked a series of specific questions about these 3 therapies.

Specific questions about each therapy included whether the patient was currently using the therapy, duration of use, frequency of use, and expenditures (total and out-of-pocket). We defined total expenditures as all expenditures by the patient and any other payer and out-of-pocket expenditures as those not covered by insurance or some other payer. Patients were queried about whether they had ever stopped using prescription medicines or specific CAM therapies because of the cost. We then asked if there was a specific main reason the patient sought the alternative therapy. Patients who reported a main reason for using a therapy were asked what that reason was and were queried about perceived efficacy of the therapy for that main reason. All patients, including those who did not report a main reason, were asked if there were any other reasons they used the therapy. Patients could report as many other reasons as applied. We also asked if their primary care physician was aware that they used the therapy and whether they started using the therapy before finding out they were HIV positive.

We collected demographic information, including level of education, race, and years of known HIV infection, as well as current employment status and income. Patients were queried about their sources of information about alternative therapies and their preferences for sources of information in the future.

Medical Chart Review. We abstracted clinical data from the computerized medical record for the 2-year period between July 1, 1995, and June 30, 1997. Demographic data were collected, including age, sex, insurance type, HIV risk factors, and duration of HIV infection. We abstracted clinical information, including all prescription medications, HIV-related complications, CD4 cell counts and viral load measurements, clinic visits and hospital admissions, history of anxiety and depression, outpatient psychiatric care, and history of painful syndromes (eg, neuropathy and back pain). We also noted whether there was documentation of alternative therapy use in the medical record. Because of concern that patients might choose alternative therapies in place of conventional therapies, we searched text of notes and problem lists for evidence that this had occurred.

Statistical Analyses

We used descriptive statistics (SAS Institute Inc, Cary, NC) to characterize our study population. Nonrespondents and respondents were compared using logistic regression models with a single covariate, with $P<.05$ as a criterion for statistical significance. We calculated yearly expenditures on supplements and marijuana by multiplying reported monthly expenditures by 12. For CAM providers, we calculated yearly expenditures by multiplying reported costs per visit by the average number of visits per year. We used descriptive statistics to examine

Table 1. Patients Reporting Use of CAM in the Past Year (n=180)*

Type of CAM	Patients, No. (%)
Supplements	
Herbal therapies	49 (27.2)
Minerals	28 (15.6)
Vitamins (not including multivitamins)	70 (38.9)
Protein or amino acid supplements	24 (13.3)
Other supplements (dehydroepiandrosterone, SPV30, and coenzyme Q)	34 (18.9)
Any herb, mineral, or vitamin supplement	122 (67.8)
CAM provider	
Acupuncturist or acupressurist	43 (23.9)
Chiropractor	21 (11.7)
Herbalist or practitioner of traditional Chinese medicine	19 (10.6)
Practitioner of homeopathic medicine	6 (3.3)
Massage therapist	68 (37.8)
Other providers (Reiki, craniosacral, or reflexology)	5 (2.8)
Any provider of CAM	81 (45.0)
Other CAM use	
Off-label prescription medications	12 (6.7)
Marijuana	43 (23.9)
Any CAM	137 (76.1)

*CAM indicates complementary and alternative medicine.

most common self-reported indications for therapies, perceived efficacy of specific therapies, and current vs ideal sources of information for patients.

Our outcomes of interest included use of CAM providers, herbs, vitamins, other supplements, and marijuana and any other CAM use. We sought to identify all correlates of CAM use for each major category of CAM. Because of inadequate statistical power, we present only descriptive statistics (Table 1) for CAM not included in these major categories. Using bivariable logistic regression, we identified all unadjusted predictors of CAM use. The best multivariable model for each type of CAM use was then selected by carrying out forward logistic regression with stepwise checks and elimination of any previously selected variables with the smallest nonsignificant partial F statistic.[8] Variables that were eliminated were examined as potential confounders using a change in the variable estimate of 10% as the criterion for confounding.[9] We searched for significant interaction terms based on clinical judgment and statistical associations. Final models were created for each type of CAM using the best models from stepwise regression with the addition of confounders. We report relative risks with 95% confidence intervals as measures of association.

The number of visits and costs of CAM nationwide were extrapolated by multiplying the number of known adult and adolescent HIV-positive persons in the United States[10] by the percentage who would be expected to use any CAM (for costs) or CAM provider (for visits) from our estimates of CAM use. We used the consumer price indexes for medical care between 1991 and 1997 to estimate costs of conventional medical care for persons with HIV in 1997 using cost data from 1990.[11]

Results

Table 2 provides a comparison of demographic data for respondents vs nonrespondents (including refusals and ineligibles). Respondents and nonrespondents did not differ significantly with regard to age, sex, insurance status, HIV risk factors, years of HIV infection, percentage of patients with CD4 cell counts less than 0.20×10^9/L (200 cells/μL), acquired immunodeficiency syndrome diagnosis, or protease inhibitor use. We report data on years of HIV infection from the medical chart review instead of the interview because we have chart data on all participants, and concordance between duration of HIV infection by patient reports and medical chart review was excellent. Because educational attainment, income, and employment status were assessed with the survey, we do not have data on nonrespondents. Both respondents and nonrespondents used a median of 16 prescription medications.

Table 1 describes the prevalence of CAM use in the study population, excluding users of multivitamins or commonly prescribed energy supplements. The most common dietary supplements were vitamins and herbal therapies. Massage therapists and acupuncture and acupressure providers were the most commonly reported CAM providers visited. Twenty-four percent of patients reported using marijuana for medicinal purposes. Forty-seven (38.5%) of 122 respondents who used supplements used more than 3 types of supplements, whereas 14 (17%) of 81 respondents who used CAM providers used more than 3 types of providers.

For respondents who used CAM, mean total (and out-of-pocket) annual expenditures were $815 ($620) for herbs, vitamins, and supplements; $510 ($340) for marijuana; and $652 ($495) for CAM providers. Mean total (and out-of-pocket) annual expenditures for all CAMs were $1159 ($939) per year. These data represent reported expenditures for the 3 most helpful CAMs in each category for a respondent. Sixteen percent of patients reported discontinuing use of prescription medications at some point because of cost. For respondents who used CAM, 20% stopped using supplements, 49% stopped seeing CAM providers, and 49% stopped using marijuana at some point because of cost.

Overall, for patients who saw CAM providers, the median visit frequency was 12 visits per year. Respondents

Table 2. Sample Demographics*

Characteristic	No. (%) Respondents (n=180)	Nonrespondents (n=95)†
Median age, y	41	39
Sex		
Male	157 (87.2)	76 (80)
Female	23 (12.8)	19 (20)
Insurance		
Private	91 (50.5)	43 (45)
Medicaid/Medicare	68 (37.8)	39 (41)
Hospital system of free care or uninsured	21 (11.7)	13 (14)
Education		
High school or less	55 (30.6)	
Vocational or some college	43 (23.9)	NA
College or professional	82 (45.6)	
Primary employment status		
Full-time worker	82 (45.6)	
Part-time worker	15 (8.3)	NA
Disabled	46 (25.6)	
Unemployed or other	37 (20.6)	
Income‡		
≤$30,000/y	108 (60.0)	NA
>$30,000/y	58 (32.2)	
Risk factor for HIV infection		
Homosexual contact	137 (76.1)	65 (68.4)
Intravenous drug use	22 (12.2)	14 (14.7)
Transfusion	5 (2.8)	1 (1.1)
Heterosexual contact	28 (15.6)	18 (18.9)
Years HIV positive		
≤5 y	86 (47.8)	57 (60.0)
>5 y	94 (52.2)	38 (40.0)
CD4 count <200	45 (25.0)	29 (30.5)
AIDS diagnosis	103 (57.2)	43 (45.3)
Using protease inhibitor	115 (63.9)	47 (49.5)

*P>.05 for all comparisons between respondents and nonrespondents. NA indicates not available from medical chart review; HIV, human immunodeficiency virus; and AIDS, acquired immunodeficiency syndrome.
†Includes all patients who were not interviewed, except hospital employees (n=14).
‡Fourteen patients (7.8%) refused to answer question.

who saw massage therapists (n=68) and acupuncturists (n=43) made a median of 10 visits per year to each of those providers; respondents who saw chiropractors (n=21) made a median of 24 visits per year; respondents who saw herbalists (n=19) made a median of 12 visits per year; and respondents who saw practitioners of homeopathic medicine (n=6) made a median of 6 visits per year. The median frequency of visits to all other CAM providers (n=5, including Reiki, craniosacral therapy, and reflexology) was 20 visits per year. In comparison, patients who saw CAM providers made a median of 7 visits per year to their primary care physicians and nurse practitioners combined. Respondents who used supplements did so frequently during an average month, reporting that 86% of the time they used supplements more than 10 days per month.

Table 3 demonstrates main and other reasons for using CAM. The most commonly reported reasons for using herbs, vitamins, and supplements were to fight infections or boost immunity (25%) and to treat weight loss, nausea, and diarrhea (23%). The most commonly reported reasons for visiting CAM providers were pain relief or neuropathy (33%) and to reduce stress and depression (27%). For the main reason supplements were used, those who used supplements (n=122) found them "extremely" or "quite a bit" helpful in 81 (81%) of 100 reports of use. For the main reason CAM providers were used, those who used CAM providers (n=81) found them "extremely" or "quite a bit" helpful in 76 (65.5%) of 116 reports of use.

Of those patients using marijuana (n=43), 44% reported using marijuana more than 10 days per month. The most commonly reported reason for using marijuana was nausea or weight loss (53%). For the main reason marijuana was used, those who used marijuana (n=43) found it "extremely" or "quite a bit" helpful in 27 (87%) of 31 reports of use.

In response to questions about bothersome symptoms in the past year, 30.6% (55/180) of patients experienced unintentional weight loss, 31.1% (56/180) of patients experienced memory or concentration problems, and 37.8% (68/180) of patients experienced bodily pain; 47.8% (86/180) of respondents experienced fatigue.

Among patients reporting fatigue as the main reason for using CAM (15 reports), 67% found the therapy "extremely" or "quite a bit" helpful. When primarily used to improve pain (57 reports), 58% found the therapy "extremely" or "quite a bit" helpful. When primarily used to reduce stress or depression (32 reports), 57% reported finding the therapy "extremely" or "quite a bit" helpful. Among patients reporting nausea or weight loss as the main reason for using CAM (32 reports), 60% found it "extremely" or "quite a bit" helpful. Few patients received either medical or CAM treatment for memory and concentration problems.

Of patients with fatigue (Figure 1), 22 (26%) of 86 had received treatment from a physician for fatigue; of those 22 patients, 17 (77%) found the medication at least moderately helpful. Only 5 of 22 patients found medical therapy "slightly" or "not at all" helpful for fatigue, and none of those sought CAM for fatigue. Of 17 patients who found medical therapy helpful, 15 (88%) also used CAM specifi-

Table 3. Main and Other Specific Reasons for Using CAM*

Reason	Reports, No. (%) CAM Supplements (n=122 Patients [171 reports])	CAM Providers (n=81 patients [183 reports])	Marijuana (n=43 Patients [53 Reports])
Pain or neuropathy	10 (5.8)	61 (33.3)	4 (7.5)
Fight fatigue or build strength	18 (10.5)	18 (9.8)	1 (1.9)
Weight loss, nausea, or diarrhea	40 (23.4)	8 (4.4)	28 (52.8)
Improve memory or concentration	6 (3.5)	5 (2.7)	0 (0)
Fight HIV or boost immunity	43 (25.1)	27 (14.8)	1 (1.9)
Relieve stress or depression	26 (15.2)	49 (26.8)	11 (20.8)
Fight other infections	9 (5.3)	4 (2.2)	0 (0)
Other	19 (11.1)	11 (6.0)	8 (15.1)

*Limited to responses for the 3 "most helpful" providers or supplements. Respondents could report 1 main reason and multiple other reasons for using each reported complementary and alternative medicine (CAM). Among 122 supplement users, there were 171 reports of reasons (100 for a main reason) specific supplements were used. Among 81 users of CAM providers, there were 183 reports of reasons (116 for a main reason) specific providers were used. Among 43 marijuana users, there were 53 reports of reasons (31 for a main reason) marijuana was used. HIV indicates human immunodeficiency virus.

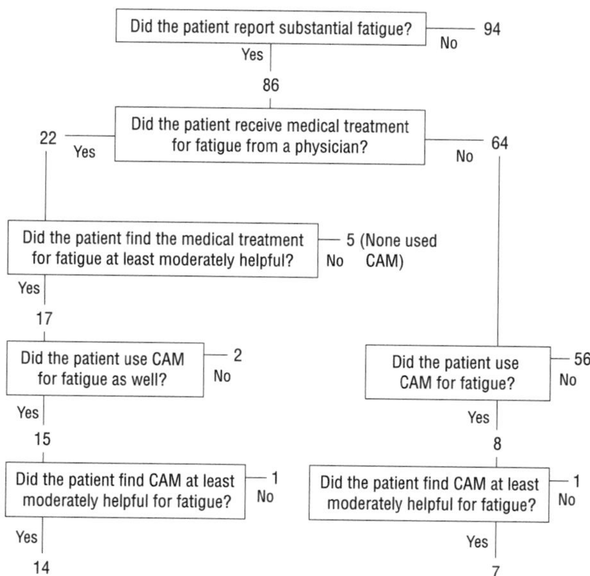

Figure 1. The integrative use of complementary and alternative medicine (CAM) for fatigue. Fatigued patients reported symptoms severe enough to keep them from their usual activities in the past year. Patients are dichotomized into those who received medical therapy from a conventional physician specifically for fatigue and those who did not. Y indicates a positive response; N, a negative response. Numbers of patients who used only CAM for fatigue or CAM plus conventional therapy are shown. Questions about specific reasons for use and perceived efficacy were limited to their 3 most helpful providers or supplements.

cally for fatigue, and 14 (93%) of 15 patients found CAM at least moderately helpful. Of 64 patients who complained of fatigue but did not receive medical therapy, 8 used CAM for fatigue, and 7 (88%) of 8 patients found CAM at least moderately helpful. We found similar patterns for use of conventional medical therapy and CAM for pain and weight loss or anorexia.

Most patients started visiting alternative providers (72.7%) and using supplements (70.9%) after learning that they were HIV positive. Users of acupuncture (87.8%) and supplements other than herbs, vitamins, and minerals (95.8%) were most likely to begin use after learning that they were HIV positive. In contrast, only 30.2% of patients reporting marijuana use began using it after learning about their HIV status. Slightly more than 67% of patients reported that their primary care physician was aware that they saw CAM providers, while 65.6% of supplement users and 69.8% of marijuana users reported that their primary physician was aware of their CAM use. For most respondents (64%) who reported that their primary care physician knew about their CAM use, we found supporting documentation in the medical record.

Respondents reported receiving information about CAM from newsletters for patients with HIV (62.2% [112/180]), friends or family members (51.1% [92/180]), physicians (47.2% [85/180]), and practitioners other than physicians (32.8% [59/180]). We queried patients about their 2 most favored sources of information on CAM. Patients reported preferring to receive CAM information from physicians (62.2% [112/180]), a consultation service at the hospital (52.2% [94/180]), and newsletters for patients with HIV (32.2% [58/180]).

We identified 3 patients (1.7%) by medical chart review who chose alternative therapies instead of conventional therapies. All 3 patients were taking other prescription medications but were not undergoing antiretroviral drug therapy. All 3 eventually accepted protease inhibitors after having a rise in their viral load. We found no documentation of patients refusing treatment or prophylaxis against opportunistic infections in favor of CAM.

Table 4. Unadjusted and Adjusted Correlates of CAM Use*

Correlate	Odds Ratio (95% CI) Unadjusted	Adjusted
CAM provider correlates		
College education	3.06 (1.66–5.64)	3.69 (1.93–7.07)
Fatigue	2.13 (1.17–3.87)	2.70 (1.41–5.18)
CAM supplement correlates†		
Memory loss	1.48 (0.78–2.81)	2.31 (1.11–4.81)
Fatigue	0.59 (0.33–1.06)	0.45 (0.22–0.95)
Weight loss	1.03 (0.55–1.94)	1.41 (0.70–2.88)
Private insurance	1.63 (0.91–2.94)	1.58 (0.83–3.02)
Marijuana correlates‡		
Weight loss	3.77 (1.84–7.74)	2.56 (1.18–5.56)
Disability	3.22 (1.55–6.72)	2.13 (0.97–4.70)
Fatigue	3.34 (1.60–6.96)	2.05 (0.91–4.59)

*CAM indicates complementary and alternative medicine; CI, confidence interval.
†Weight loss and private insurance status are included as confounders.
‡Disability status and fatigue are included as confounders.

Table 4 shows the unadjusted and adjusted odds ratios for the significant predictors of CAM use. In multivariable models, history of college education and fatigue were positively associated with CAM provider use. For patients taking supplements, history of memory loss was positively associated with use, but patients with fatigue were less likely to use supplements. History of weight loss was positively associated with marijuana use. We did not identify any significant interaction terms. A diagnosis of acquired immunodeficiency syndrome, CD4 cell count, number of HIV-related complications, duration of HIV infection, history of depression, HIV risk factors, frequency of clinic visits, and race were not statistically associated with CAM use in bivariable or multivariable models.

Comment

We found a high rate of CAM use among HIV-infected patients in our population, and most often these patients were using conventional therapy as well. However, patients who used CAM providers made more visits to these providers than to their physicians and nurses combined. Patients reported substantial benefit from the use of CAM, whether they used it alone or in combination with conventional treatment.

There are few previous data on expenditures for CAM among the HIV-infected population, a group known to experience economic hardship because of changes in employment from their debilitating disease.[12,13] In our study, costs for these visits were variable, with several patients reporting that they receive services free of charge. Several clinics in the Boston area now offer these services at low or no cost to patients with HIV and acquired immunodeficiency syndrome. Despite this availability, the mean out-of-pocket yearly expenditure was more than $900 for all alternative therapies for those using any CAM. The observation that nearly half the respondents stopped using a therapy at some point because of cost suggests that some patients may seek alternative therapies to the point of financial hardship.

There has been an intense increase in media coverage on the issue of medicinal use of marijuana in the recent past. One quarter of our population uses marijuana for medicinal purposes. To our knowledge, no recent survey has assessed prevalence of marijuana use among patients with HIV. Patients seem to be aware of the purported benefits of marijuana, using it primarily for symptoms of nausea and weight loss. We also found high perceived efficacy of marijuana, with 87% finding it "extremely" or "quite a bit" helpful regardless of the problem for which it was used. Total and out-of-pocket expenditures on marijuana were nearly as high as expenditures on CAM providers. It is unclear why some patients reported out-of-pocket costs for marijuana that differed from total costs and whether some patients were receiving subsidies for marijuana purchases.

Our findings are consistent with those of earlier studies in Boston[6] and California[5] of HIV-infected patients showing high rates for using CAM. Our findings differ from those of Greenblatt et al[14] and Anderson et al,[15] who found that only 29% to 40% of patients attending conventional medical care sites were also using CAM. These studies may have underestimated CAM use because they referred to therapies as "unorthodox" or "alternative" or because they only assessed therapies taken by mouth.[14] Because we collected our data after protease inhibitors became widely available, it seems that the availability of efficacious antiviral drugs has not diminished CAM use. Others have reported comparably high rates of CAM use in patients with long-term disease other than HIV infection, including cancer[16,17] and arthritis.[18] Our findings suggest that HIV-infected patients, like those with other long-term illness, may use CAM to a much greater degree than the general population.

Patients with HIV seem to use CAM for a variety of reasons, most importantly to relieve pain or neuropathy, to relieve stress or depression, to fight other infections, and to treat weight loss and nausea. In contrast to findings by Anderson et al[15] suggesting that many patients sought cure or antiviral effects from CAM, we found that few respondents used CAM to fight HIV specifically. This difference may be because of the availability of more potent antiviral drugs (ie, protease inhibitors) than were available to patients studied by Anderson et al in 1993. Perceived efficacy for CAM was high overall among our study patients. Patients often use CAM for a specific problem even if they received medical treatment for the same problem and had perceived the conventional therapy to be efficacious. These data are consistent with findings from previous works[1,6] demonstrating that most CAM users also sought conventional therapy for medical problems treated with CAM. Therefore, patients infected with HIV who receive care in a conventional setting seem to use CAM with conventional medical therapies in an integrative fashion.

We found a high rate of disclosure regarding CAM use between patients and physicians. Patient reports of disclosure were supported by medical record documentation in most cases. These data are in contrast to the findings by Eisenberg et al[1] in 1990, who found that 72% did not inform their physician about CAM use. The reasons for higher disclosure rates are unclear but may reflect secular trends, a change in the receptivity of physicians to discussing CAM use, or the possibility that individuals with long-term or life-threatening illness are more apt to discuss CAM with their conventional caregivers.

We estimated that mean total and out-of-pocket annual expenditures for all CAM were $1159 and $939, respectively, for users of CAM. Comparison with expenditures on conventional medical care is difficult because reliable data on out-of-pocket expenditures for medical care of patients with HIV are limited. The Boston Health Study[19] reported mean out-of-pocket expenditures of $429 per person with acquired immunodeficiency syndrome for 4 months in 1990 ($1287 annually). They reported mean total expenditures of $9093 ($27,279 annually). When adjusted for the consumer price index,[11] the comparable 1997 estimates would be $1801 out-of-pocket and $38,165 total expenditures. Current out-of-pocket expenditures may vary from this estimate because of changes in outpatient drug therapy for HIV and hospitalization rates. We estimate that 2% of total costs and 24% of out-of-pocket costs of medical care for HIV-infected patients are attributable to CAM. Given that approximately 600,000 adults and adolescents are known to be HIV-infected in the United States,[10] extrapolation to the US HIV population (assuming that 76% use CAM) would place total expenditures on CAM at approximately $529 million per year and the total number of annual visits for CAM providers (assuming 45% utilization) at 3.2 million nationwide.

Our study has several limitations. Because the study population consists primarily of homosexual males and is limited geographically to the metropolitan Boston area, our findings may not be generalizable to the entire US population. However, given that CAM use seems to be higher in the western United States, it is likely to underestimate utilization rates in the HIV population nationwide. Our small sample size may result in low statistical power to detect differences between respondents and nonrespondents. Also, we queried only patients who had already chosen to receive care in a conventional setting, making it difficult to extrapolate conclusions about the integrative nature of CAM use among all people with HIV infection. However, this is also likely to underestimate CAM use because people with HIV who reject conventional care may be expected to use CAM to a greater degree. There is potential for selection bias if patients who used CAM were more likely to complete the interview. However, we did not inform patients of the study's purpose during the recruitment process.

An additional limitation is that small numbers of users of certain types of CAM make it difficult for us to comment on perceived efficacy for specific therapies. Our data with regard to perceived efficacy may be biased because our study is cross-sectional in nature. Respondents may have ceased using therapies perceived as less helpful in the past. In addition, for patients who used several alternative therapies, we asked detailed questions about expenditures and perceived efficacy only for the 3 they believed were most helpful. This may have biased our results toward those therapies used most frequently and therefore increased our estimates for visit frequency as well as perceived efficacy. Also, patients may be more likely to perceive therapies as efficacious if they made an active choice to obtain them. In addition, our study can comment on perceived efficacy only and not on efficacy of CAM for specific problems. However, data on perceived efficacy may guide randomized controlled trials in the future. Our cost data are incomplete because we only inquired about cost for a limited number of CAMs. However, this may have resulted in an underestimation of total visits and costs because many patients used several types of CAM. In addition, our relatively small sample may not be representative of the HIV population in the United States for the reasons discussed above, so the extrapolation of our cost data should be viewed with caution.

Another potential limitation of our study is our choice of definition of CAM. We included massage and vitamins (but not daily multivitamins), which may be considered mainstream therapy by some providers of conventional medicine. These inclusions would tend to overestimate prevalence and costs of CAM use. Nonetheless, use of high-dosage vitamins and massage can be distinguished from such activities as weight training and day-spas as having specific therapeutic (if not "medicinal") goals for most patients who use them (eg, immune boosting or stress reduction). However, use of high-dosage vitamins and massage are not generally believed to be therapeutic maneuvers by conventional physicians, and massage techniques are not taught at conventional medical schools. Although data on therapeutic efficacy for some therapies (such as acupuncture for neuropathic pain) are being collected, we may have to be flexible about definitions of CAM for purposes of descriptive studies.

In this study, we did not collect data on potential adverse effects of CAM. There are several reports in the medical literature that suggest potential for harm with certain CAM therapies.[20–23] Little is known about the biologic activity of most CAM therapies, and there seems to be potential for "drug-drug" (or "drug-herb or supplement") interaction for CAM therapies that are ingested. This may be particularly problematic when patients involved in clinical trials also use CAM therapies.[24] Several groups nationally and internationally have called for regulation of CAM and prospective monitoring for adverse events.[25–28] Future studies should place emphasis on careful collection of data on adverse events.

In summary, we demonstrated a high prevalence of CAM use among patients with HIV, with high yearly visit rates and expenditures. Patients involved in conventional care use CAM to complement conventional therapies for specific symptoms or problems rather than to the exclusion of conventional care. In general, perceived efficacy of CAM is high. Clinicians are often queried about CAM and have limited information to offer patients. Until more information is available from randomized trials, perceived efficacy of therapies may be a useful way to guide patients toward therapies that seem to provide relief from refractory symptoms. Research funds should be directed toward conducting outcomes research and randomized controlled trials of specific therapies in those patient subgroups who seem to derive the most benefit. For example, studies of the antiemetic effect of marijuana and the analgesic effects of acupuncture and chiropractic might be given higher priority. These trials should include patients who are undergoing intensive pharmacological therapy for HIV to provide data on potential interactions or adverse effects.

This study was supported by National Research Service Award PE11001-09 (Dr Fairfield). Partial funding for this project was provided by the Center for Alternative Medicine Research; grant U24 AR3441 from the National Institutes of Health, Bethesda, Md; The John E. Fetzer Institute, Kalamazoo, Mich; the Friends of Beth Israel Deaconess Medical Center, Boston, Mass; the Kenneth J. Germeshausen Foundation, Boston; and the J. E. and Z. B. Butler Foundation, New York, NY.

We thank the patients of Beth Israel Deaconess Medical Center who gave their time for this study.

References

1. Eisenberg DM, Kessler RC, Foster C, Norlock FE, Calkins DR, Delbanco TL. Unconventional medicine in the United States: prevalence, costs, and patterns of use. *N Engl J Med.* 1993; 328:246–252.

2. Gevitz N. Alternative medicine and the Orthodox Canon. *Mt Sinai J Med.* 1995; 62:127–131.

3. Delbanco TL. Bitter herbs: mainstream, magic, and menace. *Ann Intern Med.* 1994; 121:803–804.

4. Murray RH, Rubel AJ. Physicians and healers: unwitting partners in health care. *N Engl J Med.* 1992;326:61–64.

5. Dwyer JT, Salvato-Schille AM, Coulston A, Casey VA, Cooper WC, Selles WD. The use of unconventional remedies among HIV-positive men living in California. *J Assoc Nurses AIDS Care.* 1995;6:17–28.

6. Cohen CJ, Mayer KH, Eisenberg DM, Orav EJ, Delbanco TL. Determinants of nonconventional treatment use among HIV-infected individuals. In: *International Conference on AIDS.* 1990; 6:285. Abstract SD781.

7. Safran C, Rury C, Rind DM, Taylor WC. A computer-based outpatient medical record for a teaching hospital. *MD Comput.* 1991; 8:291–299.

8. Kleinbaum DG, Kupper LL, Muller KE. *Applied Regression Analysis and Other Multivariable Methods.* Belmont, Calif: Duxbury Press; 1988.

9. Mickey RM, Greenland S. The impact of confounder selection criteria on effect estimation. *Am J Epidemiol.* 1989;129:125–137.

10. Centers for Disease Control and Prevention. HIV/AIDS Surveillance Report. 1997;9(No. 1). Available at: http://cdcnac.org. Accessed January 22, 1998.

11. US Department of Labor, Bureau of Labor Statistics. Consumer Price Index Web site. Available at: http://stats.bls.gov/cpihome.htm. Accessed March 2, 1998.

12. Massagli MP, Weissman JS, Seage GR III, Epstein AM. Correlates of employment after AIDS diagnosis in the Boston Health Study. *Am J Public Health.* 1994;84:1976–1981.

13. Kass NE, Munoz A, Chen B, et al. Changes in employment, insurance, and income in relation to HIV status and disease progression. *J Acquir Immune Defic Syndr.* 1994;7:86–91.

14. Greenblatt RM, Hollander H, McMaster JR, Henk CJ. Polypharmacy among patients attending an AIDS clinic: the utilization of prescribed, unorthodox, and investigational treatments. *J Acquir Immune Defic Syndr.* 1991;4:136–143.

15. Anderson W, O'Connor BB, MacGregor RR, Schwartz JS. Patient use and assessment of conventional and alternative therapies for HIV infection and AIDS. *AIDS.* 1993;7:561–566.

16. Cassileth BR, Lusk EJ, Strouse TB, Bodenheimer BJ. Contemporary unorthodox treatments in cancer medicine. *Ann Intern Med.* 1984; 101:105–112.

17. US Congress, Office of Technology Assessment. *Unconventional Cancer Treatments.* Washington, DC: Government Printing Office; 1990. Publication OTA-H-405.

18. Cronan TA, Kaplan RM, Posner L, Blumberg E, Kozin F. Prevalence of the use of unconventional remedies for arthritis in a metropolitan community. *Arthritis Rheum.* 1989;32:1604–1607.

19. Epstein AM, Seage G, Weissman JS, et al. Costs of medical care and out-of-pocket expenditures for persons with AIDS in the Boston Health Study. *Inquiry.* 1995;32:211–221.

20. Curt GA, Katterhagen G, Mahaney FX Jr. Immunoaugmentative therapy: a primer on the perils of unproved treatments. *JAMA.* 1986; 255:505–507.

21. Woolf GM, Petrovic LM, Rojter SE, et al. Acute hepatitis associated with the Chinese herbal product Jin Bu Huan. *Ann Intern Med.* 1994; 121:729–735.

22. Hirschtick RE, Dyrda SE, Peterson LC. Death from an unconventional therapy for AIDS [letter]. *Ann Intern Med.* 1994;120:694.

23. Seely DR, Quigley SM, Langman AW. Ear candles: safety and efficacy. *Laryngoscope.* 1996; 106:1226–1229.

24. Fogelman I, Lim L, Bassett R, et al. Prevalence and patterns of use of concomitant medications among participants in three multicenter human immunodeficiency virus type I clinical trials. *J Acquir Immune Defic Syndr.* 1994; 7:1057–1063.

25. Marwick C. Growing use of medicinal botanicals forces assessment by drug regulators. *JAMA.* 1995;273:607–609.

26. De Smet PA. Should herbal medicine–like products be licensed as medicines [editorial]? *BMJ.* 1995;310:1023–1024.

27. Vautier G, Spiller RC. Safety of complementary medicines should be monitored [letter]. *BMJ.* 1995;311:633.

28. Drew AK, Myers SP. Safety issues in herbal medicine: implications for the health professions. *Med J Aust.* 1997;166:538–541.

6 Medical Malpractice Implications of Alternative Medicine

David M. Studdert, LLB, ScD, MPH; David M. Eisenberg, MD; Frances H. Miller, JD; Daniel A. Curto, JD; Ted J. Kaptchuk, OMD; Troyen A. Brennan, MD, JD, MPH
From the Department of Health Policy and Management, Harvard School of Public Health (Drs Studdert and Brennan); the Center for Alternative Medicine Research, Department of Medicine, Beth Israel Deaconess Medical Center, Harvard Medical School (Drs Eisenberg and Kaptchuk); Boston University School of Law (Ms Miller); and Harvard Law School (Mr Curto), Boston, Mass.

Although use of alternative therapies in the United States is widespread and growing, little is known about the malpractice experience of practitioners who deliver these therapies or about the legal principles that govern the relationship between conventional and alternative medicine. Using data from malpractice insurers, we analyzed the claims experience of chiropractors, massage therapists, and acupuncturists for 1990 through 1996. We found that claims against these practitioners occurred less frequently and typically involved injury that was less severe than claims against physicians during the same period. Physicians who may be concerned about their own exposure to liability for referral of patients for alternative treatments can draw some comfort from these findings. However, liability for referral is possible in certain situations and should be taken seriously. Therefore, we review relevant legal principles and case law to understand how malpractice law is likely to develop in this area. We conclude by suggesting some questions for physicians to ask themselves before referring their patients to alternative medicine practitioners.

JAMA 1998;280:1610–1615

Many Americans seek medical care from practitioners of alternative medicine. (We define *alternative medicine* as medical interventions not taught widely at US medical schools or generally available at US hospitals.[1]) In 1990, chiropractors, acupuncturists, massage therapists, naturopaths, and a variety of other practitioners of alternative medicine received 425 million visits, for which patients paid $10.3 billion in out-of-pocket expenses.[1] Financial analysts have suggested that consumer spending on alternative medicine may have surged 69% since 1989,[2] and the market may be growing as fast as 30% annually.[3] Employers and insurers, including several major managed care organizations such as Oxford Health Plans and Health Net, have recently begun to respond to this demand by adding alternative therapies to their insurance products.[4–8] As well, state legislatures have enacted laws that require health insurers to include alternative treatments in the benefits they cover.[9]

Despite this activity, coordination between alternative and conventional medical care remains poor. An estimated 90% of patients using alternative medical care are not referred by their physicians (MDs or DOs) but are, instead, self-referred.[1] This lack of communication and the absence of proactive referral for alternative treatment or, when appropriate, professional advice to avoid alternative care are unfortunate from a quality perspective. Various measures to improve the coordination between physicians and alternative medicine practitioners have been proposed.[10]

Improved quality of care in this area is frustrated by a long-standing professional rivalry between organized medicine and unorthodox health care practitioners.[11,12] However, a more fundamental obstacle is physicians' lack of knowledge about the appropriateness and efficacy of alternative medicine. While anecdotal evidence abounds, only a few well-designed clinical studies have examined the efficacy of alternative medicine therapies.[13–19] Additional outcomes studies and randomized trials are only now being launched.[20]

A subset of these general doubts and concerns about alternative medicine relates to medical malpractice.[2,21–25] We believe physicians worry that they will be sued if a patient they refer to an alternative medicine practitioner suffers a poor outcome. Even when patients have independently chosen to submit to alternative treatment, physicians may be reluctant to discover or discuss this care with them for fear that, if they know about it, they will be deemed to endorse it.

To address these issues, we have examined available data on rates of claims against chiropractors, acupuncturists, and massage therapists. Next, we explore the kinds of situations in which physicians may be exposed to liability for the referrals they make. Finally, we note the approach courts have adopted in assessing the malpractice liability of alternative medicine practitioners. We conclude that malpractice concerns alone should not inhibit physicians from referring patients to alternative medicine practitioners, particularly where those practitioners are licensed and accredited. A caveat to our conclusions is that legal principles in this area are not well developed—a situation that is poised to change as conventional and unconventional medicine become increasingly integrated in health care delivery systems.[8]

Claims Experience

Alternative medicine accounts for approximately 5% of the total medical malpractice insurance market, and coverage is provided by fewer than 50 insurers.[26] We collected claims information from the leading indemnity insurers in the country serving chiropractors, massage therapists, and acupuncturists. Together these 3 groups of practitioners account for approximately two thirds of the estimated 425 million visits made annually to offices of alternative medicine practitioners.[1]

Chiropractic data were obtained from NCMIC Insurance Company (NCMIC) of Des Moines, Iowa. NCMIC insured 25,103 chiropractors in 1996, nearly half of all licensed chiropractors practicing in the United States.[27] We obtained data on claims against massage therapists from Albert H. Wohlers and Co of Park Ridge, Ill. Wohlers has provided professional indemnity insurance services to members of the American Massage Therapy Association (AMTA) since 1993 and currently insures approximately 27,000 massage therapists throughout the country—again, almost half of all licensed practitioners in this area. Acupuncture Insurance Services of Elmhurst, Ill, provided information on acupuncture claims. With approximately 1500 policyholders in 1996, it is the largest carrier of insurance for acupuncturists in the United States.

The data used to describe the claims experience of physicians are drawn from 2 sources. Information on claims paid against physicians comes from the Physician Insurers Association of America's (PIAA's) Data Sharing Project.[28] Information on claims frequency comes from the American Medical Association's annual core survey of a national sample of physicians. In contrast to our other claims data, the survey data reflect the experience of a general physician population (excluding federally employed physicians) rather than a discrete population defined by a specific insurer.[29]

To maximize comparability of the data, we specified a number of parameters: (1) a claim was defined as a formal demand for compensation arising from health care (ie, incident reports were excluded); (2) multiple claims against a single insured that related to the same incident were counted as a single claim; (3) claims against multiple practitioners relating to the same incident were counted separately; (4) all claims for which a nonzero indemnity payment was made to the plaintiff were counted as paid claims; and (5) claims were assigned to years according to file date, and payment figures were assigned to years according to closure date.

Table 1 compares the claims rates, average amount on paid claims, and percentage of claims among massage therapists, chiropractors, and primary care physicians for 1990 through 1996. Claims rates against chiropractors insuring through NCMIC have remained steady at 2 to 3 claims per 100 policyholders per year through the 1990s. The average severity of claims against chiropractors, as measured by average indemnity amounts on paid claims, increased by 81%. Conventional medicine experienced this same trend with a 47% increase. NCMIC resolved approximately half of its claims with payment, 18% more on average than did PIAA insurers. Table 2 shows the percentage of claims received by NCMIC in various injury categories during 1992 through 1996.

Table 1 also shows that rates of claims against massage therapists are less than one tenth of those against physicians and decreased in 1996. Table 3 shows the percentage of claims against AMTA members received by Wohlers in various injury categories during 1993 through 1996. Most claims (61%) relate to minor injuries, although a significant proportion (14%) relate to sexual misconduct.

Less information is available on rates of claims against other practitioners of alternative medicine. We were unable to obtain comprehensive data on claims against acupuncturists; however, some information on claims history was obtained from Acupuncture Insurance Services. Although this company insures one sixth of the 8900 licensed acupuncturists in the country,[30] it has had ongoing difficulties underwriting its policies because of its relatively small insurance pool.

After working through several offshore underwriters during the 1980s, a relatively stable relationship with a domestic underwriter was disrupted when a single acupuncturist apparently infected 35 people with hepatitis B,[31] 21 of whom filed claims (Martin Shaw, president, Acupuncture Insurance Services, oral communication, March 1997). The other major claims experienced by Lincoln in its 15 years of operation include a case of irreversible nerve damage, several burns, and 2 cases involving pneumothorax.

The best explanation for the relative infrequency and lower severity of claims against alternative medicine practitioners concerns the nature of alternative therapies. Since rates of medical injury increase with invasiveness of

Table 1. Selected Claims Information for Massage Therapy, Chiropractic, and Medicine, 1990–1996

	Claims per 100 Policy Holders			Average Indemnity Payment per Paid Claim, $			Claims Paid, %		
Year	**Massage Therapy***	**Chiropractic†**	**Medicine (Primary Care)‡**	**Massage Therapy**	**Chiropractic**	**Medicine (Primary Care)§**	**Massage Therapy**	**Chiropractic**	**Medicine (Primary Care)**
1990	. . .	2.7	7.7 (5.9)	. . .	33,625	137,900 (129,213)	. . .	49.1	31.9 (32.5)
1991	. . .	2.7	8.2 (5.7)	. . .	43,670	159,788 (148,533)	. . .	49.0	33.1 (32.0)
1992	. . .	2.8	9.1 (6.9)	. . .	40,621	183,541 (143,730)	. . .	47.5	33.2 (33.9)
1993	0.2	3.0	9.8 (7.1)	12,011	52,231	185,243 (147,084)	38.5	56.9	30.3 (30.7)
1994	0.2	2.7	9.5 (6.7)	4251	65,597	182,003 (151,001)	44.8	46.0	31.7 (30.2)
1995	0.2	2.6	9.0 (6.2)	4864	52,385	179,732 (149,028)	63.0	49.5	30.2 (30.3)
1996	0.1	2.2	. . .	4253	60,985	202,772 (166,379)	23.8	46.0	28.6 (29.9)

*Data from Albert H. Wohlers & Co, Park Ridge, Ill. Ellipses indicate data were not available prior to 1993.

†Data from the NCMIC Insurance Company, Des Moines, Iowa.

‡Data from Gonzales.[29]

§Data from PIAA Data Sharing System, Rockville, Md.

Table 2. Categories of Claims Against Chiropractors, 1992-1996*

Type of Injury	Total Claims, %	Paid Claims, %
Disk	27.1	27.6
Failure to diagnose	12.2	11.3
Fracture	13.5	10.3
Aggravation of existing condition	7.6	9.9
Cerebral vascular	5.4	2.9
Vicarious liability	3.5	4.5
Other	30.7	33.5

*Data obtained from the NCMIC Insurance Company, Des Moines, Iowa.

Table 3. Categories of Claims Against Massage Therapists, 1993-1996*

Type of Injury	Total Claims, %
Minor†	61
Major‡	5
Grave§	1
Nonphysical	15
Sexual misconduct	14
Other	4

*Data obtained from Albert H. Wohlers & Co, Park Ridge, Ill.
†Includes soft tissue injuries, minor fractures, and minor scarring with no residuals.
‡Includes fractures, serious internal injuries, serious back injuries (ie, fusions, ruptured disks, laminectomies), loss of vision in 1 eye, and serious scarring.
§Includes brain damage, quadriplegia, severe burns, fatalities, dismemberment of 1 or more major limbs, and extremely serious multiple fracture cases.

therapy,[32] fewer bases for suit are likely to present in the largely noninvasive alternative medicine setting. Moreover, injuries that do occur may not be as severe.

Another explanation may be the immature state of medical malpractice law and claims consciousness outside conventional clinical medicine—a phenomenon that may change as use and awareness of alternative therapies grow and as these therapies are progressively integrated into health care delivery systems. A third explanation may be that personal characteristics of alternative medicine practitioners and their patients or the dynamics of that patient-practitioner relationship are associated with a reduced propensity to sue, whether or not negligence occurred.

From the perspective of a physician who is concerned about the malpractice implications of referring to alternative medicine practitioners or comanaging patients with them, these findings should offer a degree of reassurance: they diminish the practical importance of situations in which practitioners might be exposed to liability for mere referral. Nonetheless, such situations can arise and should be taken seriously, particularly in light of uncertainty about how courts will decide medical malpractice cases.

Liability for Referral to Alternative Medicine Practitioners

As a general rule, a physician's mere referral of a patient to another physician, without more, does not expose the referring physician to liability.[33–35] This rule has been applied by courts throughout the country in cases involving referral among physicians. Yet in certain circumstances—alluded to in the qualification, "without more"—the rule does not hold. These exceptional situations in the context of alternative medicine can be divided into 2 categories: (1) situations in which a decision to refer the patient for alternative medical treatment is negligent and (2) situations in which the referring physician is held liable for the treating practitioner's negligence because the physician supervised the care, jointly treated the patient, or knew the practitioner to whom the physician referred the patient was incompetent.

In the first category, the referral itself falls short of the reasonable practice standard and is sufficient to form the basis of a malpractice lawsuit, regardless of the quality of care delivered by the practitioner to whom the referral is made. The law still requires that the patient suffer injury causally related to the substandard referral. But if, for example, a physician refers a patient to an alternative medicine practitioner instead of to some other, more appropriate practitioner and the referral delays, decreases, or eliminates the opportunity for the patient to receive important care, the referring physician could be held liable.[36]

Available empirical evidence on alternative medicine use suggests that this type of referral liability may be a theoretical concern more than a practical one: the most commonly used alternative therapies treat minor ailments or serious conditions for which conventional medicine can offer little in the way of therapeutic benefit.[1] Nonetheless, it does highlight an important reason why physicians who refer to alternative medicine practitioners should be familiar with the efficacy of various alternative therapies. As knowledge about the appropriateness of alternative therapies expands, courts may determine that physicians act negligently when they refer patients for particular therapies that they know or should know offer no practical benefit to the patient.[37]

Another complicating issue with regard to the choice of referral is the increasingly complex set of influences brought to bear on physician decision making. Guidelines, incentives, and restrictions aimed at influencing physicians' referral decisions are hallmarks of the managed care environment.[38,39] Managed care organizations typically seek to minimize the use of specialist care and limit expensive tests that offer little or no marginal benefit.[40,41] Analogously, a plan that covers alternative medicine services may, for example, determine that its enrollees should be referred to chiropractors rather than to orthopedic surgeons, given certain clinical indications. Were liability for this type of referral to be considered by the court, the plan's guidelines or incentives could potentially mitigate the referring physician's exposure to liability, although such "reallocation" of liability has been slow to develop because of a range of barriers to holding managed care organizations liable for malpractice.[42] Yet another complication is the increasingly common practice of using alternative medical care as an adjunct to allopathic care.

The second category of exceptions to the general rule of nonliability for referral arises when the practitioner to whom a patient is referred renders negligent care that injures the patient and for which the referring physician is then considered partially or wholly responsible. There are several situations in which courts may impute liability in this way, all of which involve *vicarious liability,* defined as liability of a person or organization for the negligence of an employed individual. (Vicarious liability includes liability of supervisors [*respondeat superior*] and apparent authority, that is, when one individual apparently represents an organization.)

First, when physician A refers a patient to physician B and then exerts authority over the way physician B treats that patient, physician A may be held liable for physician B's negligent acts. In finding vicarious liability, the law considers that physician B merely acts as physician A's agent. The question of whether an agency relationship exists and hence whether vicarious liability may be appropriate for that reason depends on the level of actual (or apparent) control maintained by the referring physician.

Courts have generally been reluctant to find that one physician controls another, setting a fairly high threshold for plaintiffs who attempt to establish liability on this basis.[35,43–45] However, referral to an allied health professional—for example, a nurse practitioner or physician assistant—presents a slightly different situation. A physician may be held liable for the negligent acts of allied health professionals, such as nurses, when the physician takes charge or supervises the care provided.[46,47] The same is true if a health care organization supervises the allied health professional. Moreover, by requiring the adoption of written protocols for collaboration, professional regulation in many states explicitly commits physicians to a supervisory role over allied health professionals such as nurse practitioners, physical therapists, and physician assistants, particularly in the area of drug prescription.[48,49]

Leading cases addressing this type of vicarious liability have considered care delivered in the operating room setting, rather than referrals[46,47,50]; they have also involved practitioners using the same approach to healing (ie, conventional medicine). Nonetheless, the manner in which alternative medicine services are integrated with conventional medical services will be important in determining whether referral involves the requisite level of actual or apparent control that courts have demanded to establish the agency relationship and so constitute an exception to the general rule of nonliability for referral.

Physicians who maintain a supervisory role over the patient's care or who refer in circumstances where the patient might reasonably expect that care will be supervised could be held to account for the negligent acts of the treating practitioner. From the perspective of physicians and health plans, the agency exception to the general rule of nonliability for referral would suggest good reasons for allowing alternative medicine practitioners to practice their craft freely once referral is made and also for ensuring that patients understand that referral initiates a new and separate patient-practitioner relationship. These recommendations would, however, be qualified if the alternative medicine practitioner is not licensed or is in an organization subordinate to the referring physician.

Second, liability may be extended to the referring physician in situations when the care given exhibits characteristics of a joint undertaking. Cases that have bound defendants together in this manner have looked for a fairly high degree of unity in the practitioners' approach to treatment.[51,52] In fact, joint undertakings typically involve practitioners who act in concert, simultaneously administering treatment to a patient, rather than being separated by the referral process.

Under current health care arrangements, it seems unlikely that this kind of situation will arise between physicians and alternative medicine practitioners. However, it could emerge as a possibility if the practitioners are employed by the same hospital or health plan and collaborate closely in providing patient care. This level of collaboration could also exist in situations where physicians and alternative medicine practitioners render care in a jointly owned or operated clinic. Similarly, as alternative medicine practitioners begin to deliver care alongside physicians in "integrated" units within a hospital or clinic, the possibility of a joint-undertaking situation does arise.

Third, the general rule of nonliability for referral may not apply when the referring physician knows that the practitioner to whom she or he refers the patient is incompetent.[34,35,53] For example, if a physician is aware that a particular acupuncturist uses unsterilized needles or that the acupuncturist has recently been the subject of serious disciplinary action by a professional board, then the physician may be considered negligent if a patient referred to that acupuncturist suffers iatrogenic injury.

While the physician's own liability is certainly a consideration in the above scenario, the courts have been far more active in holding institutions accountable in this area. Hospitals[54] and managed care organizations[55,56] have a legal obligation to be diligent in selecting, retaining, and evaluating health care professionals; this same obligation will extend to their relationship with alternative medicine practitioners. Therefore, the plan that credentials an incompetent acupuncturist may face liability as a corporation when a physician refers a patient to this practitioner for treatment, especially when it has established incentives or guidelines to facilitate this referral.

All of the above recommendations are contingent on the assumption that courts are not prepared to make presumptive judgments about the incompetence of alternative medicine practitioners, based solely on their idiosyncratic approaches to health care. If the courts were so prepared, this possibility has serious legal ramifications because it would allow liability of the referring physician to be inferred in a much wider range of cases—not merely those in which there is knowledge about a particular practitioner's incompetence. Once again, the courts do not yet appear to have considered this issue directly. However, we can find important clues about how they might deal with the situation by returning to litigation against alternative medicine practitioners and examining more closely how these cases have been decided.

Regulation and Liability of Alternative Medicine Practitioners

A widely accepted rule of medical malpractice states that "a physician is entitled to have his treatment of his patient tested by the rules and principles of the school of medicine to which he belongs, and not by those of some other school."[57–60] Although this rule is most often used as a basis for delineating different standards of care among conventional medical specialties, it has also been used to set standards for practitioners of alternative medicine in schools ranging from chiropractic to homeopathy, naturopathy (the resurgent remnants of the "drugless practitioners" of an earlier era[61]), and even Christian Science healing.[62,63] An important rationale underlying school-specific standards is that, when a patient elects or gives informed consent to receive care from a particular practitioner, the patient is presumed to have also elected to be treated with an ordinary level of skill and care common to that practitioner's field of practice.[64]

But courts have not applied a school-specific standard of care in situations where they do not recognize the school to which a defendant claims membership. How do judges make this decision? Licensure has thus far been the decisive piece of evidence in determining whether an identifiable school of medicine exists[65–67]; the regulatory apparatus that accompanies licensure defines its scope. As one court stated: "Through the enactment of this legislation, the legislature has recognized the practice . . . as a separate and distinct health care discipline."[66] Another piece of evidence likely to be important in signaling a school's identity and validity is state legislative mandates that compel insurance companies to cover certain alternative medicine treatments in all policies sold.

The chiropractic profession is the best example of an easily recognizable school of alternative medicine. Chiropractors are licensed in all 50 states and the District of Columbia (Table 4).[68] Forty-two states mandate coverage of chiropractic services in health insurance policies (Susan S. Laudicina, director of state services research, BlueCross BlueShield Association, oral communication, March 1998). Courts apply a standard of care in malpractice actions against chiropractors enunciated by experts in the chiropractic profession itself. They will rarely hear the testimony of a physician for purposes of establishing the appropriate chiropractic standard of care.[59,65,69]

Other schools of alternative medicine besides chiropractic have established systems of licensure and regulation (Table 4). Thirty-five states license acupuncturists (with 7 states mandating insurance coverage of acupuncture services), 27 states license massage therapists, 14 states license naturopaths, and 4 states license homeopaths. Few reported cases in the modern era have considered the liability of licensed practitioners of alternative medicine practicing in these areas. Nonetheless, it is entirely consistent with prevailing legal principles to expect that their conduct will be judged in the same way as chiropractic medicine.

In contrast, where practitioners of alternative medicine are unlicensed, courts tend not to recognize them as belonging to an identifiable school of medicine and hence do not apply a school-specific standard of care. Instead, the allegation of negligence will be judged according to conventional medical[70] or lay[65,67] standards of care. A court's decision to adopt either of these alternate standards, rather than standards set by the defendant practitioner's own school, has a significant bearing on case outcome: it becomes more likely that the conduct under scrutiny will be judged negligent.

Table 4. Statutory Licensure of Alternative Medicine Practitioners

Chiropractic			
Licensed in 50 states and District of Columbia*			
Massage Therapy			
AL	§34-43-2	NM	61-12C-1
AK	§17-86-102	NY	§7802
CT	§20-206	ND	43-25-01
DE	24 Del C 5306	OH	§503.42
DC	§2-3305	OR	§687.011
FL	§480.033	RI	§23-20.8-1
HI	§452.3	SC	§40-30-110
IA	§152C	TN	§63.18-201
LA	37:3556	TX	4512K
ME	32 MRS 14306	UT	58-47b-304
MD	HOcc 3-5A-04	VT	26 VSA 3405
MA	c140 §51	VA	§54.1-3029
NE	§71-1278	WA	18.108.005
NH	328-B:4		
Acupuncture			
AK	§08.06.030	NH	328-E:12
AZ	§32-2901	NJ	45:9B-8
AR	§17-102-101	NM	61-14A-4†
CA	BPC §4925†	NY	§8214
CO	§12-29.5	NC	§90-455
CT	§20-206bb	OR	§677.759†
DC	§2-3302.3	PA	63 PS §1803
FL	§457.105†	RI	§5-37.2-12
HI	§436E-3	SC	§40-47-40
IL	225 ILCS 2/15	TN	§63-1-102
IA	§148E.3	TX	4495b
LA	37:1357	UT	58-72-101
ME	32 MRS 12511	VT	26 VSA 3401
MD	HOcc 1A-201	VA	§54.1-2900
MA	c112 §152	WA	18.06.050†
MN	§147B.02	WV	§30-36-1
MT	37-13-301†	WI	451.04
NV	§634A.120†		
Naturopathy			
AK	§08.45.020	ME	32 MRS 12521
AZ	§32-1555	MT	37-26-401
CT	§20-34	NH	328-E:14
DC	§2-3309.1	OR	§685.02
FL	§462.18	UT	58-71-102
HI	§455-3	VT	26 VSA 3401
KS	§65-2872a	WA	18.36A.030
Homeopathy			
AZ	§32-2915	NE	§630A.230
CT	§20-10	WA	18.36A.030

*Mandates for coverage of chiropractic services are in force in all but 8 states (CO, HI, ID, NH, OR, SD, VT, WY) and the District of Columbia.
†Coverage of acupuncture services in health insurance products is mandated by state law.

Conclusion

Opening a professional dialogue between physicians and practitioners of alternative medicine is crucial to better health care for those patients who choose alternative therapies. This need can be expected to grow with use of alternative therapies, particularly as health insurance plans include such therapies in the benefits they offer. The larger solution lies with better education for physicians about alternative medicine and further outcome studies and randomized trials that comprehensively assess the efficacy and relative safety of alternative therapies. Some of this work has begun, spurred by such developments as the Office of Alternative Medicine at the National Institutes of Health.[71] However, clarification of the medical liability issues involved should remove a significant obstacle to integration and continuity of patient care.

Physicians who currently refer patients to practitioners of alternative medicine or who are contemplating doing so should not be overly concerned about the malpractice liability implications of their conduct. The same commonsense considerations applicable to other referrals will be a reasonably reliable guide regarding acceptable practice. However, it may be useful to ask the following questions. First, is there evidence from the medical literature to suggest that the therapies a patient will receive as a result of the referral will offer no benefit or will subject the patient to unreasonable risks? Second, is the practitioner licensed in my state? (Some added comfort can be derived from knowing that the practitioner carries malpractice insurance.) Third, do I have any special knowledge or experience to make me think that this particular practitioner is incompetent? And fourth, will this be the usual kind of referral (ie, basically at arm's length, without ongoing and intrusive supervision of the patient's management)?

If the answers to the first and third of these questions are no and the answers to the second and fourth questions are yes, then this should remove many of the concerns a physician has that the referral decision itself will be construed as negligent. This conclusion holds even if the patient suffers an injury caused by the alternative medicine practitioner's negligence. That practitioner should be held accountable for his or her autonomous actions and should be judged according to standards set by fellow practitioners.

This work was supported by grants from the National Institutes of Health (U2AR43441), the John E. Fetzer Institute, Kalamazoo, Mich, the Kenneth J. Germeshausen Foundation, Boston, Mass, and the J. E. and Z. B. Butler Foundation, New York, NY.

References

1. Eisenberg DM, Kessler RC, Foster C, et al. "Unconventional" medicine in the United States: prevalence, costs, and patterns of use. *N Engl J Med.* 1993;328:246–252.
2. Duff C. Redefining the good life: indulging in inconspicuous consumption. *Wall Street Journal.* April 14, 1997:B1.
3. Blecher MB. Alternative medicine on pins and needles no more: acupuncturists and others get mainstream nod. *Crain's Chicago Business.* January 27, 1997:4.
4. Whitaker B. Now in the H.M.O.: yoga teachers and naturopaths. *New York Times.* November 24, 1996:11.
5. Hilts PJ. Health maintenance organizations turn to spiritual healing. *New York Times.* January 2, 1996:10.
6. Blecher MB. Gold in goldenseal: healing herbs have become a cash crop. *Hospitals & Health Networks.* 1997;71(20):50–54.
7. A special background report on trends in industry and finance. *Wall Street Journal.* April 3, 1997:1.
8. Pelletier KR, Marie A, Krasner M, Haskell WL. Current trends in the integration and reimbursement of complementary and alternative medicine by managed care, insurance carriers, and hospital providers. *Am J Health Promotion.* 1997;12(2):112–123.
9. Firshein J. Picture alternative medicine in the mainstream. *Business & Health.* 1995; 13(4):28–31.
10. Eisenberg DM. Advising patients who seek alternative medical therapies. *Ann Intern Med.* 1997;127:61–69.
11. *Wilk v American Medical Association.* 719 F2d 207 (7th Cir 1983).
12. *Idaho Association of Naturopathic Physicians v FDA.* 582 F2d 850 (4th Cir 1978).
13. Bigos SJ, Bowyer OR, Beaen GR, et al. *Clinical Practice Guideline Number 14: Acute Low Back Problems in Adults.* Rockville, Md: Agency for Health Care Policy and Research, US Dept of Health and Human Services; 1994.
14. Shekelle PG, Adams AH, Chassin MR, et al. Spinal manipulation for low-back pain. *Ann Intern Med.* 1992;117:590–598.
15. Kleijnen J, Knipschild P, ter Riet G. Clinical trials of homeopathy. *BMJ.* 1991;302:316–323.
16. Linde K, Clausius N, Ramirez G, et al. Are the clinical effects of homeopathy placebo effects? a meta-analysis of placebo-controlled trials. *Lancet.* 1997;350:834–843.
17. Le Bars PL, Katz MM, Berman N, et al. A placebo-controlled, double-blind, randomized trial of an extract of *Ginkgo biloba* for dementia. *JAMA.* 1997;278:1327–1332.
18. ter Riet G, Kleijnen J, Knipschild P. Acupuncture and chronic pain: a criteria-based meta-analysis. *J Clin Epidemiol.* 1990;43:1191–1199.
19. Vickers AJ. Can acupuncture have specific effects on health? a systematic review of acupuncture antiemesis trials. *J R Soc Med.* 1996;89:303–311.
20. National Institutes of Health, Office of Alternative Medicine. Program areas: research development and investigation. Available at: http://altmed.od.nih.gov/oam/rdi. Accessed October 6, 1998.
21. Fields DH. Oxford's expanded health plan is dangerous. *New York Times.* October 17, 1996:26.
22. Can standard medicine employ "alternative" & "complementary" medicine without liability. *NCAHF Newsletter.* November 21, 1991:1.
23. Grandinetti DA. "Integrated medicine" could boost your income. *Med Econ.* 1997;74:73–75.
24. Alternative care raises questions. *National Underwriter.* November 26, 1996:18.
25. Edlin M. Changing their ways to keep up with the times. *Managed Healthcare.* June 1997: 14–18.
26. Covaleski J, Goch L. Malpractice insurers target alternatives. *Best's Review, P/C.* April 1997: 61–63.
27. Federation of Chiropractic Licensing Boards. *Official Directory: Chiropractic Licensure and Practice Statistics.* Greeley, Colo: Federation of Chiropractic Licensing Boards; 1997.
28. Physician Insurers Association of America. *PIAA Data Sharing Reports, 1997.* Rockville, Md: Physician Insurers Association of America; 1997.
29. Gonzales M. *Socioeconomic Characteristics of Medical Practice 1997.* Chicago, Ill: American Medical Association; 1997:39–44.
30. Mitchell BB. *Acupuncture and Oriental Medicine Laws.* Bethesda, Md: National Acupuncture Foundation; 1997.
31. Kent GP, Brondum J, Keenslyside RA, LaFazia LM, Scott HD. A large outbreak of acupuncture-associated hepatitis B. *Am J Epidemiol.* 1988;127:591–598.
32. Brennan TA, Leape LL, Laird NM, et al. Incidence of adverse events and negligence in hospitalized patients: results of the Harvard Medical Practice Study I. *N Engl J Med.* 1991;324:370–376.
33. *Datiz v Shoob.* 71 NY2d 867 (1988).
34. *Jennings v Burgess.* 917 SW2d 790 (Tex 1996).
35. *Reed v Bascon.* 124 Ill2d 386 (1988).
36. *Delaney v Cade.* 255 Kan199 (Super Ct 1994).
37. *Riser v American Medical International.* 620 So2d 372 (5th Cir 1993).
38. Hall MA. Rationing health care at the bedside. *New York University Law Review.* 1994; 69:693–780.
39. Orentlicher D. Paying physicians more to do less: financial incentives to limit care. *University of Richmond Law Review.* 1994;30:155–197.
40. Miller RH, Luft HS. Does managed care lead to better or worse quality of care? *Health Aff (Millwood).* 1997;16(5):7–25.
41. Morreim EH. Diverse and perverse incentives of managed care: bringing patients into alignment. *Widener Law Symposium Journal.* 1996;1:89–139.
42. Greely H. Direct financial incentives in managed care: unanswered questions. *Health Matrix.* Winter 1996;6:53–88.
43. *Graddy v New York Medical College.* 19 AD2d 426, 243 NYS2d 940 (App Div 1963).
44. *Cox v Kingsboro Medical Group.* 214 AD2d 150, 88 NY2d 904 (1995).
45. *Kavanaugh v Nussbaum.* 71 NY2d 535 (Ct App 1988)
46. *Hoffman v Wells.* 397 SE2d 696 (Ga 1990).
47. *Rudeck v Wright.* 709 P2d 621 (Mont 1985).
48. §225 Ill Comp Stat Ann 95/7, 7.5 (1997).
49. NJ Stat §45:11–49 (1997).
50. *Harris v Miller.* 335 NC 379, 438 SE2d 731 (NC Super Ct 1994).
51. *Hammer v Waterhouse.* 895 SW2d 295 (Mo App 1995).
52. *Crump v Piper.* 425 SW2d 924 (Mo 1968).
53. *Stovall v Harms.* 214 Kan 835 (Super Ct 1974).
54. *Darling v Charleston Community Memorial Hospital.* 211 NE2d 253 (Ill Super Ct 1965).
55. *Harrell v Total Health Care, Inc.* No. 71610, 1989 WL 153066 (Mo Ct App April 25, 1989), aff'd, 781 SW2d 58 (Mo 1989).
56. *McClellan v Health Maintenance Org.* 604 A2d 1053 (Pa 1992).
57. *McLauchlin v Dahlquist.* 1997 Minn App LEXIS 571 (Ct App 1997).

58. *Williams v Hotel Dieu Hospital.* 595 So2d 783 (La Ct App 1992).

59. *Brodersen v Sioux Valley Memorial Hospital.* 902 F Supp 931 (ND Iowa 1995).

60. *Wozny v Godsil.* 4747 So2d 1078 (Ala Super Ct 1985).

61. Baer HA. The potential rejuvenation of American naturopathy as a consequence of the holistic health movement. *Med Anthropol.* 1992;127:369–383.

62. *Baumgartner v the First Church of Christ Scientist.* 490 NE2d 1319 (Ill App 1986).

63. *Sutton v Cook.* 254 Ore 116 (Super Ct 1969).

64. Hobson SM. Note: the standard of admissibility of a physician's expert testimony in a chiropractic malpractice action. *Indiana Law Journal.* 1989;64:737–753.

65. *Boudreaux v Panger.* 481 So2d 1382 (La App 5th Cir 1986).

66. *Kerkman v Hintz.* 142 Wis2d 404 (1988).

67. *State of North Carolina v Howard.* 78 NC App 262; 337 SE2d 598 (Ct App 1985).

68. Cohen MH. Holistic health care: including alternative and complementary medicine in insurance and regulatory schemes. *Arizona Law Review.* 1996;38:83–164.

69. *Johnson v Lawrence.* 720 SW2d 50 (Tenn Ct App 1986).

70. *Metzler v New York State Board for Professional Medical Conduct.* 610 NYS2d 334 (NY Super Ct 1994).

71. 42 USC §283g.

2 Cultural/Social Aspects

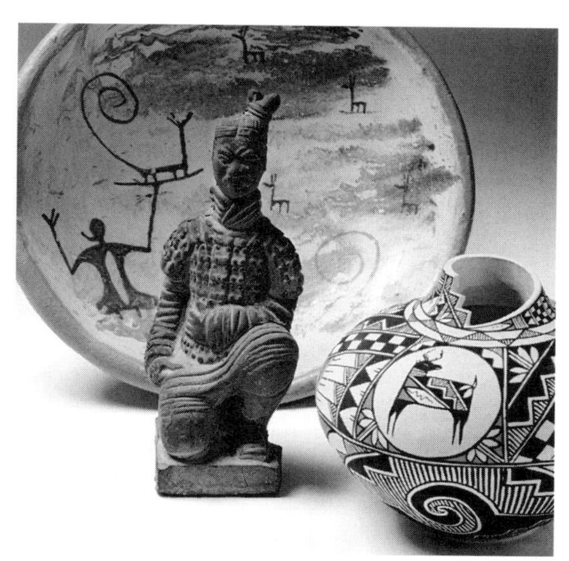

Overview

Joseph J. Jacobs, MD, MBA
From the Office of Vermont Health Access, Waterbury.

American medicine, and particularly its physicians, is being challenged by issues relating to an increasingly ethnically and culturally diverse population. First and subsequent generations of immigrants to this country bring with them traditional healing systems that reflect their own cultures, and they use them for different reasons. Health professionals, meanwhile, become acculturated to the culture of medicine in the process of their medical training. Consequently, physicians often encounter belief systems and views of health and illness that are different from their own as they try to elicit a history. A cultural divide emerges. As we rediscover the importance of the physician-patient relationship, we begin to appreciate the value of not only verbal, but also nonverbal communication in the course of a clinical transaction.

One of the principles of community-oriented primary care (a primary health care ideal popular in the 1970s) is to know one's target community. Part of that "knowing" is understanding the cultural makeup and beliefs of patients. The increasing popularity of complementary and alternative medicine (CAM) has given the clinician a renewed imperative for this understanding.

Complementary and alternative medicine is one of several indicators of a changing health care market. Increasing consumerism is changing the traditional patient role, previously characterized by willing, passive dependence on a physician, to that of an activist health consumer prepared to seek out and act on health information in a market-driven health economy. No longer are pronouncements or recommendations provided by physicians readily accepted with blind faith by the patient. Patients are now demanding and seeking better access to timely and accurate health information. Sophisticated health consumers are also willing to "vote" with their feet by going to practitioners whom they have identified as open-minded and supportive about unconventional approaches to health care. Patients trust physicians with their bodies and also want to trust physicians with their beliefs.

The American health care industry is a dynamic and pluralistic marketplace in which cost reduction has taken top priority. A managed care organization must show prospective "clients" a willingness to provide services in order to sign them up, but must also exhibit cultural sensitivity to increase market share among untapped groups of people.

This section of *Alternative Medicine: An Objective Assessment* contains a series of articles that focus on the value that culture plays in the delivery of health care.

The chapter "Navajo Use of Native Healers" by Kim and Yeong[1] surveys the use of native healers among 300 Navajo patients in an ambulatory clinic on a Navajo reservation. The findings reveal a certain "comfort level" among Navajos in their willingness to use the services of a traditional healer for common diseases; this comfort level bears no relation to age, sex, or income. The investigators note the lack of inhibition by Navajos to discuss their use of native healers and do not observe a conflict between native and conventional medicine.

The use of prayer as a health care modality has only recently begun to draw attention to its acknowledgment by physicians. There has always existed an understanding of the role that indigenous belief systems played in the coping strategies of American Indians and other native peoples. The article by Daaleman and Frey,[2] "Prevalence and Patterns of Physician Referral to Clergy and Pastoral Care Providers," demonstrates the willingness of family physicians to refer patients to pastoral care providers. The study reports that more than 80% of surveyed physicians reported referring their patients to pastoral care providers, especially for marital problems and end-of-life care. These findings reflect understanding that the spiritual dimension of patients' lives is an important component of well-being.

In "Alternative Medicine Use by Homeless Youth" by Breuner et al,[3] an intriguing study is presented on the use of unconventional medicine by this population in Seattle, Wash. It is quite surprising to discover significant use of CAM by a population of individuals who might be expected to have self-imposed limited access to basic health benefits (an issue identified by the authors, not addressed). Even though the authors acknowledge some of the methodological problems of their study, this article makes for an interesting first study on the health care-seeking behavior of this population.

Pachter et al,[4] in "Home-Based Therapies for the Common Cold Among European American and Ethnic Minority Families," provide us with a gentle reminder of the importance of folk medicine in society. They discuss the mechanism of belief and find similarities between Puerto Rican mothers and European Americans. This study points out the importance that home remedies play in modern health care in America in the same way as the Daaleman and Frey study demonstrates the value of spiritual comfort.

Patients seem particularly troubled by the occurrence of dermatological disorders. The selected group of articles in this section bear out the universality of this concern. The article "Traditional Chinese Medicine for the Treatment of Dermatological Disorders," by Koo and Arain,[5] presents an interesting overview of traditional Chinese medicine, beginning with a detailed discussion of efficacy and mechanism(s) of action, as well as toxic effects, of Chinese herbology.

Ng[6] focuses on topical traditional Chinese medicine in Singapore and describes an overview not only for dermatological use, but also other ailments, as well as topical treatments for aches, pains, and musculoskeletal injuries.

A European perspective is presented in the article by Happle,[7] "The Essence of Alternative Medicine: A Dermatologist's View From Germany." The author offers an overview of alternative medicine in Germany, along with a discussion of the elements of debate between conventional practitioners and proponents of alternative medicine. This article is particularly informative about institutional attitudes toward alternative medicine.

Satimia et al[8] provide an interesting description of treatment of dermatological disorders in rural Tanzania, where traditional healers play a major role because of the paucity of Western-trained health care professionals. This study investigated choice of health care system in this population. Individuals who were older and less educated tended to use traditional healers, while those younger and better educated tended to use modern health care methods.

Oumeish[9] presents an interesting discussion of medical practices in the Old World that are still practiced in some areas today, such as the Middle East. Descriptions of various practices may be useful to the clinician who may has patients from this part of the world.

Ubogui et al[10] continue the dermatological theme with "Thermalism in Argentina." This is a clinical description of the successful use of hot-water springs, as well as mud and algae, to treat psoriasis. The authors provide a clinical description of the treatment as well as a chemical analysis of the water used from this mineral spring. This article does not explore the cultural dimension of this practice but instead focuses on the methods and efficacy of treatment.

The final chapter in this section, "Different Modalities of Spa Therapy for Skin Diseases at the Dead Sea Area," by Halevy and Sukenik,[11] provides a historical overview and review of the literature for spa therapy in the Dead Sea. Additionally, the authors provide a postulated mechanism of action for Dead Sea spa therapy for psoriasis and psoriasis arthritis.

The articles in this section give the Western-trained physician insights into some of the cultural aspects of medicine. Awareness and understanding of these issues may enhance the artful practice of medicine for the beleaguered physician who finds technology to be less than fulfilling.

References

1. Kim C, Yeong KS. Navajo use of native healers. *Arch Intern Med.* 1998;158:2245–2249.
2. Daaleman TP, Frey B. Prevalence and patterns of physician referral to clergy and pastoral care providers. *Arch Fam Med.* 1998;7:548–552.
3. Breuner CC, Barry PJ, Kemper KJ. Alternative medicine use by homeless youth. *Arch Pediatr Adolesc Med.* 1998;152:1071–1075.
4. Pachter LM, Sumner T, Fontan A, Sneed M, Bernstein BA. Home-based therapies for the common cold among European American and ethnic minority families. *Arch Pediatr Adolesc Med.* 1998;152:1083–1088.
5. Koo J, Arain BA. Traditional Chinese medicine for the treatment of dermatologic disorders. *Arch Dermatol.* 1998;134:1388–1393.
6. Ng S. Topical traditional chinese medicine. *Arch Dermatol.* 1998;134:1395–1396.
7. Happle R. The essence of alternative medicine: a dermatologist's view from Germany. *Arch Dermatol.* 1998;134:1455–1460.
8. Satimia FT, McBride SR, Leppard B. Prevalence of skin disease in rural Tanzania and factors influencing the choice of health care, modern or traditional. *Arch Dermatol.* 1998; 134:1363–1366.
9. Oumeish OY. The philosophical, cultural, and historical aspects of complementary, alternative, unconventional, and integrative medicine in the Old World. *Arch Dermatol.* 1998; 134:1373–1412.
10. Ubogui J, Stengel FM, Kien M, Sevinsky L, Lupo LR. Thermalism in Argentina. *Arch Dermatol.* 1998;134:1411–1412.
11. Halevy S, Sukenik S. Different modalities of spa therapy for skin diseases at the Dead Sea area. *Arch Dermatol.* 1998;134:1416–1420.

7 Navajo Use of Native Healers

Catherine Kim, MD, MPH; Yeong S. Kwok, MD
From the US Public Health Service, Crownpoint, NM.

Background
Although the Indian Health Service provides extensive health care service to Navajo people, the role of native healers, or medicine men, has not been quantitatively described.

Objective
To determine the prevalence of native healer use, the reasons for use, cost of use, and the nature of any conflict with conventional medicine.

Methods
We conducted a cross-sectional interview of 300 Navajo patients seen consecutively in an ambulatory care clinic at a rural Indian Health Service hospital.

Results
Sixty-two percent of Navajo patients had used native healers and 39% used native healers on a regular basis; users were not distinguishable from nonusers by age, education, income, fluency in English, identification of a primary provider, or compliance, but Pentecostal patients used native healers less than patients of other faiths. Patients consulted native healers for common medical conditions such as arthritis, depression, and diabetes mellitus as well as "bad luck." Perceived conflict between native healer advice and medical provider advice was rare. Cost was the main barrier to seeking native healer care.

Conclusions
Among the Navajo, use of native healers for medical conditions is common and is not related to age, sex, or income but is inversely correlated with the Pentecostal faith; use of healers overlaps with use of medical providers for common medical conditions. Patients are willing to discuss use of native healers and rarely perceive conflict between native healer and conventional medicine. This corroborates other research suggesting that alternative medicine is widely used by many cultural groups for common diseases.

Arch Intern Med. 1998;158:2245–2249

Navajo traditionally received treatment for illness from native healers or "medicine men." As in a conventional medical care system, many different types of practitioner exist; these range from diagnosticians such as hand tremblers, crystal gazers, and "listeners," to individuals who perform healing ceremonies involving herbs, balms, and purgatives.[1] Native healers have been the focus of extensive ethnographic study by anthropologists, psychiatrists, and physicians[1–5] but the prevalence and frequency of use of native healers among Navajo have not been described. The Navajo are also eligible for extensive free health care services through the Indian Health Service (IHS). It is not clear if conventional medical care provided by IHS physicians conflicts with the recommendations of native healers.

To improve understanding of the use of native healers and its interaction with conventional medicine, an interview was conducted of Navajo IHS patients to determine the prevalence of use, reasons for use, characteristics of those who use native healers, cost of care, and whether native healer care conflicts with care provided by conventional physicians.

Methods

Between June 23, 1997, and September 1, 1997, consecutive adult patients seen in the ambulatory care clinic at a rural IHS hospital were interviewed. The hospital is a 39-bed hospital located on the eastern edge of the Navajo reservation in New Mexico. Its catchment area contains roughly 10,000 of the 25,351 square miles of the Navajo Nation, which is roughly the size of West Virginia. Despite its location on the edge of the reservation and the access that patients have to other nongovernmental health care facilities, almost 47,000 outpatient visits were made to the hospital during the 1992 fiscal year.[6]

Eligibility was limited to consenting patients 18 years or older who did not have cognitive or physical impairment that prevented completion of the interview. An interview rather than a self-administered questionnaire was necessary because many eligible participants cannot read or cannot speak English and therefore require a translator. The overall response rate among eligible individuals was 99%; 2 patients refused to participate and 1 patient chose to respond only to demographic questions and issues related to hospital care. Three patients were excluded secondary to dementia.

The Interview

A questionnaire was developed in focus groups consisting of the English-speaking Navajo hospital staff and a native healer. The questionnaire was then pilot tested among Navajo nursing assistants to ensure that questions were understandable, nonoffensive, and informative. The Navajo Nation Research Board, which acts as the institutional review board for research involving the Navajo tribe, reviewed and approved the study.

Two non-Navajo interviewers who were medical providers conducted the surveys in the ambulatory care clinic. The medical providers had worked at the hospital for 1 year in the continuity clinics, ambulatory care clinics, and the emergency department. The interviewer addressed the reason for the outpatient visit then asked if the patient was willing to participate in the interview. The purpose of the interview was described to potential respondents and they were assured that their responses would be kept confidential and not be entered into their medical record.

Navajo nurses and nursing assistants who knew the purpose of the interview and who spoke Navajo translated for non-English–speaking patients. The responsibilities of the Navajo nursing staff include translation between patients and health care providers. Each translator was trained to administer the interview. The interview was reviewed with each assistant individually. The questions were primarily phrased in yes/no format with open-ended questions afterward to decrease variability between translators.[7] In 3 cases, family members served as translators.

The interviews averaged 15 minutes in length and began with demographic questions on age, educational level, income, and religion. Next, respondents were asked about their interactions with medical doctors, nurse practitioners, and physician's assistants. From the patients' medical charts, the number of outpatient visits, inpatient stays made to the hospital in the last year, and the reasons for the visits were recorded. Use of conventional medicine at other locations in the last year was inquired about and the number of visits and the reasons for these visits were recorded. Patients were also asked about their satisfaction with conventional medical care for these problems. Next, patients were asked if they followed medical provider instructions all the time, most of the time, some of the time, or never.

At this point, respondents were asked about their use of native healers: whether they had ever consulted a medicine man and if so, how many times in the last year. However, no inquiry was made about the type of native healer sought or the type of ceremony performed since the native healer consultant advised that such questions might be considered intrusive. The time of their last visit to a native healer, the reasons for the visits, and satisfaction with these visits was recorded.

Then, questions were asked about barriers to medicine man care; patients were asked if the cost of native healer care, religious reasons, or trust in native healers deterred them from seeking native healer care. They were also asked if there were any other deterrents.

Finally, patients were asked about the interaction between conventional medicine and native healers: whether they had been given significant conflicting instructions about an ailment, what the nature of this conflict was, and whose instructions they chose to follow.

Statistical Analysis

The demographic characteristics of the population, prevalence and frequency of native healer use, and reasons for visits to medical providers and native healers were described using percentages for dichotomous variables and the mean and SD for continuous variables. The characteristics of patients who used a native healer were compared with those who did not, using χ^2 tests for dichotomous and categorical variables and t tests for continuous variables. To adjust for potential confounding, a multivariate logistic model was used to evaluate variables associated with use of a native healer. All statistical tests were carried out using STATA software.[8]

Results

Predictors of Use of Native Healers

Sixty-two percent of individuals interviewed had used a native healer at least once in their lifetime and 39% had used a native healer during the last year. Those who had seen a native healer in the past averaged 2 visits per year although the number of visits ranged widely. Among those who had used a native healer at some time but not during the past year had a mean time of 11 years elapsed from their last visit although the number of years also ranged widely.

Characteristics of the subjects interviewed are shown in Table 1. The age and sex distributions of subjects are similar to that of all patients seen at the Crownpoint Healthcare Facility, Crownpoint, NM, between June 23, 1997, and September 1, 1997. The median income calculated was similar to that listed by the Navajo Nation,[6] meaning 56% live below the poverty line. The rates of lifetime and recent use were not correlated with age, sex, education, income, fluency in English, identification of a primary provider, number of clinic visits or hospitalizations, or compliance with medical provider instructions in univariate analysis and multiple logistic regression analysis. There were significant differences in the rates of use among religions; use of medicine men was significantly less common among members of the Pentecostal faith ($P<.001$) than among those who identified themselves as Catholic, traditional Navajo, Native American Church, Mormon, Protestant, Christian, no religion, or Baptist. In a multivariate logistic analysis that included all variables in Table 1 as predictors, only religion was significantly associated with use of native healers (odds ratio, 0.16; 95% confidence interval, 0.057–0.483).

Table 1. Characteristics of the 300 Navajo Individuals Interviewed*

Characteristic	Used a Native Healer at Least Once	Never Used a Native Healer
Age, y		
18–29	46 (25)	29 (25)
30–49	64 (35)	45 (39)
50–65	44 (24)	30 (26)
66–90	31 (17)	10 (9)
Sex		
Female	108 (58)	72 (63)
Income, $		
<5000	60 (32)	36 (32)
5000–9999	35 (19)	27 (24)
10,000–19,999	54 (29)	32 (28)
≥20,000	35 (19)	16 (14)
Education		
<High school	51 (28)	34 (30)
Some high school	22 (12)	25 (22)
High school	67 (36)	37 (32)
Some college	36 (19)	15 (13)
College or graduate school	9 (5)	3 (3)
Requires a translator	31 (17)	14 (12)
Religion		
Christian, not specified	25 (14)	28 (24)
Traditional Navajo, only	46 (25)	6 (5)
Native American church	41 (22)	9 (8)
Pentecostal	13 (7)	36 (31)
Mormon	27 (15)	7 (6)
Baptist	10 (5)	13 (11)
Catholic	14 (8)	1 (1)
Other	9 (5)	14 (12)
No primary medical provider	96 (52)	54 (47)
Outpatient visits in prior year		
1–5	69 (37)	42 (37)
6–10	52 (32)	34 (30)
11–20	38 (21)	35 (22)
21–50	19 (10)	13 (11)

*Values are number (percentage). Because some patients chose not to respond to certain questions, numbers do not total 300.

Patterns of Use of Native Healers

Table 2 summarizes the most common reasons for visits to a medical provider and the frequency of concomitant use of native healers. Among these conditions, the use of native healers was highest for arthritis, abdominal pain, depression/anxiety, and chest pain. No patient saw a native

Table 2. Most Common Conditions for Which Treatment Is Sought*

Condition	Saw a Medical Provider	Saw a Native Healer Also	Saw a Native Healer	Saw a Medical Provider Also
Upper respiratory tract infection	83 (28)	0 (0)	. . .	. . .
Arthritis	75 (25)	18 (6)	24 (21)	18 (16)
Hypertension	70 (23)	2 (1)	. . .	. . .
Diabetes mellitus	68 (23)	8 (3)	8 (7)	8 (7)
Health care maintenance	58 (19)	0 (0)	. . .	. . .
Abdominal pain	32 (11)	9 (3)	7 (6)	5 (4)
Urinary tract infection	31 (10)	2 (1)	. . .	. . .
Back pain	23 (8)	4 (1)	10 (9)	4 (3)
Chest pain	20 (7)	5 (2)	. . .	. . .
Depression/anxiety	17 (6)	5 (2)	17 (15)	5 (4)
Pregnancy	17 (6)	0 (0)	. . .	. . .
Allergies	16 (5)	0 (0)	. . .	. . .
Skin problems	16 (5)	2 (1)	. . .	. . .
Headache	13 (4)	2 (1)	8 (7)	2 (2)
Blessing	. . .	. . .	30 (26)	0 (0)
Bad luck	. . .	. . .	20 (17)	0 (0)
"Sick"	. . .	. . .	12 (10)	0 (0)
Insomnia	. . .	. . .	9 (8)	2 (2)
Headache	. . .	. . .	8 (7)	2 (2)
Family problems	. . .	. . .	7 (6)	0 (0)

*Values are number (percentage). Because patients often had more than 1 reason per visit, percentages do not total 100. Ellipses indicate not applicable.

healer for upper respiratory tract infections, health care maintenance, pregnancy, or allergies.

Table 2 also summarizes the most common reasons for visits to a native healer and the frequency of concomitant use of a medical provider. These reasons overlapped with the most common reasons for seeing a medical provider, such as arthritis, depression/anxiety, back pain, and diabetes mellitus, but certain complaints such as family problems and insomnia were much more common reasons for visits to native healers than medical providers. Patients who saw native healers for arthritis and diabetes mellitus commonly consulted a medical provider in addition. Those who consulted a native healer for depression/anxiety and arthritis were less likely to also consult a medical provider, and medical providers were never consulted for "sickness," "blessing," "bad luck," or family problems.

Patients' ratings of self-compliance were high. Only 2 patients (1%) said they were never compliant. Seventy-eight patients (26%) stated they were sometimes compliant, 115 patients (38%) said they were usually compliant, and 104 patients (35%) said they were always compliant. Compliance did not correlate with use of native healers.

Dissatisfaction was reported infrequently for both medical provider and native healer use; roughly 10% of patients reported they were dissatisfied with care. Twenty patients (6.6%) reported being dissatisfied with the medical treatment of arthritis, but only 7 (2.3%) reported seeking native healer care due to dissatisfaction. Six patients (2%) reported being dissatisfied with the native healer treatment of arthritis, and 5 (1.6%) reported seeking medical care because of this. Dissatisfaction with the treatment of other complaints occurred only 1% of the time for both medical providers and native healers. Satisfaction with conventional medical care did not correlate with use of native healers.

Perceived conflict in medical provider and native healer instructions occurred infrequently. Twenty-one patients stated that their medical provider and the native healer gave them conflicting recommendations. When faced with conflicting advice, 15 patients stated they attempted to follow both sets of advice, 1 patient followed the medical provider's advice only, and 5 patients followed the native healer's advice only.

Barriers to Seeking Native Healer Care

Medical care provided by the IHS is free, with the exception of certain procedures such as cosmetic surgery and certain items such as dentures. In contrast, the cost of visiting a native healer was reported to vary from $1 to $3000, with an average cost per visit of $388. The average annual cost of native healer use as a proportion of the patient's self-reported annual income was 0.21, or roughly one fifth. Cost was cited by 108 patients (36%) as the reason for not seeking native healer care more frequently and was the most common barrier to native healer care. Costs are a conservative estimate as they may exclude such customary expenses as transportation, feeding all those who participate in a ceremony, and costs of materials needed such as buckskin or herbs. Cost charged to the patient did not correlate with the patient's income.

Other patients stated that lack of trust in native healers (76 patients [25%]), their religion (70 patients [23%]), unsupportive families (37 patients [12%]), lack of belief in traditional Navajo medicine (33 patients [11%]), lack of knowledge about traditional Navajo medicine (20 patients [7%]), good health (11 patients [4%]), and lack of local native healers (10 patients [3%]) also acted as deterrents to native healer care.

Comment

Patients use unconventional medicine extensively. In their 1993 national survey, Eisenberg et al[9] discovered that roughly 34% of respondents used unconventional therapy at an expense of $13.7 billion dollars per year. The rate of unconventional therapy use is as high as 50% among patients who use conventional medical care.[10] Smaller studies[11–13] have also determined that the use of unconventional therapy is widespread and used primarily for common chronic or self-limiting illnesses, but also used for diseases such as cancer, human immunodeficiency virus infection, and asthma.

We also found high rates of alternative medicine use in the Navajo population. Most patients interviewed had used native healers at some point and almost 40% used native healers on a regular basis. Those who had not used native healers within the last year generally had not used them for more than a decade. Cost was the main barrier to using native healers.

Religion was the only predictor of native healer use. Patients who belonged to an organized religion generally held traditional beliefs as well, but religion was a barrier to seeking native healer care, particularly if they were of the Pentecostal faith. "I'm a Christian now, so I don't go so much, but I used to go more often," stated one patient.

Patients consulted both native healers and medical providers for a wide range of health problems. Common conditions among the Navajo such as diabetes mellitus, arthritis, and depression or anxiety were common reasons for consulting both the medical provider and the native healer. However, certain diseases such as upper respiratory tract infections and allergies were recognized as the exclusive domain of the medical provider and other problems such as bad luck, blessings, and family difficulties were recognized as the exclusive domain of the native healer. This may reflect the fact that family problem is not a medical diagnosis and sickness and bad luck are also categorized differently in medical terminology. For diseases such as diabetes, native healer care was viewed as an adjunct rather than a substitute for medical provider care. The patients using native healers consulted native healers for depression or anxiety a greater proportion of the time than patients only using medical providers consulted medical providers for depression or anxiety. As one patient stated, "The doctors give me pills for my body, the medicine man gives me songs for my spirit."

Patients' satisfaction with care provided by the native healer or the medical provider did not seem to serve as a driving force to seeking alternate care because most patients were satisfied with the care they received. Patients who expressed dissatisfaction with medical care did not always seek native healer care for their health problems and vice versa.

The cost of visiting a native healer was the main barrier to use. More than one third of patients stated they would use native healers more often except for the cost. The costs listed may underestimate the costs actually involved as no inquiry was made regarding materials and ancillary costs of the ceremonies. Even so, native healer cost is high, sometimes exceeding 20% of the patient's annual income. The cost may vary for several reasons, particularly regarding the type of ceremony performed and the complexity of the ceremony. Certain diagnostic ceremonies such as hand trembling tend to cost significantly less than "treatment" ceremonies, which may involve the patient's entire extended family and last for days.

Many patients reported that they did not trust certain individuals claiming to be native healers. While these patients still believed in traditional Navajo medicine, they stated that they could not find a trustworthy practitioner; one patient stated, "There are a lot of quacks out there," applying the term *quacks* to those masquerading as native healers. Several patients stated that certain individuals claiming to be native healers did not bother to learn the intricacies of their trade but rather charged patients for inadequately performed services. The longer ceremonies can last as long as 9 days with different chants and rituals performed throughout, and can take years of apprenticeship to learn.[2] Patients who cited lack of trust were concerned that the quality of native healer care varied substantially from practitioner to practitioner. "I know a good one, so I use him a lot," stated one patient.

Lack of availability of local healers also acted as a barrier. No exact tally exists of the number and location of native healers, but several patients stated that the number of local healers varies at different locations on the Navajo reservation. "All the good medicine men are far away," stated one patient. "I would have to drive 3 hours to get the ceremony I need."

Participants in the survey may not accurately represent Navajo patients, as patients interviewed were exclusively drawn from those who seek care at an IHS hospital; the use of native healers may be much higher for those who do not seek conventional medical care or who seek care at a nongovernmental hospital. Also, as previously mentioned, the reservation is large and the IHS site where the interview was conducted is located at the edge of the reservation. Thus, patients interviewed may have easier access to non-Navajo sources of health care than patients who are located in the interior of the reservation. Conversely, patients located in the interior of the reservation may have easier access to native healers than the patients interviewed if there is a higher concentration of healers in the interior of the reservation. Finally, not all Navajo live on the reservation, and it is unknown how this population's access to conventional or native healer care differs from the populations mentioned above.

The fact that 2 non-Navajo medical providers conducted the interview in a hospital clinic may have led to an underestimate of patients' use of native healers. Patients may have felt uncomfortable divulging the frequency or history of use for fear of how this might influence their medical care due to the misperception that the interviewers, being non-Navajo, might be prejudiced against native healer care. Also, since patients had just received medical provider care, they may have been reluctant to state they were dissatisfied with their medical care. Similarly, they may have overestimated their compliance rates with medical care.

As with many other subpopulations in the multicultural society that composes the United States, the use of alternative medicine is common among Navajo patients. Patients usually do not perceive conflict between different health system beliefs and may use remedies prescribed by several practitioners for a single health care problem; they may perceive such an approach as more effective than using a single system. This may be rooted in the belief that disease is multifaceted, and different health care systems treat different facets effectively.[5] As one patient succinctly stated, "It is better to stand on two legs than on one." Therefore, inquiring about patients' use of native healers can significantly enhance understanding of the patients' health.

Even though use of native healers can be a religious and private issue, patients are willing to discuss their use of native healers if asked in a sensitive manner. Increased understanding of this deeply rooted system can improve communications between providers and patients and, therefore, can help medical providers improve the quality of care provided. Further research is needed to elucidate how extensive native healer use is across various areas of the Navajo reservation, what patients' expectations of their various health care providers are, their view of the success of the care provided, and how conventional care and native healer care can interact with each other to increase the overall effectiveness of care provided to the patient.

We appreciate the assistance of Albert Tolino for serving as our native healer consultant, the Navajo nursing staff for translating, including Vicky Abeita, Louise Begay, Susie Chiquito, Gloria Gray, Ann Jordan, Isabelle Mariano, Lorraine Miles, Carolyn Sam, Ella Sandoval, Janice Willie, and the Health Promotion Disease Prevention staff for their preparation of fliers and posters.

References

1. Sandner D. *Navajo Symbols of Healing*. Orlando, Fla: Harcourt Brace & Co; 1979.
2. Reichard GA. *Navajo Religion: A Story of Symbolism*. 2nd ed. Tuscon: University of Arizona Press; 1983.
3. Hammerschlag C. *The Dancing Healers*. New York, NY: HarperCollins Publications Inc; 1988.
4. Kelly KB, Francis H. *Navajo Sacred Places*. Bloomington: Indiana University Press; 1994.
5. Coulehan JL. Navajo Indian medicine: implications for healing. *J Fam Pract*. 1980;10:55–61.
6. Etcitty D. *Navajo Nation FAX 1993*. Window Rock, Ariz: Division of Economic Development, Navajo Nation; 1994.
7. Hully SB, Cummings SR. *Designing Clinical Research*. Baltimore, Md: Williams & Wilkins; 1988.
8. *Stata Statistical Software*. College Station, Tex: Stata Corp; 1997.
9. Eisenberg D, Kessler R, Foster C, Norlock FE, Calkins DR, DelBanco TL. Unconventional medicine in the United States. *N Engl J Med*. 1993;328:246–252.
10. Elder NC, Gillchrist A, Minz R. Use of alternative health care by family practice patients. *Arch Fam Med*. 1997;6:181–184.
11. Cook C, Baiseden D. Ancillary use of folk medicine by patients in primary care clinics in southwestern West Virginia. *South Med J*. 1986; 79:1098–1101.
12. MacIntyre RC, Holzemer WL. Complementary and alternative medicine and human immune deficiency virus and AIDS. *J Assoc Nurses AIDS Care*. 1997;8:25–38.
13. Hackman RM, Stern JS, Gershwin ME. Complementary and alternative medicine and asthma. *Clin Rev Allergy Immunol*. 1996; 14:321–336.

8 Prevalence and Patterns of Physician Referral to Clergy and Pastoral Care Providers

Timothy P. Daaleman, DO; Bruce Frey, PhD
From the Department of Family Medicine (Dr Daaleman) and the Office of Primary Care (Dr Frey), University of Kansas Medical Center School of Medicine, Kansas City.

Background
There is a heightened interest in spiritual and religious interventions in clinical settings, an area marked by unease and lack of training by physicians. A potential resource for generalists is specialty consultation and referral services, although little is known about the prevalence and patterns of involvement of clergy or pastoral professionals in patient care.

Objectives
To identify the prevalence and patterns of physician-directed patient referral to or recommended consultation with clergy or pastoral care providers and to describe attitudinal and demographic variables that can predict referring and nonreferring physicians.

Design
A mailed anonymous survey.

Setting
Family physicians in the United States.

Participants
Active members of the American Academy of Family Physicians whose self-designated professional activity is direct patient care. Of the 756 randomly selected physicians for participation in the study, 438 (57.9%) responded.

Main Outcome Measures
Physician reporting on their attitudes and referral behaviors, including referral frequency, and conditions or reasons for referral or nonreferral to clergy and pastoral care providers.

Results
More than 80% of the physicians reported that they refer or recommend their patients to clergy and pastoral care providers; more than 30% stated that they refer more than 10 times a year. Most physicians (75.5%) chose conditions associated with end-of-life care (ie, bereavement, terminal illness) as reasons for referral. Marital and family counseling were cited by 72.8% of physicians; however, other psychosocial issues, such as depression and mood disorders

(38.7%) and substance abuse (19.0%), were less prevalent. Physicians who reported a greater degree of religiosity had a small increased tendency to refer (*r*=0.39, *P*<.05) to these providers. In addition, physicians who were in practice for more than 15 years were more likely to refer to clergy (*P*<.01).

Conclusions

Most family physicians accept clergy and pastoral professionals in the care of their patients. In medical settings, the providers of religious and spiritual interventions have a larger and more expanded role than previously reported.

Arch Fam Med. 1998;7:548–553

In a 1993 landmark national survey that depicted the prevalence, costs, and patterns of unconventional medicine in the United States, 25% of the respondents acknowledged using prayer as a treatment modality.[1] From a physician perspective, it is unclear what role spiritual and religious interventions and providers have in clinical encounters. Although 72% of physicians are interested in training in prayer, only 33% believe in it as a legitimate medical practice.[2] Despite the opacity of these studies, religion and spirituality continue to be major and consistent factors in the lives of most Americans.[3] In health care settings, religious and spiritual beliefs[4] wield a substantial influence on patient health beliefs, and some may directly affect clinical outcomes.[5]

Family physicians are perceived as being unqualified or untrained to discuss spiritual and religious issues with patients,[6] which may be reflected through diagnostic or therapeutic uncertainty when addressing these issues. The *Diagnostic and Statistical Manual of Mental Disorders, Fourth Edition*[7] provides some background and direction for the assessment of religious or spiritual problems.[8] Although another potential resource for generalists is specialty consultation and referral services, little is known about the prevalence and patterns of involvement of clergy or pastoral professionals in patient care.

One previous study conducted in Great Britain found that general practitioners perceived an important theoretical role for the involvement of clergy in patient care; however, this role was not matched in practice.[9] In a study of family and general practitioners conducted in the United States, fewer than half (45%) of respondents reported a usual pattern of referral to clergy when their geriatric patients were in great distress or near death.[10] Although limited by sample size, an additional university medical center-based study of physicians found that 49% of physicians made no referrals to chaplain services.[11]

The heightened interest in spiritual interventions in clinical settings and the unease and lack of training in this area by physicians highlight the importance of developing an understanding of the interactions between physicians and clergy. Pastoral care providers and clergy may benefit from an awareness of expectations and reasons for receiving consultation from physicians. Physicians in turn may gain a greater insight into their own rationale for involving or not involving clergy in the care of their patients.

To address these issues, we studied family physicians nationwide about their experiences with referring patients to clergy and pastoral care providers. We used the terms *pastoral care* and *clergy* and the terms *religion* and *spirituality* interchangeably for the purposes of the study, although there are differences in how each is defined.[12] In addition, we did not distinguish between *consultation* and *referral,* despite the spectrum of physician understanding of these terms.[13] Our objectives were to identify the prevalence and patterns of physician-directed patient referral or recommended consultation to clergy or pastoral care providers and to describe attitudinal and demographic variables that can predict referring and nonreferring physicians.

Methods

Study Population

The study was reviewed and approved by the Human Subjects Committee of the University of Kansas Medical Center, Kansas City, before its initiation. Study subjects were selected from the membership list of the American Academy of Family Physicians (AAFP), Kansas City, Mo. Physicians who were active members of the AAFP (n=44,194) and whose self-designated professional activity was direct patient care were eligible for the study. The requirements for active AAFP membership include family practice residency training, unrestricted licensure, specified continuing medical education, and engagement in the practice, teaching, or administration of family practice or in the practice of emergency medicine.[14] By using these criteria, a randomized sample of 756 physicians was obtained from the AAFP.

Methods and Survey Content

A self-administered, anonymous survey was mailed to all eligible physicians during October 1997. Enclosed with each survey was a preaddressed, stamped, return envelope; a cover letter from the senior investigator explaining the nature of the survey and our affiliation with the University of Kansas Medical Center; and an invitation to participate. Approximately 2 weeks after the initial mailing, all subjects were sent a postcard reminder. Data collection was completed in December 1997.

The survey consisted of 11 fixed-response items, 5 questions that gathered demographic information, and 1 open-ended question that asked for comments. The survey was prefaced with the instruction, "Please circle the answer that most accurately describes your feelings and choices." Four survey questions, which were included to measure under what circumstances, if any, physicians refer or recommend patients to pastoral care providers and clergy, were taken from a previous survey that also studied these issues.[9] Two 5-point Likert-scale questions were used to assess physicians' attitudes toward the role of clergy in patient care. One item addressed perceived importance to patients of religion and spirituality, since this has been found to be a significant variable for determining which physicians refer or recommend geriatric patients to clergy.[10] The other attitudinal item focused on the contribution of clergy and pastoral care providers to patient care and was designed specifically for this study.

Five questions were included to measure physician religious beliefs and practices. Items were derived from questions developed by the National Opinion Research Center, Chicago, Ill[15] and the Index of Core Spiritual Experiences scale.[16] The Index of Core Spiritual Experiences scale was developed from the National Opinion Research Center, which is the oldest national survey research facility that is nonprofit and university-affiliated. The 5 questions asked about the frequency of private religious or spiritual practices and the frequency of religious service attendance and assessed subjective or intrinsic religiosity.

The final section of the survey requested data on physician characteristics, such as sex, age, length of practice, primary practice site, and religious denomination. Questions were pretested and revised after pilot testing with a group of eligible physicians at our institution. Physicians from the pilot group were excluded from the sample. Fewer than 5 minutes were needed to complete the survey.

Data Analysis

After recoding and reverse scoring the items as necessary, descriptive statistics for responses to the clergy referral questions and physician characteristics were calculated. For questions in which respondents could choose more than 1 option, each option was treated as a separate item. Returned surveys that were only partially completed by subjects were included in the data set, and individual items not completed were excluded from analysis.

To compare physicians who refer to clergy with nonreferring physicians, responses to the 6 clergy referral items were summed to create a single score that represented tendency to refer to clergy. The Cronbach α was calculated as a measure of the internal reliability of the resulting measure. Analyses of variance were conducted for age, length of practice, primary practice site, and self-reported religious denomination to compare the tendency to refer to clergy across different demographic variables. A t test was performed using the sex data set. The dependent variable in each of these tests was the total score on the clergy referral scale. A 2-sided P value of less than .05 was considered statistically significant. For any significant result in the analysis of variance, a post hoc means comparison was conducted. All analyses were performed by using the Statistical Package for the Social Sciences, version 7.5 (SPSS, Chicago, Ill).

Results

Response Rate

Of the 756 surveys that were mailed, 1 was returned as undeliverable. The response rate was 57.9% (438 of 756 physicians); 386 completed surveys were received after the first mailing. The AAFP provided demographic information about the membership, and Table 1 gives the comparison of the characteristics of the study physicians with those of the active membership of the AAFP. All proportions were statistically different from the AAFP population, but only the proportion of respondents at an urban or rural primary practice site was considered meaningfully different. Because of unequal sample sizes and proportions, we did not perform a statistical analysis.

Prevalence and Patterns of Referral to Clergy

More than 80% of physicians reported that they refer or recommend their patients to clergy and pastoral care providers. Table 2 lists the frequency of physician-directed referral to clergy during a year. Only 12.6% of the respondents reported that they never refer patients to

Table 1. Characteristics of Study Physicians and AAFP-Member Physicians*

Characteristic	Study Physicians	AAFP Membership
Sex	n=397	n=44,191
Male	80.3	79.1
Female	19.7	20.9
Age, y	n=420	n=44,123
< 30	1.2	1.1
30–40	32.7	35.8
41–55	48.6	44.5
56–65	9.9	11.9
> 65	7.6	6.6
Primary practice site	n=434	n=26,260
Urban	56.4	68.4
Rural	43.6	31.6

*Data for the American Academy of Family Physicians (AAFP) members were provided by the AAFP, Kansas City, Mo, and were current as of January 1, 1995. Data are reported as percentages unless otherwise indicated.

Table 2. Physician-Reported Referral to Clergy*

Item/Response	% of Respondents
I refer or recommend my patients to clergy and pastoral care providers (n=430).	
Yes	80.2
No	19.8
In a year, I refer or recommend consultation with clergy and pastoral care providers (n=428).	
Never	12.6
1–2 times	15.2
3–4 times	12.9
5–6 times	16.1
7–10 times	13.1
More than 10 times	30.1

*SE, ± 4.7 percentage points.

clergy, while 30.1% reported that they refer more than 10 times during a year.

Table 3 gives the indications or reasons for clergy referral. Approximately 75% of physicians chose conditions and diagnoses associated with end-of-life care (ie, terminal illness, bereavement) as reasons for referral. Marital and family counseling were cited by 72.8% of physicians; however, other psychosocial issues, such as depression and mood disorders (38.7%) and substance abuse (19.0%), were less prevalent. Table 4 lists reasons that physicians do not refer to clergy. The belief that "patients will self-refer anyway," was noted by 13.3% of physicians as the major reason for nonreferral.

Clergy Referral Scale

One response to the question asking reasons for nonreferral did not correlate well with other clergy referral items.

Table 3. Physician-Reported Indications for Clergy Referral (n=437)*

Condition or Diagnosis	% of Respondents
Bereavement	76.2
Terminal illness	74.8
Marital and family counseling	72.8
Religious or spiritual problems	64.3
Depression and mood disorders	38.7
Substance abuse	19.0
Reproductive health issues	11.0
None	10.3
Other	4.6

*SE, ± 4.7 percentage points.

Table 4. Physician-Reported Reasons for Nonreferral to Clergy (n=427)*

Reason Cited	% of Respondents
Patients will self-refer anyway	13.3
Other	7.3
Do not know the "right" clergy	6.6
Nonreligious patients would be offended	4.8
Previous bad experience with clergy	3.2
Not my responsibility to make referral	2.1

*SE, ± 4.7 percentage points.

The low percentage of respondents (38.2%) who chose the response, "I do refer or recommend to clergy," suggested that many physicians did not respond at all to this item, even if they do actually refer in practice. This item was not included in the referral to clergy scale. In addition, after an initial internal consistency analysis, we found that the overall reliability of the scale could be improved by removing the item that represented the "other condition" response option under the question that asked for conditions or diagnoses for referral. These slight revisions resulted in a Cronbach α for this scale of .82, indicating adequate reliability. The mean score of this scale was 17.91 (SD, 4.30), with a range of scores from 7 to 25.

Relation of Tendency to Refer and Level of Religious Belief

Total scores on the clergy referral scale were correlated with total scores on a scale of religiosity. High religiosity scores indicated strong intrinsic religious belief and frequent practice of private and corporate religious and spiritual behaviors (α=.87). The Pearson product moment correlation between the 2 sets of scores was .39 (P=.01), indicating a small to moderate positive correlation.

Differences in Tendency to Refer to Clergy

Among the demographic variables we assessed (ie, age, sex, primary practice site, self-reported religious denomination, and length of practice), only the length of practice demonstrated significant differences in tendency to refer to clergy. Physicians in practice from 16 to 25 years scored significantly higher than other physicians within this category (Table 5). However, a post hoc analysis with Bonferroni controls found that this group of physicians did not differ significantly from any of the other 3 categories of length of practice. We then collapsed the 4 length-of-practice groups into 2 groups: those practicing 15 years or less and those practicing 16 years or more. A *t* test showed a significant difference between these groups, with physicians who were in practice longer having a greater tendency to refer to clergy (Table 5).

Comment

Whether viewed as an alternative practice or as an integrative and complementary adjunct to conventional medical care, the role of spiritual and religious providers of care in clinical practice remains largely unexplored. Our results suggest that these providers may have a larger and more expanded role in clinical care than previously reported. More than 80% of the physicians in the present study referred or recommended consultation with clergy, with most (59.3%) referring more than 4 times a year. When queried in a different fashion, only 12.6% of physicians reported that they never refer to clergy in a given year (Table 2).

The call for research to further understand the consultation and referral process has been placed within the context of 4 domains: (1) describing the pattern of consultation and referral, (2) understanding the components of the consultation and referral decision, (3) describing the costs and outcomes of consultation and referral, and (4) developing better strategies for consultation and referral.[13] Our purpose in this study focused on the first of these domains and was 2-fold: (1) to identify the prevalence and patterns of physician-directed patient referral to or recommended consultation with clergy or pastoral care providers and (2) to describe attitudinal and demographic variables that can predict referring and nonreferring physicians.

Jones[9] studied British general practitioners and defined 4 groups of clergy referrers: 43% were nonreferrers; 44% were occasional referrers (1–6 cases per year); 9% were regular referrers (7–12 cases per year); and 4% were frequent referrers (more than 13 cases per year). In 2 studies conducted in the United States, Koenig et al[10,11] found that fewer than one half of physicians (45% and 49%) reported a usual pattern of clergy referral for their patients or initiated a referral to clergy services. Each of these studies was limited by a nonrandom study population and a sampling method that recruited subjects from a similar geographic area, which may limit the generalizability to other physician populations.

Physicians consult and refer patients for several reasons: for diagnosis, treatment, or both; for patient, relative, or referring physician reassurance; for specific examinations or specialty procedures; and for medicolegal reasons.[13] With the exception of marital and family counseling, we preferentially selected patient conditions or diagnoses rather than specific therapeutics as potential indications and reasons for referral, since patients are more likely to have seen a consultant if the referral was for advice on management of a problem, rather than for a specified treatment.[17] In our study and the study by Jones,[9] end-of-life care was the leading condition cited as a reason for clergy referral. Whether the prevalence of physician-directed clergy referral actually occurs in clinical practice remains unclear, since studies involving end-of-life care are largely silent on this topic.[18]

Approximately 73% of physicians listed marital and family counseling as a condition for referral to clergy, although fewer than half chose other psychosocial conditions (ie, depression and mood disorders, substance abuse) commonly seen in a primary care practice. This selection by physicians of religious or spiritual providers for family and marriage problems parallels patient-reported preferences. Most patients opt for religious counseling for domestic problems and nonreligious counseling for mental illness and addictive disorders.[19]

Almost two thirds (64.3%) of physicians in our survey cited religious or spiritual problems as a condition for referral. The *Diagnostic and Statistical Manual of Mental Disorders, Fourth Edition*[7] lists religious or spiritual problem as a V code (V62.89), or a condition that may be a focus of clinical attention. End-of-life care and family and marital counseling are frequently distressing experiences that can involve an unstable religious or spiritual state. The high response to each of these conditions suggests a recognition of additional and overlapping diagnoses. Perhaps physicians expressed a greater sensitivity to value-laden and culturally laden experiences by acknowledging a referral to clergy. Another explanation is that physicians may have responded to an overt patient request to address their spiritual and religious needs during the clinical encounter.

To identify physicians who refer to clergy from nonreferring physicians, we developed a scale that incorporated physician attitudes and behaviors. The measure was a reliable instrument (α=.82), which enabled us to study physi-

Table 5. Length of Physician Practice and Tendency to Refer to Clergy

Length of Practice, y	Tendency to Refer to Clergy Score, Mean ± SD	Test Value	*P*
Analysis of 4 groups			
<5 (n=65)	17.00 ± 4.49		
5-15 (n=176)	17.65 ± 4.39		
16-25 (n=100)	18.69 ± 4.11	F=2.65	.05
>25 (n=75)	18.41 ± 4.02		
Analysis of 2 groups*			
≤15 (n=241)	17.48 ± 4.41		
≥16 (n=175)	18.57 ± 4.06	*t*=2.58	.01

*Because of unequal group size, the Levene test for equality of variances was conducted. Variances were found to be statistically equal.

cian characteristics more accurately. Physician religiosity had a small to moderately positive correlation with a tendency to refer to clergy. This finding is congruent with that of Koenig and colleagues[11] who found that physicians with less religiosity referred patients to pastoral care services less often than other physicians. Among the demographic variables, only the length of practice was statistically significant for identifying referring physicians (Table 5), a finding reported in another study on the consultation and referral patterns of family physicians.[20] Physicians in practice for 16 years or longer scored higher on our scale of tendency to refer. Age, primary practice site, sex, and self-reported religious denomination were not significant variables.

Our study had several limitations. There is generally no formal documentation of the referral process to clergy and pastoral care providers in clinical practice, in contrast to the documentation of other types of consultation and referral in primary care.[13] This drawback, in addition to the absence of claims data, markedly hampers research in this area. Logs maintained by clergy[21] remain a source of data, but they are limited to institutionally based physicians and patients. Owing to the lack of these sources of data, it is difficult to validate whether our study measured actual behavior (ie, referral) or an attitude toward referring. The lack of physician economic and administrative incentives or prohibitions tied to clergy referral led us to believe that our findings reflect referral behavior, as well as attitude.

A higher proportion of our study population reported a rural primary practice site than did the general AAFP membership. Rural physicians may not have the same access as their more urban colleagues to social work and mental health professionals in their communities. In such settings, clergy and pastoral care providers may be viewed as the primary available resource in these ancillary fields. Although the higher proportion of rural practitioners could have accounted for the reported referral rates and reasons for referral in our study, the primary practice site was not found to be a significant variable in identifying a tendency to refer.

Good item construction from established measures, pilot testing and scale refinement, and a high α coefficient support the reliability and validity of our instrument scales. Although our response rate of 57.9% was modest, it is comparable with other survey studies of clinicians in active clinical practice.[22,23] The sample population was family physicians, and the generalizability of these findings to other specialties is unclear.

We found that 80.2% of physicians refer patients to clergy and pastoral care providers, with a majority (59.3%) referring more than 4 times a year. End-of-life care and marital and family counseling were cited as the major conditions for referral. More religious physicians and physicians in practice for 16 years or more tended to refer more than did other physicians. Directions for future research include studying specialty differences and the clinical decision-making process for clergy referral. There is also great promise and usefulness in outcomes-based studies, which can explore the effect of these providers on such areas as patient satisfaction, cost of care, and changes in general health and functional status.

Dr Daaleman is a Robert Wood Johnson Generalist Physician Faculty Scholar (Career Development Award).

We thank Cynda A. Johnson, MD, Jasjit S. Ahluwalia, MD, MPH, MS, and Ken Kallail, PhD for their review of the manuscript.

References

1. Eisenberg DM, Kessler RC, Foster C, et al. Unconventional medicine in the United States: prevalence, costs, and patterns of use. *N Engl J Med.* 1993;328:246–252.

2. Berman BM, Singh BK, Lao L, et al. Physicians' attitudes toward complementary or alternative medicine: a regional survey. *J Am Board Fam Pract.* 1995;8:361–366.

3. Gallup Poll. *Religion in America: 1990.* Princeton, NJ: Princeton Religion Research Center; 1990.

4. Furnham A. Explaining health and illness: lay perceptions on current and future health, the causes of illness, and the nature of recovery. *Soc Sci Med.* 1994;39:715–725.

5. King M, Speck P, Thomas A. Spiritual and religious beliefs in acute illness: is this a feasible area for study? *Soc Sci Med.* 1994; 38:631–636.

6. Daaleman TP, Nease DE. Patient attitudes regarding physician inquiry into spiritual and religious issues. *J Fam Pract.* 1994;39:564–568.

7. American Psychiatric Association. *Diagnostic and Statistical Manual of Mental Disorders, Fourth Edition.* Washington, DC: American Psychiatric Association; 1994:685.

8. Turner RP, Lukoff D, Barnhouse RT, et al. Religious or spiritual problem: a culturally sensitive diagnostic category in the *DSM-IV. J Nerv Ment Dis.* 1995;183:435–444.

9. Jones AW. A survey of general practitioners' attitudes to the involvement of clergy in patient care. *Br J Gen Pract.* 1990;40:280–283.

10. Koenig HG, Bearon LB, Dayringer R. Physician perspectives on the role of religion in the physician–older patient relationship. *J Fam Pract.* 1989;28:441–448.

11. Koenig HG, Bearon LB, Hover M, et al. Religious perspectives of doctors, nurses, patients, and families. *J Pastoral Care.* 1991; 45:254–267.

12. Daaleman TP. A cartography of spirituality in end-of-life care. *Bioethics Forum.* 1997; 13:49–52.

13. Nutting PA, Franks P, Clancy CM. Referral and consultation in primary care: do we understand what we are doing? *J Fam Pract.* 1992;35:21–23.

14. American Academy of Family Physicians. *American Academy of Family Physicians Membership & Resource Directory: 1997–1998.* Kansas City, Mo: American Academy of Family Physicians; 1997:11.

15. Davis JA, Smith TW. *General Social Surveys, 1972–1985.* Chicago, Ill: National Opinion Research Center; 1985.

16. Kass JD, Friedman R, Leserman J, et al. Health outcomes and a new index of spiritual experience. *J Sci Stud Religion.* 1991;30:203–211.

17. Bourguet C, Gilchrist V, McCord G, et al. The consultation and referral process: a report from NEON. *J Fam Pract.* 1998;46:47–53.

18. Steinmetz D, Walsh M, Gabel LL, et al. Family physicians' involvement with dying patients and their families: attitudes, difficulties, and strategies. *Arch Fam Med.* 1993;2:753–761.

19. Privette G, Quakenbos S, Bundrick CM. Preferences for religious or nonreligious counseling and psychotherapy. *Psychol Rep.* 1994; 75:539–546.

20. Brock C. Consultation and referral patterns of family physicians. *J Fam Pract.* 1977; 4:1129–1134.

21. Sharp CG. Use of the chaplaincy in the neonatal intensive care unit. *South Med J.* 1991; 84:1482–1486.

22. Tunis SR, Hayward RS, Wilson MC, et al. Internists' attitudes about clinical practice guidelines. *Ann Intern Med.* 1994;120:956–963.

23. Halm EA, Causino N, Blumenthal D. Is gatekeeping better than traditional care? a survey of physician's attitudes. *JAMA.*1997;278:1677–1681.

9 Alternative Medicine Use by Homeless Youth

Cora Collette Breuner, MD; Paul J. Barry, MSW; Kathi J. Kemper, MD, MPH

From the Departments of Pediatrics (Dr Breuner) and Health Services (Dr Kemper), University of Washington; 45th Street Clinic Youth Program (Mr Barry); and the Family Medicine Residency at Swedish Medical Center (Drs Breuner and Kemper), Seattle, Wash.

Background

Mainstream health care for homeless youth is often fragmented or unavailable.

Objective

To evaluate the use of complementary and alternative medicine (CAM) by homeless youth who use our free clinic.

Design

Self-administered cross-sectional survey.

Subjects and Methods

Subjects included homeless youth between the ages of 14 and 21 years receiving care at the 45th Street Clinic Youth Program in Seattle, Wash, between January 29, 1998, and March 5, 1998. The self-administered survey included items on demographics, health issues, use frequency of different therapists or therapies, referral sources, and perceived effectiveness of treatment.

Results

The response rate by patients was 96.3% (157/163) with an average respondent age of 18.5 years (range, 14–21 years). Complementary and alternative medicine was used by 70.1% of the subjects. Referrals most often came from friends (52.7%). The most common reason for using CAM was because it was "natural" (43.9%). Most of those who used alternative therapies (87.3%) believed they had been helped "some" or "a lot." Given a choice of providers to visit when they were ill, 51.7% would seek care from a physician, 36.9% from a CAM provider, and 11.4% would treat themselves.

Conclusions

Care with CAM is frequently used and accepted by homeless youth. Cost-effectiveness and contributions to overall health care require additional evaluation. Integrating CAM into allopathic health centers may serve as an incentive to entice youth into mainstream health care.

Arch Pediatr Adolesc Med. 1998;152:1071–1075

Adolescents are generally healthy, and morbidity rates for adult medical conditions, such as heart disease and cancer, are low. However, adolescence may be associated with preventable morbidity, mortality, and poor health habits. Accidents, suicide, and homicide are the leading causes of death, while sexually transmitted diseases, substance abuse, pregnancy, and homelessness yield substantial physical and emotional morbidity.[1]

A major role of health supervision is the periodic assessment and support of the adolescent's ability to adapt to the challenges and risks attendant to growing up. The annual health guidance and screening visits recommended by the American Medical Association's *AMA Guidelines for Adolescent Preventive Services (GAPS)*[2] and *Bright Futures*[3] provide adolescents with a sense of confidence and knowledge of good health habits. During these visits, teenagers are encouraged to develop the responsibility to make healthy choices and be actively involved in decisions regarding delivery of their own health care.[4]

Despite these recommendations, many adolescents lack access to health care. In the National Medical Education Survey of 1987, one third of adolescents (8 million) did not receive medical care. Reasons cited include lack of insurance, low income, perceived racial barriers, and general mistrust of authority.[5]

The homeless encounter similar barriers to health care. Homelessness is now a major social problem in the United States, affecting both small and large cities. Estimates of the total numbers of homeless people range from 250,000 and 3 million.[6] Homeless men, women, and children make up a growing population highly susceptible to preventable diseases, which may lead to premature death.[7] Unfortunately, their health care use is fragmented and delayed by both internal and external barriers such as cost, transience, location, and perceived acceptance.[8,9]

Homeless adolescents, a subset of this population, are among the most medically needy and underserved people in the United States.[10] Street youths have many acute and chronic health problems, such as malnutrition, respiratory tract infections, headaches, soft tissue trauma, dental problems, and mental illness.[11] Their high-risk lifestyle leads to serious individual health consequences, such as sexually transmitted diseases, substance abuse, pregnancy, and trauma.[10,12] In a recent study,[13] homeless youth were at least twice as likely as those visiting a school-based clinic to be depressed, abuse drugs, and visit the emergency department.

The formidable barriers to comprehensive health care for all adolescents are amplified for homeless youth.[14,15] Money, consent, confidentiality, and alienation frequently present hurdles to receiving services.[16] Mainstream allopathic care is often fragmented, not relevant to their needs, or inaccessible.[17–19] As a result, conventional medical care is unavailable and treatment is often delayed. Most youth are asked for identification, permanent address, proof of insurance, and parental permission for treatment when requesting health care. Vital to utilization of health care by homeless youth is an open and caring environment that is both physically and psychologically accessible to them. Many homeless youth have been exploited or deceived by adults and mistrust health professionals and the traditional health care system.[20]

Disenchantment with mainstream medicine is 1 reason more Americans are turning to complementary or alternative medicine (CAM).[21] Approximately one third of American adults use CAM for health problems.[22] Complementary or alternative medicine treatments are medical interventions not generally taught at US medical schools or not usually available at US hospitals. Examples of CAM include chiropractic, acupuncture, naturopathy, herbal medicine, massage therapy, megavitamins, homeopathy, aromatherapy, and meditation.[23] People who use alternative medicine are generally more educated and in higher economic strata.[22,24] In a study[25] of the use of alternative medicine by children, 3 major characteristics differentiated users from nonusers: the child's age (children were more likely to use CAM if they were older than 1 year), parental use of alternative medicine, and higher maternal education level. Patients with serious chronic illnesses, eg, cancer, cystic fibrosis, and juvenile arthritis, are especially likely to use CAM. Use rates for people in these groups may approach 66%.[26–28]

Little is known about the characteristics of those who use alternative therapy among underserved populations, specifically homeless adolescents, or on the perceived effectiveness of such treatments. Homeless youth could have either higher or lower use of CAM compared with the general population. Potential reasons for CAM use by homeless youth are that they are at high risk for chronic illness and addiction, mainstream care is unavailable, and they are leery of authority. Homeless youth may perceive CAM has unique advantages because it fits into their value system that includes an alternative lifestyle; a preference for the natural; and a reliance on themselves, their peers, and their street culture to solve problems rather than mainstream authorities.[19] The barriers to mainstream health care may create a direct incentive to consider CAM.[15] Alternatively, CAM use by homeless youth may be infrequent because the lack of parental role models (or even reverse effect of parental role models [ie, parental role models may negatively influence youth practices because youths rebel against parental authority, values, or examples]), low educational level, and decreased availability or promotion to this population. Another disadvantage of CAM use is that it is not reimbursed by most insurance plans and the youth may be unable to pay for it.

The extent of CAM use, conditions for which it is sought, and referral patterns among homeless youth are unknown. We evaluated patterns of CAM use by homeless youth to learn how they select health care and to enhance our ability to meet their complex health needs. Specifically, the following were our study questions: *What CAM treatments do homeless youth most commonly seek? Who refers them? Why do they use alternatives? What is the perceived effectiveness of these treatments by homeless youth?*

Subjects and Methods

To answer these questions, we performed an anonymous, cross-sectional survey in a free clinic serving homeless youth in Seattle, Wash. Subjects were eligible for the study if they were between the ages of 14 and 21 years and attended the 45th Street Clinic Youth Program between January 29, 1998, and March 5, 1998. Obviously mentally ill or acutely intoxicated subjects were excluded from the survey.

The Youth Program is a special operation of the 45th Street Clinic, a community health center whose mission is to provide health care to low-income people of all ages who otherwise could not afford it. Free primary health care for homeless and at-risk street youth is offered on a drop-in basis on Tuesday and Thursday evenings from 6 PM to 9 PM. Follow-up is provided during regular daytime clinic hours. Special focus is placed on providing a safe, supportive, and accessible environment for homeless youth that is sensitive to their needs.

The Youth Program serves 25 to 40 teenagers each evening. Of these, 20% to 30% are new patients. The program has adopted a comprehensive approach to treat its young patients.[29] Program staff includes a social worker, nurse practitioner, medical assistants, receptionist, laboratory technician, pharmacist, and counselors for mental health, drug and alcohol, and human immunodeficiency virus (HIV). A large cadre of volunteer physicians, nurse practitioners, and physician assistants provide primary clinical care. The Swedish Family Practice residency also provides 2 family practice residents and their preceptor.

Prompted by a need first expressed by the patients, the program staff explored offering CAM. The medical philosophy of the program (ie, care should be youth centered and multidisciplinary) resonated with the values of CAM (ie, patient driven and holistic). The program staff hoped that, by providing CAM, they could encourage even the hardest-to-engage youths to use the clinic. Complementary and alternative medicine also appeared to reflect the counterculture values and distrust of traditional institutions some of these youth espoused. Providers of CAM include an acupuncturist and acupuncture students from the Northwest Institute of Acupuncture and Oriental Medicine, Seattle, Wash. The program staff also includes 4 students and a preceptor from the Bastyr University Natural Health Clinic, 1 of 4 schools of naturopathy in the United States. Complementary and alternative medicine services, which are also free, can only be obtained by referral from the allopathic medical providers at the clinic.

The survey was initially tested with peer outreach workers who are former homeless youth. After modification, the survey was tested again with youth visiting the clinic. The final revised version was distributed between January 29, 1998, and March 5, 1998 (Figure 1).

The subjects read the cover letter or had it read to them by a volunteer who approached potential subjects after they registered. The cover letter explained in simple terms the reasons for the survey, the significance of the research, an assurance of anonymity, and an assurance of care even if they declined to participate. They received a coupon for a free cup of coffee or hot chocolate as an incentive for participating in the study.

The self-administered survey contained 2 pages of questions and took less than 5 minutes to complete. There were 4 demographic items: age, sex, last year of school completed, and duration of homelessness. There was 1 question concerning the health problems in the past 6 months and 1 question on the reason for the current visit.

There were 2 questions concerning the CAM treatments homeless youth may have sought in the past 6 months (herbs, vitamins, special diets, special exercise, and aromatherapy) and practitioners they may have seen (acupuncturists, naturopaths, homeopaths, and chiropractors). There was 1 question concerning who referred the youth to CAM, and 1 question on the reason for the use of alternative types of therapies. There was 1 question on the perceived efficacy of such treatments and 1 question on

1. How old are you?
2. Are you male or female?
3. How many times have you been to this clinic in the past year? (Please circle one reply.)
 1-5
 6-10
 7-14
 ≥15
4. Why did you come to the clinic tonight?
5. What was the last year of school that you finished?
6. How long have you been homeless?
7. What are three health problems that you have had in the past 6 months?
 a.
 b.
 c.
8. What remedies have you tried to treat those problems? (Please check all that apply.)
 Antibiotics or other prescription medications
 Surgery
 Psychotherapy (counseling)
 Herbal remedies (for example, echinacea, St John's wort, ephedra)
 Vitamins and minerals (B_6, zinc, vitamin C)
 Special diet (for example, vegetarian, macrobiotic)
 Special exercise
 Acupuncture
 Massage or bodywork
 Aromatherapy
 Mind body meditation, hypnosis, or biofeedback
 Reiki
 Homeopathy
 Chiropractic or craniosacral therapy
 Other:
9. In the past 6 months, how many times have you visited each of the following health care providers?

Provider	Number of Visits
Doctor or nurse practitioner	
Nurse	
Counselor or therapist	
Drug or alcohol counselor	
Chiropractor	
Acupuncturist	
Naturopath	
Massage therapist	
Psychic healer	
Other:	

10. Who told you that alternative medicine would help? (Please check all boxes that apply.)
 Friend
 Outreach worker
 Doctor or nurse practitioner
 Social worker
 Case manager
 Family member
 Other:
11. Why do you use alternative therapy? (Please check all that apply.)
 Because it is inexpensive
 Because my friends use it and recommend it
 Because I prefer natural and organic remedies
 Because it works better than traditional medicine
 Because I have had negative experiences with medical doctors
 Because alternative providers care about me more than doctor
 Other: (Please add any reasons you may have.)
12. How much do you think alternative therapy has helped you?
 A lot
 Some
 A little
 Not at all
13. If you had a sore throat and a fever, who would you want to see first? (Check one.)
 Doctor or nurse practitioner
 Naturopath
 Acupuncturist
 Other:
14. Is there anything else you would like to say about different medicines and therapies available at the 45th Street Youth Clinic? Your opinions are greatly appreciated!

Figure 1. Homeless youth alternative medicine survey.

the desired health provider if the subject had a sore throat and a fever.

Data were entered on EXCEL spreadsheet (EXCEL 7.0, Microsoft, Seattle, Wash) and analyzed using simple summary statistics.

This study was approved by the University of Washington Human Subjects Committee.

Results

Of 163 questionnaires distributed, 157 (96.3%) were returned and analyzed. The 6 excluded subjects included 5 who were older than 21 years and 1 who did not want to finish the survey. The average age of respondents was 18.5 years (range, 14–21 years); 38.2% were male. The average last year of school completed was 10.6 years, with responses ranging from 8th grade to some college. Nearly 72% of the respondents were homeless. Slightly more than 28% of the respondents had tentative housing situations or were estranged from families. Of the respondents who were homeless, 48.6% had been for less than a year, 19.4% for 1 to 2 years, and 31.8% for longer than 2 years.

More than 78% of the youth had visited the clinic in the past 6 months for an acute medical problem such as an upper respiratory tract infection, vaginal or penile discharge, diarrhea, or musculoskeletal injury. Approximately 66.2% of the respondents reported chronic health problems, including asthma, back pain, stomach pain, or headaches. About 26.1% reported mental health issues such as stress, anxiety, or depression. More than 10% were concerned about their use of drugs or alcohol. Slightly more than 40% of the respondents had visited the clinic more than 5 times in the past 6 months. The reasons for the current visit included preventative care (31.1%) such as contraception, HIV screening, and physical examinations; medical problems (46.5%); seeking CAM care (11.2%); and "came with a friend" (11.2%).

The average number of visits in the past 6 months to an allopathic medical doctor was 5.3; to a mental health or drug and alcohol counselor, 4.3; and to a CAM provider, 2.5.

In the past 6 months, 81.3% used allopathic or mainstream forms of therapy, 44.6% used mental health services, and 70.1% used CAM (Table 1). The percentages total more than 100% because respondents could check more than 1 form of treatment. The most frequently used forms of CAM therapies were vitamins (76.4%) and herbs (73.6%). Other forms of treatments frequently used were diet (40.9%), massage therapy (38.2%), exercise (31.8%), acupuncture (27.2%), meditation (26.4%), aromatherapy (21.8%), homeopathy (17.3%), and chiropractic (11.8%).

Table 1. Percentage of Therapies Used by Homeless Youth in the Past 6 Months

Type of Therapy	Subjects Reporting Use (n=157), %
Allopathic (mainstream)*	81.3
Counseling	44.6
Complementary and alternative medicine	70.1
Vitamins	76.4
Herbs†	73.6
Special diet†	40.9
Massage	38.2
Special exercise	31.6
Acupuncture	27.2
Meditation	26.4
Aromatherapy	21.8
Homeopathy	17.3
Chiropractic	11.8
Shaman, magic, psychic healer, flower tea, fasting	7.3
Reiki	4.5

*Examples of allopathic or mainstream treatment would be prescription medications or surgery.
†Examples of herbs used would be echinacea, St John's wort, or ephedra; of special diets, vegetarian or macrobiotic.

Slightly more than 7% of the youth used shamans, psychic healers, magic spells, and flower teas.

The most frequent sources of referrals to CAM treatments follow. Nearly 53% of the youth were referred by friends, 21.8% by physicians or nurse practitioners, 20.9% by outreach workers or case managers, 20.4% by family members, and 14% by social workers. A little more than 18% were self-referred.

The most common reason for using CAM was because it was natural and organic (43.9%); other reasons included low cost (28%), perceived efficacy (26.1%), negative experiences with physicians (24.2%), friends use CAM and recommend it (20%), and pervasive mistrust of physicians (19%).

A little more than 87% of the youth reported that they were helped "some" or "a lot" by CAM. In a hypothetical situation where the subject had a sore throat and a fever, 51.7% would seek care from a physician, 36.9% from a naturopath or acupuncturist, and 11.4% would treat themselves.

Comment

This is the first study of CAM use in the traditionally underserved population of homeless youth. The 70% CAM-use rate is higher than that shown in prior studies of the general adult or pediatric population. In fact, CAM use among these homeless youths is similar to that of people with cystic fibrosis.[27]

Is this prevalence unexpected? Unlike many teenagers who are seen only once a year for a sports physical, this group seeks health care at a much higher rate because of the risks inherent in their lifestyle. Their higher morbidity repeatedly brings them face-to-face with a system they mistrust yet have to rely upon. Use of CAM may allow them to take care of their own needs while maintaining their autonomy. Including CAM in an allopathic clinic may even be a selling point to encourage youth to seek health care.

These youth are usually referred by friends, verifying that the fraternity of the street is the principal support network for those whose lives have been shattered by physical and sexual abuse, family dysfunction, chaos, and alienation.[30] Friends' recommendations of CAM serves as one of the highest motivators and is greatly valued. Our study also found that mainstream physicians were an important referral source for CAM providers. A previous study[31] has shown that, despite the stereotype of nonacceptance, physicians do refer patients to a wide range of CAM providers, particularly chiropractors, acupuncturists, hypnotists, and spiritual healers. Another study[32] reported that more than half of the responding physicians recommended relaxation techniques, biofeedback, therapeutic massage, meditation, and hypnosis.

Unlike others who seek CAM out of frustration with mainstream medicine,[15] these subjects are driven by the values of organic and natural therapies. Many are vegetarian. Other important motivators include expense, caring, and perceived effectiveness. Their comments indicate that they are disaffected with materialism and technical societal values. These youth may have been disappointed by the health care system and other authorities, leading to a pervasive mistrust of anything presumed not "natural." Complementary and alternative medicine is psychologically more accessible to them than allopathic medicine because it matches their preferences for natural therapies, it is nonthreatening, and it allows them to retain a sense of control over their bodies.

These data raise at least 4 important questions: (1) If 70.1% of an underserved population is using some form of alternative treatment, is it really alternative? In our study, we included vitamins, diet, and exercise, which have been considered forms of alternative therapy in previous research.[22] Even excluding these forms of therapy, 73.6% of the respondents used herbs and 27.2% used acupuncture. (2) Since physicians are an important referral source for CAM, should there be more systematic training during and after medical school on the appropriate use of these therapies? (3) What impact do these treatments and therapies have on the overall health care costs for this high-risk population? (4) What is the overall impact of adding CAM therapies to other therapies in clinics serving underserved and vulnerable populations?

Despite these intriguing findings, this study has several limitations that need to be addressed in future studies. All participants were patients of a primary allopathic clinic. The study did not include youth who did not seek formal medical care and may have excluded those who use CAM exclusively. Seattle is replete with CAM providers and training schools: the Northwest School of Acupuncture and Oriental Medicine and the Bastyr University have clinics within the youth program. Lower access to CAM, such as in rural areas, may be associated with lower rates.

Also, there was no control group of youths attending similar clinics where there were no CAM providers on site. Adolescents attending our program may have chosen this clinic to have access to CAM. Future studies including other clinics may reveal more representative use patterns for this population.

More outcome studies need to be performed to determine the cost-effectiveness of CAM, particularly in those clinics where there is already an integrated system of CAM and allopathic care.[33] One such study[34] of a substance abuse treatment program showed that adding acupuncture helped clients recover. Such clinics already exist in Great Britain, where uniform practice aims and increased knowledge sharing has proven beneficial to their patients.[35]

Despite these limitations, our data have clinical and public health implications. The barriers to the use of mainstream health care by homeless youth include not only cost, confidentiality, and trust but also perceptions that mainstream care is not natural, organic, or compassionate. While most youth would seek care for a sore throat and fever from a physician, a substantial minority would turn to a CAM provider first. This may in part account for the delays in care so common among the homeless youth in the United States. This previously unrecognized reliance homeless adolescents have on CAM providers has implications for improving youth services. Every time alienated youths seek care from a clinic they feel is open and caring, they may get closer to mainstream health care, safer health practices, and eventually shelter and a reconnection to the community.

One of the major recommendations of the task force on homeless and runaway youth[14] is that creative multidisciplinary service strategies should be established. Integrating complementary medicine and health care services may be a beneficial intervention for this population.[36] Our study has revealed for the first time that homeless youth frequently use CAM and often prefer it to other treatments. They have different motivations for using CAM and are referred by different sources compared with previously studied populations. Important questions remain. Further research studies need to be undertaken, especially on the cost-effectiveness of an integrated comprehensive primary care clinic for underserved youth.

We thank Joanne Balintona for her help in distributing the survey, Chris Vincent, MD, for his editorial support, and Michelle Bell, PhD, for her thoughtful comments.

References

1. Ginsburg KR, Slap GB. Unique needs of the teen in the health care setting. *Curr Opin Pediatric.* 1996;8:111–118.
2. Elster A, ed. *AMA Guidelines of Adolescent Preventive Services (GAPS): Recommendations and Rationale.* Baltimore, Md: Williams & Wilkins; 1994.
3. Green M, ed. *Bright Futures: Guidelines for Health Supervision of Infants, Children, and Adolescents.* Arlington, Va: National Center for Education in Maternal and Child Health; 1994.
4. Jones R, Finlay F, Simpson N, Kreitman T. How can adolescents' health needs and concerns best be met? *Br J Gen Prac.* 1997;47:631–634.
5. Bartman BA, Moy E, D'Angelo L. Access to ambulatory care for adolescents: the role of a usual source of care. *J Health Care Poor Underserved.* 1997;8:214–226.
6. Department of Housing and Urban Development. *A Report to the Secretary on the Homeless and Emergency Shelters.* Washington, DC: Dept of Housing and Urban Development; 1984:18–19.
7. National Center of Children in Poverty. *Five Million Children: A Statistical Profile Of Our Poorest Young Citizens.* New York, NY: School of Public Health, Columbia University; 1990.
8. Plumb JD. Homelessness: care, prevention, and public policy. *Ann Intern Med.* 1997; 126:973–975.
9. Gallagher TL, Anderson RM, Koegel P, Gelberg L. Determinants of regular source of care among homeless adults in Los Angeles. *Med Care.* 1997;35:814–830.
10. Morey MA, Friedman LS. Health care needs of homeless adolescents. *Curr Opin Pediatr.* 1993; 5:395–399.
11. Deisher RW, Rogers WM. The medical care of street youth. *J Adolesc Health.* 1991; 12:500–503.
12. Kipke MD, O'Connor S, Palmer R, MacKenzie RG. Street youth in Los Angeles: profile of a group at high risk for human immunodeficiency virus infection. *Arch Pediatr Adolesc Med.* 1995;149:513–519.
13. Ensign J, Santelli J. Health status and service use: comparison of adolescents at a school-based health clinic with homeless adolescents. *Arch Pediatr Adolesc Med.* 1998; 152:20–24.
14. Farrow JA, Deisher RW, Brown R, Kulig JW, Kiple MD. Health and health needs of homeless and runaway youth. *J Adolesc Health.* 1992; 13:717–726.
15. Geber GM. Barriers to health care for street youth. *J Adolesc Health.* 1997;21:287–290.

16. Proimos J. Confidentiality issues in the adolescent population. *Curr Opin Pediatr.* 1997; 9:325–328.

17. Committee on Community Health Services, American Academy of Pediatrics. Health needs of homeless children and families. *Pediatrics.* 1996;98:789–791.

18. Sherman DJ. The neglected health care needs of street youth. *Public Health Rep.* 1992; 107:433–440.

19. Cauce AM, Paradise M, Embry L, et al. *Homeless Youth In Seattle: Youth Characteristics, Mental Health Needs, And Case Management*. Seattle, Wash: University of Washington; 1997. Technical report.

20. Council on Scientific Affairs. Health care needs of homeless and runaway youths. *JAMA.* 1989; 262:1358–1361.

21. Vincent C, Furnham A. Why do patients turn to complementary medicine? *Br J Clin Psychol.* 1996;35:37–48.

22. Eisenberg DM, Kessler RC, Foster C, Norlock FE, Calkins DR, Delbanco TL. Unconventional medicine in the United States. *N Engl J Med.* 1993; 328:246–252.

23. Jonas W. Alternative medicine and the conventional practitioner. *JAMA.* 1998;279:708–709.

24. Verhoef MJ, Sutherland LR. General practitioners' assessment of and interest in alternative medicine in Canada. *Soc Sci Med.* 1995; 41:511.

25. Spigelblatt L, Laine-Ammara G, Pless IB, Guyver A. The use of alternative medicine by children. *Pediatrics.* 1994;94:811–814.

26. Sawyer MG, Gannoni AF, Toogood IR, Antoniou G, Rice M. The use of alternative therapies by children with cancer. *Med J Aust.* 1994;160:320–322.

27. Stern RC, Canda ER, Doershuk CF. Use of nonmedical treatment by cystic fibrosis patients. *J Adolesc Health.* 1992;13:612–615.

28. Southwood TR, Malleson PN, Roberts-Thomson PJ, Mahy M. Unconventional remedies used for patients with juvenile arthritis. *Pediatrics.* 1990; 85:150–154.

29. Kemper KJ. Separation or synthesis: a holistic approach to therapeutics. *Pediatr Rev.* 1996;17:279–283.

30. Eisenstein E. Street youth: social imbalance and health risks. *J Pediatr Child Health.* 1993; 29(suppl 1):S46–S49.

31. Borkan J, Neher JO, Anson O, Smoker B. Referrals for alternative therapies. *J Fam Pract.* 1994;39:545–550.

32. Blumberg DL, Grant WD, Hendricks SR, Kamps CA, Dewan MJ. The physician and unconventional medicine. *Altern Ther Health Med.* 1995;1:31–35.

33. Jacobs JJ. Building bridges between two worlds: the NIH's Office of Alternative Medicine. *Acad Med.* 1995;70:40–41.

34. Konefal J, Duncan R, Clemence C. The impact of the addition of an acupuncture treatment program to an existing Metro-Dade county outpatient substance abuse treatment facility. *J Addict Dis.* 1994;13:71–99.

35. Patterson C, Peacock W. Complementary practitioners as part of the primary health care system: evaluation of one model. *Br J Gen Pract.* 1995;45:255–258.

36. La Valley JW, Verhoef MJ. Integrating complementary medicine and health care services into practice. *CMAJ.* 1995;153:45–59.

10 Home-Based Therapies for the Common Cold Among European American and Ethnic Minority Families

The Interface Between Alternative/Complementary and Folk Medicine

Lee M. Pachter, DO; Tracy Sumner, MA; Annette Fontan, MD; Mary Sneed, BS; Bruce A. Bernstein, PhD

From the Center for Children's Health and Development, Department of Pediatrics, Saint Francis Hospital and Medical Center, Hartford, Conn (Drs Pachter, Fontan, and Bernstein and Ms Sneed); Division of General Pediatrics, Department of Pediatrics, University of Connecticut School of Medicine, Farmington (Drs Pachter, Fontan, and Bernstein); and Department of Anthropology, University of Connecticut, Storrs (Drs Pachter and Bernstein and Ms Sumner).

Background

Most studies of alternative/complementary medicine use in children have focused on children with chronic illness and have not addressed the more common form of complementary medicine: popular home-based interventions and therapies for common low-morbidity sickness episodes. Also, there has often been a distinction between alternative/complementary medical practices used by the general population and those used by members of ethnic minority groups and commonly referred to as folk medicine or ethnomedicine.

Objective

To describe the home-based therapies and practices that parents from diverse ethnocultural backgrounds use to treat the common cold in their children.

Method

Interviews with mothers of children coming for care at a number of clinics and physicians' offices. Included were mothers from European American, African American, Puerto Rican, and West Indian–Caribbean heritages.

Results

Mean number of home-based remedies for the common cold did not differ among ethnic groups (controlling for maternal age, maternal education, number of children, and health insurance status). There were differences among groups regarding the frequency of use of specific remedies.

Conclusions

Home-based remedies for colds in childhood are commonly used. Many of the treatments are complementary to biomedical treatment (ie, antipyretics, over-the-counter cold remedies, fluids). Very few are potentially hazardous if taken in moderation. Mothers from ethnic minorities use similar amounts of home-based interventions when compared with mothers from the majority culture.

Arch Pediatr Adolesc Med. 1998;152:1083–1088

An early study of health care practices showed that 70% to 90% of self-recognized sickness episodes are managed outside of the formal health care system.[1] The increasing popularity of alternative/complementary medicine in recent years has further increased the options that patients and families have regarding health care interventions. *Health care* has been described by Kleinman[2] as a local system composed of 3 overlapping parts or sectors: (1) the professional sector, (2) the popular sector, and (3) the folk sector (Figure 1). The *professional* sector encompasses organized healing traditions, which by nature of their history and present usage are considered the dominant local healing paradigm. Western biomedicine is one such professional sector tradition, although others such as Ayurvedic and Traditional Chinese Medicine exist. The *popular* sector includes self-treatment, family care, and systems of community and socially based networks of care. Overall, most health care activities occur in this sector. The *folk* sector includes nonprofessional healers and practitioners who use alternative therapies based on paradigms external to the dominant professional (eg, biomedical) model.

It is important to appreciate the interactive and overlapping nature of these sectors. They are not exclusive options that are singularly used during a sickness episode or during health maintenance. Patients move among the 3 sectors of the health care system in both sequential and simultaneous manners. Because of this, it becomes important for biomedical clinicians to have a sense of what therapies their patients may be using in addition to the prescribed and recommended biomedical therapies and management plans. In an often-quoted study, it was shown that 1 of 3 adults interviewed by telephone reported having used at least 1 "unconventional" therapy in the past year, and 72% of those respondents did not inform their physicians about their use of alternative/complementary therapies.[3]

Alternative therapies, *alternative/complementary medicine*, and *holistic medicine* are terms connoting the vast array of therapies and techniques outside of the traditional biomedical approach that are currently very popular. They include lifestyle and mind-body techniques (eg, nutrition, exercise, environmental, meditation), biomechanical therapies (eg, massage, spinal manipulation), biochemical therapies (eg, herbs and nutritional supplements), and bioenergetic therapies (eg, therapeutic touch, acupuncture, *chi gong*, prayer, and homeopathy).[4] Although not exclusive to any one ethnic or socioeconomic group, the vast majority of users of alternative/ complementary medicine come from the majority cultural group, including the educated middle and upper socioeconomic classes.

Although not usually defined as alternative/complementary medicine, *folk medicine* or *ethnomedicine* describes various alternative practices and therapies that are used by members of a cultural minority group. Ethnic remedies and practices are common and, like alternative/complementary therapies, are often used in combination with the professional biomedical health care system. In fact, ethnomedicine can be thought of as a subset of alternative/complementary medicine.

Studies of ethnomedicine usually have been conducted in particular ethnic minority populations, for example, the study of folk remedies for asthma in a Puerto Rican community or the study of coining in Southeast Asian immigrants. Although these types of study provide important information about the beliefs and practices of patients in diverse communities, readers often get the incorrect implication that folk medicine, by nature, is only practiced in ethnic minority communities. Because of the lack of cross-cultural and cross-socioeconomic studies, it is difficult to place these beliefs and practices into a broader perspective, ie, that of alternative/complementary therapies (which usually are conducted on samples from the majority cultural groups). Indeed, many ethnic therapies become "alternative" or "holistic" therapies, but only after they have been embraced by the general population (an example being acupuncture).

A goal of culturally sensitive health care is to place cultural beliefs and practices in perspective. Different cultural groups have different ways of conceptualizing illness, but individuals from all cultural groups use the 3 sectors of the health care system, including the personal and folk

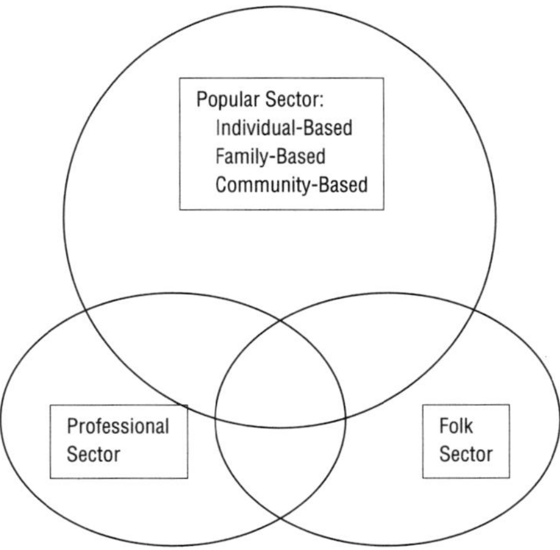

Figure 1. Kleinman's model of the health care system.[2] For an explanation of the sectors, see the Introduction.

sectors. It is the goal of the present study to identify home-based alternative and ethnic practices and approaches to a common childhood illness (the common cold) from a cross-cultural perspective. Our hypothesis is that personal, home-based practices for a common childhood sickness occur with similar frequency among families of diverse cultural groups, and that these practices are truly "complementary" to the professional biomedical system, and not an exclusive "alternative" to that system.

Subjects and Methods

Study Sample

Our study population consisted of parents who brought a child for care to 1 of 3 health care centers in the greater Hartford, Conn, area. One site was a hospital-based, inner-city pediatric clinic that serves a poor, multiethnic population; the second site was a family medicine private practice that primarily serves a Puerto Rican and African American working- and middle-class clientele; and a third site was a private pediatric practice that serves primarily a European American working- and middle-class clientele. These sites were chosen to obtain samples of respondents of different cultural affiliations and socioeconomic strata. In the greater Hartford area, the major ethnocultural groups are Puerto Rican, African American, European American (a term loosely used to describe the nonblack, non- Hispanic population, often referred to as *anglo*), and a smaller but growing number of individuals from the West Indian–Caribbean cultural area (including Jamaica, Guyana, Trinidad, Barbados, and Grand Cayman).

The study population consisted of parents (or primary caretakers) from the area's 4 predominant ethnocultural backgrounds with previous experience in child rearing. The study sample consisted of parents (or primary caregivers) who brought their children to 1 of these offices or clinics for either a well-child or an illness visit, and who had previous experience caring for a child with the common cold. Since the majority of parents and caretakers were mothers, for the remainder of the article, the term *mother* will be used.

A convenience sample of these mothers was selected at each site. Ethnocultural affiliation was determined by respondent self-report and birthplace.[5] We attempted to obtain socioeconomically varied samples for each of the ethnocultural groups (using health insurance status as a proxy for socioeconomic status).

Data Collection

Once a mother was identified as being eligible for inclusion (by ethnocultural affiliation and experience of caring for a child with a cold), she was interviewed by a research assistant (T.S., A.F., M.S.). The assistant explained that we were interested in learning about what parents do at home for common pediatric problems. They stated this to the mother as follows: "We are conducting a study of how parents manage common childhood illness. There are many things that a parent can do when their child has an illness, like a cold for example. Therapies and treatments other than those specifically recommended by a doctor or nurse are often used by people, especially when their child has a mild illness that may not require seeing or calling a doctor. We are interested in learning about these remedies and therapies."

We then asked if the parent had ever had to treat their child for a cold. If they answered affirmatively, we asked them to free-list the remedies or therapies that they have used to treat a cold.[6] The parents listed all the remedies and therapies that they could recall, as well as whether they thought the remedy was effective or not. If the parent was having trouble answering the question, the research assistant would prompt for answers by asking whether the mother had ever tried giving homemade remedies, special foods or herbs, vitamins or supplements, physical treatments, or spiritual therapies. In this way, a list was generated of all alternative remedies and therapies that the parent had tried, and the parent's estimation of the effectiveness of these remedies and therapies.

Statistical Analysis

Differences among ethnocultural groups in sociodemographic data were analyzed by analysis of variance or the χ^2 test, depending on whether the variable was continuous or discrete. The major analyses for this study were (1) differences in mean number of home-based therapies among ethnic groups, and (2) differences in specific remedies/therapies used among ethnocultural group. Differences in mean number of responses were determined through analysis of covariance, controlling for significant confounding variables (age of mother, education level of mother, number of children, and socioeconomic status). Differences in specific remedies/therapies were determined by analyzing the most common responses for each ethnocultural group.

We calculated that to find a difference of 0.67 SD in mean number of responses per group at an α level of .05 and a β level of .2, approximately 45 respondents were needed per ethnocultural group.

Results

During the study period, no mother refused to participate in this short interview while waiting to be seen by the clinician. We interviewed a total of 292 parents. Seven mothers' responses were excluded from the analysis because of missing data and 4 mothers had no previous experience in treating a child with a cold; therefore, our sample size is 281. The ethnocultural breakdown was as follows: European American, 85; African American, 68; Puerto Rican, 108; and West Indian–Caribbean, 20. All European American parents were either third-generation American (ie, respondent and both of her parents were born in the United States) or mixed second-generation American (ie, respondent and at least 1 of her parents were born in the United States).

Table 1 shows a summary of the sociodemographic characteristics of the sample. Significant differences among ethnocultural groups were seen regarding maternal age, maternal education, and percentage having private health insurance.

The mean number of home therapies for colds used per ethnocultural group (controlling for maternal age, education, insurance status, and number of children) is presented in Table 2. Since many mothers' responses to the question included biomedical home therapies, such as antipyretics and over-the-counter cold medications, we determined the mean number of responses including and excluding such therapies. There were no differences among ethnocultural group in either analysis.

The most common home therapies used per ethnocultural group are presented in Table 3. Biomedical over-the-counter therapies are listed first, followed by other home therapies and remedies. Antipyretics and miscellaneous over-the-counter medications were commonly used by all mothers. Other home therapies were used in varying degrees in different ethnocultural groups. In general, European American mothers used fluids, moisture, and heat; African American mothers, chicken soup, camphor rubs, and teas; Puerto Rican mothers, camphor rubs, chicken soup, and other fluids; and West Indian–Caribbean mothers, herbal and mint teas, camphor rubs, and chicken soup.

The listed home therapies and remedies can be grouped into the following alternative/complementary medicine categories. *Herbs and nutritional supplements* include herbal teas, mixtures, and vitamins; *physical therapies* include massage, rubs, and exercises; *prayer and spiritual* include various forms of prayer and spiritualist healing; and *humoral and hot-cold* refers to the traditional theory of balance and homeostasis as it relates to illness categorization and treatment. When responses were placed into these groupings, the following differences were noted (Table 4). European American mothers' responses commonly included interventions that fit within the hot-cold theory of illness. Examples of these include warm baths, keeping warm or dressing warmly, warm compresses, and use of steam. The most common response categories for African American mothers were herbs and nutritional supplements (vitamins and herbal teas) and physical modalities (rubs and salves). The Puerto Rican mothers' responses fit mostly into the physical treatment category (including the common use of camphor rubs), whereas 15 of the 20 West Indian–Caribbean mothers mentioned herbal teas (including senna, rosemary, milo, garlic, and bush tea, as well as unspecified herbal teas).

A small proportion of mothers (3.5% of total sample) mentioned alcohol rubs as a treatment (2 African Americans, 7 Puerto Ricans, and 1 West Indian–Caribbean). No other

Table 1. Study Sample Demographics*

	EA	AA	PR	WI/C	Significant Difference†
Maternal age, y	35.1	31.0	28.8	32.3	EA>PR and AA, PR<all
Maternal education, y	16.0	12.8	11.5	12.1	EA>all, AA>PR
No. of children	2.3	2.7	2.4	2.9	No differences
Private insurance, %	92.0	29.0	27.0	30.0	EA>all

*EA indicates European American; AA, African American; PR, Puerto Rican; and WI/C, West Indian–Caribbean.
†Analysis of variance for maternal age, education, and number of children; χ^2 for insurance status.

Table 2. Mean Number of Home Therapies per Ethnocultural Group*

	European Americans	African Americans	Puerto Ricans	West Indian–Caribbean	Difference, P†
Including antipyretics and OTC	3.8	3.2	3.5	3.2	.28
Excluding antipyretics and OTC	2.5	2.1	2.2	2.1	.51

*Controlling for maternal age, education, number of children, and insurance status. OTC indicates over-the-counter remedies.
†Analysis of covariance.

Table 3. Home Remedies and Therapies for Colds

European Americans (n=85)		African Americans (n=68)		Puerto Ricans (n=108)		West Indian–Caribbean (n=20)	
Remedy	No. (%)	Remedy	No. (%)	Remedy	No. (%)	Remedy	No. (%)
Acetaminophen	42 (49)	Acetaminophen	37 (54)	Acetaminophen	70 (65)	Acetaminophen	12 (60)
Ibuprofen	14 (17)	Ibuprofen	3 (4)	Ibuprofen	17 (16)	Ibuprofen	2 (10)
Miscellaneous OTC*	41 (48)	Miscellaneous OTC	31 (45)	Miscellaneous OTC	37 (34)	Miscellaneous OTC	5 (25)
Fluids or liquids	37 (43)	Chicken soup	22 (33)	Camphor rub	22 (20)	Herbal tea	6 (30)
Humidifier	21 (25)	Camphor rub	9 (13)	Chicken soup	21 (19)	Mint tea	4 (20)
Chicken soup	14 (16)	Tea, nonspecified	8 (12)	Ginger ale	12 (11)	Camphor rub	4 (20)
Steam or heat	12 (14)	Orange juice	7 (10)	Lipton soup†	12 (11)	Chicken soup	3 (15)
Orange juice	10 (12)	Juice, nonspecified	7 (10)	Liquid or fluids	10 (9)		
Vitamins	8 (9)	Ginger ale	7 (10)	Vitamins	9 (8)		
Elevate head	7 (8)	Liquid or fluids	5 (7)	Prayer	8 (7)		
Juice, nonspecified	7 (8)						

*OTC indicates over-the-counter remedies.
†Connotes commercially prepared soup in canned or dry form; no flavor specified.

Table 4. Frequency of Categories of Alternative Remedies

	No. (%)			
	European Americans (n=85)	African Americans (n=68)	Puerto Ricans (n=108)	West Indian–Caribbean (n=20)
Herbs or nutritional supplements	8 (9)	13 (19)	15 (14)	14 (70)
Physical (including rubs and camphor)	7 (8)	13 (19)	25 (23)	4 (20)
Prayer or spiritual	1 (1)	3 (4)	9 (8)	1 (5)
Humoral; hot-cold	20 (24)	6 (9)	8 (7)	1 (5)

remedies were identified as having significant potential for serious adverse effects if taken in moderation.

Comment

The literature regarding alternative/complementary medical practices used for childhood health and illness is scant. Much of this literature concerns alternative practices for chronic illness, such as asthma, cystic fibrosis, arthritis, and cancer. Little is known about alternative/complementary or non-physician-directed therapies for "low morbidity-high frequency" sickness episodes, or for health maintenance. One study from a pediatric outpatient department in Canada reported that 11% of families questioned had used complementary medicine, including chiropractic, homeopathy, naturopathy, and acupuncture.[7] The definition of complementary medicine in that study appeared to include only interventions that would fit into the professional or folk sectors of Kleinman's health care system model, and did not include home-based practices from the popular sector. Therefore, that study reports only the "tip of the iceberg" with regard to unconventional and alternative/complementary therapies in children. The present study specifically addressed home-based practices, which we feel constitute the majority of parent-initiated interventions.

One of our goals was to address the issues of alternative/complementary therapies in a cross-cultural perspective. It was our impression that both the medical literature and the popular press often conceptualize unconventional therapies practiced by the majority culture and ethnic minorities differently. Our goal was to determine both the difference and similarities in home health care interventions among mothers from diverse ethnocultural backgrounds. Our results show that the amount of home-based alternative/complementary therapies is similar among mothers from both the majority and minority cultural groups, even after controlling for economic and demographic differences. There was variability among cultural groups, however, in the relative frequency of specific remedies and therapies, as well as in categories of alternative/complementary therapies. Some of these differences support past literature and conventional wisdom regarding common culture-specific therapies; others do not. For example, the use of camphor rubs (such as Vicks Vaporub) has often been cited as a common therapy in the Puerto Rican community.[8, 9] Our study supports this and shows that usage of these common remedies continues to exist over time and through generations. The use of camphor rubs is not exclusive to Puerto Ricans, though, as can be documented in the literature,[10] as well as in the present study. Seven percent of the European American mothers, 13% of African American mothers, and 20% of West Indian–Caribbean mothers mentioned its use. Although camphor rubs may be considered an over-the-counter remedy in the majority European American culture, their common use in some ethnic groups assigns them the designation of folk remedy.

Our finding that humoral or hot-cold beliefs were more common in the European American group than the Puerto Rican group merits discussion. Much has been written about the hot-cold theory of disease in Hispanic-Latino or Puerto Rican folk medicine.[8, 9, 11–14] Results from this study suggest that the prevalence of humoral practices is low in this group of Puerto Rican mothers and is in fact relatively high for the group of European American respondents. Cross-cultural studies such as this place these practices in perspective and help guard against incorrect assumptions based on noncomparative data.

The observation that the most common home-based therapies included over-the-counter medications such as antipyretics and cold remedies lends further support to the belief that, in most cases, home therapies are truly complementary and not used in isolation from biomedical care. In fact, many of the home-based remedies could be recommended by physicians. If one ranks these home-based therapies on relative suitability within the biomedical model, most could fit within a broad definition of biomedical care (eg, fluids, juices, humidification). The least biomedical of the remedies would be herbal teas and camphor rubs, which were used with greater frequency in the ethnic minority groups.

The definition of what is considered an alternative vs nonalternative, home-based therapy is complex. It is important to note that *biomedicine* and *alternative/complementary medicine* are not static categories. Substantial shift, overlap, and redefinition continue to occur. Many over-the-counter remedies and environmental therapies (such as humidifiers) may have some benefit from the biomedical perspective, and some practitioners advise parents to use them under specific conditions. In these cases, they may be considered home-based but not alternative, since they were recommended by the health care practitioner. If these therapies are used without the recommendation of the health care practitioner, one might consider them alternative. Likewise, if a biomedical health care practitioner recommends a herbal tea, acupuncture, or a homeopathic remedy, are these therapies truly alternative? One can argue that in this situation they are not, whereas in other circumstances they would definitely be considered alternative. We did not specifically ask whether the remedies used were recommended by the health care practitioner. Future studies on home remedies may benefit from including questions such as, "Where did you learn about this remedy?" or "Who advised you to use this remedy?" to determine whether the therapy was truly alternative or recommended by a physician.

These data support the concept of medical pluralism: the theory that individuals draw on multiple modalities and healing traditions in their health care practices. Since patients do not often provide physicians and nurses with information about home-based or alternative/complementary therapies, it becomes crucial for providers to initiate discussion on this topic in a nonjudgmental manner.[15]

Before this study, we assumed that parents might frequently use alternative/complementary therapies for common childhood illnesses such as colds. Our data suggest that, while parents often use home-based therapies, the use of therapies that are truly alternative to biomedical practice is minimal.

One limitation of this study is its sampling design. A study of alternative medicine that relies on a clinic-based sample may underreport the use of alternative/complementary and unconventional medicine. Respondents may feel uncomfortable discussing nonbiomedical practices in a physician's office. We attempted to limit this by employing individuals not associated with the health care staff as interviewers and by explaining the reasons for the study. We do appreciate, though, that the clinical environment where the interview took place may have made candid discussion difficult. Also, by using a clinical sample, we may have missed those families who underutilize biomedical care. These families may also be high users of alternative/complementary therapies. A population-based sample would have been more optimal in this regard.

We also had a relatively small sample of West Indian–Caribbean parents, so the results from this group should be interpreted with caution. Sparse information is available in the clinical literature about this cultural group. Although they share with African Americans the stigma of minority status and the resultant discrimination, the cultures of the West Indian islands are, in many ways, distinct from traditional African American culture. We strongly recommend that researchers who work in ethnically diverse settings consider members of West

Indian–Caribbean communities separate from African Americans. Further studies within this growing community are needed to gain a better understanding of this underrepresented group.

Despite these limitations, our study suggests that parents use various home remedies during common childhood illness episodes such as colds, and that these home interventions are generally benign and truly do complement biomedical care. Furthermore, parents from different ethnocultural groups, including the majority European Americans, list similar numbers of home remedies. The use of specific remedies and categories of remedies do vary by ethnocultural affiliation, though. Health care practitioners need to be aware of the common use of home-based therapies. They should feel confident that these remedies are mostly benign and complementary to our biomedical care. Clinicians are encouraged to inquire about their use with patients and families. The importance of open communication regarding the overall treatment of sickness cannot be overstated. When physician and patient talk openly about these issues, the therapeutic environment improves, opportunities for health education increase, and the patient gains confidence in the physician as a therapeutic ally. In addition, the chance that the patient will suffer adverse effects of harmful therapies decreases, and the physician can gain important information that will help place the biomedical therapeutic plan within the patient's lifestyle and world view, thus increasing the likelihood of adherence to the clinician's therapeutic plan.

We thank Thomas Fromson, MD, and Alberto Rodriguez, MD, for allowing us to interview their patients for this study. We also thank Paul H. Dworkin, MD, and Kathi J. Kemper, MD, for their thoughtful suggestions and advice during the conceptualization of this project. We are also grateful to the parents who allowed us to interview them about this topic.

References

1. Zola IK. Studying the decision to see a doctor. *Adv Psychosom Med.* 1972;8:216–236.

2. Kleinman AK. *Patients and Healers in the Context of Culture.* Berkeley: University of California Press; 1980:49–60.

3. Eisenberg DM, Kessler RC, Foster C, Norlock FE, Calkins DR, DelBianco TL. Unconventional medicine in the United States: prevalence, costs, and patterns of use. *N Engl J Med.* 1993; 328:246–252.

4. Kemper KJ. *The Holistic Pediatrician.* New York, NY: HarperCollins Publications Inc; 1996:1–15.

5. Marín G, Marín BV. *Research With Hispanic Populations.* Newbury Park, Calif: Sage Publications; 1991:23. Sage Social Science Research Methods Series.

6. Weller SC, Romney AK. *Systematic Data Collection.* Newbury Park, Calif: Sage Publications; 1988:9–20.

7. Spigelblatt L, Laíné-Ammara G, Pless IB, Guyver A. The use of alternative medicine by children. *Pediatrics.* 1994;94:811–814.

8. Harwood A. *Ethnicity and Medical Care.* Cambridge, Mass: Harvard University Press; 1981:421–422.

9. Pachter LM, Cloutier MM, Bernstein BA. Ethnomedical (folk) remedies for childhood asthma in a mainland Puerto Rican community. *Arch Pediatr Adolesc Med.* 1995;149:982–988.

10. Snow L. *Walkin' Over Medicine.* Boulder, Colo: Westview Press; 1993.

11. Harwood A. The hot-cold theory of disease: implications for treatment of Puerto Rican patients. *JAMA.* 1971;216:1153–1158.

12. Kay M, Yoder M. Hot and cold in women's ethnotherapeutics: the American-Mexican West. *Soc Sci Med.* 1987;25:347–355.

13. Risser AL, Mazur LJ. Use of folk remedies in a Hispanic population. *Arch Pediatr Adolesc Med.* 1995;149:978–981.

14. Pachter LM. Cultural issues in pediatric care. In: Behrman RE, Kliegman RM, Arvin AM, eds. *Nelson Textbook of Pediatrics.* 15th ed. Philadelphia, Pa: WB Saunders Co; 1996: 16–18.

15. Pachter LM. Culture and clinical care: folk illness beliefs and behaviors and their implications for health care delivery. *JAMA.* 1994; 271:690–694.

11 Traditional Chinese Medicine for the Treatment of Dermatologic Disorders

John Koo, MD; Sumaira Arain, BA
From the Psoriasis Treatment Center and the Department of Dermatology, University of California, San Francisco (Dr Koo) and University of California at Berkeley (Ms Arain).

Traditional Chinese medicine (TCM) is an alternative method of therapy that can be administered in oral, topical, or injectable forms. It emphasizes the importance of using many herbs that are combined in different formulations for each individual patient. Among some segments of the patient population, it has become increasingly popular as a mode for treating dermatologic diseases. As a result, it is now worthwhile for dermatologists throughout the West to gain some familiarity with this method. Yet, dermatologists are largely unfamiliar with TCM and may possess some misconceptions. We attempt to give a general overview of TCM through the discussion of different clinical studies involving various TCMs. Some proposed mechanisms of action of TCM are also presented. A discussion of adverse effects, including hepatotoxic effects and the need for close monitoring is discussed. A warning regarding the possible contamination of TCMs is also included. Since it is not possible to discuss the application of TCM for every skin disorder, psoriasis and atopic dermatitis are used as the prototype in illustrating the use of TCM. In the future, perhaps a better understanding of TCM will be gained through more systematic analysis and controlled studies with a placebo arm. It is our hope that this article will provide an overview of the efficacy, mechanism of action, as well as adverse effects of TCM.

Arch Dermatol. 1998;134:1388–1393

Herbal medicine uses any plant part such as the root, bark, stem, seed, flowers, or leaves as a means for treatment. Many of the modern drugs now used are based on "native herbal wisdom." For example, medications like anthralin, aspirin, and alkaloids were originally herbal medications.

There are 3 basic functions that herbal medicines purportedly perform: elimination and detoxification, health management and maintenance, and health building.[1]

Herbal medical practitioners can create many different formulas for different types of applications. The formulation is contingent on the circumstances, condition being treated, type or part of the plant used, and the characteristics of the individual treated.

Most dermatologists in the United States have expertise in administering "orthodox" therapies. These dermatologists are basically knowledgeable of those therapies that are sanctioned by the Food and Drug Administration. There is usually support for these therapies in scientific medical literature, particularly literature published in the English language. However, many patients who are frustrated with orthodox medicine often decide to explore alternative therapies.

Fleischer and colleagues[2] found in a recent survey that 5% of a patient population with psoriasis have used alternative therapies, excluding the use of sunlight and nonprescription tanning equipment. Among these are dietary manipulation, herbal remedies, and vitamin therapy.

Alternative therapies have become more widely used because of increasing interest among patients. Traditional Chinese medicine (TCM) is of particular significance because it is a common choice of patients. Thus, it has become relevant for practicing dermatologists to be reasonably knowledgeable about this field. Whether administering TCM or not, it is intrinsically imperative to have an accurate perspective. In this manner, one can be properly aware of possible adverse effects from use of TCM by the patient. Many practicing dermatologists in the United States possess certain misconceptions regarding TCM because of their lack of familiarity with this field.

To begin with, some dermatologists may be still unaware of the existence of placebo-controlled studies involving TCM. There are 2 double-blind, placebo-controlled studies on TCM that have been published in the English-language medical literature. One has been conducted with children[3] and the other with adults.[4] These studies were carried out in England using TCM to treat atopic dermatitis. Many studies have also been published in Asian countries such as Japan and mainland China.

Another misconception is that detailed scientific investigation of the mechanism of action of TCM has never been conducted. Yet, several countries including China have published scientific articles on the proposed mechanism of action of TCM and further studies are being carried out.

One truly unfortunate misconception is that TCM has no adverse effects due to its natural composition. This is a misleading notion in that many people, possibly including some physicians automatically assume that natural compounds are benign. However, experienced practitioners are aware that oral TCMs have possible adverse effects such as hepatotoxicity. A common concern with topical TCM is contact dermatitis.

Our goal is to provide a general overview and understanding of this field, since a comprehensive coverage of TCM is not possible herein. A complete description of TCM would be exhaustive because of the numerous agents involved to treat almost every possible dermatologic condition.

Efficiency of TCM

Sheehan and colleagues[3] working with Luo, a Chinese herbalist in London, England, performed one of the first double-blind, placebo-controlled studies with TCM in the West. The positive findings were a surprise for many Western dermatologists. The study consisted of a double-blind, placebo-controlled trial using TCM to treat atopic dermatitis. It was performed at the Hospital for Sick Children in London.

Luo incorporated 10 herbs in the therapeutic agent.[3,5] These herbs were *Potentilla chinensis, Tribulus terrestris, Rehmannia glutinosa, Lophatherum gracile, Clematis armandii, Ledebouriella saseloides, Dictamnus dasycarpus, Paeonia lactiflora, Schizonepeta tenuifolia,* and *Glycyrrhiza glabrae*. The herbs were first ground, then placed in porous paper sachets, and boiled down into a thick concentrate and strained. This decoction was then orally administered to each patient in the form of a drink. The placebo consisted of a different assortment of herbs that had no known efficacy for the treatment of atopic dermatitis. However, the sachets were similar in taste, smell, and appearance.

At the end of the treatment period, the median decrease in erythema was 91.4% with the active herbs and 10.6% with the placebo herbs. The active herbs also contributed to an 85.7% decrease in the extent of surface involvement scores, while there was a 17.3% decrease with the placebo herbs.

During the study period there were no apparent abnormalities in liver function tests, renal function tests, and complete blood cell counts. A follow-up study (of both children and adults) was conducted a year later. Those who elected to continue with TCM maintained the benefits of the therapy with minimal adverse effects. In contrast, those who discontinued the treatment experienced a decline in their condition.[6,7] Over time many of the patients, both pediatric and adult, were able to minimize their usage of TCM and most of them eventually discontinued the treatment without a relapse. The adult patients, who continued the treatment for 1 year, did not exhibit any biochemical abnormalities. However, 2 of the pediatric subjects developed asymptomatic elevation of serum aspartate aminotransferase levels. Yet, once the medication was discontinued the elevated level normalized within 8 weeks.

Many efficacy studies have been performed, but the study by Luo is the best known in the English-language literature.[3,5] Most other studies are only published in Chinese medical journals. Many of them have never been translated into another language. Yet, the Chinese publications contain a plethora of valuable information essential for understanding TCM.

Although TCM has been used to treat a variety of skin diseases, of particular interest to us is psoriasis. Both topical and systemic use of herbs has been administered to treat psoriasis, as well as a combination of herbal medications with UV-A. This method is similar to psoralen–UV-A phototherapy.

Radix Angelicae pubescentis is a Chinese herbal medicine that is administered in combination with UV-A irradiation. A study[8] was conducted in 92 cases, 62 of these patients were successfully cleared of psoriasis. However, they exhibited relatively mild adverse effects. With long-term use it was found that there were changes in the lens.[9]

Furocoumarins, including imperatorin, isoimpertorin, and alloimperatorin are found in another Chinese herbal medicine, *Radix Angelicae dahuricae.* Psoralen compounds are formed from the combination of *Radix Angelicae dahuricae* with UV-A irradiation and DNA.[10] A study[11] involving 13 hospitals was conducted to assess the therapeutic efficacy of the oral use of *Radix Angelicae dahuricae* in combination with UV-A irradiation. The results were compared with traditional psoralen–UV-A phototherapy conducted with 8-methoxypsoralen.[11] *Radix Angelicae dahuricae* UV-A therapy was used to treat 204 patients with psoriasis. The treatment was successful in clearing psoriasis in 133 patients (46.8%) and inducing marked improvement in 121 patients (42.6%) in whom psoriasis was not completely cleared. Psoralen–UV-A phototherapy was administered in 92 patients with psoriasis. Forty patients (43.5%) were cleared whereas 43 (46.7%) exhibited marked improvement. The difference in the efficacy of treatments between psoralen–UV-A phototherapy and *Radix Angelicae dahuricae* UV-A therapy was not statistically significant. The only perceived difference was the severity of adverse effects. *Radix Angelicae dahuricae* exhibited milder adverse effects than 8-MOP. The adverse effects included nausea and dizziness.

Tripterygium wilfordii Hook and *Triptergium hypoglaucum Hutch* are 2 popular TCMs. *Tripterygium wilfordii Hook* has yielded positive therapeutic effects when used to treat various types of psoriasis. The Chinese medical literature has recorded 638 cases of plaque-type psoriasis, 37 cases of psoriatic arthritis, 16 cases of pustular psoriasis, and 5 cases of erythrodermic psoriasis that have been treated with *Tripterygium wilfordii Hook.*[12–18] Although *Tripterygium wilfordii Hook's* possible mechanism of action has been investigated to be both anti-inflammatory and immunosuppressive, there have been several negative consequences.

Some toxic effects have been observed in both animals and human subjects. Among these are gastrointestinal reaction, cutaneous/mucotaneous reactions, and abnormal menstruation. Some abnormalities in the hematopoietic system were also noted. In addition, exacerbation of latent chronic hepatitis and abnormal liver function was observed in several cases.

The clinical efficacy is similar for *Triptergium hypoglaucum Hutch* and *Tripterygium wilfordii Hook.* Chinese medical literature concludes that with the current results *Tripterygium wilfordii Hook* and *Triptergium hypoglaucum Hutch* have shown modest efficacy with an acceptable adverse effects profile.[19–21]

Another Chinese herbal medication has been analyzed in a study involving 86 patients with psoriasis with indirubin, an active ingredient found in *Indigo natualis.* Indirubin was administered in dosages varying from 100 to 300 mg/d. This was compared with ethyliminum treatment of 300 mg/d. Ethyliminum is popular in China as a "Western remedy" although it is no longer incorporated in Western medicine for psoriasis.

As a result of this study, indirubin was discovered to be more effective than ethyliminum.[22] The adverse effects of indirubin and *I natualis* were found to be mainly gastrointestinal. There was a wide range in reported adverse effects from as low as 26% to as high as 96% with some being rated as "severe."[22–26] Molecular modification of indirubin was conducted to decrease the adverse effects. Two new compounds *N*-methylisoindigotin (meisoindigo) and *N*-acetyl-indirubin were developed.[27–29]

Indigo natualis is also incorporated in *Pillulae Indigo natualis compositae*, a commercially prepared composite medicine widely marketed in China. This capsule was found to be beneficial in that it had fewer adverse effects than *I natualis* used by itself.[30]

The efficacy of oral *P Indigo natualis compositae* was evaluated in an open study. Its efficacy for psoriasis was equivalent to that of oral ethyliminum with a positive difference—fewer adverse effects.[31] As of 1993, 636 research subjects have been treated with *I nautalis* or other diindole compounds.[22–31] Among the findings published in Chinese medical literature, there is a record of 6 cases of adverse effects consisting of 3 instances of transient cases of abnormality in liver function tests, and another 3 occurrences of transient decreases in peripheral white blood cell counts.

Some TCMs that have demonstrated systemic efficacy are formulated as topical agents. This is particularly true of those medications found to be too toxic with systemic use. A plant from the southern provinces of China, *Camptotheca acuminata decne*, is one example.[32] Alkaloids with antineoplastic activities including camptotheca, 10-, 11-, or 12-hydroxycamptotheic, deoxycamptotheic, 12-chlorocamptotheic, 9-, 10-, or 11-methoxycamptothecin, and venoterpin are found in this herb.[33,34]

The efficacy of *Camptotheca acuminata decne* was studied in an open trial involving 92 cases of psoriasis. A 0.03% concentration of topical *Camptotheca acuminata decne* was compared with a 1% hydrocortisone. *Camptotheca acuminata decne* was determined to be significantly more effective. A possible weakness of this study is the choice of 1% hydrocortisone, a weak topical steroid, as a comparison. It is perhaps more appropriately considered a placebo arm of the study. Contact dermatitis was found in 9% to 15% of the subjects studied and the researchers also noticed possible enhancement of postinflammatory hyperpigmentation.

Although TCMs are commonly found in topical, oral, and photochemotherapeutic modalities, some of them are also injectable. Sometimes the injectable agent yields better results than when used in the other forms. For instance, *Radix macrotomiae seu Lithospermi* when injected resulted in a more significant therapeutic effect in treating psoriasis than in an oral formulation. An open study of 50 patients led to 13 cleared of psoriasis and 26 greatly improved without systemic adverse effects.[35]

The TCMs discussed so far are similar to Western medications in that they are marketed as capsules or tablets that are taken orally. These are the more modern, convenient, and more user-friendly prepackaged TCM preparations. They are formulated as monotherapies or in groups of herbs. However, these agents compose only a small fraction of TCM practice.

The standard TCM practice emphasizes the importance of using many herbs combined in different compositions for each individual patient. The formulation is based on the diagnosis and individual condition of the patient. Whereas Western medicine emphasizes monotherapy, standard TCM promotes herbal mixtures sometimes involving more than 10 different herbs and other agents.

According to TCM, psoriasis is subtyped into 3 main categories: "blood-heat" type, "blood deficiency-dryness" type, and "blood stasis" type. According to the subtype of psoriasis the patient has, a different mixture of herbs is suggested.

For example, when inflicted with blood stasis psoriasis the lesions are indurated and have little tendency to resolve spontaneously. There is also a purplish or dark red coloring of the tongue with occasional petechia. The pulse is often small and loose.

The principle of treatment of this type of psoriasis is to activate the blood and eliminate the stasis. The most often used prescriptions include *Herba Hedyotis diffusae, Flos carthami, Semen persicae, Ramulus euonymi, Rhizoma sparganii, Rhizoma curoumae, Pericarpium Citri reticulatae*, and *Caulis spatholob*. These are only the core ingredients that are recommended. They are ingested as decoctions. According to the needs of each patient, this list would be altered.

To treat blood deficiency-dryness a different set of herbs is considered more suitable. Among the physical manifestations of this type is the appearance of the tongue characterized by pinkish color with a thin coating. Western dermatologists do not routinely inspect the tongues or pulses of their patients with psoriasis. Thus, it is difficult to make a comparison between patients in China and those in the United States.

Since the judgment of the practitioner determines the unique herbal mixture for each individual patient, it is difficult to conduct a controlled trial. The more traditional practice of TCM involves enormous variation. Yet, a few open studies have been conducted in China comparing Western therapeutic agents with traditional approaches.

One open study[3] evaluated 206 patients with psoriasis treated with traditional approaches. They were compared with 52 patients with psoriasis treated with 600 mg/d of oral bimolanum. Both groups were found to be fairly equivalent in efficiency. Among the 52 patients treated with bimolanum there were 3 cases of leukopenia. There were no hematological or biochemical abnormalities among the 206 patients treated with TCM. Another advantage of TCM was that in a follow-up study[36] 3 years later it was found that patients treated with TCM had a significantly lower recurrence rate than those treated with oral bimolanum.

In another open study,[37] 801 patients with psoriasis were treated with a different mixture of herbs. These were *Herba serissae, Myrrha, Rhizoma zedoariae, Resina boswelliae,* and *Rhizoma sparganii*. There was an interesting 50% to 85% response rate among the 801 patients.

Another investigation involved a 6-year follow-up study of 41 patients with psoriasis treated with TCM and 106 patients treated with ethyliminum. A different mixture of herbs was administered in this study. The short-term efficacy of ethyliminum was better than that of this particular combination of Chinese medical herbs. However, the remission time was longer with TCM. Statistically there was a significant difference between the 2 groups in favor of TCM (P<.01).[37]

No discussion of TCM would be complete without considering acupuncture. It is highly doubtful as to whether acupuncture has any efficacy in a skin disorder such as psoriasis. For the last 5 years, one of us (J.K.) has traveled to mainland China every year. After interacting with prominent academic and clinical dermatology pioneers in China, the general consensus was that acupuncture is not considered efficacious for treatment of skin disease.

The medical literature has an account of only 1 controlled trial[38] of acupuncture for psoriasis. Of 56 patients, 28 received active therapy by proper placement of needles followed by electrical stimulation. The other 28 patients consisted of the placebo group. The needles were placed 1 cm away from the proper location at an insufficient depth. In addition, no electrical stimulation was applied. The treatments were administered twice weekly for 10 weeks. At the conclusion of this trial, there was no significant difference between the 2 groups. The investigators of this study[38] were led to conclude that classic acupuncture was not any more efficacious than placebo. Amazingly, the placebo group did better overall on the psoriasis area severity index evaluation. Other published reports do not have proper controls,[39] make claims without verifiable evidence,[40,41] or have been described in obscure journals.[42,43] Thus, acupuncture as a viable alternative therapy in dermatology has not been substantiated.

Mechanism of Action of TCM

The 10-herb combination of Luo as a treatment of atopic dermatitis has become widely known among Western dermatologists.[5] Consequently, several studies have been conducted to extrapolate the mechanism of action of these herbs. Currently, the focus of the investigation has been on the impact of the herbal mixture on CD23 expression.

CD23, an IgE receptor, has been implicated in the pathogenesis of atopic dermatitis. CD23 is present in 2 forms: type A, which is solely expressed on B cells, and type B, which can be induced by interleukin 4 to be expressed on a variety of cells.[44–46] In patients with atopic dermatitis, excessive expression of IgE receptor 23 has been found in monocytes.[47,48] In addition, they also have an increased expression of CD23 in their skin.[49] A possible explanation of this may be that the lymphocytes of patients with atopic dermatitis are known to produce a higher level of interleukin 4.[50,51] Some authors[5] conducted studies with the combination of the 10 herbs of Luo. They found that the herbal combination had a strong inhibitory effect on CD23 expression on peripheral blood monocytes. The placebo combination was found to have no effect on CD23 expression.

The inhibition of CD23 expression was discovered to be dose dependent. Furthermore, the mechanism of the inhibition was not due to the death of monocytes. Those peripheral mononuclear cells cultured with TCM or placebo at the same concentration as the original experiments had a similar viability to control cultures.

Xu and colleagues[52] of the Royal Free Hospital and School of Medicine in London confirmed the above findings in their publication. In addition, Xu et al found a significant reduction in HLA-DR expression. Another study from England demonstrated that the formulation of the 10 Chinese herbs when administered in vitro exhibited significant anti-oxidant activity.

Although the 10-herb formulation by Luo is well known,[3] other TCMs have also been analyzed to understand their mechanism of action. Several of these studies have been performed in countries outside of China such as Japan.

Matsumoto and colleagues[53] have been compiling data on Shor-seiryu-to, which is a TCM that is marketed in Japan as an antihistamine/antiallergy medication. Matsumoto et al found that the effectiveness of Shor-seiryu-to is due to the inhibition of histamine release based on the data from studies on rat mast cells. Another study conducted by Sakaguchi et al[54] discovered Shor-seiryu-to to have a profound effect in inhibiting 48-hour passive cutaneous anaphylactic reaction in rats. It also significantly inhibited an increase in vascular permeability induced by histamine. Shor-seiryu-to had no sedative adverse effects. This was due to Shor-seiryu-to not affecting $histamine_1$ receptors and the muscarinic cholinergic system in the brain.

Moku-boi-to is another TCM that is marketed in Japan. Data compiled through Japanese studies performed on this medicine found moku-boi-to to profoundly suppress the enhancement of capillary permeability induced by histamine, LTC_4 (leukotriene C_4), and antiserum in the rat skin. When compared with the optimal dosage of a Western anthihistamine such as diphenhydramine, moku-boi-to was equipotent in antihistaminic effect.[55] In conclusion, moku-boi-to was found to have suppressive effects on chemical mediators of inflammation such as histamine and LTC_4. In addition, it also reduces the effect of the antigen-antibody response in the skin.

Adverse Effects

It is a common misconception that natural medications, such as herbal medicine, is a safer mode of therapy because of its presumed lack of adverse effects. However, it is well documented that herbal medications used in TCM can have serious adverse systemic effects such as hepatotoxicity. Li,[56] a physician from the People's Republic of China reports that "side effects of Chinese medicinal material are not rare." In addition, "hypersensitivity, hepatic toxicity and renal damage have all been reported in China, some of which have been fatal."[57,58] There was even a report[59] from Japan of a 59-year-old woman who developed adult respiratory distress syndrome after use of TCM for seborrheic dermatitis.

Liver complications, including elevated liver function test results and acute liver failure are one of the most well-documented adverse effects of TCM. In Great Britain,[60] a 29-year-old woman was prescribed Chinese herbal treatment for eczema. She consequently developed 2 episodes of hepatitis that led to hospitalization. She had acute liver failure after the second hospitalization. This later led to her death, despite an emergency liver transplantation.[60] In response to such incidents, The Working Group on Dietary Supplements and Health Foods in the United Kingdom has taken steps to establish a reporting scheme for adverse reactions related to the use of TCM.[61]

The British governmental agency has recorded 11 cases of liver damage following the use of TCM for skin conditions from January 1991 to December 1993. In many of the cases, recovery occurred after discontinuation of the herbal medicines. Later when rechallenged with the same herbal medicine, there was a recurrence of hepatitis. Although it is difficult to establish absolute etiologic association for all 11 cases, there is an obvious circumstantial link between TCM and the consequent liver damage.

In these reported cases, there is a good chronological relationship with the absence of a viable alternative explanation for the liver damage. The herbal material was analyzed for 7 of the above 11 cases. Yet, due to the variance in the plant mixtures for each individual, no single ingredient could be extrapolated as the sole cause of the liver injury. Furthermore, the analysis of the 11 cases revealed that the liver damage was not dose related, but was most likely idiosyncratic. The authors[62] highly recommend regular liver function testing as a means for monitoring patients prescribed oral TCM.

To illustrate another case of an adverse effect of TCM,[63] consider a 42-year-old woman who developed severe cardiomyopathy following a course of TCM. She had been prescribed TCM for 2 weeks to treat her eczema. An herbal analysis, conducted later, revealed that the formulation contained more than 30 herbs. Once again, it was not possible to decisively conclude any one ingredient as the cause for the congestive cardiomyopathy.

In the hopes of determining any future adverse effects, we recommend that Chinese herbal medications be subjected to drug licensing, monitoring, and surveillance procedures. This should be done in a manner similar to what any new drug is subjected to for approval in the United States or United Kingdom.

Currently, there is an unfortunate possibility that because of the lack of quality control an herbal medication may be contaminated with undeclared prescription drugs. This may lead to adverse reactions in the patients. In St Paul, Minn, a report[62] was published that detailed the case of several patients who had been given contaminated Chinese herbal preparations. Various undeclared prescription drugs, ranging from nonsteroidal anti-inflammatory drugs to diazepam were discovered in these formulations. One particular patient developed massive gastrointestinal bleeding after ingesting a Chinese herbal medication that was later found to contain a high dose of prescription nonsteroidal anti-inflammatory medication.

Various authors have previously published analyses of Chinese herbal medications. These findings have revealed many types of contaminants. Methyltestosterone, dexamethasone, indomethacin, chlordiazepoxide, prednisolone, betamethasone, lead, diazepam, nefenamic acid, prednisone, or hydrocortisone are are some of many substances that have been found in these medications. Other possible contaminants of Chinese herbal medications include hydrochlorothiazide, chlorpheniramine, pheynlbutazone, aminopyrine, paracetamol, thiamin, caffeine, and ethaverine.

Regulation of Chinese herbal medications by governmental agencies is essential in maintaining quality control. Otherwise, there is a potential danger of undeclared prescription medications infiltrating Chinese herbal preparations and being unknowingly administered to patients.

Conclusions

Many practicing dermatologists in the United States are only familiar with orthodox Western procedures for the treatment of skin disorders. However, an increasing number of patients have begun to seek TCM as an alternative mode of therapy. It has been demonstrated in published studies that there is a real possibility that TCM has a substantial efficacy beyond a simple placebo effect. However, TCM has also been associated with notable adverse effects, some fatal. The current clinical studies in the Chinese medical literature are not a complete source of information about TCM. Many of the studies have been conducted without a placebo arm and it is difficult to interpret the results in comparison studies. This is so because the standard Western medications used for comparison in China are often not those agents currently used in Western medicine.

The individualized polypharmacy approach of TCM is intuitively sensible. This is especially in countering a complex, chronic, and often recalcitrant inflammatory process such as psoriasis or eczema in which it would be most beneficial to attack the process through many facets simultaneously. However, this approach would lead to extremely difficult scientific analysis of these medications. A more rigorous, systematic analysis and testing of therapeutic agents used in TCM may eventually lead to the development of a standard set of therapeutic agents that may be administered with reliable efficacy and good quality control.

We acknowledge the gracious and generous help from Xi-Ran Lin, MD, chairman of the Department of Dermatology, Dalian Medical University, People's Republic of China, in acquiring information regarding the relevant Chinese publications.

References

1. Dincin D. Herbalism. In: *Herbal Medicine: The Natural Way to Get Well and Stay Well*. New York, NY: Gramercy Publishing; 1979.
2. Fleischer AB, Feldman SR, Rapp SR, Reboussin DM, Exum ML, Clark AR. Alternative therapies commonly used within a population of patients with psoriasis. *Cutis.* 1996;58:216–220.
3. Sheehan MP, Atherton DJ. A controlled trial of traditional Chinese medicinal plants in widespread non-exudative atopic eczema. *Br J Dermatol.* 1992;340:13–17.
4. Sheehan MP, Rustin MHA, Atherton DJ, et al. Efficacy of traditional Chinese herbal therapy in adult atopic dermatitis. *Lancet.* 1992;340:13–17.
5. Latchman Y, Whittle B, Rustin M, Atherton DJ, Brostoff J. The efficacy of traditional Chinese herbal therapy in atopic eczema. *Int Arch Allergy Immunol.* 1994;104:222–226.
6. Sheehan MP, Atherton DJ. One year follow-up of children treated with Chinese medicinal herbs for atopic eczema. *Br J Dermatol.* 1994; 140:488–493.
7. Sheehan MP, Stevens H, Ostlere LS, Atherton DJ, Brostoff J, Rustin MHA. Follow-up of adult patients with atopic eczema treated with Chinese herbal therapy for one year. *Clin Exp Dermatol.* 1995;20:136–140.
8. Li FQ, Fang FY, Jian ZY, et al. Cases suffering from psoriasis treated with traditional Chinese medicine and long wave ultraviolet. *Chin J Phys Ther.* 1983;6:144–145.
9. Li FQ, Fang FY, Li SH. A long-term follow-up of 58 cases of psoriasis treated with traditional Chinese medicine Angelica dahuricae and long wave ultraviolet. *Chin J Physic Ther.* 1984;7:154–155.
10. Zhang GW, Li SB, Wang HJ, et al. Inhibition of Chinese herb medicine, *Angelica dahurica* (Benth et Hook) and UVA on synthesis of DNA of lymphocytes. *Chin J Dermatol.* 1980; 13:138–140.
11. Zhang GW, Wang HJ, Zhou YH, et al. Treatment of psoriasis by photochemotherapy: a comparison between the photosensitizing capsule of Angelica dahurica and 8-MOP. *Natl Med J China.* 1983;63:16–19.
12. Qin WZ. The application of *Tripterygium* in dermatology. In: *Investigative Dermatology: Integrated Traditional and Western Medicine Series.* Shanghai, Mainland China: Shanghai Science Technique Publishing; 1990:101–129.
13. Pan HY, Fu ZM, Gu X, et al. Treatment of 130 cases of psoriasis with *Tripterygium wilfordii Hook. Bull Dermatol Therap Prev Invest.* 1980;4:45–46.
14. Guan F, Wong DH. Treatment of psoriasis with *Tripterygium wilfordii Hook. J Clin Dermatol.* 1981;10:91–93.
15. Zhang JY. Treating 148 cases of psoriasis vulgaris with *Tripterygium wilfordii Hook. J Clin Dermatol.* 1982;11:118.
16. Lui XZ, Zhang KY, Yu RR. Three cases of arthropathic psoriasis treated with *Tripterygium wilfordii Hook. Chin J Dermatol.* 1982;15:29–30.
17. Chen SH. Treating 20 cases of psoriasis with *Tripterygium wilfordii Hook. Fujian J Med.* 1985;7:23.
18. Shi SY, Xu S, Yian YP. A therapeutic evaluation of *Tripterygium wilfordii Hook* in the treatment of 19 cases of psoriatic arthritis. *J Clin Dermatol.* 1988;17:294–296.
19. Long YI, Zhou GP, Luo HC. Clinical observation of the treatment of psoriasis and other dermatoses with mixture of *Triptergium hypoglaucum (levl) Hutch. Chin J Dermatol.* 1983;16:42.
20. Zheng FZ. Two cases of psoriasis arthropathica cured by *Triptergium hypoglaucum (levl) Hutch. Chin J Dermatol.* 1984;17:204.
21. Gao JC. Three cases of pustular psoriasis treated with *Triptergium hypoglaucum (levl) Hutch* and interval blood transfusion. *Chin Dermvenereol J.* 1990;4:218–219.
22. Wang MX, Wang HL, Lui WS, et al. Study of the therapeutic effect and pharmacological action of indirubin in treating psoriasis. *Chin J Dermatol.* 1982;15:157–160.
23. Yuan ZZ, Yuan X, Xu ZX. An observation on the therapeutic effect of Indigo natualis in 46 cases of psoriasis. *J Trad Chin Med.* 1982;23:43.
24. Chen LZ. Treating 23 cases of psoriasis with indirubin tablets. *J Clin Dermatol.* 1981; 10:157–158.
25. Ling MW, Chen DY, Zhu YX, et al. Treatment of 26 cases of psoriasis with indirubin. *J Clin Dermatol.* 1982;11:131–132.

26. Yan SF. A clinical observation of treating 43 cases of psoriasis with indirubin. *Yunnan J Trad Chin Med.* 1982;2:21.

27. Lin XR, Yang CM, Yang GL, et al. Treatment of psoriasis with meisoindigo. *Chin J Dermatol.* 1989;22:29–30.

28. Yang CM, Lin XR, Yang GL, et al. A study of the treatment of psoriasis with meisoindigo. *J Clin Dermatol.* 1989;18:295–297.

29. Chen NQ, Dai ZH, Wang LZ. An observation of the effectiveness of *N*-aetylindirubin in treating psoriasis. *J Clin Dermatol.* 1988;17:328.

30. Xie ZZ. Treatment of psoriasis with *Pilulae Indigo natualis* compositae. *J Trad Chin Med.* 1984;25:39–40.

31. Lu YT. Treating 159 cases of psoriasis vulgaris with *Pilualae Indigo natualis* composite. *Chin J Integ Trad West Med.* 1989;9:558.

32. Institute of Dermatology, Sichuan Province. An observation of treating 33 cases of psoriasis with camtothecin. *Sichuan Bull Chn Herb.* 1973;2:7.

33. Horwitz SB. Camptothecin. In: Sartorelli AC, Johns DG, eds. *Antineoplastic and Immunosuppressive Agents, Part II.* New York, NY: Springer-Verlag NY Inc; 1976:649–656.

34. Zeng QT. *Camptotheca acuminata decne.* In: Wang YS, ed. *The Pharmacology and Application of Chinese Traditional Medicine.* Beijing, China: Peoples Health Publishing; 1983:142–1151.

35. Lin XR. Psoriasis in China. *J Dermatol.* 1993; 20:746–755.

36. Zhao WP. Clinical observation of 206 cases of psoriasis treated with Bian Zheng Shi Zhi of traditional Chinese medicine. *J Trad Chin Med.* 1989;30:31–32.

37. Lin CH, Wang HY. Comparison of long term clinical effects of microcirculation modulating traditional drugs and ethylene diamine tetreacetylimide in the treatment of psoriasis. *J Clin Dermatol.* 1988;17:125.

38. Jerner B, Skogh M, Vahlquist A. A controlled trial of acupuncture in psoriasis: no convincing effect. *Acta Derm Venereol (Stockh).* 1997; 77:154–156.

39. Rosted P. Treatment of skin diseases with acupuncture: a review. *J Dermatol Treat.* 1995;6:241–242.

40. Jayasuriya A. Clinical acupuncture. In: *The Acupuncture Foundation of Sri Lanka.* Colombo, Sri Lanka: Tilika Press; 1980.

41. Liao SJ, Liao TA. Acupuncture treatment for psoriasis: a retrospective case report. *Acupunt Electrother Res.* 1992;17:195–208.

42. Zhao F, Wang P, Hua S. Treatment of psoriasis with acupuncture and cupping therapy. *Acupuncture.* 1990;1:16–19.

43. Zhao F, Wang P, Hua S. Treatment of psoriasis with acupuncture and cupping therapy. *Chin Acupunct Moxibust.* 1991;11:16–19.

44. Yokota A, Kikutani H, Tanaka T, et al. Two species of human Fc epsilon receptor II (FC-epsilon RII-CD23): tissue specific and IL-4–specific regulation of gene expression. *Cell.* 1988;55:611–618.

45. Vercelli D, Jabara HH, Lee BW, et al. Human recombinant interleukin 4 induces Fc epsilon R2/CD23 on normal human monocytes. *J Exp Med.* 1988;167:1406–1416.

46. Bieber T, Rieger A, Neuchrist C, et al. Induction of Fc epsilon R2/CD23 on human epidermal Langerhans cells by human recombinant interleukin 4 and gamma interferon. *J Exp Med.* 1989;170:309–314.

47. Melewicz FM, Zieger RS, Mellon MH, et al. Increased peripheral blood monocytes with Fc receptors for IgE in patients with severe allergic disorders. *J Immunol.* 1981;126:1592–1595.

48. Nakamura K, Okubo Y, Minami M, et al. Phenotypic analysis of CD23 peripheral blood mononuclear cells in atopic dermatitis. *Br J Dermatol.* 1991;125:543–547.

49. Buckley CC, Ivison C, Poulter LW, Rustin MHA. FCE R11/CD23 receptor distribution in patch test reactions to aeroallergens in atopic dermatitis. *J Invest Dermatol.* 1992;99:184–188.

50. Vollenweider S, Saurat JH, Rocken M, Hauser C. Evidence suggesting involvement of interleukin-4 (IL4) production in spontaneous IgE synthesis in patients with atopic dermatitis. *J Allergy Clin Immunol.* 1991;87:1088–1095.

51. Jujo K, Renz H, Abe J, et al. Decreased interferon gamma and increased interleukin-4 (IL4) production in atopic dermatitis promotes IgE synthesis. *J Allergy Clin Immunol.* 1992; 88:323–331.

52. Xu X-J, Banerjee P, Rustin MHA, Poulter LW. Modulation by Chinese herbal therapy of immune mechanisms in the skin of patients with atopic eczema. *Br J Dermatol.* 1997;136:54–59.

53. Matsumoto T, Ishida M, Hatta T, et al. Inhibitory effect of Sho-seiryu-to on histamine release and degranulation from rat mast cells. *ORL Tokyo.* 1991;34:289–293.

54. Sakaguchi M, Iizuka A, Yuzurihara M, et al. Pharmacological characteristics of Sho-seiryu-to: an antiallergic kampo medicine without effects on histamine H, receptors and muscarinic cholinergic system in the brain. *Meth Find Exp Clin Pharmacol.* 1996;18:41–47.

55. Shichinohe K, Shimuzu M, Kuokawa K. Effect of M-711 on experimental skin reactions induced by chemical mediators in rats. *J Vet Med Sci.* 1996;58:419–423.

56. Li LF. A clinical and patch test study of contact dermatitis from traditional Chinese medicinal materials. *Contact Dermatitis.* 1995;33:392–395.

57. Huang TK, Tao WM. Allergic and toxic drug reactions of Chinese patent medicine. *Chin Tradit Patent Med.* 1989;11:22–23.

58. Wang LX, Lu LZ. Analysis of 162 reported cases of side effects of Chinese medical material. *J Beijing Clin Pharm.* 1992;5:50–55.

59. Shiota Y, Wilson JG, Matsumoto H, et al. Adult respiratory distress syndrome induced by a Chinese medicine, Kamisyoyo-San. *Intern Med.* 1996;35:494–496.

60. Pheric-Walton L, Murray V. Toxicity of Chinese herbal remedies. *Lancet.* 1992;340:673–674.

61. Ministry of Agriculture, Fisheries and Food: Dietary Supplements and Health Foods. *Report of the Working Group.* London, England: HMSO; 1991.

62. Perharic L, Shaw D, Leon C. Possible association of liver damage with the use of Chinese herbal medicine for skin disease. *Vet Hum Toxicol.* 1995;37:562–566.

63. Ferguson JE, Chalmers RJG, Rowlands DJ. Reversible dilated cardiomyopathy following treatment of atopic eczema with Chinese herbal medicine. *Br J Dermatol.* 1997;136:592–593.

12 Topical Traditional Chinese Medicine

A Report From Singapore

See-Ket Ng, MBBS, MEd (Int Med)
From the National Skin Centre, Singapore.

Topical traditional Chinese medicine is still widely used, especially by those of Chinese descent in Singapore. This practice is likely to be similar wherever there is a sizable Chinese community. In this article I discuss the types of topical traditional Chinese medicine available in Singapore—emphasizing particularly the ingredients used in the making of them—in an attempt to dispel some myths and misconceptions about traditional oils and balms.

Arch Dermatol. 1998;134:1395–1396

The use of traditional medicated oils and ointments is still prevalent among the Chinese community in Singapore. These topical traditional Chinese medicines (TTCMs) are sold, alongside Chinese herbal medicine, in traditional Chinese medicine shops all over Singapore. Pharmacies in Singapore also almost always have a small section where these are displayed for sale.

There are many varieties of TTCM available in Singapore. Some are manufactured in Singapore. Others are imported from the surrounding region, particularly from Malaysia, Hong Kong, and China.

A common misconception—and this is due first to the myriad of preparations available, and second because of labeling, with brands like Tiger Balm, 3-Snake Oil, Dragon Balm, and Red Flower Oil—is that TTCM is a complicated, exotic art, with ingredients that are incomprehensible and often secrets. In reality, TTCM in Singapore, and this is probably also true in places where there is a sizable Chinese community, eg, in Hong Kong, Taiwan, and Chinatowns in Europe and the United States, is not at all a difficult topic.

First and foremost, it must be appreciated that brand names are just brand names, and do not indicate the type of ingredients in the TTCM, eg, Tiger Balm and 3-Snake Oil do not contain any material from these 2 animals.

Second, all these myriad of preparations can be grouped into 3 classes, according to usage. In each class, the ingredients revolve around a common theme, with only minor differences, aptly described by one retailer as "if you have seen one, you have seen them all." The 3 classes of TTCM are listed below.

Oils and Ointments for Aches and Pains

The bulk of TTCM in Singapore is used for the soothing of headaches, abdominal pain, especially in children, and rheumatic pains. These oils and ointments are also used for relief of insect bites and itchy skin lesions. A classic example of TTCM in this category is Tiger Balm. The TTCMs used for this purpose usually contain camphor and menthol and also 1 or more essential oils, the common ones being cinnamon oil, oil of clove, cassia oil, citronella oil, oil of lavender, or cajuput oil. These are compounded together in a base oil or petrolatum.

It can be appreciated therefore that these preparations are meant to be soothing. They are not an irritant to the skin. It is, however, evident that patients who are allergic to fragrances would likely react adversely to this category of TTCM. In Singapore, patients who on patch testing react positively to fragrance mix or balsam of peru would be instructed to avoid, in addition to fragance compounds, all TTCM. Nearly all TTCM in this category can be patch tested as is.

A subclass of this category of TTCM is preparations used for rheumatic pains. These would have in addition to menthol, camphor, and essential oils, methyl salicylate or oil of wintergreen. Patch testing with this subclass is best done diluted to 10% in petrolatum.

Oils and Ointments for Orthopedic Injury

This is a rather specialized category of TTCM, used to soothe and promote the healing of injury, especially bruised and contused muscle. In my mind, this is what most would consider the classic TTCM, associated with the pugilistic arts. Prototype of this category would be Tjin-Koo-Lin (balm for tendons and bones). This category usually contains, in addition to camphor, menthol, essential oils, and methyl salicylate, extracts of herbs, usually of many kinds. This is illustrated by the contents of a Tjin-Koo-Lin manufactured in Singapore (Table 1).

In a study to determine the allergenic fraction in this category of TTCM, Lee and Lam[1] found the culprit allergens to be mastic and myrrh, 2 resins frequently found in the formulation of this category of TTCM.

This may be the best time to discuss Bone-setter's herbs. This is not the TTCM that is mass produced and available from shops. These are always prepared fresh, by a bone-setter (a specialized traditional Chinese healer). Herbs are pounded, mixed with wine or honey, and wrapped around injured bones or joints after manipulation. These preparations are changed daily or every other day. The poultice is not an irritant to skin and is well tolerated by many patients. Allergic contact dermatitis is, however, not uncommon. Contact allergy commonly occurs after a few changes of the poultice. The contact dermatitis appears suddenly, is of a bright dermal erythema, and almost vasculitic in appearance. In another study, Lee and Lam[2] again showed the allergenic fraction to be myrrh. Patients often require a short course of oral steroids to settle the severe contact dermatitis.

Ointments for Skin Diseases, Usually Ringworm

The third category of TTCM is rather different from the earlier 2. These are lotions and ointments touted as efficacious for all kinds of skin diseases, particularly ringworm, which usually contain salicylic acid. One popular brand of

Table 1. Contents of a Tjin-Koo-Lin (Balm for Tendons and Bones) Manufactured in Singapore*

Wintergreen	10	*Clematis chinensis* Osbeck	3
Ethanol	10	*Acanthopanax spinosis* Mig	3
Cinnamon oil	4	*Siler divanicatum* Benth et hook fil	3
Clove oil	4	*Calamus draco* Willd	3
Nutmeg oil	4	*Gentiana tibetica* L	3
Camphor	4	*Cinnamonium loureiru* Lois	3
Rheum officinate Baill	3	*Prunus persica* Stokes	3
Sinapis alba L	3	*P mouten* Sim	3
Angelica glaora Makina	3	*Conioselinum unvittatum* Turex	3
Polypodium fortunei Kze	3	*Achyranthes bidentata B1*	3
Mannis pentadactyla Linn	3	*Commiphora myrrha* Engl	3
Carthamus tinctorius L	3	Peppermint oil	2
Cyperus iria L	3	Cassia oil	2
Piper nigrum L	3		

*Values are percentages.

this type of TTCM in Singapore contains 20% salicylic acid, which is certainly effective for tinea but may cause contact dermatitis if used on eczematous skin.

Conclusions

Topical traditional Chinese medicine, at least in Singapore, and probably also in Malaysia, Hong Kong, Taiwan, and Chinatowns everywhere, are really rather simple preparations. Topical traditional Chinese medicines serve to soothe the population, especially in the past, but are still of some popularity in our era. Topical traditional Chinese medicine is not at all a difficult, mystical art as some may think, despite the often exotic and fanciful brand names.

References

1. Lee TY, Lam TH. Allergic contact dermatitis to a Chinese orthopaedic solution Tieh Ta Yao Gin. *Contact Dermatitis.* 1993;28:89–90.
2. Lee TY, Lam TH. Myrrh is the putative allergen in Bone-setter's herbs dermatitis. *Contact Dermatitis.* 1993;29:279.

13 The Essence of Alternative Medicine

A Dermatologist's View From Germany

Rudolf Happle, MD
From the Department of Dermatology, Philipp University of Marburg, Marburg, Germany.

In Germany, alternative medicine is presently very popular and is supported by the federal government. When deliberating on the essence of alternative medicine we should simultaneously reflect on the intellectual and moral basis of regular medicine. To provide an epistemological demarcation of the 2 fields, the following 12 theses are advanced: (1) alternative and regular medicine are speaking different languages; (2) alternative medicine is not unconventional medicine; (3) the paradigm of regular medicine is rational thinking; (4) the paradigm of alternative medicine is irrational thinking; (5) the present popularity of alternative medicine can be explained by romanticism; (6) some concepts of alternative medicine are falsifiable and others are not; (7) alternative medicine and evidence-based medicine are mutually exclusive; (8) the placebo effect is an important factor in regular medicine and the exclusive therapeutic principle of alternative medicine; (9) regular and alternative medicine have different aims: coming of age vs faithfulness; (10) alternative medicine is not always safe; (11) alternative medicine is not economic; and (12) alternative medicine will always exist. The fact that alternative methods are presently an integral part of medicine as taught at German universities, as well as of the physician's fee schedule, represents a collective aberration of mind that hopefully will last for only a short time.

Arch Dermatol. 1998;134:1455–1460

Alternative medicine is presently big business in Germany. It is supported by the government, by all the major political parties, and in part even by the Federal Board of Physicians. As a consequence, numerous board-certified German dermatologists no longer follow the rules of scientific medicine but practice various irrational techniques. For example, acupuncture and homeopathy are presently included in the German fee schedule for private patients. The borderline between scientific and alternative medicine has been blurred and partly abolished.

At present, more than a hundred different methods of alternative medicine are performed in Germany. The most frequently applied methods are the following:

Acupuncture	**Electroacupuncture of Dr Voll**
Anthroposophical medicine	Hildegard medicine (named after a medieval saint)
Auriculotherapy	Homeopathy
Ayurveda	Homotoxicology
Bach flower therapy	Iris diagnosis
Bioresonance	Kirlian photography (by use of electrical current)
Clinical ecology	Orthomolecular medicine
Control of symbiosis *(symbioselenkung)*	Plantar reflex zone treatment

Two alternative doctrines, anthroposopical medicine and homeopathy, are particularly favored by the government and protected by federal law.

Because this situation appears to reflect a worldwide trend, it may be helpful to have a closer look at the present German situation and to delineate the criteria to distinguish between alternative and regular medicine. In this way, the essence of alternative medicine may become apparent.

Propagation of Alternative Medicine By Institutions

The German Federal Government has issued a law compelling medical faculties to include irrational medicine as part of the curriculum (possibilities and limitations of natural healing and homeopathy). Standardized testing of students at all German medical schools now regularly contains specific questions regarding irrational doctrines. For example, which of the following decimal potencies is the lowest and can be taken as an organotropic homeopathic potency: (A) D2; (B) D12; (C) D20; (D) D30; and (E) D100? The correct answer is (A), which is found by practicing irrationalism. The Federal Board of Physicians (Bundesärztekammer) has elaborated detailed criteria of an additional qualification for homeopathy, and similar rules regarding the qualification for acupuncture are in preparation. Veronika Carstens, MD, the wife of a former federal president, functions as head of a nationwide operating foundation that promotes irrational medicine at German universities.

The German Dermatological Society has so far followed an ambivalent strategy. In 1997, the society published a statement that "electroacupuncture of Dr Voll" is not compatible with good dermatological practice,[1] and also sent an open letter to the Ministry of Health arguing against a law protecting alternative methods.[2] On the other hand, the society has conferred the status of a sponsoring member to a major manufacturer of irrational remedies, Deutsche Homöopathie Union (Karlsruhe, Germany).[3]

Propagation of Irrational Methods By Medical Faculties

Irrational methods are presently established at many German medical faculties: Erlangen, internal medicine[4]; Giessen, anesthesiology[5]; Hannover, veterinary medicine[6]; Heidelberg, gynecology[5]; Munich, anatomy[5]; and Witten-Herdecke, anatomy.[7] For example, the Department of Anesthesiology at the Justus Liebig University of Giessen is performing ozone therapy, "control of symbiosis," and electroacupuncture of Dr Voll for the treatment of pain[5] as well as for other problems such as male pattern hair loss. At the School of Veterinarian Medicine of Hannover, the alleged effectiveness of homeopathy is measured in animal experiments.[6] The Department of Gynecology and Obstetrics at the Ruprecht-Karl University of Heidelberg is treating female infertility by auricular acupuncture, bioresonance, and homeopathy.[5] A professor of anatomy, fellow of the Medical Faculty at the Ludwig-Maximilian University of Munich, is a member of the advisory board of a manufacturer selling impressive machineries for electroacupuncture.[5] In the Department of Anatomy at the University of Witten-Herdecke, the morphological substrate of acupuncture points has been demonstrated in human skin.[7] The findings are not reproducible but this argument reflects the arrogance of scholastic medicine. In the Department of Internal Medicine at the Friedrich-Alexander University of Erlangen-Nuremberg, the Veronica and Karl Carstens Foundation has established an outpatient clinic for alternative medicine; its popularity is reported to be high.[4]

How Do Physicians Feel About Alternative Medicine?

In 1995, the Department of Psychiatry at the University of Marburg published the results of an opinion poll among physicians. Sixty percent endorsed alternative methods, 36% were using one or more of these techniques, 50% advocated inclusion of such methods into the social health plan, and 75% advocated alternative methods to be included into the curriculum at university faculties.[8] Apparently, the lack of a scientific basis does not interfere with the acceptance of a method by many physicians, including dermatologists.

For Which Complaints Do Patients Ask the Help of Alternative Physicians or Healers?

According to Lewith,[9] what brings patients into the office of alternative doctors or healers are pain, allergies, emotional problems or other psychological difficulties, and gastrointestinal tract disturbances. Most of these problems are approachable by the power of suggestion. People asking for alternative medicine tend to be young and have a rather higher level of education and income.[10] Hence, they constitute a profitable target group.

Twelve Theses on Alternative Medicine

Alternative and Regular Medicine Are Speaking Different Languages

In Germany and elsewhere, a prevailing linguistic prescriptivism has resulted in the acceptance of an irrational terminology. This is reflected by the terms *complementary, alternative, unconventional, and integrative medicine*. Physicians believing in alternative methods and those adhering to regular medicine are using the same words for different things. As a consequence, any discussion between the 2 camps tends to become absurd. For example, alternative approaches are an inherent task of scientific medicine, but that aspect is not the topic of this special issue of the *Archives*. Conversely, we use in this issue the term *alternative medicine* for all those medical methods that do not constitute an alternative to regular medicine (Table 1). To speak with each other, we need a dictionary.

An initial approach to such a glossary is presented in Table 2. For example, the euphemistic term *particular therapeutic modalities* is used in a German federal law protecting irrational doctrines such as homeopathy or anthroposophical medicine. Natural methods of healing include many that have nothing to do with nature, such as autohemotherapy, evacuation by drainage of amalgam, neural therapy, acupuncture, or electroacupuncture of Dr Voll. Extended therapeutic modalities or complementary medicine are nothing but irrational therapeutic modalities. The term *Ganzheitsmedizin* (holistic or integrative medicine) is used with either no meaning or with that of totalitarian medicine. The term *paradigm shift* means a turning away from rational thinking. Soft medicine is treatment by the power of suggestion. Allopathic means pharmacologically effective, whereas homeopathic means effective by suggestion. The term *high potency* is a poetic paraphrasing of nothing dissolved in a vehicle.

Table 2 illustrates the difficulties inherent in any dialogue between the 2 camps.

Table 1. Two Different Definitions of Alternative Medicine

Irrational Definition	Rational Definition
Methods rejected by regular medicine	Methods lacking a rational justification
Helpful complementation of regular medicine	No epistemological alternative to regular medicine
Therapeutic effects not exclusively based on suggestion	Therapeutic effects exclusively based on suggestion
Science based on a particular paradigm	No science

Table 2. Glossary for a Dialogue Between Alternative and Regular Medicine

Irrational Terminology	Rational Translation
Allopathic	Pharmacologically effective
Complementary medicine	Medicine lacking a rational justification
Extended modes of treatment	Modes of treatment lacking a rational justification
High potency	Nothing in a vehicle
Homeopathic	Effective by the power of suggestion
Integrative medicine	Totalitarian medicine
Natural healing	Therapeutic principles that do not deal with "nature"
Paradigm shift	Turning away from rational thinking
Particular therapeutic modalities	Absurd therapeutic modalities
Soft medicine	Treatment by suggestion
Unconventional medicine	Medicine exclusively based on convention

Alternative Medicine Is Not Unconventional Medicine

Many German authors adhering to scientific medicine have adopted a strange linguistic prescriptivism by applying the term *unconventional medicine* to alternative methods.[11] In fact, the regular scientific medicine should instead be called unconventional because all its concepts are continuously subject to the test of falsification. Conversely, alternative concepts usually represent doctrines announced by a master in whom one has to believe.[12] A test of falsification is either forbidden or impossible because the dogma belongs to the category of faith rather than science; consequently, alternative methods are rigid and unsuitable for further development. For obvious reasons, such methods should be considered conventional rather than unconventional.

The Paradigm of Regular Medicine Is Rational Thinking

Many physicians are convinced that the basis of regular medicine is natural science. This is not correct because modern medicine includes several fields that, either entirely or in part, do not belong to natural science, such as medical sociology, medical ethics, psychosomatic medicine, or psychiatry.[12] In fact, a paradigm common to all fields of regular medicine is rational thinking. It is difficult, however, to give an exact definition of rational thinking. Essential traits are abstraction, reproducibility of data, and the advancement of controllable terminologies and systems. According to Karl Popper,[13] scientific research means a continuous testing of all concepts and theories by the trial of falsification.[14] Another essential aspect is that rational thinking always has a moral dimension. Or, to give a rather sloppy definition—if you who are reading this article do not know what rational thinking means, you are beyond help.

The Paradigm of Alternative Medicine Is Irrational Thinking

Alternative medicine questions the crucial role of rational arguing and accepts other patterns of thinking.[15] All concepts of alternative medicine have an alogical dimension that calls for faithful acceptance. This faith excludes abstraction, testing for reproducibility of data, or double-blind studies.

Alternative medicine claims that it deals with the patients themselves, whereas regular medicine primarily concentrates on diseases. The metaphysical approach results in an irrational language using terms such as *holism*, *rejection of a particularistic ontology*, *extended modes of healing*, or *spiritual vital energy*. Some doctrines, such as homeopathy[16,17] or anthroposophical medicine,[18] fulfill the criteria of a religion, and in many ways claim to be able to explain the unexplainable.

Physicians adhering to alternative methods are often referring to Kuhn[19] who has advanced the term *paradigm shift*, or to Feyerabend[20] who coined the misleading slogan "anything goes" and wrote: "We should learn that rational research [in Popper's sense: a theory should be regarded as correct until it is falsified] is only of temporary usefulness, and that . . . free discussions belong to the prerequisites of science." Consequently, alternative physicians ask for "pluralism of sciences" and claim that rational and irrational thinking should have equal rights.[21]

The Present Popularity of Alternative Medicine Can Be Explained by Romanticism

At the beginning of the 19th century, romanticism originated in Germany as a movement against enlightenment and sober rationality. Romanticism in art and lifestyle stood for rediscovery of magic, a cult of irrationalism, and a longing for naive originality, pristine naturalness, and lack of sophisticism. In 1798, the German writer Novalis[22] enunciated:

> The world has to be romanticized. . . . By giving to the ordinary a high meaning, by rendering to the normal a mysterious aspect, by bestowing upon well-known things the dignity of the unknown, by conferring to the finite an infinite appearance, I romanticize those things. . . .

Nüchtern[23] has delineated the parallels between this movement and the revival of romanticism in our days that is a worldwide phenomenon as illustrated, for example, by the incredible variety of publications offered today in the "new age" sections of American bookshops. The present popularity of alternative medical concepts reflects a deeply rooted propensity to romanticism, as a movement against the technical conditions of modern life.

Some Alternative Concepts Are Falsifiable, and Others Are Not

Many methods of alternative medicine are falsifiable, but this does not inhibit their defenders from applying them. Other concepts belong to the category of faith rather than science and can therefore not be falsified.[14] The following examples illustrate the 2 categories.

A Falsifiable Concept: The Dogma of Potentation Through Dilution. The potency principle belongs to the field of classic homeopathy and claims that an agent becomes more powerful as it is diluted. For the irrational thinker it is essential that this dilution be performed by means of a ritualized shaking procedure.[15,16] Today it is well known that after a dilution of "D24" ($1/10^{24}$) not a single molecule of active ingredient remains in the solution. To falsify the principle of potentiation through dilution, we gathered 8 different homeopathic drugs with a potentiation of D30, dissolved in 51% alcohol, eg, *Lachesis mutus* (bushmaster), *arsenicum album*, *pyrogenium* (extract of autolytic beef meat), sulfur, *apis mellifica* (honeybee), *acidum nitricum*, *zincum metallicum*, and *Pulsatilla pratensis* (pasqueflower). As a control we prepared a bottle simply filled with 51% alcohol but having likewise undergone 30 shaking procedures, as well as a bottle containing *apis mellifica* in a dilution of 10^{-30} but prepared without any shaking procedure. The experiment consisted in removing the labels from the 10 bottles so there was no longer any possibility of discriminating between them. There were neither chemical nor physical nor biological methods to identify the name of the mother tincture as originally indicated on the label. The verum bottles avoid no longer be distinguished from the control bottles. In this way the principle of potentiation through dilution can be regarded as falsified.

Notwithstanding, some recent studies have claimed that extremely high solutions can be distinguished by their biological effects. One example is the article by Davenas et al.[24] Similarly, Reilly et al[25] claimed that in patients affected with atopic asthma, nothing dissolved in a vehicle works significantly better than the vehicle containing nothing. Many other investigations[26–28] have convincingly shown that highly diluted drugs were ineffective, but such studies have received less attention.

A Falsifiable Concept: Electroacupuncture of Dr Voll. Electroacupuncture of Dr Voll represents an amalgam of oriental mysticism and occidental electrotechnology. Two electrodes are applied to distant acupuncture points. A bottle containing an allergen or other pathogen is placed between the electrodes, and the interference of the bottle with the electrical conductive qualities of the skin is measured. In controlled studies[1,29] the method has been shown to be ineffective. Notwithstanding, even some board-certified German dermatologists are using this technique as a test for allergies, environmental intoxication, and other ailments.

A Falsifiable Concept: The Bioresonance Method. The bioresonance method is used to measure an ultrafine oscillation spectrum in the human organism that can be normalized if necessary.[30] An allergic patient is said to be treated by a mirror oscillation of the allergen.[31] Appropriately performed controlled studies,[32,33] have shown that allergens cannot be recognized by this test, and that allergies can neither be extinguished nor otherwise influenced by this method. These negative results, however, do not interfere with the popularity that the bioresonance method presently enjoys in Germany.

An Unfalsifiable Concept: The Homeopathic Drug Picture of Pulsatilla. In a homeopathic monography we read the following assertion on *Pulsatilla pratensis*: "The drug mostly corresponds to women with feminine forms, full hips, fair hair and blue eyes." Wiesenauer[35] describes the principle signs corresponding to this plant in the following way: "Girls and women, fair-skinned, blond, feminine. Nature sensitive like that of a mimosa, with a tendency to weep; depressive, capricious, faint-hearted." We may consider these statements to be nonsense, but we cannot falsify them because we are not able to prove that this rare blue flower does not correspond to a fair-haired whiney woman with feminine curves. These assertions have nothing to do with science because a test of falsification is not possible.

An Unfalsifiable Concept: Relationship Between the Spleen and Saturn. The idea that the role of the spleen within the human organism corresponds to the significance of Saturn within the planetary system is an integral part of anthroposophical medicine[18] and is believed, for example, at the University of Witten-Herdecke. This view belongs to a system of doctrines advanced by Steiner:

> Because the spleen is the first organ presenting itself to the blood . . . the ancient occultists thought that it should be best named after the star that, according to the ancient occultists and in line with their observations, presents itself as the first one in the space within the solar system; for this reason they called the spleen "Saturnian" or an "internal Saturn within man."[36]

This assertion can be rejected as an absurdity, but it is unfalsifiable because we cannot prove that there is no relationship between the spleen and Saturn. Such irrational dogmas represent a dimension inherent in many methods of alternative medicine.

Alternative Medicine and Evidence-Based Medicine Are Mutually Exclusive

If scientific evidence can be provided for the effectiveness of any unconventional approach, this method becomes a true alternative and, therefore, an integral part of regular medicine. Today it has become trendy to speak about evidence-based medicine[37] but we should not forget that this form of medicine has always been the *raison d'être* for every scientific medical journal. Some authors[38,39] pretend to adopt a neutral position by arguing that alternative methods may indeed be effective although proof is so far lacking, and that evidence-based medicine will establish some alternative methods in their full glory. This attitude, while seeming scientific, disregards 2 important points. First, other studies showing the ineffectiveness of alternative methods have already been performed, and second, alternative concepts cannot be falsified because they do not belong to the category of science. This irreconcilability of alternative and scientific medicine is often overlooked.

Placebo Effect Is an Important Factor in Regular Medicine, and the Exclusive Therapeutic Principle in Alternative Medicine

In all therapeutic measures as performed in regular medicine, the placebo effect plays an important role. In practice it is not our task to exclude it but to make appropriate usage of it.[12] In clinical trials, however, scientific medicine has to distinguish between such effects and the true efficacy of a therapeutic measure, ie, to disintegrate things and to consider them in abstraction. Conversely, the integrative principle of alternative medicine is exclusively based on the placebo effect. This view, however, will always remain controversial.[21]

Regular and Alternative Medicine Have Different Aims: Coming of Age vs Faithfulness

The aim of regular medicine is a patient who has come of age and is able to make his or her own decisions. For obvious reasons this aim often remains utopian. Rational thinking always includes the doubt, but in clinical practice we have to weigh carefully how much doubting can be tolerated by a given patient.

The aim of alternative medicine is a faithful patient who does not ask for rational explanations. The degree of absurdity of concepts to which some of our patients adhere is often amazing. This may be explained by an increasing estrangement to the faith as offered by the churches established in Germany. Apparently, an a priori need for metaphysical bonds remains unsatisfied and causes one to seeks a substitute. A similar trend appears to prevail in the United States, as illustrated, for example, by the delirium that the Hale-Bopp comet has recently evoked in some people. The fact that alternative medical approaches are not compatible with rational thinking renders such methods especially attractive. As a witty man said: "Since people decided to believe in nothing, they believe in all sorts of things."

Alternative Methods Are Not Always Safe

Similar to the methods of regular medicine, alternative approaches may be associated with severe and even life-threatening adverse effects.[40,41] This should be emphasized because such risks are frequently denied by the apologists of soft medicine. A serious aspect is the triggering of psychotic diseases by alternative approaches:[10] general chemophobia (multiple chemical sensitivity syndrome); sick building phobia; clinical ecology syndrome[42]; and amalgam phobia. In dermatological practice we are nowadays confronted rather frequently with such problems.

Alternative Medicine Is Uneconomic

Hartnack[43] analyzed applications for reimbursement as filed by private insurance companies and showed that alternative medicine is rather expensive and uneconomic. For example, the German amalgam phobia of recent years has resulted in a wave of useless diagnostic measures and unnecessary dental procedures.[10] Similarly, an Australian study[44] has shown that alternative medicine constitutes a considerable financial burden.

Alternative Medicine Will Always Exist

Alternative medicine represents the most ancient form of medicine, and it will continue to exist just as long as there are human diseases. Such methods meet the need of many people seeking some metaphysical bonds and a simple explanation of complex or inexplicable things. As a particular fact, however, alternative medicine is today an integral part of medicine as taught at German universities, as well as of the physician's fee schedule. Hopefully, this aberration of mind will only last for a short time. After this fad of collective irrationalism, alternative methods will regain their previous status as a marginal field of medicine that has nothing to do with science and cannot be reimbursed by the social health care plan.

Presented in part at the 15th Fortbildungswoche für Praktische Dermatologie und Venerologie, Munich, Germany, July 21-26, 1996.

References

1. Breit R, Meigel W. DDG-aktuell. *Hautarzt.* 1997; 48:214–220.
2. Schöpf E. *Alternative diagnostische und therapeutische Methoden als Kassenleistung: ja oder nein?* Briefwechsel des Präsidenten der DDG, Prof Dr Erwin Schöpf, mit dem Bundesministerium für Gesundheit. *Hautarzt.* 1997; 48:603–604.
3. Breit R, Meigel W. DDG-aktuell. *Hautarzt.* 1998;49:72–84.
4. Albrecht H. Muß Komplementärmedizin wissenschaftlich evaluiert werden? *Fortschr Med.* 1995;113:37–38.
5. Ostendorf GM. Die Propagierung von Außenseitermethoden an deutschen Universitäten. *Versicherungsmedizin.* 1993;3:85–90.
6. Harisch G, Kretschmer M. *Jenseits vom Milligramm.* New York, NY: Springer Publishing Co Inc; 1990.
7. Heine H. Funktionelle Morphologie der Akupunkturpunkte. *Aku.* 1988;16:4–11.
8. Gräfen U. Gut 60 Prozent der Ärzte befürworten den Einsatz komplementärer Methoden: 36 Prozent wenden sie an. *Ärzte Zeitung.* September 27, 1995:9.27.
9. Lewith G. Why do people seek treatment by alternative medicine? *BMJ.* 1985;290:28–29.
10. Ostendorf GM. Probleme der Alternativmedizin in der privaten Personenversicherung. *Versicherungsmedizin.* 1995;47:224–231.
11. Oepen I, ed. *Unkonventionelle medizinische Verfahren.* Stuttgart, Germany: Gustav Fischer Verlag; 1993.
12. Bock KD. *Wissenschaftliche und alternative Medizin: Paradigmen-Praxis-Perspektiven.* New York, NY: Springer Publishing Co Inc; 1993.

13. Popper KR. *The Logic of Scientific Discovery*. New York, NY: Basic Books Inc Publishers; 1959.

14. Lakatos I. Falsification and the methodology of scientific research programmes. In: Lakatos I, Musgrave A, eds. *Criticism and the Growth of Knowledge: Proceedings of the International Colloquium in the Philosophy of Science*. New York, NY: Cambridge University Press; 1970: 91–196.

15. Habermann E. Wissenschaft, Glaube und Magie in der Arzneitherapie: Manifestationen, Theorie und Bedarf. *Skeptiker.* 1994;7:4–14.

16. Prokop O. *Homöopathie: was leistet sie wirklich?* Frankfurt, Germany: Verlag Ullstein; 1995.

17. Burgdorf W, Happle R. What every dermatologist should know about homeopathy. *Arch Dermatol.* 1996;132:955–958.

18. Stratmann F. *Zum Einfluß der Anthroposophie in der Medizin.* Munich, Germany: W Zuckschwerdt Verlag; 1988.

19. Kuhn TS. *The Structure of Scientific Revolutions*. Chicago, Ill: The University of Chicago Press; 1962.

20. Feyerabend P. *Erkenntnis für freie Menschen*. Frankfurt, Germany: Suhrkamp Verlag; 1980:99.

21. Kiene H. Komplementärmedizin-Schulmedizin: Der Wissenschaftsstreit am Ende des 20. *Jahrhunderts*. Stuttgart, Germany: Schattauer Verlag; 1994.

22. von Hardenberg FL (alias Novalis). *Werke, herausgegeben und kommentiert von G Schulz.* Munich, Germany: CH Beck; 1969:384–385.

23. Nüchtern E. *Was Alternativmedizin populär macht.* Berlin, Germany: Evangelische Zentralstelle für Weltanschauungsfragen; 1998:26–28.

24. Davenas EF, Beauvais J, Amara M, et al. Human basophil degranulation triggered by very dilute antiserum against IgE. *Nature.* 1988; 333:816–818.

25. Reilly D, Taylor MA, Beatty NGM, et al. Is evidence for homoeopathy reproducible? *Lancet.* 1994;344:1601–1606.

26. Kainz JT, Kozel G, Haidvogl M, Smolle J. Homeopathic versus placebo therapy of children with warts on the hands: a randomized, double-blind clinical trial. *Dermatology.* 1996; 193:318–320.

27. Walach H, Haeusler W, Lowes T, et al. Classical homeopathic treatment of chronic headaches. *Cephalalgia.* 1997;17:119–126.

28. Whitmarsh TE, Coleston-Shields DM, Steiner TJ. Double-blind randomized placebo-controlled study of homoeopathic prophylaxis of migraine. *Cephalalgia.* 1997;17:608–609.

29. Gloerfeld H. *Elektroakupunktur nach Voll (EAV): ein Beitrag zur kritischen Einschätzung eines unkonventionellen Verfahrens [thesis].* Marburg, Germany: Philipp University of Marburg; 1987.

30. Ostendorf GM. Mora-und Bioresonanz-Therapie. *Münch Med Wochenschr.* 1993; 135:400–402.

31. Schulze-Werninghaus G. Paramedizinische Verfahren: Bioresonanz-Diagnostik und-Therapie. *Dtsch Dermatol.* 1994;42:891–896.

32. Kofler H, Ulmer H, Mechtler E, Falk M, Fritsch PO. Bioresonanz bei Pollinose: eine vergleichende Untersuchung zur diagnostischen und therapeutischen Wertigkeit. *Allergologie.* 1996;19:114–122.

33. Schöni MH, Schöni-Affolter F. Effekt von Bioresonanz bei Kindern mit atopischer Dermatitis: eine randomisierte Doppelblindstudie. *Schweiz Med Wochenschr.* 1996;126(suppl 78):11.

34. Zimmermann W. *Homöotherapie der Hautkrankheiten*. Regensburg, Germany: Johannes Sonntag Verlagsbuchhandlung; 1987:39.

35. Wiesenauer M. *Praxis der Homöopathie: Kurzgefaßte Arzneimittellehre für Ärzte und Apotheker.* Stuttgart, Germany: Hippokrates-Verlag; 1985:207–209.

36. Steiner R. *Eine okkulte Physiologie*. Dornach, Germany: Rudolf Steiner Verlag; 1911.

37. Evidence-based medicine, in its place. *Lancet.* 1995;346:785.

38. Walach H. Ist Homöopathie der Forschung zugänglich? (Is homeopathy accessible to research?) *Schweiz Rundschau Med.* 1994; 83:1439–1447.

39. Ernst E. Homöopathie: Argumente und Gegenargumente. *Dtsch Ärztebl.* 1997; 94:A2340–A2342.

40. Abbot NC, White AR, Ernst R. Complementary medicine. *Nature.* 1996;381:361.

41. Aberer W, Strohal R. Homeopathic preparations: severe adverse effects, unproven benefits. *Dermatologica.* 1992;182:253.

42. Ring J, Gabriel G, Vieluf D, Przybilla B. Das klinische Ökologie-Syndrom ("Öko-Syndrom"): Polysomatische Beschwerden bei vermuteter Allergie gegen Umweltschadstoffe. *Münch Med Wochenschr.* 1991;130:50–55.

43. Hartnack D. *Unkonventionelle medizinische Methoden: wirklich wirksam und preiswert?* Ulm, Germany: Universitätsverlag; 1994.

44. MacLennan AH, Wilson DH, Taylor AW. Prevalence and cost of alternative medicine in Australia. *Lancet.* 1996;347:569–573.

45. Löhr O. *Deutschlands geschützte Pflanzen*. 2nd ed. Heidelberg, Germany: Carl Winter Universitätsverlag; 1953.

14 Prevalence of Skin Disease in Rural Tanzania and Factors Influencing the Choice of Health Care, Modern or Traditional

Frederick Temba Satimia, ADDV; Sandra R. McBride, MB, BS, MRCP; Barbara Leppard, DM, FRCP
From the Regional Dermatology Training Centre, Kilimanjaro Christian Medical Centre, Moshi, Tanzania.

Objectives
To determine the prevalence of skin disease in a rural Tanzanian community and to investigate the health-seeking behavior of this community.

Design
The study was in 3 parts: (1) 120 heads of households were interviewed to determine the factors that influence the families' health-seeking behavior; (2) the 800 members of these families were examined for evidence of skin disease; and (3) a focus group discussion was held with influential members of the community to get a broader view of health-seeking behavior.

Setting
A rural village in the southwestern area of Tanzania. Individuals were interviewed and examined in their own homes.

Results
A total of 34.7% of 800 villagers had one or more skin diseases, the most common of which were tinea capitis, tinea corporis, scabies, acne, and eczema. Modern and traditional health facilities were equally used, but heads of the households older than 55 years who had never been to school and individuals who were not Christians favored traditional medicine. It was cheaper to go to a traditional healer, but modern medicine was thought to be more scientific.

Conclusions
Skin disease was a problem in this village and was perceived to be a problem by both individuals and the community. There is a need to assess the clinical and diagnostic skills of both modern and traditional health practitioners and to instigate a preventive health education program to eradicate the common infections and infestations.

Arch Dermatol. 1998;134:1363–1366

Eight hundred individuals living in a rural village in Tanzania were examined for skin disease. One hundred twenty heads of household were interviewed using a questionnaire to determine their health-seeking behavior in relation to skin disease, and a focus group discussion with influential members of the village was held to obtain a broader perspective of the community's behavior and attitude toward skin disease.

The prevalence of skin disease was 34.7%, with most of the diseases being both treatable and preventable. Approximately equal numbers of heads of household chose modern or traditional health care for their families' dermatological needs. Factors influencing this choice of treatment included the age, religion, and level of education of the head of the household (Table 1).

Background

Tanzania is similar to other sub-Saharan African countries in that it has very few dermatologists, so there is limited medical expertise in the diagnosis and treatment of skin disease. Dispensaries and health centers are not manned by doctors but by clinical officers and assistant clinical officers who have very little training in dermatology. Skin disease is common in rural communities[1] and can have a profound effect on both the individual and the community.[2]

Traditional healers are found everywhere in Africa and form the backbone of rural medical practice.[3] (See Table 1 for definitions of terms used throughout the article. Many of them are interested in skin disease,[4] and many plants and herbs have been found to be effective in the treatment of skin disease,[5] but little is known about how these remedies are used by traditional healers in Tanzania.

Chapwa Village is situated in Tunduma Ward, Mbozi District, Mbeya Region, in the Southern Highlands of Tanzania (Figure 1). The village is 18 km from Tunduma Town on the main Tunduma-Mbeya road and is well linked with other parts of Mbeya Region. It has a population of 3500 (1988 census). The main tribes are Nyumwanga, Nyika, Ndali, and Nyakyusa, each of which have different cultural characteristics. The main religion is Christianity, with several different denominations having churches in the village. Most of the houses are built with bricks; some have iron-sheet roofing, but the majority are roofed with grass.

The average temperature is between 18°C and 25°C. There are 2 seasons: the dry season, from July to October, and the wet season, from November to June. The water supply is inadequate, with many people depending on ponds and shallow wells for domestic use. The main activities of the villagers are farming (maize, beans, and ground nuts) and cattle rearing. The village has 1 primary school, but no modern health facility. The nearest health center is 18 km away in Tunduma Town. However, there are several traditional healers and 4 traditional birth attendants within the village itself.

Skin disease is among the 10 most common diseases registered at Tunduma Health Centre, and the number of patients attending there with skin disease has increased over

Table 1. Definitions

Term	Definition
Household	People sharing the same food or living under the same roof and their dependents
10-Cell leader	A person responsible for a group of 10 households
Head of household	A person who is the decision maker on health matters for a household
Traditional healer	A person using local herbs to treat disease
First choice of health facility	The first action taken when seeking treatment for skin disease
Level of education	
None	Have never attended school and are unable to read or write
Adult education	Did not attend school as a child but learned how to read and write in a special program in adulthood
Primary education and above	Attended school (at least primary school) and are able to read and write

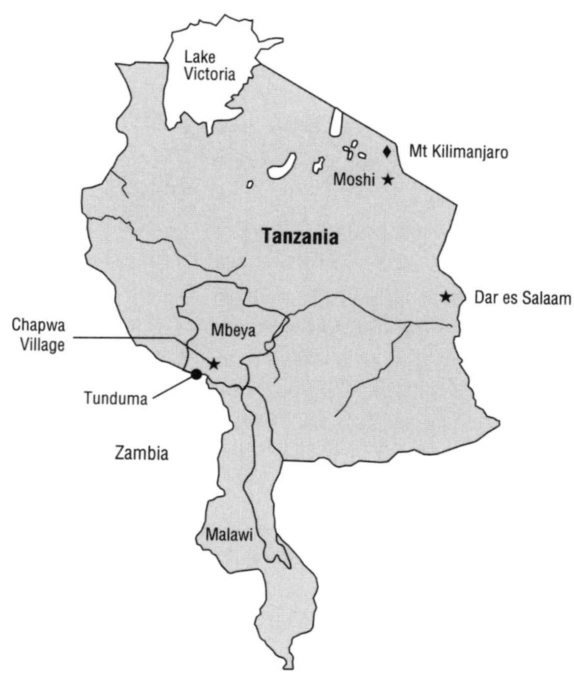

Figure 1. Map of Tanzania.

the last 3 years. There are no figures for patients attending traditional healers and no community-based data.

This study was undertaken to determine the prevalence and nature of skin disease within a rural Tanzanian community and to investigate the health-seeking behavior of this community and the factors that determine the choice of health care system within the community. It was performed with a view to developing an appropriate and effective dermatological service for the area in the future, possibly in liaison with the local traditional healers.

Subjects and Methods

Chapwa Village was randomly selected from 7 villages in Tunduma Ward by a multicluster sampling method. The sample size was determined using a method described by Kirkwood.[6] Twelve "10-cell leaders" were randomly selected, and their households provided the study population, ie, all heads of households and all members of these households. Children younger than 3 months were excluded for cultural reasons. The study was in 3 parts:

Part 1. One hundred twenty heads of households were interviewed by a research assistant using a well-structured questionnaire written in Kiswahili. Questions were asked about age, sex, marital status, level of education, occupation, knowledge about skin disease, and the factors that would influence their choice of health care for skin disease in themselves and their families.

Part 2. All members of these households older than 3 months were examined by a single researcher (F.T.S.) who had completed 1 year of dermatology training at the Regional Dermatology Training Centre, Kilimanjaro Christian Medical Centre, Moshi. Examination of the skin was performed in the individual's home after informed consent was obtained. Confidentiality and privacy were maintained as far as was possible. Individuals who were found to have skin disease were treated on the spot.

Part 3. A meeting was held with highly regarded members of the community to gain a broader perspective of the attitudes and health-seeking behavior of the villagers with regard to skin disease. The meeting was chaired by the main researcher (F.T.S.), and notes were taken by a research assistant. Participants included the village chairman, the village secretary, the village agricultural officer, 2 primary school teachers, 4 traditional birth attendants, 3 traditional healers, 4 ten-cell leaders, 2 religious leaders, and 3 other influential people in the community. Topics discussed included knowledge and superstitions about skin diseases, the types of skin diseases best treated by traditional healers, the availability of medicinal plants, and the factors that influence whether people go to traditional healers or to a modern health care facility for treatment of skin diseases.

Table 2. Study Population, by Age, Sex, and Skin Disease

			Skin Disease		
Age, y	**Males**	**Females**	**Present**	**Not Present**	**Total**
≤5	86	96	49	133	**182**
6-14	115	116	86	145	**231**
15-24	49	84	53	80	**133**
25-34	46	47	32	61	**93**
35-44	31	31	19	43	**62**
45-54	19	8	9	18	**27**
55-64	19	17	11	25	**36**
≥65	17	19	19	17	**36**
Total, No. (%)	**382 (47.8)**	**418 (52.2)**	**278 (34.7)**	**522 (65.3)**	**800**

Results

A total of 800 people were examined for the presence of skin disease; 50% of them were younger than 15 years, and there were approximately equal numbers of males and females (Table 2). The prevalence of skin disease in this community was 34.7%, with males and females equally affected. Fifty percent of all skin disease affected children younger than 15 years (Table 2). The 5 most common diseases overall were tinea capitis, scabies, acne, eczema, and tinea corporis (Table 3), but the pattern of skin diseases was different in different age groups:

Age Group, y	Most Common Skin Diseases
<2	Impetigo, atopic eczema
2-5	Tinea capitis, tinea corporis
6-13	Tinea capitis, tinea corporis, scabies
14-17	Acne, scabies
≥18	Eczema, pityriasis versicolor, tinea corporis

All patients with scabies were symptomatic, but more than half the patients with acne did not perceive it as a problem (Table 3).

Among the 120 heads of households interviewed, there were twice as many males as females, and most were older than 25 years. Almost half of the heads of households (47.5%) said that if they, or a member of their family, had a skin problem they would go to a modern health facility, and 43.3% said that they would go to a traditional healer. A few said that they would not do anything (5%) or that they would treat themselves (4.2%). Seventy percent of the heads of households older than 55 years said that they would use a traditional healer, whereas 78% of those between 15 and 34 years of age would go to a modern health

Table 3. The 5 Most Prevalent Skin Diseases and Their Relation to Symptoms

Type of Skin Disease	No. (%) Seen as a Problem	Not Seen as a Problem	Total
Tinea capitis	30 (88.2)	4 (11.8)	**34**
Scabies	32 (100)	0	**32**
Acne	12 (41.4)	17 (58.6)	**29**
Eczema	27 (96.4)	1 (3.6)	**28**
Tinea corporis	21 (75)	7 (25)	**28**
Total	**122 (80.8)**	**29 (19.2)**	**151**

Table 4. Choice of Health Facility in Relation to Level of Education of Head of Household

Health Facility	Level of Education: None	Adult Education	Primary Education and Above	Total
Traditional	22	14	16	**52**
Modern	4	7	46	**57**
Other	1	5	5	**11**
Total	**27**	**26**	**67**	**120**

facility. This difference is statistically highly significant ($P<.001$). Seventy-one percent of non-Christian heads of households prefer traditional medicine, compared with 37% of Christians; again, this is a statistically significant difference ($P<.05$). Eighty-one and a half percent of the heads of households who cannot read or write prefer traditional medicine, and 69% of those who had at least a primary school education prefer modern medicine ($P<.001$, Table 4). When asked for reasons for their choice, they said that the 2 most important ones were science and cost. Eighty-three percent of those who mentioned cost said that it was cheaper to go to a traditional healer, and 60% of those citing science said that modern medicine was more scientific and therefore likely to be more effective. Of those choosing to go to a modern health facility, 88% said they did so because it was more scientific (Table 5).

The information gained from the community meeting showed that skin disease was perceived to be a problem in the village. The diseases known to be treated by traditional healers were tinea capitis, eczema, and scabies. The plants used for treating these conditions were all easily available in and around the village.

Table 5. Reasons Given for Selecting a Particular Health Facility as the First Line of Action

Reason Given	Traditional	Modern	Other	Total
Cost related	20	1	3	**24**
Proximity	4	2	0	**6**
Science	27	50	6	**83**
Disease severity	1	3	0	**4**
Other	0	1	2	**3**
Total	**52**	**57**	**11**	**120**

Comment

In Tanzania, traditional medicine is part of the culture, although it is not as well organized as in India[7] or China.[8] Its practices are based on beliefs that were in existence thousands of years before the development and spread of modern scientific medicine.[9] People are comfortable with practices that are in harmony with their culture and are reassured when advice is given in an unhurried manner by someone who seems to understand.[10] Traditional healers are found all over Tanzania. They are accessible, affordable, culturally appropriate, and acceptable. They explain illness in terms that are familiar because they are part of the local belief system.[11] In contrast, modern health service providers hold views on health that emphasize disease; the focus is on the physical body in an attempt to be "objective and scientific."[12]

The health situation has improved in many developing countries owing to the training of personnel at the primary health care level and to the introduction of essential drug kits.[13] But modern drugs are expensive and the supply may be irregular.[14] In Abidjan, Cote d'Ivoire, 14% to 17% of urban households changed from modern to traditional medicine when the franc was devalued[15]; these figures were probably even higher in rural areas. Traditional medicine is generally cheaper than modern medicine.[16] The World Health Organization estimates that 80% of the population of most developing countries rely on traditional forms of health care as their primary source of health care.[17]

We were surprised to find that fewer than 50% of the heads of households in Chapwa Village said that they would go to a traditional healer as their first choice for treatment of skin disease. This greater than expected use of modern health facilities may be because they (1) consider skin disease a particular group of diseases that need modern medicine, (2) were reluctant to admit to using a traditional healer to personnel from a modern medical system for fear of seeming backward, or (3) were simply trying to please us. It is particularly surprising in view of the fact that the nearest health center (for modern health care) is 18 km away and that there are several traditional healers living and working in the village.

The main factors that seemed to influence the choice of health care were age and education. Heads of households who were older than 55 years and those who had not been to school mainly used traditional healers. Such findings are not surprising, since these people would have been brought up with traditional medicine and had no opportunity to learn about alternatives. Christians were more likely to use modern health care, presumably because of the possible association of traditional medicine with witch doctors. There are several Christian churches in the village, and local pastors may have a considerable influence on behavior. The cost of treatment is an important reason why people choose traditional medicine and scientific knowledge a reason for choosing modern health care.

Skin disease was a problem in Chapwa Village, and, indeed, it was perceived as a problem by the village elders; 34.7% of the population had one or more skin diseases, mainly the common infections and infestations. These diseases are both preventable and curable, so it seems that neither the traditional nor the modern health practitioners are having much impact on them. Benzyl benzoate, compound benzoic acid ointment (6% benzoic acid and 3% salicylic acid in emulsifying ointment [Whitfield ointment]), and griseofulvin, if used properly, would eradicate scabies, tinea corporis, and tinea capitis, and these drugs are meant to be available in the government drug kits. It would be interesting to compare the drugs of the traditional healers with those of the modern practitioners.

Because it is now obligatory in Tanzania for all children to attend primary school, the future heads of household will be relatively well educated and therefore more likely to seek their health care from modern health care facilities rather than from traditional healers. Since traditional medicines have been found to be useful in other countries, it would be a pity if that indigenous knowledge of herbs and plants were lost in Tanzania. Perhaps now would be a good time to integrate both traditional and modern health care systems, as has been done in rural Uganda.[18] It seems only a matter of common sense to combine the 2 to optimize skin care so that people can benefit from locally available, cheap medicines rather than buying expensive, imported pharmaceutical products. In this way, some of Tanzania's many indigenous species will be preserved and perpetuated.

Because of our findings, there are plans (1) to instigate a preventative health education program in the community, (2) to assess the diagnostic and treatment skills of both modern and traditional medical practitioners in relation to skin disease and sexually transmitted diseases, and (3) to explore the possibility of integrating traditional and modern facilities in the treatment of skin disease.

References

1. Mollel V. *Prevalence of Skin Diseases and Associated Factors in Under Five Children at Lepurko Village in Monduli District, Tanzania.* Dar es Salaam, Tanzania: Muhimbili University College of Health Sciences; 1994. ADDV Research Report.
2. George AO. Skin diseases in tropical Africa: medical, social and economic implications. *Int J Dermatol.* 1988;27:187–189.
3. Kahn MR, Nkunya MHH. *Antimicrobial activity of Tanzanian medicinal plants.* In: Proceedings of International Conference on Traditional Medicinal Plants; February 18–23, 1990; Arusha, Tanzania. Pages 48–63.
4. Ngwatu G. *Management of Skin Diseases by Traditional Healers in Mlalo Ward, Lushoto District (Tanzania).* Dar es Salaam, Tanzania: Muhimbili University College of Health Sciences; 1993. ADDV Research Report.
5. Behl PN. Ancient Indian dermatology. *Probe.* 1967;6:137.
6. Kirkwood BR. *Essentials of Medical Statistics.* Cambridge, Mass: Blackwell Scientific Publications; 1988:194–195.
7. Behl PN, Arora RB, Srivastava G. *Traditional Indian Dermatology: Concepts of Past and Present.* New Delhi, India: Skin Institute and School of Dermatology; 1992.
8. Hesketh T, Zhu WX. Traditional Chinese medicine: one country, two systems. *BMJ.* 1997; 315:115–117.
9. Akerele O. Registration and utilization of herbal remedies in some countries of East, Central and Southern Africa. In: Proceedings of International Conference on Traditional Medicinal Plants; February 18–23, 1990; Arusha, Tanzania. Page 3.
10. Parry E. The scope and limits of traditional care. *Trop Doct.* 1997;27(suppl 1):2.
11. Green EC. The participation of African healers in AIDS/STD prevention programmes. *Trop Doct.* 1997;27(suppl 1):56–59.
12. Nyamwaya D. *African Indigenous Medicine: An Anthropological Perspective for Policy Makers and Primary Health Care Managers.* Nairobi, Kenya: African Medical Research Foundation; 1992.
13. Sofowora A. Research on medicinal plants and traditional medicine in Africa. *J Altern Complement Med.* 1996;2:365–372.
14. Bodeker G. Tropical medicine and traditional methodologies: maximizing options for safe and effective health care coverage. *Trop Doct.* 1997;27(suppl 1):1–2.
15. ADB/UNICEF. *Les stratégies d'adaptation sociales des populations vulnérables d'Abidjan face à la dévaluation et à ses effects.* African Development Bank, in association with United Nations Children's Fund; 1995;34–36,87.
16. Erinosho OA, Ayonrinde A. *Traditional Medicine in Nigeria.* Lagos, Nigeria: Federal Ministry of Health; 1985.
17. World Health Organization. *WHO Guidelines for the Evaluation of Herbal Medicines.* Manila, the Philippines: WHO Regional Office; 1993.
18. Tumwesigye O. Bumetha Rukararwe: integrating modern and traditional health care in South West Uganda. *J Altern Complement Med.* 1996;2:373–376.

15 The Philosophical, Cultural, and Historical Aspects of Complementary, Alternative, Unconventional, and Integrative Medicine in the Old World

Oumeish Youssef Oumeish, MD, FAAD, FACP, FRCP(Glasg)
From Amman Clinic, Amman, Jordan.

Background
Complementary, alternative, unconventional, and integrative medicine are types of natural medicine that have been known and practiced ever since the recording of history, and in particular in the Old World. This has been rediscovered in many countries, including the New World and especially in the United States. In this review, the philosophical, cultural, and historical aspects are discussed, and the many types of alternative medical practices are mentioned.

Observations
The study of complementary medicine shows that evidence required the medical establishment to take unconventional therapies more seriously, and realize that their use alongside traditional medicine, is rapidly increasing.

Conclusions
Complementary medicine is a formal method of health care in most countries of the Old World and is expected to become integrated in the modern medical system and to be part of the medical curriculum and the teaching programs of medical institutions as well. Issues of efficacy and safety of complementary medicine have become increasingly important and supervision of the techniques and procedures used is required. More research studies are needed to understand and use this type of medicine.

Arch Dermatol. 1998;134:1373–1386

Alternative medicine is the art of offering choices, or several options, that exist and function outside the ordinary medical practice or system of any one country or culture. The styles and methods used are unconventional. Moreover, it is complementary, serving and mutually supplying the lack of therapy that exists elsewhere. It is holistic and attempts to stimulate the body's natural self-healing and self-regulating abilities. It is also favoring integration in a simple and practical pattern.

Alternative medicine was the fundamental method used by humans to preserve their health and avoid diseases since the dawn of time. It is an alternative for those who live far from medical facilities, in places where there are no physicians. Even where there are physicians, people still take the lead in their own health care. Alternative medicine can also be defined as the continuity of traditions, religious beliefs, and even quackery that nonspecialists practice in many ways to treat people. Ordinary people provided with clear and simple information can prevent and treat many common health problems in their homes, which can stop maladies earlier and provide cheaper treatment.

After all, medical knowledge should not be the guarded secret of a select few but should be freely shared by everyone. It is believed by many people that a physician is a helping factor in the cure of the disease rather than the major instrument in healing. The art of healing therefore comes from nature, from God, and not only from the physician. Thus, the physician must start from nature with an open mind and rely on God as the major source of guidance for healing.

Approaching the third millennium, and with the tremendous progress that we witness in the standard of technology and research in different sciences, especially in medicine, people still believe in complementary medicine as safer and cheaper than conventional medicine. It has a great public demand and grows in popularity, especially in the Old World, but even in developed countries like the United States,[1] where it has become increasingly prevalent[2] and is making a steady incursion into the health budget of Americans. In the United States, for example, unconventional therapy in 1990 generated expenditures estimated upward of $14 billion,[3] which doubled by 1997.

Unconventional therapies are medical practices that are not known in teaching programs or in the systems of medical institutions.[4] These therapies have branched out in the last few years to include categories such as homeopathy, balneology, climatotherapy, chiropractice, acupuncture, and many psychotherapeutic treatments.

History

A review of alternative medicine through anthropological studies on health problems shows that medical sciences were enhanced by the contribution of some universal figures and scholars who enriched the literature of such civilizations. They did this through translation, copying, collecting, and documentation of all medical material they could retrieve. However, the practice of alternative medicine, especially in the developing countries, needs supervision regarding the use of some products because of the lack of quality control and legislation. Issues of efficacy and safety of complementary medicine have become increasingly important, and supervision of the techniques and procedures is required.[5] This kind of therapy should also coincide with the ethical criteria of medical practice.

Unconventional medicine came into being early in the history of different Old World civilizations. It is of great significance not only for its intrinsic value but also because it has always been closely allied with other sciences like alchemy, the science of chemistry that has been understood and practiced throughout its long history as a main pillar for such medicine. In addition, it has to do not only with the physical domain of existence but also with the subtle spiritual domain as well.[6] That type of medicine will continue to have a magicoreligious influence. In the history of Old World civilizations, unconventional medicine was practiced mostly by experts, intelligent and highly skilled individuals. Nowadays there are many people who practice complementary medicine who pretend to cure diseases, but in fact most of them are quacks or charlatans.

Anthropological attention was first drawn to the significance of theories of illness by Forrest E. Clements in 1932.[7] His research clearly demonstrated that the explanations of illness current among most individuals of the world have little in common with those recognized by modern medical sciences and relate much more closely to the ideology of primitive religion. Studying primitive medicine leads us to the question of the theories of natural causation of illness. These theories are defined as infection, stress, organic deterioration, accident, and overt human aggression. Other theories that partially coincide with our study are the theories of supernatural causation. These are (1) theories of mystical causation that are neither apparent to the senses nor obvious to the intelligence and are mysterious, like personified ill luck or the ascription of illness to astrological influence; (2) theories of animistic causation are related to the existence of spirits that are separable from bodies; and (3) theories of magical causation explain the extraordinary powers over natural forces, incantations, and enchantment.

Medical sciences in general have been brilliantly featured in the different civilizations of the Old World. Many cultures, and in particular the Arabs, have excelled in both the Medieval ages and during the Renaissance (11th Hijri/17th AC) in teaching the medical sciences of Eastern and Arabic origin, which continued to play an important role in Western medical institutions.

The different types of complementary, alternative, unconventional, and integrative medicine in the Old World include the historical, cultural, social, traditional, and philosophical aspects of the various civilizations that prevailed mainly in Asian, African, Far Eastern, Middle Eastern, and Arabian countries. Most of that kind of medicine continues to be practiced today. Many realize that it takes into account not only the individual's physiological and biological conditions but it also includes the psychological, social, environmental, and even spiritual dimensions that may reveal the underlying factors contributing to illness.

Ancient medicine, which was mainly unconventional, was practiced by physicians who were considered to be wise men. An Arabian physician used to be called "Hakim," or "akin," and was thought to have vast experience. He was a profound philosopher, mature, and distinguished for his sound judgment. Such a physician was described (6th Hijri/12th AC) as the following:

> The physician should be of tender disposition, and wise nature, excelling in acumen, in keenness and depth of perception, being nimble of mind in forming correct views, and possessed of comprehension that is to say a rapid transition to the unknown from the known. And no physician can be of tender disposition if he fails to recognize the nobility of the human soul, nor of wise nature unless he is acquainted with logic, nor can he excel in acumen unless he is strengthened by God's aid.[8]

Although unconventional medicine was practiced according to the personal judgment and views of the physician, it was still used to reflect the beliefs of that physician. It was controlled by his/her free conscience, mind, and soul. In other words, moral courage in speech and ethical attitudes in practice constituted the philosophy of alternative medical practice and the secret of its success in ancient times.

Today medicine is becoming too divided, compartmentalized, and commercialized, and thus far from its spiritual and pure purport, meaning, and contents. However, at the same time, it was inevitable for medicine to go this way because of the major and rapid changes and progress in the research and technology of medical sciences. It also reflects the economic, social, demographic, and environmental problems that have appeared and recently been recognized in the Old World communities.[9]

Historical Review of Old World Medicine in the Pre-Arabian Era and Its Continuing Effect

Pre-Arabian medicine in the Old World was to our present understanding complementary and unconventional in most of its contexts and practices. Several civilizations that existed in the Old World were characterized by the development in various sciences and in particular medicine.

The Old Egyptian "Pharaohs" Medicine

The Old Egyptian "Pharaohs" medicine is the oldest and goes back to 4500 BC, as documented in papyrus sheets. The Egyptians were the first to perform surgery on the human body. They were also experts in embalming (mummification), using aromatics and herbs to help preserve flesh for thousands of years. They also used the infusion method to extract oils from aromatic plants to create incense, one of the oldest ways of using aromatics.

Aromatherapy began in ancient Egypt, and the medical papyri are believed to date back to 1600 BC and contain remedies for all kinds of diseases. Egyptians used oils of sweet and delicate odor and scent extracted from flowers and pine trees. In addition, they used different types of salts and alabaster to esthetically improve the skin shape. They also produced creams that contain fruit acids (glycolic acid) from sugarcane, mango, apple, and other fruits that were used by women of the royal family and the rich. They also used sour milk, which contains lactic acid, to smoothen the skin. They used many herbs in the treatment of diseases and in particular skin diseases, such as alopecia and skin infections.

The ancient healing art of reflexology was practiced thousands of years ago by Egyptians, Indians, and Chinese. Its premise is that the body has the ability to heal itself. Following illnesses, the body is in a state of imbalance, and consequently vital energy pathways are blocked, preventing the body from functioning effectively. Hence, reflexology can be used to restore and maintain the body's natural equilibrium and encourage healing. Pressure on specific parts of the body could have an anesthetizing effect on the related area. Thus, reflex areas on the feet and hands are linked to other areas and organs of the body within the same zone.

The Greeks

Greek medicine includes a lot of magic and legendary thoughts and practices. The renowned Greek physician Hippocrates wrote his famous oath and invented the theory of body composition paralleling earth's 4 elements: fire, air, water, and soil. He also described the 4 "humors" he believed that the body is composed of: blood, sputum (phlegm), and yellow and black bile. The Greeks used aromatic oils for treating diseases and also for cosmetic purposes. They also used herbal medicine, and the eminent physician Pedacius Dioscorides wrote his herbal medicine book that continues for 1200 years to be a standard Western medical reference on herbs. The Greeks also used hashish to treat glaucoma, and the diluted opium was used as a sedative and painkiller for children.

Persian Medicine

Persian medicine flourished during the reign of king Shapur I in the city of Jundishapur (near the present Persian city of Ahwaz) in the eighth Hijri/14th AC. Here a school of medicine was founded and considered the most important connection between Arabian and earlier traditional medicine. Persians believed in magicoreligious medicine and the importance of food to health.

Indian Medicine

Indian medicine was well known for the science of poisons. Indian medicine was based on the theory of the components of the human body by the following 6 balanced materials: blood, flesh, muscles, marrow, mucus, and semen.

Traditional Indian medicine, known as "Ayurveda," which means the science of longevity or "medicine of the gods," was originally a Hindu medical system and had its beginnings in the sixth century. It soon developed outside of the strictly Hindu community and was adapted by Buddhists and other religious groups. It still survives today and is undergoing a renaissance both in India and throughout the Western world. Ayurveda is basically a humoral medical system that maintains that there are 3 essential humors that cause disease if they become imbalanced—wind, bile, and phlegm. One of the main aspects of Ayurveda is aromatic massage. Indians used a lot of herbal medicine, including cannabis for anesthesia and belladonna for pain. One of the most well-known Indian medical books was *Wisdom of the Indians*, which was translated from Indian to Arabic, then from Arabic to Greek by Simon Antioch in 1070 AC.

Yoga is another kind of worship that is believed to be proceeding directly from God. It is a theological practice that leads to unification with the divine. Yoga is derived from the Sanskrit word "yug," meaning union with the divine. It is the teaching of the suppression of all activity of body, mind, and will so that the self may realize its distinction from them and attain liberation. To the Hindu believers, a yogi becomes beloved by destroying his pride. He gets rid of sorrow if he destroys anger. He acquires peace if he destroys desire. He achieves happiness if he destroys greed.

Urine therapy is also as old as 5000 years and documented in Indian literature. This therapy is based on the simple use of our own water of life: it is the drinking of urine to rejuvenate. The idea is to stop the use of certain medications and start taking a few drops of urine, or rub fresh urine into the acupressure points of the ears. Urine therapy includes external use by massaging or rubbing daily of the whole body for 4 to 8 days. Urine therapy is believed to nourish the body through the skin and regulate heartbeats. Applying fresh urine after shaving produces soft skin. It is also useful in cases of acne, psoriasis, eczema, sunburn, and pruritus. It is effective for athlete's foot, and as compressors for the body and scalp application to help hair growth. Drinking urine, especially the middle stream, is considered a tonic. It is used as gargle for a sore throat and a sedative for toothache. It is useful as an enema, a vaginal douche, eardrop and eyedrop, and also for different diseases.

Chinese Medicine

Chinese medicine started with the philosophy of Confucius who called for the ideal family ties and the promotion of social and ethical standards of societies. Classic Chinese medical cosmology, which is a branch of metaphysics that deals with the nature of the universe, existed through the ages and was naturalistic.

The pattern of Chinese medical practice mainly includes the use of herbs, dietary therapy, massage, and acupuncture. Chinese medicine is a wide subject and is practiced throughout China and East Asia by millions of people.

The Chinese used aromatics at the same time as the Egyptians. Herbal medicine was famous, and Shen Nung's herbal book, dated 2700 BC, is considered the oldest

Chinese medical book and contains details on more than 300 plants. The Chinese used aromatic herbs and burned aromatic woods and incense to show respect to God. There are now many traditional Chinese herbs that are used by people for different ailments.

Acupuncture[10,11] is considered to be the most important old and new Chinese alternative medicine worldwide. It dates back as far as 4700 years ago, as it was described by Huang Ti Nei Ching Wen in *The Yellow Emperor's Classic of Internal Medicine*,[12] considered the most important early Chinese medical book. The most interesting part of this book is the Sun Wên, "Familiar Conversations" between the emperor and his physician Ch'i Pai, because it develops in a lucid and attractive way a theory of humans in health and disease and a theory of medicine.

Acupuncture or "needling" is a method of using fine needles to stimulate the body's own healing process through the body lines of energy. A symptom manifests because the free flow of this energy is obstructed. Consequently, the aim of acupuncture is to remove these obstructions and to encourage the energy to flow smoothly. The Chinese believe that each symptom is only the end product of a series of breakdowns in the proper functioning of the body and mind. Each symptom has a route cause, which has a deeper route cause and so on until one gets back to what is termed the *constitutional factor*. In Chinese medicine each organ has responsibility for maintaining specific aspects of physical and emotional health. The acupuncture point is a precise anatomical location where the energy can be contacted by inserting a needle. Acupuncture works through the following 5 theories:

- The augmentation of immunity, which raises the level of triglycerides, prostaglandins, white blood cells, γ-globulins, and antibody levels.
- The endorphin theory, by stimulation of enkephalin secretions in the body.
- As a neurotransmitter, in which certain neurotransmitter levels (serotonin and noradrenaline) are affected.
- As circulatory theory, with the effect of constricting or dilating blood vessels through the release of histamines.
- As gate-control theory, in which the perception of pain is controlled by a part of the nervous system that regulates the impulse, which will later be interpreted as pain. This part of the nervous system is called the *gate*. If the gate is hit with too many impulses, it is overwhelmed and thus closes. This prevents some soft impulses from getting through. The first gates closing are the smallest. The nerve fibers that carry the impulses of pain are rather small nerve fibers called *C fibers*. These are the gates that close during acupuncture.

Moxibustion or moxa has a similar purpose as acupuncture. It is the ignipuncture that is based on heat and is highly recommended to treat many diseases. The practice is almost analogous to cupping, which is still used in the Old and New Worlds. It produces stimulation of key nodal points along the circulation tracts.

Acupressure was also invented by the Chinese, which is the stimulation performed with fingers rather than needles. It is based on the principles of acupuncture.

Feng shui[13] is the ancient Chinese study of the movement of invisible energy, or *chi*, which is founded on wisdom. It has been practiced for thousands of years and concerns how the environment in which we live and work has an effect on our physical, mental, emotional, and spiritual well-being. The philosophy of *feng shui* is that to change people's way of living they have to change their homes, which includes design, color, art, and different arrangements that will affect the movement of energy in the home, such as bedrooms, halls, stairs, kitchen, bathrooms, and workplaces. It also includes changes in schools and gardens. Such changes will eventually be reflected on health and create opportunities and happiness that can result in feelings of satisfaction and peace.

The "Bagua" is an ancient form of map that shows how energy moves within a defined space. It is a template divided into 9 areas that can be laid over a plan of a land, a house, an apartment, or rooms. It gives clues to how we can create new possibilities in our lives. The map is divided into the following 9 areas with a definition and meaning for each: (1) water/journey, (2) earth/relationships, (3) thunder/elders, (4) wind/fortunate blessings, (5) health (Tai Chi)/the center of all areas, (6) heaven/helpful friends, (7) lake/creativity, (8) mountain/wisdom, and (9) fire/illumination.

The *feng shui* philosophy could change people's environments if it is done gradually with the use of one's own energy. Our diets, exercises, lifestyles, personalities, and astrological profiles are all important in producing the environmental change and the positive reflections on our health that is the main goal of that philosophy.

The goal of *feng shui* is a healthy and harmonious lifestyle. The study of the movement of energy forms the basis of one of the most noted analytical systems in Chinese Culture—Wu Hsing. Wu Hsing means the 5 elements or 5 energies and is based on the theory that energy tends to move in 5 directions, ie, radiating outward, concentrating inward, rising, descending, and rotating. In the system of the 5 energies, different colors, smells, and tastes are seen as manifestations of each of these energies and so are the seasons, foods, directions, and numbers. The 5 energies are described using the names of 5 natural phenomena that typify those movements of energy: fire, earth, metal or gold, water, and wood. They control each other through a relationship known as the central cycle.[14] Every organ in our body is classified under the 5 elements, which represent material forces that were introduced by the Chinese as early as the fourth century BC—gold (*jin*), wood (*mu*), water (*tu*), and earth and fire (*hua*). Gold has the nature of quietness, wood is the evidence of growth, water is coolness, fire is heat, and earth has the quality of substance. The 5 elements[15] or energies may combine, change with seasons, and have different colors, shapes, directions, and locations.

The health of the human being is the main core of energy in our body. Every organ in our body is classified and influenced by the 5 elements (Table 1). Thus, the wood element will create liver and eye diseases, the fire will create heart and tongue diseases and so on. The philosophy of *feng shui* is still practiced by millions as an alternative medicine.

Chinese dietary therapy is based on the theory that "we are what we eat," and what we eat is important to our health and could cause illness.

Kinesiology is another practice in Chinese medicine, which is the study of the principles of mechanics and anatomy in relation to human movement. It is practiced by training that enables patients to control their biological processes.

Moreover, Chinese medicine is a holistic type of medicine. It treats the individual and reflects the unique experience of that disease. It also treats the vital energy and encourages the body, mind, and spirit to return to a harmoniously balanced state of well-being.

Table 1. Five *feng shui* Elements*

Elements	Internal Organs	Sensory Organs
Wood	Liver	Eye
Fire	Heart	Tongue
Earth	Spleen	Mouth
Gold	Lung	Nose
Water	Kidney	Ear

*See the "Chinese Medicine" section in the text for explanation of *feng shui.*

Roman Medicine

Romans took much of their medical knowledge from the Greeks. They used and improved the effect of aromatics and they also used steam, sauna, and vapor baths, and Rome became the bathing capital of the world. Using oils and massage was a continuous practice of the Romans.

They also imported herbs and aromatic products from India and Arabia through the opening up of trade routes. The Romans used to cauterize the wounds and ulcers of the cervix. They also performed the cesarean section.

The Philosophy of Ancient Arab-Islamic Unconventional Medicine

The prolonged wars between the Romans and Persian empires led to disasters and ethnic tensions among Greeks, Semites, Persians, Armenians, and Slavs with splits among Christian groups. The bubonic plague in 541 AC heralded 200 years of outbreaks. The efforts of Justinian (524–565 AC) to recover the Roman Empire did not work, and the Greeks also became weak. Learned medicine continued in large cities and in particular in Alexandria, but physicians were not so popular, and religion dominated the life of people in that era. At that time the scene was set for Islam, when Mohammed the Prophet (570–632 AC) came from the Quraysh tribe that ruled Mecca,[16] and at the age of 40 years he received God's call, and the *Holy Quran* (*Koran*) was revealed to him in visions. By the time of his death, all of Arabia had been won over to Islam, and a century later his followers had conquered half of Byzantine Asia, all of Persia, Egypt, the Maghreb (North Africa), and Spain. Islam was not a proselytizing faith and did not force people to convert. Islam granted Christians and Jews special status as "People of the Book" (Anl-al-Kitab). During the Arab- Islamic empire medicine flourished because it was promoted by Caliphs, and Baghdad, Seville, Toledo, Granada, and other cities were well known as main centers for Arab-Islamic medical sciences and culture.

Unconventional medicine in ancient Arab-Islamic civilization was characterized as metaphysical and was also sometimes gnostic, practiced by those who believed in gnosticism. It was supernatural, abstruse, and marked by unconventional imagery. It was popular, inexpensive, widely accepted, commonly liked, and approved. It related to the general public, was easy to understand, and suited the means of the majority. It was not coincidental to have a good number of universal outstanding figures of Arab-Islamic scientists who played a major role and contributed to both traditional and unconventional medicine and who were philosophers at the same time. Such a physician usually was a poet, writer, historian, mathematician, chemist, astronomer, and, above all, philosopher. He was known as the "Hakim," or "sage," who reflects the unity of the sciences as many branches of a tree whose trunk is the wisdom embodied in the sage.

Arabian physicians stressed that treating the early symptoms of a disease by unconventional means, especially herbs, will not mask the disease but expose it in the early treatable stage. They also believed in preventive medical practices such as diet, exercises, hygiene, and moderation in habits. It is of interest to remember an old saying: "A good physician tries to keep people in good health and good shape, but a lesser physician will only treat people when they get sick."

Medicine in general is considered to be one of the most illustrious and best known facets of Arab-Islamic civilization in which Arabs most excelled. It became influential in Western medical circles to such an extent that it was included in the curriculum of medical schools for many centuries. Arabic medicine was a result of Roman, Greek, Persian, and Indian theories and practices, within the general context of Islam's system of ethics. Islam was based on revelation, with its simple meaning as "submission," and "peace," or "being at one with the Divine Will." Arabic medicine was connected to philosophy and tied to numerical and astrological symbolism and influenced by magicoreligious thoughts. Arabs then established and promoted their own medical sciences in theories and practices that became highly influential in Western science and teaching.

Physicians, whether they were Muslims, Christians, or Jews, under the umbrella of Islam raised the dignity and caliber of the medical profession. The teaching in the light of edicts from the *Holy Quran* and prophetic directions led the scholars of mysticism and spiritualism to the determination between the material and the spiritual worlds. The teaching of the *Holy Quran* is also the belief in Allah (God) and the Day of Judgment after life. Faith exercises a deep effect on the spirit and the body of humans. Muslims believe that diseases are the result of the dissociation of the harmony between the body and the spirit, and faith is the exactitude that is extremely effective in keeping the harmony intact through its belief in "tawhid" (unity) of thought; thus, healing comes through faith.

During the Islamic age, Arabs raised the dignity of the medical sciences from that of a menial calling to the rank of one of the learned professions.

Unconventional Arabic Medical Practices

I mention herein some of the unconventional medical practices that were present before and during Islam, and many of them are still practiced today.

Physiognomy

Physiognomy is the ability of discovering temperament and inner characters of an individual from the outward appearance. Arabs believed that a disease would attack a person or a tribe due to an evil, which can also cause harm to certain people or a tribe. This evil can be driven away by the use of charms and magic. Those practicing physiognomy also used magic to intimidate their enemies.

Metaphysical Medicine

This type of medicine is clerical or ministerial and invisible. It was a priestly medicine practiced by clergymen, wizards, and sorcerers who were skilled in magic. Such individuals could influence the mental and physical states of others by foretelling their health condition.

Fortune-teller

A fortune-teller is one who professes to foretell the future and claims that by looking at and talking to an individual could tell secrets of the past, present, and future of that person. He/she also predicts knowledge about health, wealth, and destiny and fate. A diviner, or augurer, can also use cards arranged in different ways and to tell secrets and a person's fortune. The fortune-teller might use a cup from which a person has drunk coffee, let the cup dry for a few minutes, and then read the lines, streaks, and what shows as figures and pictures made by the remnants of coffee at the bottom and inner sides of the cup to tell the person's fortune. This reading is based on intuition, anticipation, and foreknowledge.

Geomancy

Geomancy is the art of using sand or small pieces of stones of different shapes to tell the fortune of a person. The individual who practices geomancy tosses stones or cowrie shells and interprets the arrangements to predict the future.

Palmistry

Palmistry is practiced by the chiromancer or palmist who looks at the different markings, lines, and ridges on the palm of a person to foretell his/her future, health, the length of life, and destiny.

Drive Out (or Exorcism)

Exorcism is practiced by magicians, prestidigitators, sorcerers, quacks, and charlatans to drive away bad spirits and evil from the soul and body in states of illness or catastrophies. People believed that the forces responsible for ill health were the evil spirits that transmigrate into the body by the process of metempsychosis. Many still believe in "jinn" and the evil eye (*al'ayn*), a glance that is supposed to harm those on whom it falls. The jinn (plural, jinni) could bring good as well as bad luck. They were to blame for fevers, madness, and children's diseases. Spiritual therapy is practiced in many Arabian countries and is based on the exorcism and expulsion of bad spirits from the body.

Inspiration

Inspiration is a divine influence or action put on a person to make him/her, by suggestion, believe an idea and produce an effect on him/her with that idea. Burying a green wedge in a cave in the dark during the night, inserting a gram of wheat in an eggplant and then touching a wart with it are some of the methods used. After the green wedge or eggplant is buried and forgotten, warts are believed to have been cured.

Amulets

Amulets are prescribed, prepared, and advised by certain clergymen or magicians or sometimes ordinary people who claim to possess the knowledge of the secrets of amulets. Amulets or periapts are usually made of different kinds of cloth, often silk or cotton, with different colors and in different shapes. They usually include a piece of paper with written incantations, either religious phrases or words that can work as exorcism of evil. Some amulets also contain pieces of hair from a man or his wife. They might also contain nonsense words or nothing.

The people who carry amulets believe and are told to believe that amulets are useful to bring good luck and health to them. Sometimes they are meant also to beat somebody or intimidate an enemy or make sterile women conceive. Amulets are hung around the neck or placed near the chest, abdomen, umbilicus, or pubic region and genitalia. They are also placed under the main steps of the house or bedroom or under the pillow or bed.

Precious Stones, Metals, and Crystals

Arabs believed in the healing power of gemstones, metals, and crystals. They are useful for protection of the body and soul, and drive away sickness and vanquish enemies. Each stone has its value and effect according to its size, shape, and color.

Astrology

Astrologists claim that they can read and understand the meanings behind the appearance, disappearance, and movements of certain stars. They also relate all that to the beginning of an epidemic of a disease, a disaster, or misery or happiness of a person or a tribe. Counting stars is also believed to cure some diseases such as warts.

Horoscopy

The horoscope is the diagram or map of the relative positions of planets and signs of the zodiac at a specific time. It is used by astronomers to infer individual character and personality traits and in foretelling events of a person's life as at one's birthday. This is known as astrological forecast.

Horoscopes can denote revenge, grudge, hostility, dissatisfaction, indignation, optimism, pessimism, confidence, expectation, travel, and wealth. They can tell the existence of a love affair or enemies and health status and length of life. Some people shape their lives and behave on a daily basis according to their horoscopes. They might get scared if they expect a bad event and become sick and paranoid. Good news, good luck, feeling down, and the feeling that people we consider as close friends have abandoned us are some interpretations. They might also have a funny side, known as cosmic laugh.

Cupping

Cupping is still used to treat chest infections, and in particular pneumonia and muscular pain. It is a procedure in which blood is drawn to the surface of the skin by the use of a glass vessel evacuated of air by heat. A small piece of paper is burned, placed inside glass cups, and then extinguished, so that the air inside the cups will be burned and emptied. The cups are then placed on areas such as the chest, back, buttocks, chin, and dorsum of the foot. The cups are left on a specific area for a few minutes, and eventually they will stick by negative pressure to the skin. Next they are removed, leaving raised red patches, which are rich in blood supply with the production of superficial skin inflammation that will help to reduce inflammation in deeper adjacent organs. Following that, both pain and infection will be alleviated by the effect of counterirritation.

Arabs believed that cupping could be useful to treat 72 diseases, including leprosy, toothaches, boils, gout, piles, and elephantiasis.

Cautery and Local Stimulation

This method is still used to treat some kinds of pain, alopecia, and warts. Cautery with fire by using a burnt stick and/or lighted cigarette are used to treat warts. Garlic and vinegar are used to rub an area of alopecia areata to stimulate hair growth. Garlic is rubbed and vinegar is applied to smoothen stings of bites. Cautery to the back and at certain specific sites is well known to treat sciatica and lumbago pain.

Scarification

Scarification is made by scratching or making incisions in the skin using a razor blade or knife for bloodletting. It is based on the assumption that this will get rid of poisoned blood. Scarification is practiced for snakebite, in which the limb is cuffed and fastened tight by a rope or a piece of cloth above the site of the bite to prevent the poisoned circulating blood from moving upward. The bitten area is then scarified and incised for bloodletting. Sometimes the blood is sucked and spit out. The site of the bite is then covered with a poultice.

Leech Therapy

Leeches are used to suck blood from the ears, face, neck, thighs, or legs. They are still used mainly by barbers who place the leech on the surface of the skin and leave it for 15 to 30 minutes while it sucks blood, becomes swollen, and then drops off by itself. This kind of therapy is used to reduce hypertension, relieve headache, and treat varicose veins in the lower limbs.

Compresses and Poultices

Compresses and poultices are used for different purposes in treating many illnesses. A piece of cloth is immersed in cold water and then squeezed, or some ice is wrapped with the cloth, which is then applied to the forehead, hands, forearms, thighs, and legs to reduce body temperature. Poultices are made of a mixture of herbs in a paste form such as mustard papers, cayenne, and ginger oils, then applied to the area of pain for 1 to 3 hours. The idea is to increase blood circulation in the treated area and create a counterirritation. Poultices are sometimes made of cabbage or warm bread, in which a warm piece of bread is applied to sties on eyelids to help them drain.

Steam and Vaporization Therapy

This therapy is a process in which steam from a bowl of boiling water is allowed to seep into the face or any area of the skin. It is applied for 5 to 10 minutes, and an essential oil, a menthol, or incense is added to the boiling water. The top of the head and sides of the face are covered with a towel to prevent evaporation. Vaporization is useful for colds, flu, acne lesions, and as a freshener too.

Venesection

Phlebotomy was also practiced by Arabs to treat many diseases in the belief that drawing and letting blood will get rid of the excess contaminated blood. It was usually done using a heated knife, razor blade, or a warmed needle. It was useful in the treatment of headache, hypertension, and many other conditions.

Paracentesis

A puncture in the abdomen was created by Arabs using a knife sterilized by fire. This procedure was used to treat ascites, which Arabs believed to be due to bad water in the abdomen.

Herbal Medicine

Arabs used many kinds of herbs to treat different diseases, and even now herbal medicine is still popular and practiced by some physicians, but also by many quacks. Arabian herbal medicine was famous and Arabian scientists wrote many books describing the uses, indications, and benefits of such herbs.[17,18] There are some important books and manuscripts in the Arab herbal pharmacopeia. The most renowned ones are the following:

- *The Bimaristan Law in Pharmacopoeia*, *Materitenses* that includes 12 chapters was written by Ibn Abil-Bayan in 1161 AC in Spain. This book contains 607 medications and all are mentioned in detail.
- *Al Kitab Al Jami*, about liquids and creams, was written by Abu Marwan Abd al Malik Ibn Zuhr (Avenzoar), who lived in Seville, Spain (1091–1161 AC). This book includes 230 medications that are mostly herbal and a few are of animal and mineral origin. This book gives a full description of the uses of herbs whether they are roots, seeds, or leaves.
- *Tuhfat al-Ahbab*[19] is a dictionary from an unknown author on herbs that includes 462 topics.
- *Drugs Terminology*, which is a manuscript compiled by Rabbi Moses Ben Maimon, who lived in Spain (1135–1204 AC). This manuscript contains 405 chapters and gives synonyms of medications in Arabic, Greek, Persian, and Spanish languages.
- *The Book on Drinks and Foods* is a collection of different drinks and foods compiled by Ibn-el Beithar, who lived in Damascus, Syria (1197–1248 AC). It is the most prestigious book in the Arabian pharmacopeia; it contains 260 references and the medications are classified in alphabetical order. Most Arabic medications were mentioned in Spanish pharmacopeia and were known as *Farmacopea Espanole* and *Pharmacopea Hispana*.

Examples of some herbs and fruits that were used by Arabian scientists and are still used in the European pharmacopeia are *Myrtus communis* L (myrtle), *Asarum eu-*

ropaeum (assarbacca), *Papaver somniferum* (opium), *Pimpinella anisum* (anise), and *Matricaria chamomilla* (wild chamomile).

The following are some examples of Arabian herbs, their Latin names, and uses: *Gelsenium sumpervirens* (yellow jasmine) for migraine; *Apium graveolens* (celery) for gout; *Angelica archangelica* (angelique) for rheumatism; *Alliam sativum* (garlic) for flu and influenza; *Forsythia suspensa* (lian qiao) for abcesses and folliculitis; *Morus alba* (mulberry) for cough; *Pimpinella anisum* (anise) for cough; *Galium aparine* (cleavers) for psoriasis; *Aloe vera* (aloe) for vitiligo and fungus infection; *Plantaso psyllium* (psyllium) for constipation; *Agrimonia eupatoma* (agrinomy) for diarrhea; and *Trigonella foenum-graecum* (fenugreek) for diabetes mellitus. Wallflower (gilly flower) leaves are crushed and mixed with salt for treating eczema. *Nigella sativa* mixed with olive oil is a good local moisturizer for ichthyosis and psoriasis.[20]

Polypodium leucotomos "difur" is an herb that contains a lipid hydrosoluble extract known as "calagula" or "anapsos."[21] The leaves of this herb were used first in Spain and Portugal to treat psoriasis and then vitiligo,[22] as they proved to make psoriatic[23] lesions disappear, and to repigment vitiliginous skin. The leaves are grounded or made into a paste and applied to the vitiliginous lesions and the areas are then exposed to sunlight. The herb was also used to treat eczema.

Aloe is a large genus of succulent, chiefly southern African plants of the lily family with basal leaves and spicate flowers. The dried juice or the leaves of various aloes are used as a purgative and tonics. The extract is also used as a 0.5% hydrophilic cream with or without salicylic acid to treat psoriasis. It is also used with exposure to sunlight to treat vitiligo. Aloe is believed to regenerate capillaries and promotes regrowth of hair follicles.

Psoralens as repigmenting agents for vitiligo were described as early as 1400 BC. The Indian sacred book *Atharva Veda* mentioned the effect of the plant on the skin color. Ancient Egyptians identified *Psoralea corylifolia* and *Amni majus* as psoralen, and they used it for vitiligo. Psoralens are furocoumarin compounds, photodynamically active drugs that are capable of absorbing radiant energy. They are also found in limes, lemons, celery, figs, and parsnips. Psoralens[24] were introduced into the field of dermatology by El-Mofty[25,26] in 1947 when he observed repigmentation of vitiliginous lesions after the use of powdered seeds prescribed by herbalists. The drug was then manufactured in both a lotion and tablet form as meladinine.

Khellin is produced from the seeds of the plant *Ammi visnaga*, and its chemical structure closely resembles that of psoralen,[27] used as a topical application in combination with sunlight for vitiligo.[28]

Tattooing

Tattooing is used in the Arab world as a decorative and cosmetic practice on the face and the back of hands for women, and is also a tribal tradition for men.

Henna

Henna is an Old World tropical shrub or small tree (*Lowsonia inermis*) of the loose strife family with small opposite leaves and axillary panicles of fragrant white flowers. A reddish brown or blackish dye is obtained from the leaves of the henna plants, especially in the Arab world. The powder of henna is used by women to dye hair, and used also in marriage ceremonies by painting different shapes and figures on hands and feet of women and children. Some men are using henna to dye scalp, mustache, and beard hair. Henna is also applied to the hands and feet to treat some skin diseases or as a camouflage for vitiligo and skin scars.

Kohl

Kohl is a black powder that is used widely in the Arab countries. It is used as a powder or smear to darken the edges of the eyelids similar to eyeliner. It was introduced to Europe in the 13th century by Crusaders who brought kohl from Arabia as presents to their wives and girlfriends, and is still used today. Some men from certain tribes in Arabia also use kohl as eyeliner. It is also used as a treatment for blepharitis.

Honey Therapy

The Arabs used honey as a medicine for many centuries to improve the blood circulation. It is also a laxative and relieves stomach pain. It is a protective agent for children against scurvy and rickets. Honey improves hearing and vision. It is used as an antimicrobial and antifungal in the form of creams or liquids in 10% to 50% dilutions. It is used as warm eardrops when mixed with salt to clear earwax and infection. It is used as a mouth gargle for tonsillitis and diphtheria. Honey is also mixed with hot lemon and used to ease colds and congestion. When applied to the skin it clears infections, abscesses, ulcers, and folliculitis. It has also been used to treat lice in children.

Contraceptive and Abortifacient Methods in Ancient Arabic Medicine

Oral contraceptive methods[29] included drinking water of sweet basil or weeping willow leaves, eating beans on an empty stomach, dogs fennel in "white drink," and consuming myrrh and cinnamon after menstruation.
Contraception was also performed by magical means such as stepping on the cyclamen plant or the use of suppositories and tampons, such as tar, before and after coitus. Flowers and seeds of cabbage, after menses, are also used before or after coitus. Pulp of colocynth, white bryony, iron dross, sulfur, scammony, and cabbage seeds with tar are also well-known methods of contraception.

Abortifacient methods include techniques used by men such as onion juice smeared on the penis, or smeared tar or balm oil and white lead on the penis before coitus. Other miscellaneous techniques include smearing the navel with the gallbladder of a cow plus a recipe taken orally and by insertion in the vagina. Fumigation with galbanum plant and sulfur and savin is also a time-honored method as well as avoiding simultaneous orgasms. Bodily movements and jumping backward to expel semen, spoiling the testicles with hemlock, sitting in the broth of wallflowers and Jew's mallow green sticks are still used, especially in Egypt, and introduced into the cervix and manipulated to help induce abortion.

Chiropractic Medicine

Chiropractic medicine is a system of therapy that considers that disease results from a lack of normal nerve function and uses manipulation and specific adjustment of body structures, such as bones, joints, and spinal column. It is a health care discipline that emphasizes the inherent and restorative power of the body to heal itself without the use of drugs or surgery.

It is still practiced widely in the Arab world by chiropractors who are not physicians. Even today, chiropractors use observation and knowledge and their vast experience to identify the cause of pain, whether it is a bone fracture or a joint or a spinal column problem. They usually use pieces of wooden board to splint the fracture. For example, if it is an arm fracture, a chiropractor applies an ordinary cloth bandage underneath and over the arm, then a paste made of a mixture of egg white with ground homemade soap is applied all around the fractured limb that will stick the cloth to the splint, and then the limb is hung 2 to 3 months before it is released. In a case of a badly healed fracture, the chiropractor would wrap the broken limb with a piece of cloth to protect it from burns, and then the limb is exposed to the vapor of a boiling *Inula viscosa* herb. After a few minutes there is a dramatic response, and the badly healed fractured bone releases itself and the fractured parts separate. After that, the chiropractor unites them again as previously described.

Fasting

Fasting is 1 of the 5 basic elements of Islam. It is considered one of the means of providing the ideal conditions necessary for the repair of bodily damages and for the elimination of toxins. It is an exercise in which a Muslim purifies the body and soul by feeling hunger and thus sympathizing with those who are hungry because they cannot afford to buy food. Fasting during Ramadan every year includes meditation, contemplation, and cogitation.

Circumcision

Male Circumcision. This is both a Muslim and a Jewish rite performed on male infants as a sign of inclusion in the Muslim or Jewish communities. It is usually practiced in most countries of the Old World by barbers and includes a quick cut of the foreskin (prepuce) with a sharp knife or a razor blade. It is also practiced by Arab Christians on the basis of natural hygiene.

Female Circumcision (Clitorodectomy). This is an ancient practice[30] performed in the name of tradition without ideological or religious sanction.[31,32] Evidence from the remains of female mummies dating back to 2000 BC indicates that female genital mutilation originated during the reign of the Pharaohs. Ancient Egyptian myths stressed the bisexuality of the gods, and thus circumcision may have been introduced to clarify the femininity of girls. In some African countries the clitoris is considered a masculine organ that should be removed. Circumcision is practiced in about 30 African countries that include millions of Arabs from Mauritania and the Ivory Coast in the west to Egypt, Sudan, Somalia, and Tanzania in the east. The Arabic name for circumcision is "tahara," which means "to purify." It is practiced by Africans of all religions, Muslims, Christians, and Ethiopian Jews, as well as followers of animist religions, such as the Masai.

Recent statistics from the World Health Organization show that more than 100 million women have undergone circumcision in about 40 African countries. In Egypt, almost 80% of rural women are circumcised and around 370 girls are operated on daily. Ninety percent of circumcisions are performed by traditional practitioners, mainly barbers and sometimes midwives.

The justification of clitorodectomy is based on the belief of sexual control of women and the prevention of female promiscuity. It is believed that circumcision will abolish women's sexual enjoyment, and that clitoris cutting is closely associated with virginity. The operation lasts 15 minutes, during which the girl is nude and her legs spread wide apart while she is held down by several women. A traditional practitioner offers a short prayer, takes a sharp razor, and excises the clitoris. The razor cuts from top to bottom, which often cuts part of labia minora of the vagina. Then the practitioner uses 4 acacia thorns that pierce one side and pass through the other held in place by a thread or horsehair to close the wound.

The procedure is painful and horrifying for the girl and has complications that include sudden death from bleeding or tetanus resulting from the use of unsterilized equipment such as razor blades, iron knives, and broken bottles. The child might develop severe and permanent scarring that eventually leads to difficulty in urination and menstruation. The mutilated scar might cause future fetal and maternal death when the girl marries and becomes pregnant. It also creates a psychological trauma for the victim. Other complications include recurrent infections, pain during intercourse, infertility, and spreading of the acquired immunodeficiency syndrome.

Infibulation is another type of circumcision in which the clitoris and labia minora are cut, and then the labia majora are stitched together to cover the urethral and vaginal entrances. This is practiced in Sudan, Mali, Somalia, Ethiopia, and Nigeria.

The practice of female circumcision has been recently considered torture and a form of genital mutilation. It has nothing to do with religion or morality. Governments in most African countries especially in Egypt have recently banned such practice but are faced with objections, and at least are trying to subject such procedures to medical supervision. Immigrants from African countries to the United States and Canada brought the practice of circumcision with them. Female circumcision was criminalized by the US Congress and some state governments.

Other Alternative Medical Therapies in the Old World

The Use of Water

Water has always been an important topic in medicine.[33] It has been prescribed for the treatment of edema, arthritis, psoriasis, and even sexually transmitted diseases. In contemporary practice, water is used for compressing, bathing, and cleansing the skin. One of the various uses of water in alternative medical practice is in balneology.

Balneology

The study of the medicinal uses of mineral water and the uses of water has been an integral part of human existence. Water is a natural gift and is a part of the act of purification found in the major religions. The Pharaohs, the Greeks, and the Romans developed medicinal and religious rites associated with water.[34,35] The Pharaohs worshiped the Nile River[36] because they believed it to have supernatural powers and the ability to cure diseases. The Ganges River has significance in the Hindu religion, just as the Jordan River has importance to Christianity and Judaism. Muslims and Buddhists relate washing to religious purity. Muslims believe in the performance of rituals or ablutions by washing 5 times a day before each of the daily prayers. The Hindu believes that Ganges water brings physical wellness and peace. The healing aspects of the Dead Sea water were known for ages and mentioned in both the Old Testament and *Holy Quran* (also discussed in the "Climatotherapy" section). Water from the Zamzam well in Mecca is considered holy, and millions of Muslim believers use it to cure diseases.

The effects of warm spas are activation of sweat glands, dilation of cutaneous blood vessels, and stimulation of intestinal peristalsis.[37] They have also vagotonic action and augment blood pH levels.

Thermal and mineral waters are also used as alternative therapy in many countries in the Old World. There are many health spas and clinics around the world offering a wide range of natural treatments that may be combined with a relaxing vacation. Many of these centers are used simply for restoring health. European countries have a 2000-year tradition of spa treatment. The former Soviet Union alone has 3500 spas.

Thermal and mineral waters are present in the Middle East, in particular in Jordan and Israel. Such waters are considered curative due to their physical and chemical properties and also through psychological effect.

Thermal and mineral spas are believed to help relax muscles and the mind, provide relief of muscular and joint pains, respiration, and heal infections. Water containing hydrogen, sulfur, carbon dioxide, and bromides is useful as a tranquilizer and a relaxant. Some waters are radioactive and contain high levels of iodides, iron, calcium, and magnesium, and are useful for the body as a whole. It is believed that mineral water exerts an effect on the immunological and neuropeptidergic systems of the skin beyond the antibacterial, antifungal, and keratolytic effects.[38] Water plays an important role in dermatological therapy through its hydrating, cooling, and cleansing effects, and as a vehicle for more effective delivery of active agents.[39]

Heliotherapy

The use of sunlight in the treatment of different diseases was known for many decades even before advanced technology in this field, in the form of phototherapy and photochemotherapy (psoralen–UV-A), were introduced.[40] Heliotherapy was used especially in Europe to derive benefit from the UV-A present in sunlight to treat numerous diseases. Many sanitariums were established for sunbathing to treat diseases of the chest and in particular tuberculosis and rheumatism, in addition to various skin diseases.[41] Heliotherapy is an alternative therapy for patients with skin diseases, especially psoriasis, so that the severity of the disease is dramatically reduced and they receive favorable long-term effects.

Climatotherapy at the Dead Sea

Exposure to sunlight to treat different ailments and skin conditions and the use of natural health spas and mud have been used for thousands of years to treat psoriasis and other diseases.[42,43] Skin shows marked improvement in many cases with a longer delay of relapses, less need to use conventional medications such as corticosteroids, and eventually fewer adverse effects. These were also a much less expensive method of treatment.

The Dead Sea is one of the most popular sites for climatotherapy. It is the lowest point on Earth, 400 m below sea level, and it is the world's saltiest lake, with salinity reaching 290 g/L,[44] compared with that of the Red Sea, whose salinity is only 40 g/L. The natural elements and minerals in the sea, in addition to the mud present on the shores, give the water their curative powers, as has been mentioned in the Bible and recognized by king Herod more than 2000 years ago. However, the principal factor in the cure of skin diseases, mainly psoriasis, comes from the naturally filtered UV radiation, which is greater in UV-A and low in UV-B compared with other locations[44]; this permits a prolonged exposure to sunlight with minimal phototoxicity. This filtered UV radiation is due to the thick atmospheric layer over the Dead Sea, with its vapor and haze, and to the great amount of ozone, which is minimally depleted compared with other areas. It is also due to the low humidity and warm climate, with 332 sunny days yearly in that area.[45]

The Dead Sea Spa Treatment Centres in Israel (Ein Bokek) were established years ago and have attracted thousands of patients, mainly from the Netherlands, France, Switzerland, Italy, Austria, Germany, the United Kingdom, Scandinavia, South Africa, and the United States, in addition to patients coming from within Israel.[46,47] Most of those patients seek therapy for psoriasis.

The Dead Sea Spa Treatment Village in Jordan was opened in 1991 and since then thousands of patients with psoriasis, mainly psoriasis vulgaris, and other diseases such as eczema,[48] acne, and asthma have received climatotherapy at the village, which is 35 km west of Amman, the capital of Jordan. Most patients are from western Europe, Arabia, and Jordan.

It is anticipated that the peace process between Jordan and Israel will create active cooperation, promote bilateral and regional studies, encourage research, and eventually promote health tourism in many areas, such as wellness health centers, especially in the Dead Sea region.

The Dead Sea is mentioned in the Old Testament and *Holy Quran*, and it was described by both the Greeks and Arabs and was given many names, including Sedom, Dragon, Araba, Asphilt Sea, and Lot Sea[49] (Lot, ie, the nephew of Abraham, who lived at Sodom and Gomorrah).

The Dead Sea water contains a natural tar called *bitumen*, which is why it has been called the Asphilt or tar sea. This natural tar is believed to function as an anti-inflammatory and keratolytic agent to the skin. In general, it is possible that the water of the Dead Sea functions as a major factor in slowing down the rapid turnover process of skin cells in patients with psoriasis, a possibility that should be further investigated.

The mud at the Dead Sea is rich in magnesium, natural tar (bitumen), and silicates (silicon compounds); the latter is often used as a mask for the skin.[50] The black color of mud absorbs much of the solar radiation, hence acting as a photosensitizer when applied to the skin. Mud baths are useful mainly for arthropathy because they aid in stimulating blood circulation around the affected joints; thus, mud packs are effective for individuals with psoriatic arthropathy.

In conclusion, the curative alternative factors at the Dead Sea are climate, sunlight, water, and black mud, along with their physical and psychological effects.

Naturopathic Medicine

The most popular kind of unconventional medicine is naturopathic medicine, which is a natural approach to health and healing that recognizes the integrity of the whole person. The philosophy of naturopathic medicine includes the treatment of disease through the stimulation, enhancement, and support of the inherent healing capacity of the person. There are 6 principles for this kind of medicine: (1) the healing power of naturethe body has the inherent ability to establish, maintain, and restore health; (2) identify and treat the cause—underlying causes of a disease must be discovered and removed; symptoms are not the cause of a disease, and the causes of diseases include physical, mental, emotional, and spiritual factors, which all have to be dealt with; (3) first do no harm—therapeutic action should be complementary to and synergistic with the healing process; (4) treat the whole person; (5) the physician as teacher—he/she should create a healthy interpersonal physician-patient relationship; and (6) prevention—it is the aim of the physician, and the best cure; it is the building of health rather than fighting the disease.

Hypothermia

Hypothermia is the use of cooling with direct ice or ice packs to treat bruises, swelling, joint problems, and muscular pain. It is also useful to lower the body temperature. It was first used as an anesthesia in World War I by surgeons to amputate injured limbs or operate on injured extremities.

The effects of cold include stimulation of vegetative sympathetic nervous system (sympathiotonic action), dilution of the blood, diminution of blood pH, and diminution of intestinal peristalsis.

Hyperthermia

Hyperthermia is the use of heat to treat certain skin diseases. It was used as direct cautery for many centuries to treat backache, infected skin conditions, and leishmaniasis pimples. It is also used now to treat warts. Cautery was used to seal the stumps of amputees involved in wars.

Hypnotherapy

Hypnosis is defined as an unusual or altered state of consciousness in which distortion of perception occurs as uncritical responses of the subject to motions from an objective source, a subjective source or both.[51] Hypnosis is mainly used to treat obsession, fear, anxiety, and other psychological and emotional disturbances. It is also used to discover events and incidents that happened to the patient that he/she had forgotten or occurred to others such as crimes that they witnessed.

Homeopathy

Homeopathy[52] is a system of medicine based on the theory of "like cures like." For example, a poison that causes symptoms of illness in a healthy person can treat the same symptoms in a diluted form. Substances are diluted several times to make a remedy that is safe to use, yet homeopaths believe sufficient likeness remains between the remedy and the illness to stimulate the body's self-healing abilities. It is based on the pharmacological "law of similars" that was invented in 1796 by Samuel Hahnemann, a German physician. The word derives from the Greek "homoios" and "pathos," meaning to suffer. Another example is rubbing chilblains with snow. Homeopathy also encourages people to reject strong medications.

Precious Stones and Crystals Therapy

The philosophy of diamond, crystals, and precious stones therapy is based on the belief of using energies in the healing of a disease, trauma, or an injury. It is holistic, and many claim benefits from this kind of therapy. The healing properties of gemstones, minerals, and crystals were common and used for many centuries to treat many diseases. They have different philosophical evaluation and variant effects on people. The quality, shape, and color of the gemstones are also important in their effect. Some people feel more self-confident when they wear certain stones such as amazonite. The wearing of a purple necklace is spiritual and placing it on the abdomen might cure intestinal problems. The rose quartz and the aquamarine have much to do with the mood of love. Cape amethyst, for example, was believed to be useful for arthritis when strands were wrapped around the joint. Carnelian was used to treat allergic reactions and asthma. Coral, diamond, emerald, and green and purple fluorite are used for emotional stress and hormonal imbalance, and jade for relaxation. People select precious stones according to their birthdates and they are classified according to their horoscopes. Garnet for January means fire elements or energy, and represents drive in life. Amethyst for February means fine, peaceful, intelligence, comfort, kindness, and honesty. Diamonds for April as gold, everyone's best friends and represent eternal love as the most hardest and brilliant stones. Pearls for June and rubies for July symbolizes feminine charm and love. Topaz for November represents friendship, and it has the power to improve eyesight and mental perception.

Massage and Touch Healing Powers and Therapy

Massage was used thousands of years ago by the Chinese. It was preventive, practiced on healthy individuals and not the ill. The Japanese massage called "shiatsu" was recommended for those living in the highly cultured areas in central Japan, near the Yellow River where people had more mental than physical stress. The Japanese shiatsu is finger pressure applied to specific points on the body. The word massage comes from an Arabic word meaning "stroke." It dates back 3000 years when it was practiced in China, then later by the Arabs. Massage is the manipulation of tissues of the body by stroking, rubbing, kneading, or tapping with the hands or an instrument. It is also the anointment, smear, or rubdown of the skin with oil or a specific cream. Massage art is based on the idea of touch that can heal. The Pharaohs practiced massage and touch therapy more than 4000 years ago, and so did Hippocrates, the Greek physician, in the fourth century BC. The church in the Middle Ages saw the manipulation of the body as the work of the devil and tried to prohibit massage. Massage improves body image in those with obesity and eating disorders. It improves stiffness and pain in those with arthritis by stimulating the circulation and soothing both the muscles and tendons. It is useful to treat tension, anxiety, insomnia, and both physical and mental exhaustion. Massage also helps to decrease the consumption of coffee, alcohol intake, and cigarette smoking. It also treats migraine, asthma, and paresis.

Touch is another healing power, especially for children. It is the first sense to develop in humans and may be the last to fade. Children from 6 months to 5 years having a daily 15-minute massage seem to be more alert, more responsive, and able to sleep more deeply according to Touch Research Institute in Miami, Fla. Touching has excellent effects on children's growth, development, and emotional well-being. The procedure is done by applying the light pressure of the fingertips in gentle downward strokes to the back and the chest or the palmar aspect of the fingers and/or the palms in touching and massaging the abdomen and extremities. This can be useful to treat stomach pain and get rid of gases. It is also useful for premature babies and helps in their recovery, both mental and physical. Touch has also social, educational, cultural, and humanitarian aspects.

Tattooing Therapy

Tattooing has been a well-known and practiced art for several centuries. Originally it was associated with religious ceremonies and fertility and marriage rites. It is still a common practice in Middle Eastern and Far Eastern countries, as well as in Europe and other Western countries. It is often a symbol of gang membership, and a common practice among army personnel. However, many do it for the sake of identification. Tattooing is still practiced by the Arabs as a tribal habit and decorative and beauty sign, which is done mainly on the face and hands. The techniques include the use of needles to introduce the particles of pigment into the dermis. The pigments are chosen according to the psychological factors of tattooed individuals. Blue-black is carbon, red is cinnabar, green is chromic oxide, yellow is cadmium sulfide, and brown is iron oxide. Tattoos can be in the form of lines, dots, figures, names of individuals, especially lovers, or as a sign of one's career (in the form of anchor or bower in sailors or mariners). Tattooing is also done in forms of animals, birds, dragons, or snakes since people believe tattoos protects them from evil and sickness. Tattooing is also done in certain shapes to frighten others and intimidate enemies.

Tattooing is done usually by a professional tattooer who marks or colors the skin with tattoos. The act of tattooing is an indelible mark or figure fixed on the body by insertion of one or more pigments under the skin or by production of scars using needles or scarification.

Tattooing was known for centuries as an alternative medical practice too. It was mainly performed by Buddhist monks, using a long needle to tattoo mainly the back and/or shoulders. The tattooer first puts his right hand on the tattoo place, and mutters or murmurs some kind of a prayer for a few minutes. The technique is painful but people believe that it brings them happiness and protects them from illnesses. At the same time they also believe that it has the power of a spell or incantation and talisman. They believe that tattooing acts as exorcism and protects the body from a sword, a chaser, or a bullet. This is why tattooing is applied on the face as a protection from enemy swords, or the back, chest, and abdomen for the same belief. Tattooing is also a ritual and is done in a liturgical or religious ceremony when incense, especially frankincense or cyclamen sticks are burned, and flowers are placed where the ceremony is held. Tattooing has many complications such as introducing simple pyogenic infection or tuberculosis, syphilis, infective hepatitis, or acquired immunodeficiency syndrome through unsterilized needles. Allergic reactions to the pigment and developing keloids or hypertrophic scars might also occur.

Modern tattooing for esthetic purposes features a special dye introduced to the upper part of the dermis using needles. It is practiced in the Middle Eastern countries and Europe for drawing lines or creating thicker eyebrows or eyelashes or lip lines.

Body Piercing

Body piercing is basically the technique of piercing the earlobe with a needle or a special piercing instrument to apply an ornament such as earrings or eardrops of different shapes. The ornament can be made of gold, silver, chrome, or any other metal. Nowadays ear piercing has been modified to have more than 1 piercing and more than 1 earring, and it could be 4 or more. Body piercing is known as a tribal fashion in some Arabian and African countries and is used for the nose, lips, and tongue. Today, even in the New World, some young people who reject the norms of the established societies are practicing body piercing in unusual ways. Piercing, in addition to the ears, is also done to the nose, tongue, nipples, navel, and also the vulva. This practice coincides with the way such individuals reject society by dressing unconventionally or favoring communal living.

Body piercing has adverse effects such as secondary infection and the risk of contracting acquired immunodeficiency syndrome through unclean needles.

Alternative Therapy for Insomnia

It is believed that one fifth of the world population has chronic insomnia, and difficulty sleeping without the intake of hypnotic drugs. Benzodiazepines and/or alcohol are used to help promote sleep, which can cause dependence, habit forming, or addiction after 4 to 6 weeks of continuous use.

The natural sleep process is a pattern created by the electromagnetic field produced in the brain by a combination of different radiofrequencies, which may stimulate the production of neurotransmitters or the electromagnetic field to promote the release of hormones, such as melatonin and serotonin that help promote sleep. The most common causes of insomnia are psychological in the form of worries, anxiety, fears, depression, and excitation. Sometimes the bed is too hot, too cold, too short, or has a bad mattress. Cigarette smoking late at night will create a nicotine effect that keeps one awake, or any change in sex habits.[53] The natural rhythm of sleep is disrupted in those who are frequent travelers and have jetlag, or others who develop nightmares.

Sleep loss exhibits potent effects, including decreasing cognitive abilities, alertness, and work performance. Fatigue experienced during the day following loss of sleep is risky from physical, emotional, and social standpoints. Hypnotics used to help sleep lead to daytime drowsiness, headache, poor concentration, and reduced memory in relation to place and time.

Lack of sleep affects the ability to drive or operate a machine and is followed by a hangover. Sleep can be disturbed, reduced, or completely prevented by anxiety, tension, mental exhaustion, change in bedtime habits, presence of strong light or noises, or following a heavy dinner, or in the presence of illness or due to intake of medications.

Alternative therapies for insomnia that help trigger sleep include relaxation or cogitative mental exercise. A simple exercise is, for instance, taking 3 deep breaths very slowly, exhaling fully each time, then stop breathing for as long as you can and repeat this 5 to 6 times. This breathing exercise causes a tranquilizing effect because of the accumulation of carbon dioxide in the blood. A warm bath may help, and a sound-masking device or a mask to cover the eyes are also useful methods to sleep. Drinking hot milk or hot chocolate, reading a story, listening to soft music, and to avoid thinking of daily matters could help induce sleep too. Some herbal medications are noted to help induce sleep, such as the African passion flower and passion fruit, the South American passiflora, the English *Humulus lupulus* hops and motherwort, chamomile, lemon balm, linden flowers and leaves, and wild lettuce. Children can sleep easily if stories or tales are read to them, they hear songs, or have a gentle-touch massage.

Sports as Alternative Therapies

Physical activities, exercises, and training are for pleasure and relaxation. They are outlets and help to alleviate stress, frustration, and tension. Different games and sports are also forms of self-expression, give confidence to a person, makes one feel satisfied and/or important, and encourage winners in sports to achieve more goals in life. Heavy exercises help induce sleep, some build strength of the body and soul, and some improve alertness. Spiritual, religious exercises, and devotions are also useful to treat many emotional, psychological, and physical problems, especially if they are combined with music.

I thank Hala Fattah, PhD, researcher of history, at the office of HRH Crown Prince El-Hassan bin Talal of Jordan for her assistance in editing the manuscript. I also acknowledge Inam Khayat, my secretary, for typing the manuscript.

References

1. National Institutes of Health, Office of Alternative Medicine. Alternative Medicine: *Expanding Medical Horizons.* Washington, DC: US Government Printing Office; 1994.

2. Fontanarosa PB, Lundberg GD. Complementary, alternative, unconventional, and integrative medicine. *JAMA.* 1997;278:2111–2112.

3. Eisenberg DM, Kassler RC, Foster C, et al. Unconventional medicine in the United States: prevalence, costs and patterns of use. *N Engl J Med.* 1993;328:246–252.

4. Eisenberg DM. Advising patients who seek alternative medical therapies. *Ann Intern Med.* 1997;127:61–62.

5. Anderson IB, Mullen WH, Meeker JE, et al. Penny royal toxicity: measurement of toxic metabolite levels in two cases and review of the literature. *Ann Intern Med.* 1996;124:726–734.

6. Nasr SH. *The Alchemical Tradition: Science and Civilization in Islam.* 2nd ed. London, England: The Islamic Texts Society; 1987:242.

7. Foster GM. Anthropological research perspectives on health problems in developing countries. *Soc Sci Med.* 1984;18:847–854.

8. Nizami-i A; Browne EG, trans. *Chahar Maqala.* London, England: Luzac & Co; 1921:76–77.

9. Oumeish OY, Parish LC. Community health: development and the environment. *Clin Dermatol.* 1998;16:7–9.

10. Brewington V. Acupuncture as a detoxification treatment: an analysis of controlled research. *J Subst Abuse Treat.* 1994;11:289–307.

11. Pedro E. Eastern medicine collides with western regulations at Mass Acupuncture School. *The Chronical of Higher Education.* 1993:A32.

12. Veith I. The *Yellow Emperor's Classic of Internal Medicine.* Berkeley: University of California Press; 1984:56–78.

13. Lazenby G. *The Feng Shui House Book.* New York, NY: Watson-Guptill Publications; 1998: 1–29, 56–75, 81–83.

14. Chuen MLK. *The Personal Feng Shui Manua: An Owl Book.* New York, NY: Henry Holt & Co; 1998:6, 10.

15. Lip E. *Personalize Your Feng Shui.* Singapore: Heian International Inc; 1997:5, 14, 15, 48, 54.

16. Porter R. *The Greatest Benefit to Mankind: A Medical History of Humanity.* New York, NY: WN Norton & Co; 1998.

17. Munoz P. *Indice de Sustancias Medicinnales Citadas: des en "Kitab al-kulliyyat" de Averrooes.* Granada, Spain: Estadios del Departamento de Historia de la Farmacia Legislation Farmaceutica; 1980.

18. Valver de JL. *Au Caire au XIIIe Siécle.* Cairo, Egypt: Bulletin de l'Institut d'Egypte; 1933:9–78.

19. Renaud HPJ, Colin GS. *Tuhfat al-ahbab: Glossaire de la Matieré Medicale.* Paris, France: Marcaine; 1934.

20. Awad HA. Phytotherapy in dermatology. Paper presented at: Third Congress of Pan-Arab League of Dermatologists; November 1992; Damascus, Syria.

21. Azmi A. Vitiligo repigmentation with Polypodium leucotomos. *Int J Dermatol.* 1989;28:479.

22. Corrales H, Lainez H, Pacheco J. A new agent (hydrophilic fraction of *Polypodium leucotomos*) for the management of psoriasis. In: *Proceedings of the 14th International Congress of Dermatology*; May 22–27, 1972; Padova, Venice.

23. Oumeish OY. Clinical trial of Anapsos (Difur) in vitiligo and atopic eczema: the first Jordanian trial. In: The Gulf Cooperative Council Second International Conference of Dermatology; February 5–7, 1994; Doha, Qatar.

24. Grimes P. Psoralen photochemotherapy for vitiligo. *Clin Dermatol.* 1997;15:922.

25. El-Mofty AM. A preliminary clinical report on the treatment of leucoderma with Ammi majus Linn. *J Egypt Med Assoc.* 1948;31:631–660.

26. El-Mofty AM. *Vitiligo and Psoralens.* New York, NY: Pergamon Press; 1968.

27. Abdel-Fattah A, Aboul-Ein MN, Wassel G, et al. An approach to the treatment of vitiligo by Khellin. *Dermatologica.* 1982;165:136–140.

28. Ortel B, Tanew A, Honigsmann H. Treatment of vitiligo with Khellin and ultraviolet. *J Am Acad Dermatol.* 1988;18:693–701.

29. Musallam BF. *Sex and Society in Islam: Cambridge Studies in Islamic Civilization.* 4th ed. New York, NY: Cambridge University Press; 1989:75–88.

30. Hage H, Mumna L. Female circumcision: culture or torture. *Al Raida.* 1996;13:40–41.

31. What has culture got to do with it: excising the harmful tradition of female circumcision. *Harvard Law Rev.* 1959;106:1947.

32. Abusharaf RM. A Sudanese anthropologist confronts female circumcision and its terrible tenacity: unmasking tradition. *Sciences.* 1998;38:22–27.

33. Routh HB, Bhowmik KR, Parich LC, Witkowski JA. Balneology, mineral water, and spas in historical perspective. *Clin Dermatol.* 1996;14:551–554.

34. Papalas AJ. Medical bathing in mineral springs in fifth century BC Greece. *Clio Med.* 1982; 16:81–82.

35. Major RH. *The History of Medicine.* Springfield, Ill: Charles C Thomas Publisher; 1959;31:11–12.

36. Adler AJ. Water immersion: lessons from antiquity to modern times. *Contrib Nephrol.* 1993; 102:171–186.

37. Ledo E. Mineral water and spas in Spain. *Clin Dermatol.* 1996;14:641–642.

38. Ghersetich I, Lotti T. Immunology of mineral water spas. *Clin Dermatol.* 1996;14:563–566.

39. Bernstein J. Dermatologic aspects of mineral water. *Clin Dermatol.* 1996;14:569.

40. Skin photobiology. *Lancet.* 1983;1:566–568.

41. Magnus IA. *Dermatological Photobiology.* Cambridge, Mass: Blackwell Publishers; 1976.

42. Oumeish YO. Climatotherapy at the Dead Sea in Jordan. *Clin Dermatol.* 1996;14:659–664.

43. Abels D, Even-Paz Z, Efron D. Bioclimatology at the Dead Sea in Israel. *Clin Dermatol.* 1996; 14:653–658.

44. *The Natural Resources Authority Laboratories Report.* Amman, Jordan: Ministry of Energy and Mineral Resources, The Hashemite Kingdom of Jordan; 1991:50–54.

45. Kushelevsky AP, Slifkin MA. Ultraviolet light measurements at the Dead Sea and at Beer-Sheva. *Isr J Med Sci.* 1975;11:488–490.

46. *The Meteorological Department Report.* Amman, Jordan: The Hashemite Kingdom of Jordan; 1991:66–69.

47. *Climatological Treatment of Psoriasis.* Tel Aviv, Israel: Ministry of Tourism; 1991:1–14.

48. Abels DJ, Kattan-Byron J. Psoriasis treatment at the Dead Sea: a natural selective ultraviolet phototherapy. *J Am Acad Dermatol.* 1985; 12:639–643.

49. Zuhair ZB, Oumeish YO. Climatotherapy of atopic dermatitis at the Dead Sea. Paper presented at: Third Congress of Pan-Arab League of Dermatologists; November 1992; Damascus, Syria.

50. Abed Abdul-Kader M. Geology of the Dead Sea: water and salts and evolution. *Dar al Argam.* October 1985:11–50.

51. Wilkinson JB. Hypnotherapy in the psychosomatic approach to illness: a review. *J R Soc Med.* 1981;74:525–530.

52. Woodham A, Peters D. *Homeopathy in Medical Therapies: Encyclopedia of Complementary Medicine.* London, England: Dorling Kindersley Book Publication; 1997:126.

53. Rosenfeld I. Insonmia: your passport to the land of nod. In: *The Best Treatment Textbook.* New York, NY: Simon & Schuster; 1991:160–163.

16 Thermalism in Argentina

Alternative or Complementary Dermatologic Therapy

Javier Ubogui, MD; Fernando M. Stengel, MD; María C. Kien, MD; Luis Sevinsky, MD; Liliana Rodríguez Lupo, MD
From Hospital Diego Thompson and Academia Nacional de Medicina (Dr Ubogui), Hospital CEMIC (Dr Stengel), Hospital Argerich (Dr Kien), Hospital Jose de San Martin, Buenos Aires University (Dr Sevinsky), Buenos Aires, Argentina, and Hospital Neuquén (Dr Lupo), Neuquén, Argentina.

Our study took place in the region of the Copahue Volcano in the Andes Mountain range, 1900 m above sea level. Fifty-five patients who came to the Copahue Thermal Basin Complex (Neuquén, Argentina) for treatment of psoriasis vulgaris were clinically evaluated for participation in this study. Thermal products—waters, mud, and/or algae—were the only therapeutic agents used, except for bland emollients for xerosis. Treatment for brief periods (10±3 days) resulted in notable improvement.

Arch Dermatol. 1998;134:1411–1412

Dermatologic thermalism—the therapeutic use of hot-water springs and their products (muds and algae)—offers an effective, natural, multifactorial, complementary, and nontoxic alternative to traditional treatment of psoriasis. Good results have also been described when thermalism was used as a single or adjuvant therapy for eczema, acne, and chronic skin ulcers.[1,2]

Patients and Methods

Fifty-five (31 men, 24 women) of 236 patients with psoriasis who spontaneously visited the Copahue Thermal Basin Complex (Neuquén, Argentina) during the 1987–1988 to 1990–1991 summer seasons (November through April) were evaluated for inclusion in our study. Inclusion criteria for subjects comprised moderate or severe lesions and an intention to stay at the complex for at least 7 days (average, 10 ± 3 days); all subjects accepted the therapeutic protocol and the 3 control visits; and no subject had had topical and/or systemic therapy for psoriasis in the 6 previous weeks.

The study protocol included 3 objective medical assessments—at day 0, at day 5, and on the day of discharge (day 10 ± 3 days)—and 1 subjective assessment, ie, patient opinion at discharge. Objective criteria were scaling, erythema, and thickness; designations for evaluation of these criteria were worse, no change, mild improvement, improvement, and marked improvement. Surface extension was not evaluated because no change was expected with such a short course of treatment.

Thermal therapy comprised 2 daily baths, one with thermal water (algae-rich "Green Lagoon" with volcanic water) (Table 1) and the other with mud and/or algae from the sulfurous lagoons. Sunbathing in Copahue was curtailed because of weather conditions; protocol patients did not sunbathe. In 23 patients, pretherapy and posttherapy punch biopsies were performed.

The antimicrobial properties of the Copahue volcanic water were investigated with 64 nosocomial strains. In the control Petri dish, pure medium was used (trypticase soy broth agar). Three other Petri dishes were prepared with 20% unmodified volcanic water, 20% alkalized (NaOH 3N) volcanic water, and 20% acidified (HCl 0,01N) distilled water (pH 1), respectively.

Table 1. Copahue Volcano Water Chemical Analysis*

Component	Value
Color	80†
Turbidity	2.1 NTU‡
pH	1.3†
Conductimetric residue	54,180.0
Total hardness (in $CaCO_3$)	4000.0
Cl^-	4410.0
SO_4^{2-}	13,800.0
No_3	2.0
NO_2^-	0.01
NH_4^+	1.0
Ca^{2+}	680.0
Mg^{2+}	550.0
F	200.0
As	1.7
Fe	Interference§
Mn	0.05
Pb	Interference§
Cd	0.01
Hg	0.005
Zn	Interference§
S^{2-}	1.0

*Unless otherwise indicated, values are expressed in milligrams per liter.
†These values are not measured in milligrams per liter.
‡Turbidity is measured in nephelometric turbidity units.
§The measuring apparatus could not detect/distinguish this component.

Results

On day 5, all subjects showed improvement in scaling and worsening in erythema. On day 10, there was marked improvement in erythema, xerosis, and scaling. Two subjects developed new guttate lesions, and 8 exhibited a few residual macules.

Results of the objective assessments of the subjects at 10 ± 3 days revealed marked improvement in 11 subjects, improvement in 29, and mild improvement in 15. In the subjective assessments, 20 subjects felt there was marked improvement; 21, improvement; and 14, mild improvement.

In the results of 10 of the 23 biopsies, the following histological changes were noted: (1) marked decrease of the parakeratotic corneal layer associated with orthokeratotic hyperkeratosis, increase of the granular layer, and epidermal thinning with irregularity of the rete ridges; (2) minimal reduction in the size and diameter of the dermal vessels; and (3) slight decrease of the dermal infiltrate.

The Petri dish with 20% volcanic water showed no bacterial growth. The other 3 dishes yielded positive results for organisms. Thus, the pH factor was not responsible for the antibacterial effects.

Comment

According to most authors, effective thermal treatments must last 3 to 4 weeks, and in Argentina, high costs can prevent such lengthy stays. Nonetheless, the use of mineral waters and associated products from their natural environment for the treatment of skin diseases, popularized by the Dead Sea experience,[3–5] dates back in dermatologic reports from Copahue to 1938.[6,7] The mode of action of thermalism still requires investigation, but its principle depends on the integrated actionof 2 natural systems: the microecosystem, ie, thermal products per se (water, muds, algae), and the macroecosystem, ie, the natural volcanic environment (scenery, climate, calmness).

The various minerals (salts) and trace elements present in the sulfur-rich waters and mud found at Copahue give to them strongly keratolytic, moderately antimicrobial, and mildly anti-inflammatory and immunomodulatory properties. Different types of algae release active antimicrobials and natural healing components such as calcium alginate and steroidal compounds.[1,8,9] If microorganisms play a role in psoriasis, these components may play a substantial role in healing, acting either directly on the skin microflora or on eventual upper airway-polluting foci.[10] Work from Pescara, Italy, suggests that in immune-mediated conditions, sulfur products may have anti-inflammatory effects on the epithelium.[11]

Conclusions

In patients with psoriasis vulgaris, brief thermal treatments led to improvement. In thermalism, dose implies time, number of exposures, and frequency, and when therapy is extended (4 weeks), our own as-yet unpublished observations indicate that better results can be expected.

Thermalism expands the therapeutic armamentarium and complements or potentiates the action of other therapies for psoriasis (eg, mud baths plus psoralen–UV-A). It is an effective, natural, multifactorial, complementary, and nontoxic alternative to traditional management of psoriasis, and it deserves a place in dermatologic therapy and research.

References

1. Ubogui J, Ficoseco H. Ulceras por decúbito e hidroterapia en las termas de Copahue. *Arch Argent Dermatol.* 1990;40:393–399.

2. Ubogui J, Rodríguez Lupo L, Ficoseco H, Kien C, Sevinsky L, Stengel F. Terapéutica no convencional de la psoriasis en las termas de Copahue (Neuquén, Argentina): experiencia preliminar. *Arch Argent Dermatol.* 1991; 41:25–39.

3. Abels DJ, Byron J. Psoriasis treatment at the Dead Sea: a natural selective ultraviolet therapy. *J Am Acad Dermatol.* 1985;12:639–643.

4. Abels DJ, Rose T, Bearman JE. Treatment of psoriasis at a Dead Sea dermatology clinic. *Int J Dermatol.* 1985;34:134–137.

5. Harari M, Shani J. Demographic evaluation of successful antipsoriatic climatotherapy at the Dead Sea. *Int J Dermatol.* 1997;36:304–308.

6. Alvarez G. Contribución al estudio de las termas de Copahue (Neuquén), en sus aplicaciones dermatológicas. *Bol Asoc Med Argent.* 1938;4:220.

7. Gunche F, Castillo M. *Balneoterapia Preparada y Aguas Minerales Argentinas en Dermatologia.* Buenos Aires, Argentina: Ed Sophos; 1960.

8. Accorinti J, Squadrone M, Wenzel M, Perez A. Valoración de las propiedades antimicrobianas del agua del volcán Copahue (Neuquén, Argentina). *Arch Argent Dermatol.* 1991; 41:229–237.

9. Squadrone M. Acción del agua del volcán Copahue (Neuquén, Argentina) sobre las micobacterias. *Arch Argent Dermatol.* 1992;42:97–108.

10. Noah WP. The role of microorganisms in psoriasis. *Semin Dermatol.* 1990;9:269–276.

11. Valitutti S, Castellino F, Musiano P. Effect of sulfurous (thermal) water on T lymphocyte proliferative response. *Ann Allergy.* 1990;65:463–467.

17 Different Modalities of Spa Therapy for Skin Diseases at the Dead Sea Area

Sima Halevy, MD; Shaul Sukenik, MD
From the Departments of Dermatology (Dr Halevy), and Internal Medicine (Dr Sukenik), Soroka University Medical Center, Faculty of Health Sciences, Ben-Gurion University of the Negev, Beer-Sheva, Israel.

Background
Balneology and spa therapy, although not accepted as well-established treatment modalities in dermatology, are used throughout the world. The therapeutic properties for skin and rheumatic diseases of the Dead Sea area may be attributed to unique climatic characteristics and unique natural resources. The mechanisms by which a broad spectrum of diseases are alleviated by spa therapy may involve mechanical, thermal, and chemical effects.

Objective
To review and discuss various spa therapy modalities, used at the Dead Sea area for a wide spectrum of skin diseases.

Conclusions
Existing evidence indicates the therapeutic potential of Dead Sea spa therapy modalities for psoriasis and psoriatic arthritis. A beneficial effect is hinted at for other skin diseases, but the absence of relevant methodological and clinical information precludes the drawing of any scientific conclusions. It is essential to establish therapeutic guidelines to determine the optimal treatment modality for each disease, and the optimal protocol of each treatment component, adjusted individually for each patient, with respect to remission and long-term adverse effects.

Arch Dermatol. 1998;134:1416–1420

Balneology and spa therapy, although not accepted as well-established treatment modalities in dermatology, are used throughout the world.[1–3]

The therapeutic properties for skin and rheumatic diseases[4–10] of the Dead Sea (DS) area, situated 400 m below sea level, have been known since ancient times. These therapeutic properties may be attributed to unique climatic characteristics and natural resources,[4–6] including meteorological variables, attenuation of UV,[11,12] DS water (with its unparalleled salinity and unique composition), sources of natural thermomineral waters, the DS mineral mud, increased bromine content of the air, and a high selenium content of local drinking water. The possible role of psychological influences in the DS area cannot be overlooked.

Modalities of Spa Therapy at the DS Area

Various spa therapy modalities are used at the DS area.[10,13,14] These may be classified as heliotherapy (sun exposure), thalassotherapy (bathing in DS water), balneotherapy (immersion in baths and pools of thermomineral water), pelotherapy (heated DS mud pack therapy), and climatotherapy (using atmosphere, temperature, humidity, barometric pressure, and light).[13] In many studies climatotherapy at the DS area is referred to as a therapy consisting of sun exposure (heliotherapy) and bathing in DS water (thalassotherapy). Heliotherapy is carried out over a period of 3 to 4 weeks, with a gradual increase in sun-exposure time. The sun-dosage schedule is determined in accordance with the patient's skin type. Thalassotherapy[4–6] is carried out by gradually increasing bathing time to a maximum of 1 hour per day. There are variations, modifications, and combinations of these spa therapy modalities. The DS spa therapy modalities may be combined with conventional topical medications, including emollients and noncorticosteroid preparations, salicylic acid, tar, and sulfur, in varying concentrations and combinations. Systemic drugs are not usually used during DS spa therapy for skin diseases.

Inclusion and Exclusion Criteria and Adverse Effects of DS Spa Therapy

Psoriasis is the disease most frequently treated by DS spa therapy, followed by atopic dermatitis and vitiligo. The DS spa therapy is also used for a small group of patients with other skin diseases, including acne vulgaris, dyshidrotic eczema, lichen planus, ichthyosis vulgaris, early-stage mycosis fungoides, pityriasis rubra pilaris, urticaria pigmentosa (adult type), necrobiosis lipoidica, circumscribed scleroderma, alopecia areata, lichen sclerosus and atrophicus, and granuloma annulare.[14]

Exclusion criteria for climatotherapy include systemic lupus erythematosus and other photoaggravated dermatoses, skin malignancies, acute skin infections (viral and bacterial), and immunodeficiency diseases. General contraindications include severe psychiatric conditions, acute alcoholic states, epilepsy, cardiac dysrhythmias, and inadequate balance. Contraindications for balneotherapy include severe varicose veins, nonhealed wounds, and hypersensitivity to mineral baths.[14] Patients suffering from acute and subacute dermatitis are prohibited from bathing in DS water.[10]

Adverse effects of climatotherapy, consisting mainly of sunburn and other photosensitivity reactions (8.2% and 5%, respectively), have been observed in only a few patients.[14] Exfoliative dermatitis developed in 1 case.[15] Balneotherapy may cause a thermal reaction manifested primarily by exacerbation of joint pain and fatigue.

Possible Mechanisms of the Effectiveness of Spa Therapy at the DS Area

The mechanisms by which a broad spectrum of diseases are alleviated by spa therapy have not been fully elucidated. They probably incorporate mechanical, thermal, and chemical effects.[1,8,9] Chemical effects of the DS spa therapy were evidenced by in vivo and in vitro studies,[16–21] which disclosed increased levels of minerals that may play a role in cell proliferation and differentiation.[22–24] Anti-inflammatory and immunomodulatory effects[8] involving various cell lineages, inflammatory cytokine release, and cytokine receptor modulation[25–30] may be induced by the thermal effects of spa therapy. Bathing in high concentrations of salt solutions may trigger the elution of various chemotactic and proinflammatory mediators (ie, elastase and cytokines) from the affected skin of patients with psoriasis, contact dermatitis, and atopic dermatitis.[31–33] Furthermore, bathing in tap water or salt solutions (including DS salts) has recently been associated with the increased photosensitivity of the skin to UV-B irradiation, and may contribute to the efficacy of balneophototherapy.[34,35]

Spa Therapy for Psoriasis at the DS Area

Various studies[4,14,15,36–48] have indicated that different DS spa therapy modalities are effective in the treatment of psoriasis. Most types of psoriasis, except generalized pustular psoriasis, responded to treatment.[10] Psoriatic erythroderma

Table 1. Dead Sea (DS) Spa Therapy Modalities for Psoriasis*

Source, y	No. of Patients	Type of Psoriasis	DS Spa Therapy Modality	Duration	Adjuvant Therapy	Skin Evaluation	Results, %
Azizi et al,[15] 1982	94	Plaque type	Sun exposure and bathing in the DS	4 wk	Emollients ± TNSP	3-Grade scale of response	Healing or marked improvement, 85
Abels and Kattan-Byron,[40] 1985	110	Plaque/patchy, guttate, with or without PsA	Sun exposure and bathing in the DS	14-42 d (mean, 26 d)	Emollients ± TNSP	. . .	Complete clearing or excellent improvement, 81.4
Abels et al,[41] 1995	1448	Psoriasis vulgaris	Sun exposure and bathing in the DS	28 d	Emollients	. . .	Clearing of 80–100, 88
Giryes et al,[42] 1994	80	Psoriasis vulgaris and PsA	Sun exposure and bathing in the DS, mud packs, and thermal baths	3 wk	NS	PASI score, mean ± SD reduction	91.5 ± 10.5
	38	Psoriasis vulgaris	Sun exposure and bathing in the DS				88.5 ± 11.6
Sukenik et al,[43] 1994	130	PsA	Sun exposure, bathing in the DS, mud packs, and sulfur baths	3 wk	Emollients ± TNSP	PASI score, mean ± SD reduction	93.3 ± 12.0†
	18		Sun exposure and bathing in the DS				96.0 ± 7.3†
Giryes et al,[44] 1997	69	Psoriasis vulgaris	Climatotherapy and pretreatment	NS	NS	PASI score, mean	Decrease (P<.001)
	54		Climatotherapy and no pretreatment				Decrease (P<.001)
Even-Paz et al,[45] 1996	15	Psoriasis, NS	Bathing in the DS and sun exposure (3 h)			PASI score, mean reduction	90.2
	15		Bathing in the DS and sun exposure (4.5 h)	28 d	Emollients		85.5
	15		Bathing in the DS and sun exposure (6 h)				88.9
Even-Paz et al,[46] 1996	34	Plaque type	Sun exposure			PASI score, mean reduction	72.8
	15		Bathing in the DS	4 wk	Emollients		28.4
	32		Sun exposure and bathing in the DS				83.4
Halevy et al,[47] 1997	13	Psoriasis vulgaris	DS salt baths	3 wk	Emollients	PASI score, mean ± SD reduction	34.8 ± 24.0
	12		Common salt baths				27.5 ± 18.3

*TNSP indicates topical nonsteroid preparations; PsA, psoriatic arthritis; NS, not specified; ellipses, not applicable; and PASI, psoriasis area and severity index.

†A significant reduction in the number of inflamed joints.

was successfully treated by heliotherapy in the DS area.[48] Until recently, most of these studies have consisted of clinical observations and descriptive rather than well-controlled studies. A review of the main clinical studies on DS spa therapy for psoriasis is presented later and in Table 1.

The pioneering pilot studies of Dostrovsky et al[36] and Dostrovsky and Shanon[37] elucidated the therapeutic effect of helio-balnetherapy for psoriasis in the DS area. Avrach[38] and Montgomery[39] reported a beneficial effect in large groups of patients with psoriasis (577, 1052, and 1631, respectively) treated at the DS area.

Retrospective studies[15,40,41] on 94, 110, and 1448 patients with psoriasis, respectively, treated at the DS area revealed a beneficial effect at the end of treatment in 81% to 88% of the patients, defined as complete clearing (95%–100% improvement), excellent improvement (80%–95% improvement), and marked improvement. The study groups consisted of selected patients with psoriasis,[15] patients with psoriasis enrolled in a dermatology clinic at the DS from March 1983 to June 1983,[40] and a cohort of consecutive patients with psoriasis treated at a DS psoriasis clinic.[41] Although most of the patients suffered from psoriasis vulgaris or plaque-type psoriasis, some heterogeneity with respect to the type of psoriasis was observed.[40] Furthermore, there were no uniform criteria for the extent of skin involvement prior to DS spa therapy (ie, >50 cm^2 involvement of skin area[15]; an average of 29% skin involvement[40]; and ≥7% involvement in 76% of the patients[41]). Heterogeneity with respect to the country of origin (Israeli and non-Israeli)[41] and the duration of treatment (4 weeks,[15] 14–42 days [mean, 26 days],[40] and 28 days[41]) was also observed. The treatment protocol[40] consisted of sun exposure (initial exposure of 10-20 minutes twice a day, depending on the skin type, with an increase in increments of 10 minutes each day until a maximum of approximately 6 hours a day) and bathing in the DS (initial bathing of 5 minutes, twice a day, with an increase in increments of 5 minutes every 3 days until a maximum of 30 minutes, twice a day). Topical adjuvant therapy consisted of emollients with or without nonsteroid ointments (containing salicylic acid, tar, and sulfur). In 1 of the series,[40] no significant improvement was observed in many patients until the third or fourth week. No significant associations were found with sex, previous DS spa treatments, prior hospitalization for psoriasis, prior psoralen–UV-A therapy, or history of arthritis.[41] Determination of the individual UV sensitivity index (defined as the lowest exposure time to a UV radiation source, which produced erythema with defined border 24 hours later) by Azizi et al[15] revealed a more favorable result of the DS climatotherapy in patients with psoriasis with high UV sensitivity index (≥90 seconds) compared with low UV sensitivity index (30 seconds).

A retrospective study by Giryes et al[42] disclosed a similar efficacy of climatotherapy compared with a combination of climatotherapy and balneotherapy performed for 3 weeks in patients with psoriasis vulgaris. Climatotherapy given to 38 patients without joint involvement consisted of sun exposure and bathing in the DS. A combination of climatotherapy and balneotherapy was used in 80 patients with joint involvement. The regimen of balneotherapy consisted of heated DS mud packs and thermal baths. The mean (± SD) percentage reduction of the psoriasis area and severity index (PASI) score did not differ significantly between the groups (88.5% ±11.6% and 91.5% ± 10.5%, respectively).

The therapeutic role of DS spa therapy in patients with psoriatic arthritis was also shown in a prospective controlled study by Sukenik et al.[43] The study group was treated by a combination of sun exposure, bathing in the DS, mud packs, and sulfur baths, whereas patients treated traditionally only by sun exposure and bathing in the DS served as controls. The duration of treatment was 3 weeks. The mean (± SD) percentage reduction of the PASI score in the study group (n=130) did not differ significantly from that of the control group (n=18) (93.3% ± 12.0% and 96.0% ± 7.3%, respectively). A statistically significant improvement of the joint disease was observed in both groups ($P<.001$ and $P=.02$, respectively). However, reduction of spinal pain and increased range of lumbar spine movements were only observed in the study group. Despite the small number of patients in the control group and the fact that this study was not randomized, the age of the patients, the duration of psoriasis, and psoriatic arthritis as well as the use of nonsteroidal anti-inflammatory drugs and disease remitting drugs were similar in both groups.

The results of a retrospective analysis[44] implied that antipsoriatic pretreatment did not influence clearing of psoriasis vulgaris following DS climatotherapy (sun exposure and bathing in the DS). The study group consisted of 69 patients suffering from psoriasis vulgaris who were divided into 5 groups according to the antipsoriatic regimen used 4 weeks before DS climatotherapy (topical corticosteroids, calcipotriol, tar, salicylic acid ointment, or UV radiation). Fifty-four patients, who avoided using any medications 4 weeks prior to climatotherapy, served as a control group. Patients in all 5 pretreatment groups did not differ significantly with respect to sex, age, duration of disease, and climatotherapy. The PASI scores at the end of climatotherapy were significantly lower compared with PASI scores before climatotherapy in each study group ($P<.001$). However, no significant difference was observed in the PASI scores when the pretreatment groups were compared with the control group ($P>.05$).

A recent prospective study conducted by Even-Paz et al[45] determined the best sun-exposure times for psoriasis treatment at the DS area. The study included 45 Israeli patients with psoriasis (volunteers from the Israel Psoriasis Association) treated at the DS area in July and August 1994 for 28 days. Patients were assigned to 1 of 3 sun-exposure schedules with a maximum daily sun exposure of 3.0, 4.5, or 6.0 hours, respectively. The therapy regimen consisted of sun exposure (twice daily, gradually increased from a few minutes daily to the maximum), bathing in the DS (twice daily for 20–30 minutes), and emollients (used freely). At the end of the therapy, the mean percentage reduction in the PASI score did not differ significantly among the 3 groups (90.2%, 85.5%, and 88.9%, respectively). The weekly cumulative improvement was similar for all groups. The degree of improvement did not differ significantly in patients whose initial PASI score was 20 or more. The results indicate that the daily sun exposure for treatment of psoriasis at the DS area in July and August need not exceed 3 hours.

Another prospective study conducted by Even-Paz et al[46] indicated that sun exposure was the main factor producing beneficial results for psoriasis (plaque type) in DS spa therapy, and that bathing in DS water enhanced the effect of solar radiation. The study included 81 patients with psoriasis (volunteers from the Israel Psoriasis Association) allocated to 1 of the following groups: DS water bathing only (15 patients); sun exposure only (34 patients); and sun exposure combined with DS water bathing (32 patients). The DS water bathing was performed for 20 minutes twice daily in heated indoor pools. Sun exposure was done twice daily in solaria, with a gradual increase in exposure from a few minutes to 5.5 hours daily. The duration of treatment was 4 weeks. Adjuvant treatment consisted of emollients (used freely). Previous antipsoriatic treatments were discontinued 3 weeks before arrival at the DS area. The mean percentage reduction in the PASI score (recorded by 1 physician alone, or by 2 working together) was 28.4% in patients who only bathed in the DS water, 72.8% in those only sunbathing, and 83.4% in those doing both. There was no significant seasonal difference in the results related to the sun-exposure groups.

A recent prospective double-blind controlled study by Halevy et al[47] evaluated the sole therapeutic effect of DS salt in patients with psoriasis. The study included 25 patients with psoriasis vulgaris involving 15% or more of body area randomly allocated to 2 groups who were treated with either DS salt baths (13 patients) or common salt baths (12 patients). The treatment protocol consisted of once-daily salt baths that were heated to 35°C and of 20 minutes' duration, immediately followed by washing with tap water and lubrication of the skin (white soft paraffin, twice daily) for 3 weeks. Topical and systemic antipsoriatic therapy was withdrawn for 2 and 4 weeks, respectively, before starting the salt baths. In the DS bath salt and the common salt groups the mean PASI score at the end of treatment was significantly lower than the mean PASI score before treatment ($P=.005$ and $P=.001$, respectively). However, the mean percentage reduction in the PASI score at the end of treatment was higher in patients treated by DS bath salt compared with common salt (34.8% and 27.5%, respectively; $P>.05$). A similar trend was observed 1 month after termination of the treatment protocol (43.6% and 24%, respectively; $P>.05$). The results imply a beneficial therapeutic effect to bathing with either DS bath salt or common salt as monotherapy for psoriasis vulgaris, although an enhanced beneficial effect was observed in patients treated with DS bath salts. Statistical significance was not reached, probably due to the small number of patients in our study ($P>.05$ and $P>.05$, respectively).

The studies reviewed earlier display heterogeneity with respect to study group composition (demographic variables, disease type, and severity), spa therapy modality (protocol, timing, and duration), and criteria used for assessment of disease severity and therapeutic results. Most lack relevant data regarding joint disease, previous treatments, and length of remission achieved. Evaluation of the relative effectiveness of various treatment modalities has been carried out in only a few recent studies. These limitations preclude comparative analyses of DS spa therapy for psoriasis.

Spa Therapy for Atopic Dermatitis and Other Skin Diseases at the DS Area

Two recent clinical observations[14,49] provided evidence for the therapeutic potential of DS spa therapy for atopic dermatitis. Complete clearance of lesions was recorded in 90% of 1408 patients after 4 to 6 weeks' stay at the DS area (in 97% of the patients lesions cleared after 6 weeks and in 89% after 4 weeks). A reduction in itching was recorded during the first week of stay at the DS area. The percentage of patients who improved during the spring and summer was higher than in the autumn and winter.[14] Giryes et al[49] reported the efficacy of DS climatotherapy for atopic dermatitis in 56 patients: 18 children younger than 18 years and 38 adults. The climatotherapy regimen consisted of daily sun exposure (maximum, 3–4 hours), bathing in diluted DS water or sweet water (20 minutes twice a day), and free application of emollients. Clinical evaluation was based on the index for Severity Scoring of Atopic Dermatitis. At the end of climatotherapy both groups showed a significant clearing of skin lesions, reductions in itch and sleep disturbances, and a significant decrease ($P<.001$) in the Severity Scoring of Atopic Dermatitis index.

Clinical observation of 102 patients with vitiligo treated by the DS climatotherapy[50] revealed beneficial results manifested by total or almost total repigmentation in 11% of the patients, significant repigmentation in 82.3%, partial repigmentation in 6.4%, and no change in 1% of the patients. Marked improvement was observed in 78% and 70% of the patients who stayed 4 to 6 weeks and 4 weeks, respectively, in the DS area.

Clinical observation of 86 patients treated for acne vulgaris in the DS area[14] showed a significant improvement manifested by a reduced number of comedones and pustules.

Favorable effects of DS spa therapy were reported also for dyshidrotic eczema, lichen planus, ichthyosis, parapsoriasis, mycosis fungoides stage I, pityriasis rubra pilaris, urticaria pigmentosa (adult type), necrobiosis lipoidica, circumscribed scleroderma, alopecia areata, lichen sclerosus and atrophicus and granuloma annulare.[14]

Conclusions

Existing evidence indicates the therapeutic potential of DS spa therapy modalities for psoriasis and psoriatic arthritis. A beneficial effect is hinted at for other skin diseases, but the absence of relevant methodological and clinical information precludes the drawing of any scientific conclusions.

It is essential to establish therapeutic guidelines to determine the optimal treatment modality for each disease and the optimal protocol of each treatment component (dosing, frequency, duration, maintenance, or adjuvant medications), adjusted individually for each patient, with respect to remission and long-term adverse effects.

A large spectrum of variables should be integrated into the therapeutic guidelines of DS spa therapy, including the skin disease (type, severity, and duration), the skin type, history of skin cancer, chemical photosensitivity, associated diseases, drug intake and alcohol consumption, emotional state, response to previous treatments (conventional and nonconventional), and measurements of solar UV radiation during the DS spa therapy.[51]

The use of similar definitions and criteria in studies related to DS spa therapy modalities is mandatory for analysis and determinations of cost-effectiveness of DS spa therapy for skin diseases, compared with other conventional treatment modalities.

References

1. Lotti T, Freedman D. Balneology and spa treatments in dermatology: the European point of view. *J Eur Acad Dermatol Venereol.* 1994; 3:449–450.
2. Parish LP, Witkowski JA. Dermatologic balneology: the American view of waters, spas, and hot springs. *J Eur Acad Dermatol Venereol.* 1994; 3:465–467.
3. Routh HB, Bhowmik KR, Parish LC, Witkowski JA. Balneology, mineral water, and spas in historical perspective. *Clin Dermatol.* 1996; 14:551–554.
4. Even-Paz Z, Shani J. The Dead Sea and psoriasis: historical and geographic background. *Int J Dermatol.* 1989;28:1–9.
5. Even-Paz Z, Efron D. The Dead Sea as a spa health resort. *Isr J Med Sci.* 1996; 32 (suppl 3): 4–8.
6. Even-Paz Z. Dermatology at the Dead Sea spas. *Isr J Med Sci.* 1996; 32 (suppl 3): 11–15.
7. Sukenik S, Shoenfeld Y. The Dead Sea is alive. *Isr J Med Sci.* 1996; 32 (suppl 3): 1–3.
8. Tishler M, Shoenfeld Y. The medical and scientific aspects of spa therapy. *Isr J Med Sci.* 1996; 32 (suppl 3): 8–10.
9. Sukenik S. Balneotherapy for rheumatic diseases at the Dead Sea. *Isr J Med Sci.* 1996; 32 (suppl 3): 16–19.
10. Abels DJ, Even-Paz Z, Efron D. Bioclimatology at the Dead Sea in Israel. *Clin Dermatol.* 1996; 14:653–658.
11. Kushelevsky AP, Slifkin MA. Ultraviolet measurements at the Dead Sea and at Beersheba: biometeorological considerations. *Isr J Med Sci.* 1975; 11:488–490.
12. Kushelevsky P, Kudish A. Intercomparison of global ultraviolet B and A radiation measurements in the Dead Sea region (Ein Bokek) and Beer Sheva. *Isr J Med Sci.* 1996; 32 (suppl 3): 24–27.
13. Routh HB, Bhowmik KR. Basic tents of mineral water: a glossary of concepts related to balneology, mineral water, and the spa. *Clin Dermatol.* 1996; 14:549–550.
14. Shani J, Seidel V, Hristakieva E, Stanimirovic A, Burdo A, Harari M. Indications, contraindications and possible side-effects of climatotherapy at the Dead Sea. *Int J Dermatol.* 1997; 36:481–492.
15. Azizi E, Kushlevsky A, Avrach W, Schewach-Millet M. Climate therapy of psoriasis at the Dead Sea. *Isr J Med Sci.* 1982; 18:267–270.
16. Shani J, Barak S, Levi D, et al. Skin penetration of minerals in psoriatics and guinea pigs bathing in hypertonic salt solutions. *Pharmacol Res Commun.* 1985; 17:501–512.
17. Shani J, Sharon R, Koren R, et al. Effects of Dead Sea brine and its main salts on cell growth in culture. *Pharmacology.* 1987; 35:339–347.
18. Shani J, Sulliman A, Katzir I, Brenner S. Penetration of selected Dead Sea minerals through a healthy rabbit skin, from a sustained-release transparent varnish, as a prospective treatment for psoriasis. *J Eur Acad Dermatol Venereol.* 1995; 4:267–272.
19. Shani J, Even-Paz Z, Avrach WW, et al. Topical replacement therapy of psoriasis by Dead Sea salts, evaluated by scanning electron microscopy and x-ray fluorescence. *Dermatosen.* 1991; 39:49–55.
20. Shani J, Tur E, Wald E, et al. Computerized morphometry of psoriatic keratinocytes after bathing in the Dead Sea bath solutions. *J Dermatol Treat.* 1993; 4:195–198.
21. Shani J, Barak S, Ram M, et al. Serum bromine levels in psoriasis. *Pharmacology.* 1982; 25:297–307.
22. Vorhees JJ, Duell EA. Imbalanced cyclic-AMP and cyclic GMP levels in psoriasis. *Adv Cyclic Nucleotide Res.* 1975; 5:735–738.
23. Blondell JM. The anti-carcinogenic effect of magnesium. *Med Hypotheses.* 1980; 6:863–871.
24. Petrini M, Vaglini F, Carulli G, et al. Effects of lithium and rubidium on the differentiation of mononuclear cells. *Int J Tissue React.* 1986; 8:391–392.

25. Valitutti S, Costellino F, Musiani P. Effect of sulphureous "thermal" water on T lymphocytes proliferative response. *Ann Allergy.* 1990; 65:463–468.

26. Simonelli C. Come le acque sulfuree modulano il sistema immunitario. *Current.* 1994; 1:15.

27. Wollenberg A, Richard A, Bieber T. In vitro effect of the thermal water from La Roche-Possay on the stimulatory capacity of epidermal Langerhans cells. *Eur J Dermatol.* 1992; 2:128–129.

28. Sainte-Laudy J. Etude du pouvoir anti-degranulant de l'Eau d'Avene vis-à-vis de basophiles humains sensibilises. *Int J Immunother.* 1987; 3:307–310.

29. Celerier P, Richard A, Litoux P, Dreno B. Modulatory effects of selenium and strontium salts on keratinocyte-derived inflammatory cytokines. *Arch Dermatol Res.* 1995; 287:680–682.

30. Arenberger P, Bartak P, Kemeny L, Ruzicka T. Cytokine receptor modulation: a possible balneotherapeutic effect in psoriasis. Paper presented at: Sixth International Psoriasis Symposium; July 20–24, 1994; Chicago, Ill.

31. Wiedow O, Streit V, Christophers E, Stander M. Liberation of human leukocyte elastase by hypertonic saline baths in psoriasis. *Hautartz.* 1989; 40:518–522.

32. Wiedow O, Wiese F, Streit V, Kalm C, Christophers E. Lesional elastase activity in psoriasis, contact dermatitis, and atopic dermatitis. *J Invest Dermatol.* 1992; 99:306–309.

33. Wiedow O, Wiese F, Christophers E. Lesional elastase activity in psoriasis: diagnostic and prognostic significance. *Arch Dermatol Res.* 1995; 287: 632–635.

34. Boer J, Schothorst AA, Boom B, Hermans J, Suurmond D. Influence of water and salt solutions on UVB irradiation of normal skin and psoriasis. *Arch Dermatol Res.* 1982; 273:247–259.

35. Schempp CM, Blumke C, Schopf E, Simon JC. Skin sensitivity to UV-B radiation is differentially increased by exposure to water and different salt solutions. *Arch Dermatol.* 1997; 133:1610.

36. Dostrovsky A, Sagher F, Even-Paz Z, et al. Preliminary report: the therapeutic effect of the hot springs of Zohar (Dead Sea) on some skin diseases. *Harefuah.* 1959; 57:143–145.

37. Dostrovsky A, Shanon J. Influence of helio-balneotherapy at the hot spring of Zohar (Ein-Bokek) on psoriasis: a further report. *Harefuah.* 1963; 63:127–129.

38. Avrach WW. Climatotherapy at the Dead Sea. In: *Proceedings of the Second International Symposium on Psoriasis, Stanford University.* New York, NY: Yorke Medical Books; 1976: 258–261.

39. Montgomery BJ. Bathing for psoriasis in the Dead Sea. *JAMA.* 1979; 241:227–231.

40. Abels DJ, Kattan-Byron J. Psoriasis treatment at the Dead Sea: a natural selective ultraviolet phototherapy. *J Am Acad Dermatol.* 1985; 12:639–643.

41. Abels DJ, Rose T, Bearman JE. Treatment of psoriasis at the Dead Sea dermatological clinic. *Int J Dermatol.* 1995; 34:134–137.

42. Giryes H, Halevy S, Sukenik S. Climatotherapy and balneotherapy for treatment of psoriasis vulgaris in the Dead Sea area. Paper presented at: Sixth International Psoriasis Symposium; July 20–24, 1994; Chicago, Ill.

43. Sukenik S, Giryes H, Halevy S, et al. Treatment of psoriatic arthritis at the Dead Sea. *J Rheumatol.* 1994; 21:1305–1309.

44. Giryes H, Friger M, Sarov B, Halevy S. Does pretreatment of psoriatic patients influence climatotherapy at the Dead Sea? Biology and therapy of inflammatory skin diseases. Paper presented at: International Symposium at the Dead Sea; November 2–6, 1997; Dead Sea, Israel.

45. Even-Paz Z, Efron D, Kipnis V, Abels DJ. How much Dead Sea sun for psoriasis? *J Dermatol Treat.* 1996; 7:17–19.

46. Even-Paz Z, Gumon R, Kipnis V, Abels DJ, Efron D. Dead Sea sun versus Dead Sea water in the treatment of psoriasis. *J Dermatol Treat.* 1996; 7:83–86.

47. Halevy S, Giryes H, Friger M, Sukenik S. Dead Sea bath salt for the treatment of psoriasis vulgaris: a double-blind controlled study. *Eur J Acad Dermatol Venereol.* 1997; 9:237–242.

48. Giryes H, Sukenik S, Halevy S. Clearing of psoriatic erythroderma following heliotherapy in the Dead Sea. *J Eur Acad Dermatol Venereol.* 1995; 5:44–46.

49. Giryes H, Friger M, Sarov B. Treatment of atopic dermatitis in the Dead Sea area: biology and therapy of inflammatory skin diseases. Presented at: International Symposium at the Dead Sea; November 2–6, 1997; Dead Sea, Israel.

50. Seidel V, Hristakeive E, Harari M. Climatotherpy of vitiligo at the Dead Sea. *Dtsch Dermatol.* 1994; 42:144–161.

51. Kushelevsky A, Harari M, Kudish AI, et al. Safety of solar phototherapy at the Dead Sea. *J Am Acad Dermatol.* 1998; 38:447–452.

3 Mind-Body Medicine

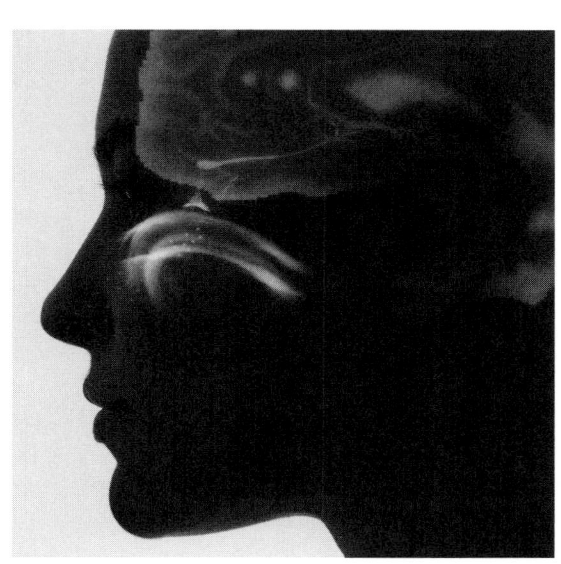

Overview

James S. Gordon, MD
From the Department of Psychiatry and Family Medicine, Georgetown University, and the Center for Mind-Body Medicine, Washington, DC.

The scientific literature on mind-body medicine includes studies that date from the late 1960s on the power of meditation and the "relaxation response" to balance sympathetic overactivity with parasympathetic stimulation, to alter many of the body's physiologic responses,[1] and to make a significant clinical difference in conditions as diverse as hypertension, chronic pain, and insomnia.[2] Studies dating from the 1970s explored the connection and mutual regulation of the nervous and immune system[3]; the findings that the same peptide receptors exist on cells of the nervous, immune and endocrine systems[4]; the effect of Western aerobic and Eastern nonaerobic exercise on mood[5-7]; the power of group support to prolong as well as improve the quality of life of people with cancer[8]; the utility of an integrated mind-body approach in reversing cardiovascular disease[9]; and the power of prayer and hands-on healing to effect changes in physiology and health status.[10,11]

Many of these findings have been published in prestigious peer-reviewed journals.[12] Some of these observations and studies have been repeated; others are being replicated. Together, they have stimulated a significant volume of basic and clinical research. This research is beginning to affect clinical practice in most major medical institutions and in the curricula of the majority of American medical schools.[13]

The chapters in this part of *Alternative Medicine: An Objective Assessment* represent another step in the evolution of the research on mind-body medicine. Although the 7 chapters, drawn from *JAMA* and the *Archives* Journals, only hint at the breadth and depth of current research, they present interesting new information and intriguing perspectives and raise important issues.

Perhaps the most straightforward of the studies in this section is the one by Garfinkel and her colleagues, "Yoga-Based Intervention for Carpal Tunnel Syndrome."[14] This study confirms, under rigorously controlled conditions, reports that have been coming out of India for more than 30 years: yoga postures, carefully chosen, well-taught, and conscientiously practiced, can make a real difference in clinical conditions—in this case, carpal tunnel syndrome. The study is not only significant in itself, but also points to the need for similarly well-designed investigations of the use of yoga and tai qi, among other physical approaches, to address significant illnesses (among them, hypertension, arthritis, diabetes, and asthma) for which they have long been used in Asia.

The study on relaxation training and breast milk secretory IgA by O'Connor and her colleagues,[15] by contrast, indicates some of the problems in evaluating mind-body approaches, as well as some of the complexity of the mind-body system. Relaxation training has long been regarded as a way to decrease stress and enhance immunity. Previously, as O'Connor et al note, it has been shown to increase salivary IgA levels in children and adults and thus, presumably, to confer enhanced immunity on them. It did not, it turned out, have the same effect on IgA levels in the breast milk of nursing mothers. The authors, who seem somewhat surprised at the outcome, raise a host of interesting questions about why this might have been the case and how, in this instance, lower IgA levels may actually have been a sign of less "subclinical infection" in those mothers who received relaxation training. Still, a mystery remains—one suitable for further exploration.

The 2 surveys presented, "Complementary Therapies for Depression" by Ernst[16] and "The Neuro-Immuno-Cutaneous-Endocrine Network: Relationship of Mind and Skin" by O'Sullivan and his colleagues,[17] give a nice sense of state of the art of alternative treatments for one condition—depression—and the breadth and depth of our understanding of the relationships between mind, immunity, endocrine functioning, and one organ, the skin.

Ernst's chapter, which gives a thorough view of much of the Western literature (but unfortunately neglects most of what has been published in Asia and the rich, if controversial, information about the use of nutritional therapies and dietary supplementation), nicely demonstrates the various degrees of scientific evidence for widely used complementary therapies. Exercise and one herbal therapy (the use of St John's wort or *Hypericum perforatum*) are, he concludes, effective treatments for mild and moderate depression, while evidence for acupuncture, massage, and relaxation is promising but not compelling. The weakness of the evidence for this latter group, as well as for such techniques as music therapy and hypnotherapy, clearly points to the need for more and better studies of these widely accepted and broadly used approaches.

The elegant overview that O'Sullivan and his colleagues provide gives a sense of the solidity of the mind-body connection. Moreover, it provides, with its well-documented emphasis on communication between neurons and immune cells in the skin, a clear picture of the many ways that this connection can serve—or undermine—the healing process.

The perspectives offered by Bilkis and Mark[18] and Thomsen[19] underscore the possible therapeutic utility of a variety of mind-body interventions for such common dermatological conditions as psoriasis, acne, and urticaria. Although the authors don't offer much data on the effectiveness of their interventions (which include relaxation, meditation, a hypnotic technique called neurolinguistic programming, prayer, and spiritual advice), these chapters do underscore the importance dermatologists give to the mind-body connection and to techniques that make use of it.

Finally, 2 of the chapters, Thomsen's and the one by Rosa and her colleagues,[20] hint at the insistent and sometimes uncritical advocacy that can cloud writings that touch on the domain of the spiritual. Thomsen's chapter, "Spirituality in Medical Practice," with its passionate and sympathetic treatment of the spiritual domain and its personal appreciation for the power of prayer, sometimes blurs the boundaries between the physician's desire to invoke spiritual help and the patient's need for it. It also neglects subtleties in the therapeutic use of the spiritual approach, including the necessity for the individual physician to be firmly grounded and modest about the spiritual practices he or she advises, and the possible negative effects of prayer.[21]

The Rosa study, "A Close Look at Therapeutic Touch," is well and tightly argued, but its results are highly overgeneralized. It concludes, quite rightly, that the practitioners of therapeutic touch who were studied were unable to detect the "human energy field" (regarded as essential to their diagnostic work) in the young experimenter. The authors don't, however, consider that therapeutic touch may work even if practitioners cannot actually feel the human energy field. They ignore some of the significant body of evidence on the physiological effects of laying on of hands.[22] And, finally, they jump to the conclusion, which this single study could hardly justify, that the claims of therapeutic touch are "groundless" and that "further use is unjustified."

The messages that should be drawn from this interesting and varied collection of chapters are less definite and dramatic than either Thomsen or Rosa and her colleagues would suggest. These chapters are, however, significant additions to the growing scientific evidence for the interconnection, indeed the interpenetration, of mind and body. They show that some techniques can have an obvious and powerful effect, that others may work, but not necessarily in the way that proponents claim, and that still others, which are widely used, are as yet awaiting scientific proof. These studies remind us, too, that we are very much at the beginning of a scientific exploration of this promising, exciting, controversial, and still incompletely defined field.

References

1. Benson H, Beary JF, Carol MP. The relaxation response. *Psychiatry*. 1974;37:37–46.
2. Gordon JS. Self-care as primary care: the power of the mind. In: *Manifesto for a New Medicine: Your Guide to Healing Partnerships and the Wise Use of Alternative Therapies.* Reading, Mass: Addison-Wesley;1996:92–129.
3. Ader R. *Psychoneuroimmunology*. New York NY: Academic Press; 1981.
4. Pert C, Dienstfrey H. The neuropeptide network. *Ann N Y Acad Sci.* 1988;521:189–194.
5. Jin P. Efficacy of tai chi, brisk walking, meditation, and reading in reducing mental and emotional stress. *J Psychosom Res.* 1992; 36:361–370.
6. Tse SK, Bailey DM. Tai chi and postural control in the well elderly. *Am J Occup Ther.* 1992; 46:295–300.
7. Griest JH. Running as a treatment for depression. *Compr Psychiatry*. 1979;20:41–54.
8. Spiegel D, Bloom JR, Kraemer HC, Gottheil E. Effect of psychosocial treatment on survival of patients with metastatic breast cancer. *Lancet*. 1989;2:881–891.
9. Ornish D, Scherwitz LW, Doody RS, et al. Effects of stress management training and dietary training in treating ischemic heart disease. *JAMA*. 1983;249:54–59.
10. Byrd R. Positive therapeutic effects of intercessory prayer on a coronary care unit population. *South Med J.* 1988;81:826–829.
11. Grad D. Some biological effects of the laying on of hands (a review of experiments with animals and plants). *J Am Soc Psychical Res.* 1975; 59:95–126.
12. Gordon JS. Notes. In: *Manifesto for a New Medicine: Your Guide to Healing Partnerships and the Wise Use of Alternative Therapies.* Reading, Mass: Addison-Wesley;1996:300–328.
13. Wetzel MS, Eisenberg DM, KaptchukTJ. Courses involving complementary and alternative medicine at US medical schools. *JAMA*. 1998;280:784–787.
14. Garfinkel MS, Singhal A, Katz WA, et al. Yoga-based intervention for carpal tunnel syndrome: a randomized trial. *JAMA*. 1998;280:1601–1603.
15. O'Connor M E, Schmidt W, Carroll-Pankhurst C, et al. Relaxation training and breast milk secretory IgA. *Arch Pediatr Adolesc Med.* 1998; 152:1065–1070.
16. Ernst E. Complementary therapies for depression: an overview. *Arch Gen Psychiatry.* 1998; 55:1026–1032.
17. O'Sullivan R, Lipper F, Lerner E. The neuro-immuno-cutaneous endocrine network: relationship of mind and skin. *Arch Dermatol.* 1998; 134:1431–1435.
18. Bilkis M, Mark K. Mind body medicine: practical applications in dermatology. *Arch Dermatol.* 1998;134:1437–1431.
19. Thomsen R. Spirituality in medical practice. *Arch Dermatol.* 1998;134:1443–1446.
20. Rosa L, Rosa E, Sarner L, Barrett S. A close look at therapeutic touch. *JAMA*. 1998;279:1005–1010.
21. Dossey L. Be careful what you pray for or you just might get it. In: *What We Can Do About the Unintentional Effects of Our Thoughts, Prayers and Wishes.* San Francisco, Calif: HarperCollins; 1998.
22. Gordon JS. The healing path. In: *Manifesto for a New Medicine: Your Guide to Healing Partnerships and the Wise Use of Alternative Therapies.* Reading, Mass: Addison-Wesley; 1996:221–222.

18 Yoga-Based Intervention for Carpal Tunnel Syndrome

A Randomized Trial

Marian S. Garfinkel, EdD; Atul Singhal, MD; Warren A. Katz, MD; David A. Allan, MD, PhD; Rosemary Reshetar, EdD; H. Ralph Schumacher, Jr, MD
From the Department of Medicine, Division of Rheumatology, University of Pennsylvania School of Medicine (Drs Garfinkel, Singhal, Katz, and Schumacher), the Arthritis-Immunology Center, Veterans Affairs Medical Center (Dr Schumacher), University of Pennsylvania Health System/Presbyterian Medical Center (Drs Katz and Allan), and the American Board of Internal Medicine (Dr Reshetar), Philadelphia, Pa. Dr Garfinkel is now with Cooper Health System and Center for Health and Wellness, Cherry Hill, NJ. Dr Singhal is now in private practice in Mesquite, Tex. Dr Reshetar is now with the Educational Testing Service, Princeton, NJ.

Context
Carpal tunnel syndrome is a common complication of repetitive activities and causes significant morbidity.

Objective
To determine the effectiveness of a yoga-based regimen for relieving symptoms of carpal tunnel syndrome.

Design
Randomized, single-blind, controlled trial.

Setting
A geriatric center and an industrial site in 1994-1995.

Patients
Forty-two employed or retired individuals with carpal tunnel syndrome (median age, 52 years; range, 24–77 years).

Intervention
Subjects assigned to the yoga group received a yoga-based intervention consisting of 11 yoga postures designed for strengthening, stretching, and balancing each joint in the upper body along with relaxation given twice weekly for 8 weeks. Patients in the control group were offered a wrist splint to supplement their current treatment.

Main Outcome Measures
Changes from baseline to 8 weeks in grip strength, pain intensity, sleep disturbance, Phalen sign, and Tinel sign, and in median nerve motor and sensory conduction time.

Results
Subjects in the yoga groups had significant improvement in grip strength (increased from 162 to 187 mm Hg; *P*=.009) and pain reduction (decreased from 5.0 to 2.9 mm; *P*=.02), but changes in grip strength and pain were not significant for

control subjects. The yoga group had significantly more improvement in Phalen sign (12 improved vs 2 in control group; *P*=.008), but no significant differences were found in sleep disturbance, Tinel sign, and median nerve motor and sensory conduction time.

Conclusion

In this preliminary study, a yoga-based regimen was more effective than wrist splinting or no treatment in relieving some symptoms and signs of carpal tunnel syndrome.

JAMA. 1998;280:1601–1603

Carpal tunnel syndrome (CTS) is a common problem in the workplace and causes significant morbidity. In addition to its potentially debilitating physical aspects, CTS has a negative financial impact resulting from lost time from work and increasing medical expenses.[1] Traditionally, CTS has been treated with wrist splints, anti-inflammatory agents, avoidance of occupational duties, career changes, injection therapy, and surgery. However, many of these options have provided less than satisfactory symptom relief.[1]

Yoga and relaxation techniques have been used to help alleviate musculoskeletal symptoms.[2] However, except for a previous study on osteoarthritis of the hand,[3] to our knowledge, these methods have not been studied in a prospective controlled trial. Our previous investigation showed significant improvement in range of motion, decreased tenderness, and decreased hand pain during activity in patients with osteoarthritis who followed a supervised program of yoga and relaxation.

The purpose of this study was to evaluate whether a program of yoga and relaxation techniques might offer an effective treatment alternative for patients with CTS. Yoga was proposed to be helpful because stretching may relieve compression in the carpal tunnel, better joint posture may decrease intermittent compression, and blood flow may be improved to decrease ischemic effects on the median nerve. In this article, we report the results of a randomized controlled trial examining the effects of an intervention using supervised yoga and relaxation techniques specifically designed for patients with CTS.

Methods

Subject Selection

Approximately 400 potential subjects were recruited through advertisements in the city newspaper and notices posted at study sites. After initial screening by telephone, 72 interested, available, and suitable patients with characteristic symptoms of CTS were interviewed in person and examined; 51 subjects met the criteria for inclusion in the study.

Entry criteria included the presence of at least 2 of 5 of the following clinical findings: positive results on Tinel sign, positive results on Phalen sign, pain in the median nerve distribution, sleep disturbances resulting from hand symptoms, and numbness or paresthesias in the median nerve distribution. All potential subjects were required to have abnormal median nerve conduction latencies on neuroelectrical testing.[4] All subjects were required to agree not to change medications, receive other new treatments, or change work duties during the study. Exclusion criteria were previous surgery for CTS, rheumatoid arthritis or other recognized inflammatory arthritis, CTS related to systemic disease (such as hypothyroidism), and pregnancy.

The study took place at Ralston House, the Geriatric Center of the University of Pennsylvania in Philadelphia, and at QVC Corporation, an industrial site in West Chester, Pa. Participants from QVC were actively employed and were compensated to arrive 1 hour before their shift began. Ralston House participants included employed and retired subjects. The study was approved by the institutional review boards of Presbyterian Medical Center, Philadelphia, Pa, and the University of Pennsylvania Medical Center. Written informed consent was obtained from study subjects.

Interventions

Subjects were randomized into 2 groups by having them select sealed envelopes containing a group assignment. Subjects in the control group were offered a standard wrist splint with a metal insert (if not already in use) to supplement their current treatment. Subjects in the yoga-based intervention group received a program focused on upper body postures: improving flexibility; correcting alignment of hands, wrists, arms, and shoulders; stretching; and increasing awareness of optimal joint position during use. We used the Iyengar approach to hatha yoga, which emphasizes proper structural alignment of the body and is based on the teachings of yoga master B. K. S. Iyengar.[3,5] The method of study is orderly and progressive, and postures are adjusted to meet the physical conditions of the subjects. With education in the postures (asanas), habitual poor posture can improve. As musculoskeletal alignment improves, the ability to perform the asanas also should improve. Potential benefits of this method include improvements in strength, coordination, and flexibility and an increased sense of well-being.

The sequence of postures used in this study was designed to focus on the upper body for subjects with CTS. The exercises were performed while the subject was sitting and standing and were designed to take each joint in the upper body through its full range of motion with strengthening, stretching, and balancing each part.[5] Instructions for the 11 asanas used and the relaxation technique are shown in Table 1.

Every session ended with relaxation using the relaxation response of savasana (corpse pose), which is proposed to help counteract the energy-draining effects of prolonged stress and chronic pain.[5] During relaxation, the body remains still and movement is not possible.

The yoga program was given for 1 to 1 1/2 hours twice weekly by 1 instructor (M.S.G.) for 8 weeks.

Measurements

Subjects reported the approximate number of hours of disturbed sleep per night during the previous week. Subjects indicated the intensity of pain for the previous week on a visual analog scale of 0 to 10, with 10 indicating the greatest level of pain.[6] Phalen[7] sign (90 seconds) and Tinel sign[8] were assessed, with results recorded as positive or negative for each involved wrist. Patterns of paresthesia and numbness were recorded on hand diagrams. Grip strength was measured with a sphygmomanometer cuff that was rolled, taped, and inflated to 20 mm Hg. The subject was encouraged to squeeze with maximum strength and the best of 3 efforts was recorded for each hand.

An electroneurometer[4] (NERVEPACE, NeuMed [Neurotron Medical], Lawrenceville, NJ) was used to measure the distal latency of the median nerve across the wrist. This electroneurometer has been validated to show comparable specificity to standard nerve conduction studies.[9] All tests were assessed at baseline and were repeated at the end of 8 weeks. The assessments all were conducted by 1 physician (A.S.) who was blinded to the patient's group assignment and the intervention.

Statistical Analysis

Differences between the pretest and posttest changes were examined using repeated-measures analysis of variance for within-group differences in improvement for continuous measures of grip strength and nerve conduction times (sensory and motor) for each involved wrist, and for pain intensity for each subject. Paired difference *t* tests were conducted to examine pretest vs posttest differences on continuous variables within each group. χ^2 Tests were used to examine the relationship between group membership and categorically coded variables of improvement on Phalen sign, Tinel sign, and sleep disturbance. The $P<.05$ level of significance was used. Post hoc analysis was carried out to calculate the appropriate sample size to detect clinically meaningful differences in each of the proposed tests. For variables measured on a continuous scale this sample size would yield a power of 80%, and for variables measured on a categorical scale power would be 64%.

Results

Of the 51 subjects who met inclusion criteria and were randomized, 9 dropped out or were excluded (Figure 1). Final data were analyzed for 42 subjects (67 unique wrists with CTS), 22 (35 wrists) in the yoga group and 20 subjects (32 wrists) in the control group (Table 2).

Table 3 shows a comparison between pretest and posttest results for pain, grip strength, and nerve conduction time (sensory and motor) in the yoga-treated and control groups. Patients in the yoga-treated group had statistically significant improvements for grip strength and pain reduction. Trends toward improvement also were observed within the yoga-treated group in pretest to posttest measures of motor nerve conduction time, Phalen sign, Tinel sign, and sleep disturbance, although these trends were not statistically significant. Both groups also showed trends toward improvement in sensory and motor nerve conduction times, but no significant differences between pretest and posttest values were found. Results of repeated-measures analyses for between-group differences were not statistically significant for any of the variables. Improvement on Tinel sign, Phalen sign, and reported sleep disturbance were more common in the yoga-treated group, but were statistically significant only for improvement in Phalen sign (Table 4).

Comment

Occupationally related health problems such as CTS are the leading cause of lost earnings in the workplace.[10] As a result of cumulative trauma disorders, businesses sustain substantial losses annually due to medical expenses and lost productivity. In this study, a program of yoga-based simple stretching and postural alignment, which does not

Table 1. Yoga Postures Used for Carpal Tunnel Syndrome*

1. Sitting with extension of the trunk (dandasana). Sit on a chair with the trunk upright. Press hands into the seat. Press shoulder blades into the back. Move shoulders back and down.
2. Hands in prayer position (namaste). Press palms and fingers of each hand together, with fingers away from their position of ulnar deviation. Release and repeat, pressing palms together with fingers spread as widely as possible. Repeat by pressing metacarpals of each finger. Pull fingers back into hyperextension, increasing distance between fingers of each hand.
3. Arms extended overhead (urdhva hastasana). Stretch arms and fingers forward and up, with hands facing vertically. Open palms, keep fingers together and lock the elbows. Lift sides of the body. Keep arms straight.
4. Arms extended overhead with fingers interlocked (parvatasana). Interlock fingers with the right thumb base over the left, with the base of the fingers in contact. Turn palms out and stretch arms forward and up. Lock elbows and keep arms straight. Raise trunk by lifting the arms and pull arms further back. Lower arms. Repeat with left thumb over the right.
5. Arms interlocked in front of the body (garudasana). Bend elbows, crossing arms in front of the chest with the forearms stretching up and thumbs facing the head. Cross left elbow over the right. Move right hand toward the head and the left hand away; cross hands and place fingers of the right hand on left palm. Stand and raise elbows to shoulder level and bend them. Stretch hands and fingers. Release arms and stand straight.
6. Chair twists (bharadvajasana). Sit sideways on a chair, with right hip and thigh against the back of chair. Stretch the trunk up and pull shoulders back. Keep knees and feet together, turn toward the back of chair. Place hands on back of chair. Pull left hand to bring left side toward back of chair and push with right hand to turn right side away. Turn body then the head to look over right shoulder.
7. Standing, mountain pose (tadasana). Stand straight in bare feet, facing forward, feet together, toes and heels in line, with big toes and centers of the inner ankles touching. Balance weight evenly on inner and outer edges of both feet and heels and soles. Lift knee caps into the joints. Raise upper chest and collarbones.
8. 90-Degree forward bend to wall (half uttanasana). Stand with feet 1 foot apart. Stretch the arms over head. Bend from the hips, extending entire body toward the wall, hands touching the wall. Stretch forward.
9. Arms extended overhead with palms together in prayer position (virabhadrasana 1, arms only). Stand in tadasana. Stretch arms to sides at shoulder level keeping fingers together. Turn arms circularly in their sockets, palms facing the ceiling. Keeping arms straight, extend them over the head until they are parallel. While moving arms upward, stretch the sides of chest and armpits. Take arms back, and bring them closer together; join palms, with the fingers stretching upward. Lock elbows.
10. Dog pose with chair, with special emphasis on hand placement (urdhva mukha svanasana). Stand, feet hip width apart, facing the seat of a chair. Bend, placing palms on the seat, shoulder width apart. Straighten arms and lift waist, hips, and knees a few inches above chair. Turn arms out and curve trunk back between them. Bring coccyx, sacrum, and lumbar spine forward, keeping buttocks tight. Stretch front of the body from the pubis. Raise sternum and ribs. Hold shoulders back. Press shoulder blades and dorsal spine in.
11. Hands joined in prayer position behind the back (namaste). Stand in tadasana. Join palms behind the back, fingers pointing down and in line. Turn hands toward the trunk and then up. Raise them as high as possible between the shoulder blades. Join heels of the hands and press little fingers into the dorsal spine. Stretch fingers up. Turn upper arms outward and press shoulders back and down.
12. Relaxation. Lie flat on the back. Keep arms slightly away from thighs, palms up, heels together, and toes apart. Close eyes. Breathe deeply. Concentrate on soft, slow exhalation. Relax lower jaw, tongue, and pupils of the eyes. Relax completely and exhale slowly. Remain in pose for 10 to 15 minutes.

*Hold positions 1 through 11 for 30 seconds and breathe through the nose. Do not tense the throat and keep the shoulders away from the ears. Repeat each position. The Iyengar system of hatha yoga emphasizes structural alignment. These postures are described in abbreviated form. A detailed description of the yoga intervention is available on request from the author.

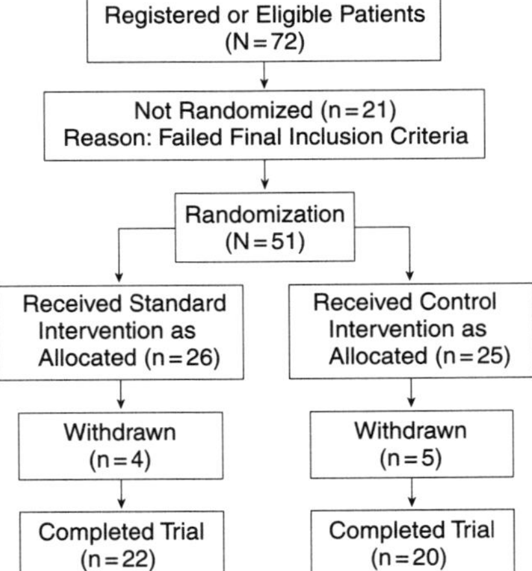

Figure 1. Progress through the various stages of a randomized controlled trial, including flow of participants, withdrawals, and timing of primary and secondary outcome measures.

Table 2. Characteristics of Study Subjects by Group

Characteristic	Yoga Group* (n=22)	Control Group (n=20)
Age, mean (median)	48.9 (45)	48.7 (42)
[range], y	[17–68]	[18–70]
Sex		
Women	16	12
Men	5	8
Race		
Black	3	3
White	18	17
Smokers	2	5

*Demographic data missing for 1 subject. Data are presented as number of subjects unless otherwise indicated.

Table 3. Comparison Between Grip Strength, Pain, and Sensory and Motor Nerve Conduction Times*

Variable	n†	Mean (SD) Pretest	Posttest	Improvement	P Value‡
Grip strength, mm Hg					
Yoga	33	161.6 (70.4)	187.4 (68.8)	25.8 (41.4)	.009
Controls	29	183.9 (69.5)	190.5 (68.2)	6.6 (41.1)	.37
Pain, visual analog scale (1–10)					
Yoga	22	5.0 (2.8)	2.9 (2.2)	2.1 (3.1)	.02
Controls	20	5.2 (2.1)	4.3 (2.2)	0.9 (2.8)	.16
Median nerve sensory conduction, ms					
Yoga	35	4.40 (1.5)	3.97 (1.5)	.42 (1.8)	.18
Controls	32	4.66 (1.4)	4.36 (1.6)	.29 (1.5)	.28
Median nerve motor conduction, ms					
Yoga	33	4.79 (1.3)	4.27 (1.4)	.52 (1.7)	.08
Controls	29	4.78 (1.1)	4.52 (1.1)	.26 (0.8)	.09

*Repeated measures analysis for each of the variables (grip strength, pain, and sensory and motor conduction time) showed none of the test results was significant at the .05 level for between-group differences.

†Data are presented as number of involved wrists for grip strength and median nerve conduction times, and as number of subjects for pain.

‡P values are 2-tailed and reflect paired differences within groups.

Table 4. Improvement in Phalen Sign, Tinel Sign, and Sleep Disturbance*

Variable	Yoga Group	Control Group	χ^2	P Value
Phalen sign				
Improved	12	2		
Same	18	19	9.72	.008
Worsened	2	7		
Tinel sign				
Improved	7	3		
Same	22	21	1.88	.39
Worsened	4	6		
Sleep disturbance				
Improved	4	2		
Same	13	14	2.68	.26
Worsened	0	2		

*Data are presented as number of involved wrists for Phalen sign and Tinel sign, and as number of subjects for sleep disturbance.

require drugs, expensive equipment, or surgery, reduced pain and improved grip strength for patients with CTS.

Yoga classes such as the one used in this study can improve awareness of proper postures and use of the upper extremities. Although not studied here, we propose that a properly supervised program may be helpful not only to treat symptoms, but also to prevent recurrences or the onset of symptoms.

Our study was designed as a preliminary study and as such has several limitations including small sample size, lack of generalizability, and the use of a simple wrist splint as a control. We did not obtain data on medication use, time lost from work, or patient compliance with wrist splint use or other therapies.

Although not systematically studied, many subjects in the yoga group reported that they maintained improvement in their CTS symptoms 4 weeks after conclusion of the program. Further studies are needed to ascertain whether a single course of yoga intervention with occasional reinforcement can be effective for long-term relief. Programs could be initiated at workplaces with a high incidence of CTS, perhaps with 2 classes per week for 8 to 10 weeks, with monthly follow-up sessions to monitor home practice. Continued evaluations of outcomes are needed to evaluate long-term effects of yoga on CTS symptoms, lost time from work, and patient satisfaction.

This study was supported by grant 91-07-14 from the Commonwealth of Pennsylvania.

References

1. Pascarelli E, Quilter D. *Repetitive Strain Injury: A Computer User's Guide*. New York, NY: John Wiley & Sons Inc; 1994:55–57.

2. Garfinkel MS. *The Effect of Yoga and Relaxation Techniques on Outcome Variables Associated With Osteoarthritis of the Hands and Finger Joints* [dissertation]. Philadelphia, Pa: Temple University; 1992.

3. Garfinkel MS, Schumacher HR Jr, Husain A, Levy M, Reshetar RA. Evaluation of a yoga based regimen for treatment of osteoarthritis of the hands. *J Rheumatol*. 1994;21:2341–2343.

4. Atroshi I, Johnsson R. Evaluation of portable nerve conduction testing in the diagnosis of carpal tunnel syndrome. *J Hand Surg Am*. 1996;21:651–654.

5. Iyengar BKS. *Light on Yoga*. London, England: Allen & Unwin; 1966:544.

6. Huskisson EC. Measurement of pain. *J Rheumatol*. 1982;9:768–769.

7. Phalen GS. The carpal tunnel syndrome: seventeen years' experience in diagnosis and treatment of six hundred fifty-four hands. *J Bone Joint Surg Am*. 1966;48:211–228.

8. Mossman SS, Blau JN. Tinel's sign and the carpal tunnel syndrome. *BMJ*. 1987;294:680.

9. Steinberg DR, Gelberman RH, Rydevik B, Lundborg G. The utility of portable nerve conduction testing for patients with carpal tunnel syndrome: a prospective clinical study. *J Hand Surg Am*. 1992;17:77–81.

10. Thompson R. Workers' comp costs: out of control. *Nation's Business*. July 1992;80:1–6.

19 Relaxation Training and Breast Milk Secretory IgA

Mary E. O'Connor, MD, MPH; Wendy Schmidt, OTR/L, MPA; Cindie Carroll-Pankhurst, PhD; Karen N. Olness, MD

From the Department of Pediatrics (Drs O'Connor and Olness and Ms Schmidt) and the Mandel School of Applied Social Sciences (Dr Carroll-Pankhurst), Case Western Reserve University, Rainbow Babies and Childrens Hospital (Drs O'Connor and Olness), Cleveland, Ohio.

Objective

To evaluate the hypothesis that breast-feeding women who participate in relaxation training will have increased secretory IgA (sIgA) levels in their breast milk compared with women not receiving training.

Design

Nonrandomized control trial of a convenience sample.

Setting

Women were recruited from the postpartum floor of a university teaching hospital. The intervention took place in the women's homes.

Participants

Women in the first 48 hours after delivery who were planning to breast-feed their healthy newborn infants for at least 8 weeks were approached for enrollment. Women were excluded if they had previous experience with relaxation training. At 4 to 6 weeks postpartum, we enrolled 38 women still breast-feeding their infants.

Interventions

Women were allocated into 3 groups. Women in group 1 were taught relaxation and had breast milk samples collected before and after the teaching. Women in group 2 had conversation with similar breast milk sample collection, and women in group 3 had 1 breast milk sample collected. Women in group 1 were encouraged to practice the relaxation once or twice a day for 2 weeks, and a second visit was made to all mothers with repeated breast milk collections. Women who were still breast-feeding at 6 to 8 weeks after study end had a final breast milk sample collected. Breast milk was analyzed for secretory IgA levels. Stress was assayed using the *Symptom Checklist-90-R* and open-ended questions.

Results

There was no difference in sIgA levels among the 3 groups at any time. Women who reported stress present between

visit 1 and visit 2 increased their sIgA levels at the final sample collection (+0.16 g/L) compared with women who reported no stress (–0.09 g/L; *P*=.03). The ratings of success in relaxation in women in group 1 were related to the following sIgA levels in sample 4: poor relaxation, 0.67 g/L; fair relaxation, 0.41 g/L; good relaxation, 0.35 g/L; and very good, 0.30 g/L (*P*=.006).

Conclusions

Self-reported stress appears to increase breast milk sIgA levels. Success at relaxation was inversely related to sIgA levels in the group learning relaxation.

Arch Pediatr Adolesc Med. 1998;152:1065–1070

Breast-feeding is recognized around the world as the optimum method of infant feeding. It has numerous advantages in promoting the health, development, and psychological outcomes of children. Documented benefits of breast-feeding include decreased instances of wheezing-associated illnesses,[1] decreased ear infections[2,3] and other infectious diseases,[4] decreased development of allergies,[4] increased maternal-infant bonding,[4,5] and improved intellectual development.[6]

Breast-feeding provides important protections from infectious diseases for infants in the developed and developing worlds. One mechanism of this protection is the effect of the immunologic components of breast milk on the infant.[7] These immunologically important substances include the immunoglobulins, lysozyme, lactoferrin, macrophages, *Lactobacillus bifidus* growth factor, and others. Of the immunoglobulins, IgA is the most prominent. Secretory IgA (sIgA) is found in very high levels in colostrum, which then decline within 4 to 6 weeks postpartum, but sIgA remains present for the duration of lactation.

The stimulus for production of sIgA in breast milk is unclear. Secretion may occur, in part, as a response to past or present maternal infections. In children, secretion of salivary IgA has been shown to be modified through relaxation training that included the suggestion to increase the infection-fighting substances in their saliva.[8] This example of the self-regulation of IgA depends on communication between the nervous and immune systems. Accordingly, research in this area falls into the realm of complementary and alternative medicine. Our hypothesis was that relaxation training and suggestion to breast-feeding women would increase the sIgA levels in their breast milk. Increased levels in breast milk might improve the immunity of breast-fed infants.

Subjects and Methods

Subjects

This prospective study was approved by the Institutional Review Board of University Hospitals of Cleveland, Cleveland, Ohio. A convenience sample of healthy breast-feeding women, aged 20 to 40 years, delivered of healthy, full-term infants at University Hospitals, was visited within 48 hours of delivery by 1 of the investigators (M.E.O'C.). The investigator explained the study to the new mothers and asked permission to call them 4 to 6 weeks after delivery to determine if they were still breast-feeding and interested in participating in the study. Women whose home addresses were nearest to the hospital were called first. Women were called until the researchers' slots were filled for the week. The women were assigned to 1 of the following 3 study groups: relaxation intervention (14 women; group 1), attention control (15 women; group 2), and nonintervention control (9 women; group 3). Assignments for a given week were made on the basis of availability of the 2 investigators who made the home visits (nonrandomized control trial). One investigator (K.N.O.), skilled in relaxation training, visited all of the group 1 mothers; another (M.E.O'C.) visited all the groups 2 and 3 mothers.

Methods

At the first home visit, informed consent was obtained, and a baseline sample of 10 mL of breast milk was obtained by breast pump or hand expression. Any mother who did not have a breast pump was given a manual breast pump. Basic demographic questions were answered regarding maternal and infant health, number of children, profession of parents, and breast-feeding supplements. Each mother completed the *Symptom Checklist-90-R (SCL-90-R)* scale at the first visit. The *SCL-90-R* is a 90-item self-reported questionnaire designed to reflect psychological symptoms. It includes a global score and subscales of depression and anxiety. Norms exist for healthy women, but not specifically for a postpartum population.[9] Group 1 mothers underwent relaxation training followed by a second breast milk sample collection of 10 mL. During this training, the suggestion was given to mothers to increase breast milk IgA levels. This suggestion was given in a similar manner to all mothers; however, the suggestions to aid relaxation were individualized depending on the preference of each mother. This training was audiotaped. The tape was left with mothers who were asked to listen to the tape twice daily or to perform the relaxation from their memory twice daily. Group 2 mothers had conversation with the investigator for 20 to 25 minutes about hobbies, jobs, infant care, or other issues, followed by a second breast milk sample of 10 mL. Group 3 mothers had no further intervention.

Between the first and second home visits, all women were called and asked about their health and their infants' health. Those in group 1 were encouraged to continue the relaxation practice. Two weeks after the initial home visit, a second visit was made by the same investigator. A baseline sample of breast milk was obtained as previously. Questions about maternal and infant health and stresses in the 2-week interval were asked of all mothers. Mothers in group 1 practiced the relaxation in the presence of the investigator and collected a second 10-mL breast milk sample. Mothers in group 1 were encouraged to continue relaxation practice twice daily. The investigator subjectively graded the success of the mothers in relaxing on a scale of 1 to 4 (poor to very good). Mothers in group 2 had conversation with the investigator for 20 to 25 minutes, followed by a second 10-mL breast milk collection. At the end of the visit, after the sample collection, a relaxation tape was also given to each mother in groups 2 and 3. The investigator explained how to use the tape but did not demonstrate use of the tape. Each mother was encouraged to listen to the tape and practice the relaxation daily.

Six to 8 weeks later, all women were called to determine if they were still breast-feeding and whether they were still listening to the audiotape or using the relaxation techniques. Those women who were still breast-feeding were asked to collect and freeze a 10-mL sample of breast milk. Analyses of sIgA levels this time were performed for the 3 original assigned groups and for 2 groups determined by whether the mothers were using the relaxation technique.

Laboratory Analysis

Breast milk samples were labeled with a sample number, transported chilled, and then frozen at –20°C. Laboratory personnel were unaware of the identity of the participants and could not associate sample number with the participants.

The IgA concentration in the breast milk was measured using radial immunodiffusion with a commercially available kit (Sanofi Diagnostics Pasteur, Inc, Chaska, Minn) that incorporated standards of known IgA concentration to generate a standard curve for IgA vs diffusion diameter. A calculated correction was made according to the kit instructions to account for the dimeric structure of sIgA, because the standards provided were for monomeric IgA.

Data Analysis

Data were entered using commercially available software (Epi Info Version 6.0, Centers for Disease Control and Prevention, Atlanta, Ga) and analyzed using 2 commercially available packages (Epi Info Version 6.0 and SPSS for Windows, SPSS Institute, Chicago, Ill). Significance testing was performed using χ^2 analysis, Student *t* tests, and analysis of variance.

Results

Relaxation training was conducted in a comfortable room of the subjects' homes. Although most sessions were conducted in a quiet atmosphere, several were complicated by dogs wandering around the home, cats jumping on the investigator during the sessions, and crying infants. Excerpts from investigators' notes are included in Table 1.

One hundred six women who were approached while hospitalized agreed to a telephone call at 4 to 6 weeks postpartum. Of the women called, 38 agreed to participate and were enrolled. Major reasons for not wanting to participate when called included returning to work, too busy, and no longer breast-feeding their infant for most feedings.

The demographic information on the women enrolled in the study is listed in Table 2. The only differences among the 3 groups is that group 3 had more mothers insured with Medicaid (P=.006), and group 2 had more women for whom this was their first infant (P=.04). There were no differences in the scores on the *SCL-90-R* among the 3 groups when analyzed using the General Severity Index (total score) or the Anxiety and Depression subscales (Table 3). The mean scores were all within the normal range for healthy women.[9] There was no relationship between whether the mother had older children or previous breast-feeding experience and the presence of stress as defined by the open-ended question.

Table 4 shows the mean sIgA levels. There were no differences in the sIgA levels among the groups at any of the 5 times tested. During the 2 weeks of the study, 5 of the 14 women in group 1 had practiced the relaxation less than once daily, and 9 had practiced between 1 and 2 times daily. During the second home visit for group 1, relaxation success was evaluated. The sIgA levels in group 1 varied with relaxation success. The women rated very good, good, fair, and poor at relaxation had levels of 0.30, 0.35, 0.41, and 0.67 g/L, respectively (P=.006). Women in all groups who reported any stress at the second visit (n=14) had a significant increase in their sIgA level (+0.16 g/L) in the final sample when compared with the women (n=22) reporting no stress (–0.09 g/L; P=.03). There was no difference in self-reported stress across 3 groups.

At the telephone calls at 6 to 8 weeks after the second visit, 16 women were still using the relaxation techniques by listening to the relaxation tape or practicing relaxation without listening to the tape. Twenty-two women were not using the relaxation at all. This was not different among the groups. The sIgA levels in the final breast milk samples from women in each of the intervention groups were not significantly different, nor were there significant differences

Table 1. Relaxation Training Observations

Visit 1: "The subject said she had not had any previous relaxation training. She described excellent visual, auditory, and olfactory imagery. She appeared very relaxed during the training."
Visit 2: "The subject said she had been practicing about once a day and used the tape 3 times only because the tape recorder broke. She noted that she likes to imagine a beautiful pink color flowing through each of her muscles and relaxing them. I watched her infant lying on the sofa beside her as I guided her through the relaxation review. My impression was that she was very relaxed and comfortable."

Visit 1: "The subject held the baby during the relaxation training, which was interrupted several times by her 3-year-old son. The session included progressive relaxation, focusing on a favorite place, suggestions to increase breast milk IgA, and future positive programming about her family. This was tape-recorded and she was given the tape. It was evident that she had not relaxed during this first session."
Visit 2: "The subject said she has practiced 15 minutes each day and that this effort made her aware just how difficult it is to find 15 minutes in the day for relaxation. She used the tape for each practice. During our practice today a babysitter was with her son. She became very relaxed and, at the conclusion, said she didn't notice any sounds, including cars on the street outside."

Visit 1: "The subject did well during the relaxation training and said she enjoyed it."
Visit 2: "The subject said she listened to the tape a couple of times and then preferred to do the relaxation practice on her own. She has been practicing daily. When I arrived the baby was a little fussy and in her arms. As soon as she began to do the relaxation he fell soundly asleep and remained asleep during the review period. She also appeared very relaxed."

Table 2. Demographic Characteristics of Women*

Variable	Group 1 (n=14)	Group 2 (n=15)	Group 3 (n=9)
Age, mean ± SD, y	32.4 ± 4.2	29.0 + 4.1	29.1 ± 4.7
Race			
White	11 (78)	14 (93)	8 (89)
African American	3 (21)	0	1 (11)
Education			
High school only	0	2 (13)	2 (22)
Some college	1 (7)	0	2 (22)
College degree	5 (38)	5 (33)	2 (22)
Postgraduate degree	7 (50)	8 (53)	3 (33)
Marital status			
Married or living with infant's father	14 (100)	14 (93)	8 (89)
Single	0	1 (7)	1 (11)
Insurance			
Private	14 (100)	15 (100)	6 (67)†
Medicaid	0	0	3 (33)†
Worked before pregnancy	12 (86)	15 (100)	7 (78)
First child	4 (28)	10 (67)	2 (23)‡
Full breast-feeding	14 (100)	14 (93)	7 (78)

*Unless otherwise indicated, data are given as number (percentage) of mothers. Percentages have been rounded and may not total 100. See the "Subjects" subsection of the "Subjects and Methods" section for a description of the groups.
†P=.006.
‡P=.04.

Table 3. Scores on the *SCL-90-R**

	Mean Scores		
	Group 1 (n=14)	Group 2 (n=15)	Group 3 (n=9)
General Severity Index, total	0.29	0.40	0.35
Anxiety subscale	0.17	0.24	0.30
Depression subscale	0.72	0.67	0.62

*The norms (SD) for healthy women are 0.36 (0.35) for the General Severity Index; 0.37 (0.43) for the Anxiety subscale; and 0.46 (0.52) for the Depression subscale. Higher scores are associated with psychological pathology. *SCL-90-R* indicates *Symptom Checklist-90-R*.[9]

Table 4. Mean Values for sIgA Levels*

Sample No.	sIgA Level, Mean ± SD, g/L† Group 1 (n=14)	Group 2 (n=15)	Group 3 (n=9)
1	0.35 ± 0.07 (12)	0.37 ± 0.08 (15)	0.38 ± 0.07 (9)
2	0.34 ± 0.08 (14)	0.38 ± 0.05 (15)	...
3	0.32 ± 0.04 (13)	0.36 ± 0.06 (15)	0.35 ± 0.05 (8)
4	0.37 ± 0.11 (13)	0.38 ± 0.08 (15)	...
5	0.47 ± 0.29 (10)	0.33 ± 0.05 (9)	0.49 ± 0.42 (5)

*Collection of samples is described in the "Methods" subsection of the "Subjects and Methods" section of the text. Group 3 mothers did not collect samples 2 and 4. sIgA indicates secretory IgA.
†Numbers in parentheses indicate number of mothers providing samples.

between those who had and those who had not been using relaxation techniques.

Comment

Breast-Feeding and the Immune System

The decreased incidence of infectious diseases in breast-fed infants in the developed world is an important contribution to the health of children. Of the numerous substances present in breast milk that play a role in this, the immunoglobulins are of major importance. Levels of sIgA are much higher than levels of IgG and IgM found in breast milk. Secretory IgA is present in high concentration in colostrum, falls in concentration as the amount of milk produced increases, and reaches a plateau at about 4 to 6 weeks postpartum.[10] Secretory IgA levels remain present for the duration of lactation, although the total amount of sIgA ingested by the infant on a daily basis gradually decreases. Secretory IgA levels in breast milk do not differ between right and left breast or by time of day.[11] The plasma cells in the breast secrete IgA specific to the antigens encountered in the maternal gastrointestinal and respiratory tract systems. This secretion of sIgA into breast milk and its transfer to the infant help to overcome the normal delay in production of immune factors by the infant.[7]

This mechanism has been demonstrated by Fishaut et al,[12] who found increased respiratory syncytial virus (RSV)–specific IgA in breast milk of mothers during the winter (RSV season). One of 2 mothers with culture-proven RSV disease showed an increase in RSV-specific IgA levels in her breast milk in the 3 weeks after infection. Studies of sIgA to *Shigella* antigen in breast milk suggest that the enteromammary system has a long memory, in this case secreting *Shigella*-specific antigens in breast milk in 24 (46%) of 52 Houston, Tex, women. These women had no history of recent *Shigella* infection, and there were no recent *Shigella* outbreaks in Houston during the years before this study.[13]

IgA and Relaxation

In the 1980s, Olness et al[8] showed that healthy children could increase their salivary IgA secretion after training with relaxation and the suggestion that they increase the infection-fighting substances. The increase in salivary IgA levels was seen immediately after a 20-minute relaxation session.[8] Hewson-Bower[14] replicated these studies in her dissertation, and also examined whether children who practiced relaxation imagery and stress reduction would have fewer upper respiratory tract infections. After an observation period during which each child was monitored for the usual individual frequency of upper respiratory tract infections, she randomized children into experimental (14 weeks of relaxation imagery and stress reduction) and control (14 weeks of attention control) groups. Salivary IgA levels were monitored frequently. Hewson-Bower found increased levels of salivary IgA and a highly significant reduction in the frequency of upper respiratory tract infections for the group that practiced relaxation imagery and stress reduction techniques.

Chronic and acute stresses related to employment have been shown to increase salivary IgA levels in some studies.[15,16] The amount of increase was not correlated with actual or perceived workload. These results may be attributable to several variables that have an impact on the direction and magnitude of the effects of stress in modulating the immune responses of humans. These variables include intrinsic host factors such as age, sex, genes, amount of sleep, quality and quantity of antigenic stimulation or exposure to infectious agents, and temporal relationship between behavioral and antigenic stimulation. Boyce et al[17] studied the effects of stressors on the immune responses of children. They concluded that some children manifest an intrinsic high immune reactivity and others a low reactivity, and that health effects of psychologically stressful events are best predicted by an interaction between the intensity of environmental stressors and the immunologic biological reactivity of the individual host.[17] Only a subset of people within any given population may be truly at risk under conditions of environmental stress and adversity.

Stress, Breast Milk, and sIgA

Stress and fatigue can have an effect on maternal breast milk production.[18] There are numerous anecdotal instances of women facing acute stress with a sudden decrease in their milk production. The mechanism of this—whether it is an effect on prolactin, oxytocin, or other hormones—is unclear.

Groer et al[19] evaluated levels of cortisol and sIgA levels in maternal breast milk in an attempt to associate stress with breast-feeding outcomes. They found that levels of cortisol (a physiologic marker of stress) and sIgA were inversely related, ie, higher stress as measured by increased cortisol levels was correlated with decreased sIgA levels in breast milk. They hypothesized that cortisol may suppress the immunoglobulin production by plasma cells in the breast. This is opposite to the relationship that we found between self-reported stress and sIgA levels in the final sample. In a small group of 17 mothers, Dillon and Totten[20] found no relationship between levels of salivary IgA and sIgA in breast milk. Using multiple regression models, they found that infant upper respiratory tract infection was related to the mother's salivary IgA level, age, maternal upper respiratory tract infections, and coping humor. There are few other data on the relationships in postpartum women between levels of salivary and breast milk IgA and stress.

In our study, the lack of effect of relaxation on sIgA levels in maternal breast milk may have been related to improper timing of the breast milk collection. Breast milk collection time was modeled on data for salivary IgA. However, breast milk sIgA may be produced much more slowly and may have needed to be measured during the 2½ to 3 hours after relaxation. Success at relaxation was found to be inversely related to sIgA levels. However, the numbers of women in this section of the study are very small.

It is generally agreed that adults require about 2 months of daily practice to become proficient in self-conditioning relaxation. An example is the standard 9 weeks of training for 30 minutes a day that is provided to Swedish athletes competing in the winter biathlon, who are trained to relax quickly and to reduce their heart rates.[21] Nonetheless, during coaching in relaxation, most adults will demonstrate physiologic changes such as reduced pulse rate, increased peripheral temperature, or reduced electrodermal activity. One third of the women in our study practiced the relaxation technique less than once a day. It is likely that they would have benefited from longer and more frequent practice sessions. One half of the mothers reported months later that they had continued the practice and found themselves increasingly proficient in achieving rapid relaxation during periods of stress.

Our subjects clearly varied in their mental imagery preferences. Some described excellent visual imagery, whereas others preferred auditory or olfactory imagery. Inasmuch as we attempted to use the same relaxation coaching for each subject, we did not allow sufficiently for individual differences and preferences as one would in a typical clinical situation.

Our study showed an effect of self-reported stress on sIgA levels in breast milk at final collection. Mothers who were stressed at the second visit may have continued to be stressed through the final sample collection 6 to 8 weeks later, although we did not measure this. This may have accounted for the increased sIgA levels in the final sample. This would be consistent with data seen in stressed employees studied by Kugler et al[16] and Zeier et al.[15] However, stress as measured by the *SCL-90-R* did not correlate with the sIgA levels in human milk. The *SCL-90-R* may not be a good measure of postpartum stress. There are no norms for postpartum women.[9] Self-reported stress was evaluated at visit 2 by asking the open-ended question, "Has anything stressful happened to you in the past 2 weeks (between visit 1 and visit 2)?" This resulted in a myriad of answers, including surgery, relatives visiting, relatives leaving, husbands gone, and illnesses. This was coded as any stress present or no stress present. This may have been a better measure of stress than a questionnaire with preset questions. The changes in sIgA levels associated with stress were not seen at the time of the second visit, but 6 to 8 weeks later. Stressed mothers may transfer more immunologically active substances to their infants.

Although there are advantages to conducting a study involving breast milk sampling in the home, it is not possible to control for environmental factors as one might in a research study unit. Nonetheless, some of the environmental factors, ie, dogs, cats, and active toddlers, were more disconcerting to the investigators than to the subjects.

The increased breast milk IgA levels in subjects not practicing relaxation is paradoxical, yet consistent with other studies of humoral immunity and stress. Kiecolt-Glaser and Glaser[22] have noted that higher antibody titers to herpesviruses, ie, Epstein-Barr virus and cytomegalovirus, appear to reflect poorer cellular immune system control of herpesvirus latency. In a study of 45 geriatric residents randomly assigned to relaxation, to participation in social contact, or to no intervention, subjects in the relaxation group showed a statistically significant decrease in herpesvirus antibody titers.[23] This was interpreted as an enhanced ability of the immune system to control viral replication. Our results may reflect increased subclinical infection and the efforts of the immune system to resist this infection via increased antibody production. In subjects practicing relaxation, reduction of stress may be associated with less subclinical infection, less antibody production, and lower IgA levels. In children, evidence of individual differences in immune reactivity exists.[17] Inasmuch as we did not select or assign subjects on the basis of immune reactivity, this variable could also explain observed differences.

The ideal system for the study of immunomodulation does not exist. To move toward a clinical intervention that is practical, research would benefit from a biofeedback system capable of providing minute-to-minute evidence of immune status. For example, humoral immunomodulation research would be more meaningful if there were techniques for monitoring the amount of various immunoglobulins in saliva, tears, or breast milk minute to minute.

Conclusions

Our research presents some intriguing data on the relationship between stress and sIgA levels in breast milk. Some of the data are very consistent with previous work on the effect of stress and the immune system. Because our study is small, it needs to be replicated in a larger group of women with better measures of stress and with collections of breast milk at varying times.

In US culture, the first several months after childbirth are recognized as times of fatigue and stress for the mother. It is important to continue studies to understand how maternal stress affects breast milk production, quality of breast milk, duration of breast-feeding, and infant growth and development.

This study was supported in part by funding from Health Frontiers, Kenyon, Minn.

Presented at Seventh Annual Meeting of the Psychoneuroimmunology Research Society, Boulder, Colo, June 5, 1997; and the meeting of the Second International Academy of Breastfeeding Medicine, Boston, Mass, October 29, 1997.

Manual breast pumps were donated by Medela Inc, McHenry, Ill. We thank the mothers for their participation in this study; Elizabeth Studer, RN, MSN, IBCLC, for data entry; and Michael Tosi, MD, for supervision of the laboratory assays.

References

1. Wright AL, Holberg CJ, Taussig LM, Martinez FD. Relationship of infant feeding to recurrent wheezing at age 6 years. *Arch Pediatr Adolesc Med.* 1995;149:758–763.
2. Duncan B, Ey J, Holberg CJ, Wright AL, Martinez FD, Taussig LM. Exclusive breast-feeding for at least 4 months protects against otitis media. *Pediatrics.* 1993;91:867–872.
3. Paradise JL, Elster BA, Tan L. Evidence in infants with cleft palate that breast milk protects against otitis media. *Pediatrics.* 1994;94:853–860.
4. Work Group on Breastfeeding, American Academy of Pediatrics. Breastfeeding and the use of human milk. *Pediatrics.* 1997;100:1035–1039.
5. Slusser W, Powers NG. Breastfeeding update, I: immunology, nutrition, and advocacy. *Pediatr Rev.* 1997;18:111–119.
6. Horwood LJ, Fergusson DM. Breastfeeding and later cognitive and academic outcomes. *Pediatrics* [serial online]. 1998;101:e9.
7. Goldman AS, Chheda S, Garofalo R. Evolution of immunologic functions of the mammary gland and postnatal development of immunity. *Pediatr Res.* 1998;43:155–162.
8. Olness K, Culbert T, Uden D. Self-regulation of salivary immunoglobulin A by children. *Pediatrics.* 1989;83:66–71.
9. Derogatis LR. *SCL-90–R: Symptom Checklist-90–R: Administration, Scoring, and Procedures Manual.* Minneapolis, Minn: National Computer Systems Inc; 1994:19–26.
10. Ogra SS, Ogra PL. Immunologic aspects of human colostrum and milk. *J Pediatr.* 1978; 92:546–549.
11. Peitersen B, Bohn L, Andersen H. Quantitative determination of immunoglobulins, lysozyme, and certain electrolytes in breast milk during the entire period of lactation, during a 24–hour period, and in milk from the individual mammary gland. *Acta Paediatr Scand.* 1975; 64:709–717.
12. Fishaut M, Murphy D, Neifert M, McIntosh K, Ogra PL. Bronchomammary axis in the immune response to respiratory syncytial virus. *J Pediatr.* 1981;99:186–191.
13. Cleary TG, West MS, Ruiz-Palacios G, et al. Human milk secretory immunoglobulin A to Shigella virulence plasmid-coded antigen. *J Pediatr.* 1991;118:34–38.
14. Hewson-Bower B. *Psychological Treatment Decreases Colds and Flu in Children by Increasing Salivary Immunoglobulin* [PhD thesis]. Perth, Western Australia: Murdoch University; 1995.
15. Zeier H, Brauchli P, Joller-Jemelka HI. Effects of work demands on immunoglobulin A and cortisol in air traffic controllers. *Biol Psychol.* 1996; 42:413–423.
16. Kugler J, Reintjes F, Tewes V, Schedlowski M. Competition stress in soccer coaches increases salivary immunoglobin A and salivary cortisol concentrations. *J Sports Med Phys Fitness.* 1996;36:117–120.
17. Boyce WT, Chesterman EA, Martin N, Folkman S, Cohen F, Wara D. Immunologic changes occurring at kindergarten entry predict respiratory illnesses after the Loma Prieta earthquake. *J Dev Behav Pediatr.* 1993;14:296–303.
18. Lawrence RA, ed. *Breastfeeding: A Guide for the Medical Profession.* 4th ed. St Louis, Mo: Mosby–Year Book Inc; 1994:395–396.
19. Groer MW, Humenick S, Hill PD. Characterizations and psychoneuroimmunologic implications of secretory immunoglobulin A and cortisol in preterm and term breast milk. *J Perinat Neonat Nurs.* 1994;7:42–51.
20. Dillon KM, Totten MC. Psychological factors, immunocompetence, and health of breast-feeding mothers and their infants. *J Genet Psychol.* 1989;150:155–162.
21. Unestahl LE. The use of sport psychology in Scandinavia. In: Klavora P, Daniel J, eds. *Coach, Athlete, and Sports Psychologist.* Champaign, Ill: Human Kinetics; 1979:248–271.
22. Kiecolt-Glaser JK, Glaser R. Stress and immune function in humans. In: Ader R, Felten D, Cohen N, eds. *Psychoneuroimmunology.* Orlando, Fla: Academic Press Inc; 1991: 849–867.
23. Kiecolt-Glaser JK, Glaser R, Williges D, et al. Psychosocial enhancement of immunocompetence in a geriatric population. *Health Psychol.* 1985;4:25–41.

20 Complementary Therapies for Depression

An Overview

Edzard Ernst, MD, PhD, FRCP(Edin); Julia I. Rand, MBBS, MSc; Clare Stevinson, BSc, MSc
From the Department of Complementary Medicine, School of Postgraduate Medicine and Health Sciences, University of Exeter, Exeter, England.

Depression is one of the most common reasons for using complementary and alternative therapies. The aim of this article is to provide an overview of the evidence available on the treatment of depression with complementary therapies. Systematic literature searches were performed using several databases, reference list searching, and inquiry to colleagues. Data extraction followed a predefined protocol. The amount of rigorous scientific data to support the efficacy of complementary therapies in the treatment of depression is extremely limited. The areas with the most evidence for beneficial effects are exercise, herbal therapy (*Hypericum perforatum*), and, to a lesser extent, acupuncture and relaxation therapies. There is a need for further research involving randomized controlled trials into the efficacy of complementary and alternative therapies in the treatment of depression.

Arch Gen Psychiatry. 1998;55:1026–1032

Depression is a frequently occurring psychiatric disorder with a prevalence of approximately 5% in the general population.[1,2] It is estimated that at least one third of all individuals are likely to experience an episode of depression during their lifetime.[3] Depression results in high personal, social, and economic costs through suffering, disability, deliberate self-harm, and health care provision. Despite the availability of drug and psychotherapeutic treatments, much depression remains undiagnosed or inadequately treated.[4] This state of affairs has stimulated the development of educational campaigns and treatment consensus statements.[5,6]

Complementary and alternative medicine (CAM) is often negatively defined, for example, as "a system of health care which lies for the most part outside the mainstream of conventional medicine."[7] A more inclusive definition[8] has been adopted by the Cochrane Collaboration: "complementary medicine is diagnosis, treatment, and/or prevention which complements mainstream medicine by contributing to a common whole, by satisfying a demand not met by orthodoxy, or by diversifying the conceptual frameworks of medicine."

Complementary and alternative therapies (CATs) are popular. In 1991, 34% of the US adult population used at least 1 such therapy for 1 year.[9] This figure has now risen to 40%.[10] Twenty percent of those suffering from depression had used an unconventional therapy within the past year.[9] Depression is among the 10 most frequent indications for using CATs, and relaxation, exercise, and herbal remedies are the 3 most prevalent CATs tried for this condition.[10] Forty-two percent of 115 Danish psychiatric inpatients had used CATs at least once, with herbal medicine being the most frequent type.[11] Herbal remedies, homeopathy, acupuncture, massage, relaxation, and unconventional psychotherapeutic approaches have been reported[12] as the most prevalent CATs among psychiatric patients.

The response to the question of why people turn toward CAM is as fascinating as it is complex. No simple, uniform answer can be identified as the list of motivations will vary depending on which (patient) group one asks. Generally speaking, however, people opt for CAM because they want to leave no option untried and look for treatments devoid of adverse effects.[13] Another important reason is that CATs are viewed as less authoritarian and more empowering, offering more patient conetrol.[14] Astin[10] found that CAM users are, on average, better educated and report poorer health than nonusers. Interestingly, they do not usually turn to CAM as a result of being dissatisfied with orthodox medicine, and only 5% use CAM as a true alternative to conventional medicine.

Lay books on CAM[15–18] promote a wide range of CATs for depression (Table 1). In view of such promotion and CAM's popularity, the need for more information arises.[21] The aim of this article, therefore, is to review the published evidence regarding the effectiveness of CAT in the treatment of depression. As we will see, the trial data are almost invariably burdened with numerous limitations. Small sample size, selection bias, uncertainty about the diagnosis, lack of blinding, lack of adequate outcome measures, failure to control for nonspecific therapeutic effects, failure to control for confounders, inadequate duration, and personal belief of the investigator in the treatment are the most frequent drawbacks.

Computerized literature searching without language restrictions was carried out to identify all randomized controlled trials (RCTs) relating to CATs used for depression. The following databases were searched: MEDLINE (literature from 1966–1996), EMBASE (literature from 1986–1996), CISCOM (Centralized Information Service for Complementary Medicine; search performed in January 1997), and the Cochrane Library (accessed March 1997 [Issue 1]). A wide range of search terms was used, reflecting the diversity of CATs: acupuncture, affective disorders, Alexander technique, alternative medicine, aromatherapy, art therapy, Bach (flower remedies), balneology, chiropractic, color therapy, complementary medicine, depression, depressive disorders, energy, essential oils, exercise, healing, herbal medicine, hydrotherapy, hypnosis, kinesiology, laughter, manipulation, massage, music, naturopathy, osteopathy, oxygen, polarity, qigong, reflexology, relaxation, therapeutic touch, and tragerwork. The reference lists of all articles thus found were also searched. Furthermore, inquiries were made to colleagues for any further publications and our files were searched.

Ideally, only RCTs would be selected for this review. However, as the search revealed that few RCTs have been conducted, less-rigorous studies are referred to in cases in which no RCTs are available. Articles discussing the following mainstream treatments for depression were excluded: cognitive therapy, light therapy for seasonal affective disorder, and partial sleep deprivation. Articles with no factual data were also excluded. All studies admitted to this review were read in full by two of us (E.E. and J.I.R.). Data were extracted according to a predefined checklist. Discrepancies were settled through discussion.

Acupuncture

Acupuncture is an ancient Chinese treatment. Based on the belief that 2 types of "energies" flow in "meridians" throughout the body and that an imbalance of these energies constitutes illness, acupuncturists insert needles into points located on meridians with the aim of correcting the imbalance and restoring health. Western acupuncturists are critical of these Taoist theories and attribute acupuncture's alleged benefits to neurophysiological effects.[22] Hence, the putative mechanism for acupuncture in

Table 1. Therapies Frequently Cited for the Treatment of Depression in Lay Books*

Therapy	Description
Acupuncture	Therapy usually involving sticking needles into acupoints along "meridians" to restore the body's flow of "energy."
Alexander technique	Movement therapy to reduce muscular tension, involves retraining of posture and movement patterns.
Aromatherapy	Use of aromatic plant oils, which usually are massaged into the skin.
Applied kinesiology	Diagnostic and therapeutic technique based on the assumption that muscle groups are related to distant parts and organs of the body.
Autogenic training	A form of self-hypnosis involving a series of visual and sensory exercises.
Bach flower remedies	Treatment with remedies designed by Edward Bach, MB,BS, MRCS, LRCP, DPH, similar to those of homeopathy.
Color therapy	The use of different colored light for therapy based on the assumption that certain colors have specific effects on diseases.
Exercise	Treatment through different forms of regular physical activity, usually supervised by a physiotherapist.
Healing	Also called spiritual or faith healing, healers believe to channel "energy" from a higher force toward the patient with a view to restore health and well-being.
Herbalism	Treatment of diseases with plants, parts of plants, or plant extracts.
Homeopathy	Treatment based on the "like cures like" principle, often with highly dilute remedies.
Hypnotherapy	Use of hypnosis as an adjunct to medical treatments.
Massage	Manual stroking of the body surface with a view of relaxing muscles and mind.
Naturopathy	Drugless therapy to enhance the body's own healing powers using the treatment modalities supplied by nature.
Oxygen therapy	Treatment with oxygen: several variants exist, eg, injecting oxygen into the arteries or veins or treating blood with oxygen in vitro before reinjection.
Qigong	Traditional Chinese regimen involving movements and breathing techniques with a view of balancing the body's flow of "energies."
Tragerwork	Treatment with gentle rhythmic touch and movement exercises, also known as psychophysical integration.

*See books by the Burton Goldberg Group,[15] McCarthy,[16] and Olsen,[17] and the article published in Reader's Digest.[18] For good introductory text to these treatments see Cassileth[19] and Fugh-Berman.[20]

depression is provided through studies[23] showing that the level of endorphins can be increased through needling. Acupuncture is normally carried out in specialized clinics either by physicians or (more often) by nonmedically qualified therapists (NMQTs). One session would typically last for 20 minutes, and a series of 6 to 12 treatments may be required.

Case series[24,25] indicate that acupuncture is promising for treating depression. Several uncontrolled[26,27] and controlled[28] clinical trials provide data in support.

Electroacupuncture appears to have greater efficacy than traditional acupuncture, and the preliminary results[29] of a trial comparing standard electroacupuncture and computer-controlled electroacupuncture have been published. These indicate that the computer-controlled electroacupuncture treatment produced greater clinical improvement than electroacupuncture ($P<.05$) as measured by the grading system commonly used in China for the assessment of therapeutic effects.

Two RCTs[30,31] compare the effects of electroacupuncture and amitriptyline hydrochloride in depressed patients. Patients suffering from depression (defined according to National Survey and Coordination Group of Psychiatric Epidemiology standards) were grouped at random to receive 5 weeks of therapy with either electroacupuncture (n=27) or the tricyclic antidepressant amitriptyline hydrochloride (n=20; average daily dose, 142 mg).[30] A comparison of Hamilton Depression Scale scores before and after treatment showed a significant reduction (from 29 to 13 and 29 to 14, respectively) in the scores for both groups ($P<.01$). At the end of the treatment period, there was no statistically significant difference between the 2 groups.

An RCT[31] involving 241 depressed patients compared treatment with electroacupuncture or amitriptyline hydrochloride for 6 weeks. Hamilton Depression Scale scores showed a significant reduction after treatment in both groups (from 35 to 8 and 35 to 10, respectively). There was no significant intergroup difference after 6 weeks. Follow-up of 148 patients for 2 to 4 years revealed no significant difference in the depression recurrence rate between the 2 groups.

Herbal Medicine

Medical herbalism (also termed *phytotherapy* in Europe) is the treatment of illness with plants, parts of plants, or plant extracts. It has a long history in all medical cultures, and many of our modern drugs have been derived from botanical sources. Each plant contains a whole array of compounds, and it is sometimes difficult to define which and how many of these contribute to which pharmacological effect. The mechanism of action can thus be complex, but may be understood or researched by conventional pharmacological methods. While the general public usually view plant-based medicines as devoid of adverse effects, this notion can be dangerously misleading.[32] In continental Europe, phytotherapy is an integral part of physicians' prescribing. In the United States and the United Kingdom, herbal medicine is mostly in the hands of NMQTs.

Scattered references[33,34] occur in the ethnobotanical literature to plants used by indigenous peoples to treat depression. In China, herbal remedies are often used in combination with conventional western drug therapy.[35] However, only few trials, usually of poor methodological quality, investigate Chinese herbal therapies for depression. A similar situation exists in Japan where traditional herbal mixtures are used for depression, but their effects have not yet been scientifically tested.[36]

Lay books on CAM[15–18] claim a variety of plants to be helpful in depression, eg, wild oats, lemon balm, ginseng, wood betony, basil, and St John's Wort. Yet, only for St John's Wort (*Hypericum perforatum*) does a substantial body of evidence exist. It has recently been reviewed[37,38] in English. The meta-analysis by Linde et al[38] identified 23 RCTs involving a total of 1757 outpatients suffering from mild to moderate depression. Fifteen of these trials were placebo controlled, and 8 compared *H perforatum* with orthodox antidepressants. The overall responder rate ratio showed that *H perforatum* was significantly superior to placebo (2.67; 95% confidence interval, 1.78–4.01). *H perforatum* was found to have an efficacy similar to that of standard antidepressants. Compared with the antidepressant groups, the *H perforatum* groups had lower dropout rates (7.7% vs 4%) and numbers of patients reporting adverse effects (35.9% vs 19.8%). A recent comparative analysis (C. S. and E. E., unpublished data, June 1998) of adverse effects concluded that "Hypericum seems to be at least as safe and possibly safer than conventional antidepressant drugs."

Exercise

Many categories of physical exercise exist, eg, leisure-time and work-related physical activity or single bout and regular exercise. Their physiological responses may differ considerably. For the purpose of the following discussion, it is helpful to distinguish between regular endurance (mostly aerobic) exercise and power (mostly anaerobic) exercise. For the treatment of depression, exercise can be carried out either under supervision (eg, by a physiotherapist) or independently at home. In practice, a combined approach is usually the best.

A large body of evidence[39] (>1000 trials) exists relating to exercise and depression and numerous reviews[40–53] on the topic have recently been published. A meta-analysis of 80 studies[50] (regardless of their methodological quality) produced an overall mean exercise effect size of –0.53 (range, –3.88 to 2.05). This suggests that the depression scores decreased by approximately one half of an SD more in the exercise groups than in the comparison groups. The antidepressant effect occurred with all types of regular exercise, independent of sex or age, and it increased with the duration of therapy. Overall, exercise was as effective as psychotherapy.

The available evidence suggests that any type of exercise alleviates depression. Martinsen and Stephens[49] identified 8 experimental exercise-intervention trials in clinically depressed patients, and exercise was associated with reductions in depression scores in all of the studies. Two further RCTs[54,55] were identified via our search strategy. In the first study[54] moderately depressed elderly subjects were randomly allocated to walking exercises, social-contact control condition, or a waiting-list control group. After 6 weeks, the first 2 groups showed a significant decrease in Beck Depression Inventory scores compared with baseline. The second RCT[55] involved 124 depressed subjects allocated to aerobic exercise, low-intensity exercise, or to a no exercise-intervention group. All subjects continued their usual psychiatric treatment. No significant difference was found in the Beck Depression Inventory scores between the groups after 12 weeks. However, the control group had been significantly more depressed at baseline.

Aromatherapy

Aromatherapists (normally NMQTs) use a combination of gentle massage techniques and essential oils from plants. These oils are thought to have specific pharmacological effects after transdermal resorption. One treatment would last about 30 minutes, and a series of 6 to 12 treatments would usually be recommended.

Although aromatherapy is advocated for improving mood in depression,[56] and is perceived as helpful by some patients,[57] there is very little objective evidence. In a small pilot study,[58] 12 depressed men were exposed to citrus fragrance in the air and compared with 8 patients who were not exposed to the fragrance. Both groups were taking antidepressants. It was reported that the dose of antidepressants in the experimental group could be markedly reduced. The study was not randomized and involved only a small number of patients with varying dose and type of antidepressants. At present, it is not possible to draw any firm conclusions about the value of aromatherapy for depression.

Dance and Movement Therapy

A dance therapist (usually an NMQT) aims to involve patients through encouragement to express themselves in movement and therefore enhance well-being. Treatments can be organized as group sessions, adding an additional element of social interaction. Typically, a session lasts 30 to 40 minutes, and regular (eg, weekly) repetitions are normally recommended.

Little scientific evidence is available for the role of dance and movement therapy.[59] Only 2 studies[60,61] were found, neither involving large numbers or of rigorous design. Twenty hospitalized psychiatric patients and 20 normal control subjects were divided into 4 groups.[60] Half of the psychiatric patients and half of the controls received 1 dance and movement therapy session, and the other subjects received no intervention. After therapy, only the psychiatric patients showed a significant reduction in depression as measured by the Multiple Affect Adjective Checklist self-rating scale ($P<.001$). In the second study,[61] 12 inpatients with major depression were randomly assigned to movement therapy sessions on 7 of 14 days. Five of the patients showed a reduction in depression scores on movement therapy days compared with days with no therapy ($P<.05$). Both studies suffer from methodological limitations. Thus, insufficient evidence exists to assess the effect of dance and movement therapy in depression.

Homeopathy

Homeopathy is based on the "like cures like" principle that suggests that a remedy (often, but not always, plant based), which causes certain symptoms in a healthy individual, can be used as a treatment for patients presenting with such symptoms. Furthermore, homeopaths believe that, by "potentizing" (stepwise dilutions combined with vigorous shaking) a remedy, it will get not less, but more, potent. They assume that even dilutions devoid of molecules of the original remedy will have powerful clinical effects.[62] Homeopathy is practiced by both physicians and NMQTs. A first consultation will usually last in excess of 1 hour.

There is a dearth of investigations into homeopathy for depression. The literature consists mainly of unsubstantiated treatment suggestions or case reports.[63,64] The thorough review by Kleijnen et al[65] and a recent meta-analysis by Linde et al[66] of clinical trials of homeopathy detected only 1 study related to depression. It[67] compared homeopathic treatment with diazepam in mixed anxiety and depressive states. This open trial was of low methodological quality, but produced a result in favor of homeopathy. A working group of the European Union located 377 reports of trials f homeopathy, which included no further studies in depression.[68] The value of homeopathy as a treatment of depression is, therefore, presently unknown.

Hypnotherapy

Hypnotherapy is a state of focused attention or altered consciousness. All current theories of hypnosis are provisional and incomplete.[69] Hypnotherapy cannot cure disease, but can be a useful adjunct to conventional treatments. Therapy sessions vary in length and rate of repetitions. Hypnotherapy is practiced both by physicians and NMQTs.

The literature on the subject consists only of anecdotal accounts and case reports.[69,70] Our literature searches discovered no controlled clinical trials. It has been suggested[71] that hypnotherapy may facilitate the process of cognitive therapy by aiding the restructuring of negative thought patterns. Again, this has not been substantiated. The value of hypnotherapy for depression is, therefore, not known at present.

Massage Therapy

There are several different forms and traditions of massage therapy.[72] In the context of this article, massage uses typically a gentle manual stroking technique over the body (usually the back). This has a number of complex physiological and psychological effects, not least of which is relaxation of both the musculature and the mind.[72] A treatment, usually carried out by an NMQT, would normally last for 20 to 30 minutes and a series of approximately 6 twice weekly sessions would constitute a typical prescription.

Most publications relating to massage and depression were found to consist of anecdotal accounts and case studies.[73,74] A recent review[75] of massage therapy uncovered only a few controlled trials. An RCT[76] allocated 122 intensive care unit patients to receive either massage, massage with 1% lavender (*Lavendula vera*) oil, or rest periods.

Those who received the massage with lavender oil reported a greater improvement in mood as measured by a self-rating 4-point scale. The study did not involve patients with depression, was short-term, and used a crude outcome measure. It is thus not possible to draw firm conclusions from its results.

In a well-conducted RCT,[77,78] 72 hospitalized children and adolescents, half with adjustment disorder and half with depression, either received 30-minute back massages (n=52) daily for 5 days or watched a relaxing video (n=20) for the same period. Profile of mood states depression scores were significantly lower immediately after massage compared with pretreatment values (P=.005). In addition, the premassage profile of mood states scores significantly declined during the 5-day treatment period (P=.01), and the massage group was less depressed than the control group at the end of the study. Because of the small sample size and the short treatment period, the data are insufficient to judge the value of massage for depression.

Music Therapy

Music therapy is the active or passive use of music to promote health and well-being. During treatment, patients perform music or listen to music carefully chosen and supervised by a trained music therapist (usually an NMQT). The type of music will depend on the personality and condition of the patient.

A limited amount of work relates to the effects of music therapy on depression.[79] The results of an observational study[80] using psychodynamic music therapy methods with depressed inpatients suggest that there may be a beneficial effect. One RCT[81] involved 30 elderly patients (aged 61–86 years) with depression. They were randomly allocated to either a home-based music therapy program, a self-administered music therapy program, or a nonintervention waiting list (control group). After 8 weeks, the Geriatric Depression Scale scores of the 2 music groups were significantly better than those of the control group (P<.05). There is a need for further trials with larger numbers to determine whether this result can be replicated.

Relaxation Therapy

Relaxation therapy is an umbrella term for several techniques primarily aimed at decreasing physical and mental tension. Such treatments may include elements of meditation, yoga, and other mind-body therapies. They would normally be carried out by NMQTs.

Three RCTs[82–84] investigating the effects of relaxation therapy were found. In the first study, 30 psychiatric outpatients with depression, all taking medication, were randomized to 3 groups.[82] Two of the groups were given different forms of relaxation therapy during 3 days, while the third group acted as a control. Compared with controls, both relaxation-therapy groups showed a significant improvement in symptom scores (P<.05). However, a symptom score list was used that had not been validated, the sample size was small, and the treatment period short.

In an RCT[83] involving 37 moderately depressed patients assigned to cognitive behavior therapy, relaxation therapy, or tricyclic antidepressants, the first 2 interventions resulted in significantly better mean Beck Depression Inventory scores than the pharmacological treatment (P<.01). The results should be viewed with caution because of the small sample size, lack of control for the nonspecific effects of attention from professionals, and reported noncompliance with the medication regime.

An RCT[84] in 30 moderately depressed adolescents showed that relaxation training or cognitive behavior therapy resulted in a greater improvement than no intervention. Again, the sample size was small and there was no control for nonspecific effects.

On balance, therefore, relaxation treatments are promising, but further research and replications are required.

Conclusions

Because of the nature of the evidence relating to CAM and depression, a qualitative overview seemed preferable to a systematic review. Collectively, the above data suggest that exercise and *H perforatum* are effective symptomatic treatments for mild to moderate depression. The evidence for acupuncture, massage, and relaxation is promising, but not compelling.

Acupuncture and electroacupuncture can stimulate the synthesis and release of the monoamines serotonin and noradrenaline-norepinephrine in animals.[85] This is the postulated mechanism for the perceived beneficial effect of acupuncture in depression. The evidence available on the efficacy of electroacupuncture in the treatment of depression has mainly come from 1 research group at the Institute of Mental Health, Beijing, China. The limited number of RCTs suggest a beneficial effect of a similar magnitude to that produced by amitriptyline hydrochloride. Electroacupuncture is reported to produce fewer and less-severe adverse effects than standard antidepressants. However, there is a need for the results to be replicated in rigorously designed RCTs using clear diagnostic criteria for patient entry, specified randomization procedures, and control for nonspecific responses resulting from the time and attention received during the acupuncture therapy.

Despite the potential of plant extracts as psychoactive substances, *H perforatum* is the only herb that has been investigated rigorously. The results show promising effects in patients with mild to moderate depression. However, they need to be followed up by further studies with more clearly defined diagnostic groups, groups of patients with major depression, standardized preparations, trials longer than 8 weeks, and comparison with antidepressant doses within the normal therapeutic range.[86,87] *H perforatum* is associated with a markedly better adverse effect profile than standard antidepressants.[88] This could lead to better compliance, quality of life, and efficacy.

The results of exercise-intervention studies indicate that there is an overall association between exercise and reduction in the symptoms of mild to moderate depression. However, many studies suffer from significant methodological flaws that make it difficult to draw firm conclusions.[46] Many of the investigations are not of RCT design, involve only small numbers of subjects, are not controlled for the nonspecific effects of exercise, such as attention from trainers and social interaction where a group is involved, do not give full details of the exercise intervention, and use a variety of mainly self-reporting depression scales without objective blinded assessment. As with other CATs, it is unclear how long the antidepressive effects (if any) would persist.

A number of mechanisms by which exercise may improve mood have been proposed.[41,46] These include physiological effects, such as changes in endorphin and monoamine levels; psychological effects, such as subject expectation, diversion from stressful stimuli, the effects of receiving attention, improved self-image, and feelings of control; and sociological factors, such as the benefits of social interaction and support. Although some longitudinal epidemiological evidence[89,90] indicates that there may be a strong link between exercise and a reduction in depression levels, it is necessary to investigate this possibility further via high quality RCTs.

Few clinical studies are available regarding the effectiveness of other CATs in the treatment of depression. The data that do exist are generally of poor methodological quality. There are some indications that aromatherapy, massage, music therapy, and relaxation techniques may be of value. These areas thus warrant further investigation. No data exist regarding the efficacy of other therapies such as Alexander technique, Bach flower remedies, color therapy, kinesiology, naturopathy, polarity, tragerwork, qigong, and reflexology.

In CAM, there is heated debate about which research methods might be appropriate. Some claim that this area of medicine is so different that it defies standard research methods. This, however, has repeatedly been demonstrated to be wrong (as shown by White et al[91] and Vickers et al[92]). Clearly, the optimal method has to be chosen according to the research question and not to some vague ideological underpinning. If the question relates to testing the efficacy of a given treatment for depression, the RCT is unquestionably the design option that best excludes bias (eg, as summarized by Ernst,[93] Sibbald and Roland,[94] and Ernst[95]).

In conclusion, apart from *H perforatum* and exercise, little rigorous scientific evidence exists regarding the effectiveness of CATs in depression. In view of the public's demand for CAT, investigation of these therapeutic options by well-designed RCTs is important.

References

1. Bebbington P, Hurry J, Tennant C, Sturt E, Wing JK. Epidemiology of mental disorders in Camberwell. *Psychol Med.* 1981;11:561–579.
2. Weissman MM, Leaf PJ, Tischler GL, Blazer DG, Karno M, Livingston-Bruce M, Florio LP. Affective disorders in 5 US communities. *Psychol Med.* 1988;18:141–153.
3. Rorsman B, Gräsbeck A, Hagnell O, Lanke J, Öhman R, Öjesjö L, Otterbeck L. A prospective study of first-incidence depression: the Lundby Study, 1957–72. *Br J Psychiatry.* 1990; 156:336–342.
4. Freeling P, Rao BM, Paykel ES, Sireling LI, Burton RH. Unrecognised depression in general practice. *BMJ.* 1985;290:1880–1883.
5. Hirschfeld RMA, Keller MB, Panico S, Arons BS, Barlow D, Davidoff F, Endicott J, Froom J, Goldstein M, Gorman JM, Guthrie D, Marek RG, Maurer TA, Meyer R, Phillips K, Ross J, Schwenk TL, Sharfstein SS, Thase ME, Wyatt RJ. The National Depressive and Manic-Depressive Association consensus statement on the undertreatment of depression. *JAMA.* 1997; 277:333–340.
6. Paykel ES, Priest RG. Recognition and management of depression in general practice: consensus statement. *BMJ.* 1992;305:1198–1202.
7. Downer SM, Cody MM, McCluskey P, Wilson PD, Arnott SJ, Lister TA, Slevin ML. Pursuit and practice of complementary therapies by cancer patients receiving conventional treatment. *BMJ.* 1994;309:86–89.
8. Ernst E, Resch KL, Mills S, Hill R, Mitchell A, Willoughby M, White A. Complementary medicine: a definition [letter]. *Br J Gen Pract.* 1995; 45:506.
9. Eisenberg DM, Kessler RC, Foster C, Norlock FE, Calkins DR, Delbanco TL. Unconventional medicine in the United States. *N Engl J Med.* 1993; 328:246–252.
10. Astin JA. Why patients use alternative medicine: results of a national study. *JAMA.* 1998;279:1548–1553.
11. Raben H, Aggernæs KH. Psykiatriske patienters brug af alternativ behandling. *Ugeskr Laeger.* 1991;153:782–784.

12. Pfeifer S. Alternative Heilmethoden bei psychischen Erkrankungen. *Schweiz Arch Neurol Psychiatry.* 1993;144:501–516.

13. Ernst E, Willoughby M, Weihmayr TH. Nine possible reasons for choosing complementary medicine. *Perfusion.* 1995;11:356–359.

14. Vincent C, Furnham A. Why do patients turn to complementary medicine? an empirical study. *Br J Clin Psychol.1996*;35:37–48.

15. Strohecker J, executive ed. *Alternative Medicine: The Definitive Guide.* Puyallup, Wash: Burton Goldberg; 1994.

16. McCarthy M, ed. *Natural Therapies.* London, England: Thorsons; 1994.

17. Olsen K. *The Encyclopedia of Alternative Health Care: The Complete Guide to Choices in Healing.* London, England: Piatkus Ltd; 1991.

18. Kennedy D, managing ed. *Natural Remedies: Health and Healing the Natural Way.* London, England: Reader's Digest Assoc Ltd; 1995.

19. Cassileth BR. *The Alternative Medicine Handbook.* New York, NY: WW Norton & Co Inc; 1997.

20. Fugh-Berman A. *Alternative Medicine: What Works.* Tucson, Ariz: Odonian Press; 1996.

21. Mental Health Foundation. *Knowing Our Own Minds.* London, England: Mental Health Foundation; 1997.

22. Filshie J, White A, eds. *Medical Acupuncture: A Western Scientific Approach.* Edinburgh, Scotland: Churchill Livingstone Inc; 1998.

23. Han JS, Terenius L. Neurochemical basis for acupuncture analgesia. *Annu Rev Pharmacol Toxicol.* 1982;22:193–220.

24. Liu G, Jia Y, Zhan L, Luo H. Electroacupuncture treatment of presenile and senile depressive state. *J Tradit Chin Med.* 1992;12:91–94.

25. Lorini G, Fusari A. Agopuntura e psichiatria: nota preliminare. *Minerva Med.* 1977;68:711–715.

26. Polyakov SE. Acupuncture in the treatment of endogenous depressions. *Zh Neuropat Psikhiatr Korsakova.* 1988;21:36–44.

27. Tao DJ. Research on the reduction of anxiety and depression with acupuncture. *Am J Acupunct.* 1993;21:327–329.

28. Yang X. Clinical observation on needling extrachannel points in treating mental depression. *J Tradit Chin Med.* 1994;14:14–18.

29. Luo H, Jia Y, Feng X, Zhao X, Tang LC. Advances in clinical research on common mental disorders with computer controlled electro-acupuncture treatment. In: Tang L, Tang S, eds. *Neurochemistry in Clinical Application.*New York, NY: Plenum Press; 1995:109–122.

30. Luo H, Jia Y, Zhan L. Electro-acupuncture vs amitriptyline in the treatment of depressive states. *J Tradit Chin Med.* 1985;5:3–8.

31. Lou H, Jia Y, Wu X, Dai W. Electro-acupuncture in the treatment of depressive psychosis. *Int J Clin Acupunct.* 1990;1:7–13.

32. Ernst E. Harmless herbs? a review of the recent literature. *Am J Med.*1998;104:170–178.

33. Bhat RB, Jacobs TV. Traditional herbal medicine in Transkei. *J Ethnopharmacol.* 1995;48:7–12.

34. Singh V, Kapahi BK, Srivastava TN. Medicinal herbs of Ladakh especially used in home remedies. *Fitoterapia.* 1996;67:38–48.

35. Saku M. The current clinical practice of herbal medicine in psychiatry in mainland China: a review of literature. *Jpn J Psychiatry Neurol.* 1991;45:825–832.

36. Sarai K. Oriental medicine as therapy for resistant depression: use of some herbal drugs in the Far East (Japan). *Prog Neuropsychopharmacol Biol Psychiatry.* 1992;16:171–180.

37. Ernst E. St John's Wort, an anti-depressant? a systematic, criteria-based review. *Phytomedicine.*1995;2:67–71.

38. Linde K, Ramirez G, Mulrow CD, Pauls A, Weidenhammer W, Melchart D. St John's Wort for depression: an overview and meta-analysis of randomised clinical trials. *BMJ.* 1996; 313:253–258.

39. Hughes JR. Psychological effects of habitual aerobic exercise: a critical review. *Prev Med.* 1984;13:66–78.

40. Byrne A, Byrne DG. The effect of exercise on depression, anxiety, and other mood states: a review. *J Psychosom Res.* 1993;37:565–574.

41. Casper RC. Exercise and mood. *World Rev Nutr Diet.* 1993;71:115–143.

42. Ernst E. Run away from depression. *Eur J Phys Med Rehabil.* 1995;5:181–182.

43. Glenister D. Exercise and mental health: a review. *J R Soc Health.* 1996;116:7–13.

44. Gleser J, Mendelberg H. Exercise and sport in mental health: a review of the literature. *Isr J Psychiatry Relat Sci.* 1990;27:99–112.

45. LaFontaine TP, DiLorenzo TM, Frensch PA, Stucky-Ropp RC, Bargman EP, McDonald DG. Aerobic exercise and mood: a brief review, 1985–1990. *Sports Med.* 1992;13:160–170.

46. Leith LM. *Foundations of Exercise and Mental Health.* Morgantown, WVa: Fitness Information Technology; 1994:17–44.

47. Martinsen EW. The role of aerobic exercise in the treatment of depression. *Stress Med.* 1987; 3:93–100.

48. Martinsen EW. Benefits of exercise for the treatment of depression. *Sports Med.* 1990; 9:380–389.

49. Martinsen EW, Stephens T. Exercise and mental health in clinical and free-living populations. In: Dishman RK, ed. *Advances in Exercise Adherence.*Champaign, Ill: Human Kinetics; 1994:55–72.

50. North TC, McCullagh P, Tran ZV. Effect of exercise on depression. *Exerc Sport Sci Rev.* 1990; 18:379–415.

51. Raglin JS. Exercise and mental health: beneficial and detrimental effects. *Sports Med.* 1990; 9:323–329.

52. Veale DMWC. Exercise and mental health. *Acta Psychiatr Scand.* 1987;76:113–120.

53. Weyerer S, Kupfer B. Physical exercise and psychological health. *Sports Med.* 1994;17:108–116.

54. McNeil JK, LeBlanc EM, Joyner M. The effect of exercise on depressive symptoms in the moderately depressed elderly. *Psychol Aging.* 1991; 6:487–488.

55. Veale D, le Fevre K, Pantelis C, de Souza V, Mann A, Sargeant A. Aerobic exercise in the adjunctive treatment of depression: a randomised controlled trial. *J R Soc Med.* 1992; 85:541–544.

56. Mojay G. Oils for depression. *Int J Aromatherapy.* 1994;6:18–23.

57. Alexander B. *The Place of Complementary Therapies in Mental Health: A User's Experiences and Views.* Nottingham, England: Nottingham Patients' Council Support Group; 1993.

58. Komori T, Fujiwara R, Tanida M, Nomura J, Yokoyama MM. Effects of citrus fragrance on immune function and depressive states. *Neuroimmunomodulation.* 1995;2:174–180.

59. Ritter M, Low KG. Effects of dance/movement therapy: a meta-analysis. *Arts Psychother.* 1996; 23:249–260.

60. Brooks D, Stark A. The effect of dance/movement therapy on affect: a pilot study. *Am J Dance Ther.* 1989;11:101–112.

61. Stewart NJ, McMullen LM, Rubin LD. Movement therapy with depressed inpatients: a randomised multiple single-case design. *Arch Psychiatr Nurs.* 1994;8:22–29.

62. Ernst E, Hahn EG, eds. *Homoeopathy: A Critical Appraisal.* Oxford, England: Butterworth-Heinemann; 1998.

63. Spence DS. Day-to-day management of anxiety and depression. *Br Homoeopathic J.* 1990; 79:39–44.

64. Davidson JRT, Morrison RM, Shore J, Davidson RT, Bedayn G. Homeopathic treatment of depression and anxiety. *Altern Ther Health Med.* 1997;3:46–49.

65. Kleijnen J, Knipschild P, ter Riet G. Clinical trials of homoeopathy. *BMJ.* 1991;302:316–323.

66. Linde K, Claudius N, Ramirez G, Melchart D, Eitel F, Hedges LV, Jonas W. Are the clinical effects of homoeopathy placebo effects? a meta-analysis of placebo-controlled trials. *Lancet.*1997;350:834–843.

67. Heulluy B. *Essai randomisé ouvert de L 72 (spécialté homéopathique) contre diazépam 2 dans les états anxiodépressifs.* Metz, France: Laboratoires Lehning; 1985.

68. Homeopathic Medicine Research Group. *Overview of Data From Homeopathic Medicine Trials.* Brussels, Belgium: European Commission; 1996.

69. Kirsch I, Lynn SJ. Dissociating the wheat from the chaff in theories of hypnosis: reply to Kihlstrom (1998) and Woody and Sadler (1998). *Psychol Bull.* 1998;123:198–202.

70. Mow KE. Treatment of psychoneurosis and depression with medical hypnoanalysis: San Antonio Conference, September 22–25, 1994. *Med Hypnoanalysis J.* 1994;9:167–176.

71. Deltito J, Baer L. Hypnosis in the treatment of depression: research and theory. *Psychol Rep.* 1986;58:923–929.

72. Vickers A. *Massage and aromatherapy.* London, England: Chapman & Hall; 1996.

73. Bortoft J. Massage for mental health. *Therapist.* 1996;4:38–40.

74. Hilliard D. Massage for the seriously mentally ill. *J Psychosoc Nurs Ment Health Serv.* 1995; 33:29–30.

75. Ernst E, Fialka V. The clinical effectiveness of massage therapy: a critical review. *Forschende Komplementärmed.* 1994;1:226–232.

76. Dunn C, Sleep J, Collett D. Sensing an improvement: an experimental study to evaluate the use of aromatherapy, massage, and periods of rest in an intensive care unit. *J Adv Nurs.* 1995;21:34–40.

77. Field T, Morrow C, Valdeon C, Larson S, Kuhn C, Schanberg S. Massage reduces anxiety in child and adolescent psychiatric patients. *J Am Acad Child Adolesc Psychiatry.* 1992;31:125–131.

78. Field T. Massage therapy for infants and children. *Dev Behav Pediatr.* 1995;16:105–111.

79. Aldridge D. Music therapy research, I: a review of the medical research literature within a general context of music therapy research. *Arts Psychother.* 1993;20:11–35.

80. Reinhardt A, Ficker F. Erste Erfahrungen mit Regulativer Musiktherapie bei psychiatrischen Patienten. *Psychiatr Neurol Med Psychol.* 1983;35:604–610.

81. Hanser SB, Thompson LW. Effects of music therapy strategy on depressed older adults. *J Gerontol.* 1994;49:265–269.

82. Broota A, Dhir R. Efficacy of two relaxation techniques in depression. *J Pers Clin Stud.* 1990;6:83–90.

83. Murphy GE, Carney RM, Knesevich MA, Wetzel RD, Whitworth P. Cognitive behavior therapy, relaxation training, and tricyclic antidepressant medication in the treatment of depression. *Psychol Rep.* 1995;77:403–420.

84. Reynolds WM, Coats KI. A comparison of cognitive-behavioral therapy and relaxation training for the treatment of depression in adolescents. *J Consult Clin Psychol.* 1986; 54:653–660.

85. Han JS. Electroacupuncture: an alternative to antidepressants for treating affective diseases? *Int J Neurosci.* 1986;29:79–92.

86. de Smet PAGM, Nolen WA. St John's Wort as an antidepressant. *BMJ.* 1996;313:241–242.

87. Kendrick T. Commentary on "Meta-analysis: hypericum extracts (St John's Wort) are effective in depression." *Evidence-based Med.* 1997;2:24.

88. Ernst E, Rand JI, Barnes J, Stevinson C. Adverse effects profile of the herbal antidepressant St John's Wort. *Eur J Clin Pharmacol.* In press.

89. Camacho TC, Roberts RE, Lazarus NB, Kaplan GA, Cohen RD. Physical activity and depression: evidence from the Alameda County Study. *Am J Epidemiol.* 1991;134:220–231.

90. Farmer ME, Locke BZ, Moscicki EK, Dannenberg AL, Larson DB, Radloff LS. Physical activity and depressive symptoms: the NHANES I epidemiolgic follow-up study. *Am J Epidemiol.* 1988;128:1340–1351.

91. White AR, Resch KL, Ernst E. Methods of economic evaluation in complementary medicine. *Forschende Komplementärmed.* 1996; 3:196–203.

92. Vickers A, Cassileth B, Ernst E, Fisher P, Goldman P, Jonas W, Kang SK, Lewith G, Schulz K, Silagy C. How should we research unconventional therapies? a panel report from the Conference on Complementary and Alternative Medicine Research Methodology, National Institutes of Health. *Int J Technol Assess Health Care.*1997;13:111–121.

93. Ernst E. Klinische Studien: was ist Goldstandard [editorial]? *Perfusion.* 1997;4:125.

94. Sibbald B, Roland M. Why are randomised controlled trials important. *BMJ.* 1998;316:201.

95. Ernst E. RCT: relatively clear triumph [editorial]. *Perfusion.* 1998;11:121.

"We are always slow in admitting great changes of which we do not see the steps."—Charles Darwin[1]

21 The Neuro-Immuno-Cutaneous-Endocrine Network: Relationship of Mind and Skin

Richard L. O'Sullivan, MD; Graeme Lipper, MD; Ethan A. Lerner, MD, PhD
From the Department of Psychiatry, Massachusetts General Hospital Psychiatric Neuroscience Program (Dr O'Sullivan), and the Department of Dermatology, Massachusetts General Hospital–Harvard Cutaneous Biology Research Center (Drs Lipper and Lerner), Charlestown, Mass, and the Departments of Psychiatry (Dr O'Sullivan) and Dermatology (Drs Lipper and Lerner), Harvard Medical School, Boston, Mass.

Skin does more than present one's "face" to the world; it plays a vital role in the maintenance of physical and mental health. As our most ancient interface, skin retains the ability to respond to both endogenous and exogenous stimuli, sensing and integrating environmental cues while transmitting intrinsic conditions to the outside world. As such, it has long been a target for the application of both medical and nonmedical therapies of healthy and diseased states. Our understanding of how the skin and topical therapies affect health is in its infancy. Conversely, we know little of how our internal systems affect our skin. By exploring an elaborate web of neuro-immuno-cutaneous-endocrine (NICE) phenomena, we seek to shed light on the generally acknowledged, but inadequately defined, relationship between mental and physical health. We use skin as our window, noting some of the biological mediators linking nervous, immune, cutaneous, and endocrine functions. It is likely that these mediators are important in homeostasis, and that they affect several dermatologic and psychiatric conditions.

Arch Dermatol. 1998;134:1431–1435

A view of integrated mind, brain, and body connections in wellness and disease has been appreciated for centuries. Yet the conventional medical community still trivializes this complex set of relationships, and has alienated many patients. Notably, US patients visited alternative practitioners 425 million times in 1990—40 million more times than they visited their primary care physician.[2] Clearly, increasing numbers of consumers are seeking something other than conventional medical care.

While modern medicine is often focused on acute disease, many individuals living with chronic illnesses, such as cancer, acquired immunodeficiency syndrome, arthritis, pain syndromes, and chronic fatigue, are looking elsewhere for help, abandoning traditional medicine completely. Others combine conventional therapies with alternative techniques, such as homeopathy, acupuncture, diet modification, chiropractic, aromatherapy, and other interventions aimed at perceived "mind-body" links.[3,4] Surprise cures and responses often remain unexplained and are attributed to complex mind-body forces[4,5]; yet, as these associations are described, the biological substrate to these mysteries is gaining further definition. Alternative or "holistic" medicine approaches typically lack the accepted empirically derived scientific foundations of "Western" medicine. These approaches, however, have a core unifying theme: the interconnectedness of mind and body.[5] Furthermore, alternative therapies highlight the capacity of humans to respond to a range of interventions, including touch, sound, mental imagery, and fragrances.[6–9] Interest in alternative therapies that incorporate mind-body concepts has grown among conventional scientists and clinicians. However, while awareness of links between mental and physical well-being grows, objectively quantifying and describing mechanisms to account for these links remains a formidable empirical task.[10–12] To date, the science lags behind the practice, and explanatory models are in their rudimentary stages. One such model—the neuro-immuno-cutaneous-endocrine (NICE) network—is a simple construct featuring 4 organ systems intimately involved in the bridge between body and mind. These intimately linked systems share a language of neuropeptides, cytokines, glucocorticoids, and other effector molecules: common words used in a dynamic web of dialogue.

Bidirectionality of Mind-Body Influences

From Body to Mind: Afferent Pathways in the NICE System

Few investigators and clinicians would question the impact of conventional sensory stimuli on mood and cognitive function, but only now are scientists beginning to characterize the "hidden" senses and pathways that may profoundly influence daily health and subjective well-being. For instance, physical afferent stimuli to skin, such as traction, rubbing, and scratching, can result in local stimulation, irritation, and inflammation. Immunocompetent cells stimulated by these conditions may cross the blood-brain barrier and secrete their cytokines and other inflammatory mediators, thereby directly modulating the central nervous system (CNS) as well as the local skin environment. The CNS may respond by releasing neurotransmitters and, perhaps, initiate motor behaviors directed at the skin, such as scratching and picking. As one example of such a physical connection, immobilization-induced stress in male Syrian hamsters resulted in a wide range of stress-induced end-organ effects. Plasma testosterone levels, sebaceous lipogenesis, and epithelial cell proliferation were reversibly reduced.[13] A cutaneous-endocrine connection has been demonstrated in male Wistar rats anesthetized with pentobarbital that responded to nociceptive pinch stimulation of bilateral hindpaws with significantly increased plasma levels of luteinizing hormone, testosterone, and corticosterone.[14,15] In vivo paracrine interactions between the immune and peripheral nervous systems have also been demonstrated. Using a rat model of adjuvant-induced local joint inflammation, the existence and activation of a local anti–nociceptive system in response to the stress of a cold water swim has been shown. β-Endorphin was produced by macrophages, lymphocytes, and plasma cells infiltrating the inflamed synovial tissue. This model suggests that immune cells, by producing neuroendocrine peptides such as β-endorphin, may actually initiate or modify the perception of pain. It is possible that the immune system might constitute a sixth sense by converting stimuli from environmental factors (viruses, bacteria, trauma, tissue necrosis, etc) into "biochemical information in the form of neurotransmitters, hormones, and cytokines."[16] If these factors can induce or modify pain perception, it is conceivable that they could alter other sensory perceptions,[17,18] such as those inherent in the perception of beauty or unattractiveness. Perhaps these factors mediate, in part, some of the behavioral components in cycles associated with pruritus-induced[19–22] scratching, neurotic excoriations, compulsive skin picking, and trichotillomania. Furthermore, many "mind-skin" types of conditions, such as self-cutting, burning, skin piercing, and so-called self-mutilation, may be postulated to be mediated, in part, through similar mechanisms via pain- and anxiety-reducing components.

From Mind to Body: Efferent Pathways

Efferent pathways provide a link between higher cortical, limbic, and CNS functions and the diverse organ systems of the body. For instance, pathways linking higher cortical function to the hypothalamic pituitary axis have been established.[16] Additional evidence has accumulated to suggest numerous efferent links between the CNS and the immune system. For instance, certain areas of primary and secondary lymphoid organs, such as lymph nodes and the spleen, are innervated with noradrenergic sympathetic neuronal fibers. Finally, lymphocytes and macrophages express a wide range of hormone, neuropeptide, and steroid receptors.[22]

The discovery of such concrete pathways of neuroimmune modulation dovetails with the observation that chronic or repetitive mental stress seems to alter immune response.[23] Clinical examples of this phenomenon abound. For instance, patients often note an exacerbation of latent herpetic infections in the context of feeling anxious or "worn down." Psychological stresses in students during examination periods may affect antibody production to hepatitis vaccine.[24] Stress effects on delayed-type hypersensitivity responses, including modification of delayed-type hypersensitivity responses in depression and other nervous conditions, have also been described.[25] A compromised immune system induced by environmental stimuli and nervous system responses may predispose certain individuals to cutaneous malignancies associated with viruses (eg, Kaposi sarcoma associated with human herpesvirus and human immunodeficiency virus infection; human papillomavirus associated with cervical carcinoma).

Skin as a Neuroimmunoendocrine Interface: NICE

Dermatologists and other clinicians have long recognized neuropsychological connections between skin appearance, perception of beauty, and health. Simple observations of normal expressions of these connections, such as blushing associated with strong emotions or pallor and sweating due to fear and anxiety, are well known.[26] Pathological expressions of the association between nervous system perturbations and skin disease are commonly seen in clinical practice.[27] Stressful life events may exacerbate psoriasis, acne, eczema, and urticaria.[21,28,29] In a survey of 5600 patients with psoriasis, Farber and Nall[28] found that more than 30% of the patients believe that stress triggers their psoriatic flares, and in a companion study of 2144 patients with psoriasis, 40% of the patients associated the appearance of psoriatic plaques with concurrent life stressors.[29] One report, based on a survey of patients seen in a dermatology clinic, noted that approximately 40% of the patients also had concurrent psychiatric symptoms.[30] Thus, the perceived association between mental and physical well-being is strong. But how does "stress" translate into tangible cutaneous manifestations?

Traditionally, the concept of stress has been linked to physical mechanisms of cutaneous damage, such as scratching, picking, rubbing, and poor hygiene. In contrast, science has been unable to explain how an abstraction such as psychogenic stress could generate structural and functional changes predisposing skin to disease. However, recent evidence of concrete neuroanatomical links between CNS and skin reveals that some of these conceptual connections can be anatomically demarcated, thereby shedding light on the pathophysiological mechanisms of skin disease. The nervous and the immune systems share specific communication molecules that originate in both systems.[31] In skin, Langerhans cells and the proximity of calcitonin gene–related peptide (CGRP) to both Langerhans cells and neurons led to consideration of bidirectional communication in skin between the immune and the nervous systems. Expression of neurotrophic factors and neuropeptide receptors by Langerhans cells gives further support to the theory that there is a functional relationship between these cells and epidermal nerves.[32,33] These neuropeptides modulate bidirectional communication between the nervous and the immune systems[34,35] and provide firm evidence for a mind-body connection in the skin. The application of techniques of in situ immunohistochemistry and confocal microscopy has led to the characterization of elaborate networks of cutaneous nerves containing numerous neuropeptides, many of which have intriguing properties such as vasodilatation, edema formation, and epithelial cell proliferation. A wealth of data concerning the function and distribution of these cutaneous neuropeptides has accumulated, fueling research aimed at uncovering structural and functional evidence linking stress to skin disease.

Cutaneous Neuropeptides

Neuropeptides are ubiquitous in the skin and constitute a diverse group of molecules functioning as neurotransmitters, neuromodulators, potential growth factors, and hormones. Immunohistochemical staining for various neuropeptides in the skin has shown that these molecules are present in both cutaneous nerve fibers and all cutaneous cells examined, including keratinocytes, immunocytes, fibroblasts, Langerhans cells, and endothelial cells. Comments on select neuropeptides in skin follow, with more details provided in reviews and primary articles.[22] Interest has developed on the physiological and pathogenic roles of vasodilatory cutaneous neuropeptides, such as CGRP, the nociceptive neurotransmitter substance P (SP), vasoactive intestinal peptide (VIP), neuropeptide Y, and the more recently characterized pituitary adenylate cyclase activating peptide. When injected intradermally, these substances are known to induce vasodilatation, and intradermal SP produces classic wheal and flare reactions.[22] Epidermal growth factor was, in retrospect, one of the first neuropeptides described. Recent studies suggest that it has a role in the development of psoriasis. The skin contains other neuropeptides with less well-defined cutaneous functions, including somatostatin, neurokinin A, neurotensin, atrial natiuretic peptide, galanin, and α-melanocyte-stimulating hormone.[22,36,37] In addition to reports on the neuropeptide properties of α-melanocyte-stimulating hormone, an expanding literature on its role in immune responses has developed. Substance P is one of the cutaneous neuropeptides under investigation for its potential role in the pathogenesis of skin disease. It is part of the peptide family of tachykinins and has been identified mainly by its role in nonciceptive pathways, but it also has a putative role in tissue repair. Substance P immunoreactivity is strongest in perivascular sites and in the papillary dermis, yet changes in this distribution have inconsistently been reported for lesional and nonlesional skin in common dermatoses, such as atopic dermatitis[37] and psoriasis.[38] Substance P receptors are found on mast cells, neutrophils, and macrophages,[22] and SP is chemotactic for mononuclear and polymorphonuclear leukocytes,[39] suggesting a link between neurogenic stimuli and infiltration of the skin by inflammatory cells. Cultured normal human keratinocytes contain specific SP-binding sites,[40] suggesting a link between this neuropeptide and keratinocyte activity. Calcitonin gene–related peptide has been implicated in disorders of the cutaneous microvasculature. The digital cutaneous microvasculature in patients with Raynaud phenomenon shows a deficiency of CGRP-containing nerves in the distal digital skin.[41] Human suction blister injury produces an increase in PGP (a pan-neuronal marker protein) and CGRP-immunoreactive nerves as compared with controls 6 hours after injury, suggesting a relationship between epidermis, blood vessels, and nerve fibers during the tissue healing process.[42] A similar increase in CGRP-immunoreactive fibers was noted in the skin of shaved rats that had been stimulated by pinching or ice water, suggesting that cutaneous stimulation can cause a rapid rise in CGRP content. Calcitonin gene–related peptide probably has crucial immunomodulatory effects in vivo, as revealed by the intimate relationship between Langerhans cells and CGRP-containing nerve fibers and the observation that CGRP inhibits Langerhans cell antigen presentation.[43] Other neuropeptides likely involved in cutaneous physiology and pathophysiology include VIP and pituitary adenylate cyclase activating peptide; both peptides demonstrate potent vasodilatory activity when intradermally injected, and in vitro evidence suggests that VIP may be both mitogenic for cultured human keratinocytes and immunosuppressive, dampening experimental delayed hypersensitivity reactions.[44] Pituitary adenylate cyclase activating peptide, a member of the VIP-secretin-glucagon family of ligands, shares some of VIP's cutaneous activities, including potent vasodilatation and immunomodulatory function.[45] This brief survey of cutaneous neuropeptides suggests that these molecules likely play a key role as intermediary signals connecting the neuroendocrine system with immune and organ-specific processes. The neuroendocrine system may relay higher cortical "signals" via an array of processes, some circuitous and involving a cascade of steps (such as nitric oxide induction in cells adjacent to target cells), while other connections may be more direct. Shedding light on these complex pathways may be the first step toward a better understanding of how abstract cortical processes (stress) can lead to concrete manifestations, such as inflammatory disorders of the skin (atopic dermatitis, psoriasis, vitiligo, alopecia areata, etc). Although this section has focused on neuropeptides, these molecules are a small subset of intercellular messengers that likely influence cellular function in vivo. Investigation into the distributions and roles of nonpeptidergic neurotransmitters, such as catecholamines, steroids, nitric oxide, endorphins, and other small molecules, will contribute to our understanding in this area.[46–48] Additional factors, such as mechanical tension on both a microlevel and a macrolevel, appear to modulate local cellular function.[49]

NICE Smells

While we have focused on the role of skin as an interface between environment, body, and mind, it is likely that other sensory modalities have equally profound effects on physical and mental health. How, for instance, does olfactory input influence the body and mind? Odors, scents, and fragrances have long been used in a host of rituals, including religious rites, and as primitive protective agents against infection. For example, medieval physicians wore scented masks as protection against infection with the plague.[50] Acupuncture for reducing pain and bolstering the immune system is frequently used in conjunction with olfactory stimulation with incense. Furthermore, a body of literature suggests that in both therapeutic agents and appearance-enhancing cosmetics, certain odors, whether within a topical medium or delivered ambiently, can influence mood, anxiety, cognition, immune function, and, possibly, skin health.[8,51,52] Since odor molecules, like medications, stimulate signal transduction pathways via ligand-receptor interactions in peripheral and central pathways,[53] it is conceivable that olfactory administration of medications in the form of fragrances could alter nervous and immune function. Aromatherapy, or the use of fragrances to enhance well-being and treat sickness, is a well-established technique of "alternative medicine."[3,7–9,50]

The anatomical basis for olfactory and limbic system interconnections has been described.[53] Although the mechanism of action is unclear, odor may effect mind processes via the interaction of fragrance molecules on olfactory mucosal cells with information transfer via olfactory pathways to limbic and hypothalamic structures.[53] Therefore, olfactory approaches may yield a direct route into limbic system structures and thus modulate many basic human functions.[53,54] Pleasing, as opposed to disagreeable, odors have a strong, immediate, and powerful effect on humans and social interactions. Even odorific molecules not consciously recognized, such as pheromones, are recognized as influential, primal means of communication among virtually all species, humans included.[54,55] Odor identification, recognition, and discrimination have important survival and reproductive value,[55] and deficits in olfaction have been noted in several neuropsychiatric disorders, including Alzheimer disease, Parkinson disease, schizophrenia, and depression.[52–54,56–58]

Since many dermatologic treatments are topical, the addition of specific olfactory cues may maximize the therapeutic value of these agents, particularly when the agents are used for conditions with strong presumptive mind-body connections (eg, allergic dermatitis, psoriasis, eczema, pruritus, urticaria atopic dermatitis, and inflammmatory dermatoses).[7,21,51,52]

Conclusions and Further Directions

The process of mapping the tangled web connecting physical and mental well-being is underway. Could pharmacologic agents be developed for oral, topical, or intranasal (fragrant) delivery to be used in combination with techniques of tactile stimulation to ameliorate disease processes or to make persons feel better about themselves? Can these intervention pathways act at various in–roads of the NICE system to affect this still ill-defined proposed circuit?

Capsaicin has been used to alter cutaneous neuropeptide content (depletion of SP and other neuromediators from nerve terminals), thereby dampening local and systemic neuropeptide-mediated effects, such as vasodilatation, pruritus, and subjective pain.[59] As individual neuropeptides and their functions are further characterized, specific agonists and antagonists may prove to have specific anti-inflammatory and vasoactive properties. For instance, a topically applied CGRP agonist may improve symptomatic Raynaud phenomenon. Topical application of vasoactive neuropeptides might produce a long-lived "natural blush." Selective neuropeptide agonists and antagonists may find utility as tools for the manipulation of local and systemic immune responses. Perhaps these compounds could modify ascending nociceptive and tactile pathways, mitigating painful impulses, while amplifying pleasurable tactile sensations.

If stressful environmental experiences can hamper immune function, could beneficial environmental manipulations improve immune function, thereby ameliorating immune-related skin conditions? For example, just as β-blockers are used by many individuals to decrease autonomic arousal due to anxiety associated with a speech or musical performance, could an analogous approach decrease the likelihood of a stress-induced herpetic episode?

An even more powerful mood-modifying effect could be attained by simultaneously manipulating tactile, mental/visual imagery, olfactory modalities, and, while not discussed herein, aural stimuli. Such an approach is fundamental to holistic medicine, which emphasizes synergistic treatment using multiple methods of CNS stimulation, such as biofeedback, herbal medicine, and mechanical manipulation.

In a similar fashion, a cosmetic application containing compounds designed to induce cutaneous flushing, while enhancing tactile sensation, coupled with a pleasing fragrance, may enhance an individual's subjective well-being. Conversely, blockade of erythema or flushing by topical application of inhibitors of nitric oxide production or other vasocontrictor molecules could have analogous cosmetic applications. Although topical medications are used for a host of conditions in dermatology, no topical psychiatric medications have been developed. Perhaps this area holds promise for future development.

Restorative fragrances, whether in cosmetics or perfumes, have only begun to be applied in settings other than cosmesis. Cosmetics are typically used to enhance appearance, a sense of youthfulness, and self-esteem. Studies noted herein have suggested that scents have positive effects on function, mood, and anxiety. Because many skin conditions have a multifactorial origin, including psychiatric components, combined treatment with psychotropic scents and creams in conjunction with visualization and autohypnotic techniques may prove beneficial in select clinical settings.[6–8,51,53,58,59]

In conclusion, an attempt has been made to synthesize literature from various disciplines regarding NICE connections relevant to mind-body interactions in dermatology. Neuropeptides and other still poorly characterized messengers may serve as important communication molecules mediating nervous, immune, and skin health. Appearance, although often relegated to a minor concern in overall health, plays a crucial role in the maintenance of self-esteem and mental and physical health. Dermatologists play a critical role in maintaining and improving skin health and appearance and can play a pivotal role in recognizing and exploiting these interactions clinically. The interconnections described herein suggest a window into brain functioning, immune system, and skin health that we are only starting to fathom. Some of the studies outlined above suggest that seemingly trivial perturbations, such as tactile nociceptive and olfactory stimulation, might have profound neuroendocrine effects. The simplest of tamperings may ultimately influence the very substrate of the human mind.

The authors would like to thank John Parrish, MD, Richard Granstein, MD, Rebecca Campen, MD, Ned Cassem, MD, Scott Rauch, MD, and Nancy Etcoff, PhD, for helpful comments on earlier drafts of the manuscript for this article.

References

1. Darwin C. *Origin of Species*. New York, NY: PF Collier; 1909.
2. Eisenberg DM, Kessler RC, Foster C, Norlock FE, Calkins DR, Delbanco TL. Unconventional medicine in the United States: prevalence, costs, and patterns of use. *N Engl J Med.* 1993; 328:246–252.
3. Gordon JS. Alternative medicine and the family physician. *Am Fam Physician.* 1996; 54:2205–2212.
4. Kent J, Coates TJ, Pelletier KR, O'Regan B. Unexpected recoveries: spontaneous remission and immune functioning. *Adv Inst Adv Health.* 1986;6:66–73.
5. Locke SE, Colligan D. *The Healer Within: The New Medicine of Mind and Body*. New York, NY: Dutton; 1986.
6. Field T, Morrow C, Valdeon C, Larson S, Kuhn C, Schanberg S. Massage reduces anxiety in child and adolescent psychiatric patients. *J Am Acad Child Adolesc Psychiatry.* 1992; 31:125–131.
7. Buchbauer G, Jirovetz L. Aromatherapy: use of fragrances and essential oils as medicaments. *Flavour Fragrance J.* 1994;9:217–222.
8. Knask SC. Ambient odor's effect on creativity, mood, and perceived health. *Chem Senses.* 1992;17:27–35.
9. Komori T, Fujiwara R, Tanida M, Nomura J. *Potential antidepressant effects of lemon odor in rats.* 1995;5:477–480.
10. O'Leary A. Stress, emotion, and human immune function. *Psychol Bull.* 1990; 108:363–382.
11. Pennisi E. Neuroimmunology: tracing molecules that make the brain-body connection. *Science.* 1997;275:930–931.
12. Brambilla F. Psychoneuroimmunology: a scientific domain of the future or a dream from the past? *CNS Spectrums.* 1998;31:41–51.
13. Tsuchiya T, Horii I. Epidermal cell proliferative activity assessed by proliferating cell nuclear antigen (PCNA) decreases following immobilization-induced stress in male Syrian hamsters. *Psychoneuroimmunology.* 1996;21:111–117.
14. Tsuchiya T, Nakayama Y, Sato A. Somatic afferent regulation of plasma corticosterone in anesthetized rats. *Jpn J Physiol.* 1991;41:169–176.
15. Tsuchiya T, Nakayama Y, Sato A. Somatic afferent regulation of plasma luteinizing hormone and testosterone in anesthetized rats. *Jpn J Physiol.* 1992;42:539–547.
16. Blalock JE. The syntax of immune neuroendocrine communication. *Immunol Today.* 1994;15:504–511.
17. Stefano GB, Salzet B, Fricchione GL. Enkelytin and opioid peptide association in invertebrates and vertebrates: immune activation and pain. *Immunol Today.* 1998;19:265–268.
18. Etcoff N. *Survival of the Prettiest: The Science of Beauty*. New York, NY: Doubleday & Co Inc. In press.
19. Christenson G, O'Sullivan RL. Trichotillomania: rational treatment options. *CNS Drugs.* 1996; 6:23–34.
20. O'Sullivan RL, Phillips KA, Keuthen NJ, Wilhelm S. Near fatal skin picking from delusional body dysmorphic disorder responsive to fluvoxamine. *Psychosomatics.* In press.
21. Gupta MA, Gupta AK, Schork NJ, Ellis CN. Depression modulates pruritus perception: a study of pruritis in psoriasis, atopic dermatitis, and chronic idiopathic urticaria. *Psychosom Med.* 1994;56:36–40.
22. Lotti T, Hautmann G, Panconesi E. Neuropeptides in skin. *J Am Acad Dermatol.* 1995;33:482–496.
23. Manuck SB, Cohen S, Rabin BS, et al. Individual differences in cellular immune response to stress. *Psychol Sci.* 1991;2:111–115.
24. Solomon GF. Whither psychoneuroimmunology? a new era of immunology, of psychosomatic medicine, and of neuroscience. *Brain Behav Immun.*1993;7:352–366.
25. Hickie I, Hickie C, Lloyd A, et al. Impaired in vivo immune responses in patients with melancholia. *Br J Psychiatry.* 1993;162:651–657.
26. Wilkin JK. The red face: flushing disorders. *Clin Dermatol.* 1993;11:211–223.
27. Koblenzer CS. Psychologic aspects of aging and the skin. *Clin Dermatol.* 1996;14:171–177.
28. Farber EM, Nall ML. The natural history of psoriasis in 5,600 patients. *Dermatologica.* 1974; 148:1–18.
29. Farber EM, Bright RD, Nall ML. Psoriasis: a questionnaire of 2144 patients. *Arch Dermatol.* 1968;98:248–459.
30. Wessly SC, Lewis GH. The classification of psychiatric morbidity in attenders at a dermatology clinic. *Br J Psychiatry.* 1989;155:686–691.
31. Weidermann CJ. Shared recognition molecules in the brain and lymphoid tissues: the polypeptide mediator network of psychoneuroimmunology. *Immunol Lett.* 1987;16:371–378.

32. Tsuchiya T, Kishomoto J, Granstein RD, Nakayama Y. Quantitative analysis of cutaneous calcitonin gene–related peptide content in response to acute cutaneous mechanical or thermal stimuli and immobilization-induced stress in rats. *Neuropeptides.* 1996;30;149–157.

33. Torii, H, Hosoi J, Asahina A, Granstein RD. Calcitonin gene–related peptide and Langerhans cell function. *J Invest Dermatol Symp Proc.* 1997;2:82–86.

34. Blalock JE. A molecular basis for bidirectional communication between the immune and neuroendocrine systems. *Physiol Rev.* 1989;69:1–32.

35. Reichlin S. Neuroendocrine-immune interactions. *N Engl J Med.* 1993;329:1246–1253.

36. Karanth SS, Springall DR, Kuhn DM, Levene MM, Polak JM. An immunocytochemical study of cutaneous innervation and the distribution of neuropeptides and protein gene product 9.5 in man and commonly employed laboratory animals. *Am J Anat.* 1991;191:369–383.

37. Ostiere LS, Cowen T, Rustin MH. Neuropeptides in the skin of patients with atopic dermatitis. *Clin Exp Dermatol.* 1995;20:462–467.

38. Pincelli C, Fantini F, Giardino L, et al. Autoradiographic detection of substance P receptors in normal and psoriatic skin. *J Invest Dermatol.* 1993;101:301–304.

39. Payan DG, Brewster DR, Missirian-Bastian A, Goetzl EJ. Substance P recognition by a subset of human T lymphocytes. *J Clin Invest.* 1984; 74:1532–1539.

40. von Restorff B, Kemeny L, Michel G, Ruzicka T. Specific binding of substance P in normal human keratinocytes. *J Invest Dermatol.* 1992;98:510.

41. Bunker CB, Goldsmith PC, Leslie TA, Hayes N, Foreman JC, Dowd PM. Calcitonin gene–related peptide, endothelin-1, the cutaneous microvasculature and Raynaud's phenomenon. *Br J Dermatol.* 1996;134:399–406.

42. Terenghi G, Chen S, Carrington AL, Polak JM, Tomiinson DR. Changes in sensory neuropeptides in dorsal root ganglion and spinal cord of spontaneously diabetic BB rats: a quantitative immunohistochemical study. *Acta Diabetol.* 1994;31:198–204.

43. Hosoi J, Murphy GF, Egan CL, et al. Regulation of Langerhans cell function by nerves containing calcitonin gene–related peptide. *Nature.* 1993;363:159–163.

44. Girolomoni G, Tigelaar RE. Peptidergic neurons and vasoactive intestinal peptide modulate experimental delayed-type hypersensitivity reactions. *Ann N Y Acad Sci.* 1992;650:9–12.

45. Ichinose M, Asai M, Imai K, Savada M. Enhancement of phagocytosis in mouse macrophages by pituitary adenylate cyclase activating polypeptide (PACAP) and related peptides. *Immunopharmacology.* 1995;30:217–224.

46. Levins PC, Carr D, Fisher JE, Momtaz K, Parrish JA. Plasma beta-endorphin and beta-lipotropin response to ultraviolet radiation. *Lancet.* 1983; 16:166.

47. Wintzen M, Yaar M, Burbach PH, Gilchrest BA. Pro-opiomelanocortin gene product regulation in keratinocytes. *J Invest Dermatol.* 1996; 106:673–678.

48. Qureshi AA, Lerner LH, Lerner EA. From bedside to the bench and back: nitric oxide and the cutis. *Arch Dermatol.* 1996;132:889–893.

49. Ingber DE. Tensegrity: the architectural basis of cellular mechanotransduction. *Am Rev Physiol.* 1997;59:575–579.

50. Stoddart DM. *The Scented Ape: The Biology and Culture of Human Odour*. New York, NY: Cambridge University Press; 1990.

51. Redd WH, Manne SL, Peters B, Jacobsen PB, Schmidt H. Fragrance administration to reduce anxiety during MR imaging. *J Magn Reson Imag.* 1994;4:623–626.

52. Steiner J, Lidar-Lifschitz D, Perl E. Taste and odor: reactivity in depressive disorders: a multidisciplinary approach. *Percept Mot Skills.* 1993;7:1331–1346.

53. Doty RL. *Olfactory Dysfunction in Neurodegenerative Disorders: Smell and Taste in Health and Disease*. New York, NY: Raven Press; 1991:735–751.

54. Kirk-Smith MD, Van-Toller C, Dodd G. Unconscious odour conditioning in human subjects. *Biol Psychol.* 1983;17:221–231.

55. Stern K, McClintock MK. Regulation of ovulation by human pheromones. *Nature.* 1998; 392:177–179.

56. Matsunami H, Buck LB. A multigene family encoding a diverse array of putative pheromone receptors in mammals. *Cell.* 1997;90:775–784.

57. Bertollo DN, Cowen MA, Levy AV. Hypometabolism in olfactory cortical projection areas of male patients with schizophrenia: an initial positron emission tomography study. *Psychiatry Res.* 1996;60:113–116.

58. Martzke JS, Kopala LC, Good KP. Olfactory dysfunction in neuropsychiatric disorders: review and methodological considerations. *Biol Psychiatry.* 1997;42:721–732.

59. Lotti T, Teofoli P, Tsampau D. Treatment of aquagenic pruritus with topical capsaicin cream. *J Am Acad Dermatol.* 1994;30:232–235.

22 Mind-Body Medicine

Practical Applications in Dermatology

Michael R. Bilkis, MD, MSC; Kenneth A. Mark, MD
From the New York University Medical Center, New York, NY.

It is only recently that Western physicians are rediscovering the link between thought and health. The spectrum of causative factors in inflammatory dermatoses are often multifactorial. Stress and negative thoughts are major factors in dermatologic conditions. This article begins with some basic information on the ways that thoughts affect health. Practical methods of intervention including meditation, journal writing, affirmations, prayer, biofeedback, and hypnosis are presented.

Arch Dermatol. 1998;134:1437–1441

Have you ever wondered how your thoughts affect your health? Did you know that you can improve your health by changing the way you think and respond to events in your life? This article covers the basics of several different techniques in mind-body medicine. Additionally, 2 pathways are presented that represent the ways thoughts can affect health. Metaphors are used to help explain certain principles and treatments.

It is extremely important for all physicians to have an understanding of the basic principles of mind-body interactions because it has been shown that there are direct connections between the central nervous system and the immune system.[1] These connections include

> compartmentalized innervation with noradrenergic sympathetic fibers of primary and secondary lymphoid organs, neuropeptide

and neurotransmitter receptors on immune cells and cytokine production by activated immune cells that can influence brain function.[1]

Additionally, it has been found that Langerhans cells have neuropeptide receptors and also express neurotrophic factors, suggesting that there is bidirectional communication between the two.[2] Therefore, it is reasonable to conclude that the immune system may be influenced by thoughts and other functions of the brain. If this is so, then we can also conclude that most of the common dermatologic problems such as adult acne, rosacea, eczema, psoriasis, and other nonspecific inflammatory disorders may be directly influenced by the patient's thoughts and emotions. While most dermatologic problems are multifactorial in origin, in this article we only discuss the causative role of thoughts and emotions in the development of disease. In some patients, this may be the primary causative component, while in others it may be a tertiary or minor component. In all cases, however, knowledge of mind-body interactions and mind-body interventions can be useful in improving a patient's dermatologic condition and, in most cases, their quality of life.

To begin, construct a picture in your mind that sees every human being as consisting of 3 distinct bodies: physical, mental, and emotional. The 3 are intimately connected and changes in one will produce changes in the others. Each body vibrates at a different energetic frequency, therefore any changes in these bodies will occur at its specified rate. For example, the mind operates at the highest frequency. Throughout the day, the mind creates many thoughts and most people will quickly jump from one thought to the next and back again without much difficulty. The emotional body operates at a lower vibrational rate than the mind, and changes of state in the emotional body occur at a slower rate than in the mental body. A good example of the ease with which shifts occur in the emotional body is a child. If the child is happily playing and something occurs that upsets the child, he/she will freely express displeasure, usually by crying. A few moments later, tears are replaced by a smile. Whereas, the physical body operates at the lowest vibrational rate and changes in the physical body occur at a much slower rate than changes in the other two. To understand this concept better, consider the reaction of a person who sees a car heading straight for him/her and almost gets hit by it. The first reaction probably is the thought, "Oh no!" Fear quickly follows the recognition of danger, which releases hormones, including adrenaline, and the person moves out of the way. Once the event is over, the person may think, "I am OK" and the fear may slowly be replaced by feelings of gratitude. Finally, slowest of all, the physical body begins to return to a relaxed parasympathetic state.

Normally, all 3 bodies respond to and easily return to baseline following changes from external stimuli. Pathologic manifestation occurs when there is a problem with the ease in which the mental body returns to baseline. For a pathway that may explain how negative thoughts can lead to pathologic changes in the physical body see Figure 1. A negative thought form can be metaphorically thought of as a "demon" who has taken up residence in a person's consciousness. It constantly makes itself known and whenever the person acknowledges it and feeds into it, the demon grows stronger. For many people, this thought eventually grows so strong that they may develop the belief that it is true and unchangeable. As thought forms become beliefs, emotions become frozen in a negative state, and the body enters a chronic sympathetic state often termed *stress*. As a result, the normal homeostatic mechanisms fail and disease appears. The type of disease that manifests is dependent on the degrees of change in the body and the genetic predisposition of the individual.

Negative thoughts are one of the more prevalent contributors to stress. Stress is the result of a person's response to external stimuli and not the events themselves. From the viewpoint of traditional Chinese medicine, when stress is internalized, the flow of vital life energy throughout all 3 bodies is impeded.[3] This vital life energy is called *chi* in Chinese, *ki* in Japanese, and *prana* in Sanskrit (India). To better understand the effects of stress on a person's chi, imagine that a healthy person is like a deep river, flowing smoothly on its course. A person on the shore throwing rocks of all different sizes into the river represents stressful events. As the number of rocks increases, the river's flow becomes more turbulent. This corresponds to turbulence in the flow of chi and the appearance of physical problems. Therefore, treatment plans must include a method of preventing the accumulation of more stress and, moreover, a plan for removing the stress that is already in place.

There are many different techniques in mind-body medicine for achieving these goals. Figure 2 illustrates a pathway for reversing the disease process and creating health. In dermatology, disease usually falls into several major categories such as acquired inflammatory dermatoses, congenital dermatoses, and noninflammatory dermatoses/tumors. Based on observations in the office, stress appears to be one of the most prevalent components in the

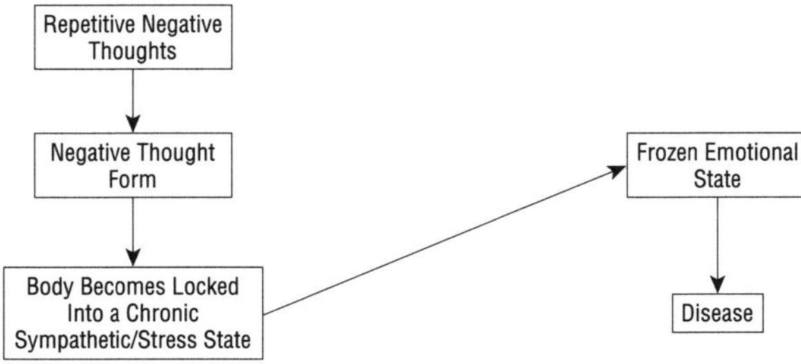

Figure 1. Thought-disease pathway.

Affirmation

Positive Thought Form

Negative Thought Form

Positive Thought Form

Fleeting Negative Thoughts

Release of Frozen Emotional State

Body Relaxes and Moves Into a Parasympathetic State

Health

Figure 2. Thought-healing pathway.

cause and severity of most inflammatory skin conditions. Through the use of mind-body techniques for the reduction of stress, most inflammatory dermatologic conditions can be helped to some extent. Acquired inflammatory dermatoses are the most amenable to mind-body techniques because their life cycle is one that waxes and wanes. Other dermatologic problems can also improve, to some degree, with mind-body techniques. In all cases, however, the quality of life of the patient can be greatly improved with mind-body techniques.

We divide mind-body techniques into 2 major categories: techniques practiced by the patient and techniques used by the practitioner with the patient. The first category includes meditation, affirmations, journal writing, prayer, exercise, reading spiritual books, and biofeedback. The second category includes hypnosis and Neurolinguistic Programming (NLP, explained later). The techniques listed above that are practiced by the patient represent the categories of the mind-body techniques that are easy to do and readily available. There are many classes and books available that list a myriad of other techniques and spiritual practices.

Meditation

Meditation is the practice of bringing one's total focus into the present moment. The first reports in American literature of the physical effects of meditation were made by Herbert Benson, MD, a cardiologist at Harvard Medical School, Boston, Mass. Benson observed that after 20 minutes of meditation participants' heart rate, breathing rate, blood pressure, oxygen consumption, carbon dioxide production, and serum lactic acid levels all decreased, while skin resistance increased and blood flow was altered. He called this phenomenon the "relaxation effect."[4] Similar physiological responses have been found to occur with other techniques such as hypnosis, progressive muscular relaxation, and autogenic training.[5]

One of the simplest forms of meditation involves sitting comfortably and focusing on the breath. For most Westerners, this means sitting in a chair with the feet flat on the floor and the hands in the lap. A word or phrase is then repeated over and over for a specified length of time. This word or phrase is called a mantra. Most people will find that their mind will wander at times and they will begin thinking of different things. It is important that, when one becomes aware of the wandering, he/she lets go of the superfluous thoughts and returns to following the breath and repeating the mantra. A meditator must be willing to let go of extraneous thoughts, without judgment, and return to his/her point of focus.[6] Since focus is the key to meditation, it can take many forms—sitting quietly, painting, playing an instrument, participating in a sport, or working out at the gym. During any of these activities, the person's mind becomes clear of everything but what he/she is doing at that specific moment. The goal of meditation is to bring one's full awareness into the present moment and simply be. When this occurs, not only can a person induce relaxation but he/she also can begin to bring the benefits of meditation into all aspects of his/her life.[7]

Affirmations

Affirmations are statements made in the present tense, containing only positive statements, and expressed in the first-person singular. The use of affirmations provides a simple and effective vehicle to access the "thought-healing pathway" as illustrated in Figure 2. Many of our dermatology patients look at themselves in the mirror and have decided that their problem is so awful that they are embarrassed to go out in public. Some of these patients may even have a minor skin problem, yet they refuse to believe that the problem is minor or that it is safe to be seen in public. These beliefs started out as repetitive negative thoughts (Figure 1). The use of affirmations occupies the consciousness with positive thoughts, leaving no room for negative thoughts. By repetitively using affirmations, the patient is unable to subvocalize the 2 opposing thoughts at the same time. With time, the patient's neurologic pathways shift and the positive thoughts can predominate. For example, a patient who has spider veins states that she is disfigured and cannot wear shorts. One possible affirmation for her to say may be, "I am beautiful in every way." It is not important for her to believe what she is saying; the belief comes later. The important thing is for her to say the positive words. Our advice to our patients is to use the affirmation every morning and also whenever they become aware of the presence of the negative thoughts. The repeated use of affirmations provides a powerful tool for eliminating negative self-talk, which is a major contributor to stress and turmoil in people's lives.[8]

Journal Writing

Journal writing is the next, most simple technique to use for self-help. As with affirmations, writing in a journal requires no classes and the only skills needed are reading and writing. Patients are instructed to set aside the same time each day for their journal writing. At the start of a session, it is important to sit quietly for a few moments and take some breaths to become centered. The next step is to write whatever comes to mind, without stopping to think about what is being written. The final step is to read over the entry. Writing in a journal helps unlock the unconsciousness and bring repressed emotions and thoughts up into consciousness. It also creates a new perspective for the patient to approach his/her challenges. Studies of college students and executives have shown that immune function can be improved through the use of a journal. In addition, when the test subjects stopped writing in their journals, their immune function returned to the prestudy baseline after about 6 months.[9] The following comments were made by 2 patients regarding their journal writing experience.
"Whenever I write in my journal, I feel like the problems I was having are now in my book and no longer in my body."
"I feel lighter . . . like a load has been lifted from me."

Prayer

Dossey in his book *Healing Words*[10] defines prayer as communication with the Absolute (this is the name he chose to represent God). In this book, he states that there are more than 300 experiments using prayer involving living organisms, from microbes to humans, and that about half of the studies show that prayer can cause a statistically significant change in the test subjects. The studies he quotes in his book show that all types of prayer are equally effective, including prayers that specify an outcome vs nonspecific types of prayer such as, "Thy will be done." The studies showed differences in an individual's ability to evoke a positive effect from prayer. In essence some people were better "prayers" than others. It appears that the more effective prayers were more able to alter their state of consciousness and enter a more meditative or prayerfulness state than those who were less effective prayers. It is helpful to suggest to patients that prayer be approached like a meditation, in which the object of the meditation is the prayer itself. With this approach the prayer experience can be intensified. Most studies on prayer have been performed with microscopic organisms like bacteria and fungi.[11] One of the most profound studies of prayer and health was reported by cardiologist Byrd.[12] In his study, a computer assigned the 393 patients admitted to the coronary care unit to either a group that was prayed for by outside prayer groups or to a control group. This study was done according to a strict double-blind protocol.

The results of this study showed that the prayed-for patients differed significantly from the control group in the following areas:

- They were 5 times less likely than the control group to require antibiotics (3 compared with 16 patients).
- They were 3 times less likely to develop pulmonary edema (6 compared with 18 patients).
- None of the prayed-for group required intubation while 12 in the control group did.
- Fewer patients in the prayed-for group died, although this was the only result that was not statistically significant.[13]

While the results seem difficult to believe, the study was well designed. If the focus of the study were a medication, then it might be heralded as a new miracle drug. This study had some flaws, which Dossey discusses in *Healing Words*.[10] The flaws, however, are overshadowed by the positive implications, if even part of the study's results are true.

Biofeedback

Biofeedback is a technique that uses machinery to measure autonomic functions such as heart rate or muscle tension. The patient uses various imagery exercises and learns how to consciously alter these autonomic functions. In the rheumatology literature, the use of biofeedback has been shown to be beneficial in the treatment of Raynaud disease and phenomenon. In this study, patients were taught biofeedback first as a relaxation technique and then as a method of increasing the skin temperature in their fingers. All patients in the study were able to elevate their baseline fingertip temperature. The results suggested that biofeedback is useful in the treatment of Raynaud disease and phenomenon, and that "further studies were required to completely evaluate the efficacy and clinical significance of biofeedback."[9]

Hypnosis and NLP

The essential goal of both hypnosis and NLP (Richard Bandler & Associates Seminars Group International, Hopatcong, NJ) is to help a patient access resources that he/she has available in his/her subconscious and use them to change his/her behavior. Milton Erickson is considered to be the father of modern hypnosis and was a firm believer that everyone is born possessing all the resources needed to create new behaviors. The problem is that most people have set up conscious and unconscious blocks that thwart their healing process. Erickson used hypnosis to help his patients bypass these blocks and overcome their problems. Richard Bandler and John Grinder studied the works of Erickson and other therapists who had the reputation of being miracle workers when it came to curing patients with behavioral disorders. They found that Erickson and other therapists used certain language patterns when working with their patients. Bandler and Grinder developed specific language models based on their study that achieved success for various mental conditions. In the 1970s, they began to teach these models in conjunction with hypnosis and called their new technology Neurolinguistic Programming.[11,13]

Neurolinguistic Programming is a process-oriented science as opposed to the content-oriented science of traditional psychotherapy. This means that an NLP practitioner only needs to know the type of problem that the patient is having and what the patient desires as the outcome of the session. The actual details of the situation and the patient's history is unimportant to make therapeutic changes. One of us (M.R.B.), for instance, had a patient who became very stressed at work and her acne flare up corresponded with the start of a new job. During the session, he helped the patient create a relaxed state and associate this relaxed state with events that previously triggered her stress. The specific details of what caused her stress at work were not important to help her overcome and feel better about the situation.

The first author (M.R.B) has used hypnosis and NLP for several types of problems: treatment of neurogenic skin problems, stress reduction, improvement of self-image and quality of life as a result of a skin problem, and as anesthesia for minor surgical procedures/sclerotherapy. The following are examples of treatments with the NPL techniques that the first author used with some of his patients. The explanations of the actual procedures have been simplified and, for the sake of brevity, examples of the language patterns used are not included.

Patient 1, an aspiring actress and model in her middle 20s, complained of constantly picking at her skin that created marks and scars. This problem was distressing to her. She denied any pruritus. The essence of the first author's work with his patient was to suggest that she develop new behaviors that provided the same benefit as the unwanted behavior. Moreover, it was suggested that these new behaviors be fully evaluated by her subconscious so that the negative aspects are minimized. All negative behaviors have some sort of reward for the person engaged in that behavior. If we simply "command" the person to stop the unwanted action, then they may develop an even worse behavior or resume the old one. After 1 session with her, the patient completely stopped picking at her skin. This remission lasted for about 1 year when she returned complaining that the problem was back. Once again, hypnosis was used and the condition resolved itself after 1 hypnosis session.

Patient 2, a 30-year-old white woman, complained of a scar on her left thigh. The scar was flat, brown, and 3 × 1 cm. Objectively, this was not a terrible problem. Subjectively, however, she stated that the scar was so horrible and disfiguring that she could not expose it in public. For example, she stated that if she needed to use a communal dressing room, she would either wait until it was empty or stand in a corner with her hip facing the wall before removing her pants. A common reaction to a patient with this type of problem might be to try to convince her that the scar is barely noticeable and she should stop obsessing about it. Had that been done, she would have looked for a new physician because her point of view would not have been acknowledged. Instead, it was acknowledged how awful this problem was for her and NLP techniques were used to neutralize her emotional reaction to the scar. On the follow-up visit 1 month later, she said that while she did not like having the scar, she no longer had any problems exposing it in public. In this case, the use of NLP did not improve the appearance of the problem; it did, however, greatly improve the patient's quality of life.

Patient 3 (a woman) was treated with sclerotherapy and patient 4 (a woman) was treated for multiple electrodessicated and curreted dermatosis papulosa nigra. In both cases, a hypnotic induction was done and suggestions of anesthesia were given. Patient 3 stated that there was no pain compared with the severe leg cramping she had experienced during previous sclerotherapy sessions. Patient 4 also experienced no pain while the procedure was performed. A 1.5-cm seborrheic keratosis was even electrodessicated and curreted from her cheek without any memory of it ever happening. As an aside, patient 4 has had many sessions for the treatment of her dermatosis papulosa nigra and on her all subsequent visits hypnotic anesthesia was induced in less than 1 minute.

Conclusions

In this article, we have offered some illustrations of how a person's health and thoughts are connected and how stress plays a role in the origin and exacerbation of health problems. The old mechanistic viewpoint of health and disease, as started by Rene Descartes, is now known to be obsolete. The connection between our thoughts and health has been well established thanks to the work of many health care practitioners, including Larry Dossey, MD, Bernie Seigal, MD, Herbert Benson, MD, Dean Ornish, MD, Jon Kabat-Zin, PhD, Joan Borysenko, MD, and others. The field of mind-body medicine is vast and offers the dermatologist an opportunity to treat his/her patients on more levels than simply prescribing medications for symptomatic relief. Our responsibility as physicians is to promote health in addition to combating disease. In almost all cases, the medications we prescribe will help alleviate the symptoms, yet they do little to induce a remission. Through the use of mind-body medicine, improved nutrition, exercise, and general improvement in lifestyle, we as physicians can play a pivotal role in teaching our patients how to be healthy.

Our special thanks to Hilary Bilkis, MS, LMT, for proofreading and editing the manuscript.

References

1. Lotti T, Hautmann G, Panconesi E. Neuropeptides in skin. *J Am Acad Dermatol.* 1995;33:482–496.
2. Torii H, Yan Z, Hosoi J, Granstein R. Expression of neurotrophic factors and neuropeptide receptors by Langerhans cells and the Langerhans cell-like cell line XS52: further support for a functional relationship between Langerhans cells and epidermal nerves. *J Invest Dermatol.* 1997;109:586–591.
3. Beinfield H, Korngold E. *Between Heaven and Earth: A Guide to Chinese Medicine.* New York, NY: Ballantine Books; 1991.
4. Benson H, Beary JF, Carol MP. The relaxation response. *Psychiatry.* 1974;37:37–46.
5. Kutz I, Borysenko JZ, Benson H. Meditation and psychotherapy: a rationale for the integration of dynamic psychotherapy: the relaxation response, and mindfulness training. *Am J Psychiatry.* 1985;142:1–8.
6. Hanh TN. *Peace Is Every Step.* New York, NY: Bantam Books; 1991.
7. Levine B. *Your Body Believes Every Word You Say.* Lower Lake, Calif: Aslan Publishing; 1991.
8. Siegel MD. *Peace, Love and Healing.* New York, NY: Harper Perennial; 1990:224–225.
9. Yocum DE, Hodes R, Sundstrom WR, Cleeland CS. Use of biofeedback training in the treatment of Raynaud's disease and phenomenon. *J Rheumatol.* 1985;12:90–93.
10. Dossey L. *Healing Words.* San Francisco, Calif: Harper Collins Publishers; 1993.
11. Bandler R, Grinder J. *Trance-formations.* Mohab, Utah: Real People Press; 1981.
12. Byrd R. Positive therapeutic effects of intercessary prayer in a coronary care unit population. *South Med J.* 1988;81:826–829.
13. Bandler R, Grinder J. *Frogs to Princes.* Mohab, Utah: Real People Press; 1979.

23 Spirituality in Medical Practice

Robert J. Thomsen, MD
From the Los Alamos Medical Center, Los Alamos, NM.

Body, mind, and spirit are integrally connected. Medical training in the Western world has been strong concerning the more easily measured physical aspects, and on the mental needs it has been virtually mute on how to minister to the spiritual needs of our patients. Learning the spiritual aspects of medical care is not a typical part of the medical school curriculum, and yet it is emerging as something that our patients want and expect us to do as part of our caring for them. Herein I discuss the role of spirituality in medical practice, how it relates to alternative medical practices, methods to use to grow spiritually, and ways to apply your spirituality to medical practice.

Arch Dermatol. 1998;134:1443–1446

Why are you in the field of health care? Is it for the prestige? Interesting problems to solve? Financial security? To satisfy the demands of family? To help people who are ill? These are questions that everyone who entered medical school has consciously or subconsciously addressed, but questions that we rarely consider in the midst of a demanding practice. To answer them we must examine our core values and be honest with ourselves about our motivation for being in the health care field. If helping people who are ill is a primary reason for you, then the rest of this article may make some sense. If it is not, then it will seem total bunk and you may as well not read further.

We will assume, then, that helping people is a primary goal for you, and that earnestly pursuing that goal provides you with satisfaction. Let us contemplate for a moment on some of the sources of dissatisfaction in our role as a health care provider. Many may come immediately to mind, such as paperwork, insufficient time to interact with patients, patient dissatisfaction, failure of patients to follow through with our recommendations, and finally, the limitations on our abilities to really help a person.

Our Human Limitations

We work hard to stay current with the newest surgical methods, new physical therapy modalities, the newest medications, and better ways to use the old medications. The volume of literature about the technical aspects of medicine is more than enough to totally consume all efforts to stay current. And yet we know in our hearts that even this would not be enough. There are some problems that are just not fixable by our skills and tools. There is a limit.

We all have tried to care for people who, despite our best efforts, skills, and intentions, just are not getting better. We have prescribed all the right medicines. We have done all the right tests. We are missing something. Unfortunately, we are not able to help everyone to the extent we want. We are frustrated and saddened when a disease like melanoma defeats our efforts to control it.

There are times too, puzzling times, when we know that we cannot help, and yet the patient gets better anyway, despite what we have done. Why? The answer eludes us, but obviously there is more to our care than we are capable of understanding. This is what we sometimes call psychosomatics. This is the territory of spirituality.

What Is Spirituality?

Spirituality is difficult to define. It can be regarded as that part of a person's being that involves the intangible nonphysical world. It is influenced by our core value systems, our psychological makeup, our religious beliefs, and our emotional subconscious memories. Spirituality cuts across all the major world religions. Each of us can probably think of spiritual people who do not participate in organized religion, and we can think of people who attend worship services regularly who are not particularly spiritual. There is a rapidly growing body of literature on spirituality. For example, Dossey[1] in his book discusses in detail the role of prayer in medical practice.

How are we to understand how spirituality works? It is impossible to really measure prayer or other aspects of spiritual practice.

Our Scientific Understanding

But must we understand how something works to use it skillfully? No. Just as we can learn the use of tools without knowing how they work, like a microwave oven, CD player, automobile, or computer, we can also apply skills of spirituality to our medical practice without understanding them. It takes knowing how and when to use certain skills to make them effective tools for us.

In every aspect of medical care there comes a time, a level of understanding, when, if we are absolutely honest we say, I do not know why. The reality is that science-based medicine can only go so far in caring for people. The unspoken scientific paradigm that permeates modern medical care says that everything can be explained by the scientific model if only we do more research. That is a flawed model. Everything cannot be explained. The Heisenberg uncertainty principle says that at a certain level we will never be able to know with certainty how the physical world works. There is something more. It can be called faith, and that is where spirituality is applied.

Just as we use the electrocautery machine effectively, so too we use other skills effectively; eg, a friendly smile, a handshake, a warm pat on the shoulder, or a prayer. Many of these techniques are eloquently discussed in a book by Shelley and Shelley[2] in a chapter entitled "Zen and the Art of Patient Maintenance." We can scarcely imagine the benefit of such skills to a patient. There are no double-blind studies for testing this, but we know instinctively that it is crucial.

Relationship of Spirituality to Alternative Health Care

Why do patients seek alternate forms of health care? Although alternative therapies can be expensive, especially when not covered by health insurance, they are not usually as expensive as conventional treatments. The alternative therapies are generally regarded as "natural" and therefore benevolent. People want to avoid the drugs with potentially harmful adverse effects, preferring treatments perceived as less toxic, although they may be less effective. Alternative treatments often sound true and relate more directly to people's personal experiences. For example, we can relate to the need to flush the toxic wastes from our liver since we flush the toxic wastes from our toilets.

The treatments in many alternative health care systems are based on intuitive reasoning. Intuition appeals to our spirituality directly for guidance and validation, and so frequently alternative health care practitioners will refer to spirituality and draw on spiritual foundations for validation and credibility. Alternative therapies and spirituality are often, then, linked—to the extent that we accept or reject the alternative health care method we accept or reject spirituality. The practitioner who claims to be scientifically based becomes unwilling to apply spirituality because that would appear to mean accepting alternative therapies. In reality alternative therapies have no monopoly on spirituality, and spirituality is as much the provence of science-based medicine as any other area. One way that our scientific paradigm refers to spirituality is in the term *psychosomatics*.

Psychosomatic Medicine

Psychosomatic illness is readily accepted as valid,[3] but there is no good way in the scientific paradigm to deal with it. It does not readily become the subject of scientific investigation because it cannot be quantified and measured easily. When we cannot explain something we tend to refer to it as psychosomatic, and leave it at that. We acknowledge the spiritual, but deny it at the same time, because we have had no training or experience in what to do in that arena. By ignoring the psychosomatic we neglect the spiritual sides of our patients.

Although there are limits on our scientific skills, there are other skills that can be developed to help our patients' spiritual skills. The rest of this article looks at some practical ways to develop spiritual skills.

Methods to Spirituality

In the following sections I examine what you can do by and for yourself to grow spiritually and progress on your own spiritual path; what you can do spiritually for the patients in your medical practice; what you can do spiritually with your patients; and what you can help the patient do for himself/herself in the area of spirituality.

For Ourselves

There are many methods to develop and practice a spiritual life. There are some practices that are virtually universal to all major religions such as worship, prayer, meditation, and fasting, although there are obvious cultural differences. I would suggest reading the book *Celebration of Discipline: The Path of Spiritual Growth* by Foster.[4] Foster is a Quaker with profound suggestions for living a spiritual life.

There is a caveat. There is potential for abuse of power. Spirituality should be used for good, but can be used in many ways for evil purposes. Seek the good. We little realize the power we have.

To help others spiritually you must be as integrated and centered as you can be. Of course, perfection is not attainable. It takes time and effort to develop spiritually. The spiritual life is a journey, and that journey is different for each and every individual. Seek your own journey, and be aware of where you think you are on that path. Develop the skills for your spiritual journey through study, prayer, meditation, worship, and community.

Study. Select carefully the materials you choose. There are many to choose from, but they should have proved the test of time. Read the Hebrew Bible, the New Testament, the Koran, the Way of Life of Lao-Tzu, the Talmud, the writings of the desert fathers, and other classics of religion. Nurture the spiritual part of your intellect as much as you would the scientific. But remember that the intellect is not enough.

Prayer. You must develop a prayer life. But what exactly is prayer? There are many forms of prayer, some are appropriate in the medical setting and some are not. I like to think of prayer as a conversation with God. In a conversation you must do your share of listening, and so it is with prayer. Prayer is not just talking. Listen in prayer as much as you talk. Include praise and thanksgiving in prayers before you ask for things. Intercessory prayer is the type of prayer that asks for something—the team to win, the person to be healed, or the car not to break down. Be careful with intercessory prayer to ask for things that are possible. We cannot ask that purple be green, or that triangles have 4 sides.

I like the serenity prayer very much that says,

> God, grant me serenity to accept the things I cannot change, courage to change the things I can, and the wisdom to know the difference; living one day at a time, enjoying one moment at a time; accepting hardship as a pathway to peace; taking, as Jesus did, this sinful world as it is, not as I would have it; trusting that You will make all things right if I surrender to Your will; so that I may be reasonably happy in this life and supremely happy with You forever in the next. Amen.

I also like the prayer of St Francis:

> Lord, make us instruments of your peace.
> Where there is hatred, let us sow love;
> where there is injury, pardon;
> where there is discord, union;
> where there is doubt, faith;
> where there is despair, hope;
> where there is darkness, light;
> where there is sadness, joy.

Grant that we may not so much seek
to be consoled as to console;
to be understood as to understand;
to be loved as to love.
For it is in giving that we receive;
it is in pardoning that we are pardoned; and
it is in dying that we are born to eternal life.

Meditation. Meditation means opening our subconscious, our soul, to the influences of higher powers. It is distinct from prayer, but similar, and there are many forms of meditation practice. Herbert Benson,[5] MD, has taught the relaxation response for many years. In this simple but effective form of meditation you concentrate solely on breathing and emptying the mind of other distractions. There are many sources of instruction in meditation, including books and seminars.

Worship. True worship involves prayer and meditation, but it also involves participating in spirituality with others, and there is great power in doing this.

Community. You must seek help. Just as you cannot learn medicine from a book you also cannot learn spirituality. This is not easy for physicians, who are constantly looked to and relied on as the authority figures. But all of the previous activities alone will not be sustained and directed without the help and support of a religious community. Now that "community" may be a spiritual advisor, or a pastor, or a rabbi, or it may be a Bible study group or congregation, but our spiritual growth needs to be nurtured by others, or it will be nothing. So seek the help of like-minded people. Seek for them and you will find them.

For the Patient

Admit that we are not omnipotent. The more honestly we admit this the more content we will be. Sincere humility will be appreciated by most patients, and be regarded as a strength rather than a weakness. Hubris, the opposite of humility, is probably the base cause for most lawsuits.

Pray for your patients. The most powerful thing we can do in our medical practice is to pray. Prayer helps us be the vessel and agent for the higher power to bring needed healing, and it helps us to be open to what the specific techniques of healing should be, whether it be prayer, or a healing service, or sweat lodge, or the latest corticosteroid cream, or methotrexate, or psoralen–UV-A. Prayer turns the ultimate responsibility for the patient's welfare over to a higher power, relieving us of the burden of being more than we can be.

I do not believe that it is necessary to ask patients for permission to pray for them. Ask in your prayers for help and guidance so that your medical skills might be best applied to the situation. Ask for what is best for the patient. Usually we think we know but sometimes what we think is best turns out not to be. The "Thy will be done" prayer is as effective as directed prayer.

In the morning as you look at the schedule for the day you might pray for specific people. Pray that they be improved, pray that they lose their anger, and pray that they understand their medical problem. Pray for yourself; that you might be a good listener to your patient's problems, that you apply the correct therapies, and that you be alert to the signs and symptoms of disease.

In the evening when office hours are over take a copy of your schedule and pray for the people you have seen. Pray that they may understand their problems and be motivated to do the right things. Pray for their other needs—the patient whose father is dying or whose wife just had a mastectomy or who is having trouble with his/her parents. Ask for healing of their whole self, not only their specific problems.

With the Patient

Know your patient. One aspect of American society that complicates dealing spiritually with a patient is the plurality of our religious beliefs and practices. Many of our patients have well-developed spiritual lives, but many are antagonistic to spirituality. Many have half-baked poorly organized inconsistent belief systems. Trying to pray with a person who is an avowed militant agnostic is not going to be a beneficial experience for either of you. It takes time and trust to know who you are dealing with. It cannot be done quickly, but it can be done.

One way to know your patients is to notice the jewelry that they are wearing. The cross necklace that a person is wearing may start a conversation about his/her beliefs.

Maugans[6] has proposed the mnemonic device "SPIRIT"ual history to help in remembering what to ask. S stands for Spiritual belief system; P, Personal spirituality; I, Integration with a spiritual community; R, Ritualized practices and Restrictions; I, Implications for medical care; and T, Terminal events planning. This spiritual history may take many visits to collect.

Pray. Offer to pray with or for the patient. This must be done with care and tact, but when properly done will be a powerful way to help. When people know that they are prayed for they receive a strength that is not measurable or explainable, but is real. You may tell the patient what you will be praying for, or just simply that you are praying for him/her.

Declare Your Spirituality. I believe it is inappropriate to actively proselytize in the office setting. To try to persuade someone to your personal beliefs is a misuse of the power entrusted to us as physicians. However, I think it is appropriate to indicate in some way our spiritual persuasion, perhaps by wearing a lapel pin cross or by a Star of David on the wall. These stand as silent invitations to discussion that the patient can accept or reject without potential repercussions from you. They give patients permission to bring up their spiritual concerns.

For the Patient to Do

Offer instruction in prayer or meditation. Patients may not know how to pray. With your experience in spiritual discipline you can teach and guide them. Tailor the advice to the spiritual background of the patient. If you force your spirituality on the patient it will not work. He/she will seek another physician. If you offer your spirituality, it can be received with joy.

Let your patients tell you what to do. Listen to their inner voice. Most of the time it will be the correct one.

Give your patient permission to pursue other forms of health care. Many will pursue alternate forms of health care whether you let them or not. Knowing them and what they are doing gives you all the more effectiveness in their care. And granting permission to be open with us also gives us more credibility in the patient's eyes. Now we are caring for them and giving them every chance to get better, not just the chances that our methods might give.

For You to Do Now

Where to start: Seek ye first the kingdom of God. If you do not have a background in spiritual concerns and are not part of a religious community, then begin your spirituality now. Now is the acceptable time. Do not put this off. You can do it. Say a prayer now. Even if it does not help a single patient it will help you. Pray. Meditate. Study. Worship. Seek community.

Seek reconciliation with other forms of alternative health care in your community to learn spirituality from them. If they reject you, it may be because they have been so long and so often rejected by the medical monolithic establishment that they are shy of consorting with it. I have experienced the hostility and rejection of alternative health care workers who have been hurt by rejection from the medical establishment. Give them time and earn their trust. This can only be done through genuine respect. What if you do not have genuine respect? Work on it and find it. Apply the tests of sincerity and effectiveness. Reject the shysters. Be honest and open with those who sincerely believe in what they are doing. Belief is a powerful thing.

Conclusions

Throughout the ages there have been men and women who were both highly religious people and highly skilled healers, and they applied their spirituality to their healing practices. But there has been an ever increasing split between those talents. Religious and spiritual ways of thinking have been steadily removed from scientific-based medical practice as we have come to know it in the 20th century. Thus, we have a tendency to dismiss the skills of a shaman just because modern scientific medicine is not being applied.

Can science-based medicine recapture the role of healer? Are we healers or are we applied medical technicians? How do we view ourselves? If we do not think of ourselves as healers we become technicians, manipulating the tools of our trade, and we cease to be real and complete healers. As technicians we will lose the respect that we had as healers.

Each of us is capable of becoming a healer, although that power comes not through our own power or initiative. We are capable of bringing peace and comfort to people who seek our help and advice, and this extends beyond the prescribing of medications and the dispensing of advice. It means caring for people and their concerns, of taking time to set an example for them.

Why seek spirituality? Because it works. How does it work? I do not know. I do not know at the molecular level how cortisone works, or what electrons look like. They work whether I understand them or not, and so does spirituality. When the spiritual needs of patients are sincerely met they will do better and receive better care. More important, the health care giver, the physician, is also going to be more whole, more healthy, and more integrated in body, mind, and spirit. Spirituality is an area to pursue both for your patients and you.

References

1. Dossey L. Healing Words: *The Power of Prayer and the Practice of Medicine*. San Francisco, Calif.: Harper San Francisco; 1987.

2. Shelley WB, Shelley ED. *Advanced Dermatologic Therapy.* Philadelphia, Pa: WB Saunders Co; 1987:4–9.

3. Koblenzer CS. *Psychocutaneous Disease*. Orlando, Fla: Grune & Stratton Inc; 1987.

4. Foster RJ. *Celebration of Discipline: The Path of Spiritual Growth*. San Francisco, Calif: Harper & Row Publishers; 1978.

5. Benson H. *The Relaxation Response*. Philadelphia, Pa: Avon Books; 1976.

6. Maugans TA. The SPIRITual history. *Arch Fam Med*. 1996;5:11–16.

24 A Close Look at Therapeutic Touch

Linda Rosa, BSN RN; Emily Rosa; Larry Sarner; Stephen Barrett, MD
From the Questionable Nurse Practices Task Force, National Council Against Health Fraud Inc (Ms L. Rosa), and the National Therapeutic Touch Study Group (Mr Sarner), Loveland, Colo; and Quackwatch Inc, Allentown, Pa (Dr Barrett). Ms E. Rosa is a sixth-grade student at Loveland, Colo.

Context
Therapeutic Touch (TT) is a widely used nursing practice rooted in mysticism but alleged to have a scientific basis. Practitioners of TT claim to treat many medical conditions by using their hands to manipulate a "human energy field" perceptible above the patient's skin.

Objective
To investigate whether TT practitioners can actually perceive a "human energy field."

Design
Twenty-one practitioners with TT experience for from 1 to 27 years were tested under blinded conditions to determine whether they could correctly identify which of their hands was closest to the investigator's hand. Placement of the investigator's hand was determined by flipping a coin. Fourteen practitioners were tested 10 times each, and 7 practitioners were tested 20 times each.

Main Outcome Measure
Practitioners of TT were asked to state whether the investigator's unseen hand hovered above their right hand or their left hand. To show the validity of TT theory, the practitioners should have been able to locate the investigator's hand 100% of the time. A score of 50% would be expected through chance alone.

Results
Practitioners of TT identified the correct hand in only 123 (44%) of 280 trials, which is close to what would be expected for random chance. There was no significant correlation between the practitioner's score and length of experience (r=0.23). The statistical power of this experiment was sufficient to conclude that if TT practitioners could reliably detect a human energy field, the study would have demonstrated this.

Conclusions

Twenty-one experienced TT practitioners were unable to detect the investigator's "energy field." Their failure to substantiate TT's most fundamental claim is unrefuted evidence that the claims of TT are groundless and that further professional use is unjustified.

JAMA. 1998;279:1005–1010

Therapeutic touch (TT) is a widely used nursing practice rooted in mysticism but alleged to have a scientific basis. Its practitioners claim to heal or improve many medical problems by manual manipulation of a "human energy field" (HEF) perceptible above the patient's skin. They also claim to detect illnesses and stimulate recuperative powers through their intention to heal. Therapeutic Touch practice guides[1–6] describe 3 basic steps, none of which actually requires touching the patient's body. The first step is centering, in which the practitioner focuses on his or her intent to help the patient. This step resembles meditation and is claimed to benefit the practitioner as well. The second step is assessment, in which the practitioner's hands, from a distance of 5 to 10 cm, sweep over the patient's body from head to feet, "attuning" to the patient's condition by becoming aware of "changes in sensory cues" in the hands. The third step is intervention, in which the practitioner's hands "repattern" the patient's "energy field" by removing "congestion," replenishing depleted areas, and smoothing out ill-flowing areas. The resultant "energy balance" purportedly stems disease and allows the patient's body to heal itself.[7]

Proponents of TT state that they have "seen it work."[8] In a 1995 interview, TT's founder said, "In theory, there should be no limitation on what healing can be accomplished."[9] Table 1 lists some claims made for TT in published reports.

Table 1. Claims Made for Therapeutic Touch

Calms colicky infants,[9] hospitalized infants,[10] women in childbirth,[11] trauma patients,[12] and hospitalized cardiovascular patients[13,14]
Promotes bonding between parents and infants[15]
Increases milk let down in breast-feeding mothers[16]
Helps children make sense of the world[17]
Protects nurses from burnout[18] and effects changes in their lifestyle[19]
Helps to evaluate situations where diagnosis is elusive[9]
Relieves acute pain,[20] especially from burns[21]
Relieves nausea,[22,23] diarrhea,[5] tension headaches,[24] migraine headaches,[21] and swelling in edematous legs and arthritic joints[7]
Decreases inflammation[25]
Breaks fever[21]
Remedies thyroid imbalances[5]
Helps skin grafts to seed[9]
Promotes healing of decubitus ulcers[7]
Alleviates psychosomatic illnesses[5]
Increases the rate of healing for wounds, bone and muscle injuries, and infections[26]
Relieves symptoms of Alzheimer disease,[27] acquired immunodeficiency syndrome,[5] menstruation,[28] and premenstrual syndrome[21]
Is an innovative means of social communication[29]
Is effective with the aged,[30,31] asthmatic or autistic children, stroke patients, and coma patients[9]
Supports people with multiple sclerosis and Raynaud disease[32]
Treats measles[33] and many different forms of cancer[34]
Comforts the dying[35–37]
Helps to bring some dead back to life[2]

Background

Professional Recognition

Proponents state that more than 100,000 people worldwide have been trained in TT technique,[38] including at least 43,000 health care professionals,[2] and that about half of those trained actually practice it.[39] Therapeutic Touch is taught in more than 100 colleges and universities in 75 countries.[5] It is said to be the most recognized technique used by practitioners of holistic nursing.[40] Considered a nursing intervention, it is used by nurses in at least 80 hospitals in North America,[33] often without the permission or even knowledge of attending physicians.[41–43] The policies and procedures books of some institutions recognize TT,[44] and it is the only treatment for the "energy-field disturbance" diagnosis recognized by the North American Nursing Diagnosis Association.[45] *RN*, one of the nursing profession's largest periodicals, has published many articles favorable to TT.[46–52]

Many professional nursing organizations promote TT. In 1987, the 50,000-member Order of Nurses of Quebec endorsed TT as a "bona fide" nursing skill.[32] The National League for Nursing, the credentialing agency for nursing schools in the United States, denies having an official stand on TT but has promoted it through books and videotapes,[3,53,54] and the league's executive director and a recent president are prominent advocates.[55] The American Nurses' Association holds TT workshops at its national conventions. Its official journal published the premier articles on TT[56–59] as well as a recent article designated for continuing education credits.[60] The association's immediate past president has written editorials defending TT against criticism.[61] The American Holistic Nursing Association offers certification in "healing touch," a TT variant.[62] The Nurse Healers and Professional Associates Cooperative, which was formed to promote TT, claims about 1200 members.[39]

The TT Hypothesis

Therapeutic Touch was conceived in the early 1970s by Dolores Krieger, PhD, RN, a faculty member at New York University's Division of Nursing. Although often presented as a scientific adaptation of "laying-on of hands,"[63–68] TT is imbued with metaphysical ideas.

Krieger initially identified TT's active agent as *prana*, an ayurvedic, or traditional Indian, concept of "life force." She stated,

> Health is considered a harmonious relationship between the individual and his total environment. There is postulated a continuing interacting flow of energies from within the individual outward, and from the environment to the various levels of the individual. Healing, it is said, helps to restore this equilibrium in the ill person. Disease, within this context, is considered an indication of a disturbance in the free flow of the pranic current.

Krieger further postulated that this "pranic current" can be controlled by the will of the healer.

> When an individual who is healthy touches an ill person with the intent of helping or healing him, he acts as a transference agent for the flow of prana from himself to the ill person. It was this added input of prana . . . that helped the ill person to overcome his illness or to feel better, more vital.

Others associate all this with the Chinese notion of *qi*, a "life energy" alleged to flow through the human body through invisible "meridians." Those inspired by mystical healers of India describe this energy as flowing in and out of sites of the body that they call *chakras*.

Soon after its conception, TT became linked with the westernized notions of the late Martha Rogers, dean of nursing at New York University. She asserted that humans do not merely possess energy fields but *are* energy fields and constantly interact with the "environmental field" around them. Rogers dubbed her approach the "Science of Unitary Man,"[69] which later became known as the more neutral "Science of Unitary Human Beings." Her nomenclature stimulated the pursuit of TT as a "scientific" practice. Almost all TT discussion today is based on Rogers' concepts, although Eastern metaphysical terms such as *chakra*[2,70] and *yin-yang*[71] are still used.

The HEF postulated by TT theorists resembles the "magnetic fluid" or "animal magnetism" postulated during the 18th century by Anton Mesmer and his followers. Mesmerism held that illnesses are caused by obstacles to the free flow of this fluid and that skilled healers ("sensitives") could remove these obstacles by making passes with their hands. Some aspects of mesmerism were revived in the 19th century by Theosophy, an occult religion that incorporated Eastern metaphysical concepts and underlies many current New Age ideas.[72] Dora Kunz, who is considered TT's codeveloper, was president of the Theosophical Society of America from 1975 to 1987. She collaborated with Krieger on the early TT studies and claims to be a fifth-generation "sensitive" and a "gifted healer."[20]

Therapeutic Touch is set apart from many other alternative healing modalities, as well as from scientific medicine, by its emphasis on the healer's intention. Whereas the testing of most therapies requires controlling for the placebo effect (often influenced by the recipient's belief about efficacy), TT theorists suggest that the placebo effect is irrelevant. According to Krieger,

> Faith on the part of the subject does not make a significant difference in the healing effect. Rather, the role of faith seems to be psychological, affecting his acceptance of his illness or consequent recovery and what this means to him. The healer, on the other hand, must have some belief system that underlies his actions, if one is to attribute rationality to his behavior.[65]

Thus, the TT hypothesis and the entire practice of TT rest on the idea that the patient's energy field can be detected and intentionally manipulated by the therapist. With this in mind, early practitioners concluded that physical contact might not be necessary.[13] The thesis that the HEF extends beyond the skin and can be influenced from several centimeters away from the body's surface is said to have been tested by Janet Quinn, PhD, and reported in her 1982 dissertation.[14] However, that study merely showed no difference between groups of patients who did or did not have actual contact during TT. Although Quinn's work has never been substantiated, nearly all TT practitioners today use only the noncontact form of TT.

As originally developed by Krieger, TT did involve touch, although clothes and other materials interposed between practitioner and patient were not considered significant.[56] It was named TT because the aboriginal term *laying-on of hands* was considered an obstacle to acceptance by "curriculum committees and other institutional bulwarks of today's society."[66] The mysticism has been downplayed, and various scientific-sounding mechanisms have been proposed. These include the therapeutic value of skin-to-skin contact, electron transfer resonance, oxygen uptake by hemoglobin, stereochemical similarities of hemoglobin and chlorophyll, electrostatic potentials influenced by healer brain activity, and unspecified concepts from quantum theory.[66,67]

Therapeutic Touch is said to be in the vanguard of treatments that allow "healing" to take place, as opposed to the "curing" pejoratively ascribed to mainstream medical practice. Therapeutic Touch supposedly requires little training beyond refining an innate ability to focus one's intent to heal; the patient's body then does the rest.[5] Nurses who claim a unique professional emphasis on caring are said to be specially situated to help patients by using TT.[56,59] Nonetheless, proponents also state that nearly everyone has an innate ability to learn TT, even small children and juvenile delinquents on parole.[2,17,32]

Proponents describe the HEF as real and perceptible. Reporting on a pilot study, Krieger claimed that 4 blindfolded men with transected spinal cords "could tell exactly where the nurse's hands were in their HEFs during the Therapeutic Touch interaction."[5] In ordinary TT sessions, practitioners go through motions that supposedly interact with the patient's energy field, including flicking "excess energy" from their fingertips.[3]

Therapeutic Touch is claimed to have only beneficial effects.[39] However, some proponents warn against overly lengthy sessions or overtreating certain areas of the body. This caution is based on the notion that too much energy can be imparted to a patient, especially an infant, which could lead to hyperactivity.[5,73,74]

Literature Analysis

Although TT proponents refer to a voluminous and growing body of valid research,[63,75,76] few studies have been well designed. Some clinical studies, mostly nursing doctoral dissertations, have reported positive results, principally with headache relief, relaxation, and wound healing.[5,13,14,23,24,26,28,30,68,77–86] However, the methods, credibility, and significance of these studies have been seriously questioned.[41,87–95] One prominent proponent questions the validity of the typical placebo control used in these studies.[96]

Two of the authors (L.R. and L.S.) have conducted extensive literature searches covering the years 1972 through 1996. Using key words such as *therapeutic touch*, *touch therapies*, *human energy field*, *quackery*, and *alternative medicine*, we have searched MEDLINE, *Index Medicus*, CINAHL, *Dissertation Abstracts*, *Masters Abstracts*, *Science Citation Index*, *Government Publications Index*, *Books in Print*, *National Union Catalog*, *Reader's Guide to Periodical Literature*, and *Alternative Press Index*. We attempted to obtain a full copy of each publication and every additional publication cited in the ones we subsequently collected. During 1997, we continued to monitor the journals most likely to contain material about TT.

These methods have enabled us to identify and obtain 853 reports (or abstracts), of which 609 deal specifically with TT, 224 mention it incidentally, and 20 discuss TT predecessors. Ninety-seven other cited items were either nonpublished or were published in obscure media we could not locate. Only 83 of the 853 reports described clinical research or other investigations by their authors. Nine of these studies were not quantitative. At most, only 1 (the study by Quinn[14]) of the 83 may have demonstrated independent confirmation of any positive study.[97] (That study was conducted by a close associate of the original researcher.) To our knowledge, no reported study attempted to test whether a TT practitioner could actually detect an HEF.

Of the 74 quantitative studies, 23 were clearly unsupportive. Eight reported no statistically significant results,[16,58,98–103] 3 admitted to having inadequate samples,[22,56,104] 2 were inconclusive,[11,105] and 6 had negative findings.[106–111] Four attempted independent replications but failed to support the original findings.[112–115] To our knowledge, no attempt to conduct experiments to reconcile any of these unsupportive findings has been reported.

In 1994, the University of Colorado Health Sciences Center (UCHSC), Denver, empaneled a scientific jury in response to a challenge to TT in its nursing curriculum. After surveying published research, the panel concluded that "there is not a sufficient body of data, both in quality and quantity, to establish TT as a unique and efficacious healing modality."[116]

A few months later, a University of Alabama at Birmingham research team declared that their own imminent study (financed by a $335,000 federal grant) would be "the first real scientific evidence" for TT.[117,118] This project compared the effects of TT and sham TT on the perception of pain by burn patients. The final report to the funding agency noted statistically significant differences in pain and anxiety in 3 of 7 subjective measurements, but there was no difference in the amount of pain medication requested.[119]

With little clinical or quantitative research to support the practice of TT, proponents have shifted to qualitative research, which merely compiles anecdotes.[120] This approach, which involves asking subjects what they feel and drawing conclusions from their descriptions,[17,43,121–128] was sharply criticized by UCHSC's scientific panel.[116]

Both TT theory and technique require that an HEF be felt in order to impart any therapeutic benefit to a subject. Thus, the definitive test of TT is not a clinical trial of its alleged therapeutic effects, but a test of whether practitioners can perceive HEFs, which they describe, in print and in our study, with such terms as *tingling*, *pulling*, *throbbing*, *hot*, *cold*, *spongy*, and *tactile as taffy*. After doing its own survey, the UCHSC panel declared that no one had "even any ideas about how such research might be conducted."[115] This study fills that void.

Methods

In 1996 and 1997, by searching for advertisements and following other leads, 2 of us (L.R. and L.S.) located 25 TT practitioners in northeastern Colorado, 21 of whom readily agreed to be tested. Of those who did not, 1 stated she was not qualified, 2 gave no reason, and 1 agreed but canceled on the day of the test.

The reported practice experience of those tested ranged from 1 to 27 years. There were 9 nurses, 7 certified massage therapists, 2 laypersons, 1 chiropractor, 1 medical assistant, and 1 phlebotomist. All but 2 were women, which reflects the sex ratio of the practitioner population. One nurse had published an article on TT in a journal for nurse practitioners.

There were 2 series of tests. In 1996, 15 practitioners were tested at their homes or offices on different days for a period of several months. In 1997, 13 practitioners, including 7 from the first series, were tested in a single day.

The test procedures were explained by 1 of the authors (E.R.), who designed the experiment herself. The first series of tests was conducted when she was 9 years old. The participants were informed that the study would be published as her fourth-grade science-fair project and gave their consent to be tested. The decision to submit the results to a scientific journal was made several months later, after people who heard about the results encouraged publication. The second test series was done at the request of a Public Broadcasting Service television producer who had heard about the first study. Participants in the second series were informed that the test would be videotaped for possible broadcast and gave their consent.

During each test, the practitioners rested their hands, palms up, on a flat surface, approximately 25 to 30 cm apart. To prevent the experimenter's hands from being seen, a tall, opaque screen with cutouts at its base was placed over the subject's arms, and a cloth towel was attached to the screen and draped over them (Figure 1).

Each subject underwent a set of 10 trials. Before each set, the subject was permitted to "center" or make any other mental preparations deemed necessary. The experimenter flipped a coin to determine which of the subject's hands would be the target. The experimenter then hovered her right hand, palm down, 8 to 10 cm above the target and said, "Okay." The subject then stated which of his or her hands was nearer to the experimenter's hand. Each subject was permitted to take as much or as little time as necessary to make each determination. The time spent ranged from 7 to 19 minutes per set of trials.

To examine whether air movement or body heat might be detectable by the experimental subjects, preliminary tests were performed on 7 other subjects who had no training or belief in TT. Four were children who were unaware of the purpose of the test. Those results indicated that the apparatus prevented tactile cues from reaching the subject.

The odds of getting 8 of 10 trials correct by chance alone is 45 of 1024 (P=.04), a level considered significant in many clinical trials. We decided in advance that an individual would "pass" by making 8 or more correct selections and that those passing the test would be retested, although the retest results would not be included in the group analysis. Results for the group as a whole would not be considered positive unless the average score was above 6.7 at a 90% confidence level.

Results

Initial Test Results

If HEF perception through TT was possible, the experimental subjects should have each been able to detect the

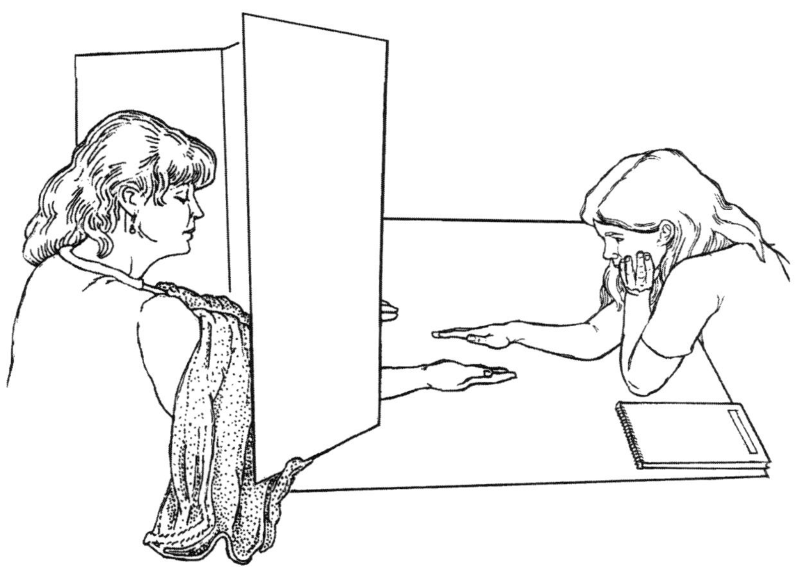

Figure 1. Experimenter hovers hand over one of subject's hands. Draped towel prevents peeking. Drawing by Pat Linse, Skeptics Society.

experimenter's hand in 10 (100%) of 10 trials. Chance alone would produce an average score of 5 (50%).

Before testing, all participants said they could use TT to significant therapeutic advantage. Each described sensory cues they used to assess and manipulate the HEF. All participants but 1 certified massage therapist expressed high confidence in their TT abilities, and even the aforementioned certified massage therapist said afterward that she felt she had passed the test to her own satisfaction.

In the initial trial, the subjects stated the correct location of the investigator's hand in 70 (47%) of 150 tries. The number of correct choices ranged from 2 to 8. Only 1 subject scored 8, and that same subject scored only 6 on the retest.

After each set of trials, the results were discussed with the participant. Because all but 1 of the trials could have been considered a failure, the participants usually chose to discuss possible explanations for failure. Their rationalizations included the following: (1) The experimenter left a "memory" of her hand behind, making it increasingly difficult in successive trials to detect the real hand from the memory. However, the first attempts (7 correct and 8 incorrect) scored no better than the rest. Moreover, practitioners should be able to tell whether a field they are sensing is "fresh." (2) The left hand is the "receiver" of energy and the right hand is the "transmitter." Therefore, it can be more difficult to detect the field when it is above the right hand. Of the 72 tests in which the hand was placed above the subjects' right hand, only 27 (38%) had correct responses. In addition, 35 (44%) of 80 incorrect answers involved the allegedly more receptive left hand—consistent with randomness. Moreover, practitioners customarily use both hands to assess. (3) Subjects should be permitted to identify the experimenter's field before beginning actual trials. Each subject could be given an example of the experimenter hovering her hand above each of theirs and told which hand it is. Since the effects of the HEF are described in unsubtle terms, such a procedure should not be necessary, but including it would remove a possible post hoc objection. Therefore, we did so in the follow-up testing. (4) The experimenter should be more proactive, centering herself and/or attempting to transmit energy through her own intentionality. This contradicts the fundamental premise of TT, since the experimenter's role is analogous to that of a patient. Only the practitioner's intentionality and preparation (centering) are theoretically necessary. If not so, the early experiments (on relatively uninvolved subjects, such as infants and barley seeds), cited frequently by TT advocates, must also be discounted. (5) Some subjects complained that their hands became so hot after a few trials that they were no longer able to sense the experimenter's HEF or they experienced difficulty doing so. This explanation clashes with TT's basic premise that practitioners can sense and manipulate the HEF with their hands during sessions that typically last 20 to 30 minutes. If practitioners become insensitive after only

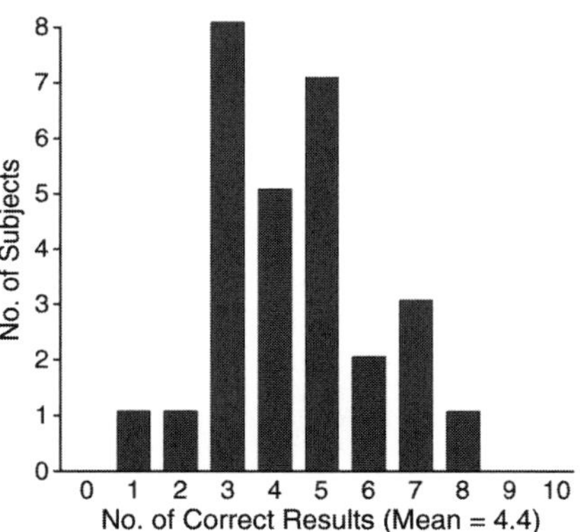

Figure 2. Distribution of test results.

Table 2. Statistical Analysis

Statistical Function	Initial Test (n=15)	Follow-up Test (n=13)
Mean (95% confidence interval)	4.67 (3.67–5.67)	4.08 (3.17–4.99)
SD	1.74	1.44
α (1-tailed test)	.05	.05
t statistic	−0.7174	−2.222
Upper critical limit of Student *t* distribution	1.761	1.782
Alternative hypothesis, μ=6.67	0.9559	0.9801
Alternative hypothesis, μ=7.50	0.999644	0.999953

brief testing, the TT hypothesis is untestable. Those who made this complaint did so after they knew the results, not before. Moreover, only 7 of the 15 first trials produced correct responses.

Follow-up Test Results

The 1997 testing was completed in 1 day and videotaped by a professional film crew. Each subject was allowed to "feel" the investigator's energy field and choose which hand the investigator would use for testing. Seven subjects chose her left hand, and 6 chose her right hand.

The test results were similar to those of the first series. The subjects correctly located the investigator's hand in only 53 (41%) of 130 tries. The number of correct answers ranged from 1 to 7. After learning of their test scores, one participant said he was distracted by the towel over his hands, another said that her hands had been too dry, and several complained that the presence of the television crew had made it difficult to concentrate and/or added to the stress of the test. However, we do not believe that the situation was more stressful or distracting than the settings in which many hospital nurses practice TT (eg, intensive care units). Figure 2 shows the distribution of test results.

Our null hypothesis was that the experimental results would be due to chance (μ=5). Our alternative hypothesis was that the subjects would perform at better than chance levels. The *t* statistic of our data did not exceed the upper critical limit of the Student *t* distribution (Table 2). Therefore, the null hypothesis cannot be rejected at the .05 level of significance for a 1-tailed test, which means that our subjects, with only 123 of 280 correct in the 2 trials, did not perform better than chance.

Our data also showed that if the practitioners could reliably detect an HEF 2 of 3 times, then the probability that either test missed such an effect would be less than .05. If the practitioners' true detection rate was 3 of 4, then the probability that our experiment missed it would be less than 3 in 10,000. However, if TT theory is correct, practitioners should always be able to sense the energy field of their patients. We would also expect accuracy to increase with experience. However, there was no significant correlation between the practitioners' scores and the length of time they had practiced TT (r=0.23). We conclude on both statistical and logical grounds that TT practitioners have no such ability.

Comment

Practitioners of TT are generally reluctant to be tested by people who are not proponents. In 1996, the James Randi Educational Foundation offered $742,000 to anyone who could demonstrate an ability to detect an HEF under conditions similar to those of our study. Although more than 40,000 American practitioners claim to have such an ability, only 1 person attempted the demonstration. She failed, and the offer, now more than $1.1 million, has had no further volunteers despite extensive recruiting efforts.[129]

We suspect that the present authors were able to secure the cooperation of 21 practitioners because the person conducting the test was a child who displayed no skepticism.

Conclusion

Therapeutic touch is grounded on the concept that people have an energy field that is readily detectable (and modifiable) by TT practitioners. However, this study found that 21 experienced practitioners, when blinded, were unable to tell which of their hands was in the experimenter's energy field. The mean correct score for the 28 sets of 10 tests was 4.4, which is close to what would be expected for random guessing.

To our knowledge, no other objective, quantitative study involving more than a few TT practitioners has been published, and no well-designed study demonstrates any health benefit from TT. These facts, together with our experimental findings, suggest that TT claims are groundless and that further use of TT by health professionals is unjustified.

Ms E. Rosa designed and conducted the tests and tabulated her findings. Mr Sarner did the statistical analysis. He and Ms L. Rosa recruited the test subjects, performed the literature analysis, and drafted this report. Dr Barrett added background material and edited the report for publication.

The television program "Scientific American Frontiers" showed excerpts from the second test series on November 19, 1997.

Lisa Feldman Barrett, PhD, Department of Psychology, Boston College, graciously helped with our statistical analyses.

References

1. Boguslawski M. The use of Therapeutic Touch in nursing. *J Continuing Educ Nurs*. 1979; 10(4):9–15.
2. Krieger D. *Therapeutic Touch Inner Workbook*. Santa Fe, NM: Bear; 1997:162.
3. Quinn JF. *Therapeutic Touch: Healing Through Human Energy Fields: Theory and Research* [videotapes and study guide]. New York, NY: National League for Nursing; 1994: 42–2485–42–2487, 42–2493.
4. Krieger D. *Living the Therapeutic Touch: Healing as a Lifestyle*. New York, NY: Dodd Mead; 1987.
5. Krieger D. *Accepting Your Power to Heal: The Personal Practice of Therapeutic Touch*. Santa Fe, NM: Bear; 1993.
6. Chiappone J. *The Light Touch: An Easy Guide to Hands-on Healing*. Lake Mary, Fla: Holistic Reflections; 1989:14.
7. Quinn JF, Strelkauskas AJ. Psycho immunologic effects of Therapeutic Touch on practitioners and recently bereaved recipients: a pilot study. *ANS Adv Nurs Sci*. 1993;15(4):13–26.
8. Jarboux D. Nurse knows Therapeutic Touch "works.". *Boulder Sunday Camera*. January 2, 1994:3E.
9. Putnam ZE. Using consciousness to heal. Massage *Ther J*. Fall 1995:47–48, 50, 52, 54, 56, 58, 60.
10. Leduc E. Therapeutic Touch. *Neonat Network*. 1987;5(6):46–47.
11. Krieger D. Therapeutic Touch during childbirth preparation by the Lamaze method and its relation to marital satisfaction and state anxiety of the married couple. In: Krieger D. *Living the Therapeutic Touch: Healing as a Lifestyle*. New York, NY: Dodd Mead; 1987:157–187.
12. Glazer S. The mystery of "Therapeutic Touch." *Washington Post*. December 19–26, 1995;Health section:16–17.
13. Heidt PR. Effect of Therapeutic Touch on anxiety level of hospitalized patients. *Nurs Res*. 1981;30(1):32–37.
14. Quinn JF. *An Investigation of the Effects of Therapeutic Touch Done Without Physical Contact on State Anxiety of Hospitalized Cardiovascular Patients* [dissertation]. New York: New York University; 1982.
15. Thayer MB. Touching with intent: using Therapeutic Touch. *Pediatr Nurs*. 1990; 16(1):70–72.
16. Mersmann CA. *Therapeutic Touch and Milk Let Down in Mothers of Non-nursing Preterm Infants* [dissertation]. New York: New York University; 1993.
17. France NEM. The child's perception of the human energy field using Therapeutic Touch. *J Holistic Nurs*. 1993;11:319–331.
18. Meehan MTC. The Science of Unitary Human Beings and theory-based practice: Therapeutic Touch. In: Barrett EAM, ed. *Visions of Rogers' Science-Based Nursing*. New York, NY: National League for Nursing; 1990:67–81. Publication 15–2285.
19. Peters PJ. *The Lifestyle Changes of Selected Therapeutic Touch Practitioners: An Oral History* [dissertation]. Minneapolis, Minn: Walden University; 1992.
20. Boguslawski M. Therapeutic Touch: a facilitator of pain relief. *Top Clin Nurs*. 1980;2(1):27–37.
21. Satir F. Healing hands. *Olympian*. July 19, 1994.
22. Brown PR. *The Effects of Therapeutic Touch on Chemotherapy-induced Nausea and Vomiting: A Pilot Study* [master's thesis]. Reno: University of Nevada; 1981.
23. Sodergren KA. *The Effect of Absorption and Social Closeness on Responses to Educational and Relaxation Therapies in Patients With Anticipatory Nausea and Vomiting During Cancer Chemotherapy* [dissertation]. Minneapolis: University of Minnesota; 1993.
24. Dollar CE. *Effects of Therapeutic Touch on Perception of Pain and Physiological Measurements From Tension Headache in Adults: A Pilot Study* [master's thesis]. Jackson: University of Mississippi Medical Center; 1993.
25. Quinn JF. Holding sacred space: the nurse as healing environment. *Holistic Nurs Pract*. 1992;6(4):26–36.
26. Wirth DP. The effect of non-contact Therapeutic Touch on the healing rate of full thickness dermal wounds. *Subtle Energies*. 1990;1(1):1–20.
27. Woods DL. *The Effect of Therapeutic Touch on Disruptive Behaviors of Individuals With Dementia of the Alzheimer Type* [master's thesis]. Seattle: University of Washington; 1993.
28. Misra MM. *The Effects of Therapeutic Touch on Menstruation*. [master's thesis]. Long Beach: California State University; 1993.
29. Putnam ZE. The woman behind Therapeutic Touch: Dolores Krieger, PhD, RN. *Massage Ther J*. Fall 1995:50, 52.
30. Simington JA, Laing GP. Effects of Therapeutic Touch on anxiety in the institutionalized elderly. *Clin Nurs Res*. 1993;2:438–450.
31. Quinn JF. The Senior's Therapeutic Touch Education Program. *Holistic Nurs Pract*. 1992;7(1):32–37.
32. Krieger D. Therapeutic Touch: two decades of research, teaching and clinical practice. *Imprint*. 1990;37:83, 86–88.
33. Fiely D. Field of beams. *Columbus Dispatch*. August 20, 1995:1B-2B.
34. Calvert R. Dolores Krieger, PhD, and her Therapeutic Touch. *Massage Magazine*. 1994;47:56–60.
35. Mueller Jackson ME. The use of Therapeutic Touch in the nursing care of the terminally ill person. In: Borelli MD, Heidt PR, eds. *Therapeutic Touch: A Book of Readings*. New York, NY: Springer; 1981:72–79.
36. Brunjes CAF. Therapeutic Touch: a healing modality throughout life. *Top Clin Nurs*. 1983;5(2):72–79.
37. Messenger TC, Roberts KT. The terminally ill: serenity nursing interventions for hospice clients. *J Gerontol Nurs*. 1994;20(11):17–22.
38. Maxwell J. Nursing's new age? *Christianity Today*. 1996;40(3):96–99.
39. Kauffold MP. TT: healing or hokum? debate over "energy medicine" runs hot. *Chicago Tribune Nursing News*. November 19, 1995:1.

40. Keegan L. Holistic nursing. *J Post Anesth Nurs.* 1989;4(1):17–21.

41. Bullough VL, Bullough B. Therapeutic Touch: why do nurses believe? *Skeptical Inquirer.* 1993;17:169–174.

42. Dr Quinn studies Therapeutic Touch. *University of Colorado School of Nursing News.* May 1989:1.

43. Cabico LL. *A Phenomenological Study of the Experiences of Nurses Practicing Therapeutic Touch* [master's thesis]. Buffalo, NY: D'Youville College; 1992.

44. Rosa LA. When magic gets to play science. *Rocky Mountain Skeptic.* 1993;10(6):10–12.

45. Carpenito LJ. *Nursing Diagnosis: Application to Clinical Practice.* 6th ed. Philadelphia, Pa: Lippincott; 1995:355–358.

46. Sandroff R. A skeptic's guide to Therapeutic Touch. *RN.* 1980;43(1):24–30, 82–83.

47. Raucheisen ML. Therapeutic Touch: maybe there's something to it after all. *RN.* 1984; 47(12):49–51.

48. Haddad A. Acute care decisions: ethics in action. *RN.* 1994;57(11):21–22, 24.

49. Swackhamer AH. It's time to broaden our practice. *RN.* 1995;58(1):49–51.

50. Schmidt CM. The basics of Therapeutic Touch. *RN.* 1995;58(6):50, 52, 54.

51. Ledwith SP. Therapeutic Touch and mastectomy: a case study. *RN.* 1995;58(7):51–53.

52. Keegan L, Cerrato PL. Nurses are embracing holistic healing. *RN.* 1996;59(4):59.

53. Moccia P, ed. *New Approaches to Theory Development.* New York, NY: National League for Nursing; 1986;15–1992.

54. Barrett EAM, ed. *Visions of Rogers' Science-Based Nursing.* New York, NY: National League for Nursing; 1990;15–2285.

55. Moccia P. Letter to the editor. *Time.* 1994; 144(24):18.

56. Krieger D. Therapeutic Touch: the imprimatur of nursing. *Am J Nurs.* 1975;75:784–787.

57. Krieger D, Peper E, Ancoli S. Therapeutic Touch: searching for evidence of physiological change. *Am J Nurs.* 1979;79:660–662.

58. Macrae JA. Therapeutic Touch in practice. *Am J Nurs.* 1979;79:664–665.

59. Quinn JF. One nurse's evolution as a healer. *Am J Nurs.* 1979;79:662–664.

60. Mackey RB. Discover the healing power of Therapeutic Touch. *Am J Nurs.* 1995; 95(4):27–33.

61. Joel LA. Alternative solutions to health problems. *Am J Nurs.* 1995;95(7):7.

62. Hover-Kramer D. Healing Touch certificate program continues to bring the human dimension to the nation's nurses. *Beginnings.* 1992; 12(2):3.

63. Cowens C, Monte T. *A Gift for Healing: How You Can Use Therapeutic Touch.* New York, NY: Crown Publishing Group; 1996.

64. Krieger D. The response of in-vivo human hemoglobin to an active healing therapy by direct laying on of hands. *Human Dimensions.* Autumn 1972:12–15.

65. Krieger D. Therapeutic Touch and healing energies from the laying on of hands. *J Holistic Health.* 1975;1:23–30.

66. Krieger D. Therapeutic Touch: an ancient, but unorthodox nursing intervention. *J N Y State Nurs Assoc.* 1975;6(2):6–10.

67. Krieger D. Healing by the laying-on of hands as a facilitator of bio-energetic change: the response of in-vivo human hemoglobin. *Int J Psychoenergy Syst.* 1976;1(1):121–129.

68. Krieger D. The relationship of touch, with intent to help or to heal, to subjects' in-vivo hemoglobin values: a study in personalized interaction. In: *Proceedings of the Ninth ANA Nurses Research Conference.* New York, NY: American Nurses' Association; 1973:39–59.

69. Rogers ME. *An Introduction to the Theoretical Basis of Nursing.* Philadelphia, Pa: Davis; 1970.

70. Karagulla S, Kunz D. *The Chakras and the Human Energy Field: Correlations Between Medical Science & Clairvoyant Observation.* Wheaton, Ill: Theosophical Publishing House; 1989.

71. Randolph GL. The yin and yang of clinical practice. *Top Clin Nurs.* 1979;1(1):31–42.

72. Brierton TD. Employers' New Age training programs fail to alter the consciousness of the EEOC. *Lab Law J.* 1992;43:411–420.

73. Emery CE. Therapeutic Touch: healing technique or New Age rite? *Providence Sun Journal-Bulletin.* November 27, 1994:A1, A24.

74. Knaster M. Dolores Krieger's Therapeutic Touch. *East/West.* 1989;19(8):54–57, 59, 79–80.

75. Colorado State Board of Nursing. *Subcommittee to Investigate the Awarding of Continuing Education Units to Nurses for the Study of Therapeutic Touch and Other Non-traditional and Complementary Healing Modalities. Recommendations.* Denver: Colorado State Board of Nursing; 1992.

76. Mulloney SS, Wells-Federman C. Therapeutic Touch: a healing modality. *J Cardiovascul Nurs.* 1996;10(3):27–49.

77. Brown CC, Fischer R, Wagman AMI, Horrom N, Marks P. The EEG in meditation and Therapeutic Touch healing. *J Altered* States *Conscious.* 1977;3:169–180.

78. Quinn JF. Therapeutic Touch as energy exchange: testing the theory. *Adv Nurs Sci.* 1984;6(1):42–49.

79. Guerrero MA. *The Effects of Therapeutic Touch on State-Trait Anxiety Level of Oncology Patients* [master's thesis]. Galveston: University of Texas; 1985.

80. Keller EAK, Bzdek VM. Effects of Therapeutic Touch on tension headache pain. *Nurs Res.* 1986;35(2):101–106.

81. Meehan MTC. Theory development. In: Barrett EAM, ed. *Visions of Rogers' Science-Based Nursing.* New York, NY: National League for Nursing; 1990;15–2285:197–207.

82. Kramer NA. Comparison of Therapeutic Touch and Casual Touch in stress reduction of hospitalized children. *Pediatr Nurs.* 1990;16:483–485.

83. Shuzman E. *The Effect of Trait Anxiety and Patient Expectation of Therapeutic Touch on the Reduction in State Anxiety in Preoperative Patients Who Receive Therapeutic Touch* [dissertation]. New York: New York University; 1993.

84. Sies MM. *An Exploratory Study of Relaxation Response in Nurses Who Utilize Therapeutic Touch* [master's thesis]. East Lansing: Michigan State University; 1993.

85. Wirth DP, Richardson JT, Eidelman WS, O'Malley AC. Full thickness dermal wounds treated with Therapeutic Touch: a replication and extension. *Complementary Ther Med.* 1993;1:127–132.

86. Gagne D, Toye RC. The effects of Therapeutic Touch and relaxation therapy in reducing anxiety. *Arch Psych Nurs.* 1994;8:184–189.

87. Schlotfeldt RM. Critique of: Krieger D. The relationship of touch, with intent to help or heal, to subjects' in-vivo hemoglobin values: a study in personalized interaction. In: *Proceedings of the Ninth ANA Nurses Research Conference.* New York, NY: American Nurses' Association; 1973:59–65.

88. Walike BC, Bruno P, Donaldson S, et al. "...[A]ttempts to embellish a totally unscientific process with the aura of science...." *Am J Nurs.* 1975;75:1275, 1278, 1292.

89. Levine ME. "The science is spurious...." *Am J Nurs.* 1979;79:1379–1380.

90. Clark PE, Clark MJ. Therapeutic Touch: is there a scientific basis for the practice? *Nurs Res.* 1984;33(1):38–41.

91. Meehan MTC. Therapeutic Touch. In: Bulechek GM, McCloskey JC, eds. *Nursing Interventions: Essential Nursing Treatments.* 2nd ed. Philadelphia, Pa: Saunders; 1992:201–212.

92. Fish S. Therapeutic Touch: can we trust the data? *J Christian Nurs*. 1993;10(3):6–8.

93. Meehan MTC. Therapeutic Touch and postoperative pain: a Rogerian research study. *Nurs Sci Q* 1993;6(2):69–78.

94. Bandman EL, Bandman B. *Critical Thinking in Nursing*. Norwalk, Conn: Appleton & Lange; 1995.

95. Meehan MTC. Quackery and pseudo-science. *Am J Nurs*. 1995;75(7):17.

96. Meehan MTC.... And still more on TT. *Res Nurs Health*. 1995;18:471–472.

97. Rosa LA. *Survey of Therapeutic Touch "Research."* Loveland, Colo: Front Range Skeptics; 1996.

98. Tharnstrom CAL. *The Effects of Non-contact Therapeutic Touch on the Parasympathetic Nervous System as Evidenced by Superficial Skin Temperature and Perceived Stress* [master's thesis]. San Jose, Calif: San Jose State University; 1993.

99. Parkes BS. *Therapeutic Touch as an Intervention to Reduce Anxiety in Elderly Hospitalized Patients* [dissertation]. Austin: University of Texas; 1985.

100. Mueller Hinze ML. *The Effects of Therapeutic Touch and Acupressure on Experimentally-Induced Pain* [dissertation]. Austin: University of Texas; 1988.

101. Bowers DP. *The Effects of Therapeutic Touch on State Anxiety and Physiological Measurements in Preoperative Clients* [master's thesis]. San Jose, Calif: San Jose State University, 1992.

102. Olson M, Sneed NV. Anxiety and Therapeutic Touch. *Issues Ment Health Nurs*. 1995; 16:97–108.

103. Fedoruk RB. *Transfer of the Relaxation Response: Therapeutic Touch as a Method for Reduction of Stress in Premature Neonates* [dissertation]. Baltimore: University of Maryland; 1984.

104. Hogg PK. *The Effects of Acupressure on the Psychological and Physiological Rehabilitation of the Stroke Patient* [dissertation]. Alameda: California School of Professional Psychology; 1985.

105. Snyder M, Egan EC, Burns KR. Interventions for decreasing agitation behaviors in persons with dementia. *J Gerontol Nurs*. 1995; 21(7):34–40, 54–55.

106. Schweitzer SF. *The Effects of Therapeutic Touch on Short-term Memory Recall in the Aging Population: A Pilot Study* [master's thesis]. Reno: University of Nevada; 1980.

107. Randolph GL. Therapeutic and physical touch: physiological response to stressful stimuli. *Nurs Res*. 1984;33(1):33–36.

108. Nodine JL. *The Effects of Therapeutic Touch on Anxiety and Well-being in Third Trimester Pregnant Women* [master's thesis]. Tucson: University of Arizona; 1987.

109. Post NW. *The Effects of Therapeutic Touch on Muscle Tone* [master's thesis]. San Jose, Calif: San Jose State University; 1990.

110. Straneva JAE. *Therapeutic Touch and In Vitro Erythropoiesis* [dissertation]. Bloomington: Indiana University; 1992.

111. Bush AM, Geist CR. Testing electromagnetic explanations for a possible psychokinetic effect of Therapeutic Touch in germinating corn seed. *Psycholog Rep*. 1992;70:891–896.

112. Edge H. The effect of laying on of hands on an enzyme: an attempted replication. Paper presented at: 22nd Annual Convention of the Parapsychology Association; August 15–18, 1979; Moraga, Calif.

113. Meehan MTC. *The Effect of Therapeutic Touch on the Experience of Acute Pain in Postoperative Patients* [dissertation]. New York: New York University; 1985.

114. Hale EH. *A Study of the Relationship Between Therapeutic Touch and the Anxiety Levels of Hospitalized Adults* [dissertation]. Denton: Texas Women's University; 1986.

115. Quinn JF. Therapeutic Touch as energy exchange: replication and extension. *Nurs Sci Q*. 1989;2(2):79–87.

116. Claman HN, Freeman R, Quissel D, et al. *Report of the Chancellor's Committee on Therapeutic Touch*. Denver: University of Colorado Health Sciences Center; 1994.

117. Butgereit B. Therapeutic Touch: UAB to study controversial treatment for Pentagon. *Birmingham News*. November 17, 1994:1A, 10A.

118. Turner JG. *Tri-Service Nursing Research Grant Proposal* [revised abstract]. 1994. Grant No. MDA905–94–Z-0080.

119. Turner JG. *The Effect of Therapeutic Touch on Pain & Anxiety in Burn Patients* [grant final report]. Tri-Service Nursing Research Program; November 14, 1996. Grant No. N94020.

120. Lionberger HJ. Therapeutic Touch: a healing modality or a caring strategy. In: Chinn PL, ed. *Nursing Research Methodology: Issues and Implementation*. Rockville, Md: Aspen Publishers; 1986:169–180.

121. Lionberger HJ. *An Interpretive Study of Nurses' Practice of Therapeutic Touch* [dissertation]. San Francisco: University of California; 1985.

122. Polk SH. *Client's Perceptions of Experiences Following the Intervention Modality of Therapeutic Touch* [master's thesis]. Tempe: Arizona State University; 1985.

123. Hamilton-Wyatt GK. *Therapeutic Touch: Promoting and Assessing Conceptual Change Among Health Care Professionals* [dissertation]. East Lansing: Michigan State University, 1988.

124. Heidt PR. Openness: a qualitative analysis of nurses' and patients' experiences of Therapeutic Touch. *Image J Nurs Sch*. 1990;22:180–186.

125. Thomas-Beckett JG. *Attitudes Toward Therapeutic Touch: A Pilot Study of Women With Breast Cancer* [master's thesis]. East Lansing: Michigan State University; 1991.

126. Clark AJ, Seifert P. Client perceptions of Therapeutic Touch. Paper presented at: Third Annual West Alabama Conference on Clinical Nursing Research; 1992.

127. Samarel N. The experience of receiving Therapeutic Touch. *J Adv Nurs*. 1992; 17:651–657.

128. Hughes PP. *The Experience of Therapeutic Touch as a Treatment Modality With Adolescent Psychiatric Patients* [master's thesis]. Albuquerque: University of New Mexico; 1994.

129. James Randi Educational Foundation. Available at: http://www.randi.org. Accessed March 15, 1997.

4 Diet, Nutrition, Lifestyle

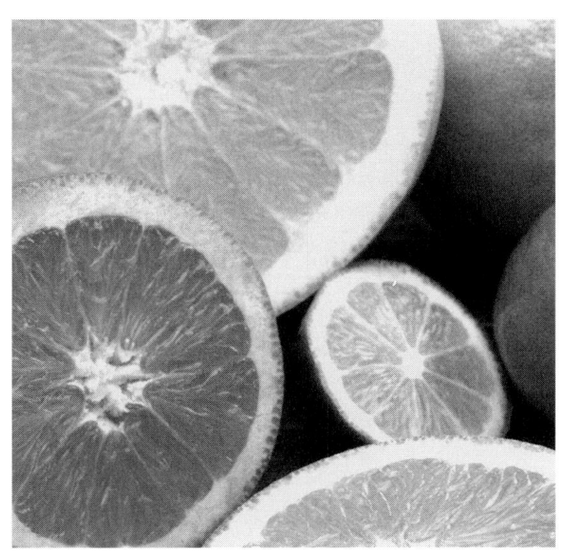

Overview

Marc S. Micozzi, MD, PhD
From the College of Physicians of Philadelphia, University of Pennsylvania School of Medicine.

Human diet and nutrition is coming of age as a component of contemporary medical practice just as medicine is rediscovering the roots of ancient healing traditions (today called complementary or alternative medicine) that have incorporated diet and nutrition as fundamental components of health promotion and disease management for centuries or even millennia.[1]

With serious large-scale investigations of the role of diet and nutrition during the last 15 years,[2,3] medicine has moved beyond the prevention and cure of frank malnutrition to learning about the potential for optimal nutrition in health promotion and about the role of therapeutic nutrition in disease management. Accordingly, earlier scientific challenges to establishing recommended daily allowances (RDAs) of micronutrients are giving way to new challenges regarding the discovery of optimal dietary intake and micronutrient nutrition in terms of developing a clinically useful scientific database.[4]

With respect to medical technology and clinical practice, medicine is also moving forward from the seminal clinical nutrition work of Rhoads[5] on intravenous hyperalimentation for support of the critically ill, to learning optimal formulations of foods, diets, dietary supplements, and "nutraceuticals" for ambulatory patients.

Medical practice is refining understanding of iron supplementation to reconcile old knowledge about the role of iron supplementation in the avoidance of dietary deficiency in menstruating, pregnant, and lactating women to accommodate new evidence about the role of excess body iron stores in the etiology of cancer, heart disease, and possibly other chronic diseases.[6] Ironically, as illustrated in the chapter by Goodwin and Tangum,[7] "Battling Quackery," now-discredited concerns about the possible dangers of a range of micronutrient supplementation among the medical profession did not prevent medicine from embracing wholeheartedly the prescription of iron (one micronutrient that might be truly dangerous). The CDC is now revising its dietary guidelines for iron intake downward for most people.[8]

The current regulatory climate at the Food and Drug Administration has now moved herbal remedies into the category of dietary supplements, together with micronutrients, which are now included under the Dietary Supplement Health and Education Act of 1994.[9] After establishing in medical science clear data about the micronutrient levels required for human nutrition and about the biological effects of phytochemicals isolated from plants, new emphasis is now being placed on the total diet and on the synergic effects of combinations of phytochemicals naturally occurring in plants used for centuries as medicines in the form of herbal remedies.

Curiously, in traditional Chinese medicine, practice is not based on distinctions between micronutrients and phytochemicals, or between "foods" and "drugs," but on the consumption of plants as foods that are "good medicine" (in various formulations) and that promote health or manage disease. In biomedicine, decisions were made to label some biologically active constituents as micronutrients (based on valid scientific criteria), while those left over are called phytochemicals.

People eat foods, not nutrients. Many human foods are plants. Given emerging understanding of human evolutionary biology (and evolutionary or "Darwinian" medicine), it comes as no surprise that plants are rich sources of foods and medicines for humans due to their relative abundance of biologically active constituents, as micronutrients and phytochemicals. Evolution is a process by which plant and animal organisms adapt to the environment in which they evolve. In this perspective, plants in turn contain biologically active constituents for the same reason that some molds contain antibacterial agents. They compete with one another in nature.

In similar perspective, many plants contain abundant antioxidants because they are in the sun all day. Likewise, other phytochemicals evolve to meet the requirements of plant physiology and metabolism. Plants have always been a predominant part of the terrestrial environment in which humans evolved. Geologic evidence suggests that plants evolved before people did. To some extent, it may be considered that human physiology and metabolism evolved and is adapted to obtain foods and medicines from plants (which in turn contain many modern micronutrients and phytochemicals).

Human culture, society, and civilization also evolve to provide sustenence to human populations. Just as human societies have always learned to use and obtain foods from plants (containing what subsequently have been called nutrients), humans also have learned for millennia to obtain medicine from plants. First, hunter-gatherers gathered foods and medicines from among plants; then, over the past 10,000 years, agricultural domestication permitted selective cultivation of plant foods and medicines.

Given this evolutionary biological perspective, medicine must closely examine the issues of "mega-vitamin" therapy vs the biological effects of micronutrients in physiologic doses. It is likely that human physiology and metabolism are not equipped to handle micronutrients at levels higher than possibly could be seen in nature. Therefore, the medical management of mega-dose nutrients may mimic clinical use of powerful pharmaceuticals also not found in nature. The challenges and opportunities for therapeutic nutrition are many, as illustrated in the following chapters in this section,[10–14] but undoubtedly will benefit from the application of medical standards of investigation and practice. The use of diet, nutrition, and natural products in general must be elevated above the standards of the local health food marketplace in the interests of both public health and medical practice.

References

1. Micozzi MS, ed. *Fundamentals of Complementary and Alternative Medicine.* 2nd ed. New York, NY: Churchill Livingstone. In press.
2. Moon T, Micozzi MS, eds. *Nutrition and Cancer Prevention: Investigating the Role of Micronutrients.* New York, NY: Marcel Dekker; 1989:608.
3. Micozzi MS, Moon T, eds. *Macronutrients: Investigating Their Role in Cancer.* New York, NY: Marcel Dekker; 1992:496.
4. Micozzi MS. Foods, micronutrients and reduction of human cancer. In: Micozzi MS, Moon T, eds. *Macronutrients: Investigating Their Role in Cancer.* New York, NY: Mancel Dekker;1989:213–241.
5. Rhoads JE. Development of surgical nutrition at the University of Pennsylvania. *JPEN J Parenter Enter Nutr.* 1980;4:464–466.
6. Stevens R, Jones DY, Micozzi MS, Taylor PR. Body iron stores and the risk of cancer. *N Engl J Med.* 1988;319:1047–1052.
7. Goodwin JS, Tangum MR. Battling quackery: attitudes about micronutrients supplements in American academic medicine. *Arch Intern Med.* 1998;158:2187–2191.
8. Stevens RL, Graubard BR, Micozzi MS, Neriishi K, Blumberg BS. Moderate elevation of body iron level and increased risk of cancer occurrence and death. *Int J Cancer.* 1994;56:364–369.
9. Dietary Supplement Health and Education Act (DSHEA). 1994;S.784.ENR.
10. Clarke R, Smith DA, Jobst KA, Refsum H, Sutton L, Ueland PM. Folate, vitamin B_{12}, and serum total homocysteine levels in confirmed Alzheimer disease. *Arch Neurol.* 1998;55:1449–1455.
11. Diaz-Arrastia R. Hypohomocysteinemia: a new risk factor for Alzheimer disease? *Arch Neurol.* 1998;55:1407–1408.
12. Tur E, Brenner S. Diet and pemphigus: in pursuit of exogenous factors in pemphigus and fogo selvagem. *Arch Dermatol.* 1998;134:1406–1410.
13. Vining EPG, Freeman JM, Ballaban-Gil K, et al. A multicenter study of the efficacy of the ketogenic diet. *Arch Neurol.* 1998;55:1433–1437.
14. Roach ES. Alternative neurology: the ketogenic diet. *Arch Neurol.* 1998;55:1403–1404.

25 Battling Quackery

Attitudes About Micronutrient Supplements in American Academic Medicine

James S. Goodwin, MD; Michael R. Tangum, MD
From the Center on Aging, The University of Texas Medical Branch, Galveston.
Arch Intern Med 1999;158:2187–2191

Throughout the 20th century American academic medicine has resisted the concept that supplementation with micronutrients might have health benefits. This resistance is evident in several ways: (1) by the uncritical acceptance of news of toxicity, such as the belief that vitamin C supplements cause kidney stones; (2) by the angry, scornful tone used in discussions of micronutrient supplementation in the leading textbooks of medicine; and (3) by ignoring evidence for possible efficacy of a micronutrient supplement, such as the use of vitamin E for intermittent claudication.

Part of the resistance stems from the fact that the potential benefits of micronutrients were advanced by outsiders, who took their message directly to the public, and part from the fact that the concept of a deficiency disease did not fit in well with prevailing biomedical paradigms, particularly the germ theory. Similar factors might be expected to color the response of academic medicine to any alternative treatment.

In *The Crime of Galileo,* historian Giorgio de Santillana[1] presents a revisionist view of the great scientist's struggle with the Catholic church. According to de Santillana, Galileo's crime was not his propounding a heliocentric universe; it was that he wrote in Italian; he communicated his revolutionary ideas about astronomy directly to the public. Previous scientists wrote in Latin, limiting their audience to other scholars. Within this small community, controversial ideas could be entertained. Copernicus' proposal of a heliocentric universe 70 years before Galileo's treatises had elicited no attempts at suppression by the church. The 17th-century church represented the intellectual establishment, and Galileo's persecutors included some of the finest minds of his time. Galileo was punished not for writing heresy, not for threatening paradigms, but for bypassing the intellectual establishment and taking his exciting ideas directly to the people. The establishment, threatened not so much by his ideas as by his methods, did what it could to destroy his credibility.

In addition, Galileo did not respect professional boundaries. He was a mathematician, and yet his writings dealt with phenomena considered within the purview of philosophers, a profession of considerably higher status than mathematics.[2] Thus, he was considered a usurper as well as a popularizer. In what follows we argue that the reaction of academic medicine to the concept of micronutrient supplementation can best be understood in light of the foregoing description of Galileo. Our thesis is that throughout much of the 20th century, American academic medicine was resistant to the concept that micronutrient supplementation might prove beneficial, and that the cause of this resistance was similar to that which faced Galileo. This resistance is evident in several ways: (1) by uncritical acceptance of bad news about micronutrient supplements; reports of toxic effects were rarely questioned and widely quoted; (2) by the scornful, dismissive tone of the discussions about micronutrient supplementation in textbooks of medicine, a tone avoided in most medical controversies; and (3) by the skeptical reaction greeting any claim of efficacy of a micronutrient, relative to other therapies; indeed, most claims were simply ignored.

Note that in each of the areas mentioned above we examine the reaction to micronutrients relative to other therapies. It is not proof of bias to be concerned about toxicity or to be skeptical of claims of efficacy. Bias occurs when concern and skepticism are applied selectively. Also note that we are not proposing to prove that any particular micronutrient supplement is indeed efficacious. Some readers of earlier drafts of this article have concluded that we are apologists for megavitamins. We are not. Rather, the vitamin controversy is one of a series of examples we have used to discuss the forces that influence medical practice other than those stemming directly from scientific discovery.[3–7]

Herein we rely on the multiple editions of 2 major American medical textbooks: *A Textbook of Medicine*[8] and *Principles of Internal Medicine.*[9] Each has been published in 12 different editions between 1950 and 1992. They can be presumed to represent established opinions and can be used to sample how medical opinion changes over time.[3]

Uncritical Acceptance of News of Toxicity: The Example of High-Dose Vitamin C

To illustrate the uncritical acceptance of bad news, we focus on the discussion of one particular toxic effect—kidney stones resulting from megadose vitamin C.

It is well known that high-dose ascorbate ingestion can cause kidney stones.[10–13] In a casual survey of 20 of our physician colleagues, all were aware of the association. But where does this common knowledge come from? A search of the medical literature found no articles in refereed journals reporting instances of high-dose vitamin C causing kidney stones. Instead, review articles cite book chapters that in turn cite abstracts, letters, and other review articles. Take, for example, a 1984 article entitled "Toxic Effects of Water-Soluble Vitamins"[13] that noted that excessive intake of vitamin C may cause kidney stones and cited 7 references to buttress that statement.[14–20] Of these 7 citations, 5 were textbooks or monographs,[14,15,17–19] 1 was a letter to the *Lancet,*[20] and 1 was a case report not related to either ascorbate or kidney stones.[16] Of the 5 books, 2[15,18] cite a total of 2 additional references to substantiate the claim that high-dose vitamin C causes kidney stones; one was a letter[21] and another a chapter.[22] This chapter in turn cites the same *Lancet* letter[20] and an article in the *Medical Letter,*[23] which is without citations. Nowhere in the trail of citations is there related any fundamental information on whether or how frequently high-dose vitamin C leads to kidney stones. Instead, authors simply make the statement that vitamin C may cause kidney stones and as proof cite other authors who have said the same thing.

What is the actual evidence about vitamin C intake and kidney stones? In 3 case-control studies[24–26] there was no clear association between ascorbate intake or excretion and stone formation. In a prospective observational study[27] of 45,000 men with no history of kidney stones, those men consuming 1500 mg or more of ascorbate daily from diet and supplements had 78% the rate of kidney stone formation of those consuming less than 250 mg daily. This reduction was not statistically significant, but certainly does not support the idea that high-dose ascorbate increases the risk of kidney stones.

The story of vitamin C and kidney stones is not unique. A major component of medical writing on vitamin supplements focused on toxic effects,[10–13] under such titles as "The Vitamin Craze"[10] and "Toxic Effects of Vitamin Overdosage."[11] The 1987 and 1991 editions of Harrison's[9] contain the statement that " . . . disorders of vitamin excess may now be more common than vitamin deficiency." Once again, no evidence is cited to support this statement.

Scornful, Dismissive Tone: The Example of Daily Multiple Vitamin Supplementation

In Harrison's the practice of routine use of multiple vitamins was condemned in the 1950s, 1960s, and 1970s. The following are a few representative quotations:

The [recommended daily] allowances can be met by ingestion of a variety of readily available foods without supplementation emphasis in original . . . the present custom of massive vitamin supplementation on the part of the American public . . . may lead to carelessness in the selection of foods, with resultant amino acid or mineral deficiencies . . . Failure to understand these principles has resulted in much useless supplementation of patients with a great variety of preparations containing vitamin (1950, 1954, 1958, and 1962 editions).

. . . the indiscriminate use or "routine" prescription of vitamin preparations is indefensible, it is poor medical practice . . . (1962 edition).

This practice [prescription of multiple vitamins] is undesirable in three counts. It is wasteful; the use of unnecessary medication is to be deplored; and such use of vitamins lulls many patients and a few doctors into neglecting needed diagnostic studies. . . . well people do not need supplemental vitamins in their diets. . . . There is no justification for the widespread marketing of multivitamins to families for their purported value in preventing colds or infections. This effect cannot be documented. The tendency among food merchants to increase the vitamin content of breakfast cereals to therapeutic levels is an insidious marketing device that cannot be justified (1970 edition).

The attitude toward supplementation with multiple vitamins in Cecil's[8] was more complex, evolving over time. The editions published prior to 1960 contained positive statements, for example: "even a liberal well-balanced diet should be supplemented with all the vitamins known to be essential to human nutrition" (1944, 1947, 1951, 1955, and 1959 editions).

In 1963 the positive comments were eliminated, and the treatment of multiple vitamin supplements became similar to that in Harrison's. For example: "For normal persons consuming foods of a normal diet, multivitamins are not necessary . . . the use of preparations containing not only a number of vitamins but also several minerals is poor medical practice" (1963 edition).

Once again, let us review some of the words: "massive, carelessness, useless, indiscriminate, false, indefensible, wasteful, insidious, unnecessary, deplored, and poor medical practice." Over the last several decades there have been many areas of medical practice about which uncertainty and controversy exist, and these are well covered in the various editions of these 2 textbooks; they include the drug treatment of hyperlipidemia and hyperglycemia, surgical vs medical treatment of angina, and indications for tonsillectomy or hysterectomy. But in none of these discussions does one encounter the contemptuous descriptions found in the discussions of multiple vitamins.

Ignoring Claims of Efficacy: The Example of Vitamin E for Intermittent Claudication

The proposal that vitamin E functioned as an antioxidant in vivo was first raised by several groups of investigators in the early 1940s, and this hypothesis received considerable support from experimental evidence.[28] The easy availability of vitamin E formulations led to considerable human experimentation, much of it self-experimentation, looking for beneficial effects in a wide variety of diseases. A prime example is the use of vitamin E for intermittent claudication.

Exercise-induced claudication of the legs was first described by Erasistratus in the fourth century BC.[29] In modern literature Charcot[30] clearly defined the syndrome and named it intermittent claudication. Medical textbooks throughout the 20th century describe its clinical presentation, course, etiology, and treatment. During the 1940s and 1950s, several clinicians published reports that high-dose vitamin E supplementation was beneficial in intermittent claudication. These reports followed the usual progression from case reports to quasi-experimental design trials, to controlled prospective trials with controls either matched or randomized and with varying degrees of blinding.[31]

Several themes were apparent from these reports. First, high doses of vitamin E were required; the most successful studies used 400 or 800 mg daily, or 50 to 100 times greater than the current recommended daily allowance.[11] Second, the therapeutic effect was delayed, generally becoming evident only after 3 months. This delayed effect distinguished the effect of vitamin E from a placebo effect, which typically is seen early and decays over time.[32] Third, the effect of vitamin E was marked, frequently increasing exercise tolerance several-fold.[31] Four randomized, controlled, double-blinded trials[33–36] have been published. Three[34–36] found efficacy. The fourth,[33] which was negative, was criticized for its relatively brief (12-week) duration and the low levels of bioavailable vitamin E intake.[34,37]

Once again, examining the treatment of a comparison therapy may be helpful. Vasodilating agents have also been in use for intermittent claudication since the late 1940s. There have been a large number of randomized controlled trials of various agents.[38–44] Overall, about half the trials produced a statistically significant effect with treatment, and the magnitude of the effects were similar to or smaller than those found for vitamin E.

Nevertheless, vitamin E was not mentioned in the discussions of therapies for intermittent claudication in any of the 13 editions of Cecil's or the 12 editions of Harrison's published from 1947 to 1992. Both texts in their early editions emphasized a number of specific exercises and physical manipulations; the space devoted to this decreased over time. All editions of the texts discussed surgery, and all discussed the use of vasodilators.

The lack of discussion of vitamin E for intermittent claudication in the 2 major textbooks is paralleled by the dearth of medical publications citing this treatment. A MEDLINE search from 1980 through 1994 found 173 articles referenced under intermittent claudication and vasodilators, 83 articles under intermittent claudication and pentoxifylline, and 5 articles under intermittent claudication and vitamin E.

It is instructive to read some of the early trials of vitamin E treatment for claudication. Vitamin E was associated with marked decreases in the rate of leg amputation and even overall mortality, in addition to decreasing claudication.[33,45,46] It is perfectly possible, perhaps even probable, that those dramatic results, which may have been produced by advocates, would not be reproduced in more rigorous trials. We do not know. To our knowledge, no trials of vitamin E in intermittent claudication have been published in the last 20 years. Only recently, with the growth of studies on the potential role of free radicals in atherogenesis, has vitamin E made it onto the radar screen of academic medicine.

Why the Resistance?

Negative attitudes about micronutrients did not evolve recently; they have deep roots. The resistance of the medical community to the concept that scurvy, beri-beri, and rickets were caused by vitamin deficiencies has been well documented.[47–51] Consider this statement from a 1919 report of the British Medical Research Committee:

> It is difficult to implant the idea of disease as due to deficiency. Disease is so generally associated with positive agents—the parasite, the toxin, the *materies morbi*—that the thought of the pathologist turns naturally to such positive associations and seems to believe with difficulty in causation prefixed by a minus sign.[51]

The pathologists who dominated academic medicine in the late 19th and early 20th centuries lacked the vocabulary to integrate the public health observations of vitamin deficiency into a pathophysiology dominated by the germ theory.[49,50] A popular term used to describe vitamin deficiency disease, *negative causality*, evidenced the pathologists' awkwardness in grappling with the idea.[47,49,50]

This awkwardness is reminiscent of the concept of incommensurability put forth by Feyerabend[52] and Kuhn.[53] We have previously discussed how treatments that do not make sense can be rejected in favor of less effective or more toxic therapies that better fit in with the current understanding of pathophysiology.[3,4]

There are many factors that influence the adoption of new medical treatments other than strict consideration of efficacy, toxic effects, and cost.[5,6,54–57] For example, the financial incentives conferred by patent protection that stimulate the aggressive marketing of new pharmaceuticals were lacking in the case of micronutrients.[55] However, these factors do not explain the anger and scorn illustrated in the quotations from medical textbooks given earlier. Where did the emotion come from? Why did academic medicine deploy the language of denunciation against proponents of vitamin supplements?

For answers we return to the idea with which we introduced this discussion. Galileo is one of the heroes of present day science. We see him as a role model, the man of science battling the forces of unreason. It is therefore extremely ironic, and not a little unsettling, to consider the possibility that, in the fight between academic medicine and the various proponents of micronutrient supplements, the role of academic medicine was more analogous to the 17th-century curia than it was to Galileo. But one senses some of the same vehemence, the same anger directed against "popularizers" of the benefits of micronutrients that must have greeted Galileo. He was not persecuted by an ignorant mob of religious zealots; his enemies were the intellectual and scholarly elite, whom he had bypassed, usurped, and rendered irrelevant.

Of course, this was precisely the course followed by many of the proponents of the benefits of micronutrients, the most famous of whom was Linus Pauling, the chemist who intruded into clinical matters. It is instructive to reread the review articles and editorials published in the 1970s ridiculing and condemning the ideas of Pauling. He was treated as a dangerous enemy, although a few years before his death, like Galileo, he was rehabilitated to the status of a genius with controversial ideas.

Many readers might object at this point, arguing that Pauling was wrong in his advocacy of megadose vitamin C to prevent upper respiratory tract infections. That issue is unresolved,[58–60] and misses the point. Defenders of the 17th-century curia could argue that Galileo was wrong too. He thought the planetary orbits were circular. Pauling's conceptual breakthrough was to postulate that micronutrients might be beneficial in levels higher than the minimum required to avoid classic deficiency syndromes. This idea is now a respectable hypothesis, but 20 years ago it was quackery.

Conclusions

Why is it important or necessary to determine if there has been bias against micronutrient supplements? First, it is always important to talk about bias in science, whether such discussions are couched in the terminology of paradigms and paradigm shifts or whether more earthy language is used. The practice of medicine, and to a lesser extent the practice of science, takes place in and is strongly influenced by social context.[7,61] This context influences everything we do as physicians—which diseases we recognize and which we ignore, which treatments we use, and which we reject.[4] The more we learn about why we do what we do, the more likely we are to avoid errors in the future.

In most areas of investigative medicine, investigators are either right or wrong, or correct or incorrect in their scientific observation and conclusions. But in an area subject to bias the investigator is given no leeway. One error, or perhaps one poorly documented truth, and he/she is at risk of being stigmatized as a quack. Positive results are viewed with suspicion, and are usually accompanied by editorials urging caution; negative results are published in the best journals, with a celebratory tone to the accompanying editorials. What if high-dose vitamin E reduces cardiovascular disease; what if supplemental antioxidants lower the risk of cataracts; what if supplemental folate reduces atherosclerosis and birth defects? For that matter, what if spinal manipulation works better than medications for low back pain or if yoga and relaxation exercises can prevent headache? What is wrong about medical investigators getting excited about these possibilities, just as we get excited about the potential for cytokine antagonists in the therapy of acquired immunodeficiency syndrome or Alzheimer disease?

There are only 3 important questions when evaluating a potential treatment.[5] Does it work? What are the adverse effects? How much does it cost? Ideally, issues such as the theory underlying the treatment or the guild to which the proponents of the treatment belong should be irrelevant to the fundamental questions of efficacy, toxicity, and cost. The history of the response of academic medicine to micronutrient supplementation suggests that we have not attained that ideal.

This work was supported by a Geriatric Leadership Academic Award (AG00618) from the National Institute on Aging, Bethesda, Md.

We thank Malcolm Brodwick, PhD, Donald Burke, MD, David Chiriboga, PhD, Ronald Carson, PhD, Thomas Cole, PhD, Frederick Goodwin, MD, Jean Goodwin, MD, and Ellen Moore, PhD, and Marilyn Brodwick, MPH, for their many helpful suggestions.

References

1. de Santillana G. *The Crime of Galileo.* Chicago, Ill: University of Chicago Press; 1955.

2. Biagioli M. *Galileo Courtier: the Practice of Science in the Culture of Absolutism.* Chicago, Ill: University of Chicago Press; 1993.

3. Goodwin JS, Goodwin JM. Failure to recognize efficacious therapy: the history of aspirin treatment for rheumatoid arthritis. *Perspect Biol Med.* 1981;25:78–92.

4. Goodwin JS, Goodwin JM. The tomato effect: rejection of highly efficacious therapies. *JAMA.* 1984;251:2387–2390.

5. Goodwin JS. The empirical basis for the discovery of new therapies. *Perspect Biol Med.* 1991; 35:20–36.

6. Goodwin JS, Hunt WC, Key CR, Samet JM. Changes in surgical treatments: the example of hysterectomy versus conization for cervical carcinoma in situ. *J Clin Epidemiol.* 1990;43:977–982.

7. Goodwin JS. Culture and medicine: the influence of puritanism on American medical practice. *Perspect Biol Med.* 1995;38:567–577.

8. Cecil RL, ed. *A Textbook of Medicine.* Philadelphia, Pa: WB Saunders Co; 1927.

9. Harrison TR, ed. *Principles of Internal Medicine.* Philadelphia, Pa: Blakiston Co; 1950.

10. Herbert V. The vitamin craze. *Arch Intern Med.* 1980;140:173.

11. Toxic effects of vitamin overdosage. *Med Lett Drugs Ther.* 1984;26:73–74.

12. Woolliscroft JO. Megavitamins: fact and fancy. *Dis Mon.* 1983;29:1–56.

13. Alhadeff L, Gualtiers T, Lipton M. Toxic effects of water-soluble vitamins. *Nutr Rev.* 1984;42:33–40.

14. Wentzler R. *The Vitamin Book.* New York, NY: Doubleday & Co Inc; 1979.

15. Ivey M. *Handbook of Non-Prescription Drugs.* 6th ed. Washington, DC: American Pharmaceutical Association; 1979:141–174.

16. Sugarman AA, Clark CG. Jaundice following the administration of niacin. *JAMA.* 1974; 228:202.

17. Rudman D. Nutritional disorders. In: Isselbacher KJ, Adams RD, Braumwald E, Petersdorf RG, Wilson JD, eds. *Harrison's Principles of Internal Medicine,* 9th ed. New York, NY: McGraw-Hill Book Co; 1980:396–403.

18. Danford DE, Munro HN; Gilman AG, Goodman LS, Gilman E, eds. *The Pharmacologic Basis of Therapeutics.* New York, NY: Macmillan Publishing Co Inc; 1980:1560–1582.

19. Pauling L.; Williams RJ, Kalita DK, eds. *A Physicians' Handbook on Orthomolecular Medicine.* New Canaan, Conn: Keats Publishing Inc; 1977:45–50.

20. Briggs MH, Garcia-Webb P, Davies P. Urinary oxalate and vitamin C supplements. *Lancet.* 1973;2:201.

21. McLeod DC, Nahata MC. Inefficacy of ascorbic acid as a urinary acidifier. *N Engl J Med.* 1977; 296:1413.

22. Herbert V. The rationale of massive-dose vitamin therapy: megavitamin therapy—hot fictions vs cold facts. In: White PL, Selvey N, eds. *Proceedings of the Western Hemisphere Nutrition Congress IV.* Anton, Mass: Publishing Sciences Group; 1974:84–91.

23. Vitamin C: were the trials well controlled and are the large doses safe. *Med Lett.* 1971;13:46–48.

24. Cowley DM, McWhinney BC, Brown JM, Chalmers AH. Chemical factors important to calcium nephrolithiasis: evidence for impaired hydroxycarboxylic acid absorption causing hyperoxaluria. *Clin Chem.* 1987;33:243–247.

25. Power C, Barker DJ, Nelson M, Winter PD. Diet and renal stones: a case-control study. *Br J Urol.* 1984;56:456–459.

26. Fellstrom B, Danielson BG, Karlstrom B, Lithell H, Ljunghall S, Vessby B. Dietary habits in renal stone patients compared with healthy subjects. *Br J Urol.* 1989;63:575–580.

27. Curhan GC, Willett CS, Rimm EB, Stampfer MJ. A prospective study of vitamins B6 and C and the risk of kidney stones in men. *J Urol.* 1996; 155:1848–1851.

28. Green J, Bunyan J. Vitamin E and the biological antioxidant theory. *Nutr Abst Rev.* 1969; 39:321–345.

29. Mettler CC. *History of Medicine.* Philadelphia, Pa: Blakiston Co; 1947:521–522.

30. Charcot JMC. Sur la claudication intermittente observé dans un cas d'oblitèration complète de l'une des artéres iliaques primitives. *C R Soc Biol (Paris).* 1858;5:225–228.

31. Marks J. Clinical appraisal of the therapeutic value of α-tocopherol. *Vitam Horm.* 1962;20:573.

32. Wolf S. The pharmacology of placebos. *Pharmacol Rev.* 1959;11:689–704.

33. Hamilton M, Wilson GM, Armitage P, Boyd JT. The treatment of intermittent claudication with vitamin E. *Lancet.* 1953;1:367–370.

34. Livingstone PD, Jones C. Treatment of intermittent claudication with vitamin E. *Lancet.* 1958;2:602.

35. Williams HTG, Clein LJ, Macbeth RA. Alpha-tocopherol in the treatment of intermittent claudication: a preliminary report. *CMAJ.* 1962;87:538–541.

36. Westheim AS, Brox D, Selvo AW. D-α-tocopherol VFD claudicatio intermittens: en klinsk undersokelse. *Tidsskr Nor Laegeforen.* 1975; 95:13–15.

37. Kleijnen J. Vitamin E and cardiovascular disease. *Eur J Clin Pharmacol.* 1989;37:541–544.

38. De Felice M, Gallo P, Masotti G. Current therapy of peripheral obstructive arterial disease: the nonsurgical approach. *Angiology.* 1990;41:1–11.

39. Hentzer E. Treatment of peripheral arterial insufficiency with inositoli nicotinas (Hexanicit). *Scand J Clin Lab Invest Suppl.* 1967;99:226–232.

40. Reich T. Cyclandelate: effect on circulatory measurements and exercise tolerance in chronic arterial insufficiency of the lower limbs. *J Am Geriatr Soc.* 1977;25:202–205.

41. Trubestein G, Balzer K, Bisler H, et al. Buflomedil in arterial occlusive disease: results of a multicenter study. *Angiology.* 1984;35:500–505.

42. Trubestein G, Bohme H, Heidrich H, et al. Naftidrofuryl in chronic arterial disease: results of a controlled multicenter study. *Angiology.* 1984;35:701–708.

43. Adhoute G, Bacourt F, Barral M, et al. Naftidrofuryl in chronic arterial disease: results of a six-month controlled multicenter study using Naftidrofuryl tablets 200 mg. *Angiology.* 1986;37:160–167.

44. Cameron HA, Waller PC, Ramsay LE. Placebo-controlled trial of ketanserin in the treatment of intermittent claudication. *Angiology.* 1987; 38:549–555.

45. Haeger K. The treatment of peripheral occlusive arterial disease with alpha tocopherol as compared with vasodilator agents and antiprothrombin (dicumarol). *Vasc Dis.* 1968;5:199–213.

46. Boyd AM, Marks J. Treatment of intermittent claudication. *Angiology.* 1963;14:198–208.

47. Maltz A. Physicians' skepticism towards vitamins: the issue of negative causality. *Soc Hist Med Bull.* 1987;40:41–44.

48. Carter KC. The germ theory, beri beri and the deficiency theory of disease. *Med Hist.* 1977; 21:119–136.

49. Ihde AJ, Becker SL. Conflict of concepts in early vitamin studies. *J Hist Biol.* 1971;4:1–33.

50. Follis RH. Cellular pathology and the development of the deficiency disease concept. *Bull Hist Med.* 1960;34:291–317.

51. Medical Research Committee. *Report on the Present State of Knowledge Concerning Accessory Food Factors (Vitamines).* London, England: Medical Research Committee; 1919. Special report No. 38.

52. Feyerabend P. *Farewell to Reason.* London, England: Versa Press; 1987.

53. Kuhn TS; Asquith PD, Nickles T, eds. *Commensurability, Comparability, Communicability.* East Lansing, Mich: Philosophy of Science Association; 1983; 2:669–688.

54. Greer AL. Adoption of medical technology. *Int J Technol Assess Health Care.* 1985;1:669–680.

55. Root-Bernstein RS. The development and dissemination of non-patentable therapies. *Perspect Biol Med.* 1995;39:110–117.

56. De Vet HC, Kessels AG, Leffers P, Knipschild PG. A randomized trial about the perceived informativeness of new empirical evidence. *J Clin Epidemiol.* 1993;46:509–517.

57. Antman EM, Lau J, Kupelnick B, Mosteller F, Chalmers TC. A comparison of results of meta-analyses of randomized trials and recommendations of clinical experts. *JAMA.* 1992; 268:240–248.

58. Chalmers TC. Effects of ascorbic acid on the common cold. *Am J Med.* 1975;58:532–536.

59. Weisburger JH. Vitamin C and disease prevention. *J Am Coll Nutr.* 1995;14:109–111.

60. Heila H. Vitamin C, the placebo effect, and the common cold: a case study of how preconceptions influence the analysis of results. *J Clin Epidemiol.* 1996;49:1079–1084.

61. Foucault M. *The Birth of the Clinic: An Archeology of Medical Perception.* Smith S, trans. New York, NY: Pantheon Books; 1973.

26 Folate, Vitamin B_{12}, and Serum Total Homocysteine Levels in Confirmed Alzheimer Disease

Robert Clarke, MD; A. David Smith, DPhil; Kim A. Jobst, DM; Helga Refsum, MD; Lesley Sutton, BSc; Per M. Ueland, MD

From the Clinical Trial Service Unit and Epidemiological Studies Unit, Nuffield Department of Clinical Medicine (Dr Clarke), Oxford Project to Investigate Memory and Ageing (OPTIMA), University Department of Pharmacology, University of Oxford, and Radcliffe Infirmary Trust (Drs Smith and Jobst and Ms Sutton), Oxford, England; and Department of Pharmacology, University of Bergen, Bergen, Norway (Drs Refsum and Ueland).

Background

Recent studies suggest that vascular disease may contribute to the cause of Alzheimer disease (AD). Since elevated plasma total homocysteine (tHcy) level is a risk factor for vascular disease, it may also be relevant to AD.

Objective

To examine the association of AD with blood levels of tHcy, and its biological determinants folate and vitamin B_{12}.

Design

Case-control study of 164 patients, aged 55 years or older, with a clinical diagnosis of dementia of Alzheimer type (DAT), including 76 patients with histologically confirmed AD and 108 control subjects.

Setting

Referral population to a hospital clinic between July 1988 and April 1996.

Main Outcome Measures

Serum tHcy, folate, and vitamin B_{12} levels in patients and controls at entry; the odds ratio of DAT or confirmed AD with elevated tHcy or low vitamin levels; and the rate of disease progression in relation to tHcy levels at entry.

Results

Serum tHcy levels were significantly higher and serum folate and vitamin B_{12} levels were lower in patients with DAT and patients with histologically confirmed AD than in controls. The odds ratio of confirmed AD associated with a tHcy level in the top third (≥14 μmol/L) compared with the bottom third (≤11 μmol/L) of the control distribution was 4.5 (95% confidence interval, 2.2–9.2), after adjustment for age, sex, social class, cigarette smoking, and apolipoprotein E *ϵ4*. The corresponding odds ratio for the lower third compared with the upper third of serum folate distribution was 3.3

(95% confidence interval, 1.8–6.3) and of vitamin B_{12} distribution was 4.3 (95% confidence interval, 2.1–8.8). The mean tHcy levels were unaltered by duration of symptoms before enrollment and were stable for several years afterward. In a 3-year follow-up of patients with DAT, radiological evidence of disease progression was greater among those with higher tHcy levels at entry.

Conclusions

Low blood levels of folate and vitamin B_{12}, and elevated tHcy levels were associated with AD. The stability of tHcy levels over time and lack of relationship with duration of symptoms argue against these findings being a consequence of disease and warrant further studies to assess the clinical relevance of these associations for AD.

Arch Neurol. 1998;55:1449–1455

Alzheimer disease (AD) and vascular dementia—the 2 major subtypes of dementia—have distinct pathological features, but these frequently coexist,[1] and the combination results in more severe symptoms of dementia.[2,3] In addition to the established role of cerebral infarction in vascular dementia,[4] recent studies have suggested that cardiovascular disease,[5,6] atherosclerosis, and abnormalities in the cerebral microvasculature[7–10] may also be relevant to the cause of AD. Furthermore, the ϵ*4* allele of apolipoprotein E (apoE) is a risk factor not only for AD[11] but also for cardiovascular disease, and the presence of both may interact in the cause of AD.[7,12]

These findings have prompted us to investigate whether elevated serum total homocysteine (tHcy) levels, a risk factor for vascular disease,[13,14] may also be relevant to AD. Moderately elevated levels of tHcy are common in the population and increase with aging,[15,16] and have been reported in patients with clinical diagnoses of dementia of Alzheimer type (DAT) or vascular dementia.[17,18] In the present study, we examined the association of histologically confirmed AD with serum tHcy levels using a case-control design. We studied the nutritional (folate and vitamin B_{12})[15] and genetic (*MTHFR* [methylenetetrahydrofolate reductase] polymorphisms)[19] determinants of tHcy levels, and their relation to AD. We also assessed whether differences in tHcy levels at study recruitment were related to the clinical course by using atrophy of the medial temporal lobe as a marker of disease progression.[20]

Subjects and Methods

Subjects and Clinical Investigations

Between July 1988 and April 1996, 228 patients from the Oxfordshire Health Authority area in England who had varying degrees of cognitive dysfunction were referred to the Oxford Project to Investigate Memory and Ageing (OPTIMA).[21] Patients younger than 55 years (n=9) or for whom blood samples were not available for tHcy measurements (n=28) were excluded.

Among the 191 remaining patients, 76 of the 103 on whom an autopsy was performed had a histological diagnosis of AD using Consortium to Establish a Registry for Alzheimer's Disease (CERAD) criteria[22] for definite or probable AD, 12 had vascular dementia, and 15 had other causes of dementia. A further 88 living patients had a clinical diagnosis of probable or possible DAT according to National Institute of Neurological Disorders and Stroke–Alzheimer's Disease and Related Disorders Association criteria,[23] and these were combined with the 76 histopathologically confirmed AD cases to give 164 patients with a clinical diagnosis of DAT. Among the AD cases, histological evidence of concomitant cerebrovascular disease was defined by the presence of 1 or more infarcts in the cortex, thalamus, or basal ganglia in addition to the typical histological features of AD. These patients were compared with 108 elderly volunteer controls without symptoms of memory impairment (17 of whom were patients' relatives) who were recruited by leaflets or by lectures given at retirement association clubs or from general practices in the Oxfordshire Health Authority area during the same period. All subjects underwent a detailed clinical history, physical examination, assessment of cognitive function (Cambridge Examination for Mental Disorders of the Elderly [CAMDEX],[24] from which the Cambridge Cognitive Examination [CAMCOG] and Mini-Mental State Examination [MMSE] scores were derived) annually. X-ray cranial computed tomography scans were performed annually using both the standard axial angle and the temporal lobe–oriented angle, as described previously.[21] The minimum thickness of the medial temporal lobe at the level of the brainstem was measured from hard copies of the temporal lobe–oriented scan by 2 independent observers who were unaware of the diagnosis and previous scans. A Dementia Severity Rating score was derived from the CAMDEX at the time of assessment and scored as follows: none, 0; minimal, 0.5; mild, 1; moderate, 2; and severe, 3. Informed consent was obtained for all individuals to participate in the study, which had local ethics committee approval.

Biochemical Measurements

Nonfasting blood samples were taken at the first visit and stored at –70°C. Vitamin B_{12} level was measured using a radioimmunoassay; serum folate and red blood cell folate levels were determined by microbiological assays on fresh samples. Levels of tHcy were determined by high-performance liquid chromatography with fluorescence detection.[25] The intraclass correlation coefficient of tHcy between replicate samples taken at 2-month intervals on 7 occasions during a 1-year period in 96 healthy elderly subjects was 0.88.[26] ApoE genotypes[27] and the 677C→T mutation in the *MTHFR* gene[19] were determined by standard methods. All measurements were obtained in a blind manner to each other and to the diagnoses.

Statistical Analyses

The odds ratio (OR) of AD was examined using logistic regression analysis for the top third and middle third compared with the bottom third of the tHcy concentration distribution in the control population. For folate and vitamin B_{12}, the OR of AD for the bottom third and middle third were compared with the top third of the distribution in the control population. In the regression analysis models, age and years of full-time education were entered as continuous variables, and sex, social class (manual or nonmanual employment), cigarette smokers (ever or never smokers), and apoE $\epsilon 4$ allele status (present or absent) were entered as dichotomous variables. The confidence interval (CI) for each OR was estimated by treating these as "floating absolute risks."[28]

Results

Study Populations

Characteristics of the study populations are shown in Table 1. The clinically diagnosed DAT patients and controls were well matched for age, sex, and smoking status (Table 1). The subset of patients with histologically confirmed AD were older than the controls, and both case populations had a lower social class distribution than controls. The disease severity among the patients is reflected by the low cognitive scores (MMSE and CAMCOG). Fifty-nine (36%) of the patients with clinically diagnosed DAT and 43 (57%) of the patients with histologically confirmed AD had a Dementia Severity Rating score (maximum 3) of 2 or greater at the first visit. Forty-one (25%) of the patients with clinically diagnosed DAT and histologically confirmed AD were residents in institutions at the first visit. Among the patients with histologically confirmed AD, the median interval between the first visit and death was 29 months (95% CI, 2–69 months).

Serum Homocysteine

The mean serum tHcy levels at the first visit were significantly higher in patients with clinically diagnosed DAT and histologically confirmed AD than in Table 1. The cumulative frequency plots (Figure 1) show a shift in the distribution of tHcy concentrations to higher values in patients with clinically diagnosed DAT and histologically confirmed AD compared with controls. Seventy-four patients (45%) with clinically diagnosed DAT and 45 patients (59%) with histologically confirmed AD had a tHcy value in the top third (≥14 μmol/L) of the control distribution.

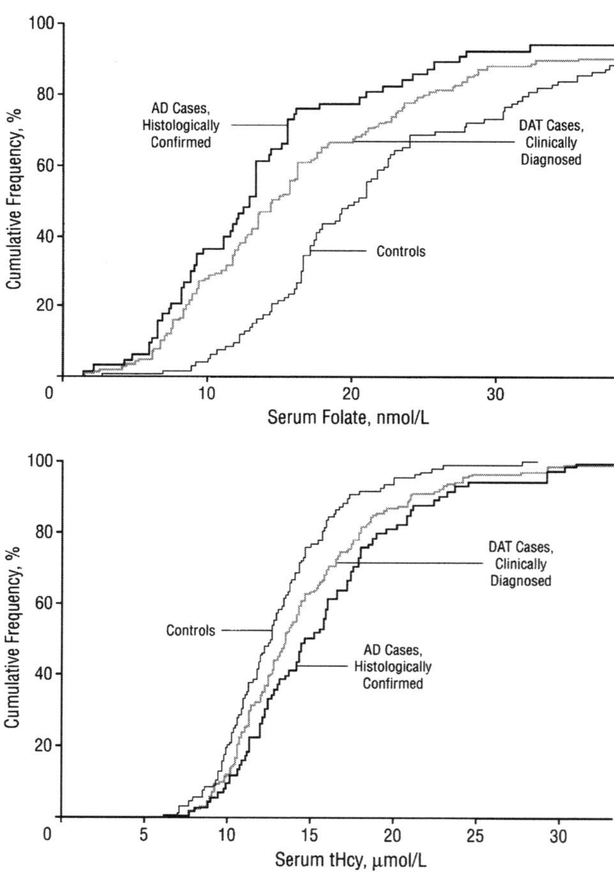

Figure 1. Cumulative frequency distributions of serum folate (top) and serum total homocysteine (tHcy) (bottom) levels in patients with histologically confirmed Alzheimer disease (AD) and clinically diagnosed dementia of Alzheimer type (DAT) and in control subjects.

Table 1. Characteristics at Presentation in Controls and in Patients With Alzheimer Disease*

Variable	Controls (n=108)	Patients With Alzheimer Disease: Clinically Diagnosed (n=164)	Patients With Alzheimer Disease: Histologically Confirmed (n=76)
Clinical variables			
Age, mean (SD), y	72.8 (8.8)	73.2 (8.6)	76.6 (8.0)†
Sex, % male	43	39	37
Current smokers, %	21	21	24
Social class: grades 1 and 2, %	80	46†	49†
Full-time education, mean (SD), y	11.4 (1.5)	10.4 (2.0)†	10.3 (2.3)†
CAMCOG score (maximum 107), mean (SD)	97.8 (4.9)	55.2 (26.5)†	45.1 (27.5)†
MMSE score (maximum 30), mean (SD)	28.5 (1.7)	16.2 (8.0)†	12.8 (8.1)†
Minimum medial temporal lobe thickness, mean (SD), mm	13.5 (3.0)	9.9 (2.9)†	9.3 (2.9)†
Biochemical variables, mean (SD)			
Total homocysteine, μmol/L	13.2 (4.0)	15.3 (8.4)‡	16.3 (7.4)†
Serum folate, nmol/L	22.9 (10.0)	17.6 (10.7)†	15.2 (9.5)†
Red blood cell folate, nmol/L	991 (407)	866 (446)‡	737 (386)†
Vitamin B_{12}, pmol/L	253 (100)	236 (112)	215 (79)‡
Creatinine, μmol/L	93 (19)	90 (18)	90 (20)
Albumin, g/L	45 (4)	43 (3.8)†	42 (4)†
Hemoglobin, g/L	136 (15)	133 (14)	131 (15)‡
Genotypes			
ApoE ϵ*4* allele frequency, %	14	38†	44†
MTHFR homozygous mutant frequency, %	9	7	5

*CAMCOG indicates Cambridge Cognitive Examination; MMSE, Mini-Mental State Examination; ApoE, apolipoprotein E; and *MTHFR*, methylenetetrahydrofolate reductase.

†*P*<.001 vs controls.

‡*P*<.05.

To identify possible confounders for this association, we looked at the influence of several variables on tHcy levels. Among controls, tHcy level was positively correlated with age (r=0.32, P=.001), male sex (r=0.27, P=.004), cigarette smoking (r=0.23, P=.02), and creatinine level (r=0.44, P<.001), and was inversely associated with levels of serum folate (r=–0.34, P=.001), vitamin B_{12} (r=–0.32, P=.002), and red blood cell folate (r=–0.21, P=.05). There was no association between tHcy and apoE ϵ*4*, or the *MTHFR* mutation, or with social class or years of full-time education in the control population. Among the DAT cases, years of full-time education were inversely related with social class grades 1 to 6 (r=–0.58, P<.001), but tHcy levels were unrelated to social class (r=0.03, P=.72) or years of full-time education (r=–0.10, P=.28). The mean (SD) tHcy levels were 15.5 (7.5) μmol/L in social class grades 1 and 2 and 15.1 (9.0) μmol/L in grades 3 to 6.

Table 2 shows that the associations of tHcy levels with both clinically diagnosed DAT and histologically confirmed AD were independent of age, sex, smoking status, apoE ϵ*4*, and social class. When social class was replaced by years of education in the multivariate analysis, an OR of 4.6 (95% CI, 1.8–5.5) was found for histologically confirmed AD in subjects with tHcy levels in the top third of the distribution; the OR was 3.6 (95% CI, 1.7–5.7) when both social class and years of education were adjusted for simultaneously. In addition, when the analyses were confined to cases (n=38) and controls (n=88) from social classes 1 and 2, the corresponding OR of AD associated with tHcy level in the top third of the distribution was 6.5 (95% CI, 2.6–16.5).

The OR of histologically confirmed AD for the top third compared with the bottom third of tHcy values was 5.1 (95% CI, 1.8–14.0) when both folate and vitamin B_{12} were also included in the regression analysis model. Among the histologically confirmed AD cases, the 31 patients with concomitant histological evidence of cerebrovascular disease had a mean (SD) tHcy level of 16.3 (5.8) μmol/L (P<.001 vs controls), and the 45 who had confirmed AD alone had a mean (SD) tHcy level of 16.3 (8.4) μmol/L (P<.001 vs controls).

Among the 26 patients with histopathologically diagnosed non-AD dementia, the mean (SD) tHcy level was 20.0 (9.6) μmol/L in 12 with vascular dementia (P<.001 vs controls), 18.4 (7.7) μmol/L in 3 with Parkinson disease, 18.7 (7.7) μmol/L in 2 with glioblastoma, 11.0 (3.2) μmol/L in 2 with Huntington disease, and 12.0 (3.2) μmol/L in the

Table 2. Odds Ratios of Clinically Diagnosed Dementia of Alzheimer Type (DAT) and of Histologically Confirmed Alzheimer Disease (AD) by Total Homocysteine (tHcy) and Vitamin Levels*

	Clinically Diagnosed DAT		Histologically Confirmed AD	
Tertiles	**Adjusted for Age and Sex**	**Adjusted for Age, Sex, Smoking, Social Class, and ApoE ϵ4**	**Adjusted for Age and Sex**	**Adjusted for Age, Sex, Smoking, Social Class, and ApoE ϵ4**
tHcy, μmol/L				
I ≤11.0	1.0 (0.6–1.6)	1.0 (0.6–1.8)	1.0 (0.5–1.9)	1.0 (0.4–2.7)
II 11.1–14.0	1.1 (0.7–1.7)	1.1 (0.7–1.9)	1.3 (0.7–2.3)	1.0 (0.4–2.3)
III >14.0	1.9 (1.2–2.9)	2.0 (1.1–3.4)	3.3 (2.1–5.2)	4.5 (2.2–9.2)
Folate, nmol/L				
III >24.2	1.0 (0.6–1.6)	1.0 (0.5–1.7)	1.0 (0.5–2.1)	1.0 (0.3–3.1)
II 17.2–24.2	0.8 (0.5–1.4)	0.7 (0.4–1.5)	0.6 (0.2–1.6)	0.4 (0.1–1.5)
I ≤17.1	2.5 (1.7–3.8)	2.3 (1.4–3.8)	5.0 (3.1–8.2)	3.3 (1.8–6.3)
Vitamin B_{12}, pmol/L				
III >280	1.0 (0.6–1.6)	1.0 (0.5–1.9)	1.0 (0.5–2.1)	1.0 (0.3–3.8)
II 200–280	1.3 (0.8–2.0)	1.7 (1.0–3.0)	2.1 (1.2–3.6)	5.6 (2.6–11.9)
I ≤199	1.4 (0.9–2.2)	1.4 (0.8–2.5)	1.8 (1.0–3.2)	4.3 (2.1–8.8)

*Data are given as odds ratios (confidence intervals). ApoE indicates apolipoprotein E. The confidence intervals for the odds ratios have been estimated by treating these as "floating absolute risks," which take account of the variance in the reference category.[28] The cut points selected were based on the tertile levels in the control subjects.

7 remaining patients with various histopathological findings. Two of the 3 patients with Parkinson disease who had elevated tHcy levels were taking levodopa. The OR of vascular dementia associated with a tHcy concentration in the top third (≥14 μmol/L) compared with the bottom third (≤11 μmol/L) of the control distribution was 4.5 (95% CI, 1.6-12.8) after adjustment for age, sex, social class, smoking status, and apoE ϵ4, which was similar to that for AD.

Serum Folate and Vitamin B_{12}

The mean serum folate and vitamin B_{12} levels at the first visit were significantly lower in AD patients than in controls (Table 1). There was a marked shift in the distribution of folate concentrations to lower values in both clinically diagnosed DAT and histologically confirmed AD patients compared with controls (Figure 1). Ninety-eight patients (60%) with DAT and 58 patients (76%) with confirmed AD had serum folate concentrations in the bottom third of the control distribution. Among the 12 patients with vascular dementia, the mean (SD) folate levels were 13.8 (11.3) nmol/L (P=.01 vs controls) and mean vitamin B_{12} levels were 231.7 (83.4) pmol/L (P=.52 vs controls).

Possible confounders of the association of folate level with histologically confirmed AD were also examined. Among the controls, serum folate levels were lower in smokers compared with nonsmokers (P<.05). Controls had a higher social class distribution than the patients, but there was no significant difference in folate (or tHcy) concentrations between manual and nonmanual employment classes. After including years of education in addition to social class and all the other confounders shown in Table 2, the OR of AD comparing the bottom third with the top third of serum folate distribution was 2.3 (95% CI, 1.2–4.4). The strength of association between vitamin B_{12} levels and confirmed AD was similar to that for tHcy (Table 2). After the addition of tHcy to the multivariate model, the ORs for confirmed AD for the lower third compared with the upper third of control concentrations of serum folate or vitamin B_{12} were no longer significant: 1.6 (95% CI, 0.8–3.2) and 2.2 (95% CI, 0.8–5.2), respectively.

ApoE and *MTHFR* Polymorphisms

The apoE ϵ4 allele frequency was 38% in DAT and 44% in AD cases, compared with 14% in controls. After adjusting for differences in age, sex, smoking status, and social class, the OR of confirmed AD for the presence of 1 or more apoE ϵ4 alleles compared with none was 7.9 (95% CI, 3.3–18.8). Moreover, the strength of the association of apoE ϵ4 was unchanged by the inclusion of tHcy in the multivariate analysis. There was no significant difference in the prevalence of the *MTHFR* gene 677C→T mutation, whether expressed as the proportion homozygous (5% vs 9%) or as allele frequency (22% vs 30%), in patients with histologically confirmed AD compared with controls.

Influence of Duration of Memory Impairment on Homocysteine and Vitamin Levels

To assess whether the prior duration of dementia could explain the observed biochemical changes, 72 histologically confirmed AD patients with available data were classified by tertiles of duration of memory impairment (as reported by an informant) before their first visit when the blood samples were taken (Table 3). The disease severity was substantially greater in those with a longer duration of memory impairment, but there was no significant trend in the mean levels of any of the biochemical variables with increasing duration of symptoms. The biochemical findings were also unaltered by duration of illness among patients with clinically diagnosed DAT (data not shown).

Stability of Homocysteine Concentrations Over Time

Replicate tHcy measurements were obtained at sequential annual follow-up visits in 30 patients with DAT. The mean tHcy level was 14.1 μmol/L at first visit, 13.6 μmol/L at year 1, 13.6 μmol/L at year 2, and 13.3 μmol/L at year 3, and the correlation coefficients at these intervals with baseline levels were 0.85, 0.83, and 0.78, respectively. Similar estimates of stability in tHcy measurements were obtained in 34 controls with correlation coefficients with baseline tHcy concentrations of 0.78, 0.74, and 0.73 at years 1 through 3, respectively.

Homocysteine and Vitamin Levels and Disease Progression

To assess whether differences in tHcy and vitamin levels at the first visit were related to disease progression, we compared the results in 43 patients with clinically diagnosed DAT for whom we had computed tomographic scans and MMSE scores from 4 annual visits (Table 4). At the first visit, the mean age-corrected minimum thickness of the medial temporal lobes in subjects for each of the tertiles of tHcy did not differ. After 3 years, there was significantly greater radiological evidence of disease progression, as assessed by medial temporal lobe thickness, among those with tHcy levels in the middle and upper tertiles compared with those in the lower tertile, who showed little atrophy (Table 4). The association between blood levels of folate and vitamin B_{12} at the first visit and disease progression showed a similar trend, but the differences were not statistically significant (data not shown). The mean (SD) MMSE scores when classified by low, middle, and upper tertiles of tHcy declined from 22 (5), 22 (6), and 19 (8) at the first visit to 13 (6), 15 (9), and 12 (9) after 3 years, but the variance was too large to distinguish any difference from no effect.

Comment

Elevated tHcy levels within the range of those associated with vascular disease[14] have been previously reported in patients with clinically diagnosed DAT and in patients with vascular dementia[17,18] and several studies have demonstrated inverse associations between clinically diagnosed DAT and folate and vitamin B_{12} levels.[17,18,29–34] Similar associations also have been shown for cognitive impairment in the elderly.[35] We observed that there were significant associations of histologically confirmed AD and of vascular dementia with moderately elevated blood levels of tHcy and with reduced blood levels of folate and vitamin B_{12}. The cumulative frequency plots (Figure 1) showed a more marked case-control difference for the distribution of serum folate levels than that for serum tHcy levels, but the relative importance of these associations requires further study. The finding that patients with elevated tHcy levels (Table 4) at the first visit had more rapid atrophy of the medial temporal lobe during a 3-year follow-up than those with lower tHcy levels warrants confirmation in other prospective studies.

The crucial question is whether the observed associations are a cause or consequence of the disease. It could, for example, be argued that dementia leads to a reduced dietary intake of folate and vitamin B_{12}, causing an elevation in tHcy levels. We cannot refute this possibility in this case-control study, but we found no evidence that the duration of memory impairment before the blood sample was taken influenced the biochemical variables. Patients who were symptomatic for more than 4 years before their first visit and whose mean MMSE score was 8 showed no significant difference in the blood levels of tHcy, folate, or vitamin B_{12} from those whose symptoms had been present for less than 2 years and who had a mean MMSE score of 16 (Table 3). Furthermore, the high correlation observed in the DAT cases and controls between baseline tHcy concentrations and those obtained a few years later suggests that the biochemical differences between patients and controls were not due to a progression of the disease during this period. Thus, we suggest that the low vitamin levels and high tHcy levels either existed before the start of AD or developed early in the disease phase. Either way, the abnormality in these biochemical markers may be relevant to the clinical course of AD and should be considered in clinical trials as possible targets for therapeutic intervention. Daily supplementation with 0.5 to 5 mg of folic acid and about 0.5 mg of cyanocobalamin would be expected to reduce homocysteine levels found in typical Western populations on

Table 3. Clinical and Biochemical Variables in Patients With Histologically Confirmed Alzheimer Disease by Duration of Memory Impairment at Presentation*

	Clinical Variables, Mean (SD) or %			Biochemical Variables, Mean (SD)			
Tertiles of Duration of Memory Impairment, y	MMSE Score (Maximum 30)	Minimum Medial Temporal Lobe Thickness, mm	Dementia Severity Rating (Maximum 3) % 2 or 3	Total Homocysteine, μmol/L	Serum Folate, nmol/L	Red Blood Cell Folate, nmol/L	Vitamin B_{12}, pmol/L
I <2	16 (8)	9.9 (2.3)	33	18.8 (10.8)	17.6 (12.2)	749 (466)	216 (82)
II 2–4	14 (8)	9.5 (2.4)	56	15.4 (5.7)	12.9 (5.7)	722 (398)	201 (63)
III >4	8 (6)	8.7 (3.6)	88	14.8 (4.1)	14.0 (7.3)	706 (242)	235 (89)
Test for linear trend *P*	<.001	<.001	<.001	.06	.19	.72	.42

*MMSE indicates Mini-Mental State Examination.

Table 4. Changes in Minimum Medial Temporal Lobe Thickness (MMTL) Over a 3-Year Period by Total Homocysteine (tHcy) Levels at Presentation in Patients With Clinically Diagnosed Dementia of Alzheimer Type

	Baseline			Follow-up*				
				Ratio of Age-Adjusted Baseline MMTL Values, %				
Tertiles of tHcy in Controls, μmol/L	No. (n=43)	Absolute MMTL Values, Mean (SD), mm	Age-Adjusted MMTL Values, Mean (SD) (Multiple of Median)†	Year 0	Year 1:0	Year 2:0	Year 3:0	Trend by Years of Follow-up, *P*
I ≤11.0	15	10.0 (2.5)	0.71 (0.16)	100	101	99	95	.07
II 11.1–14.0	11	11.6 (2.7)	0.83 (0.16)	100	93	81	68	.04
III >14.0	17	10.4 (2.5)	0.77 (0.17)	100	97	93	81	.03
Test for difference by tertiles of tHcy‡		.20	.31	. . .	.12	.06	.02	

*The follow-up data are adjusted for age and expressed as a ratio of the values at presentation. Ellipses indicate data are not applicable.

†Details of how the age-adjusted values were derived have been previously described.[21]

‡Analysis of variance, probability greater than F. Ellipses indicate data are not applicable.

average by about one third.[36] Large-scale clinical trials in high-risk populations are now needed to determine whether lowering blood homocysteine levels reduces the risk of AD and of other dementias.

The chief strength of the present study is the longitudinal assessment of dementia cases with subsequent histopathological confirmation of the types of dementia, so overcoming the inaccuracies of clinical diagnosis. A limitation of this study was that control subjects had a higher overall social class than the patients. However, there were no differences in the mean tHcy or folate levels between manual and nonmanual classes or by years of education in the patients. In addition, when either social class or years of education, or both together, were taken into account in the multivariate analyses, and when the analyses were confined to a subset where most of the controls were recruited, the ORs of AD were still highly significant. A further limitation of this study is the lack of data on recent dietary intake and vitamin supplements in patients compared with controls.

Although the mechanisms underlying the observed associations remain to be established, certain hypotheses should be considered. The association of low folate and vitamin B_{12} levels with AD may be related to their effects on methylation reactions in the brain[37] or may be mediated by their effects on tHcy levels.[15] Homocysteine may have a neurotoxic effect by activating the *N*-methyl-D-aspartate receptor, leading to cell death,[38] or it might be converted into homocysteic acid, which also has an excitotoxic effect on neurons.[39] In addition, elevated tHcy levels are a strong risk factor for vascular disease.[13,14] This might explain the association in the patients with confirmed AD who also had histological evidence of cerebrovascular disease. However, the association with tHcy was also observed in patients with AD and no macroscopic cerebrovascular disease. Perhaps microvascular disease associated with tHcy could play a role in the cause of "pure" AD. We have previously suggested that the onset of AD is triggered by some kind of "insult."[20] This insult could be a consequence of microvascular disease or ischemia in a critical region of the brain, such as the hippocampus, which shows marked vascular abnormalities in AD.[10] The CA_1 pyramidal neurons in the hippocampus are particularly vulnerable to ischemia,[40] and these same neurons show the highest density of neurofibrillary tangles and are selectively depleted in AD.[31,41] Thus, microinfarcts, arising as a consequence of elevated tHcy levels, may result in the deposition of β-amyloid plaques and neurofibrillary tangles that are the pathologic hallmarks of dementia.

Despite the plausible mechanisms, further work is required to establish whether the observed associations are causal. Our data show that elevated tHcy levels and low folate and vitamin B_{12} levels are common in patients with AD. The stability of tHcy levels and lack of relationship with duration of symptoms argue against these associations being a consequence of disease and warrant further studies to determine the relevance of these associations to the onset and progression of AD.

This work was supported by a grant from Bristol-Myers Squibb, Princeton, NJ.

We thank the patients, caregivers, volunteers, and referring clinicians in the Oxford Region. Richard Doll, FRS, Richard Peto, FRS, Rory Collins, and Marc Budge, FRACP, provided helpful comments. We acknowledge Lin Barnetson, Elizabeth King, Amy Smith, Jean Barton, Carole Johnston, and Nicholas Hindley and colleagues in the Neuropathology and Neuroradiology Departments at the Radcliffe Infirmary, Oxford, England, for their help in this project.

References

1. Esiri M, Wilcock GK. Cerebral amyloid angiopathy in dementia and in old age. *J Neurol Neurosurg Psychiatry.* 1986;49:1221–1226.
2. Nagy ZS, Esiri MM, Jobst KA, et al. The effects of additional pathology on the cognitive deficit of Alzheimer's disease. *J Neuropathol Exp Neurol.* 1997;56:165–170.
3. Snowden DA, Greiner LH, Mortimer JA, Riley KP, Greiner PA, Markesbery WR. Brain infarction and the clinical expression of Alzheimer's disease: the Nun Study. *JAMA.* 1997; 277:813–817.
4. Esiri MM, Wilcock GK, Morris JH. Neuropathological assessment of the lesions of significance in vascular disease. *J Neurol Neurosurg Psychiatry.* 1997;63:749–753.
5. Hachinsky V. Preventable senility: a call for action against the vascular dementias. *Lancet.* 1992;340:645–647.
6. Launer LJ, Masaki K, Petrovitch H, Foley D, Havlick RJ. The association between midlife blood pressure levels and late-life cognitive function: the Honolulu-Asia Aging Study. *JAMA.* 1995;274:1846–1851.
7. Hoffman A, Ott A, Breteler MM, et al. Atherosclerosis, apolipoprotein E, and prevalence of dementia and Alzheimer's disease in the Rotterdam Study. *Lancet.* 1997;345:151–154.
8. Kalaria RN. The blood brain barrier and cerebral microcirculation in Alzheimer disease. *Cerebrovasc Brain Metab Rev.* 1992;4:226–260.
9. de la Torre JC, Mussivand T. Can disturbed brain microcirculation cause Alzheimer's disease? *Neurol Res.* 1993;15:146–153.
10. Buee L, Hof PR, Bouras C, et al. Pathological alterations of the cerebral microvasculature in Alzheimer's disease and related dementing disorders. *Acta Neuropathol Berl.* 1994; 87:469–480.
11. Roses AD. Apolipoprotein E alleles as risk factors in Alzheimer diseases. *Annu Rev Med.* 1996;47:387–400.
12. Kalaria RN. Arteriosclerosis, apolipoprotein E, and Alzheimer's disease. *Lancet.* 1997;349:1174.
13. Clarke R, Daly L, Robinson K, et al. Hyperhomocysteinemia: an independent risk factor for vascular disease. *N Engl J Med.* 1991;324:1149–1155.
14. Boushey CJ, Beresford SA, Omenn GS, Motulsky AG. A quantitative assessment of plasma homocysteine as a risk factor for vascular disease: probable benefits of increasing folic acid intakes. *JAMA.* 1995;274:1049–1057.
15. Selhub J, Jacques PF, Wilson PWF, Rush D, Rosenberg IH. Vitamin status and intake as primary determinants of homocysteinemia in an elderly population. *JAMA.* 1993;270:2693–2698.
16. Nygard O, Vollset SE, Refsum H, et al. Total plasma homocysteine and cardiovascular risk profile: the Hordaland Homocysteine Study. *JAMA.* 1995;274:1526–1533.
17. Nilsson K, Gustafson L, Faldt R, et al. Hyperhomocysteinemia: a common finding in a psychogeriatric population. *Eur J Clin Invest.* 1996;26:853–859.
18. Joosten E, Lesaffre E, Riezler R, et al. Is metabolic evidence for vitamin B-12 and folate deficiency more frequent in elderly patients with Alzheimer's disease. *J Gerontol.* 1997;52:76–79.
19. Frosst P, Blom HJ, Milos R, et al. A candidate genetic risk factor for vascular disease: a common genetic mutation in methylene tetrahydrofolate reductase. *Nat Genet.* 1995;10:111–113.
20. Jobst KA, Smith AD, Szatmari M, et al. Rapidly progressing atrophy of medial temporal lobe in Alzheimer's disease. *Lancet.* 1994;343:829–830.
21. Jobst KA, Smith AD, Szatmari M, et al. Detection in life of confirmed Alzheimer's disease using a simple measurement of medial temporal lobe atrophy by computed tomography. *Lancet.* 1992;340:1179–1183.
22. Mirra SS, Heyman A, McKeel D, et al. The Consortium to Establish a Registry for Alzheimer's Disease (CERAD), 2: standardization of the neuropathologic assessment of Alzheimer's disease. *Neurology.* 1991;41:479–486.
23. McKhann G, Drachman D, Folstein M, Katzman R, Price D, Stadlan EM. Clinical diagnosis of Alzheimer's disease: report of the NINCDS-ADRDA work group under the auspices of the Department of Health and Human Services Task Force of Alzheimer's Disease. *Neurology.* 1984; 34:939–944.
24. Roth M, Huppert FA, Tym E, et al. *CAMDEX: The Cambridge Examination for Mental Disorders of the Elderly.* Cambridge, England: Cambridge University Press; 1988.
25. Ueland PM, Refsum H, Stabler SP, Malinow MR, Andersson A, Allen RH. Total homocysteine in plasma or serum: methods and clinical applications. *Clin Chem.* 1993;39:764–779.
26. Clarke R, Woodhouse P, Ulvik A, et al. Variability and determinants of plasma total homocysteine levels in an elderly population. *Clin Chem.* 1998;44:102–107.

27. Wenham PR, Price WH, Blandell G. Apolipoprotein E genotyping by one-stage PCR. *Lancet.* 1991;337:1158–1159.

28. Easton DF, Peto J, Babiker AG. Floating absolute risk: an alternative to relative risk in survival and case-control analysis avoiding an arbitrary reference group. *Stat Med.* 1991;10:1025–1035.

29. Renvall MJ, Spindler AA, Ramsdell JW, Paskvan M. Nutritional status of free-living Alzheimer's patients. *Am J Med Sci.* 1989;298:20–27.

30. Kristensen MO, Gulmann NC, Christensen JEJ, Ostergaard K, Rasmussen K. Serum cobalamin and methylmalonic acid in Alzheimer dementia. *Acta Neurol Scand.* 1993;87:475–481.

31. Ball MJ, Fisman M, Hachinski V, et al. A new definition of Alzheimer's disease: a hippocampal dementia. *Lancet.* 1985;1:14–16.

32. Cole MG, Prchal JF. Low serum vitamin B_{12} in Alzheimer-type dementia. *Age Ageing.* 1984; 13:101–105.

33. Karnaze DS, Carmel R. Low serum cobalamin levels in primary degenerative dementia: do some patients harbor atypical cobalamin deficiency states? *Arch Intern Med.* 1987;147:429–431.

34. Nijst TQ, Wevers RA, Schoonderwaldt HC, Hommes OR, de Haan AF. Vitamin B^{12} and folate concentrations in serum and cerebrospinal fluid of neurological patients with special reference to multiple sclerosis and dementia. *J Neurol Neurosurg Psychiatry.* 1990;53:951–954.

35. Riggs KM, Spiro A, Tucker K, Rush D. Relations of vitamin B^{12}, vitamin B^{6}, folate, and homocysteine to cognitive performance in the Normative Aging Study. *Am J Clin Nutr.* 1996;63:306–314.

36. Clarke R, Frost C, Leroy V, Collins R. Lowering blood homocysteine with folic acid based supplements: meta-analysis of randomised trials: Homocysteine Lowering Trialist's Collaboration. *BMJ.* 1998;316:894–898.

37. Bottiglieri T, Hyland K, Reynolds EH. The clinical potential of adometionine (*S*-adenosylmethionine) in neurological disorders. *Drugs.* 1994; 48:137–152.

38. Lipton SA, Kim WK, Choi YB, et al. Neurotoxicity associated with dual actions of homocysteine at the *N*-methyl-D-aspartate receptor. *Proc Natl Acad Sci U S A.* 1997;94:5923–5928.

39. Beal MF, Swartz KJ, Finn SF, Mazurek MF, Kowall NW. Neurochemical characterization of excitoxin lesions in the cerebral cortex. *J Neurosci.* 1991;11:147–158.

40. Schmidt-Kastner R, Freund TF. Selective vulnerability of the hippocampus in brain ischemia. *Neuroscience.* 1991;40:599–636.

41. West MJ, Coleman PD, Flood DG, Troncoso JC. Differences in the pattern of hippocampal neuronal loss in normal ageing and Alzheimer's disease. *Lancet.* 1994;344:769–772.

27 Hyperhomocysteinemia

A New Risk Factor for Alzheimer Disease?

Ramon Diaz-Arrastia, MD, PhD
From the Department of Neurology, University of Texas, Southwestern Medical Center at Dallas.

Arch Neurol. 1998;55:1407–1408

Judging by the number of citations in the medical literature, the lay press, and the Internet, homocysteine is the favorite amino acid of the late 1990s. This is primarily because of the recognition during the past several years that hyperhomocysteinemia is an important risk factor for vascular disease, independent of long-recognized factors such as hyperlipidemia, hypertension, and smoking. A wealth of epidemiological data has accumulated in support of the hypothesis initially advanced by Kilmer McCully in 1969,[1] which was based on autopsy findings from 2 children with elevated plasma homocysteine levels. By now, more than 20 case-control and cross-sectional studies, involving more than 15,000 patients, have validated this correlation.[2] A recent meta-analysis by Boushey et al[3] estimated that 10% of the risk of coronary artery disease in the general population is due to homocysteine.[3] Of particular importance to neurologists is the increased prevalence of cerebrovascular disease in patients whose homocysteine concentrations were in the upper quartile.[4] What is not yet clear is whether intervention to lower plasma homocysteine levels is effective in decreasing the risk of vascular disease, although well-designed multicenter trials are under way to answer this important question.

Given the association between elevated homocysteine levels and cerebrovascular disease, it is not surprising that hyperhomocysteinemia was found in case-control studies to be associated with vascular dementia. More surprising have been several recent reports,[5] the most convincing of which is published in this issue of the *Archives*, that elevated serum homocysteine is also related to Alzheimer disease (AD).[6] In that article, Clarke et al[6] use a case-control approach to study a well-defined group of patients selected by the Oxford Project to Investigate Memory and Ageing (OPTIMA). A critical feature of their study, which was missing from earlier reports, is that in almost half of their cases the diagnosis of AD was proven pathologically, thus excluding the trivial explanation that the association was related to the clinical misdiagnosis of vascular dementia as AD. They found that patients in the upper third of the serum homocysteine distribution had at least a 2-fold elevated risk of developing AD, a correlation that became stronger when only pathologically confirmed cases were included in the analysis. This increased risk is not explained by differences in socioeconomic status, smoking, or apolipoprotein E (apoE) ϵ4 haplotype. Interestingly, the increased risk for AD due to hyperhomocysteinemia was similar to that for vascular dementia.

Clarke et al[6] also found an inverse correlation between serum folate and vitamin B_{12} levels and the risk of AD. The magnitude of the association was similar to that found between homocysteine and AD, and it is likely that decreased levels of these vitamins is functionally related to hyperhomocysteinemia. Because tetrahydrofolate and cyanocobalamin are required by enzymes that metabolize homocysteine, there is a ready biochemical explanation for this epidemiological association. It also raises a trivial explanation for their results: is it possible that as patients became demented their diet deteriorated, suggesting that low vitamin levels and hyperhomocysteinemia are the result rather than the cause of the dementia? The authors did not include a nutritional questionnaire in their data collection battery, making it difficult to conclusively settle this issue. They partly address this problem by demonstrating that homocysteine and vitamin levels were stable for several years in patients while their dementia progressed, and by the lack of a relationship between severity of cognitive impairment and homocysteine levels. Definitive resolution of this issue will likely require a prospective trial.

If the association between AD and homocysteinemia is confirmed, there will be important implications concerning the pathogenesis of AD. Hyperhomocysteinemia will be the second biochemical factor, the other being apoE ϵ4, which increases the risk of both vascular disease and AD. Since apoE may bind amyloid precursor protein and amyloid β peptide, a mechanistic hypothesis explaining how the ϵ4 allele leads to the deposition of plaques, in a manner independent of vascular disease, can be readily envisioned.[7] It is harder to come up with a similar hypothesis to explain the association between homocysteine and AD, although as Clarke et al point out, homocysteine and its metabolite, homocysteic acid, have acute neurotoxic effects on neurons.[8] The possibility must also be considered that microvascular disease and AD share some pathogenic mechanisms, and that the different pathologic features that characterize the 2 conditions result from the interaction of other genetic or environmental factors, which so far are incompletely understood. Is the line separating vascular dementia from AD fuzzier than has been believed during the past decades?

There are other issues left unanswered by the present study. The authors did not find an association between AD and the C677→T mutation in methylenetetrahydrofolate reductase (MTHFR), a common mutation that is known to result in elevations in homocysteine and produce atherosclerosis, particularly in patients with marginal folate intake. If homocysteine is in fact a risk factor for AD, there should be an association with this mutation. Failure to find it may be owing to the relatively low number of homozygous patients in their study, and it suggests that a cross-sectional study should be done to look at this issue. This is part of a larger question of whether the elevations in homocysteine levels are totally explained by differences in folate, vitamin B_{12}, or vitamin B_6 concentrations, or whether other genetic or environmental factors predispose to hyperhomocysteinemia despite adequate vitamin concentrations. Furthermore, is the difference in homocysteine levels explained by differences in diet, or are there differences in absorption, metabolism, or clearance of the vitamins? Finally, Clarke et al[6] measured homocysteine concentrations in randomly obtained serum samples. Would fasting samples provide a more accurate reflection of a patient's risk? Or should blood samples be obtained after patients receive methionine loading or consume a high-protein meal? These issues have been addressed in assessing patients for vascular disease risk, and given the present results it seems important to also study them in patients at risk for AD.

One of the reasons why homocysteine has attracted so much attention is that it is potentially a readily reversible risk factor. Polyvitamin therapy with folic acid, pyridoxine hydrochloride, and cyanocobalamin are effective in lowering homocysteine levels in most people. It has been suggested that supplementation of cereal and grain products with low doses of folic acid may prevent much cardiovascular disease.[9] In the United States, cereals and grains have been fortified with folic acid since January 1, 1998, with the goal of reducing the incidence of neural tube defects. The level of supplementation chosen is estimated to increase daily folic acid intake by less than 150 μg, and while this degree of supplementation may be sufficient to prevent most neural tube defects, it is unlikely to lower serum homocysteine levels substantially. How much folate is needed to lower homocysteine levels in patients at risk?

Is pyridoxine and cyanocobalamin supplementation also needed, and at what dose? Do patients with the C677→T MTHFR mutation require higher doses? What about patients using drugs known to elevate homocysteine levels, such as methotrexate or anticonvulsant agents? What are the risks of polyvitamin therapy in aging populations? These important questions require study, some of which is ongoing on patients at risk for vascular disease. Similar studies should also be started on patients at risk for AD.

Like all seminal research, the article by Clarke et al[6] raises as many questions as it answers. Given the intense public interest in medicine and nutrition, many patients will not wait for definitive studies, and practicing physicians will be faced with the need to give advice based on limited information. Although it may be premature to advocate population-wide programs to screen for hyperhomocysteinemia, neurologists may want to add measurements of homocysteine levels to the battery of blood tests[10] that are routinely done in usually futile searches for reversible factors that predispose to dementia.

References

1. McCully KS. Vascular pathology of homocysteinemia: implications for the pathogenesis of arteriosclerosis. *Am J Pathol.* 1969;56:111–128.

2. Welch GN, Loscalzo J. Homocysteine and atherothrombosis. *N Engl J Med.* 1998; 338:1042–1050.

3. Boushey CJ, Beresford SA, Omenn GS, Motulsky AG. A quantitative assessment of plasma homocysteine as a risk factor for vascular disease: probable benefits of increasing folic acid intakes. *JAMA.* 1995;274:1049–1057.

4. Selhub J, Jacques PF, Bostom AG, et al. Association between plasma homocysteine concentrations and extracranial carotid-artery stenosis. *N Engl J Med.* 1995;332:286–291.

5. McCaddon A, Davies G, Hudson P, Tandy S, Cattell H. Total serum homocysteine in senile dementia of Alzheimer type. *Int J Geriatr Psychiatry.* 1998;13:235–239.

6. Clarke R, Smith AD, Jobst KA, Refsum H, Sutton L, Ueland PM. Folate, vitamin B_{12}, and serum total homocysteine levels in confirmed Alzheimer disease. *Arch Neurol.* 1998; 55:1449–1455.

7. Hyman BT, Tanzi R. Molecular epidemiology of Alzheimer's disease. *N Engl J Med.* 1995; 333:1283–1284.

8. Lipton SA, Kim WK, Choi YB, et al. Neurotoxicity associated with dual actions of homocysteine at the *N*-methyl-D-aspartate receptor. *Proc Natl Acad Sci U S A.* 1997; 94:5923–5928.

9. Malinow MR, Duell PB, Hess DL, et al. Reduction of plasma homocysteine levels by breakfast cereal fortified with folic acid in patients with coronary heart disease. *N Engl J Med.* 1998;338:1009–1015.

10. Corey-Bloom J, Thal LJ, Galasko D, et al. Diagnosis and evaluation of dementia. *Neurology.* 1995;45:211–218.

28 Diet and Pemphigus

In Pursuit of Exogenous Factors in Pemphigus and Fogo Selvagem

Ethel Tur, MD; Sarah Brenner, MD
From the Department of Dermatology, Tel Aviv Sourasky Medical Center, Tel Aviv University, Sackler School of Medicine, Tel Aviv, Israel.

Individuals with a genetic predisposition to pemphigus will develop the disease only when one or more additional factors are present. The nature of these factors is as yet unknown, but our starting point was that certain drugs (penicillamine, captopril, and rifampicin) are recognized as such factors. Since some nutrients have chemical compositions similar to these known causative drugs, these nutrients may act similarly and, therefore, nutritional factors should also be suspected. As when drugs are involved, elimination of the inciting ingredients may be crucial for management of the disease. This article discusses the possible role of nutritional ingredients in the disease process of pemphigus, including fruit, leaves, roots, seeds, and even water. Possible causative candidates are thiol, thiocyanate, phenols, and tannins.

Arch Dermatol. 1998;134:1406–1410

Because the variability in the incidence and age of onset of pemphigus cannot be explained by genetics, environmental factors are implied. Susceptibility to autoimmune diseases is multifactorial[1]; not all individuals with a proven susceptible genotype will develop autoimmunity. In many diseases, it appears that autoimmunity is preceded by some environmental insult. Tissue damage may be the key event that either allows for release of sequestered antigens from immunologically privileged sites or causes local inflammation resulting in lymphokine release and subsequent expression of antigens, or both. Sinha et al[1] note that perhaps the biggest challenge in the future will be the search for the environmental events that trigger self-reactivity.

It has been established that exogenous factors in the form of drugs, in particular thiol-containing drugs,[2,3] play a role in the induction of pemphigus. This points to the possibility of finding other offenders, such as food products with chemical compositions similar to these drugs.[4–9] We suggest that diet factors are involved in the pemphigus disease process and that, potentially, morbidity can be reduced if these factors are identified and avoided.

Dietary Factors in Pemphigus

Thiol

When a thiol group is included in the molecular structure of a drug, the drug is capable of inducing pemphigus. Thiol groups are part of the molecular structure of certain plants; therefore, when these plants are ingested, they may have the same effects as thiol-containing drugs. Indeed, 3 compounds of garlic (allylmercaptan, allylmethylsulfide, and allylsulfide) were shown to induce acantholysis in vitro.[5] Garlic belongs to the *Allium* group of plants, as do onion, shallot, chive, and leek, all of which also contain a thiol group. In the mountainous (Himalayan) zones of India there are many wild species of *Allium* L, and these appear at tribal markets.[10] Evidence for involvement of thiol-containing foods in autoimmunity is provided by case reports indicating induction of pemphigus by garlic[7] and leek.[6] Elimination of these foods from the diet induced remission, and readministration caused exacerbation.

Isothiocyanates (Mustard Oils)

A distinct group of thiol-containing plants comprises those with thioglucosides—isothiocyanate-producing glucosides (by enzymatic hydrolysis). They are of the mustard family of plants that includes 3200 species in 375 genera and is of worldwide distribution.[11] Mustard (*Brassica nigra*) is a member of the Cruciferae family, as are horseradish, winter cress, turnip, broccoli (which contains both mustard oils, namely, isothiocyanates and allyl isothiocyanates), radish, cabbage, brussel sprouts, and cauliflower. The seeds of mustard (containing 30% fat) are used in French mustard, spices, and oils, and seed and root extracts yield allergenic mustard oils—isothiocyanates.[12] Depending on the chemical structure, the compounds are immunologically reactive (allyl and benzyl isothiocyanate) or irritants (phenyl isothiocyanate): they may either cause antibody-mediated acantholysis or be incorporated into the epidermis leading to nonimmunologic biochemical acantholysis in a manner similar to thiol-bearing drugs.[13]

The caper family (Capparidaceae), a tropical relative of the mustard family, is another source of thioglucosides.[12] Usually, several thioglucosides coexist in a single plant, and they are distributed throughout the plant in varying amounts during its growth cycle. Synthetic oil of mustard contains allyl isothiocyanate as the principal ingredient. Allyl isothiocyanate is widely used for flavoring of food products, especially seasoned sauces. It is an irritant to mucous membranes and produces blisters if left in contact with the membranes long enough.[14]

Phenols

Pemphigus may be topically induced as well: pemphigus erythematosus has been induced by allergic contact dermatitis caused by tincture of benzoin,[15] and contact with chromate has also caused pemphigus.[16] The possibility of induction of pemphigus by contact with phenols has been described.[17] Some phenolic compounds such as phenylisothiocyanate contain sulfur, and others do not. Following our previous publications,[4–9] we received several letters from patients with pemphigus who experimented with foods and experienced variations in the symptoms of their disease with elimination or readministration of phenol-rich foods.

Urushiol. The mechanism by which urushiol elicits allergic contact dermatitis probably begins with covalent binding of the pentadecylcatechols to skin proteins.[18] A similar reaction might be the first step in the sequence of events leading to acantholysis. Plants containing urushiol (3′,5′-pentadecylcatechol) belong to the Anacardiaceae family that includes the genus *Toxicodendron* (poison ivy, poison oak, and poison sumac), the most prominent genus in causing allergic skin reactions. There are many related cross-reacting species such as mango,[19,20] pistachio, and cashew that belong to the same family.

Other Phenolic Compounds. Aspartame, an artificial sweetener, is a phenolic compound, as are many other food additives such as preservatives, colorings, and flavorings. Sodium benzoate, tartrazine (yellow dye No. 5), vanillin, eugenol, caffeic acid, vitamins C and E, and cinnamic acid are all phenols. Cinnamic acid is present in apple, grape, orange, pineapple, and tomato juices. Cinnamon spice is derived from the inner bark of *Cinnamonium zeylanicum,* the phenol-containing cinnamon tree, and many other species of *Cinnamonium* are also used as spices. Eugenol, for example, an oil distilled from *Cinnamonium* green leaves, is used as a flavoring for sweets and foods.

Pinene, another phenol-containing substance, is used to flavor baked goods, beverages, candy, condiments, chewing gum, and ice cream. It is also found in tomatoes, potatoes, mangoes, and bananas. Phenol-containing piperine constitutes 5% to 9% of the content of black pepper.

Firewoods used for smoking and grilling foods are another source of phenol. Ingested phenolics are secreted in the milk and therefore appear in cows' milk. For example, gossypol is a phenolic constituent of cottonseed, and when cows are fed cottonseed, this fat-soluble compound appears in all the milk-fat products made from those cows' milk. Indole is another phenol found in milk.

Tannins

Tannins are naturally occurring plant polyphenolic compounds with considerable biologic activity. The astringency of many fruits during the early part of growth is due to high tannin content that declines as the fruit ripens. Certain woods, root materials, barks, leaves, and even hairs are also sources of tannin.

Previously, we pointed out the possible role of tannins in the induction or promotion of pemphigus.[8] Some of the possible effects of tannins are listed below:

- Precipitating interaction with proteins
- Alveolar macrophage stimulation
- Interaction with drugs
- Platelet activation
- Effect on nutrition
- Enzyme inhibition
- Release of neutrophil chemotactic factor
- Metal ion deprivation

There is also evidence suggesting that tannins inhibit copper utilization.[21] Interestingly, the well-known pemphigus inducer penicillamine is a chelating agent for copper. Polyphenols induce apoptosis.[22] Tannins also induce binding of IgA paraprotein to red blood cells in a manner analogous to tanning (waterproofing and preserving animal skins to make leather) with phenolic plant extracts. Tannins react with structures on or in the red blood cell membrane.[23] Tannin is frequently used as a cross-linking agent,[24] and similar cross-linkage in the epidermis may possibly be the mechanism through which these compounds induce pemphigus. Similarly, the first step in drug-induced acantholysis involves binding of the drug to the cell membrane.

Tannic acid has often been used in electron microscopy as a stain for carbohydrate-rich cell surfaces. Tannic acid stains the cell surface and intercellular material in squamous epithelium and the desmosomes.[25] Tannins may activate platelets and are implicated in the epithelial injury of bronchi by cotton dust. Some are carcinogens, linked to nasal sinus cancer in woodworkers, squamous cell carcinoma of the oral mucosa, and gastrointestinal malignancies. Tannin has been shown to produce a cytotoxic effect on human peripheral blood lymphocytes in vitro, although this effect is dependent on increasing concentrations and time of exposure.[26]

Other factors affecting tannin activity include the steric structure of both the tannin and the protein, absorption, and the composition and size of the protein on which the tannins act. Temperature, pH, and the presence of metal ions, calcium, and other chemical compounds will also influence tannin activity.

Intake of Tannins. *Examples of Foods Containing Tannin.* Cassava (*Manihot esculenta* Crantz), also known as manioc, mandioca, Brazilian arrowroot, and yucca, is an important dietary staple in many forms for more than 500 million people in South America, Africa, and Asia.[27] Cassava roots and leaves contain cyanogenic and noncyanogenic glycosides. Cassava leaves (both red and white varieties) also contain condensed tannins. The tannin content of oven-dried (70°C for 3 days in an air oven) cassava leaves is from 0.2 to 3 g/100 g, depending on the variety of cassava, and that of blanched leaves (100°C for 5 minutes) is 0.15 to 0.22 g/100 g.[28]

Mango also contains high amounts of tannin in the pulp and skin, though this varies with the different kinds of mango. India is the largest producer of mango, with over 60 varieties grown there. The cashew tree produces apples (not a true fruit botanically) in addition to the nuts, and these apples are rich in tannins and are used to make juice and alcoholic drinks in Brazil.

The guarana plant is a perennial climbing shrub native to Brazil and other wooded Amazon regions. In recent years, products manufactured from guarana have been imported into the United States. The fruit is reddish and contains glossy brown seeds. Some Indian tribes grate fresh seed and swallow it with water, and some make a fermented drink. Sometimes it is dry roasted and then ground with cassava. This mixture of 2 high-tannin foods might have important implications. The greatest use of guarana presently is as a soft drink, which is imported to the United States. Guarana contains a high caffeine level as well as tannin. The total tannin content of air-dried guarana is 12.1% (proanthocyanidins and prototannins).[29] The seeds before any treatment contain 6% tannin.

Fruits such as the kola nut, betel nut, black walnut, raspberry, cherry, cranberry, and blackberry are all high in tannin content. Avocado, banana, apple, and pear are also rich in tannins, as are peach, persimmon, eggplant, and grape skins. Coffee and cocoa seeds and the roots of ginger, ginseng, and garlic are tannin rich, as are the leaves of cassava, tea, maté, and rosemary, the stems of vanillin, and the shells of carob. Provisions such as beer, wine, and soft drinks contain tannin additives. Tannin is also added to candy, ice cream, baked goods, and even nutritional supplements.

Stimulants and Masticatories. Certain plants that are used for recreational and social ingestion and also as aphrodisiacs and medications are rich in tannins (Table 1). To this category belong the guarana from Brazil, betel nut or areca nut (*Areca catechu*) from Malaya, which is popular in India and in many other countries in that region and in South Africa, and the kola nut from west Africa. The appeal of exotic products has led to their spread to North America as well, where they are now sold in sundries shops and grocery stores. Guarana and kola nut are also rich in caffeine and are used as stimulants.[30] Chewed betel nuts release tannins and thiocyanate. Immature nuts contain 38% to 47% tannin, mainly polymerized leukocyanidins, but the percentage decreases as the fruit matures, and processing reduces the level to 8% to 15%.

Betel nut addiction afflicts at least 10% of the human race.[30] The betel *quid* is a package of fresh betel leaf (*Piper betle* vine), the undersurface of which is smeared with lime, containing pieces of betel nut and tobacco. Spices are sometimes added too, as well as mustard. The leaves that are used for chewing contain 1% to 1.3% tannin and other phenols. The leaf yields 0.62% to 2.4% volatile oil, which is 75% phenolic.[30]

The nut itself, aqueous extracts of it, and specific constituents in the nut can be mutagenic and carcinogenic.[31] Several phenolics from the chewed plant products can generate free radicals that can exert a cytotoxic effect on the oral mucosa.[32] It is a common practice to keep pieces of the nut or betel quid in the mouth for prolonged periods of time. Betel nut constitutes 50% of the betel quid by weight, and a person may consume the equivalent of 20 to 30 nuts and 200 leaves of betel vine per day.

One method of preservation of the fresh betel nuts involves blanching them in boiling calcium chloride. The calcium (lime) component of the betel quid may take part in pemphigus pathogenesis because the reaction of pemphigus autoantibodies is enhanced by calcium supplementation.

Another ingredient of the betel quid, katha, is derived from the heartwood of the cutch tree (*A catechu*), and contains 11.7% to 14.2% tannin. It is a potent tanning agent; 0.45 kg of cutch is equal to 3.2 kg to 3.6 kg of oak bark for tanning purposes. It is also used as an antioxidant in vegetable oils. An aqueous solution of *A catechu* bark containing catechin and tannin, prepared as a tincture or powder, has been used in the United States as an astringent coloring in liquors, soft drinks, ice cream, candy, and baked goods.

Table 1. Tannin and Caffeine Content of Some Masticatories and Stimulants*

Substance	Tannin Content	Caffeine Content
Guarana	12	3–5
Coffee beans	0.7	1–2
Roasted coffee beans	1.7	. . .
Dry tea leaves	3.7	1–4
Kola nuts (*Cola nitida, Cola acuminata,* family Sterculiaceae)	3.9–4.4	1.5–3.2
Maté	7–11	1.0–1.5
Betel nut (*Areca catechu* L)	8–15	Negligible
Betel leaf (*Piper betle*)	1.0–1.3	Negligible
Katha (derived from *catechu*)	11.7–14.2	Negligible
Cassava leaves	0.15–3.0	Negligible

*Tannin and caffeine contents are measured as a percentage of dry weight. Ellipses indicate not available.

The expression of antigens that are markers of epithelial differentiation may be regulated by substances such as retinoic acid or calcium. Moreover, these antigens may be involved in cell-to-cell adhesion in the epidermis.[33] Thus, the same food compounds that play a role in carcinogenesis of the mouth may play a role in cell-to-cell adhesion leading to the development of pemphigus. However, a combination of factors is needed: carcinogenicity has been shown to occur as a result of chewing a mixture of pepper leaf, betel, and lime but not the betel nut without lime.[30]

Interestingly, chronic exposure to cashew nut oil has been shown to cause oral carcinoma in women who refrain from tobacco and betel nut habits.[34] In addition, oral submucous fibrosis, a precancerous condition, is prevalent among cashew workers in south India.[35] Chromosome breakage observed among betel nut chewers has been attributed to the joint action of betel nut–derived alkaloids, polyphenols and/or tannins, and nitrosamines in the saliva.

Kola nuts (*Cola nitida* and *Cola acuminata,* family Sterculiaceae) were carried to America from Africa with the slave trade in the 17th century[30] and spread due to the reputation of the seeds as stimulants. Tannin levels in *C nitida* are 3.9% to 4.4%, and total polyphenol levels are 6.7%, particularly catechol and epicatechol. Kola nuts are consumed fresh wherever they are grown throughout the world, and aqueous extracts or concentrates are used as flavorings in soft drinks, particularly with extracts of coca leaves.

Table 2. Tannin and Calcium Content in Spices, and Average Daily Consumption per Individual in India

Spice	Tannis, g/100g	Calcium, g/100g	Spice Consumed, g/d*	Tannins Consumed in Each Spice, mg/d
Garlic (*Allium sativum*)	0.12	0.11	2.49 ± 2.78	3.0
Dry ginger (*Zingiber officinale*)	0.54	1.47	0.04 ± 1.31	0.2
Red chillies (*Capsucum annum*)	0.90	0.06	3.08 ± 2.06	24.6
Asafoetida (*Ferula foetida*)	0.80	1.01	0.06 ± 0.10	0.5
Coriander (*Coriandrum sativum*)	0.82	0.65	1.37 ± 1.30	11.3
Cumin seeds (*Cuminum cyminum*)	0.90	0.92	0.80 ± 0.77	7.2
Black pepper (*Piper nigrum*)	0.94	0.38	0.33 ± 0.30	3.1
Ajowan (*Carum copticum*)	1.26	1.26	0.11 ± 0.17	1.4

*Values are expressed as mean ± SD.

Nuts such as peanuts and pistachios may contribute to pemphigus induction because people who eat them have a habit of sucking the shells. These shells have high tannin content.

Drinks. Tannin is the main component of tea,[36] and coffee also contains a substantial amount of tannin.[37] Maté, also called yerba maté, Brazilian tea, or Paraguay tea, is a tealike beverage popular in many South American countries. It is brewed from dried leaves of an evergreen tree, *Ilex paraguarensis,* and contains caffeine (1%–1.5%) and tannin (7%–11%). The plant grows wild in southern Brazil, where pemphigus is endemic in the Parana and Paraguay river basins.[38]

Fruit juice, beer, wine, and liquor are all sources of tannin. Tannins are used in the clarification of wine and beer. Distilled liquor contains spices and flavoring agents such as vanillin and cinnamon that contain tannins. But the most intriguing issue is water. Possible constituents and effects of water have been discussed in detail in a previous publication.[9] South American pemphigus foliaceus (endemic pemphigus, fogo selvagem) affects individuals of all ages and has a familial prevalence where it is endemic in areas of Brazil. This has prompted a search for environmental factors.[33]

Most patients with fogo selvagem live in close proximity to rivers. Many of these rivers contain high levels of tannin caused by decomposing leaves and other vegetable matter from the lush surrounding forests. Along these rivers, fogo selvagem occurs in regions where the weather is hot and humid. These conditions are needed for tannins to decompose, fitting our hypothesis that tannins in the water are an important factor in pemphigus.

The number of new cases of fogo selvagem is highest at the end of the rainy season and lowest during the dry summer. Rainfall causes a rise of the waters; large quantities of organic materials are then carried by the stream, and the amount of tannins dissolved in the water increases. Furthermore, variations of annual rainfall result in differences in the tannin content, and this may account for the observation that new fogo selvagem cases occur in clusters.[39]

A possible lead toward a means for controlling pemphigus lies in the fact that chlorination of water results in the formation of the hypochlorite ion that combines with phenolic compounds even in high dilutions. This might account for the disappearance of fogo selvagem following urbanization, which usually involves treating of the water.

Spices. Spices have a high tannin content, ranging from 0.12 g/100 g to 1.26 g/100 g (Table 2). Spices of the Umbelliferae family (ajowan, coriander, and cumin) and black pepper have the highest content of tannin. All over India, where pemphigus is prevalent, spices constitute an important part of the daily diet.[40] Among spices, red chillies account for the highest daily tannin consumption by individuals in India, followed by coriander, cumin seeds, black pepper, and garlic. It is noteworthy that patients showing positive skin-prick test results to fresh fruits and vegetables also exhibited positive skin-prick reactions to spice (mustard included).[41]

Calcium ions are necessary for the reaction of tannins, tannins' action resulting in elevated intracellular calcium ion concentration. Interestingly, dry ginger, ajowan, and asafoetida, which are spices with high tannin content, also have high calcium levels.[41]

Food Coloring. Several food coloring products have high tannin content. Mangosteen, a tropical fruit that originated in Southeast Asia, was introduced into the Americas centuries ago. Its skin contains 13% tannin and is used as a coloring for food. The use of the catechu bark as food coloring was discussed earlier. It is also used as an antioxidant in vegetable oils.

Nutritional Supplements. Several popular nutritional supplements contain high concentrations of tannins. Some preparations are bark extracts containing proanthocyanidins and other polyphenols. There are also grape seed extracts containing flavonoids, tea extracts with high levels of tannins, and mixtures of extracts with high tannin levels.

Conclusions

In summary, inferences that diet plays a role in pemphigus induction may be drawn from a wide variety of facts: (1) The molecular structure of many food ingredients is similar to that of known pemphigus-inducing drugs. (2) Case reports[6,7] indicate the connection. (3) Tannins and phenols are known to interact with proteins. (4) Seasonal variations in pemphigus incidence coincide with seasonal tannin variations in diet. (5) Yearly variations in pemphigus outbreaks coincide with yearly tannin variations. (6) Incidence of fogo selvagem drops as populations move into urban areas with chlorinated water supplies.

Finding the exogenous stressors is the first step toward their elimination. The second step is unfolding the sequence of events and the interaction between these stressors. The task is enormous and includes many variables, as even changes in the mode of preparation of the same foods might eliminate the deleterious effects of certain constituents.

We suggest that foods containing thiol, phenolic compounds, and polyphenols have a role in pemphigus. But which of the multitude of these compounds are involved, their mode of action, and under what conditions their effect is exerted still remains to be unveiled.

References

1. Sinha AA, Lopez MT, McDevitt HO. Autoimmune diseases: the failure of self tolerance. *Science*. 1990;248:1380–1387.
2. Ruocco V, Sacerdoti G. Pemphigus and bullous pemphigoid due to drugs. *Int J Dermatol*. 1991; 30:307–312.
3. Esposito C, Ruocco V, Cozzolino A, Lo Schiavo A, Lombardi ML, Porta R. Are acantholysis and transglutaminase inhibition related phenomena? *Dermatology*. 1996;193:221–225.
4. Brenner S, Wolf R. Possible nutritional factors in induced pemphigus. *Dermatology*. 1994; 189:337–339.
5. Brenner S, Ruocco V, Wolf R, de Angelis E, Lombardi ML. Pemphigus and dietary factors. *Dermatology*. 1995;190:197–202.
6. Chorzelski TP, Hashimoto T, Jablonska S, et al. Can pemphigus vulgaris be induced by nutritional factors? *Eur J Dermatol*. 1996;6:284–286.
7. Ruocco V, Brenner S, Lombardi ML. A case of diet-related pemphigus. *Dermatology*. 1996; 192:373–374.
8. Tur E, Brenner S. Contributing exogenous factors in pemphigus. *Int J Dermatol*. 1997; 36:888–893.
9. Tur E, Brenner S. The role of the water system as an exogenous factor in pemphigus. *Int J Dermatol*. 1997;36:810–816.
10. Negi KS, Pant KC. Less-known wild species of *Allium* L. (*Amaryllidaceae*) from mountainous regions of India. *Econ Botany*. 1992;46:112–114.
11. Mitchell JC, Jordan WP. Allergic contact dermatitis from the radish, *Raphanus sativus*. *Br J Dermatol*. 1974;91:183–189.
12. Dannaker CJ, White IR. Cutaneous allergy to mustard in a salad maker. *Contact Dermatitis*. 1987;16:212–214.
13. Mobini N, Ahmed AR. Immunogenetics of drug-induced bullous diseases. *Clin Dermatol*. 1993;11:449–460.
14. Gaul LE. Contact dermatitis from synthetic oil of mustard. *Arch Dermatol*. 1964;90:158–159.
15. Lynfield YL, Pertschuk LP, Zimmerman A. Pemphigus erythematosus provoked by allergic contact dermatitis. *Arch Dermatol*. 1973; 108:690–693.
16. Tsankov N, Stransky L, Kostowa M. Induzierter Pemphigus durch beruflichen Kontakt mit Basochrom. *Dermatosen*. 1990;38:91–93.
17. Tsankov N, Dimitrowa J, Obreschkowa E, Lasarowa A. Induziert Pemphigus durch das Pestizid Phosphamid. *Z Hautkr*. 1987; 62:196–201.
18. Epstein WL. The poison ivy picker of Pennypack Park: the continuing saga of poison ivy. *J Invest Dermatol*. 1987;88(suppl):7S–11S.
19. Fisher AA. The notorious poison ivy family of *Anacardiaceae* plants. *Cutis*. 1977;20:570.
20. Catalano PN. Mango sap and poison ivy dermatitis. *J Am Acad Dermatol*. 1993;9:522.
21. Kies C, Umoren J. Inhibitors of copper bioutilization: fiber, lead, phytate and tannins. *Adv Exp Med Biol*. 1989;258:81–93.
22. Sakagami H, Kuribayashi N, Iida M, et al. Induction of DNA fragmentation by tannin- and lignin-related substances. *Anticancer Res*. 1995; 15:2121–2128.
23. Hunt AF, Reed MI. Tannic acid and chromic chloride–induced binding of protein to red cells: a preliminary study of possible binding sites and reaction mechanisms. *Med Lab Sci*. 1990;47:189–194.
24. Muzykantov VR, Smirnov MD, Zaltzman AB, Samokhin GP. Tannin-mediated attachment of avidin provides complement-resistant immunoerythrocytes that can be lysed in the presence of activator of complement. *Anal Biochem*. 1993;208:338–342.
25. Davina JHM, Lamers GEM, van Haelst UJGM, Kenemans P, Stadhouders AM. Tannic acid binding of cell surfaces in normal, premalignant, and malignant squamous epithelium of the human uterine cervix. *Ultrastruct Pathol*. 1984;6:275–284.
26. Vincentini-Diaz VEP, Takahashi CS. Action of an extract of *Stryphnodendron obovatum* Benth seed on rat bone marrow and on human lymphocytes. *Rev Bras Genet*. 1993;16:175–185.
27. Okezie BO, Kosikowski FV. Cassava as a food. *Crit Rev Food Sci Nutr*. 1982;17:259–275.
28. Awoyinka AF, Abegunde VO, Adewusi SRA. Nutrient content of young cassava leaves and assessment of their acceptance as a green vegetable in Nigeria. *Plant Foods Hum Nutr*. 1995; 47:21–28.
29. Marx F. Analysis of guarana seeds, II: studies on the composition of the tannin fraction. *Z Lebensm Unters Forsch*. 1990;190:429–431.
30. Morton JF. Widespread tannin intake via stimulants and masticatories, especially guarana, kola nut, betel vine, and accessories. *Basic Life Sci*. 1992;59:739–765.

31. van Wyk CW, Stander I, Padayachee A, Grobler-Rabie AF. The areca nut chewing habit and oral squamous cell carcinoma in South African Indians: a retrospective study. *S Afr Med J.* 1993;83:425–429.

32. Stich HF, Mathew B, Sankaranarayanan R, Nair MK. Remission of precancerous lesions in the oral cavity of tobacco chewers and maintenance of the protective effect of beta-carotene or vitamin A. *Am J Clin Nutr.* 1991; 53:298S-304S.

33. Sampaio SAP, Rivitti EA, Aoki V, Diaz LA. Brazilian pemphigus foliaceus, endemic pemphigus foliaceus, or fogo selvagem (wild fire). *Dermatol Clin.* 1994;12:765–776.

34. Rajendran R, Anil S, Vijayakumar T. A rare human model for oncogenesis. *Singapore Dent J.* 1988;13:49–52.

35. Varghese I, Rajendran R, Sugathan CK, Vijayakumar T. Prevalence of oral submucous fibrosis among cashew workers of Kerala-south India. *Indian J Cancer.* 1986;23:101–104.

36. Bokuchava MA, Skobeleva NI. The biochemistry and technology of tea manufacture. *Crit Rev Food Sci Nutr.* 1980;12:303–370.

37. Savolainen H. Tannin content of tea and coffee. *J Appl Toxicol.* 1992;12:191–192.

38. Maté. In: *Encyclopaedia Britannica,* Vol 14. Chicago, Ill: William Benton; 1970:1053.

39. Hans-Filho G, dos Santos V, Katayama JH, et al. An active focus of high prevalence of fogo selvagem on an Amerindian reservation in Brazil. *J Invest Dermatol.* 1996;107:68–75.

40. Pradeep KU, Geervani P, Eggum BO. Common Indian spices: nutrient composition, consumption and contribution to dietary value. *Plant Foods Hum Nutr.* 1993;44:137–148.

41. Niinimaki A, Hannuksela M, Makinen-Kiljunen S. Skin prick tests and in vitro immunoassays with native spices and spice extracts. *Ann Allergy Asthma Immunol.* 1995;75:280–286.

29 A Multicenter Study of the Efficacy of the Ketogenic Diet

Eileen P. G. Vining, MD; John M. Freeman, MD; Karen Ballaban-Gil, MD; Carol S. Camfield, MD; Peter R. Camfield, MD; Gregory L. Holmes, MD; Shlomo Shinnar, MD PhD; Robert Shuman, MD; Edwin Trevathan, MD; James W. Wheless, MD; and The Ketogenic Diet Multi-Center Study Group

The affiliations of the authors appear in the acknowledgment section at the end of the chapter.

Arch Neurol. 1998;55:1433–1437

Objective

To determine the efficacy of the ketogenic diet in multiple centers.

Design

A prospective study of the change in frequency of seizures in 51 children with intractable seizures who were treated with the ketogenic diet.

Setting

Patients were enrolled from the clinical practices of 7 sites. The diet was initiated in-hospital and the patients were followed up for at least 6 months.

Patients

Fifty-one children, aged 1 to 8 years, with more than 10 seizures per week, whose electroencephalogram showed generalized epileptiform abnormalities or multifocal spikes, and who had failed results when taking at least 2 appropriate anti-epileptic drugs.

Intervention

The children were hospitalized, fasted, and a 4:1 ketogenic diet was initiated and maintained.

Main Outcome Measures

Frequency of seizures was documented from parental calendars and efficacy was compared with prediet baseline after 3, 6, and 12 months. The children were categorized as free of seizures, greater than 90% reduction, 50% to 90% reduction, or lower than 50% reduction in frequency of seizures.

Results

Eighty-eight percent of all children initiating the diet remained on it at 3 months, 69% remained on it at 6 months, and 47% remained on it at 1 year. Three months after initiating the diet, frequency of seizures was decreased to greater than 50% in 54%. At 6 months, 28 (55%) of the 51 initiating the diet had at least a 50% decrease from baseline, and at 1 year, 40% of those starting the diet had a

greater than 50% decrease in seizures. Five patients (10%) were free of seizures at 1 year. Age, sex, principal seizure type, and electroencephalogram were not statistically related to outcome.

Conclusion

The ketogenic diet is effective in substantially decreasing difficult-to-control seizures and can successfully be administered in a wide variety of settings.

Arch Neurol. 1998;55:1433–1437

The ketogenic diet is an individually calculated and rigidly controlled, high-fat, low-protein, low-carbohydrate diet used for the treatment of difficult-to-control seizures. Originally developed in the 1920s, this diet was designed to mimic the biochemical changes associated with starvation.[1] In that era, when few anticonvulsants were available, 60% to 75% of children placed on the diet had a more than 50% decrease in their seizures and 30% to 40% of those had a greater than 90% decrease in the frequency of seizures.[2] When the clinical efficacy of diphenylhydantoin was reported in 1938, attention turned to new anticonvulsant development and therapy.

As new anticonvulsant medications became available, the diet was used less frequently and lack of experience led to the widespread opinion that the diet did not work and was difficult to tolerate.[3] However, a few centers continued to occasionally use the diet.[4] In the early 1990s Kinsman et al[5] reported a series of 57 patients, refractory to the newer medications including valproate, who were treated with the classic diet. Their results were similar to the older studies.

Since 1994, when a flurry of media coverage focused attention on the ketogenic diet,[6] clinicians have shown a renewed interest in its use.[3,7] With funding from the Charlie Foundation to Cure Pediatric Epilepsy (Santa Monica, Calif), physician-nurse-dietician teams from 8 medical centers were trained to provide the ketogenic diet and jointly developed a standardized protocol to prospectively enroll children on the ketogenic diet, to compare outcomes, and to determine factors such as age or type of seizures associated with success or failure. Adverse events associated with the diet were also evaluated. This article is the results of that study.

Patients and Methods

Children aged 1 to 8 years, having more than 10 seizures per week of any type, whose electroencephalogram (EEG) demonstrated generalized epileptiform abnormalities or multifocal spikes, and who had failed at least 2 appropriate anti-epileptic drugs were eligible for the study and were consecutively enrolled. Children with partial seizures only, those whose EEG showed a single epileptic focus, and those who had evidence of metabolic or degenerative disease were to be excluded from the study group, as were families with psychosocial issues that might preclude compliance. This protocol was approved by the individual centers' institutional review boards and informed consent was obtained from each family.

Children were admitted to the hospital, fasted for 36 hours, and started on the classic 4:1 diet (ratio of grams of fat to grams of protein plus carbohydrate) according to the Johns Hopkins protocol.[3,8,9]

Table 1 summarizes the protocol. For 1 to 2 days before fasting the family is instructed to decrease their child's intake of carbohydrates and starches. Fasting is begun after dinner, the evening before admission. Whenever possible, carbohydrate-free anticonvulsant medications should be used. On day 1 the child is admitted to the hospital. Fluids (free of caffeine and carbohydrate) are limited to 60 to 75 mL/kg of body weight with an upper limit of 1200 mL/d. Blood glucose is measured by a fingerstick method using a reagent strip (Dextrostix) every 6 hours unless the level falls below 2.2 mmol/L (40 mg/dL) in which case it is measured every 2 hours. Symptoms simulating hypoglycemia warrant an immediate blood glucose test. Symptoms, or glucose levels lower than 1.3 mmol/L (<25 mg/dL), warrant giving 30 mL of orange juice and measuring the blood glucose level again. Symptomatic hypoglycemia during this fasting is uncommon, even in small children.

On day 2 lack of energy and lethargy are common during the second 24 hours of fasting. Hunger is uncommon. On the evening of day 2, after 48 hours of fasting, one third of the calculated ketogenic diet is given as an "eggnog." The diet is generally calculated on the basis of a given number of calories per kilogram to be provided in a given day, divided into 3 equal meals. Usually a 4:1 ratio is used. A 4:1 ratio eggnog would contain 60 g of 36% cream, 25 g of egg, vanilla, and saccharine for flavor. This would yield 245 calories, approximately 4 g of protein, 2 g of carbohydrate, and 24 g of fats (24:6 or 4:1 ratio). Therefore, if 120 mL of a

Table 1. Protocol for the Ketogenic Diet

Before diet
Minimize carbohydrates for 1–2 d
Fasting is begun after dinner the evening before admission
Day 1
Admit to the hospital
Use carbohydrate-free anticonvulsant medications
Fasting continues
Restrict fluids (free of caffeine and carbohydrates) to 60–75 mL/kg of body weight (maximum 1200 mL)
Dextrostix (a fingerstick method using a reagent strip) every 6 h; if <40 mg/dL, then every 2 h
If symptoms, or glucose levels below 1.3 mmol/L (25 mg/dL), give 30 mL of orange juice; measure the blood glucose level again
Continue fasting
Day 2
Continue fasting
Dinner (after 48 h of fasting) give one third of the calculated ketogenic diet meal as an "eggnog"; for example, if 120 mL of eggnog would be normal meal, then 60 mL given
Excess ketosis (nausea or vomiting) may be relieved with small amounts of orange juice
Day 3
Breakfast and lunch: one third of the calculated diet as eggnog
Dinner: two thirds of allowance as eggnog
Day 4
Breakfast and lunch: two thirds of allowance as eggnog
Dinner is the first full ketogenic meal
Severe ketosis/acidosis managed with additional carbohydrate-free fluids and the diet is continued
Day 5
The child receives a full ketogenic breakfast and is discharged
Every child should receive a sugar-free, fat-soluble vitamin supplement and additional calcium

4:1 ratio eggnog would usually serve as a meal for a given child, one third would be 60 mL of the eggnog and two thirds would be 120 mL of the eggnog. Although most children will have reached large ketones on reagent strip for urinalysis (>160 mmol/dL while receiving Ketostix) by this time, we begin feeding even if this degree of ketosis is not reached. Excess ketosis may be manifested by nausea or vomiting and may be relieved with small amounts of orange juice followed by continuation of the protocol.

On day 3 one third of the calculated diet is given as eggnog for breakfast and lunch. Two thirds is given beginning with dinner. As the body is shifting to the use of ketones as the primary energy source, general lack of energy and lethargy persist; they will be regained over the ensuing 2 weeks.

On day 4 the child continues two thirds of the calculated diet as eggnog, and dinner is the first full meal. Occasionally, the child becomes too ketotic or acidotic as evidenced by failure to drink, Kussmaul breathing, pallor, or limpness. In such an event the child is rehydrated with carbohydrate-free fluids and the diet is continued.

On day 5 the child receives a full ketogenic breakfast and is discharged. Each day while the child is hospitalized, the parents (and older children) are involved in classes to learn the rationale behind the diet, the calculation of meals, the weighing of foods, the reading of labels, and the management of the diet during the usual childhood infections. Every child should receive a sugar-free, fat-soluble vitamin supplement, and additional calcium.

After discharge parents are instructed to measure urinary ketones daily in the morning. The diet is individually adjusted (calories or ratio) by telephone to provide maximum control of seizures, maintain the child in large ketones as measured on reagent strip for urinalysis ketosis, and to avoid both significant weight gain and weight loss. We do not routinely monitor blood glucose or electrolytes after discharge, nor do we follow up on serum lipid levels, except for research purposes. We do not alter or abandon the diet even if the lipid levels are elevated.

After 1 month on the diet, if seizures had decreased or were eliminated, anticonvulsant medication could be decreased. Frequency of seizures was tabulated from the baseline parental calendars and from parental calendars collected at the time of follow-up at 3, 6, and 12 months.

Demographic, baseline, and study data were recorded on customized data collection forms and transferred to a Paradox for Windows (Borland International Inc, Scott's Valley, Calif) database. The percentage of decrease from the initial baseline frequency of seizures is reported for all children entering the protocol. Independent variables (age, sex, type of seizures, or EEG) were analyzed using Yates corrected χ^2 and all P values are 2-tailed. Kaplan-Meier survival analysis was based on percentage of decrease from baseline and examined the probability of remaining on the diet for a year. Adverse events related to the diet were also noted at the follow-up visits.

Results

Fifty-one patients, 34 males and 17 females, mean age 4.7 years (range, 1.3–8.6 years) were enrolled in the study between January 1, 1994, and December 30, 1995. The children had been treated with an average of 7 medications and were having an average of 230 seizures per month (range, 11–1880 seizures) during the baseline period. Twenty of the 51 children had tonic-clonic seizures, 19 had myoclonic seizures, 14 had atonic and/or drop seizures, 10 had tonic seizures, 8 had absence, 6 had complex partial seizures, 5 atypical absence, 2 partial seizures with secondary generalization, and 1 each had infantile spasms, simple partial seizures, and clonic seizures. Seizures for 8 children were unclassified. Many children had more than 1 type of seizure.

Three months after initiation of the diet, 45 (88%) of 51 remained on the diet (Table 2). Six were free of seizures; an additional 7 children, for a total of 13 (25%) of 51 had a greater than 90% decrease in seizures, and 15 (29%) of 51 had a 50% to 90% decrease. Only 6 children (12%) had discontinued the diet.

Six months after initiation of the diet, 15 (29%) of 51 children had a greater than 90% decrease in seizures and 12 (24%) of 51 had a 50% to 90% decrease. Fourteen children (27%) had discontinued the diet, and 2 were lost to follow-up.

One year after initiation of the diet 24 (47%) of 51 remained on the diet, 11 (22%) had a greater than 90% decrease in seizures (5 were free of seizures) and 9 (18%) of 51 had a 50% to 90% decrease in seizures. Four children remained on the diet despite a less than 50% decrease in seizures, usually because the seizures were of less frequency or severity, or because the child was receiving less medication. Longitudinal observation showed that 20 (71%) of 28 children who had better than 50% seizure control at 3 months remained on the diet at 12 months. Most of the 23 who had discontinued the diet did so because they had a lower than 50% decrease in seizures. Four (8%) of the 51 children were lost to follow-up during the first year.

Figure 1 illustrates the Kaplan-Meier survival curves for the probability of remaining on the diet in relation to the success of the diet in controlling seizures. It shows a statistically significant difference in the probability of remaining on the diet between the children who had a greater than 50% decrease in seizures and those who had a lower than 50% decrease in the frequency of seizures (Wilcoxon, $P<.001$). There was little difference with respect to the probability of remaining on the diet between those whose seizures were totally controlled, more than 90% controlled, and 50% to 90% controlled.

There was no statistically significant difference ($P<.05$) in outcome (<50% control of seizures vs >50% control of seizures at 3, 6, or 12 months) using c2 for the following variables: age, sex, primary type of seizures, presence or absence of normal background, focal EEG changes, or generalized spike-wave abnormalities. There was a marginally significant difference ($P=.04$) for children who had a pattern of multifocal spikes. These children did less well at 3 months. There was no significant difference at 6 or 12 months.

Table 2. Outcomes of the Ketogenic Diet*

Initiated Diet	3 mo	6 mo	12 mo
No. on diet	45 (88)	35 (69)	24 (47)
>90% Control of seizures†	13 (25)	15 (29)	11 (22)
50%–90% Control of seizures	15 (29)	12 (24)	9 (18)
<50% Control of seizures	17 (33)	8 (16)	4 (8)
Discontinued diet	6 (12)	14 (27)	23 (45)
Lost to follow-up	0	2	4

*N=51. Values are number (percentage).
†Number free of seizures were the following: 6 (3 months), 6 (6 months), and 5 (12 months).

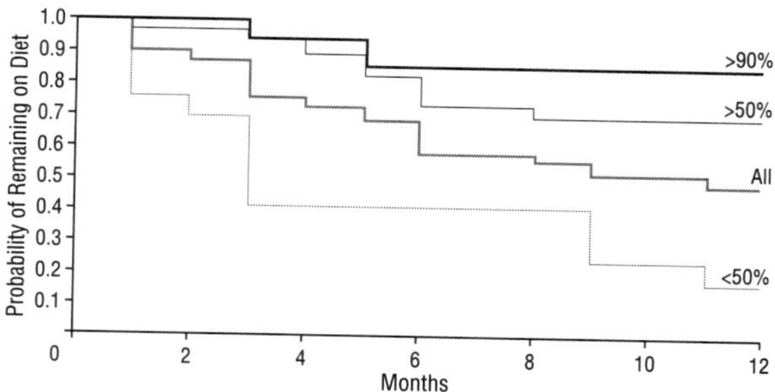

Figure 1. Kaplan-Meier survival curves for the probability of remaining on the diet in relation to the success of the diet in controlling seizures. The curves show a statistically significant difference in the probability of remaining on the diet between the children who had a greater than 50% decrease in the frequency of seizures (Wilcoxon, $P<.001$). There was little difference with respect to the probability of remaining on the diet between those whose seizures were totally controlled, more than 90% controlled, and 50% to 90% controlled.

While the number of patients at each center was small, each center entered at least 6 children; each had at least 1 child become free of seizures; and each had at least 1 child on the diet at 12 months. Only one center had no children with greater than 50% improvement at 1 year. There was no substantial difference between any of the 7 centers in the efficacy of the diet or in the percentage of children remaining on the diet at 3, 6, and 12 months.

Adverse events attributed to the diet were similar between centers and included lethargy (2), severe dehydration or acidosis (2), behavioral changes (4), increase in infections (2), severe constipation (4), and vomiting (2). The diet was discontinued in 6 children during the first 3 months, in an additional 8 by 6 months, and in a total of 23 by 1 year. Reasons given for discontinuation were medical intolerance or illness (6), "too restrictive" (4), insufficient control of seizures (12), and other (1).

Comment

Seven epilepsy groups scattered across the continent, some academic medical centers, some private practices, each with differences in available support staff and differences in prior experience with the diet, entered children in a joint protocol to evaluate the efficacy of the ketogenic diet. An eighth center initiated the study but withdrew for personnel reasons. This protocol was not used and cannot be generalized to all children with epilepsy. Children with partial seizures, those with a single EEG focus, and those with evidence of a degenerative disease were excluded from the protocol, as were families who were believed to be incapable of carrying out this rigorous diet.

This study was neither randomized nor blinded. While we recognize that the placebo effect can be significant, we believe that when 40% of the children with difficult-to-control seizures have a greater than 50% decrease in seizures 1 year after initiating the diet, this is unlikely to be due to placebo effect. In one potentially comparable study[10] of the efficacy of felbamate in the Lennox-Gastaut syndrome, felbamate-treated patients had a 34% decrease in the frequency of atonic seizures (reported by parents), compared with a 9% decrease in the patients who received placebo. Four (11%) of 37 children receiving felbamate were noted to be free of seizures, vs 1 (3%) of 35 receiving placebo. However, these results were based on only 3 months of therapy. In our study, 10% of the children who started the diet continued to be free of seizures over the year that they were followed up. It is also possible to theorize that these children simply became free of seizures based on the natural history of their disorder. However, given this population, and extrapolating from the work of Huttenlocker and Hapke,[11] such a resolution of intractable seizures within such a short time would be highly unlikely.

The rate of success was similar between the different centers and similar to studies published 4 and 5 decades ago.[2] Although recently new and effective anticonvulsant medications have become available, seizures continue to remain difficult to control for many children. Even today, for these children, the success rate of the ketogenic diet exceeds that of most new anticonvulsant medications.[12] Most children benefiting from the diet showed a substantial decrease in seizures during the first 3 months on the diet, but many continued to have even better control over the second 3 months on the diet.

Treatment of epilepsy should consider both the control of the seizures and the adverse effects of the treatment. Figure 1 shows that if effective, children can and will stay on the diet. Mattson and et al[13] used retention time on the medication to evaluate the relative efficacy and adverse effects of different anticonvulsant regimens. Kinsman et al[5] used a similar technique in their study of the ketogenic diet. In this multicenter study of the ketogenic diet, 24 (47%) of the original 51 children remained on the diet for 1 year. Four additional patients were lost to follow-up. A lack of efficacy may be tolerated for a short time (3 months) when 33% of those still on the diet had lower than 50% seizure control. However, at 12 months, only 17% of those still on the diet had a lower than 50% decrease in seizures, suggesting that it was not worth tolerating the diet without considerable control of seizure. As noted by Nordli and DeVivo,[14] "the question is not "Does the ketogenic diet have a role in the treatment of epilepsy?" but rather, "How can we maximize using the ketogenic diet and learn from it to benefit all children with epilepsy?"

We agree. Even though we now know that the diet works, we still do not know how it works, but then, we also do not know how most anticonvulsants work. Perhaps the resurgence of interest in the ketogenic diet will stimulate research to find how this dramatically different approach to control seizures affects difficult-to-control epilepsy, and thus may lead to new insights into this still devastating condition. Many questions remain about the ketogenic diet, including the effects on lipids, cognition, and behavior. We, and others, are continuing to investigate some of the many questions that the renewed interest in the diet is causing to be generated.

Conclusions

In a prospective, multicenter trial of the efficacy of the ketogenic diet, the diet was found to be effective in decreasing frequency of seizures in children with difficult-to-control seizures. The degree of effectiveness was similar between institutions, similar across different types of seizures, and similar to the reports from the last 5 decades. Further evaluation of this promising old modality of therapy is warranted.

From The Johns Hopkins Medical Institutions, Baltimore, Md (Drs Vining and Freeman); Montefiore Medical Center, Bronx, NY (Dr Ballaban-Gil); Dalhousie University, IWK Grace Health Centre, Pediatric Neurology, Halifax, Nova Scotia (Drs C. S. Camfield and P. R. Camfield); Children's Hospital, Boston, Mass (Dr Holmes); Montefiore Medical Center, Albert Einstein College of Medicine, Bronx (Dr Shinnar); Comprehensive Epilepsy Center, University of Kentucky College of Medicine, Kentucky Clinic, Lexington (Dr Trevathan); and the Department of Neurology, University of Texas Medical School, Houston (Dr Wheless). Dr Shuman is in private practice in Mishawaka, Ind.

This study was supported by the Charlie Foundation to Cure Pediatric Epilepsy, Santa Monica, Calif, and The Johns Hopkins Children's Center Telethon Funds, Baltimore, Md.

The Ketogenic Multi-Center Study Group

The Johns Hopkins Medical Institutions, Baltimore, Md: Eileen P. G. Vining, MD; John M. Freeman, MD; Jane Casey, RN, LCSW; Sophie Hsieh, RN; Regina Homer; Millicent Kelly, RD, LD; Cathy Park, RN; Diana Pillas; Paula Pyzik; Traci D. Swink, MD.

Scottish Rite Children's Medical Center, Atlanta, Ga: Edwin Trevathan, Raymond Cheng, MD; Linda McCarty, RN; MD; Linda Trevathan, RN; Caroline Silzle.University of Kentucky, Lexington: Edwin Trevathan, MD; Linda Trevathan, RN.

Boston Children's Hospital, Boston, Mass: Gregory L. Holmes, MD; Joan Anderson; Marilyn Kuehn.

Dalhousie University, IWK Grace Health Centre, Halifax, Nova Scotia: Carol Camfield, MD; Peter R. Camfield, MD; Mary Height; Edyth Smith.

Private practice, Mishawaka, Ind: Robert M. Shuman, MD; Rhonda Hammond, RN; Elaine Huffman; Cindy Tansek, RD.

Montefiore Medical Center, Bronx, NY: Karen Ballaban-Gil, MD; Shlomo Shinnar, MD, PhD; Candace Callahan, RN; Christine O'Dell, RN, MSN; Miriam Pappo, RD.

University of Texas Medical School, Houston: James W. Wheless, MD; M. Suzanne Berryman, MS, RD, LD, CS; Gretchen Matuszak, MS, RD, LD; Wendy Weisenfluh, RN, MN.

References

1. Wilder RM. The effect of ketonemia on the course of epilepsy. *Mayo Clin Bull.* 1921;2:307.
2. Swink TD, Vining EPG, Freeman JM. The ketogenic diet: 1997. *Adv Pediatr.* 1997; 44:297–329.
3. Wheless J. The ketogenic diet:fa(c)t or fiction. *J Child Neurol.* 1995;10:419–423.
4. DeVivo DC. How to use other drugs (steroids) and the ketogenic diet. In: Morselli PL, Pippenger CE, Penry JK, eds. *Antiepileptic Drug Therapy in Pediatrics.* New York, NY: Raven Press; 1983:283–292.
5. Kinsman SL, Vining EP, Quaskey SA, Mellits D, Freeman JM. Efficacy of the ketogenic diet for intractable seizure disorders: review of 58 cases. *Epilepsia.* 1992;33:1132–1136.
6. *An Introduction to the Ketogenic Diet: A Treatment for Pediatric Epilepsy* [videotape]. Santa Monica, Calif: Charlie Foundation; 1994.
7. Prasad AN, Stafstrom CF, Holmes GL. Alternative epilepsy therapies: the ketogenic diet, immunoglobulins, and steroids. *Epilepsia.* 1996;37:S81–S95.
8. Freeman JM, Kelly MT, Freeman JB. *The Epilepsy Diet Treatment: An Introduction to the Ketogenic Diet.* New York, NY: Demos; 1994.
9. Livingston S. *The Diagnosis and Treatment of Convulsive Disorders in Children.* Springfield, Ill: Charles C Thomas Publisher; 1954.
10. Felbamate Study Group in Lennox-Gastaut Syndrome. Efficacy of felbamate in childhood epileptic encephalopathy (Lennox-Gastaut syndrome). *N Engl J Med.* 1993;328:29–33.
11. Huttenlocker PR, Hapke RJ. A follow-up study of intractable seizures in childhood. *Ann Neurol.* 1990;28:699–705.
12. Walker MC, Sander JWAS. The impact of new antiepileptic drugs on the prognosis of epilepsy: seizure freedom should be the ultimate goal. *Neurology.* 1996;46:912–914.
13. Mattson RH, Cramer JA, Collins JF, et al. Comparison of carbamazepine, phenobarbital, phenytoin and primidone in partial and secondary generalized tonic-clonic seizures. *N Engl J Med.* 1985;313:145–151.
14. Nordli DR, DeVivo DC. The ketogenic diet revisited: back to the future. *Epilepsia.* 1997; 38:73–749.

"In some respects at least, myths and science fulfill a similar function: they both provide human beings with a representation of the world and of the forces that are supposed to govern it. They both fix the limits of what is considered as possible. . . . Whether mythic or scientific, the view of the world that man builds is always largely a product of his imagination."—François Jacob, *The Possible and the Actual*

30 Alternative Neurology

The Ketogenic Diet

E. S. Roach, MD
From the Department of Neurology, University of Texas Southwestern Medical Center, Dallas.
Arch Neurol. 1998;55:1403–1404

This month several journals of the American Medical Association include articles on the general theme of alternative medicine, a loosely defined assortment of techniques such as magnetic therapy, acupuncture, therapeutic touch, herbal medicine, and biofeedback that are unified by their relative lack of rigorous scientific validation. In conjunction with the alternative medicine theme, this issue of the *Archives* features an article by Vining and colleagues[1] summarizing their multicenter study of the ketogenic diet for children with epilepsy.

In many ways, the ketogenic diet is far removed from the realm of alternative medicine. The ketogenic diet, after all, has a decades long history, a clear biochemical rationale, and a well-defined therapeutic objective. But the diet could also serve as a prototype for how to approach questions such as therapeutic dietary manipulation; if the alternative methods are to ever be fully accepted by mainstream scientific medicine, there must be more convincing evidence of a scientifically feasible rationale and of clinical effectiveness.

What, exactly, distinguishes alternative medicine and complementary medicine (the use of alternative methods in conjunction with standard medical treatments) from conventional scientific medicine? The distinction does not lie in the specific treatments recommended by practitioners of alternative medicine, for there are numerous examples in scientific medicine of vitamins, nutrients, or dietary changes being used to alter the course of a disease. Ultimately, it is the rigor with which ideas are evaluated, not the nature of the treatment itself, that separates alternative from scientific medicine.

As in traditional medicine, an alternative medical concept begins as a hypothesis, a model on which methods of diagnosis and treatment can be built. Given a clear rationale, it is not intrinsically wrong to suggest that a newly touted herbal agent might help a particular illness. After all, some now well-accepted treatments in conventional medicine had similar humble origins and were initially controversial. But with conventional medicine, a new concept is usually questioned until it is either validated or rejected. Many proponents of alternative medicine, in contrast, seem unwilling or unable to go beyond the hypothesis stage and subject their ideas to the often brutal process of objective inquiry.

At its finest, conventional medical science provides a framework in which to develop and test theories of disease and ensure that treatments based on these models are both safe and effective. While clinical trials are certainly not foolproof, such studies are the best method now available. But many widely accepted methods of traditional medicine did not go through rigorous clinical trials before being used in patient care. Bed rest or back mobilizing exercises are often recommended for patients with acute low back pain, for instance, but a recent controlled trial[2] showed that simply continuing regular activity leads to quicker recovery than either bed rest or exercise. Sadly, we in conventional medicine sometime fall into the same traps as the alternative practitioners, promoting a therapy or a diagnostic procedure that may seem intuitively reasonable without sufficient testing of its effectiveness.

Whether the product of traditional or of alternative medicine, new procedures and treatments should be studied sufficiently to ensure safety and efficacy before being recommended for routine patient care. That the scientific method can be applied to alternative methods was well illustrated by a recent study[3] of the ability of touch therapists to sense a human "energy field." Although detection and modification of an energy field is the canon of touch therapy, this study proved that even experienced practitioners could not detect such a human energy field.

There are many reasons to be concerned about inadequately studied methods. First, just because a treatment is based on dietary changes, herbal products, or physical manipulation does not necessarily mean it is innocuous. There are well-documented episodes of vertebral artery dissection following chiropractic manipulation,[4] for example, and vitamins and other "natural" compounds can be toxic. Another concern is that some individuals might put their faith entirely in an alternative approach while ignoring proven treatments. By failing to require adequate testing of unconventional treatments, we might risk discarding a potential advance as a passing fad without first proving its effectiveness. One might argue that the ketogenic diet falls into this category—although used to treat epilepsy for years, the diet may have been abandoned partly because its effectiveness had not been as carefully defined as that of the drugs that replaced it years ago.

Finally, what about the cost of alternative treatments? These remedies are often not covered by agencies or insurance plans, but it would be naive to discount their costs, because money spent on these programs could be directed toward established therapies, preventive care, or to the family's other needs. Should not the disciples of alternative medicine be as accountable for the cost-effectiveness of their methods as those in traditional medicine?

Many parents are initially drawn to the ketogenic diet because they assume that a diet must somehow be more natural and less risky than a medication. They soon find that there is nothing at all normal or natural about the ketogenic diet! But it is a reasonable option, particularly for children who have not responded to medication or who have excessive adverse effects from medication. Vining and colleagues[1] have contributed a wealth of useful information on the ketogenic diet. If the ketogenic diet can be systematically examined, then other forms of nontraditional therapy could and should also be investigated. Those who champion new tests and treatments ultimately have an obligation to study these procedures thoroughly before promoting them for general use with patients.

References

1. Vining EPG, Freeman JM, Ballaban-Gil K, et al. A multicenter study of the efficacy of the ketogenic diet. *Arch Neurol.* 1998;55:1433–1437.
2. Malmivaara A, Hakkinen U, Aro T, et al. The treatment of acute low back pain: bed rest, exercise, or ordinary activity? *N Engl J Med.* 1995;332:351–355.
3. Rosa L, Rosa E, Sarner L, Barrett S. A close look at therapeutic touch. *JAMA.* 1998; 279:1005–1010.
4. Zimmerman AW, Kumar AJ, Gadoth N, et al. Traumatic vertebrobasilar occlusive disease in childhood. *Neurology.* 1978;28:185–18.

5 Herbal Therapies

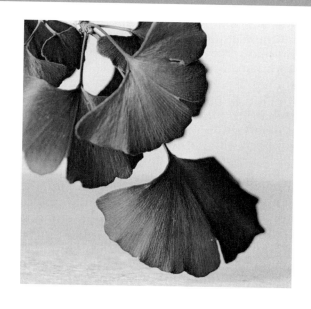

31 Herbs as Medicines

Lisa Corbin Winslow, MD; David J. Kroll, PhD
From the HealthONE Center for Health Sciences Education (Dr Winslow), the Division of General Internal Medicine (Dr Winslow), and the School of Pharmacy (Dr Kroll), University of Colorado Health Sciences Center, Denver.

Herbs and related products are commonly used by patients who also seek conventional health care. All physicians, regardless of specialty or interest, care for patients who use products that are neither prescribed nor recommended. Some herbs have been extensively studied, but little is known about others. When a patient asks for advice regarding the use of a particular herb, how should a physician respond? Similarly, how does a physician determine if a patient's symptoms are caused by a "remedy"? This review attempts to answer these questions by investigating pertinent definitions, the history of herbs in medicine, epidemiology and prevalence of herbal use, and relevant psychosocial issues.

Arch Intern Med. 1998;158:2192–2199

While a complete review of specific herbs is impossible in this setting (>20,000 herbal and related products are used in the United States),[1] the potential benefits and hazards of some of the more popular herbal products in use are examined (Table 1).

History

The earliest evidence of humans' use of plants for healing dates back to the Neanderthal period.[3] In the 16th century, botanical gardens were created to grow medicinal plants for medical schools.[4] Herbal medicine practice flourished until the 17th century when more "scientific" pharmacological remedies were favored.[5]

In the United States, the history of herbal use begins in the early colonial days when health care was provided by women in the home. Initially, they used homemade botanical remedies and later purchased similar products as "patent medicines." In the early 19th century, scientific methods became more advanced and preferred, and the practice of botanical healing was dismissed as quackery. In the 1960s, with concerns over the iatrogenic effects of conventional medicine and desire for more self-reliance, interest in "natural health" and the use of herbal products increased.[5] Recognition of the rising use of herbal medicines and other nontraditional remedies led to the establishment of the Office of Alternative

Table 1. Definitions of Terms Used in This Article

Term	Definition
Herb (urb, hurb) n	1. A flowering plant whose stem above ground does not become woody and persistent. 2. Such a plant when valued for its medicinal properties, flavor, scent, or the like.[2] A broader definition also includes fungi, fruits, roots, vegetables, and all plants; occasionally, enzymes, minerals, and hormones are also included when referring to "herbal medicine."[1] For this review, an herb refers to any plant, plant product, or mixtures of plants or plant products, in any form
Herbalist	One who prescribes plants for medicinal use
Botanical, natural, herbal, traditional, and plant medicine	All refer to the use of plants for medicinal purposes
Alternative medicine	Refers to herbal medicine, chiropractors, acupuncture, or reflexology, etc—ie, anything not taught in a medical school but used for health care
Conventional medicine	The practice of medicine as taught in a western medical school
Kampo	Japanese traditional medicine, including the use of herbs
Ayurvedic medicine	Type of herbal medicine practiced in India

Table 2. Conventional Medicines Derived From Plants

Atropine (*Atropa belladonna*)	Physostigmine (*Physostigma venenosum*)
Digoxin (*Digitalis purpurea*)	Senna (*Cassia acutifolia*)
Colchicine (*Colchicum autumnale*)	Ephedrine (*Ephedra sinica*)
Quinine (*Cinchona officinalis*)	Cocaine (*Erythroxylon coca*)
Codeine (*Papaver somniferum*)	Salicylin (*Salix purpurea*)
Vincristine (*Catharanthus roseus*)	Capsaicin (*Capsicum frutescens*)
Ipecac (*Cephaelis ipecacuanha*)	Scopolamine (*Datura fastuosa*)
Taxol (*Taxus brevifolia*)	Reserpine (*Rauvolfia serpentina*)

Table 3. Representative Epidemiological Studies of Herbal Medicine Use*

Source, y	Patient Population	Prevalence of Herbal Use, %	"Risk Factors" for Use	Notes
Brown and Marcy,[9] 1991	Kaiser Permanente, Portland, Ore (n=100)	93	Married, larger household, higher income, health food store patron, or see an alternative healer	Access to conventional care not a deterrent to use
Eisenberg et al,[8] 1993	US telephone survey (n=1539)	3	For all alternative methods: nonblack, aged 25-49 y, higher education, and higher income	83% Also seeing conventional MD, 72% did not inform conventional MD of alternative medicine use
Kassler et al,[10] 1991	University HIV clinic (114)	22	No differentiating risk factors in this population	20% Did not inform MD of herb use, 24% could not identify herb used, and 16% enrolled in clinical trials

*MD indicates medical doctor; HIV, human immunodeficiency virus.

Medicine by the National Institutes of Health (Bethesda, Md) in 1992. Worldwide, herbal use again became popular; in 1974 the World Health Organization (Geneva, Switzerland) encouraged developing countries to use traditional plant medicines to "fulfill a need unmet by modern systems."[5]

Thirty percent of all modern drugs are derived from plants.[3] Some of the more familiar ones are listed in Table 2.[4,6,7]

Epidemiology

Estimates of the prevalence of herbal medicine use differ, with studies concluding that between 3% and 93% of the US population uses herbs (Table 3).[7–10] The variability of these estimates is due to discrepant definitions of herbs (Table 1) as well as different inclusions of the length of use (ie, ever vs in the last 12 months).

Internationally, the use of botanical medicines is generally higher. For example, 70% of "Western" doctors in

Japan prescribe kampo drugs daily.[11] Eighty percent of the world's population relies primarily on traditional medicines for their health care needs.[5,12] It is certain that physicians are seeing patients who are using herbs, and, as is discussed, this use can affect the patient's health problems and effects of conventional treatments.

Economics and Reimbursement

The amount of money spent on herbal remedies is significant. Americans spent $553 million in 8000 health food stores in 1994,[13] and from all sources, the estimate of US "medical" herb sales is $1.2 billion in 1996.[14] Sales of herbal medicines are growing by 20% a year, and herbs are the largest growth area in retail pharmacy, far exceeding growth in the conventional drug category.[15]

Costs to the individual and costs of individual products can also be substantial, albeit variable. An epidemiological study[10] of patients positive for human immunodeficiency virus found that the average herbal user was spending $18 per month on herbs (range, $0–$175). Individual products have variable costs, dependent on both the product and its source (homegrown, imported, from a health food store, or from an herbalist). In another study[16] of herb use among patients with the acquired immunodeficiency syndrome (AIDS), one product recommended by a health food store sold for almost $150 for a month's supply.

Insurance plans and managed care organizations are beginning to offer reimbursement for alternative treatments. In fact, coverage of chiropractic treatment is mandated by law in at least 45 states, acupuncture in 7 states, and naturopathy in 2 states.[17] Insurance plans that cover alternative health care often require physician referral for these services, highlighting the importance of physician awareness. One managed care company, Oxford Health Plans, Norwalk, Conn, is planning to cover alternative treatments, including some that use herbal remedies, basing their decision on a survey showing that 33% of its 1.5 million members had sought alternative treatment in the last 2 years. American Western Life Insurance Company, San Mateo, Calif, has a "prevention plus" plan that covers herbal medicines. Industry analysts expect many other insurance plans to follow suit to compete for this untapped multibillion dollar market.[17] Although reimbursement for herbal medicines is in its infancy, it is expected to grow tremendously along with the continued boom in sales of herbal products and alternative health care in general. In Germany, herbs prescribed by physicians are covered by insurance, whereas over-the-counter herbs are not; and German physicians are much more knowledgeable about their use.[14] Physicians must become familiar with herbal medicine, as more insurance companies will expect their physicians to make referrals or suggest herbal products.

Why Do People Use Herbal Medicines?

There are multiple reasons patients turn to herbal therapies. Often cited is a "sense of control, a mental comfort from taking action,"[9] which helps explain why many people taking herbs have diseases that are chronic or incurable, such as diabetes, cancer, arthritis, or AIDS. In such situations, they often believe that conventional medicine has failed them. When patients use home remedies for acute, often self-limited conditions, such as a cold, sore throat, or bee sting, it is often because professional care is not immediately available, too inconvenient, costly, or time consuming.[9,18]

In rural areas, there are additional cultural factors that encourage the use of botanicals, such as the concept of an interplay between the environment and culture, a "man-earth" relationship.[12] Religious beliefs, which can be traced to the medieval doctrine of signatures, are also prominent: "The good Lord has put these yerbs here for man to make hisself with. They is a yerb, could we but find it, to cure every illness [sic]."[19] People believe that where an area gives rise to a particular disease, it will also support plants that can be used to cure it.[5]

Natural plant products are perceived to be healthier than manufactured medicines.[12] Additionally, reports of adverse effects of conventional medications are found in the lay press at a much higher rate than reports of herbal toxicities, in part because mechanisms to track adverse effects exist for conventional medicines whereas such data for self-treatment is harder to ascertain. Even physicians often dismiss herbs as harmless placebos,[10] and many consumers and physicians alike mistakenly believe that anything in a pill form has been approved by the US Food and Drug Administration (FDA).[1]

Regulation: Dietary Supplement and Health Education Act

In 1993, the FDA began scrutinizing the herbal and supplement industry, which triggered a massive letter-writing campaign organized by health food stores that encouraged consumers to "write your congressman or kiss your supplements goodbye." Under pressure, the FDA compromised its plans, creating the supplement category, which includes vitamins, minerals, and herbs and created the Dietary Supplement and Health Education Act (DSHEA) signed October 1994. The DSHEA requires no proof of efficacy, no proof of safety, and sets no standards for quality control for products labeled as supplements. Although the DSHEA requires that

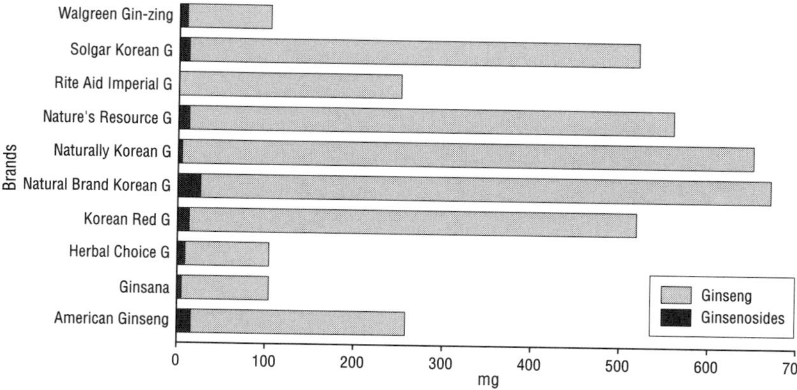

Figure 1. *Consumer Reports*[1] analyzed 10 popular brands of ginseng and found the amount of ginsenosides (black bar) was widely variable in each brand. The amount of ginseng (gray bar) were listed on the packages, but ginsenoside content (active ingredient) was not. Reprinted with permission from *Consumer Reports.*

supplements not promise a specific cure on the label, they may claim effect. Now, if questions arise, the burden lies with the FDA to prove a product unsafe, rather than a company proving its product safe. Manufacturers must put a message on the label stating that claims have not been reviewed by the FDA, but this statement can be subtle.[1] In contrast, regulating agencies in Germany, France, the United Kingdom, and Canada enforce standards of herb quality and safety assessment on manufacturers.[20,21]

Because of the lack of requirements for quality control, safety, and efficacy, consumers cannot determine if an herb's active ingredients are actually in the product, if the ingredient is bioavailable, if the dosage is appropriate, if the next bottle they buy will have the same components, or what else is in the pill besides the claimed ingredients.[1]

Quality Control

Any particular herb or mixture can vary from manufacturer to manufacturer and from batch to batch; an herb that is not toxic or therapeutic in one form or strength may be helpful or harmful in a different preparation.

Potency of various compounds is affected by growing conditions, storage, handling, and preparation such that potency of various products from the same plant can vary 10,000-fold.[1] Manufacturers use varying methods for processing the same herbs; for example, the plant can be ground up and put into pill form, or pharmaceutical methods can be used to extract the desired compound, assay the composition, and make tablets of consistent strength.[1]

Consumer Reports[1] looked at the composition of 10 different ginseng products on the market in 1995. The amount of ginseng per tablet was listed on the labels, but the amount of ginsenosides, thought to be the active components, was not listed. They found striking differences between the products (Figure 1), which could have an impact if a patient changed from one brand to another, especially as ginseng does have dose-dependent adverse effects.

Labels may be incorrect, accidentally or intentionally. The same common name may be applied to different plants recommended for different illnesses.[22] Some products labeled as ginseng actually also contain mandrake (scopolamine) or snakeroot (reserpine) because of the high cost of pure ginseng.[23] Additives may be used, yet not listed on labels; they may be the source of the therapeutic effect. Examples include steroids, nonsteroidal anti-inflammatory agents, prescription antibiotics, sedatives, and narcotics.[1,24–26]

Herbs can be misidentified or the wrong part of the plant may be picked. Such an error was the cause of an outbreak of belladonna poisoning attributable to an herbal tea in New York City,[1] and a similar misidentification led to digitalis poisoning from a mislabeled plantain extract.[27]

Heavy metals are often found in herbal preparations from other countries as they are thought to help cure without being absorbable. However, there are multiple reports in the literature of poisoning with lead, arsenic, cadmium, copper, and mercury found in herbal preparations from foreign countries.[28–34] Also problematic with herbs imported from foreign sources is that written instructions, if any, are often in foreign languages.[32]

Efficacy and Safety Studies

Controlled studies of herbal medicines are not profitable. There is little motivation for manufacturers to conduct randomized, placebo-controlled, double-blinded clinical trials to prove efficacy because (1) they are not required to do so and (2) they cannot patent the product to recoup the estimated $350 million it costs to prove a new drug effective and safe.[13] An entirely new drug must be created, or a novel extraction procedure or pharmaceutical dosage form must be discovered as a result of undertaking the study to produce patentable and thus profitable studies.

Despite these limitations, some scientific studies are being performed. Such studies often originate in other countries where the funding constraints are not as problematic, and where regulatory authorities require some basic assessment of safety and efficacy.

With the resultant lack of solid scientific analysis in the United States, claims for benefits are thus mainly supported solely with anecdotal case reports that fail to consider the natural history of the disease or the placebo effect. Toxic effects, if any, are seldom reported.

Toxicities

It is important to acknowledge that all conventional drugs have potential toxicities. However, in contrast to herbal products, conventional drugs undergo trials and postapproval surveillance that define these toxicities, giving practitioners data on that to weigh risks and benefits of treatment. The therapeutic window and dosage are also defined, as are the constituents of the medicine. Because of rigorous quality control, each pill has the same ingredients as another. Adverse reactions to herbal medicines are probably underrecognized and underreported.[35]

Physicians should become familiar with some of the more common herbal toxicities to determine if an herb is causing a patient's problems; the easiest way is to keep a shelf reference in the office.[21,36,37] Additionally, one can seek case reports in the literature, send the remedy in question to a laboratory (at university hospital settings, call the toxicology laboratory) that can analyze a particular herb for its constituents and possible contaminants, or consult Poisindex (a list of plants considered unsafe by the FDA is available). The FDA also posts recent warnings on herbal products on their Internet page (http://www.fda.gov). With mild toxicities, such as gastrointestinal upset or mildly elevated values on liver function tests, the physician can try stopping the herbal treatment and see if the problem resolves and consider a rechallenge for recurrence.

Table 4 outlines toxicities of some of the more popular herbs, listed by organ system.

There has been little evaluation of interactions between regulated drugs and herbs, but knowledge of some adverse reactions (and therapeutic actions) of herbal medicines can help one predict drug interactions. For example, herbs containing cardiac glycosides may potentiate effects of digoxin; herbs with diuretic effects may potentiate digoxin toxicity via potassium loss. Herbs that can cause hypertension or hypotension can interfere with prescription antihypertensive agents; hypoglycemic herbs can interfere with glycemic control in a patient with diabetes. Some herbs interfere with prescription medications by altering their metabolism. For example, *Eucalyptus* can induce microsomal liver enzymes[51] while flavonoids from *Echinacea purpurea* are known to inhibit the cytochrome P-450 3A4 and sulfotransferase drug-metabolizing enzymes.[52,53]

Not only might herbal therapy be toxic, but using an herbal remedy over a proven conventional therapy can be dangerous, too. Many oncologists have seen patients with early-stage cancers who eschewed curative conventional care in favor of herbal medicines. After these herbal treatments failed, the patients returned to the oncologists with incurable metastatic diseases. In fact, studies[54] have shown that patients who use herbs and other alternative therapies are more likely to abandon potentially beneficial conventional therapy when faced with an illness. Patients may also continue detrimental behaviors, such as smoking tobacco or drinking large amounts of alcohol, with the rationalization that the herbal remedy they are taking will be protective.

An herb that may be safe in small doses may become dangerous in higher doses. The risk of overdose is higher in herbal preparations than conventional medicines because of the already mentioned product variability. Consider the patient who assumed if "some is good, more is better" with respect to a copper-containing supplement he was taking. As he began to feel worse, he increased the dose. By the time he came to the attention of conventional health providers, he was unable to eat and was wasted and jaundiced, and had acquired Wilson disease.[13] Patients may assume herbs such as garlic and nutmeg to be safe, as they are commonly used in cooking without adverse effect. However, herbs in extract form are often much more potent than the traditionally used form, and can be harmful (Table 4).

Commonly Used Herbs

Of the 20,000 available products, which is the physician most likely to encounter? A 1995 survey of 163 US health food retail stores revealed that the top 10 selling herbs were echinacea (*Echinacea purpurea* and *angustifolia*), garlic (*Allium sativum*), goldenseal (*Hydrastis canadensis*), ginseng

Table 4. Reported Adverse Effects of Some Common Herbs*

Organ System	Toxic Effects	Herb	Comments
Gastrointestinal	Hepatotoxic (from asymptomatic enzyme elevation to fulminant necrosis)	Chinese herbal teas[35, 36, 38]; mistletoe[10, 35]; germander[37–41]; chaparral[42–44]; or comfrey[10, 36]	First reported case of hepatic veno-occlusive disease was caused by comfrey
	Nausea/vomiting	Dandelion, garlic, ginseng, or chaparral[10, 22]	. . .
	Diarrhea	Herbal teas[36, 38, 45]; aloe, ligustrum, dandelion, prunella, garlic, or ginseng[10]	. . .
Hematologic	Anticoagulant/antiplatelet	Yarrow, red clover, tang-kuei, pau d'arco, tang-kuei, or salvia[10, 22, 46]	. . .
Central nervous system	Nervousness, agitation, insomnia, mood changes, depression, confusion, or hallucinations	Ginseng[47]	With long-term use and higher doses
	Cholinergic toxicity	Jimson weed[33]	Contains atropine, scopolamine, hyoscyamine
	Hallucinogenic	Catnip, hops, kava kava, khat, lobelia, mandrake, nutmeg, jimson weed, valerian, or yohimbe[33]	. . .
	Sedation	Peony, salvia, or tang-kuei[10]	. . .
	Seizures, psychosis, or coma	Ephedra[48]	. . .
Pulmonary	Pulmonary hypertension	Chinese herbal teas[35]	. . .
Allergic/immunologic	Contact dermatitis	Propolis, garlic, echinacea[10]; or melaleuca oil[49]	. . .
	Systemic lupus erythematosus	Alfalfa[35]	
Endocrinologic	Gynecomastia, vaginal bleeding	Ginseng[35]	Contains estrogen
	Goiters, hyperthyroidism, and hypothyroidism	Kelp[10]	Contains iodine
	Inhibition of iodine uptake	Garlic[10]	. . .
	Hypoglycemia	Atractylodes, scrofularia, lycium, or burdock[10]	. . .
Renal	Diuresis	Burdock, astragalus, peony, or dandelion[10]	. . .
	Hypertension, sodium and water retention, or hypokalemia	Licorice[10, 35, 50]	*Glycyrrhiza glabra; Glycyrrhiza radix* can have same effects and is found in 74% of Chinese herbal teas
Cardiovascular	Hypotension	Astragalus, codonopsis, prunella, scrofularia, or salvia[10]	. . .
	Hypertension	Ginseng[10]	. . .
	Hypertension, coronary spasm, palpitations, or tachycardia	Ephedra[48]	. . .

*Ellipses indicate not applicable.

(Asian *Panax ginseng* and American *Panax quinquefolius*), ginkgo (*Ginkgo biloba*), saw palmetto (*Serenoa repens*), aloe (*Aloe species*), ma huang (*Ephedra sinica*), Siberian ginseng (*Eleutherococcus senticosus*), and cranberry (*Vaccinium macrocarpon*).[55] More recent trends suggest that St John's wort (*Hypericum perforatum*), valerian (*Valeriana officinalis*), and feverfew (*Tanacetum parthenium*) will likely earn a top 10 designation when 1998 data become available.

Patients decide which herbs to use in a variety of ways. Because of the requirements that herbal medicines must not directly claim cures on the label, manufacturers have become creative with marketing. Products are given names that allude to their effects, such as "Insomnia," "PMS," "Sleep," and "Get Trim." Pamphlets, books, and other advocacy literature not subject to labeling guidelines are shelved near herbs. Patients also get information through word of mouth, encouraged by anecdotal reports from friends. An herbalist who has training in the use of plants for healing may be consulted.

Advice can be found from health food store workers. An undercover 1993 FDA study asked clerks what to buy "for my immune system," "high blood pressure," or "something that works on cancer." From 129 clerks surveyed, 120 specific and highly variable recommendations were received.[1] Phillips et al,[16] in 1995, surveyed 20 Birmingham, Ala, area health food stores for their recommendations for AIDS. Combination products (with names like "Immunace," "Immunaction," or "Immunectar") were most frequently recommended; ginseng-containing products were recommended second (and were the most expensive). Pharmacists, on the other hand, are unlikely to give specific recommendations on herbal products sold in their stores, and say they do not know much about them.[1] In fact, only 5% of the US herbal market is actually sold in pharmacies.[20]

People can also explore the Internet to discover information about herbs. Internet sources are often perceived as "published" and therefore entirely factual. However, most sites merely list herbs and their uses, few mention regulations, safety, or efficacy. Even an herb with well-recognized toxicities, such as ephedra, may have no cautionary statement. A few sample Web sites are listed below:

- FDA: Access to "MEDWATCH," with herb warnings under "special nutritionals adverse event monitoring system" link. Available at: http://www.fda.gov. The direct address to the searchable database is http://www.vmcfsan.fda.gov/~dms/aems.html.
- ASPET Herbal and Medicinal Plant Interest Group: A site for an herb discussion group among classic pharmacologists; also with some interesting links. Available at: http://www.faseb.org/aspet/H&MIG3.htm#top.
- American Botanical Council: A respected organization dedicated to dissemination of factual herbal information. Herb Research Foundation: A nonprofit organization supported by the American Botanical Council. Available at: http://www.herbs.org.
- Botanical.com: Contains the 1931 text "A Modern Herbal," also the "Ask Dr Weil" column, who integrates Western medicine and herbs: somewhat biased toward herbs; however, with emphasis on anecdotes. Available at: http://www.botanical.com.
- Herbal Information Center: Brief overviews on common herbs; few warnings; mostly geared to sell. Available at: http://www.kcweb.com/herb/herbmain.htm.
- HerbNet: Links to other herb sites; mostly advertisements but some good information can be found. Available at: http://www.herbnet.com.
- Herbal Resource Inc: Primarily a sales site but occasionally references are noted. Biased and misleading, even stating that "there are no side effects from herbs." Available at: http://www.herbsinfo.com.
- University of Washington Medicinal Herb Garden: Nice pictures of herbs; cross-reference to MEDLINE abstracts, excellent resource. Available at: http://www.nnlm.nlm.nih.gov/pnr/uwmhg/.

When patients or practitioners want nonbiased information on a commonly used herb, they are advised to buy a book that bases advice on published and critically reviewed literature. A comprehensive literature search will ensure the most scientific, peer-reviewed information is being reviewed, but this process is often time consuming and, thus, impractical. Beginning in 1978, the German equivalent of the FDA went as far as to publish a series of herb recommendations, the Commission E Monographs, which detail dosages and indications for herbs whose efficacy is supported by the literature, and these have recently become available in the United States. However, the extrapolation of these European findings (usually conducted with well-characterized, pharmaceutical herbal preparations) to herbs available in the United States is complicated by the relative lack of regulatory standards in this country, as described earlier.

The great variation in US herb quality is unfortunate in light of the known pharmacological actions in humans of well-characterized botanical preparations. If one can put the question of US regulation aside, comments can thus be made on the efficacy of some of the best-selling herbs mentioned above.

Valerian (*Valeriana officinalis*) ranks as one of the most well characterized of the widely used herbs. Listed in The National Formulary until 1950, valerian has been described in human studies as possessing sedative and anxiolytic activity[56] and is often combined with other sedative herbs like hops (*Humulus lupulus*).

In the case of *Ginkgo biloba*, which contains ginkgolides that antagonize platelet-activating factor, human studies were greatly facilitated by the availability of a high-quality extract (EGb 761) from the manufacturer, Willmar Schwabe, in Karlsrube, Germany. The efficacy of *Ginkgo biloba* extract in improving or delaying cognitive deficits was recently demonstrated in a multicenter US trial of 309 patients with early-stage Alzheimer dementia. Improvements in 2 of 3 clinical parameters of cognitive function were observed as early as at 12 weeks of *Ginkgo* extract, Egb 761, when compared with placebo.[57] Understandably, *Ginkgo* should be used with care in this population due to the prevalence of prescription anticoagulant therapy.

Ginseng is another widely used herb touted in Chinese traditional medicine as an "adaptogen" that allows the body to respond to physical and emotional stress. The best data to date support a role for ginseng as a vasodilator and in serving a cardioprotective role in the presence of oxygen free radicals.[58] The mechanism of these effects is likely due to certain ginsenosides present in *Panax ginseng* that appear to stimulate nitric oxide synthase and increase nitric oxide production and release.

For the practicing internist, the most interesting data come from efficacy comparisons between herbs and prescription medications. For example, limited data suggest that saw palmetto compares favorably with finasteride in the management of benign prostatic hyperplasia.[59] In treating mood disorders, St John's wort has been shown to be equally efficacious to the older, tricyclic antidepressants.[60] However, it should be stressed that these studies were performed with highly characterized botanical preparations under the guidance of trained physicians. The wisdom of herbal self-treatment, as is often the case in the United States, is discussed in the following section, along with more information about specific herbs the internist is likely to encounter.

Pharmacological Basis for Use or Avoidance of Herbal Medicines

Given the previously detailed shortcomings of herbal preparations in the United States, the question arises whether any herbs possess pharmacological activity distinct from prescription or over-the-counter drugs that might therefore warrant their cautious use. Such herbs are few. The most commonly used herb in the United States and Europe, *Echinacea purpurea,* may be one. Unlike over-the-counter decongestants or antihistamines, alkylamide and polysaccharide constituents of echinacea possess significant in vitro and in vivo immunostimulation due to enhanced phagocytosis and nonspecific T-cell stimulation.[61] However, to our knowledge, only a few clinical trials have been done with echinacea, and only a handful were well designed. One well-designed, double-blind study randomized 100 patients with acute flulike illness to an echinacea extract or placebo and showed that echinacea decreased the duration of symptoms from 10 to 7 days. Another study, with 647 students from the University of Cologne given echinacea or placebo prophylactically during flu season, showed a 15% reduction in the number of colds in the group given echinecea. Neither study used commonly available preparations of echinacea.[37]

Most herbs fall into the category of agents that share pharmacological mechanisms of action with already existing prescription or over-the-counter drugs. Based on a logical consideration of the current state of herb standardization and pharmacokinetic evaluation, the patient would be best steered toward a regulated pharmaceutical preparation capable of a predictable pharmacological response. For example, powdered ginger root has been tested in humans for prophylaxis against motion sickness compared with dimenhydrate (Dramamine).[62] While one study[63] reported 1.8 mg of ginger superior to 100 mg of dimenhydrate, a follow-up study failed to show any efficacy of ginger. Other examples of herbs possessing actions similar to existing, regulated drugs are feverfew for migraines,[64] valerian for anxiety,[65] and garlic for hypercholesterolemia.[66]

Of greater concern to the physician is when patients use herbs with redundant pharmacological activity for diseases not recommended for self-treatment. Miller[67] heightened the public's awareness of the antidepressant actions of St John's wort, an herb containing the potential monoamine oxidase inhibitor hypericin. While St John's wort has shown promising antidepressant action,[60] it is unlikely that patients can make a diagnosis of endogenous depression, much less differentiate their condition from medical conditions mimicking depression. In addition, there remains concern for hypertensive reactions resulting from concomitant ingestion of high tyramine-containing foods and St John's wort, and hypericin is well known to cause photosensitivity.[68] With St John's wort, the question is not whether the herb has therapeutic efficacy but rather issues of safety and appropriateness of the disease as a candidate for self-treatment.

Similarly, the use of saw palmetto for benign prostatic hypertrophy presents another dilemma. While hydrophobic extracts of *Serenoa repens* berries indeed possess 5α-reductase inhibitory and androgen receptor antagonistic activities in vitro,[69] it is unwise for men to self-diagnose benign prostatic hypertrophy, with the clear risk of potentiating the growth of undiagnosed prostatic carcinoma.

Conclusions

Herbal remedies are commonly used by patients who access conventional health care. Few have been shown to have beneficial effects beyond those of conventionally regulated products, and they may be costly, adulterated with dangerous additives, inherently toxic, or cause the patient to forgo potentially curative care.

All medicines can be toxic under specific circumstances; there is always a risk that an adverse reaction will present a hazard to a patient. With licensed medicines, however, regulations ensure the risk is small and monitor the medicine's efficacy, safety, and quality. No such controls over herbal medicines exist.[36] As stated by Brown and Marcy,[9] the hazards of self-treatment are no less serious because of the presence of similar hazards in conventional medicine.

If a patient presents with a problem that might be due to an herb, the physician should discontinue the product and watch for resolution. Reference books, Poisindex, or MEDLINE should be consulted to see if such an adverse reaction has been described. The FDA has implemented MEDWATCH, a toll-free number to which adverse effects of herbs can be reported (800 332-1088).[70] If necessary, herbs can be sent to laboratories for content analysis, either to a toxicology laboratory or a pharmacology department. Botany departments at major universities can also be a source of information.

If patients ask if "herbal medicines" in general are safe or effective, they should be counseled about the lack of regulations for quality, safety, or efficacy, the differences in preparations from different manufacturers, and the lack of mechanism for reporting adverse effects. Curious patients can be directed to read the books mentioned, and cautioned against biased information that they may receive from health food store employees, pamphlets shelved near herbs, and the Internet.

If patients mention a friend who was helped by a certain remedy or an advertisement that was seen depicting a dramatic success with a certain herb, they should be counseled on the dangers of anecdotal reports. Patients take our recommendations of conventional medicines because we suggest it, not because we present them with reams of data from randomized controlled trials; thus, it is not unexpected that their approach to the use of unconventional medicine is the same.

Patients with chronic conditions such as AIDS or cancer should also be warned that some of the adverse effects of herbals are often similar to symptoms of problems associated with their disease or treatment, thus making it difficult to discern if the disease or the "remedy" is the problem.

Classically trained physicians cannot ignore herbal medicines anymore. We must realize that patients are using herbal medicines, and insurance companies are beginning to cover the costs and are even asking us to oversee the use of herbs in certain situations. We must all become educated about these products, and at the very least know where to find information when we need it.

Asking patients about supplement use during the initial history is thus imperative. Patient disclosure of herb use may provide an opportunity for the physician to redirect the patient toward effective conventional health care. By taking a complete drug and supplement history, a dialogue can be initiated to rationally compare the appropriateness of herbal remedies and regulated pharmaceuticals in relation to the severity of the condition. Until herbs in this country are more strictly regulated, however, no classically trained physician should recommend an herbal product to a patient. For the herb-using patient who views conventional medicine with ambivalence, the physician can foster a more open and communicative relationship by demonstrating an objective understanding of both alternative and conventional approaches.

References

1. Herbal roulette. *Consumer Reports.* November 1995:698–705.
2. *The American College Dictionary.* New York, NY: Random House Inc; 1957:565.
3. Kleiner SM. The true nature of herbs. *Phys Sports Med.* 1995;23:13–14.
4. Akerele O. Nature's medicinal bounty: don't throw it away. *World Health Forum.* 1993; 14:390–395.
5. Trevelyan J. Herbal medicine. *Nurs Times.* 1993; 89:36–38.
6. Aliotta G, Capasso G, Pollio A, Strumia S, De Santo NG. Early contributors to nephrology: Joseph Jacob Plenck. *Am J Nephrol.* 1994; 14:377–382.
7. Frate DA, Croom EM, Frate JB, Juergens JB. Self-treatment with herbal and other plant-derived remedies: rural Mississippi, 1993. *MMWR Morb Mortal Wkly Rep.* 1995; 44:204–207.
8. Eisenberg DM, Kessler RC, Foster C, Norlock FE, Calkins DR, Delbanco TL. Unconventional medicine in the United States. *N Engl J Med.* 1993; 328:246–252.
9. Brown JS, Marcy SA. The use of botanicals for health purposes by members of a prepaid health plan. *Res Nurs Health.* 1991; 14:339–350.
10. Kassler WJ, Blanc P, Greenblatt R. The use of medicinal herbs by human immunodeficiency virus-infected patients. *Arch Intern Med.* 1991; 151:2281–2288.
11. Ross C. New life for old medicine. *Lancet.* 1992;342:486–487.
12. Gesler WM. Therapeutic landscapes: medicinal issues in light of the new cultural geography. *Soc Sci Med.* 1992;34:735–746.
13. Marwick C. Growing use of medicinal botanicals forces assessment by drug regulators. *JAMA.* 1995;273:607–609.
14. Tyler VE. What pharmacists should know about herbal remedies. *J Am Pharm Assoc.* 1996; 36:29–37.
15. The right stuff: *Drug Store News* picks the categories taking off in '94. *Drug Store News.* 1994;16:15.
16. Phillips LG, Nichols MH, King WD. Herbs and HIV: the health food industry's answer. *South Med J.* 1995;988:911–913.

17. Whitaker B. Now in the HMO: yoga teachers and naturopaths. *New York Times.* November 24, 1996:11.

18. Gill GV, Redmond S, Garratt F, Paisey R. Diabetes and alternative medicine: cause for concern. *Diabet Med.* 1994;11:210–213.

19. Price E. Root digging in the Appalachians: the geography of botanical drugs. *Geogr Rev.* 1960;50:1–20.

20. Tyler VE. *Herbs of Choice: The Therapeutic Use of Phytomedicinals.* Binghampton, NY: Pharmaceutical Products Press; 1994.

21. Newall CA, Anderson LA, Phillipson JD. *Herbal Medicines: A Guide for Health-Care Professionals.* London, England: The Pharmaceutical Press; 1996.

22. Saxe T. Toxicity of medicinal herbal preparations. *Am Fam Phys.* 1987;35:135–142.

23. Siegel R. Kola, ginseng, and mislabeled herbs. *JAMA.* 1978;237:24.

24. Abt AB, Oh JY, Huntington RA, Burkhart KK. Chinese herbal medicines induced acute renal failure. *Arch Intern Med.* 1995;155:211–212.

25. DuPont R, Bogema S. Benzodiazapines in a health-catalog product. *JAMA.* 1990;264:695.

26. Capobianco DJ, Brazis PW, Fox TP. Proximal-muscle weakness induced by herbs. *N Engl J Med.* 1993;329:1430.

27. *The Denver Post.* June 13, 1997.

28. Holtan N, Hall S, Knight F, et al. Nonfatal arsenic poisoning in three Hmong patients: Minnesota. *MMWR Morb Mortal Wkly Rep.* 1984;33:347–349.

29. Levitt C, Paulson D, Duvall K, et al. Folk remedy associated lead poisoning in Hmong children: Minnesota. *MMWR Morb Mortal Wkly Rep.* 1988;32:555–556.

30. Smitherman J, Harber P. A case of mistaken identity: herbal medicine as a cause of lead toxicity. *Am J Ind Med.* 1991;20:795–798.

31. Markowitz, SB, Nunez CM, Klitzman S, et al. Lead poisoning due to Hae Ge Fen: the porphyrin content of individual erythrocytes. *JAMA.* 1994;271:932–934.

32. Shaw D, House I, Kolev S, Murray V. Should herbal medicines be licensed? *BMJ.* 1995; 11:451–452.

33. Baker D, Brender J, Davis K. Cadmium and lead exposure associated with pharmaceuticals imported from Asia: Texas. *MMWR Morb Mortal Wkly Rep.* 1989;38:612–614.

34. Yeoh TS, Lee As, Lee HS. Absorption of mercuric sulphide following oral administration in mice. *Toxicology.* 1986;41:107–111.

35. D'Arcy PF. Adverse reactions and interactions with herbal medicines, I: adverse reactions. *Adverse Drug React Toxicol Rev.* 1991; 10:189–208.

36. Tyler VE. *The Honest Herbal. Binghampton,* NY: Pharmaceutical Products Press; 1993.

37. Schulz V, Hänsel R, Tyler VE. *Rational Phytotherapy: A Physician's Guide to Herbal Medicine.* New York, NY: Springer-Verlag NY Inc; 1997.

38. Ridker PM. Toxic effects of herbal teas. *Arch Environ Health.* 1987;42:133–136.

39. Ridker PM. Health hazards of unusual herbal teas. *Am Fam Phys.* 1989;39:153–156.

40. Larrey D, Vial T, Pauwels A, et al. Hepatitis after germander (*Teucrium chamaedrys*) administration: another instance of herbal medicine hepatoxicity. *Ann Intern Med.* 1992;117:129–132.

41. Castot A, Larrey D. Hepatitis observed during a treatment with a drug or tea containing wild Germander: evaluation of 26 cases reported to the Regional Centers of Pharmacovigilance. *Gastroenterol Clin Biol.* 1992;16:916–922.

42. Katz M, Saibil F. Herbal hepatitis: subacute hepatic necrosis secondary to chaparral leaf. *J Clin Gastroerterol.* 1990;12:203–206.

43. Clark F, Reed R. Chaparral-induced toxic hepatitis: California and Texas 1992. *MMWR Morb Mortal Wkly Rep.* 1992;41:812–814.

44. Smith BC, Desmond PV. Acute hepatitis induced by ingestion of the herbal medication chaparral. *Aust N Z J Med.* 1993;23:526.

45. Anderson T, Konracki S, Lyman D, Parkin W. Diarrhea from herbal tea: New York, Pennsylvania. *MMWR Morb Mortal Wkly Rep.* 1978;27:248–249.

46. Makheja A, Vanderhoek J, Martyn B. Inhibition of platelet aggregation and thromboxane synthesis by onion and garlic. *Lancet.* 1979;1:781.

47. Siegal RK. Ginseng abuse syndrome. *JAMA.* 1979;241:1614–1615.

48. Perrotta DM, Coody G, Culmo C. Adverse events associated with ephedrine-containing products: Texas, December 1993–September 1995. *JAMA.* 1996;276:1711–1712.

49. Knight TE, Hausen BM. Melaleuca oil (tea tree oil) dermatitis. *J Am Acad Dermatol.* 1994; 30:423–427.

50. Itami N, Yamamoto K, Andoh T, Akutsu Y. Herbal medicine can induce hypertension. *Nephron.* 1991;59:339–340.

51. Liu G. Pharmacological actions and clinical use of Fructus Shizandrae. *Chin Med J.* 1989; 102:740–749.

52. Eaton EA, Walle UK, Lewis AJ, Hudson T, Wilson AA, Walle T. Flavonoids, potent inhibitors of the human form phenolsulfotransferase: potential role in drug metabolism and chemoprevention. *Drug Metab Dispos.* 1996;24:232–237.

53. Schubert W, Eriksson U, Edgar B, Cullberg G, Hedner T. Flavonoids in grapefruit juice inhibit the in vitro hepatic metabolism of 17–beta-estradiol. *Eur J Drug Metab Pharmacokinet.* 1995;20:219–224.

54. Cassileth BR. The social implications for questionable cancer therapies. *Cancer.* 1989; 63:1247–1250.

55. Brevoort P. The US botanical market: an overview. *Herbal Gram.* 1996;36:49–57.

56. Houghton PJ. Valerian. *Pharm J.* 1994;253:95–96.

57. LeBars PL, Katz MM, Berman N, Itil TM, Freedman AM, Schatzberg AF. A placebo-controlled, double-blind randomized trial of an extract *Ginkgo biloba* for dementia. *JAMA.* 1997;278:1327–1332.

58. Gillis CN. Panax ginseng pharmacology: a nitric oxide link? *Biochem Pharmacol.* 1997;54:1–8.

59. Bach D, Schmitt M, Ebeling L. Phytopharmaceutical and synthetic agents in the treatment of benign prostatic hyperplasia (BPH). *Phytomedicine.* 1997;4:309–313.

60. Linde K, Ramirez G, Mulrow CD, Pauls A, Weidenhammer W, Melchart D. St John's wort for depression: an overview and meta-analysis of randomised clinical trials. *BMJ.* 1996; 313:253–258.

61. Bauer VR, Jurcic K, Puhlmann J, Wagner H. Immunologic in vivo and in vitro studies on Echinacea extracts. *Arzneimittelforschung.* 1988;38:276–281.

62. Mowrey DB, Clayson DE. Motion sickness, ginger, and psychophysics. *Lancet.* 1982; 1:655–657.

63. Stewart JJ, Wood MJ, Wood CD, Mims ME. Effects of ginger on motion sickness susceptibility and gastric function. *Pharmacology.* 1991; 42:111–120.

64. Knight DW. Feverfew: chemistry and biological activity. *Natl Prod Rep.* 1995;12:271–276.

65. Cavadas C, Araujo I, Cotrim MD, et al. In vitro study on the interaction of Valeriana officinalis L. extracts and their amino acids on GABA-A receptor in rat brain. *Arzneimittelforschung.* 1995;45:753–755.

66. Holzgartner H, Schmidt U, Kuhn U. Comparison of the efficacy and tolerance of a garlic preparation vs benzfibrate. *Arzneimittelforschung.* 1992;42:1473–1477.

67. Miller S. A natural mood booster. *Newsweek.* May 5, 1997:74–75.

68. Duran N, Song PS. Hypericin and its photodynamic action. *Photochem Photobiol.* 1986; 43:677–680.

69. Sultan C, Terraza A, Devillier C, et al. Inhibition of androgen metabolism and binding by a liposterolic extract of Serenoa repens B in human foreskin fibroblasts. *J Steroid Biochem Mol Biol.* 1984;20:515–519.

70. Kessler DA. Introducing MEDWATCH: a new approach to reporting medication and device adverse effects and product problems. *JAMA.* 11993;269:2765–2768.

32 Herbal Medicinals

Selected Clinical Considerations Focusing on Known or Potential Drug-Herb Interactions

Lucinda G. Miller, PharmD, BCPS
From the Department of Pharmacy Practice, Texas Tech University Health Sciences Center, Amarillo.

Herbal medicinals are being used by an increasing number of patients who typically do not advise their clinicians of concomitant use. Known or potential drug-herb interactions exist and should be screened for. If used beyond 8 weeks, *Echinacea* could cause hepatotoxicity and therefore should not be used with other known hepatoxic drugs, such as anabolic steroids, amiodarone, methotrexate, and ketoconazole. However, *Echinacea* lacks the 1,2 saturated necrine ring associated with hepatoxicity of pyrrolizidine alkaloids. Nonsteroidal anti-inflammatory drugs may negate the usefulness of feverfew in the treatment of migraine headaches. Feverfew, garlic, Ginkgo, ginger, and ginseng may alter bleeding time and should not be used concomitantly with warfarin sodium. Additionally, ginseng may cause headache, tremulousness, and manic episodes in patients treated with phenelzine sulfate. Ginseng should also not be used with estrogens or corticosteroids because of possible additive effects. Since the mechanism of action of St John wort is uncertain, concomitant use with monoamine oxidase inhibitors and selective serotonin reuptake inhibitors is ill advised. Valerian should not be used concomitantly with barbiturates because excessive sedation may occur. Kyushin, licorice, plantain, uzara root, hawthorn, and ginseng may interfere with either digoxin pharmacodynamically or with digoxin monitoring. Evening primrose oil and borage should not be used with anticonvulsants because they may lower the seizure threshold. Shankapulshpi, an Ayurvedic preparation, may decrease phenytoin levels as well as diminish drug efficacy. Kava when used with alprazolam has resulted in coma. Immunostimulants (eg, *Echinacea* and zinc) should not be given with immunosuppressants (eg, corticosteroids and cyclosporine). Tannic acids present in some herbs (eg, St John wort and saw palmetto) may inhibit the absorption of iron. Kelp as a source of iodine may interfere with thyroid replacement therapies. Licorice can offset the pharmacological effect of spironolactone. Numerous herbs (eg, karela and ginseng) may affect blood glucose levels and should not be used in patients with diabetes mellitus.

Arch Intern Med. 1998;158:2200–2211

The herbal market in the United States is experiencing unprecedented growth. Herbal medicinal sales increased nearly 59% in 1997.[1] In 1997, 60 million Americans stated that they had used herbs in the previous year, accounting for $3.24 billion in sales.[2] It has been noted that 70% of patients do not reveal their herbal use to their allopathic practitioners (ie, physicians and pharmacists).[3] Hence, not only is the potential for drug-herb interactions unmonitored but the concomitant use may not even be acknowledged. This phenomenon is fraught with peril and is the subject of this article.

It is paramount for clinicians to be aware of known or potential drug-herb interactions to adequately treat their patients. The selection criteria for this article were (1) relatively commonly used herbs and (2) herbs with known or potential drug-herb interactions. Frequently used herbs will be presented first, and their use with known efficacy studies with associated drug-herb interactions will be outlined. Second, drugs with narrow therapeutic margins and drugs with the known or potential drug-herb interactions with commonly used herbal medicinals will be reviewed in the context of concomitant use. With both of these approaches, most of the known or potential important drug-herb interactions will be addressed.

Commonly Used Herbal Medicinals and Associated Drug-Herb Interactions

Chamomile

Chamomile is used for its mild sedative effects but has also been noted to have antispasmodic and antiseptic activity.[4] In a study of its sedative effects, chamomile was effective in inducing a deep sleep in 10 (83%) of 12 recipients who were about to undergo cardiac catheterization.[5] Unfortunately, allergic reactions seem to commonly occur with symptoms that include abdominal cramps, tongue thickness, tight sensation in throat, angioedema of lips and eyes, diffuse pruritus, generalized urticaria, upper airway obstruction, and pharyngeal edema.[6,7] Many of these patients were also allergic to ragweed, which serves as an IgE marker for cross-allerginicity. Chamomile contains coumarin, which is reported to exert an antispasmodic effect.[8] However, this effect has not yet translated into any coagulation disorders despite its widespread human use. Because chamomile's effect on the coagulation system has not yet been studied, it is unknown if a clinically significant drug-herb interaction exists with known anticoagulants such as warfarin. If used concomitantly, close monitoring is advised.

Echinacea

Three kinds of *Echinacea* exist: *Echinacea angustifolia*, *Echinacea pallida*, and *Echinacea purpurea*. The Germans recommend using the above-ground parts of *E purpurea* (not the roots) or the roots of *E angustifolia*. In vitro stimulation of phagocytosis has been reported with *E purpurea* attributed to immunologically active polysaccharides; therefore, it is touted as an anti-infective via immunostimulation.[9–12] Symptoms of immunostimulation (eg, shivering, fever, and muscle weakness) ensue after parenteral administration but generally are not observed following oral administration in which the most common adverse effect is an unpleasant taste.[13] Purportedly, tachyphylaxis ensues if *Echinacea* mechanisms are used for more than 8 weeks although the mechanism of this phenomenon has not been determined.[14] Since hepatotoxic effects may be associated with persistent use, it should not be taken with other known hepatotoxic drugs (eg, anabolic steroids, amiodarone, methotrexate, or ketoconazole). However, the magnitude of this hepatoxicity has been questioned since *Echinacea* lacks the 1, 2 unsaturated necrine ring system associated with hepatoxicity of pyrrolizidine alkaloids.

Feverfew

Feverfew's most common use is for migraines. Seventeen patients who used feverfew daily as migraine prophylaxis enrolled in a double-blind, placebo-controlled trial in which 8 patients continued to receive feverfew while 9 received placebo.[15] Those who received placebo (ie, untreated patients) had a significant increase in the frequency and severity of headache (mean ± SEM, 3.13 ± 0.77 headaches every 6 months when taking placebo vs 1.69 ± 0.57 headache every 6 months when taking feverfew), nausea, and vomiting, whereas there was no change in the group receiving feverfew. In a larger study of 72 patients preceded by a 1-month single-blind, placebo run-in, feverfew was associated with a 24% reduction in the mean number and severity of attacks (3.6 attacks with feverfew vs 4.7 attacks with placebo over a 2-month period; $P<.005$) although the duration of the individual attacks was unaltered.[16] Feverfew has been shown to suppress 86% to 88% of prostaglandin production but does not inhibit cyclooxygenase.[17] Nonsteroidal anti-inflammatory drugs (NSAIDs) may reduce the effectiveness of feverfew perhaps mediated by its prostaglandin inhibition effects.[18] Feverfew is contraindicated to those allergic to other members of the family Compositae (Asteraceae) such as chamomile, ragweed, or yarrow.[17] Not all products contain an adequate amount (0.2%) of parthenolide, a possible component for activity, therefore this bears validation.[19] Postfeverfew syndrome involves nervousness, tension, headaches, insomnia, stiffness, joint pain, and tiredness.[20] Feverfew has been shown to inhibit platelet activity.[21,22] Hence, it is advised to avoid use of feverfew in patients receiving warfarin or other anticoagulants.

Garlic

Although touted by the herbal industry to possess various properties (including but not limited to antispasmodic, antiseptic, bacteriostatic, antiviral activities, as well as a promoter of leukocytosis), the most recent use of garlic (*Allium sativum*) has targeted its hypotensive and hypocholesterolemic activity.[23] Numerous animal studies have documented garlic's hypotensive effects, with a usual onset of action of 30 minutes.[24–26] However, this was not sustained for more than 2 hours in the rat model.[24–26] In a review of human experiments, Kleijnen et al[27] observed that studies were not well designed and suffered from small enrollments with no treatment groups including more than 25 patients. They noted that blinding of the studies was nearly impossible because of garlic's characteristic odor, which correlated with the sulfide component. Furthermore, the dosages needed were unacceptably high (at least 7 garlic cloves daily) and often were associated with adverse effects, such as gastrointestinal upset, allergic reactions, and dermatitis.[27,28] In a meta-analysis of 8 trials evaluating 415 subjects, 3 trials demonstrated a significant reduction in systolic blood pressure and 4 studies found a decrease in diastolic blood pressure.[29] While garlic may have some benefit in patients with mild hypertension, there is still insufficient evidence to recommend its routine use in clinical practice.

Garlic has also been studied for its possible use in hypercholesterolemia. In a study of 47 ambulatory patients, garlic powder administered for 12 weeks was found to decrease diastolic blood pressure from 102 to 91 mm Hg after 8 weeks ($P<.05$) and to 89 mm Hg after 12 weeks ($P<.01$) with concomitant decreases in serum cholesterol (14%; 6.93-6.18 mmol/L [268-239 mg/dL] at 8 weeks; $P<.05$) and triglyceride levels (18%; 1.93–0.45 mmol/L [171–40 mg/dL]; $P<.05$) (SDs not provided).[30] In a controlled trial and a meta-analysis of garlic use for patients with moderate hyperlipidemia, garlic's effects were modest at 300 mg, 3 times daily.[31] Garlic was associated with a mean reduction in total cholesterol concentration of 0.65 mmol/L. Hence, garlic's effectiveness for hypercholesterolemia can be expected to be even less than that associated with hypertension.

Nonetheless, adverse effects present a concern with the use of garlic. Its use is associated with inhibition of spermatogenesis in rats.[32] This inhibition is thought to be secondary to the reduction in cholesterol and trigcycleride levels, seemingly conflicting notions when considering the supposed lack of effectiveness of garlic for hyperlipidemia.[32] When used for hyperlipidemia in 308 patients, garlic was also associated with decreased platelet aggregation.[33] In a study of 6 healthy adults, decreased platelet aggregation was noted within 5 days of oral administration, theorized to be secondary to inhibition of epinephrine-induced in vitro platelet aggregation.[34] While these authors did not feel that the effect was of clinical significance, dysfunctional platelets have resulted in spontaneous spinal epidural hematoma in an 87-year-old man.[35] Furthermore, several practitioners have noted elevated international normalized ratios (INRs) and prothrombin times in patients previously stabilized while taking warfarin; therefore, extreme caution is advised if these preparations must be used concomitantly.

Ginger

Ginger (*Zingiber officinale*) has been used as an antinauseant and antispasmodic agent. It has been subjected to placebo-controlled trials. In one such study, 8 volunteers received 1 g of powdered ginger root and then 1 hour later, were put in a dark room with their heads placed supinely 30° forward.[36] Their vestibular system was then stimulated by irrigating the left ear for 40 seconds with water that was at 44°C with recording of provoked nystagmus via electronystagmography. Ginger root was found to reduce induced vertigo significantly better than placebo with no subjects experiencing nausea, whereas 3 patients administered placebo did experience nausea. In a study of 36 patients, ginger was compared with 100 mg of dimenhydrinate while patients were subjected to a motor-driven revolving chair designed to produce motion sickness.[37] None of the subjects receiving placebo or dimenhydrinate could stay in the chair for 6 minutes, whereas half of the patients receiving ginger stayed for the full time. Further study concluded that ginger exerts a gastric mechanism unlike dimenhydrinate, which has a central nervous system mechanism.[38] Sixty women were enrolled in a study of ginger, metoclopramide hydrochloride, and placebo effectiveness to treat postoperative nausea and vomiting after they had undergone major gynecological surgery.[39] Ginger and metoclopramide treatment were similarly significantly more efficacious than placebo. Ginger therapy has also been found effective in a study of 80 naval cadets unaccustomed to sailing in heavy seas who were subjected to voyages in high seas.[40] The cadets maintained symptom reports relating to kinetosis (ie, seasickness).[40] In keeping hourly scores for 4 consecutive hours following ingestion of either 1 g of ginger or placebo, use of ginger was found to be significantly ($P<.05$) better than placebo in reducing vomiting and cold sweating, as well as in reducing nausea and vertigo.[40] The onset of action was 25 minutes and the duration of action was 4 hours.[37] These successes have led some to investigate ginger's effectiveness in hyperemesis gravidarum. Powdered ginger root given to patients in daily 1-g doses was found to be significantly ($P=.035$) better than placebo treatment in diminishing or eliminating symptoms of hyperemesis gravidarum (relief score of 4.1 with ginger vs 0.9 for those receiving placebo).[41] However, enthusiasm for this indication has been tempered by the finding of possible mutagenesis in *Escherichia coli*.[42,43] Furthermore, ginger has been found to be a potent inhibitor of thromboxane synthetase, which prolongs bleeding time.[44] Obviously, this result has adverse implications for pregnant patients but also provides the basis for the recommendation to avoid concomitant use with warfarin if at all possible.

Ginkgo

Ginkgo biloba is one of the most popular plant extracts in Europe and has recently received approval in Germany for treatment of dementia.[45] *Ginkgo* is composed of several flavonoids, terpenoids (eg, ginkgolides), and organic acids believed to synergistically act as free radical scavengers.[46] Since excessive peroxidation and cell damage have been observed in Alzheimer disease, it is hoped that *Ginkgo* will prove effective.[47] In an intent-to-treat analysis of 2020 patients, *Ginkgo* was found to decrease the Alzheimer's Disease Assessment Scale-Cognitive subscale score 1.4 points better than the placebo group ($P=.04$) with a Geriatric Evaluation by Relative's Rating Instrument score of 0.14 points better as well ($P=.004$).[48] No significant difference in adverse effects was noted leading the investigators to conclude that *Ginkgo* was safe and capable of stabilizing and perhaps improving cognitive performance in patients with dementia and was of sufficient magnitude to be recognized by caregivers.

Ginkgo is considered relatively safe with few documented adverse effects, which seem to be limited to mild gastrointestinal upset and headache. However, spontaneous hyphema in a 70-year-old man taking a 40-mg tablet of concentrated *G biloba* extract has been reported.[49] Furthermore, spontaneous bilateral subdural hematomas have also occurred secondary to *Ginkgo* ingestion.[50] This condition has been attributed to ginkgolide B, a potent inhibitor of platelet-activating factor that is needed to induce arachidonate-independent platelet aggregation.[51] Hence, concomitant use with aspirin or any of the NSAIDs, as well as anticoagulants, such as warfarin and heparin, is ill advised. Of additional concern is the presence of *Ginkgo* toxin in both the *Ginkgo* leaf and seed, which is a known neurotoxin.[52] While the investigators concluded that the amount of toxin was too low to exert a detrimental effect, it would be prudent to avoid use in known epileptic patients because it may diminish the effectiveness of administered anticonvulsants (eg, carbamazepine, phenytoin, and phenobarbital). Additionally, concomitant use with medications known to decrease the seizure threshold, such as tricyclic antidepressants, would also be ill advised. It is encouraging that *Ginkgo* did not interact or adversely affect concomitant therapy with cardiac glycosides or hypoglycemic drugs in a study of 112 outpatients with cerebral insufficiency.[53]

Ginseng

Wide variation exists among ginseng products. Ginsenoside extraction methods have found *Panax quinquefolius* in American ginseng, *Panax ginseng* in Oriental ginseng, and *Panax pseudoginseng* var *notoginseng* in Sanchi ginseng.[54] Panax-type ginsenosides were not detected in Siberian ginseng that instead contains *Eleutherococcus senticosus*. This distinction is important since properties vary according to the specific product. For example, the eleutherosides have been associated with falsely elevated digoxin levels in the absence of digoxin toxic effects presumably because of an interaction with the digoxin assay.[55] The ginseng identity issue is further compounded by the finding of tremendous content variation in products labeled as containing ginseng.[56] Using a spectrodensitometer and thin-layer chromatographic assay to quantify the panoxide and saponin content, only 25% of the commercially available products actually contained ginseng.[56] Nevertheless, ginseng enjoys widespread popularity and has been touted as an adaptogen, perhaps augmenting adrenal steroidogenesis via the pituitary gland.[57] In contradiction to this hypothesis is the finding of immunomodulatory effects of ginseng in mice (as measured by IgG and IgM responses to either a primary or secondary challenge with sheep red blood cells) with stimulation of interferon production in vitro.[58] The immunomodulatory effect of ginseng was confirmed in a sheep erythrocyte study in mice in which cell-mediated immunity and natural killer cell activity were increased following administration of 10 mg/d per mouse for 4 days.[59] Additionally, ginseng has had favorable results in a double-blind, placebo-controlled study of 36 newly diagnosed patients with type 2 diabetes.[60] A 200-mg dose improved the subjective ratings of mood, vigor, and well-being, which was associated with increased physical activity and reduced weight. A lower fasting blood glucose level was also associated with ginseng treatment but not with placebo (mean ± SEM, 7.4 mmol/L ± 1.1 and 8.3 mmol/L ± 1.3, respectively). The hypoglycemic effects have been attributed to ginsenoside Rb2 and more specifically to panaxans I, J, K, and L.[61–65] Certainly more studies are warranted regarding ginseng's use in the population with diabetes.

Ginseng's adverse effect profile includes hypertension, insomnia, vomiting, headache, and epistaxis.[66,67] Stevens-Johnson syndrome was noted in a 27-year-old law student from China following use of 2 tablets (unspecified milligram amount) of ginseng for 3 days, resulting in moderate infiltration of the dermis by mononuclear cells.[68] Oral administration of 200 mg of ginseng for an unspecified time to a 72-year-old woman resulted in vaginal bleeding attributed to a moderate estrogen effect.[69] Vaginal bleeding has also been reported following use of ginseng face cream for 1 month when an endometrial biopsy specimen demonstrated a disordered proliferative pattern.[70] Mastalgia with diffuse breast nodularity has been reported in a 70-year-old woman after 3 weeks of use of a ginseng powder; her condition resolved after she discontinued using ginseng.[71] Neonatal androgenization secondary to ginseng has been debated in the literature in cases in which maternal use of ginseng was identified as the cause of androgenization of the child.[72,73] However, others contend the entity in question was in fact a botanically distinct species, Siberian ginseng, that when studied in rats at equivalent doses is not associated with androgenicity.[74] Given the wide variety of ginseng products available, it would be prudent to avoid the use of ginseng during pregnancy until the issue is adequately resolved.

Drug interactions have been noted with the use of ginseng. A 47-year-old man with a St Jude-type mechanical heart valve in the aortic position had been stabilized while receiving warfarin for 5 years but became destabilized following administration of ginseng.[75] The patient's INR decreased to 1.5 after 2 weeks of ginseng, which had been preceded by an INR of 3.1. Following the discontinuation of ginseng therapy, the INR returned to 3.3 within 2 weeks. The mechanism underlying this drug-herb interaction is unknown but may be related to the antiplatelet components in *P ginseng*.[76] Concomitant use with warfarin, heparin, aspirin, and NSAIDs should be avoided. Several case reports have documented headache, tremulousness, and manic episodes in patients treated with phenelzine when they started a regimen of ginseng.[77,78] Central nervous system stimulant activity has been observed in a 2-year study of 133 ginseng users in which nervousness and sleeplessness were noted.[79] The author of that study likens this ginseng effect to that of corticosteroid toxic effects, suggesting a steroid mechanism of action for ginseng. As a consequence, it would be wise to avoid use of ginseng in patients with manic-depressive disorders and psychosis. Additionally, ginseng may augment corticosteroid toxic effects in predisposed patients. However, ginseng's effect on blood glucose levels may not be congruent with that expected of corticosteroids (ie, hyperglycemia).

Saw Palmetto

While touted for its use as a diuretic, urinary antiseptic, and for its anabolic properties, the most common use for saw palmetto is for benign prostatic hypertrophy. The hexane extract of saw palmetto has been identified as the active ingredient with predominantly antiandrogenic activity and in vivo estrogenic activity demonstrated in rats.[80] Saw palmetto has also been shown to inhibit both dihydrotestosterone binding at the androgen receptors and 5-α-reductase activity on testosterone, both being mechanisms thought to be influential in the management of benign prostatic hypertrophy.[81] In 2 double-blind trials both objective (eg, frequency of nocturia and urine flow rate) and subjective (eg, dysuria intensity and patient's self-rating) data indicated significant (P<.01) improvement when saw palmetto (320 mg/d) was compared with placebo.[82,83] For example, the flow rate was mean ± SEM, 5.35 ± 1.51 mL/s before treatment and was 8.05 ± 2.47 mL/s after treatment (50.5% improvement; P<.001).[82] In a 3-year trial of 309 patients, saw palmetto increased urinary flow rate to 6.1 mL/s with a 50% decrease in residual urine volume vs finasteride that demonstrated a 30% decrease in symptom scores over 3 years, with only a slight improvement in urine flow and no change in residual volume.[84] A comparative study evaluating saw palmetto, doxazosin or terazosin (α_1-adrenergic blocking agent), finasteride (a 5-α-reductase inhibitor), and flutamide (an antiandrogen) in the treatment of benign prostatic hypertrophy is needed.

Adverse effects appear minimal and are characterized mostly by gastrointestinal upset.[83] While no drug-herb interactions have been documented to date, it would be prudent to avoid concomitant use with other hormonal therapies (eg, estrogen replacement therapy and oral contraceptives), which may provide an additive effect.

St John Wort

Hypericum perforatum is commonly referred to as St John wort. It is licensed in Germany for the treatment of anxiety, depression, and sleep disorders, with more than 2.7 million prescriptions written for it in 1993 (the seventh most popular preparation in Germany).[85] St John wort contains at least 10 constituents or groups of components that may contribute to its pharmacological effects, including naphthodianthroms, flavonoids, xanthose, and bioflavonoids.[86] Therefore, standardizing the product according to its *Hypericum* content confers no guarantee of the pharmacological equivalence of products. Hence, the usual dose has been touted as being 2 to 4 g of herb, equating this measurement with 0.2 to 1.0 mg of total hypericin, which is a questionable conversion. The mechanism of action is uncertain and has been purportedly characterized as a monoamine oxidase inhibitor (MAOI) (quercitrin content) or a selective serotonin reuptake inhibitor.[87] However, MAOI properties of *Hypericum* extracts have not been confirmed and may not be of a magnitude to be clinically significant; therefore, it may not be necessary to avoid concomitant use with tyramine-containing foods (eg, Swiss cheese, Chianti, or sauerkraut).[88] The Office of Alternative Medicine of the National Institutes of Health is now undertaking a study to define its characteristics and effectiveness. However, in a meta-analysis of randomized clinical trials enrolling 1757 patients, *Hypericum* extracts were found to be significantly superior to placebo (22.3% responded to placebo, compared with 55.1% to St John wort) and were similarly effective as standard antidepressants with fewer adverse effects (20% vs 53%, with standard antidepressants such as amitriptyline, or imipramine hydrochloride).[89]

The most prominent adverse effect associated with St John wort is photosensitivity attributed to its hypericin component.[90] Hence, fair-skinned individuals should be particularly cautious. Concomitant use with other known photosensitizers, such as piroxicam or tetracycline hydrochloride, should be avoided. Until the MAOI status of St John wort has been defined, it would also be prudent to avoid concomitant use with known MAOIs, such as phenelzine or with betasympathomimetic amines (eg, ma huang or pseudoephedrine hydrochloride). Similarly, symptoms of serotonism (eg, headache, sweating, dizziness, and agitation) may be encountered if used concomitantly with selective serotonin reuptake inhibitors (eg, fluoxetine and paroxetine) if St John wort is found to have selective serotonin reuptake inhibitor effects as well.

Valerian

In a study of 8 volunteers with mild insomnia, an aqueous extract of 450 or 900 mg of valerian was compared with placebo in a double-blind, repeated-measures, random study.[91] A significant decrease in sleep latency was noted with 450 mg of valerian compared with placebo (mean ± SEM, 15.8 ± 2.2 minutes vs 9.0 ± 1.5 minutes; $P<.01$).[91] The higher dose of valerian (900 mg) was not associated with any further improvement in sleep latency.[91] These findings concur with another study of 128 patients that notes not only significantly decreased sleep latency but also that patients felt sleepier waking in the morning.[92] Valerian has not been noted to change sleep stages or electroencephalographic spectra and has been characterized as a mild hypnotic substance.[93] Purportedly, valerian does not interact with alcohol but this finding has been disputed, leading some to warn against its use with alcohol.[94] Furthermore, valerian has been shown to prolong thiopental- and pentobarbital-induced sleep.[55,95,96] Hence, valerian should not be used with barbiturates.

Allopathic Medications and Associated Drug-Herb Interactions

The first drugs to be addressed will be those with a narrow therapeutic window. Given their toxicities and the potential adverse sequelae if blood levels fall outside the therapeutic range, those drugs can be quickly and acutely affected by concomitant herbal therapies. A summary of herb-drug interactions affecting commonly used drugs is provided in Table 1.

Drugs With A Narrow Therapeutic Window

Digoxin

Numerous herbs containing cardiac glycosides have been identified as containing digoxinlike substances. These include *Adonis vernalis* (adonis, false hellebore, pheasant's eye), *Apocynum androsaemifolium* (dogbane, milkweed, and wild ipecac), *Apocynum cannabinum* (dogbane, milkweed, and wild ipecac), *Asclepias tuberosa* (pleurisy root), *Convallaria majalis* (lily of the valley), *Cystisus scoparius* (broom), *Digitalis lanata* (yellow foxglove), and *Digitalis purpurea* (purple foxglove). Other herbal medicinals include *Eleutherococcus senticosus*

Table 1. Summary of Drug-Herb Interactions of Commonly Used Drugs

Drug	Interaction
Alprazolam	Excessive sedation may result if used concomitantly with kava
Corticosteroids	The immunostimulating effects of *Echinacea, Astragalus,* licorice, alfalfa sprouts, vitamin E, and zinc may offset the immunosuppressive effects of corticosteroids
Cyclosporine	The immunostimulating effects of *Echinacea, Astragalus,* licorice, alfalfa sprouts, vitamin E, and zinc may offset the immunosuppressive effects of cyclosporine
Digoxin	Additive effects possible with herbs containing cardiac glycosides; hawthorn purportedly potentiates digoxin; licorice may cause hypokalemia, hence predisposing the patient to digoxin's toxic effects; plantain may be adulterated with foxglove, hence elevating digoxin blood levels; Siberian ginseng and kyushin may interfere with digoxin assays; uzara root may exert additive digoxin-type cardiac effects
Diuretics	Sodium-sparing herbal aquaretics (eg, dandelion, uva-ursi) may offset antihypertensive effects of diuretics (eg, hydrochlorothiazide and furosemide); gossypol may exacerbate hypokalemia secondary to diuretics (eg, hydrochlorothiazide and furosemide)
Hypoglycemics (eg, sulfonylureas)	Chromium may decrease insulin requirements; karela has been shown to decrease dosage requirements for chlorpropamide
Iron	Tannin-containing herbs (eg, chamomile, feverfew, St John wort) may interact with iron, hence inhibiting iron absorption
Levothyroxine	Horseradish and kelp may suppress thyroid function, complicating thyroid function
Nonsteroidal anti-inflammatory drugs	Additive gastrointestinal irritation may be encountered with herbs known to irritate the gastrointestinal tract (eg, gossypol and uva-ursi)
Phenelzine (and other MAO* inhibitors)	Concomitant use with ginseng, yohimbine, and *Ephedra* may result in insomnia, headache, and tremulousness; St John wort and licorice may have MAO inhibitor activity and should not be used concomitantly with known MAO inhibitors
Phenobarbital	Thujone-containing herbs (eg, wormwood and sage) may lower seizure threshold, hence increasing anticonvulsant dosage requirements; gamolenic acid–containing herbs (eg, evening primrose oil and borage) lower seizure thresholds and may increase anticonvulsant dosage requirements.
Phenytoin	Same as for phenobarbital plus Shankhapulshpi may shorten the half-life and diminish effectiveness of phenytoin
Spironolactone	Licorice may offset the effects of spironolactone
Warfarin	Garlic, ginger, *Ginkgo,* and feverfew may augment the anticoagulant effect of warfarin; ginseng may decrease the effectiveness of warfarin

*MAO indicates monoamine oxidase.

(Siberian ginseng), kyushin (Chinese medicine), *Leonurus cardiaca* (motherwort), *Scilla maritima* (white squill), *Scrophularia nodosa* (figwort), *Strophantus kombe* (strophanthus), and *Uzarae radix* (uzara root). Reports have documented the various problems encountered with these entities. Various lots of plantain (used as an herbal laxative) have been adulterated with potentially toxic woolly foxglove resulting in a Food and Drug Administration advisory.[97,98] Foxglove was included in a product called Chomper, of the Cleanse Thyself line, Aris and Shine Company, Mount Shasta, Calif. While the company voluntarily recalled suspected batches, the Food and Drug Administration did report that 1 young woman had an abnormal heart rate with heartblock. Similarly, patients who present with ventricular tachycardia, unifocal and multiform premature ventricular contractions, and atrioventricular dissociation suggestive of digoxin toxic effects but who have not ingested digoxin should be asked if they have taken plantain. This incident speaks to the lack of good manufacturing practices of some herbal medicinal companies.

Licorice has been advocated for gastrointestinal complaints, particularly peptic ulcer disease.[99] However, in 1 case it was associated with pseudoaldosteronism that resulted in hypertension but both the pseudoaldosteronism and the hypertension resolved 2 weeks after the patient stopped using licorice.[100,101] Its active component has been identified as glycyrrhizic acid, known to inhibit 11-β-hydroxysteroid dehydrogenase and should be included in a differential diagnosis of factitious mineralocorticoid excess.[102–104] Licorice's mineralocorticoid effects can be offset with the use of spironolactone.[105] Potassium loss has been associated with the use of licorice with chronic ingestion resulting in acute flaccid tetraparesis and hypokalemia.[106] In this case, a 35-year-old man ingested 20 to 40 g/d of licorice tablets for 2 years, developing acute myopathy and complete paralysis of the proximal muscles of his arms and shoulder girdles, weakness of the muscles of his forearms and hands, weakness of his proximal leg muscles, and moderate weakness of his posterior and anterior neck muscles along with a serum potassium level of 2.1 mmol/L. With potassium repletion and discontinuation of the licorice regimen, the paralysis completely resolved within 3 days. However, an accelerated loss of potassium may result in increased sensitivity to digoxin treatment.

A Chinese medicine containing kyushin has been documented to cross-react with digoxin assays. A patient taking digoxin, 0.25 mg/d, for congestive heart failure had a serum digoxin level of 2.5 mmol/L with no symptoms of digoxin intoxication.[107] Kyushin contains chan su, the dried venom of the Chinese toad *Bufo bufo gargarizans cantor,* which purportedly has digoxinlike actions.[108] It was determined that 1 tablet of kyushin had digoxinlike immunoreactivity equivalent to 1.9 µg (TDX analyzer, Abbott Laboratories, North Chicago, Ill) and 72 µg of digoxin (Enymun-Test, Boehringer, Mannheim, Germany). Thus, patients with spuriously elevated digoxin levels without associated signs and symptoms of digoxin toxicity should be approached cautiously and questioned regarding herbal therapies.

Additional entities may also interfere with digoxin activity and monitoring. *Uzarae radix* (uzara root) in large doses has been found to have digoxin-type cardiac effects so that additive effects may be encountered.[109] Ginseng may falsely elevate digoxin levels.[9] (Hawthorn berries purportedly potentiate the action of digoxin.[110] No clinical studies have validated this assertion. Animal studies suggest hawthorn may possess β-blocking activities; however, others contend that hawthorn's cardiac effects may be secondary to angiotensin-converting enzyme inhibitor properties.[111]

Phenobarbital

Several herbal medicinals may lower the seizure threshold, thus offsetting beneficial effects from known anticonvulsants such as phenobarbital. Such herbs may contain thujone. Thujones are apparently present in wormwood (used as an appetite stimulant and for intestinal spasmodic disorders) and sage (used to treat flatulent dyspepsia, gingivitis, stomatitis, and galactorrhea).[112] The mechanism of this proconvulsant effect is unknown. However, it would be prudent to avoid concomitant use with anticonvulsants and with drugs known to lower the seizure threshold (eg, tricyclic antidepressants).

Evening primrose oil contains gamolenic acid (GLA) that lowers the seizure threshold.[113] Recently, evening primrose oil has gained popularity as a remedy for premenstrual syndrome, which purportedly has been associated with low GLA levels.[113] Evening primrose oil is touted as a good source of GLA. Evening primrose oil has also been used for diabetic neuropathy (with a purported reduced ability to desaturate essential fatty acids with resulting deficits in neuronal membrane structure), multiple sclerosis (although results have been contradictory), Sjögren syndrome (a feature of essential fatty acid deficiency is exocrine gland atrophy typical of Sjögren) and attention deficit/hyperactivity disorder.[113] Hyperactive children supposedly have abnormal levels of essential fatty acid; however, no improvements in behavioral patterns were noted in one trial with evening primrose oil.[114] Similarly, starflower (borage) has also been touted as a source of GLA. Borage is used herbally as a diaphoretic, expectorant, anti-inflammatory, and galactogogue.[115] It has been used for fevers, coughs, and depression and is reputed to act as a restorative agent on the adrenal cortex.[116] Borage oil is used as an alternative source to evening primrose oil for GLA. In human studies, it was found to attenuate cardiovascular reactivity to stress induced by a reduction in systolic blood pressure and heart rate and increased task performance although the underlying mechanism of action is unknown.[117] However, borage does contain low concentrations of unsaturated pyrrolizidine alkaloids known to cause hepatotoxic effects (eg, comfrey).[118] Therefore, do not use borage with other hepatotoxic drugs, such as anabolic steroids, phenothiazines, or ketoconazole. Neither evening primrose oil nor borage should be used concomitantly with other drugs known to lower the seizure threshold (eg, tricyclic antidepressants and phenothiazines).

Phenytoin

The effectiveness of phenytoin has been adversely affected by Shankhapulshpi, an Ayurvedic preparation for epilepsy that contains[119] *Convolvulus pluricaulis* (chois), the leaves, *Centella asiatica* (urban), the whole plant, *Nardostachys jatamansi* (DC), rhizome, *Nepeta hinostana* (haines), the whole plant, *Nepeta elliptica* (Royle), the whole plant, and *Onosma bracteatum* (wall), the leaves and flowers.

After observing 2 patients experience loss of seizure control, investigators evaluated the effect of Shankhapulshpi on phenytoin.[120] They found with multidose administration of Shankhapulshpi (1 teaspoonful 3 times per day), the antiepileptic activity of phenytoin as well as the plasma levels were decreased. Phenytoin levels decreased from 9.62 ± 2.93 µmol/L when administered alone to 5.10 ± 0.67 µmol/L when coadministered with Shankhapulshpi (P<.01). Additionally, coadministration of Shankhapulshpi resulted in diminution of phenytoin's antiepileptic effectiveness measured using maximal electroshock seizure induced by administering a 150-mA current for 0.2 seconds to animals (abolition of tonic hind limb extension was interpreted as protection from maximal electroshock seizure, reflecting antiepileptic activity).[120] Thus, loss of seizure control with no changes in phenytoin dosing or pharmacokinetics should compel the clinician to explore the possibility of the patient self-administering this Ayurvedic preparation. Additionally, as with phenobarbital, thujone, evening primrose oil, and starflower may exert similar deleterious effects as outlined earlier with phenobarbital.

Warfarin

Warfarin is an anticoagulant with a narrow therapeutic window with potentially fatal consequences if either bleeding complications arise or if subtherapeutic levels occur, thus not protecting the patient from thromboembolic events. Several herbs may interact with warfarin. As previously discussed, ginseng may decrease the effectiveness of warfarin. A 47-year-old man with a St Jude-type mechanical heart valve had received warfarin therapy for 5 years with a therapeutic INR 4 weeks before he started taking ginseng. Within 2 weeks, his INR declined to 1.5 but returned to 3.3 within 2 weeks of discontinuing the ginseng regimen.[75] Fortunately, no thrombotic events occurred during this subtherapeutic period, but this result certainly highlights the potential lethality of this drug-herb interaction. Conversely, dan-shen (*Salvia miltiorrhiza*), a Chinese folk medicine remedy, has been noted to significantly increase maximum concentration (C_{max}) (mean ± SD, 5500 ± 1636 ng/mL to 10,976 ± 3.975; P=.01) and time as maximum concentration (T_{max}) (mean ± SD, 3.6 ± 0.8 hours to 7.2 ± 1.7 hours; P=.001) and decrease the volume of distribution (142.5 ± 75.20 to 54.5 ± 18.9 mL; P<.005) and elimination half-life (31.8 ± 6.4 to 16 ± 2.6 hours; P=.001) of warfarin.[121] Because of its coumarin constituents, excessive use is not recommended with known anticoagulants such as warfarin.[122] Herbs that may interfere with warfarin treatment include arnica, celery, chamomile, dan-shen, dong quai, fenugreek, feverfew, garlic, ginger, *Ginkgo,* and ginseng.

When used for hyperlipidemia for 308 patients, garlic was also associated with decreased platelet aggregation.[33] In a study of 6 healthy adults, decreased platelet aggregation was noted within 5 days of oral administration theorized to be secondary to inhibition of epinephrine-induced in vitro platelet activity.[34] While these authors did not feel the effect was of clinical significance, dysfunctional platelets have been implicated in spontaneous spinal epidural hematoma in an 87-year-old man who ingested 4 cloves of garlic daily (approximately 2000 mg) for an unspecified time.[35] Caution is advised if these preparations must be used concomitantly.

Ginger has been found to be a potent inhibitor of thromboxane synthetase with potential effects on bleeding time.[44] While not quantified and fully characterized, it is an effect that could become clinically significant if used long-term. This mechanism theoretically could cause excess bleeding if used concomitantly with warfarin. Caution is advised.

Feverfew may also inhibit platelet activity via neutralization of sulfydryl groups that may cause an increase in bleeding time and an associated increase in bleeding tendencies.[21] A dose-dependent and irreversible inhibition of eiconsanoid generation has been demonstrated when levels range from 5 to 50 µg/mL.[123,124] However, others contend that this platelet effect is of no clinical consequence and that platelets of all patients whether presently taking feverfew or having discontinued its use for 6 months have normal characteristic responses to adenosine diphosphate.[125] Therefore, until this potential drug-herb interaction is further defined, concomitant use with warfarin should be avoided.

Concomitant use of warfarin and *Ginkgo* is not recommended. Spontaneous bilateral subdural hematomas have occurred secondary to *Ginkgo* ingestion.[50] These hematomas have been attributed to ginkgolide B, a potent inhibitor of platelet-activating factor that is needed to induce arachidonate-independent platelet aggregation.[51] Hence, concomitant use with aspirin or any of the NSAIDs as well as anticoagulants such as warfarin and heparin are ill advised.

Additional Drugs With Known or Potential Drug-Herb Interactions With Commonly Used Herbal Medicinals

Alprazolam

Kava is used as a sedative to enhance sleep. Long-term use is not advised because tolerance has been shown to develop rapidly in animals.[126] Additionally, long-term use has led to *kawaism,* which is characterized by dry, flaking, discolored skin and reddened eyes.[127,128] The toxicity of kava is increased if taken with alcohol.[129]

α-Pyrone, the active component of kava, has been found to have weak effects on γ-aminobutyric acid and benzodiazepine receptors in vitro, although this has been disputed.[130–132] Synergism between α-pyrones and other actve sedatives with γ-aminobutyric acid was verified in 1994 by a German study group.[133] However, concomitant use with benzodiazepines is ill advised based on a case of coma following concomitant use. A 54-year-old man was hospitalized in a lethargic and disoriented state.[134] His medications included alprazolam, cimetidine, and terazosin hydrochloride; his alcohol levels were negative and his drug screen was positive for benzodiazepines. He became more alert after several hours and stated that he had been taking kava for 3 days; he denied overdosing on kava or alprazolam.[134] The kava–alprazolam drug interaction was identified as the cause.

Corticosteroids and Cyclosporine

The theoretical concern underlying this drug-herb interaction is that immunostimulating herbs will offset or minimize the immunosuppressive effects of corticosteroids and cyclosporine. *Echinacea* is classified as an *immunotonic* agent because of its ability to augment basophils, mast cells, and white blood cell counts.[134,135] *Astragalus* stimulates T-cell activity and ginseng is thought to nourish major immune system glands but in an unspecified manner.[136] Licorice root supposedly stimulates interferon production and pau d'arco with its antioxidant and anti-inflammatory activity has been recommended for use by herbalists for immunodeficiencies.[137,138] Alfalfa sprouts and some vitamin E products contain toxic amino acid L-canavanine that has been implicated in cases of systemic lupus erythematosus and other autoimmune diseases.[139]

Zinc

Zinc gluconate lozenges have been found useful in treating the common cold. In a randomized, double-blind, placebo-controlled study, time to complete resolution of symptoms was significantly shorter in the patients treated with zinc than the placebo group (median, 4.4 days compared with 7.6 days; $P<.001$). Patients treated with zinc had significantly fewer days with coughing (median, 2.0 days compared with 4.5 days; $P=.04$) and headache, (2.0 days compared with 3.0 days; $P=.02$) but were not significantly different in resolution of fever, muscle ache, scratchy throat, or sneezing.[140] Twenty percent of patients experienced nausea and 80% had a bad-taste reaction.[140]

Mechanisms of action have yet to be determined but in vitro studies suggest that zinc may induce interferon production.[141] Other proposed zinc mechanisms include the ability of zinc to prevent formation of viral capsid protein thereby inhibiting in vitro replication of several viruses including rhinovirus.[142,143] This immunostimulating effect may be in opposition to immunosuppressive effects desired with the use of corticosteroids and/or cyclosporine. Therefore, zinc and other immunostimulating herbs should be avoided in autoimmune disorders (eg, rheumatoid arthritis and systemic lupus erythematosus) and in cases in which patients are using immunosuppressive therapies (eg, corticosteroids and cyclosporine) to avoid competing effects on the immune system.

Diuretics

Goldenseal is an aquaretic, but is referred to by most herbalists as a diuretic.[144] Other herbal diuretics include agrimony, artichoke, boldus, broom, buchu, burdock, celery seed, zea, coughgrass, dandelion, elder, guaiacum, juniper, pokeroot, shepherd's purse, squill, uva-ursi, and yarrow.[145] The differentiation between a diuretic and an aquaretic is of clinical significance because with diuretics, sodium is excreted with the water whereas with aquaretics, sodium is not excreted. Therefore, aquaretics are not well suited for the treatment of edema and hypertension and may in fact worsen it. If taken with a diuretic (eg, hydrochlorothiazide) or any allopathic antihypertensive drug, it is conceivable that the antihypertensive effects will be diminished or offset as sodium is retained.

Gossypol

Gossypol inhibits lactate dehydrogenase X found in sperm and male gonadal cells, hence exerting contraceptive activity.[146] It has also been found to inhibit implantation and maintenance of a healthy pregnancy by adversely affecting luteinizing hormone levels and so has been studied in female fertility control.[147] However, it has been associated with renal loss of potassium resulting in hypokalemia.[146] Furthermore, this potassium loss cannot be reversed with potassium supplementation or with the use of the potassium blocker triamterene.[148] Hence, concomitant use with allopathic drugs known to promote potassium loss (eg, hydrochlorothiazide and furosemide) should be avoided. Additionally, use with digoxin whose effects are potentiated in hypokalemia should be avoided as well.

Iron/Tannin Complex With Iron-Inhibiting Iron Absorption
Tannin-containing herbs include chamomile, plantain, black cohosh, saw palmetto, feverfew, St John wort, hawthorn, valerian, nettle, and gossypol.[149]

The tannins complex has iron-inhibiting absorption.[149] While the interaction between iron and tannins has not yet been clinically observed, it is of sufficient concern to merit caution when the 2 components are used together. If a patient is not responding adequately to iron therapy, the clinician should inquire regarding concomitant use of herbal medicinals as described earlier.

Levothyroxine
Horseradish is used herbally as an antiseptic with circulatory and digestive stimulation effects and as a diuretic.[150] Traditionally, it has been used for pulmonary and urinary tract infections, urinary stones, and edematous conditions; it has been used externally for application to inflamed joints or tissues.[150] However, it may depress thyroid function and should not be used with levothyroxine or other thyroid replacements.[150] Patients with aberrant thyroid function tests should be questioned regarding herbal use of horseradish.

Kelp
Kelp diets promoted for weight loss have caused myxedema in patients sensitive to iodide and, unfortunately, neither baseline serum triidothyronine and thyroxine concentrations nor the degree of serum iodide elevations were of prognostic value in predicting which patients would develop myxedema.[151] Kelp contains 0.7 mg of iodine per tablet and may result in hyperthyroidism after 6 months of use as demonstrated in a 72-year-old woman who ingested a commercially available kelp product.[152] Her hyperthyroidism resolved 6 months after she discontinued using the product. Therefore, concomitant use of kelp with levothyroxine or other thyroid replacements may result in hyperthyroidism. Additionally, concomitant use with known stimulants (eg, amphetamines, methylphenidate, or ma huang) could be dangerous.

Nonsteroidal Anti-inflammatory Drugs
The NSAIDS should not be used with herbal medicinals that are known to cause gastrointestinal damage. Gossypol has been associated with tissue congestion, mucosal sloughing, mucosal necrosis, and ileus and intestinal wall hemorrhage.[153] Other gastric irritants include *Arctostaphylos uva-ursi, Ruta graveolens, Cetraria islandica, Sanguinaria canadensis, Chamaelirium luteum, Schinus terebinthifolia, Coffea arabica, Schinus molle, Cola acuminata, Symplocarpus foetidus, Cola nitida, Trillium erectum,* and *Quillaja saponaria*.[154,155]

Hence, a patient complaining of unexpected gastrointestinal upset should be questioned regarding herbal medicinal use and concomitant use with known gastrointestinal irritants, such as NSAIDs, should be avoided.

Phenelzine and Other MAOIs
The effect of phenelzine and other MAOIs may be potentiated by numerous herbal medicinals. *Panax ginseng* is one such agent. A 64-year-old woman treated with phenelzine developed insomnia, headache, and tremulousness following the addition of ginseng (Natrol High ginseng tea).[156] In the second case, a 42-year-old woman whose major depressive illness was being treated with phenelzine experienced headaches, irritability, and vague visual hallucinations with concomitant use of ginseng.[157] Yohimbine and ma huang (*Ephedra*) may be implicated as well. St John wort was once purported to have MAOI activity and thus should not be used with other MAOIs, but more recent data call into question the clinical significance of its MAOI activity.[88,158] Licorice (*Glycyrrhiza glabra*) may also adversely interact with MAOIs. Glycyrrhizin is 10 times more active as an MAOI as hypericin and has been identified as containing isoliquiritigenin, glycoumarin, licochalcone A, licochalcone B, and (-)-medicarpin (MAOIs).[159] So, while it is relatively common to advise patients of dietary precautions when taking MAOIs, counseling regarding herbal medicinals should be included as well.

Spironolactone
Licorice may offset spironolactone's effects. Licorice is advocated as an antispasmodic and anti-inflammatory herb for use in gastritis and peptic ulcer disease. The hemisuccinate derivative of glycyrrhetainic acid, a component of licorice, is carbenoxolone, which is used allopathically for duodenal and gastric ulcers.[160] Licorice renders the patient unable to convert 11-deoxycortisol or deoxycorticosterone into the active glucocorticoids, cortisol, and corticosterone, respectively.[161] This acquired 11-β-hydroxylase deficiency results in sodium retention, hypertension, and hypokalemia.[161] Within 10 days to 3 weeks of the discontinuation of the licorice regimen, the blood pressure will return to baseline.[100,162,163] Given the underlying mechanism of licorice's effect on hypertension, spironolactone's antihypertensive effects may be diminished by licorice. Conversely, hypertension caused by licorice may be effectively treated with spironolactone.

Hypoglycemics

Numerous herbal medicinals have been shown to affect blood glucose levels including chromium, fenugreek, garlic, ginger, ginseng, *Gymnema sylvestre,* nettle, and sage for patients with hypoglycemia and devil's claw, ginseng, licorice, and ma huang for patients with hyperglycemia. Karela (*Momordica charantia*) has been shown to improve glucose tolerance.[164,165] When taken in conjunction with chlorpropamide, the dose of the latter needed to be reduced, although this report specified neither the starting or adjusted final dose.[166] Some claim chromium increases insulin activity and reduces the amount of insulin required to control blood glucose.[167] However, in a prospective, double-blind, placebo-controlled, cross-over study of 28 patients receiving chromium picolinate, 200 mg/d, or placebo for 2 months, no statistically significant difference (P>.05) was noted in blood glucose control.[168] Ginseng, whose activity has been attributed to 2% to 3% ginsenosides has been associated with hyperglycemic properties as well.[63] There have been no reports of ginseng-induced hypoglycemic or hyperglycemic incidents in humans to date reported in the literature. The use of these herbal medicinals in patients with diabetes, especially those with brittle diabetes, should be avoided.

Estrogen Replacement Therapy

Theoretically, concomitant use of phytoestrogens with estrogen replacement may result in symptoms of estrogen excess such as nausea, bloating, hypotension, breast fullness or tenderness, migraine headache, and edema. Phytoestrogens are naturally occurring plant or food substances that are functionally similar to estradiol.[169] While more than 500 plant species contain phytoestrogens, the more common herbs include dong quai, red clover, alfalfa, licorice, black cohosh, and soybeans.[170,171] To date, no incidents of estrogen excess have been reported following concomitant use, but prudence would dictate avoiding simultaneous use if at all possible.

Comment

Standardization and monitoring for adulteration is needed to limit the present problem of wide interproduct and intraproduct (lot-to-lot) variation in composition of active constituents. Clearly, more scientifically based studies evaluating efficacy and safety issues on the use of herbal medicinals are needed. Such studies will no doubt prove to be a double-edged sword in which some herbal medicinals will fall into disfavor while others will provide the basis for new and effective drugs. Additionally, studies directed at drug-herb interactions would serve public safety. Perhaps a request for proposals from the Office of Alternative Medicine funded by the National Institutes of Health would be appropriate to promote such an agenda. However, since such studies are lacking, it is hoped that this overview of known and potential drug-herb interactions in the context of known efficacy studies of selected herbal medicinals will serve to alert the clinician to their possibility in his or her practice. Because 33% of American patients are taking herbal medicinals, clinicians should include them in their routine drug histories.[2]

References

1. Richman A, Witkowski J. Herbs by the numbers. *Whole Foods Magazine.* 1997:20, 22, 24, 26, 28.
2. Johnston BA. One-third of nation's adults use herbal remedies. *Herbalgram.* 1997;40:49.
3. Eisenberg DM, Kessler RC, Foster C, Norlock FE, Calkins DR, Delbanco TL. Unconventional medicine in the United States: prevalence, costs, and patterns of use. *N Engl J Med.* 1993; 328:246–252.
4. Newall CA, Anderson LA, Phillipson JD. Chamomile monograph. In: Newall CA, Anderson LA, Phillipson JD, eds. *Herbal Medicinals: A Guide for Health-Care Professionals.*London, England: Pharmaceutical Press; 1996:69–73.
5. Mann C, Staba EJ. The chemistry, pharmacology and commercial formulations of chamomile. In: Craker LE, Simon JE, eds. *Herbs, Spices and Medicinal Plants: Recent Advances in Botany, Horticulture and Pharmacology.* Vol 1. Binghamton, NY: Hayworth Press Inc; 1986:235–280.
6. Casterline CL. Allergy to chamomile tea. *JAMA.* 1980;4:330–331.
7. Benner MH, Lee HJ. Anaphylactic reaction to chamomile tea. *J Allergy Clin Immunol.* 1973; 52:307–308.
8. Robbers JE, Speedie MK, Tyler VE. Terpinoids. In: Robbers JE, Speedie MK, Tyler VE, eds. *Pharmacognosy and Pharmacobiotechnology.* Baltimore, Md: Williams & Wilkins; 1996:80–107.
9. Bauer R, Khan IA, Wray V, Wagner H. Structure and stereochemistry of new sesquiterpene esters from *Echinacea purpurea. Helv Chim Acta.* 1985;68:2355–2358.
10. Wagner H, Suppner H, Schafer W, Zenk M. Immunologically active polysaccharides of *Echinacea purpurea* cell cultures. *Phytochemistry.* 1988;27:119–126.
11. Tubaro A, Tragni E, DelNegro P, Galli CL, Loggia RD. Anti-inflammatory activity of a polysaccharidic fraction of *Echinacea angustifolia. J Pharm Pharmacol.* 1987;39:567–569.

12. Stimpel M, Proksch A, Wagner H, Lohmann-Matthes ML. Macrophage activation and induction of macrophage cytotoxicity b purified polysaccharide fractions from the plant *Echinacea purpurea. Infect Immun.* 1984; 46:845–849.

13. Parnham MJ. Benefit-risk assessment of the squeezed sap of the purple coneflower (*Echinacea purpurea*) for long-term oral immunostimulation. *Phytomedicine.* 1996; 3:95–102.

14. Blumenthal M, Gruenwald J, Hall T, Riggins R, Rister R, eds. *German Commission E Monographs: Therapeutic Monographs on Medicinal Plants.* Austin, Tex: American Botanical Council; 1998.

15. Johnson ES, Kadam NP, Hylands DM, Hylands PJ. Efficacy of feverfew as prophylactic treatment of migraine. *BMJ.* 1985;291:569–573.

16. Murphy JJ, Heptinstall S, Mitchell JRA. Randomized, double-blind, placebo-controlled trial of feverfew in migraine prevention. *Lancet.* 1988;2:189–192.

17. Collier JOH, Butt NM, McDonald-Gibson WJ, Saeed SA. Extract of feverfew inhibits prostaglandin biosynthesis. *Lancet.* 1980; 2:922–923.

18. Newall CA, Anderson LA, Phillipson JD. Feverfew monograph. In: Newall CA, Anderson IA, Phillipson JD, eds. *Herbal Medicinals: A Guide for Health-Care Professionals.* London, England: Pharmaceutical Press; 1996:119–121.

19. Hepinstall S, Awang DV, Dawson BA, Kindach K, Knight DW, May J. Parthenolide content and bioactivity of feverfew: estimates of commercial and authenicated feverfew products. *J Pharm Pharmacol.* 1992;44:391–395.

20. Baldwin CA, Anderson LA, Phillipson JD. What pharmacists should know about feverfew. *J Pharm Pharmacol.* 1987;239:237–238.

21. Heptinstall S, Groenewegen WA, Spangenberg P, Loesche W. Extracts of feverfew may inhibit platelet behavior via neutralization of sulphydryl groups. *J Pharm Pharmacol.* 1987; 39:459–465.

22. Makheja AN, Bailey J. The active principle in feverfew [letter]. *Lancet.* 1981;2:1054.

23. Reuter HD. *Allium sativum* and *Allium ursinum,* part 2: pharmacolocy and medicinal applications. *Phytomedicine.* 1995;2:73–91.

24. Foushee DB, Ruffin J, Banerjee U. Garlic as a natural agent for the treatment of hypertension: a preliminary report. *Cytobios.* 1982; 34:145–152.

25. Malik ZA, Siddiqui S. Hypotensive effect of freeze-dried garlic sap in dog. *J Pak Med Assoc.* 1981;31:12–13.

26. Ruffin J, Hunter SA. An evaluation of the side effects of garlic as an antihypertensive agent. *Cytobios.* 1983;37:85–89.

27. Kleijnen J, Knipschild P, Riet GT. Garlic, onions and cardiovascular risk factors: a review of the evidence from human experiments with emphasis on commercially available preparations. *Br J Clin Pharmacol.* 1989;28:535–544.

28. Bleumink E, Doeglas HMG, Klokke AH, Nater JP. Allergic contact dermatitis to garlic. *Br J Dermatol.* 1972;87:6–9.

29. Silagy CA, Neil AW. A meta-analysis of the effect of garlic on blood pressure. *J Hypertens.* 1994;12:463–468.

30. Aue W, Eiber W, Hertkorn E, et al. Hypertension and hyperlipidemia: garlic helps in mild cases. *Br J Clin Pract.* 1990;69(suppl): 3–6.

31. Neil HAW, Silagy CA, Lancaster T, et al. Garlic powder in the treatment of moderate hyperlipidemia: a controlled trial and meta-analysis. *J R Coll Physician.* 1996;30:329–334.

32. Dixit VP, Joshi S. Effects of chronic administration of garlic (*Allium sativum* Linn) on testicular function. *Indian J Exp Biol.* 1982;20:534–536.

33. Cooperative Group for Essential Oil of Garlic. The effect of essential oil of garlic on hyperlipidemia and platelet aggregation: an analysis of 308 cases. *J Tradit Chin Med.* 1986;6:117–120.

34. Bordia A. Effect of garlic on human platelet aggregation in vitro. *Atherosclerosis.* 1978; 30:355–360.

35. Rose KD, Croissant PD, Parliament CF, Levin MP. Spontaneous spinal epidural hematoma with associated platelet dysfunction from excessive garlic ingestion: a case report. *Neurosurgery.* 1990;26:880–882.

36. Grontved A, Hentzer E. Vertigo-reducing effect of ginger root. *J Otolaryngol.* 1986; 48:282–286.

37. Mowrey DB, Clayson DE. Motion sickness, ginger and psychophysics. *Lancet.* 1982; 1:655–657.

38. Holtmann S, Clarke AH, Scherer H, Hohn M. The anti-motion sickness mechanism of ginger. *Acta Otolaryngol (Stockh).* 1989;108:168–174.

39. Bone ME, Wilkinson DJ, Young JR, et al. Ginger root: a new antiemetic: the effect of ginger root on postoperative nausea and vomiting after major gynecological surgery. *Anesthesia.* 1990;45:669–671.

40. Grontved A, Brask T, Kambskard J, Hentzer E. Ginger root against seasickness: a controlled trial on the open sea. *Acta Otolaryngol (Stockh).* 1988;105:45–49.

41. Fischer-Rasmussen W, Kjaer SK, Dahl C, Asping U. Ginger treatment of hyperemesis gravidarum. *Eur J Obstet Gynecol Reprod Biol.* 1990; 38:19–24.

42. Nakamura H, Yamamoto T. Mutagen and antimutagen in ginger: *Zingiber officinale. Mutat Res.* 1982;109:119–126.

43. Nakamura H, Yamamoto T. The active part of the (6)-gingerol in mutagenesis. *Mutat Res.* 1983;122:87–94.

44. Backon J. Ginger: inhibition of thromboxane synthetase and stimulation of prostacyclin: relevance for medicine and psychiatry. *Med Hypothesis.* 1986;20:271–278.

45. Cott J. Natural product formulations available in Europe for psychotropic indication. *Psychopharmacol Bull.* 1995;31:745–751.

46. Sastre J, Millan A, de la Asuncion G, et al. A *Ginkgo biloba* extract (Egb 761) prevents mitochondrial aging by protecting against oxidative stress. *Free Radic Bio Med.* 1998;24:298–304.

47. Benzi G, Moretti A. Are reactive oxygen species involved in Alzheimer's disease? *Neurobiol Aging.* 1995;16:661–674.

48. LeBars PL, Katz MM, Berman N, et al. A placebo-controlled, double-blind, randomized trial of an extract of *Ginkgo biloba* for dementia. *JAMA.* 1997;278:1327–1332.

49. Rosenblatt M, Mindel J. Spontaneous hyphema associated with ingestion of *Ginkgo biloba* extract [letter]. *N Engl J Med.* 1997;336:1108.

50. Rowin J, Lewis SL. Spontaneous bilateral subdural hematomas associated with chronic *Ginkgo biloba* ingestion have also occurred. *Neurology.* 1996;46:1775–1776.

51. Chung KF, McCusker M, Page CP, Dent G, Guinoit P, Barnes PJ. Effect of ginkgolide mixture in antagonizing skin and platelet responses to platelet activating factor in man. *Lancet.* 1987;1:248–251.

52. Arenz A, Klein M, Fiehe K, et al. Occurrence of neurotoxic 4'-o-methylpyridoxine in *Ginkgo biloba* leaves, *Ginkgo* medications and Japanese *Ginkgo* food. *Planta Med.* 1996; 62:548–551.

53. Vorberg G. *Ginkgo biloba* extract: a long-term study of chronic cerebral insufficiency in geriatric patients. *Clin Trials J.* 1985;22:149–157.

54. Lui J, Staba EJ. The ginsenosides of various ginseng plants and selected products. *J Nat Prod.* 1989;43:34–36.

55. McRae S. Elevated serum digoxin levels in a patient taking digoxin and Siberian ginseng. *CMAJ.* 1996;155:293–295.

56. Liberti LE, Marderosian AD. Evaluation of commercial ginseng products. *J Pharm Sci.* 1978; 10:1487–1489.

57. Ng TB, Li WW, Yeung HW. Effects of ginsenosides, lectins and *Momordica charantia* insulin-like peptide on corticosterone production by isolated rat adrenal cells. *J Ethnopharmacol.* 1987;21:21–29.

58. Jie YH, Cammisuli S, Baggiolini M. Immunomodulatory effects of *Panax ginseng:* CA Meyer in the mouse. *Agents Actions Suppl.* 1984; 15:386–391.

59. Singh VK, Agarwal SS, Gupta BM. Immunomodulatory activity of *Panax ginseng* extract. *Planta Med.* 1984;50:462–465.

60. Sotaniemi EA, Haapakkoski E, Rautio A. Ginseng therapy in non-insulin-dependent diabetic patients. *Diabetes Care.* 1995; 18:1373–1375.

61. Yokozawa T, Kobayashi T, Oura H, Kawashima Y. Studies on the mechanism of the hypoglycemic activity of ginsenoside-Rb2 in streptozotocin-diabetic rats. *Chem Pharm Bull.* 1985; 33:869–872.

62. Oshima Y, Kkonno C, Hikino H. Isolation and hypoglycemic activity of panaxans I, J, K and L, glycans of *Panax ginseng* roots. *J Ethnopharmacol.* 1985;14:255–259.

63. Konno C, Murakami M, Oshima Y, Hikino H. Isolation and hypoglycemic activity of panaxans Q,R,S,R and U: glycans of *Panax ginseng* roots. *J Ethnopharmacol.* 1985;14:69–74.

64. Konno C, Sugiyama K, Kano M, Takahashi M, Hikino H. Isolation and hypoglycemic activity of panaxans A, B, C, D and E: glycans of *Panax ginseng* roots. *Planta Med.* 1984;50:436–438.

65. Tokmoda M, Shimada K, Kkonno C, Sugiyama K, Hikino H. Partial structure of panaxan A: a hypoglycemic glycan of *Panax ginseng* roots. *Planta Med.* 1984;50:436–438.

66. Baldwin CA. What pharmacists should know about ginseng. *Pharm J.* 1986;237:583–586.

67. Hammond TG, Whitworth JA. Adverse reactions to ginseng [letter]. *Med J Aust.* 1981; 1:492.

68. Dega H, Laporte J, Frances C, Herson S, Choisidow O. Ginseng as a cause for Stevens-Johnson syndrome [letter]? *Lancet.* 1996; 347:1344.

69. Greenspan EM. Ginseng and vaginal bleeding [letter]. *JAMA.* 1983;249:2018.

70. Hopkins MP, Androff L, Benninghoff AS. Ginseng face cream and unexplained vaginal bleeding. *Am J Obstet Gynecol.* 1988; 159:1121–1122.

71. Palmer BV, Montgomery ACV, Monteriro JCMP. Ginseng and mastalgia. *BMJ.* 1978;1:1284.

72. Koren G. Maternal use of ginseng and neonatal androgenization [letter]. *JAMA.* 1991; 265:1828.

73. Awang DVS. Maternal use of ginseng and neonatal androgenization [letter]. *JAMA.* 1991;265;1828.

74. Waller DP, Martin AM, Farnswort NR, Awang DVC. Lack of androgenicity of Siberian ginseng [letter]. *JAMA.* 1992;267:2329.

75. Janetzky K, Morreale AP. Probable interactions between warfarin and ginseng. *Am J Health Syst Pharm.* 1997;54:692–693.

76. Kuo SC, Teng CM, Lee JG, Ko FN, Chen SC, Wu TS. Antiplatelet components in *Panax ginseng. Planta Med.* 1990;56:164–167.

77. Shader RI, Greenblatt DJ. Phenelzine and the dream machine-ramblings and reflections [editorial]. *J Clin Psychopharmacol.* 1985;5:65.

78. Jones BD, Runikis AM. Interactions of ginseng with phenelzine. *J Clin Psychopharmacol.* 1987; 7:201–202.

79. Siegel RK. Ginseng abuse syndrome. *JAMA.* 1979;241:1614–1615.

80. Elghamry MI, Hansel R. Activity and isolated phytoestrogen of shrub palmetto fruits (*Serenoa repens* Small): an estrogenic plant. *Experientia.* 1969;24:828–829.

81. Sultan C. Inhibition of androgen metabolism and binding by a liposterolic extract of *Serenoa repens* B in human foreskin fibroblasts. *J Steroid Biochem Mol Biol.* 1984;20:515–519.

82. Champault G, Patel JC, Bonnard AM. A double-blind trial of an extract of the plant *Serenoa rerpens* in benign prostatic hyperplasia. *Br J Clin Pharmacol.* 1984;18:461–462.

83. Tasca A. Treatment of obstruction in prostatic adenoma using an extract of *Serenoa repens:* double-blind clinical test vs placebo. *Minerva Urol Nefrol.* 1985;37:887–891.

84. Bach D, Schmitt M, Ebeling L. Phytopharmaceutical and synthetic agents in the treatment of benign prostatic hyperplasia (BPH). *Phytomedicine.* 1997;3–4:209–213.

85. Lohse MJ, Muller-Oerlinghausen B. Psychopharmaka. In: Schwabe U, Pffrath D, eds. *Arzeiverordnungreport '94.* Stuttgart, Germany: Gustav Fischer; 1994:354–370.

86. Wagner H, Bladt S. Pharmaceutical quality of Hypericum extracts. *J Geriatr Psychiatry Neurol.* 1994;7(suppl 1):65–68.

87. Sparenberg B, Demisch L, Holzl J. Investigations of the antidepressive effects of St. John's wort. *Pharm Ztg Wiss.*1993:6P50–54.

88. Bladt S, Wagner H. Inhibition of MAO by fractions and constituents of *Hypericum* extract. *J Geriatr Psychiatry Neurol.* 1994;(suppl1): S57–S59.

89. Linde K, Ramirez G, Mulrow CD, Pauls A, Weidenhammer W, Melchart D. St John's wort for depression: an overview and meta-analysis of randomized clinical trials. *BMJ.* 1993; 313:253–258.

90. McGuffin M, Hobbs C, Upton R, Goldberg A, eds. *Botanical Safety Handbook.* New York, NY: CRC Press Inc; 1997:62–63.

91. Leathwood PD, Chauffard F. Aqueous extract of valerian reduces latency to fall asleep in man. *Planta Med.* 1985;51:144–148.

92. Leathwood PD, Chauffard F, Heck E, Munoz-Box R. Aqueous extract of valerian root improves sleep quality in man. *Pharmacol Biochem Behav.* 1982;17:65–71.

93. Balderer G, Borbely AA. Effect of valerian on human sleep. *Psychopharmacology (Berl).* 1985;87:406–409.

94. Brown D. Valerian: clinical overview. *Townsend Lett Doctors.* 1995:150–51.

95. Hiller KO, Zetler G. Neuropharmacological studies on ethanol extracts of *Valeriana officinalis* L: behavioural and anticonvulsant activities. *Physiother Res Int.* 1996;10:145–151.

96. Capasso A, DeFeo V, DeSimon F, Sorrentino L. Pharmacological effects of aqueous extracts from *Valeriana adscendens. Physiother Res Int.* 1996;10:309–312.

97. Food and Drug Administration. *FDA warns consumers against dietary supplement products that may contain digitalis mislabeled as plantain.* June 12, 1997.

98. Blumenthal M. Industry alert: plantain adulterated with digitalis. *HerbalGram.* 1997;40:28–29.

99. Evans WC. Saponins, cardioactive drugs and other steroids. In: Evans WC, ed. *Pharmacognosy.* 14th ed. Philadelphia, Pa: WB Saunders Co; 1996:293–321.

100. Wash LK, Bernard JD. Licorice-induced pseudoaldosteronism. *Am J Hosp Pharm.* 1975;32:73–74.

101. Walker BR, Edwards CRW. Licorice-induced hypertension and syndromes of apparent mineralocorticoid excess. *Endocrinol Metab Clin North Am.* 1994;23:359–377.

102. Stewart PM, Wallace AM, Valentino R, Burt D, Shackleton CHL, Edwards CRW. Mineralocorticoid activity of liquorice: 11–beta-hydroxysteroid dehydrogenase deficiency comes of age. *Lancet.* 1987;2:821–824.

103. Gomez-Sanchez EP, Gomez-Sanchez CE. Central hypertensivnogenic effects of glycyrrhizic acid and carbenoxolone. *Am J Physiol.* 1992;236:1125–1130.

104. Farese RV, Biglieri EG, Shackleton CHL, Rony I, Gomez-Fontes R. Licorice-induced hypermineralocorticoidism. N *Engl J Med.* 1991; 325:1223–1227.

105. Salassa RM, Mattox VR, Rosevear JW. Inhibition of the mineralocorticoid activity of licorice by spironolactone. *J Clin Endocrinol Metab.* 1962; 22:1156–1159.

106. Corse FM, Galgani S, Gasparini C, Piazza G. Acute hypokalemic myopathy due to chronic licorice ingestion: report of a case. *J Neurol Sci.* 1983;4:493–497.

107. Fushimi R, Tachi J, Amino N, Myiai K. Chinese medicine interfering with digoxin immunoassays [letter]. *Lancet.* 1989;1:339.

108. Suga T. Chemistry and pharmacology of Chansu, Taisha. *Chin Med J (Engl).* 1973;suppl 10:762–773.

109. Schliche H, ed. *Phytotherapy in Paediatrics: Handbook for Physicians and Pharmacists.* Stuttgart, Germany: Medpharm GmbH Scientific Publishers; 1997:143.

110. Hobbs C, Foster S. Hawthorn: a literature review. *HerbalGram* 1990;22:19–33.

111. Racz-Kotilla E. Hypotensive and beta-blocking effect of procyanidins of *Crataegus monogyna. Planta Med.* 1980;39:239–241.

112. Bisset NG, ed. *Herbal Drugs and Phytopharmaceuticals: A Handbook for Practice on a Scientific Basis.* Stuttgart, Germany: Medpharm GmbH Scientific Publishers; 1994:46,441.

113. Newall CA, Anderson LA, Phillipson JD. Evening primrose monograph. In: JD Newall CA, Anderson LA, Phillipson JD, eds. *Herbal Medicines: A Guide for Health-Care Professionals.* London, England: Pharmaceutical Press; 1997:110–113.

114. Barber JH. Evening primrose oil: a panacea? *Pharm J.* 1988;240:723–725.

115. Newall CA, Anderson LA, Phillipson JD. Borage monograph. In: Newall CA, Anderson LA, Phillipson JD, eds. *Herbal Medicines: A Guide for Health-Care Professionals.* London, England: Pharmaceutical Press; 1997:49.

116. Hoffman D. *The Herb User's Guide: The Basic Skills of Medical Herbalism.* Wellingborough, England: Thorsons; 1987.

117. Mills DE. Dietary fatty acid supplementation alters stress reactivity and performance in man. *J Hum Hypertens.* 1989;3:111–116.

118. Larsen L. Unsaturated pyrrolizidines from Borage *(Borage officinalis)* a common garden herb. *J Nat Prod.* 1984;45:747–748.

119. Dandekar UP, Chandra RS, Dalvi SS, et al. Analysis of a clinically important interaction betwween phenytoin and Shankhapulshpi, an Ayurvedic preparation. *J Ethnopharmacol.* 1992;35:285–288.

120. Swinyard EA. Woodhead JH. Experimental detection quantification and evaluation of anticonvulsants. In: Woodbury DM, Penry JK Pippenger CE, eds. *Antiepileptic Drugs.* New York, NY: Raven Press; 1982:111–126.

121. Lo ACT, Chan K, Yeung JHK, Woo KS. The effects of danshen on pharmacokinetics and pharmacodynamics of warfarin rats. *Eur J Drug Metab Pharmacokinet.* 1992;17:257–262.

122. Newall CA, Anderson LA, Phillipson JD. German chamomile monograph. In: Newall CA, Anderson LA, Phillipson JD, eds. *Herbal Medicines: A Guide for Health-Care Professionals.* London, England: Pharmaceutical Press; 1997:69–71.

123. Sumner H, Salan U, Knight DW, Hoult JR. Inhibition of 5–lipoxygenase and cyclo-oxygenase in leukocytes by feverfew: involvement of sesquiterpene lactones and other components. *Biochem Pharmacol.* 1992;43:2313–2320.

124. Gorenewegen WA, Heptininstall S. A comparison of the effects of an extract of feverfew and parthenolide, a component of feverfew, on platelet activity in-vitro. *J Pharm Pharmacol.* 1990;42:553–557.

125. Biggs MJ, Johnson EW, Persaud NP, Ratcliffe DM. Platelet aggregation in patients using feverfew for migraine [letter]. *Lancet.* 1982; 2;776.

126. Duffield PH, Jamieson D. Development of tolerance to kava in mice. *Clin Exp Pharmacol Physiol.* 1991;18:571–578.

127. Ruzo P. Kava-induced dermatopathy: a niacin deficiency? *Lancet.* 1990;335:1442–1445.

128. Norton SA, Ruze P. Kava dermopathy. *J Am Acad Dermatol.* 1994;31:89–97.

129. Jamieson DD, Duffield PH. Positive interaction of ethanol and kava resin in mice. *Clin Exp Pharmacol Physiol.* 1990;17:509–514.

130. Davies LP, Drew CA, Duffield P, Johnston GA, Jamieson DD. Kava pyrones and resin: studies on GABAA, GABAB and benzodiazepine binding sites in rodent brain. *Pharmacol Toxicol.* 1992;71:120–126.

131. Davies LP, Drew CA, Duffield P. Kava pyrones and resin: studies on GABAA, GABAB and benzodiazepine binding sites in rodent brain. *Pharmacol Toxicol.* 1992;71:120–126.

132. Jussofie A, Schmiz A, Hiemke C. Kavapyrone-enriched extract from Piper methysticum as modulator of GABA binding sites in different regions of rat brain. *Psychopharmacology (Berl).* 1994;116:469–474.

133. Almeida JC, Grimsley EW. Coma from the health food store: interaction between kava and alprazolam. *Ann Intern Med.* 1996; 125:940–941.

134. Stimpel M, Proksch A, Wagner H, Lohmann-Matthes ML. Macrophage activation and induction of macrophage cytotoxicity by purified polysaccharide fractions from the plant *Echinacea purpurea. Infection Immun.* 1984; 46:845–849.

135. See DM, Broumand N, Sahl T, Tilles J. In vitro effects of echinacea and ginseng on natural killer and antibody dependent cell cytotoxicity in healthy subjects and chronic fatigue syndrome or acquired immunodeficiency syndrome patients. *Immunopharmacology.* 1997;35:229–235.

136. Jin R, Wan LL, Mitsuishi T. Effects of shi-ka-ma and Chinese herbs in mice treated with antitumor agent mitocycin C. *Chung Kuo Chung Hsi I Chieh Ho Tsa Chih.* 1995;15:101–103.

137. Utsunomiya T, Kobayashi M, Pollard RB, Suzuki F. Glycyrrhizin, an active component of licorice roots, reduces morbidity and mortality in mice infected with lethal doses of influenza virus. *Antimicrob Agents Chemother.* 1997; 41:551–556.

138. Dinnen RD, Ibibuzaki K. The search for novel anticancer agents: a differentiation-based assay and analysis of a folklore product. *Anticancer Res.* 1997;17:1027–1033.

139. Herbert V, Kasdan TS. Alfalfa, vitamin E, and autoimmune disorders. *Am J Clin Nutr.* 1994; 60:639–640.

140. Mossad SB, Macknin ML, Medendorp SV, Mason P. Zinc gluconate lozenges for treating the common cold. *Ann Intern Med.* 1996; 125:81–88.

141. Salas M, Kirchner H. Induction of interferon-gamma in human leukocyte cultures stimulated by Zn2±. *Clin Immunol Immunopathol.* 1987; 45:139–142.

142. Korant BD, Butterworth BE. Inhibition by zinc of rhinovirus protein cleavage: interaction of zinc with capsid polypeptides. *J Virol.* 1976; 18:298–306.

143. Gesits FC, Bateman JA, Hayden FG. In vitro activity of zinc salts against human rhinoviruses. *Antimicrob Agents Chemother.* 1987; 31:622–624.

144. Tyler V. Kidney, urinary tract and prostate problems. In: Tyler V, ed. *Herbs of Choice.* Binghamton, NY: Pharmaceutical Products Press Inc; 1994:73–86.

145. Newall CA, Anderson LA, Phillipson JD. Diuretic herbal ingredients. In: Newall CA, Anderson LA, Phillipson JD, eds. *Herbal Medicines: A Guide for Health-Care Professionals.* London, England: Pharmaceutical Press; 1997:281.

146. Olin BF, ed. Gossypol monograph. *Lawrence Review of Natural Products.* St Louis, Mo: Facts and Comparisons Inc; 1998.

147. Lin YC, Fukaya T, Rikihisa Y, Walton A. Gossypol in female fertility control: ovum implantation and early pregnancy inhibited in rats. *Life Sci.* 1985;37;39–47.

148. Liu Z, Hinton E, Cao J, Zhu C, Li B. Effects of potassium salt or a potassium blocker on gossypol-related hypokalemia. *Contraception.* 1988; 37:111–117.

149. Pizarro F, Olivares M, Hertrampf E, Walter T. Factors which modify the nutritional state of iron: tannin content of herbal teas. *Arch Latinoam Nutr.* 1994;44:277–280.

150. Newall CA, Anderson LA, Phillipson JD. Horseradish monograph. In: Newall CA, Anderson LA, Phillipson JD, eds. *Herbal Medicines: A Guide for Health-Care Professionals.* London, England: Pharmaceutical Press; 1997:168.

151. Anonymous. Kelp diets can produce myxedema in iodide-sensitive individuals. *JAMA.* 1975; 233:9–10.

152. Shilo S, Hirsch HJ. Iodine-induced hyperthyroidism in a patient with a normal thyroid gland. *Postgrad Med J.* 1986;62:661–662.

153. Waller DP, Zaveveld LJD, Farnsworth NR. Gossypol: pharmacology and current status as a male contraceptive. In: Wagner H, Hikino H, Farnsworth NR, eds. *Economic and Medicinal Plant Research.*London, England: Academic Press Inc; 1985:87–112.

154. De Smet PAGM. *Adverse Reactions of Herbal Drugs.* Vol 2. New York, NY: Springer-Verlag NY Inc; 1993.

155. De Smet PAGM. *Adverse Reactions of Herbal Drugs.* Vol 3. New York, NY: Springer-Verlag NY Inc; 1997.

156. De Smet PAGM. *Adverse Reactions of Herbal Drugs.* Vol 1. New York, NY: Springer-Verlag NY Inc; 1992.

157. d'Arcy PF. Adverse reactions and interactions with herbal medicines: part 2. *ADR Toxicol Rev.* 1992;12:147–162.

158. De Smet PAGM, Nolen WA. St John's wort as an antidepressant. *BMJ.* 1996;313:241–242.

159. Duke JA. Commentary-novel psychotherapeutic drugs: a role for ethnobotany. *Psychopharmacol Bull.* 1995;31:177–182.

160. Reynolds JEF, ed. *Martindale: The Extra Pharmacopoeia.* 29th ed. London, England: Pharmaceutical Press; 1989.

161. Gomez-Sanchez CE, Gomez-Sanchez CE, Yamakita N. Endocrine causes of hypertension. *Semin Nephrol.* 1995;15:1–15.

162. Blachley JD, Knochel JP. Tobacco chewer's hypokalemia: licorice revisited. *N Engl J Med.* 1980;302:74–75.

163. Beretta-Piccoli C, Salvade G, Crivelli PL, Weidmann P. Body sodium and blood volume in a patient with licorice-induced hypertension. *J Hypertens.* 1985;3:19–23.

164. Leatherdale BA, Panesar RK, Singh G, Atkins TW, Bailery CJ, Bignell AHC. Improvement in glucose tolerance due to *Momordica charantia* (karela). *BMJ.* 1981;282:1823–1824.

165. Gupta SS, Seth CB. Effect of *Momordica charantia* linn (karela) on glucose tolerance in albino rats. *J Indian Med Assoc.* 1962;39:581–584.

166. Aslam M, Stockley IH. Interaction between curry ingredient (karela) and drug (chlorpropamide) [letter]. *Lancet.* 1979;1:7607.

167. Anderson RA. Chromium, glucose tolerance and diabetes. *Biol Trace Elem Res.* 1992; 32:19–24.

168. Lee NA, Reasner CA. Beneficial effect of chromium supplementation on serum triglyceride levels in NIDDM. *Diabetes Care.* 1994; 17:1449–1452.

169. Kincheloe L. Gynecological and obstetric concerns regarding herbal medicinal use. In: Miller LG, Murray WJ, eds. *Herbal Medicinals: A Clinician's Guide.* Binghamton, NY: Pharmaceutical Products Press; 1998:285–314.

170. Costello C. Estrogenic substances from plants. *J Am Pharm Assoc (Wash).* 1950;39:177–180.

171. Holt S. Phytoestrogens for a healthier menopause. *Altern Ther Health Med.* 1997;1:187–193.

33 Herbal Medicine for the Treatment of Cardiovascular Disease

Clinical Considerations

Nick H. Mashour, MD; George I. Lin, MD; William H. Frishman, MD
From the Department of Medicine, The Albert Einstein College of Medicine, Bronx, NY (Dr Mashour); the Department of Family Medicine, Columbia Presbyterian Medical Center, New York, NY (Dr Lin); and the Departments of Medicine and Pharmacology, New York Medical College/Westchester Medical Center, Valhalla, NY (Dr Frishman).

Herbs have been used as medical treatments since the beginning of civilization and some derivatives (eg, aspirin, reserpine, and digitalis) have become mainstays of human pharmacotherapy. For cardiovascular diseases, herbal treatments have been used in patients with congestive heart failure, systolic hypertension, angina pectoris, atherosclerosis, cerebral insufficiency, venous insufficiency, and arrhythmia. However, many herbal remedies used today have not undergone careful scientific assessment, and some have the potential to cause serious toxic effects and major drug-to-drug interactions. With the high prevalence of herbal use in the United States today, clinicians must inquire about such health practices for cardiac disease and be informed about the potential for benefit and harm. Continuing research is necessary to elucidate the pharmacological activities of the many herbal remedies now being used to treat cardiovascular diseases.

Arch Intern Med. 1998;158:2225–2234

Since the beginning of human civilization, herbs have been an integral part of society, valued for both their culinary and medicinal properties. Herbal medicine has made many contributions to commercial drug preparations manufactured today including ephedrine from *Ephedra sinica* (ma-huang), digitoxin from *Digitalis purpurea* (foxglove), salicin (the source of aspirin) from *Salix alba* (willow bark), and reserpine from *Rauwolfia serpentina* (snakeroot), to name just a few. A naturally occurring β-adrenergic blocking agent with partial agonism has been identified in an herbal remedy.[1] The recent discovery of the antineoplastic drug paclitaxel from *Taxus brevifolia* (pacific yew tree) stresses the role of plants as a continuing resource for modern medicine.

However, with the development of patent medicines in the early part of the 20th century, herbal medicine has been losing ground to new synthetic medicines touted by scientists and physicians to be more effective and reliable. Nevertheless, about 3% of English-speaking adults in the United States still report having used herbal remedies in the preceding year.[2] This figure is probably much higher for non–English-speaking Americans. Despite this heavy use of herbal medicines in the United States, health practitioners often fail to ask about their use when taking clinical histories. It is imperative that physicians become more aware of the wide array of herbal medicines available, as well as learning more about their beneficial and adverse effects.[3]

Part of the problem for both consumers and physicians has been the paucity of scientific data on herbal medicines used in the United States.[4] As a result, those who wish to obtain factual information regarding the therapeutic use or potential harm of herbal remedies would have to obtain it from books and pamphlets, most of which base their information on traditional reputation rather than relying on existing scientific research. One may wonder why the herbal industry never chose to simply prove its products safe and effective. The answer is primarily economical. With the slim chance of patent protection for the many herbs that have been in use for centuries, pharmaceutical companies have not provided financial support for research on the merits of herbal medicine.[5] At the same time, the National Institutes of Health have only been able to offer limited funding for this purpose.

This review examines herbal medicines that affect the cardiovascular system both in terms of efficacy and safety as gleaned from the scientific literature that is available. These herbs are categorized under the primary diseases they treat. However, most herbal medicines have multiple cardiovascular effects that frequently overlap. The purpose of this organization is to simplify, not to pigeonhole herbs under specific diseases. In general, the dilution of active components in herbal medicines results in fewer adverse and toxic effects in comparison with the concentration of active components in the allopathic medicines. However, these adverse effects and drug interactions should not be overlooked; cardiovascular disease is a serious health hazard and no herbal remedy regimen should be initiated without careful consideration of its potential impact (Table 1).

Congestive Heart Failure

A number of herbs contain potent cardioactive glycosides, which have positive inotropic actions on the heart. The drugs digitoxin, derived from either *D purpurea* (foxglove) or *Digitalis lanata,* and digoxin, derived from *D lanata* alone, have been used in the treatment of congestive heart failure for many decades. Cardiac glycosides have a low therapeutic index, and the dose must be adjusted to the needs of each patient. The only way to control dosage is to use standardized powdered digitalis, digitoxin, or digoxin. When 12 different strains of *D lanata* plants were cultured and examined, their total cardenolide yield ranged from 30 to almost 1000 nmol/1 g.[6] As is evident, treating congestive heart failure with nonstandardized herbal drugs would be dangerous and foolhardy.

Some common plant sources of cardiac glycosides include *D purpurea* (foxglove, already mentioned), *Adonis microcarpa* and *Adonis vernalis* (adonis), *Apocynum cannabinum* (black Indian hemp), *Asclepiascurassavica* (redheaded cotton bush), *Asclepias friticosa* (balloon cotton), *Calotropis precera* (king's crown), *Carissa spectabilis* (wintersweet), *Cerebra manghas* (sea mango), *Cheiranthus cheiri* (wallflower), *Convallaria majalis* (lily of the valley, convallaria), *Cryptostegia grandiflora* (rubber vine), *Helleborus niger* (black hellebore), *Helleborus viridus, Nerium oleander* (oleander), *Plumeria rubra* (frangipani), *Selenicerus grandiflorus* (cactus grandiflorus), *Strophanthus hispidus* and *Strophanthus kombe* (strophanus), *Thevetia peruviana* (yellow oleander), and *Urginea maritima* (squill).[5,7–15] Even the venom glands of the animal *Bufo marinus* (cane toad) contain cardiac glycosides.[8] Recently, the digitalislike steroid in the venom of the *B marinus* toad was identified as a previously described steroid, marinobufagenin. Marinobufagenin demonstrated high digoxinlike immunoreactivity and was antagonized with an antidigoxin antibody.[16]

Accidental poisonings and even suicide attempts with ingestion of cardiac glycosides are abundant in the medical literature.[17–21] Some herbal remedies (eg, Siberian ginseng) can elevate synthetic digoxin drug levels and cause toxic effects.[22] In the United States, there are about 15,000 intoxications due to accidental or intentional ingestion of poisonous plants annually.[23] In 1993, 2388 toxic exposures in the United States were reported to be due to plant glycosides. Of these, the largest percentage were attributed to oleander (ie, 25%).[24] In the case of oleander, all plant tissues, including the seeds, roots, stems, leaves, berries, and blossoms, are considered extremely toxic.[19] In

Table 1. Herbs for Cardiovascular Conditions With Severe Adverse Reactions or Notable Drug Interactions*

Herbal Medicine	Adverse Reaction/Drug Interaction	Treatment
Natural cardiac glycosides (>20 plant sources)	Ventricular tachyarrhythmia, bradycardia, and heart block	Digoxin-specific Fab antibody
Veratrum (hellebore)	Bradycardia, A-V dissociation, hypotension, and (rarely) seizures	ECG changes responsive to atropine
Crataegus (hawthorn)	Potentiates digitalis activity	NA
Salvia miltiorrhiza (dan-shen)	Potentiates warfarin activity	NA
Aesculus hippocastanum (horse chestnut)	Renal and hepatic toxic effects	Dialysis to reduce toxic levels

*A-V indicates arteriovenous anastomosis; ECG, electrocardiographic; and NA, data not applicable.

fact, death in humans has been reported following ingestion of as little as 1 oleander leaf.[25] The clinical manifestations of oleander intoxication, as well as other natural glycosides, is virtually identical to digoxin overdose. Morbidity and mortality are mainly related to cardiotoxic adverse effects that usually include life-threatening ventricular tachyarrhythmias, bradycardia, and heart block. The diagnosis should rely on the clinical presentation of unexplained hyperkalemia, and cardiac, neurologic, and gastrointestinal symptoms.[19]

The diagnosis can be further supported by the detection of the substance digoxin in a radioimmunoassay for digoxin. However, the extent of cross-reactivity between the cardiac glycosides from herbal sources and antibodies used in the radioimmunoassays has not been clearly defined.[26] For this reason, digoxin assays may serve to confirm the suspected diagnosis but not to quantify the severity. Once the diagnosis has been established, the use of digoxin-specific Fab antibody fragments may be helpful in the treatment of severe intoxication. Other modalities, such as dialysis, cannot be easily facilitated because, like digoxin, natural glycosides are distributed extensively into peripheral tissues.

Hypertension

The root of *R serpentina* (snakeroot), the natural source of the alkaloid reserpine, has been a Hindu Ayurvedic remedy since ancient times. In 1931, Indian literature first described the use of *R serpentina* root for the treatment of hypertension and psychoses; however, the use of *Rauwolfia* alkaloids in Western medicine did not begin until the mid 1940s.[27] Both standardized whole root preparations of *R serpentina* and its reserpine alkaloid are officially monographed in the United States Pharmacopeia.[28] A powdered whole root of 200 to 300 mg orally is equivalent to 0.5 mg of reserpine.[29]

Reserpine was one of the first drugs used on a large scale to treat systemic hypertension. It acts by irreversibly blocking the uptake of biogenic amines (norepinephrine, dopamine, and serotonin) in the storage vesicles of central and peripheral adrenergic neurons, thus leaving the catecholamines to be destroyed by the intraneuronal monoamine oxidase in the cytoplasm. The depletion of catecholamines accounts for reserpine's sympatholytic and antihypertensive actions. Reserpine's effects are long lasting, since recovery of sympathetic function requires synthesis of new storage vesicles, which takes days to weeks. Reserpine lowers blood pressure by decreasing cardiac output, peripheral vascular resistance, heart rate, and renin secretion. With the introduction of other antihypertensive drugs with fewer central nervous system adverse effects, the use of reserpine has diminished. The daily oral dose of reserpine should be 0.25 mg or less, and as little as 0.05 mg if given with a diuretic. Using the whole root, the usual adult dose is 50 to 200 mg/d administered once daily or in 2 divided doses.[27–29]

Rauwolfia alkaloids are contraindicated for use in patients with previously demonstrated hypersensitivity to these substances, in patients with a history of mental depression (especially with suicidal tendencies), in patients with active peptic ulcer disease or ulcerative colitis, and in patients receiving electroconvulsive therapy. The most common adverse effects are sedation and inability to concentrate and perform complex tasks. Reserpine may cause mental depression, sometimes resulting in suicide, and its use must be discontinued at the first sign of depression. Reserpine's sympatholytic effect and its enhancement of parasympathetic actions account for its well-described adverse effects: nasal congestion, increased gastric secretion, and mild diarrhea.[27–30]

Stephania tetrandra is an herb sometimes used in traditional Chinese medicine to treat hypertension. Tetrandrine, an alkaloid extract of *S tetrandra,* has been shown to be a calcium ion channel antagonist, paralleling the effects of verapamil. Tetrandrine blocks T and L calcium channels, interferes with the binding of diltiazem and methoxyverapamil at calcium-channel binding sites, and suppresses aldosterone production.[31,32] A parenteral dose (15 mg/kg) of tetrandrine in conscious rats decreases mean, systolic, and diastolic blood pressures for more than 30 minutes; however, an intravenous 40-mg/kg dose killed the rats by myocardial depression. In stroke-prone hypertensive rats, an oral dose of 25 or 50 mg/kg produced a gradual and sustained hypotensive effect after 48 hours without affecting plasma renin activity.[33] In addition to its cardiovascular actions, tetrandrine has reported antineoplastic, immunosuppressive, and mutagenic effects.[31]

Tetrandrine is 90% protein-bound with an elimination half-life of 88 minutes, according to dog studies; however, rat studies have shown a sustained hypotensive effect for more than 48 hours after a 25- or 50-mg oral dose. Tetrandrine causes liver necrosis in dogs orally administered 40 mg/kg of tetrandrine 3 times weekly for 2 months, reversible swelling of liver cells with a 20-mg/kg dose, and no observable changes with a 10-mg/kg dose.[31] Given the evidence of hepatotoxicity, many more studies are necessary to establish a safe dosage of tetrandrine in humans.

More recently, tetrandrine has been implicated in an outbreak of rapidly progressive renal failure, termed *Chinese herb nephropathy*. Numerous individuals developed the condition after using a combination of several Chinese herbs as part of a dieting regimen. It has been hypothesized that the cause may be attributed to misidentification of *S tetrandra;* nonetheless, questions still remain as to the role of tetrandra in the development of this serious toxic effect.[34–37]

The root of *Lingusticum wallichii* is used in traditional Chinese medicine as a circulatory stimulant, hypotensive drug, and sedative.[38] Tetramethylpyrazine, the active constituent extracted from *L wallichii*, inhibits platelet aggregation in vitro and lowers blood pressure by vasodilation in dogs. With its actions independent of the endothelium, tetramethylpyrazine's vasodilatory effect is mediated by calcium channel antagonism and nonselective antagonism of α-adrenergic receptors. Some evidence suggests that tetramethylpyrazine acts on the pulmonary vasculature.[31] Currently, there is insufficient information to evaluate the safety and efficacy of this herbal medicinal.

Uncaria rhynchophylla is sometimes used in traditional Chinese medicine to treat hypertension. Its indole alkaloids, rhynchophylline and hirsutine, are thought to be the active principles of *U rhynchophylla's* vasodilatory effect. The mechanism of *U rhynchophylla's* actions is unclear. Some studies point to an alteration in calcium ion flux in response to activation, whereas others point to hirsutine's inhibition of nicotine-induced dopamine release.[31] One in vitro study has shown *U rhynchophylla* extract relaxes norepinephrine-precontracted rat aorta through endothelium-dependent and -independent mechanisms. For the endothelium-dependent component, *U rhynchophylla* extract appears to stimulate endothelium-derived relaxing factor and/or nitric oxide release without involving muscarinic receptors.[39] Also, in vitro and in vivo studies have shown that rhynchophylline can inhibit platelet aggregation and reduce platelet thromboses induced with collagen or adenosine diphosphate plus epinephrine.[31] Safety and efficacy cannot be evaluated at this time because of a lack of clinical data.

Veratrum (hellebore) is a perennial herb grown in many parts of the world. Varieties include *Veratrum viride* from Canada and the eastern United States, *Veratrum californicum* from the western United States, *Veratrum album* from Alaska and Europe, and *Veratrum japonicum* from Asia. All *Veratrum* plants contain poisonous alkaloids known to cause vomiting, bradycardia, and hypotension. Most cases of *Veratrum* poisonings are due to misidentification with other plants. Although once a treatment for hypertension, the use of *Veratrum* alkaloids has lost favor owing to a low therapeutic index and unacceptable toxicity, as well as the introduction of safer antihypertensive drug alternatives.[40]

Veratrum alkaloids enhance nerve and muscle excitability by increasing sodium ion conductivity. They act on the posterior wall of the left ventricle and the coronary sinus baroreceptors, causing reflex hypotension and bradycardia via the vagus nerve (Bezold-Jarisch reflex). Nausea and vomiting are secondary to the alkaloids' actions on the nodose ganglion.[40]

The diagnosis of *Veratrum* toxicity is established by history, identification of the plant, and strong clinical suspicion. Clinical symptoms usually occur quickly, often within 30 minutes.[41] Treatment is mainly supportive and directed at controlling bradycardia and hypotension. *Veratrum*-induced bradycardia usually responds to treatment with atropine; however, the blood pressure response to atropine is more variable and requires the addition of pressors. Other electrocardiographic changes, such as atrioventricular dissociation, may also be reversible with atropine.[42] Seizures are a rare complication and may be treated with conventional anticonvulsants. For patients with preexisting cardiac disease, the use of β-agonists or pacing may be necessary. Nausea may be controlled with phenothiazine antiemetics. Recovery usually occurs within 24 to 48 hours.[40]

Evodia rutaecarpa (wu-chu-yu) is a Chinese herbal drug that has been used as a treatment for hypertension. It contains an active vasorelaxant component called rutaecarpine that can cause endothelium-dependent vasodilation in experimental models.[43]

Angina Pectoris

Crataegus hawthorn, a name encompassing many *Crataegus* species (such as *Crataegus oxyacantha* and *Crataegus monogyna* in the West and *Crataegus pinnatifida* in China) has acquired the reputation in modern herbal literature as an important tonic for the cardiovascular system that is particularly useful for angina. *Crataegus* leaves, flowers, and fruits contain a number of biologically active substances, such as oligomeric procyanins, flavonoids, and catechins. From current studies, *Crataegus* extract appears to have antioxidant properties and can inhibit the formation of thromboxane as well.[44,45]

Also, *Crataegus* extract antagonizes the increases in cholesterol, triglyceride, and phospholipid levels in low-density lipoprotein (LDL) and very low-density lipoprotein in rats fed a hyperlipidemic diet; thus, it may inhibit the progression of atherosclerosis.[46] This hypocholesterolemic action may be due to an up-regulation of hepatic LDL receptors resulting in greater influx of plasma cholesterol into the liver. *Crataegus* also prevents cholesterol accumulation in the liver by enhancing cholesterol degradation to bile acids, as well as suppressing cholesterol biosynthesis.[47]

According to another study, *Crataegus* extract, in high concentrations, has a cardioprotective effect on ischemic-reperfused hearts without causing an increase in coronary blood flow.[48] On the other hand, oral and parenteral administration of oligomeric procyanins of *Crataegus* has been shown to lead to an increase in coronary blood flow in both cats and dogs.[49,50] Double-blind clinical trials have demonstrated simultaneous cardiotropic and vasodilatory actions of *Crataegus*.[51] In essence, *Crataegus* increases coronary perfusion, has a mild hypotensive effect, antagonizes atherogenesis, and has positive inotropic and negative chronotropic actions.[46,52] In a recent multicenter, placebo-controlled, double-blind study, an extract of *Crataegus* was shown to clearly improve the cardiac performance of patients with New York Heart Association class II heart failure. In this study, the primary parameter analyzed was the heart rate product (systolic blood pressure × heart rate).[53] Recent studies have suggested that the mechanism of cardiac action for *Crataegus* species may be due to the inhibition of the 3′, 5′-cyclic adenosine monophosphate phosphodiesterase.[54]

Hawthorn is relatively devoid of adverse effects. In fact, in comparison with other inotropic drugs such as epinephrine, amrinone, milrinone, and digoxin, *Crataegus* has a potentially reduced arrhythmogenic risk because of its ability to prolong the effective refractory period, while the other drugs mentioned previously all shorten this parameter.[55,56] Also, it should be noted that concomitant use of hawthorn with digitalis can markedly enhance the activity of digitalis.[5,57] Undoubtedly, more studies are needed to show that hawthorn can be used safely and effectively.

Because of its resemblance to *Panax ginseng* (Asian ginseng), *Panax notoginseng* has acquired the common name of pseudoginseng, especially since it is often an adulterant of *P ginseng* preparations. In traditional Chinese medicine, the root of *P notoginseng* is used for analgesia and hemostasis. It is also often used in the treatment of patients with angina and coronary artery disease.[38] *Panax notoginseng* has been described as a calcium ion channel antagonist in vascular tissue. More specifically, its pharmacological action may be as a novel and selective calcium ion antagonist that does not interact with the L-type calcium ion channel but rather may interact with the receptor-operated calcium ion channel.[58]

Although clinical trials are lacking, in vitro studies using *P notoginseng* suggest possible cardiovascular effects. One study that used purified notoginsenoside R1, extracted from *P notoginseng*, on human left umbilical vein endothelial cells showed a dose- and time-dependent synthesis of tissue-type plasminogen activating factor without affecting the synthesis of plasminogen activating inhibitor. Thus, fibrinolytic parameters were enhanced.[59] Another study suggests that *P notoginseng* saponins may inhibit atherogenesis by interfering with the proliferation of smooth muscle cells.[60] In vitro and in vivo studies using rats and rabbits demonstrate that *P notoginseng* may be useful as an antianginal drug, since it dilates coronary arteries in all concentrations. The role of *P notoginseng* in the treatment of hypertension is less certain, since *P notoginseng* causes vasodilation or vasoconstriction depending on the concentration and target vessel.[61] The results of these in vitro and in vivo studies are encouraging; however, clinical trials will be necessary to make a more informed decision regarding the use of *P notoginseng*.

Salvia miltiorrhiza (dan-shen), a relative of the Western sage *Salvia officinalis,* is native to China. In traditional Chinese medicine, the root of *S miltiorrhiza* is used as a circulatory stimulant, sedative, and cooling drug.[38] *Salvia miltiorrhiza* may be useful as an antianginal drug because it has been shown to dilate coronary arteries in all concentrations, similar to *P notoginseng.* Also, *S miltiorrhiza* has variable action on other vessels depending on its concentration, so it may not be as helpful in treating hypertension.[61] In vitro, *S miltiorrhiza,* in a dose-dependent fashion, inhibits platelet aggregation and serotonin release induced by either adenosine diphosphate or epinephrine, which is thought to be mediated by an increase in platelet cyclic adenosine monophosphate caused by *S miltiorrhiza*'s inhibition of cyclic adenosine monophosphate phosphodiesterase.[62] *Salvia miltiorrhiza* appears to have a protective action on ischemic myocardium, enhancing the recovery of contractile force on reoxygenation.[63] More recently, *S miltiorrhiza* has been shown to protect myocardial mitochondrial membranes from ischemia-reperfusion injury and lipid peroxidation because of its free radical-scavenging effects.[64] Qualitatively and quantitatively, a decoction of *S miltiorrhiza* was as efficacious as the more expensive isolated tanshinones.[59]

Clinical trials will be necessary to evaluate the safety and efficacy of *S miltiorrhiza.* Of note, it has been observed clinically that when *S miltiorrhiza* and warfarin sodium are coadministered, there is an increased incidence in warfarin-related adverse effects; in rats *S miltiorrhiza* was shown to increase the plasma concentrations of warfarin as well as the prothrombin time.[65]

Atherosclerosis

In addition to its use in the culinary arts, garlic (*Allium sativum*) has been valued for centuries for its medicinal properties. Garlic is one of the herbal medicines that has been examined more closely by the scientific community. In recent decades, research has focused on garlic's use in preventing atherosclerosis. Garlic, like many of the other herbal medicines discussed previously, has demonstrated multiple beneficial cardiovascular effects. A number of studies have demonstrated these effects that include lowering blood pressure, inhibiting platelet aggregation, enhancing fibrinolytic activity, reducing serum cholesterol and triglyceride levels, and protecting the elastic properties of the aorta.

Consumption of large quantities of fresh garlic (0.25 to 1.0 g/kg or about 5–20 average sized 4-g cloves in a person weighing 78.7 kg) has been shown to produce the beneficial effects mentioned earlier.[66] In support of this, a recent double-blind cross-over study was conducted on moderately hypercholesterolemic men that compared the effects of 7.2 g of aged garlic extract with placebo on blood lipid levels. This study found that there was a maximal reduction of 6.1% in total serum cholesterol levels and 4.6% in LDL cholesterol levels with garlic compared with placebo.[67]

However, despite positive evidence from numerous trials, some investigators have been hesitant to outright endorse the routine use of garlic for cardiovascular disease because many of the published studies had methodological shortcomings,[66,68–72] perhaps because constituent trials were small, lacking statistical power. Also, inappropriate methods of randomization, lack of dietary run-in period, short duration, or failure to undertake intention-to-treat analysis may explain the cautious acceptance of previous meta-analyses.[73] In fact, one recent study found no demonstrable effect of garlic ingestion on lipid and lipoprotein levels. This study used a cross-over design protected by a washout period to reduce between-subject variability as well as close assessment and reporting of dietary behavior, which had been lacking in previous trials.[74] Another study found no effect of garlic on cholesterol absorption, cholesterol synthesis, or cholesterol metabolism.[71] As is evident, the precise extent of garlic's impact on atherosclerosis remains controversial; larger, more rigorously designed trials may be necessary to better determine its utility in preventing cardiovascular disease.

Garlic has also been studied in hypertensive patients as a blood pressure-lowering agent. Similar to its lipid effects, no conclusive studies have been conducted and many methodological shortcomings exist in study designs. The results of one meta-analysis that considered 8 different trials suggest some clinical use for patients with mild hypertension, but there is insufficient evidence to recommend its use as routine clinical therapy.[68] Garlic has also been shown to possess antiplatelet activity. In the past, this action was mostly documented in vitro.[75] A new study examined the effect of the consumption of a fresh clove of garlic on platelet thromboxane production and showed that after 26 weeks, serum thromboxane levels were reduced about 80%.[76] This may prove to be beneficial in the prevention of thrombosis in the future. Recently, the effect of long-term garlic intake on the elastic properties of the aorta was also studied. Participants in the trial (limited to those aged 50–80 years) consumed 300 mg/d of standardized garlic powder for more than 2 years. The results showed that the pulse-wave velocity and standardized elastic vascular resistance of the aorta were lower in the garlic group than in the control group. Consequently, long-term garlic powder intake may have a protective effect on the elastic properties of the aorta related to aging.[77] In these ways, garlic has shown numerous beneficial cardiovascular effects that need to be investigated further to determine its therapeutic utility.

Intact cells of garlic bulbs include an odorless, sulfur-containing amino acid known as *allinin.* When garlic is crushed, allinin comes into contact with allinase, which converts allinin to allicin. Allicin has potent antibacterial properties, but it is also highly odoriferous and unstable. Ajoenes, self-condensation products of allicin, appear to be responsible for garlic's antithrombotic activity. Most authorities now agree that allicin and its derivatives are the active constituents of garlic's physiological activity. Fresh garlic releases allicin in the mouth during the chewing process. Dried garlic preparations lack allicin but contain allinin and allinase. Since allinase is inactivated in the stomach, dried garlic preparations should be coated with enteric so that they pass through the stomach into the small intestine where allinin can be enzymatically converted to allicin. Few commercial garlic preparations are standardized for their allicin yield based on allinin content, hence making their effectiveness less certain.[5] However, one double-blind, placebo-controlled study involving 261 patients for 4 months using one 800-mg tablet of garlic powder daily, standardized to 1.3% allinin content, demonstrated significant reductions in total cholesterol (12%) and triglyceride levels (17%).[78]

Aside from a garlic odor on the breath and body, moderate garlic consumption causes few adverse effects. However, consumption in excess of 5 cloves daily may result in heartburn, flatulence, and other gastrointestinal disturbances. Some people have reported allergic reactions to garlic, most commonly allergic contact dermatitis. Patch testing with 1% diallyl disulfide is recommended when garlic allergy is suspected.[79] Because of its antithrombotic activity, garlic should be used with caution in people taking oral anticoagulants concomitantly.[5,80]

The resin of *Commiphora mukul* (gugulipid), a small, thorny tree native to India, has long been used in Ayurvedic medicine to treat lipid disorders. The primary mechanism of action of gugulipid is through an increase in the uptake and metabolism of LDL cholesterol by the liver.[81] In a double-blind, cross-over study completed in 125 patients taking gugulipid compared with 108 patients taking clofibrate, the average decrease in serum cholesterol and triglyceride levels was 11% and 16.8%, respectively, with gugulipid compared with 10% and 21.6%, respectively, with clofibrate. In general, hypercholesterolemic patients responded more favorably to gugulipid therapy than hypertriglyceridemic patients.[82] Moreover, it was shown in another randomized, double-blind trial that *C mukul* also decreased LDL cholesterol levels by 12.5% and the total cholesterol–high-density lipoprotein cholesterol ratio by 11.1%, whereas the levels were unchanged in the placebo group.[83]

Besides being potentially as effective in lowering blood lipid levels as modern hyperlipidemic drugs, gugulipid may even be safer. In the trial mentioned previously, compliance was greater than 96%, with only the adverse effects of headache, mild nausea, and hiccups noted.[83] However, it has been shown that gugulipid may affect the bioavailability of other cardiovascular drugs, namely, propranolol hydrochloride and diltiazem hydrochloride. Gugulipid significantly reduced the peak plasma concentration and area under the curve of both these drugs, which may lead to diminished efficacy or nonresponsiveness.[84] Undoubtedly, gugulipid is a natural lipid-lowering drug with potential for therapeutic use, but rigorous, larger clinical trials will be necessary to further evaluate its safety and efficacy before it can be endorsed as an alternative therapy for hyperlipidemia and prevention of atherosclerosis.

Maharishi amrit kalash-4 and *Maharishi amrit kalash*-5 are 2 complex herbal mixtures with significant antioxidant properties that have been shown to inhibit LDL oxidation in patients with hyperlipidemia. In experimental studies, the herbal mixtures have also been shown to inhibit enzymatic- and nonenzymatic-induced microsomal lipid peroxidation and platelet aggregation.[85]

Cerebral and Peripheral Vascular Disease

Having existed for more than 200 million years, *Ginkgo biloba* (maidenhair tree) was apparently saved from extinction by human intervention, surviving in Far Eastern temple gardens while disappearing for centuries in the West. It was reintroduced to Europe in 1730 and became a favorite ornamental tree.[38,86] Although the root and kernels of *G biloba* have long been used in traditional Chinese medicine, the tree gained attention in the West during the 20th century for its medicinal value after a concentrated extract of *G biloba* leaves was developed in the 1960s. At least 2 groups of substances within *G biloba extract* (GBE) demonstrate beneficial pharmacological actions. The flavonoids reduce capillary permeability as well as fragility and serve as free radical scavengers. The terpenes (ie, ginkgolides) inhibit platelet-activating factor, decrease vascular resistance, and improve circulatory flow without appreciably affecting blood pressure.[57,87] Continuing research appears to support the primary use of GBE for treating cerebral insufficiency and its secondary effects on vertigo, tinnitus, memory, and mood; also, GBE appears to be useful for treating peripheral vascular disease, including diabetic retinopathy and intermittent claudication.[5,57,87–91]

In a randomized, placebo-controlled, double-blind study, EGb 761, which is a standardized extract of *G biloba* with respect to its flavonol glycoside and terpene lactone content, was shown to significantly decrease the areas of ischemia as measured by transcutaneous partial pressure of oxygen during exercise. Because of its rapid anti-ischemic action, EGb 761 may be valuable in the treatment of intermittent claudication and peripheral artery disease in general.[92]

Also, studies have been examining the cardioprotective efficacy of EGb 761 in regard to its anti–free radical action in myocardial ischemia–reperfusion injury. In vitro studies with animal models have shown that this compound may exert such an effect.[93,94] A clinical study of 15 patients undergoing coronary bypass surgery demonstrated that oral EGb 761 therapy may limit free radical–induced oxidative stress occurring in the systemic circulation and at the level of the myocardium during these operations.[95] It remains to be studied whether extracts of *G biloba* may be used as pharmacological adjuvants to limit tissue damage and metabolic alterations following coronary bypass surgery, coronary angioplasty for acute myocardial infarctions, or even in managing coronary thrombosis.

Although approved as a drug in Europe, *Ginkgo* is not approved in the United States and is instead marketed as a food supplement, usually supplied as 40-mg tablets of extract. Since most of the investigations examining the efficacy of GBEs used preparations such as EGb 761 or LI 1370, the bioequivalence of other GBE products has not been established. The recommended dosage in Europe is one 40-mg tablet taken 3 times daily with meals (120 mg/d).[5,87] Adverse effects due to GBE are rare but can include gastrointestinal disturbances, headache, and allergic skin rash.[5,87]

Known mostly as a culinary spice and flavoring agent, *Rosmarinus officinalis* (rosemary) is listed in many herbal sources as a tonic and all-around stimulant. Traditionally, rosemary leaves are said to enhance circulation, aid digestion, elevate mood, and boost energy. When applied externally, the volatile oils are supposedly useful for arthritic conditions and baldness.[5]

Although research on rosemary is scant, some studies have focused on antioxidant effects of diterpenoids, especially carnosic acid and carnosol, isolated from rosemary leaves. In addition to having antineoplastic effects, antioxidants in rosemary have been credited with stabilizing erythrocyte membranes and inhibiting superoxide generation and lipid peroxidation.[96,97] Essential oils of rosemary have demonstrated antimicrobial, hyperglycemic, and insulin-inhibiting properties.[98,99] Rosemary leaves contain high amounts of salicylates, and its flavonoid pigment diosmin is reported to decrease capillary permeability and fragility.[57,100,101]

Despite the conclusions derived from in vitro and animal studies, the therapeutic use of rosemary for cardiovascular disorders remains questionable, because few, if any, clinical trials have been conducted using rosemary. Because of the lack of studies, no conclusions can be reached regarding the use of the antioxidants of rosemary in inhibiting atherosclerosis. Although external application may cause cutaneous vasodilation from the counterirritant properties of rosemary's essential oils, there is no evidence to support any prolonged improvement in peripheral circulation.[5] While rosemary does have some carminative properties, it may also cause gastrointestinal and kidney disturbances in large doses.[5,101] Until more studies are done, rosemary should probably be limited to its use as a culinary spice and flavoring agent rather than as a medicine.

Venous Insufficiency

The seeds of horse chestnut, *Aesculus hippocastanum*, have long been used in Europe to treat venous disorders such as varicose veins. The saponin glycoside aescin from horse chestnut extract (HCE) inhibits the activity of lysosomal enzymes thought to contribute to varicose veins by weakening vessel walls and increasing permeability, which result in dilated veins and edema.[5] In fact, recent research has shown that *A hippocastanum* inhibits only against hyaluronidase but not elastase, and this activity is linked mainly to the saponin escin.[102] In animal studies, HCE, in a dose-dependent fashion, increases venous tone, venous flow, and lymphatic flow. It also antagonizes capillary hyperpermeability induced by histamine, serotonin, or chloroform. This extract has been shown to decrease edema formation of lymphatic and inflammatory origin. Horse chestnut extract has antiexudative properties, suppressing experimentally induced pleurisy and peritonitis by inhibiting plasma extravasation and leukocyte emigration, and its dose-dependent antioxidant properties can inhibit in vitro lipid peroxidation.[103,104] Randomized, double-blind, placebo-controlled trials with HCE show are eduction in edema, measured using plethysmography.[105,106]

In another recent randomized, placebo-controlled study, the efficacy and safety of class 2 compression stockings and dried HCE were compared. Both HCE and the compression stockings decreased lower leg edema after 12 weeks of therapy; the results showed an average 43.8-mL reduction with HCE and 46.7-mL with compression stockings, while the placebo group showed an increase of 9.8 mL. Both HCE and compression therapy were well tolerated, with no serious adverse effects. This study may indicate that both of these modalities are reasonable alternatives for the effective treatment of patients with chronic venous insufficiency.[107] Also, HCE has been shown to markedly improve other symptoms associated with chronic venous insufficiency, such as pain, tiredness, itching, and tension in the swollen leg, in a case-observation study.[108] Aside from effects on venous insufficiency, prophylactic use of HCE has been thought to decrease the incidence of thromboembolic complications of gynecological surgery. However, since this issue is still controversial,[109] this does not appear to be the case.[109]

Standardized HCE is prepared as an aqueous alcohol extract of 16% to 21% of triterpene glycosides, calculated as aescin. The usual initial dosage is 90 to 150 mg/d of aescin, which may be reduced to 35 to 70 mg/d if clinical benefit is seen.[5] Standardized HCE preparations are not available in the United States, but nonstandardized products may be available.

Some manufacturers promote the use of topical preparations of HCE for treatment of varicose veins as well as hemorrhoids; however, at least one study has demonstrated poor aescin distribution at sites other than the skin and muscle tissues underlying the application site.[110] Moreover, the involvement of arterioles and veins in the pathophysiology of hemorrhoids makes the effectiveness of HCE doubtful, since HCE has no known effects on the arterial circulation. For now, research studies have yet to confirm any clinical effectiveness of topical HCE preparations.

Although adverse effects are uncommon, HCE may cause gastrointestinal irritation. Parenteral aescin has produced isolated cases of anaphylactic reactions, as well as hepatic and renal toxic effects.[5,111–113] In the event of toxicity, aescin can be eliminated via dialysis, with elimination dependent on protein-binding.[114] Horse chestnut extract is also one of the components of venocuran, a drug marketed as a treatment for venous disorders. In 1975, venocuran was determined to cause a pseudolupus syndrome characterized by recurrent fever, myalgia, arthralgia, pleuritis, pulmonary infiltrates, pericarditis, myocarditis, and mitochondrial antibodies in the absence of nuclear antibodies after prolonged treatment.[115,116] Venocuran has since been withdrawn from the market; however, the nature of its pathophysiologic action is still unknown.

Like *A hippocastanum, Ruscus aculeatus* (butcher's broom) is also known for its use in treating venous insufficiency. *Ruscus aculeatus* is a short evergreen shrub found commonly in the Mediterranean region. Two steroidal saponins, ruscogenin and neurogenin, extracted from the rhizomes of *R aculeatus* are thought to be its active components.[101] In vivo studies on hamster cheek pouch reveal that topical *Ruscus* extract dose dependently antagonizes histamine-induced increases in vascular permeability.[117] Moreover, topical *Ruscus* extract causes dose-dependent constriction of venules without appreciably affecting arterioles.[118] Topical *Ruscus* extract's vascular effects are also temperature dependent and appear to counter the sympathetic nervous system's temperature-sensitive vascular regulation: venules dilate at a lower temperature (25°C), constrict at near physiologic temperatures (36.5°C), and further constrict at higher temperatures (40°C); arterioles dilate at 25°C, are unaffected at 36.5°C, and remain unaffected or constrict at 40°C, depending on *Ruscus* concentration.[119] Based on the influence of prazosin, diltiazem, and rauwolscine, the peripheral vascular effects of *Ruscus* extract appear to be selectively mediated by effects on calcium channels and α_1-adrenergic receptors with less activity at α_2-adrenergic receptors.[117,118] Also, *R aculeatus* exhibits strong antielastase activity and has little effect on hyaluronidase in direct contrast to *A hippocastanum*. This activity may contribute to their efficacy in the treatment of venous insufficiency since these enzyme systems are involved in the turnover of the main components of the perivascular amorphous substance.[102]

Several small clinical trials using topical *Ruscus* extract support its role in treating venous insufficiency. One randomized, double-blind, placebo-controlled trial involving 18 volunteers showed a beneficial decrease in femoral vein diameter (median decrease, 1.25 mm) using duplex B-scan ultrasonography. The decrease was measured 2.5 hours after applying 4 to 6 g of a cream containing 64 to 96 mg of *Ruscus* extract.[120] In another small trial (N=18) it was shown that topical *Ruscus* extract may be helpful in reducing venous dilation during pregnancy.[121] Oral agents may be useful as topical drugs for venous insufficiency, although the evidence is less convincing.[122]

Although capsule, tablet, ointment, and suppository (for hemorrhoids) preparations of *Ruscus* extract are available in Europe, only capsules are available in the United States. These capsules contain 75 mg of *Ruscus* extract and 2 mg of rosemary oil.[101] Aside from occasional nausea and gastritis, adverse effects from using *R aculeatus* have rarely been reported, even in high doses.[57] Nevertheless, one should be wary of any drug that has not been thoroughly tested. Although there is ample evidence to support the pharmacological activity of *R aculeatus*, there is still a relative deficiency of clinical data to establish its actual safety and efficacy. Until more studies are completed, no recommendations regarding dosage can be offered.

Arrhythmia

In traditional Chinese medicine, arrhythmias are categorized by the characteristic symptoms of palpitations and abnormal pulse. Numerous Chinese herbal medicines are identified to have antiarrhythmic effects, such as xin bao, ci zhu wan, bu xin dan, and several others.[123] However, few clinical trials have been conducted to study their effects and safety. Xin bao is one agent that has begun to be examined. The mechanism of action of xin bao is thought to be through its stimulation and increased excitability of the sinuatrial node.[124] In one observational study, the effects of xin bao were documented in 87 patients with sick sinus syndrome. Xin bao was administered orally 2 to 3 times per day for 2 months. Patients with major symptoms of sick sinus syndrome, which included dizziness, palpitations, and chest pressure, improved significantly after treatment.[124] No serious adverse effects were noted. This study suggests a possible role of xin bao in the treatment of sick sinus syndrome. However, more scientific research on xin bao and other antiarrhythmic Chinese herbs mentioned previously are necessary before any recommendations can be made for their routine use in patients with sick sinus syndrome or other arrhythmias.

Comment

With the high prevalence of herbal medicine use in the United States, health practitioners should remember to inquire about such health practices when taking clinical histories and remain informed of the beneficial or harmful effects of these treatments. Continuing research is necessary to elucidate the pharmacological activities of the many cardiopotent herbal medicines and to stimulate future pharmaceutical development of therapeutically beneficial herbal drugs. However, such research is currently lacking in the United States and requires more support from government agencies before the full potential of these types of treatments can be determined. At the same time, legal surveillance of herbal medicine use with low safety margins should be instituted for the sake of public health; this is especially imperative for those herbs with adverse cardiovascular reactions[125] and drug interactions. As more information becomes available regarding the safety and efficacy of herbal medicines through new clinical trials, research-supported claims may one day become available to consumers and physicians in a manner similar to the allopathic medicines.

References

1. Wu B-N, Huang Y-C, Wu H-M, Hong S-J, Chiang L-C, Chen I-J. A highly selective (α_1-adrenergic blocker with partial β_2 agonist activity derived from ferulic acid, an active component of *Ligusticum wallichii* Franch. *J Cardiovasc Pharmacol.* 1998;31:750–757.
2. Eisenberg DM, Kessler RC, Foster C, et al. Unconventional medicine in the United States. *N Engl J Med.* 1993;328:246–252.
3. Astin JA. Why patients use alternative medicine: results of a national study. *JAMA.* 1998; 279:1548–1553.
4. Ernst E: Harmless herbs. a review of the recent literature. *Am J Med.* 1998;104:170–178.
5. Tyler VE. *Herbs of Choice: The Therapeutic Use of Phytomedicinals.* New York, NY: Pharmaceutical Product Press; 1994.
6. Stuhlemmer U, Kreis W, Eisenbeiss M, Reinhard E. Cardiac glycosides in partly submerged shoots of *Digitalis lanata. Planta Med.* 1993; 59:539–545.
7. Dickstein ES, Kunkel FW. Foxglove tea poisoning. *Am J Med.* 1980;69:167–169.
8. Radford DJ, Gillies AD, Hinds JA, Duffy P. Naturally occurring cardiac glycosides. *Med J Aust.* 1986;144:540–544.
9. Cheung K, Hinds JA, Duffy P. Detection of poisoning by plant-origin cardiac glycoside with the Abbott Tdx analyzer. *Clin Chem.* 1989; 35:295–297.
10. Moxley RA, Schneider NR, Steinegger DH, Carlson MP. Apparent toxicosis associated with lily-of-the-valley (*Convallaria majalis*) ingestion in a dog. *J Am Vet Med Assoc.* 1989; 195:485–487.

11. Bossi M, Brambilla G, Cavilla A, et al. Threatening arrhythmia by uncommon digitalic toxicosis [in Italian]. *G Ital Cardiol.* 1981; 11:2254–2257.

12. Hayes BE, Bessen HA, Wightman WD. Oleander tea: herbal draught of death. *Ann Emerg Med.* 1985;14:350–353.

13. Ansford AJ, Morris H. Fatal oleander poisoning. *Med J Aust.* 1981;1:360–361.

14. Shaw D, Pearn J. Oleander poisoning. *Med J Aust.* 1979;2:267–269.

15. Tumcok Y, Kozan O, Cadvar C, et al. Urginea maritima (squill) toxicity. *J Toxicol Clin Toxicol.* 1995;33:83–86.

16. Bagrov AY, Roukoyatkina NI, Pinaev AG, Dmitrieva RI. Effects of two endogenous Na+, K(+)-ATPase inhibitors, marinobufagenin and ouabain, on isolated rat aorta. *Eur J Pharmacol.* 1995;274:151–158.

17. Nishoka SA, Resende ES. Transitory complete atrioventricular block associated to ingestion of *Nerium oleander. Rev Assoc Med Bras.* 1995; 41:60–62.

18. Rich SA, Libera JM, Locke RJ. Treatment of foxglove extract poisoning with digoxin-specific Fab fragments. *Ann Emerg Med.* 1993; 22:1904–1907.

19. Safadi R, Levy I, Amitai Y, Caraco Y. Beneficial effect of digoxin-specific Fab antibody fragments in oleander intoxication. *Arch Intern Med.* 1995;155:2121–2125.

20. Galey FD, Holstege DM, Plumlee KH, et al. Diagnosis of oleander poisoning in livestock. *J Vet Diagn Invest.* 1996;8:358–364.

21. Langford SD, Boor PJ. Oleander toxicity: an examination of human and animal toxic exposure. *Toxicology.* 1996;109:1–13.

22. McRae S. Elevated serum digoxin levels in a patient taking digoxin and Siberian ginseng. *CMAJ.* 1996;155:293–295.

23. Geehr E. Common toxic plant ingestions. *Emerg Med Clin North Am.* 1984;2:553–563.

24. Litovitz TL, Clark LR, Soloway RA. 1993 Annual Report of the American Association of Poison Control Centers Toxic Exposure Surveillance System. *Am J Emerg Med.* 1993;12:546–584.

25. Szabuniewicz M, McGrady JD, Camp BJ. Treatment of experimentally induced oleander poisoning. *Arch Int Pharmcodyn.* 1971;189:12–21.

26. Osterloh J, Herold S, Pond S. Oleander interference in the digoxin radioimmunoassay in a fatal ingestion. *JAMA.* 1982;247:1596–1597.

27. Oates JA. Antihypertensive agents and the drug therapy of hypertension. In: Hardman JG, Limbird LE, Molinoff PB, et al, eds. *Goodman and Gilman's The Pharmacological Basis of Therapeutics.* 9th ed. New York, NY: McGraw-Hill Book Co; 1996:781–808.

28. Rauwolfia alkaloids. *USP DI: Drug Information for the Health Care Professional.* Vol 1. 18th ed. Rockville, Md: US Pharmacopeial Convention; 1998:2486.

29. *Physician's Desk Reference.* 43rd ed. Montvale, NJ: Medical Economics Co; 1989:1648.

30. Brunton LL. Agents affecting gastrointestinal water flux, emesis and antiemetics, bile acids and pancreatic enzymes. In: Hardman JG, Limbird LE, Molinoff PB, et al, eds. *Goodman and Gilman's The Pharmacological Basis of Therapeutics.* 9th ed. New York, NY: McGraw-Hill Book Co; 1996:917–936.

31. Sutter MC, Wang YX. Recent cardiovascular drugs from Chinese medicinal plants. *Cardiovasc Res.* 1993;27:1891–1901.

32. Rossier MF, Python CP, Capponi AM, et al. Blocking T-type calcium channels with tetrandrine inhibits steroidogenesis in bovine adrenal glomerulosa cells. *Endocrinology.* 1993; 132:1035–1043.

33. Kawashima K, Hayakawa T, Miwa Y, et al. Structure and hypotensive activity relationships of tetrandrine derivatives in stroke-prone spontaneously hypertensive rats. *Gen Pharmacol.* 1990;21:343–347.

34. Vanherweghem JL. A new form of nephropathy secondary to the absorption of Chinese herbs [in French]. *Bull Mem Acad R Med Belg.* 1994; 149:128–135.

35. Schmeiser HH, Bieler CA, Wiessler M, Van Ypersele DE, Strihou C, Cosyns JP. Detection of DNA adducts formed by aristolochic acid in renal tissue from patients with Chinese herbs nephropathy. *Cancer Res.* 1996;56:2025–2028.

36. Bieler CA, Stiborova M, Wiessler M, et al. 32P-post-labelling analysis of DNA adducts formed by aristolochic acid in tissues from patients with Chinese herbs nephropathy. *Carcinogenesis.* 1997;18:1063–1067.

37. Violin C. Belgian (Chinese herb) nephropathy: why? *J Pharm Belg.* 1997;52:7–27.

38. Ody P. *The Complete Medicinal Herbal.* New York, NY: Dorling Kindersley; 1993.

39. Kuramochi T, Chu J, Suga T. Gou-teng (from *Uncaria rhynchophylla* Miquel)-induced endothelium-dependent and -independent relaxations in the isolated rat aorta. *Life Sci.* 1994;54:2061–2069.

40. Jaffe AM, Gephardt D, Courtemanche L. Poisoning due to ingestion of *Veratrum viride* (false hellebore). *J Emerg Med.* 1990; 8:161–167.

41. Quatrehomme G, Bertrand F, Chauvet C, Ollier A. Intoxication from *Veratrum album. Hum Exp Toxicol.* 1993;12:111–115.

42. Festa M, Andreeto B, Ballaris MA, Panio A, Piervittori R. Un caso di avvelenamento da Veratro. *Minerva Anestesiol.* 1996; 62:195–196.

43. Chiou W-F, Shum AY-C, Liao J-F, Chen C-F. Studies of the cellular mechanisms underlying the vasorelaxant effects of rutaecarpine, a bioactive component extracted from an herbal drug. *J Cardiovasc Pharmacol.* 1997; 29:490–498.

44. Bahorun T, Trotin F, Pommery J, et al. Antioxidant activities of *Crataegus monogyna* extracts. *Planta Med.* 1994;60:323–328.

45. Vibes J, Lasserre B, Gleye J, et al. Inhibition of thromboxane A2 biosynthesis in vitro by the main components of *Crataegus oxyacantha* (Hawthorn) flower heads. *Prostaglandins Leukot Essent Fatty Acids.* 1994;50:173–175.

46. Shanthi S, Parasakthy K, Deepalakshmi PD, Devaraj SN. Hypolipidemic activity of tincture of *Crataegus* in rats. *Indian J Biochem Biophys.* 1994;31:143–146.

47. Rajerdan S, Deepalakshmi PD, Parasakthy K, Devaraj H, Devaraj SN. Effect of tincture of *Crataegus* on the LDL-receptor activity of hepatic plasma membrane of rats fed an atherogenic diet. *Atherosclerosis.* 1996;123:235–241.

48. Nasa Y, Hashizume H, Hoque AN, Abiko Y. Protective effect of *Crataegus* extract on the the cardiac mechanical dysfunction in isolated perfused working rat heart. *Arzneimittelforschung.* 1993;43:945–949.

49. Roddweig C, Hensel H. Reaction of local myocardial blood flow in nonanesthesized dogs and anesthesized cats to the oral and parenteral administration of a *Crataegus* fraction (oligomere procyanidines) [in German]. *Arzneimittelforschung.* 1977;27:1407–1410.

50. Taskov M. On the coronary and cardiotonic action of *crataegus. Acta Physiol Pharmacol Bulg.* 1997;3:53–57.

51. Blesken R. *Crataegus* in cardiology [in German]. *Fortschr Med.* 1992;110:290–292.

52. Petkov V. Plants and hypotensive, antiatheromatous and coronarodilating action. *Am J Chin Med.* 1979;7:197–236.

53. Weikl A, Assmus KD, Neukum-Schmidt A, et al. *Crataegus* special extract WS 1442: assessment of objective effectiveness in patients with heart failure (NYHA II). *Fortschr Med.* 1996; 114:291–296.

54. Schussler M, Holzl J, Fricke U. Myocardial effects of flavonoids from *Crataegus* species. *Arzneimittelforschung.* 1995;45:842–845.

55. Joseph G, Zhao Y, Klaus W. Pharmacologic action profile of *Crataegus* extract in comparison to epinephrine, amirinone, milrinone, and digoxin in the isolated perfused guinea pig heart [in German]. *Arzneimittelforschung.* 1995;45:1261–1265.

56. Popping S, Rose H, Ionescu I, Fischer Y, Kammermeier H. Effect of a hawthorn extract on contraction and energy turnover of isolated rat cardiomyocytes. *Arzneimittelforschung.* 1995;45:1157–1161.

57. Mawrey DB. *Herbal Tonic Therapies.* New Canaan, Conn: Keats Publishing Inc; 1993.

58. Kwan CY. Vascular effects of selected antihypertensive drugs derived from traditional medicinal herbs. *Clin Exp Pharmacol Physiol.* 1995; 22:297–299.

59. Zhang W, Wojta J, Binder BR. Effect of notoginsenoside R1 on the synthesis of tissue-type plasminogen activator and plasminogen activator inhibitor-1 in cultured human umbilical vein endothelial cells. *Arterioscler Thromb Vasc Biol.* 1994;14:1040–1046.

60. Lin SG, Zheng XL, Chen QY, Sun JJ. Effect of *Panax notoginseng* saponins on increased proliferation of cultured aortic smooth muscle cells stimulated by hypercholestoremic serum. *Chung Kuo Yao Li Hsueh Pao.* 1993;14:314–316.

61. Lei XL, Chiou GC. Cardiovascular pharmacology of *Panax notoginseng* (Burk) FH Chen and *Salvia miltiorrhiza. Am J Chin Med.* 1986; 14:145–152.

62. Wang Z, Roberts JM, Grant PG, et al. The effect of a medicinal Chinese herb on platelet function. *Thromb Haemost.* 1982;48:301–306.

63. Yagi A, Fujimoto K, Tanonaka K, et al. Possible active components of tan-shen (*Salvia miltiorrhiza*) for protection of the myocardium against ischemia-induced derangements. *Planta Med.* 1989;55:51–54.

64. Zhao BL, Jiang W, Zhao Y, Hou JW, Xin WJ. Scavenging effects of *Salvia miltiorrhiza* on free radicals and its protection for myocardial mitochondrial membranes from ischemia-reperfusion injury. *Biochem Mol Biol Int.* 1996; 38:1171–1182.

65. Chan K, Lo AC, Yeung JH, Woo KS. The effects of Danshen (*Salvia miltiorrhiza*) on warfarin pharmacodynamics and pharmacokinetics of warfarin enantiomers in rats. *J Pharm Pharmacol.* 1995;47:402–406.

66. Kleijnen J, Knipschild P, Ter Riet G. Garlic, onions and cardiovascular risk factors: a review of the evidence from human experiments with emphasis on commercially available preparations. *Br J Clin Pharmacol.* 1989;28:535–544.

67. Steiner M, Khan AH, Holbert D, Lin RI. A double-blind cross-over study in hypercholesterolemic men that compared the effect of aged garlic extract and placebo administration on blood lipids. *Am J Clin Nutr.* 1996; 63:866–870.

68. Silagy CA, Neil HA. A meta-analysis of the effect of garlic on blood pressure. *J Hypertens.* 1994;12:463–468.

69. Silagy C, Neil A. Garlic as a lipid lowering agent: a meta-analysis. *J R Coll Physicians Lond.* 1994; 28:39–45.

70. Kendler BS. Garlic (*Allium sativum*) and onion (*Allium cepa*): a review of their relationship to cardiovascular disease. *Prev Med.* 1987; 16:670–685.

71. Isaacsohn JL, Moser M, Stein EA, et al. Garlic powder and plasma lipids and lipoproteins: a multicenter, randonized, plcebo-controlled trial. *Arch Intern Med.* 1998;158:1189–1194.

72. Jain AK, Vargas R, Gotzkowsky S, McMahon FG. Can garlic reduce levels of serum lipids? a controlled clinical study. *Am J Med.*1993; 94:632–635.

73. Neil HA, Silagy CA, Lancaster T, et al. Garlic powder in the treatment of moderate hyperlipidaemia: a controlled trial and meta-analyses. *J R Coll Physicians Lond.* 1996;30:329–334.

74. Simons LA, BalaSubramaniam S, Von Konigsmark M, Parfitt A, Simons J, Peters W. On the effect of garlic on plasma lipids and lipoproteins in mild hypercholesterolemia. *Atherosclerosis.* 1995;113:219–225.

75. Bordia A, Verma SK, Srivastava KC. Effect of garlic on platelet aggregation in humans: a study in healthy subjects and patients with coronary artery disease. *Prostaglandins Leukot Essent Fatty Acids.* 1996;55:201–205.

76. Ali M, Thomson M. Consumption of a garlic clove a day could be beneficial in preventing thrombosis. *Prostaglandins Leuko Essent Fatty Acids.* 1995;53:211–212.

77. Breithaupt-Grogler K, Ling M, Boudoulas H, Beliz GG. Protective effect of chronic garlic intake on elastic properties of aorta in the elderly. *Circulation.* 1997;96:2649–2655.

78. Mader FH. Treatment of hyperlipidaemia with garlic powder tablets: evidence from the German Association of General Practitioners' Multicentric Placebo-Controlled Double-Blind Study. *Arzneimittelforschung.* 1990; 40:1111–1116.

79. Delaney TA, Donnelley AM. Garlic dermatitis. *Australas J Dermatol.* 1996;37:109–110.

80. Rose KD, Croissant PD, Parliament CF, Levin MB. Spontaneous spinal epidural hematoma with associated liver dysfunction from excessive garlic ingestion: a case report. *Neurosurgery.* 1990;26:880–882.

81. Singh V, Kaul S, Chander R, Kapoor NK. Stimulation of low density lipoprotein receptor activity in liver membrane of guggulsterone treated rats. *Pharmacol Res.* 1990;22:37–44.

82. Nityanand S, Srivastava JS, Asthana OP. Clinical trials with gugulipid: a new hypolipidemic agent. *J Assoc Physicians India.* 1989; 37:323–328.

83. Sing RB, Niaz MA, Ghosh S. Hypolipidemic and antioxidant effects of *Commiphora mukul* as an adjunct to dietary therapy in patients with hypercholesterolemia. *Cardiovasc Drugs Ther.* 1994;8:654–664.

84. Dalvi SS, Nayak VK, Pohujani SM, Desai NK, Kshirsagar NA, Gupta KC. Effect of gugulipid on bioavailability of diltiazem and propranolol. *J Assoc Physicians India.* 1994;42:454–455.

85. Sundaram V, Hanna AN, Lubow GP, Koneru L, Falko JM, Sharma HM. Inhibition of low-density lipoprotein oxidation by oral herbal mixtures *Maharishi Amrit Kalash*-4 and *Maharishi Amrit Kalash*-5 in hyperlipidemic patients. *Am J Med Sci.* 1997;314:303–310.

86. Huxtable RJ. The pharmacology of extinction. *J Ethnopharmacol.* 1992;37:1–11.

87. Z'Brun A. Ginkgo: myth and reality [in German]. *Schweiz Rundsch Med Prax.* 1995;84:1–6.

88. Kleinjen J, Knipschild P. *Ginkgo biloba* for cerebral insufficiency. *Br J Clin Pharmacol.* 1992; 34:352–358.

89. Allard M. Treatment of the disorders of aging with *Ginkgo biloba* extract [in French]. *Presse Med.* 1986;15:1540–1545.

90. LeBars PL, Katz MM, Berman N, et al, for the North American Study Group. A placebo-controlled, double-blind, randomized trial of an extract of *Ginkgo biloba* for dementia. *JAMA.* 1997;278:1327–1332.

91. Doly M, Droy-Lefaix MT, Braquet P. Oxidative stress in diabetic retina. *EXS.* 1992; 62:299–307.

92. Mouren X, Calliard P, Schwartz F. Study of the antiischemic action of EGb 761 in the treatment of peripheral arterial occlusive disease by $TcPO_2$ determination. *Angiology.* 1994; 45:413–417.

93. Tosaki A, Droy-Lefaix MT, Pali T, Das DK. Effects of SOD, catalase, and a novel antiarrhythmic drug, Egb 761, on reperfusion-induced arrhythmias in isolated rat hearts. *Free Radic Biol Med.* 1993;14:361–370.

94. Haramaki N, Aggarwal S, Kawabata T, Droy-Lefaix MT, Packer L. Effects of natural antioxidant EGb 761 on myocardial ischemia-reperfusion injury. *Free Radic Biol Med.* 1994;16:789–794.

95. Pietri S, Seguin JR, D'Arbigny P, Drieu K, Culcasi M. Egb 761 pretreatment limits free radical-induced oxidative stress in patients undergoing coronary bypass surgery. *Cardiovasc Drugs Ther.* 1997;11:121–131.

96. Offord EA, Mace K, Ruffieux C, et al. Rosemary components inhibit benzo[a]pyrene induced genotoxicity in human bronchial cells. *Carcinogenesis.* 1995;16:2057–2062.

97. Haraguchi H, Saito T, Okamura N, Yagi A. Inhibition of lipid peroxidation and superoxide generation by diterpenoids from Rosmarinus officinalis. *Planta Med.* 1995;61:333–336.

98. Larrondo JV, Agut M, Calvo-Torras MA. Antimicrobial activity of essences from labiates. *Microbios.* 1995;82:171–172.

99. Al-Hader AA, Hasan ZA, Aqel MB. Hyperglycemic and insulin release inhibitory effects of *Rosmarinus officinalis. J Ethnopharmacol.* 1994;43:217–221.

100. Swan AR, Dutton SP, Truswell AS. Salicylates in foods. *J Am Diet Assoc.* 1985;85:950–960.

101. Tyler VE. *The Honest Herbal: A Sensible Guide to the Use of Herbs and Related Remedies.* 3rd ed. New York, NY: Pharmaceutical Product Press; 1993.

102. Facino RM, Carini M, Stefani R, Aldini G, Saibene L. Anti-elastase and anti-hyaluronidase activities of saponins and sapogenins from *Hedera helix, Aesculus hippocastanum,* and *Ruscus aculeatus:* factors contributing to their efficacy in the treatment of venous insufficiency. *Arch Pharm (Weinheim).* 1995; 328:720–724.

103. Guillaume M, Padioleau F. Veinotonic effect, vascular protection, antiinflammatory and free radical scavenging properties of horse chestnut extract. *Arzneimittelforschung.* 1994; 44:25–35.

104. Rothkopf M, Vogel G. New findings on the efficacy and mode of action of the horse chestnut saponin escin [in German]. *Arzneimittelforschung.* 1976;26:225–235.

105. Diehm C, Vollbrecht, Amendt K, Comberg HU. Medical edema protection: clinical benefit in patients with chronic deep vein incompetence: a placebo controlled double-blind study. *Vasa.* 1992;21:188–192.

106. Bisler H, Pfeifer R, Kluken N, Pauschinger P. Effects of horse chestnut seed extract on transcapillary filtration in chronic venous insufficiency [in German]. *Dtsch Med Wochenschr.* 1986; 111:1321–1329.

107. Diehm C, Trampisch HJ, Lange S, Schmidt C. Comparison of leg compression stocking and oral horse chestnut seed extract therapy in patients with chronic venous insufficiency. *Lancet.* 1996;347:292–294.

108. Greeske K, Pohlmann BK. Horse chestnut seed extract: an effective therapy principle in general practice: drug therapy in chronic venous insufficiency [in German]. *Fortschr Med.* 1996; 114:196–200.

109. Schorr DM, Gruber UF. Prophylaxis of thromboembolic complications in gynecological surgery [in German]. *Geburtshilfe Frauenheilkd.* 1977;37:291–296.

110. Lang W. Studies on the percutaneous absorption of 3H-aescin in pigs. *Res Exp Med (Berl).* 1977;169:175–187.

111. Takegoshi K, Tohyama T, Okunda K, et al. A case of Venoplant-induced hepatic injury. *Gastroenterol Jpn.* 1986;21:62–65.

112. Voigt E, Junger H. Acute posttraumatic renal failure following therapy with antibiotics and beta-aescin [in German]. *Anaesthesist.* 1978; 27:81–83.

113. Hellberg K, Ruschewski W, De Vivie R. Drug induced acute renal failure after heart surgery [in German]. *Thoraxchir Vask Chir.* 1975; 23:396–399.

114. Lang W. Dialysability of aescin [in German]. *Arzneimittelforschung.* 1984;34:221–223.

115. Grob PJ, Muller-Schoop JW, Hacki MA, Joller-Jemelka HI. Drug-induced pseudolupus. *Lancet.* 1975;2:144–148.

116. Walli F, Grob PJ, Muller-Schoop J. Pseudo-(venocuran-) lupus: a minor episode in the history of medicine [in German]. *Schweiz Med Wochenschr.* 1981;111:1398–1405.

117. Bouskela E, Cyrino FZ, Marcelon G. Possible mechanisms for the inhibitory effect of Ruscus extract on increased microvascular permeability induced by histamine in hamster cheek pouch. *J Cardiovasc Pharmacol.* 1994;24:281–285.

118. Bouskela E, Cyrino FZ, Marcelon G. Possible mechanisms for the venular constriction elicited by Ruscus extract on hamster cheek pouch. *J Cardiovasc Pharmacol.* 1994; 24:165–170.

119. Bouskela E, Cyrino FZ, Marcelon G. Effects of Ruscus extract on the internal diameter of arterioles and venules of the hamster cheek pouch microcirculation. *J Cardiovasc Pharmacol.* 1993; 22:221–224.

120. Berg D. Venous constriction by local administration of ruscus extract [in German]. *Fortschr Med.* 1990;108:473–476.

121. Berg D. Venous tonicity in pregnancy varicose veins [in German]. *Fortschr Med.* 1992; 110:67–68,71–72.

122. Weindorf N, Schultz-Ehrenburg U. Controlled study of increasing venous tone in primary varicose veins by oral administration of *Ruscus aculeatus* and trimethylhespiridinchalcone [in German]. *Z Hautkr.* 1987;62:28–38.

123. Zhou ZY, Jin HD. *Clinical Manual of Chinese Herbal Medicine.* New York, NY: Churchill Livingstone Inc; 1997.

124. Chen ZY. Use of Xin Bao in the treatment of 87 patients with sick sinus syndrome. *Chin Modern Develop Trad Med.* 1990;10:529–531.

125. Jones TK, Lawson BM. Profound neonatal congestive heart failure caused by maternal consumption of blue cohosh herbal medication. *J Pediatr.* 1998;132:550–552.

34 Echinacea Root Extracts for the Prevention of Upper Respiratory Tract Infections

A Double-blind, Placebo-Controlled Randomized Trial

Dieter Melchart, MD; Ellen Walther; Klaus Linde, MD; Roland Brandmaier, MD; Christian Lersch, MD, PhD

From the Center for Complementary Medicine Research (Drs Melchart and Linde and Ms Walther) and Medizinische Klinik, Technische Universität (Dr Lersch); and Biometrisches Zentrum für Therapiestudien (Dr Brandmaier), Munich, Germany.

Objective

To investigate the safety and efficacy of 2 extracts of echinacea for preventing upper respiratory tract infections.

Design

Three-armed, randomized, double-blind, placebo-controlled trial.

Setting

Four military institutions and 1 industrial plant.

Participants

Three hundred two volunteers without acute illness at time of enrollment.

Interventions

Ethanolic extract from *Echinacea purpurea* roots, *Echinacea angustifolia* roots, or placebo, given orally for 12 weeks.

Main Outcome Measure

Time until the first upper respiratory tract infection (time to event). Secondary outcome measures were the number of participants with at least 1 infection, global assessment, and adverse effects.

Results

The time until occurrence of the first upper respiratory tract infection was 66 days (95% confidence interval [CI], 61–72 days) in the *E angustifolia* group, 69 days (95% CI, 64–74 days) in the *E purpurea* group, and 65 days (95% CI, 59–70 days) in the placebo group (*P*=.49). In the placebo group, 36.7% had an infection. In the treatment groups, 32.0% in the *E angustifolia* group (relative risk compared with placebo, 0.87; 95% CI, 0.59–1.30) and 29.3% in the *E purpurea* group (relative risk compared with placebo, 0.80; 95% CI, 0.53–1.31) had an infection. Participants in the treatment groups believed that they had more benefit from the med-

ication than those in the placebo group (*P*=.04). Adverse effects were reported by 18 subjects in the *E angustifolia* group, 10 in the *E purpurea* group, and 11 in the placebo group.

Conclusion

In this study a prophylactic effect of the investigated echinacea extracts could not be shown. However, based on the results of this and 2 other studies, one could speculate that there might be an effect of echinacea products in the order of magnitude of 10% to 20% relative risk reduction. Future studies with much larger sample sizes would be needed to prove this effect.

Arch Fam Med. 1998;7:541–545

Herbal medicines have widespread use all over the world. It has been estimated that in 1994, Europe spent $6 billion, Japan spent $2.1 billion, and the United States and Canada spent $1.5 billion on herbal medicine.[1] One of the most popular medicinal plants is echinacea (family Compositae). The use of echinacea goes back to the North American Indians, who used it both topically and in systemic administration for ailments such as burns, snakebites, pain, cough, and sore throat.[2] Nowdays, echinacea is most often used for treating and preventing uncomplicated upper respiratory tract infections such as the common cold.

Most people, including many physicians, are not aware that products commonly summarized under the name echinacea can be chemically completely different preparations. This is due to (1) the use of 3 different species of echinacea (*Echinacea purpurea, Echinacea pallida,* and *Echinacea angustifolia*); (2) the use of different plant parts (herb, roots, or both); (3) different methods of extraction (pressed juice, alcoholic extraction); and (4) the addition of other plant extracts. Depending on these factors, echinacea products can contain highly variable amounts of a variety of bioactive ingredients including caffeic acids, alkamids, polysaccharides, and glycoproteins.[3] While several studies have shown in vitro and in vivo effects on immunological parameters,[3] a clear mechanism of action or a single active principle has not been identified so far.

Despite widespread use, the efficacy of echinacea products is controversial.[4] In Germany the evaluation committee for herbal products at the former German Federal Institute for Drugs, the Commission E, has published positive assessments for 2 echinacea preparations, *E purpurea* herb and *E pallida* root, while the evidence for other extracts was seen as insufficient.[5] Data on which these assessments are based are not fully accessible. A systematic review in 1994 identified a total of 26 controlled clinical trials.[6] Overall there seemed to be some evidence that echinacea products can be effective for immunomodulation, but the quality of most of the available trials was insufficient.

Unspecific upper respiratory tract infections (common cold) are a major source of morbidity worldwide and additional effective methods for their prevention and treatment would be valuable. In Germany the use of echinacea products for these purposes is widespread.[7] Three randomized trials have been previously published that investigated the preventative action of 3 different echinacea products (2 of them combinations with other plant extracts).[8–10] One of the trials had found a statistically significant effect over placebo,[8] 1 found a trend,[9] and 1 had a nonsignificant result.[10] Our objective was to investigate if 2 extracts from the roots of *E angustifolia* and *E purpurea,* which form part of a variety of products that are marketed in Germany but have not been subjected to randomized clinical trials, are more effective than placebo in the prevention of upper respiratory tract infections in healthy volunteers.

Participants and Methods

Design

The study was randomized (stratified for participants with up to 3 and more than 3 colds in the last year; computer-generated randomization list, block size 15; concealment by consecutively numbered medication), double-blind, and placebo-controlled. The study was approved by the local ethics committee and performed according to the guidelines for good clinical practice in the European Union.

Setting and Recruitment

The study was performed at 4 military sites (1 university, 1 health service school, and 2 regular military bases) and 1 industrial plant in and around the city of Munich, Germany. Information on the study was spread through posters and information events; interested persons were asked to contact the study center to arrange a date for individual information and the eligibility checkup.

Participants

Volunteers aged 18 to 65 years and free of acute illness at the time of enrollment and who gave written informed consent could participate. Exclusion criteria were as follows: acute respiratory tract infection or other infections within the last 7 days; serious progressive disease such as tuberculosis, multiple sclerosis, or acquired immunodeficiency syndrome; systemic intake of corticosteroids, antibiotics, or immunostimulants in the previous 2 weeks; allergy to the Compositae family; and in the case of women, pregnancy. Participants were recruited in the winter of 1993-1994 (centers 1 and 2) and the winter of 1994-1995. They did not receive payment for their participation.

Interventions

Participants were instructed to take 50 drops (about 20 µL equals 1 drop) of the trial preparation 2 times daily for 12 weeks from Monday to Friday. The trial preparation was packaged in 100-mL brown glass bottles that were filled either with ethanolic extracts (plant extract ratio 1:11 in 30% alcohol) from the roots of *E angustifolia, E purpurea,* or placebo (colored ethanolic solution).

Evaluation

At the time of study enrollment subject characteristics (Table 1) were documented and the participants were asked to fill out 2 questionnaires regarding quality of life (Profile of Mood States [German version][11] and Activities of Daily Living[12]). Subjects who reported more than 3 upper respiratory tract infections in the previous 12 months were offered additional blood samples (obtained between 7 and 9 AM) for white blood cell counts and measurement of lymphocyte subpopulations at baseline and after 4, 8, and 12 weeks. Control visits were scheduled after 4 and 8 weeks for handing out new medication, asking about eventual infections, and monitoring compliance and adverse effects. At the final visit patients were asked if they believed that they benefited from the medication, were questioned about tolerability, and completed a second quality of life questionnaire. In the second recruitment phase (centers 3-5) a question was added in which the patients were asked whether they believed that they received the true treatment or the placebo.

The participants had to contact the study physicians in case of any symptoms of an upper respiratory tract infection. The physician documented findings (regarding lymph nodes, throat, tongue, and temperature) and the symptoms reported by the patients (runny nose, cough, headache, pains in legs and arms, pain in throat or ears, shivering or sweating, well-being, and ability to perform normal activities) on a 4-step scale using a standardized form. To be classified as an upper respiratory tract infection at least 2 mild symptoms or 1 moderate symptom had to be present and the clinical picture had to fit the diagnosis according to the physician. The severity of the infection was classified subjectively by the physician as well as retrospectively based on the symptom scores. All necessary treatments had to be documented. Patients were given a symptom diary to evaluate the duration of symptoms. Participants who did not present immediately in case of an infection but reported an episode at 1 of the control visits were asked to rate the maximum intensity of their symptoms retrospectively and give the dates when the infection occurred.

Sample Size Calculation

For reasons of sensitivity the time until occurrence of the first upper respiratory tract infection (time to event) was predetermined as the primary outcome measure for the statistical analysis instead of the number of patients with at least 1 infectious episode (incidence or relative risk, which were considered to be the most clinically relevant outcomes). A sample size calculation was performed using the nomogram by Day and Graham.[13] Under the assumption that an infection would occur in 40% of placebo subjects and in 25% of the treatment groups, the required sample size per group was 125 (α=.05, β=.20). Assuming a dropout rate of about 20%, the total sample size was aimed at 450.

Statistical Analysis

Data were analyzed under blind conditions for 3 populations ("as randomized," "intent to treat," and "per protocol"; see Figure 1) using SAS (SAS Institute, Cary, NC) (for the main outcome measure; log rank test, intent-to-treat population) and SPSS (SPSS Inc, Chicago, Ill) software (all other data; Kruskal-Wallis and χ^2 tests for exploratory inference statistics). A predefined subgroup analysis was performed for participants who had reported more than 3 infections in the previous 12 months.

Results

A total of 302 volunteers were enrolled in the study. Seven participants only attended the enrollment date; 6 participants in 1 center dropped out of the study and the emergency envelopes with the allocation codes were broken by

Table 1. Characteristics of Participants (Intent-to-Treat Population)*

	Echinacea angustifolia (n=100)	*Echinacea purpurea* (n=99)	Placebo (n=90)
Female sex	30 (30)	21 (21)	32 (36)
Mean ± SD age, y	28.9 ± 9.6	30.5 ± 11.1	29.1 ± 10.5
Mean ± SD weight, kg	77.2 ± 13.4	76.2 ± 13.4	75.3 ± 12.1
History of chronic disease	12 (12)	13 (13)	8 (9)
Office workers	95 (95)	87 (88)	83 (93)
Smokers	29 (29)	29 (29)	28 (31)
Regular sports activity	31 (31)	30 (30)	19 (21)
Following specific diets	1 (1)	3 (3)	1 (1)
≥4 infections last year	23 (23)	22 (22)	17 (19)
Had previously taken an echinacea product	46 (47)	43 (44)	41 (46)

*All data are presented as number (percentage) unless otherwise indicated.

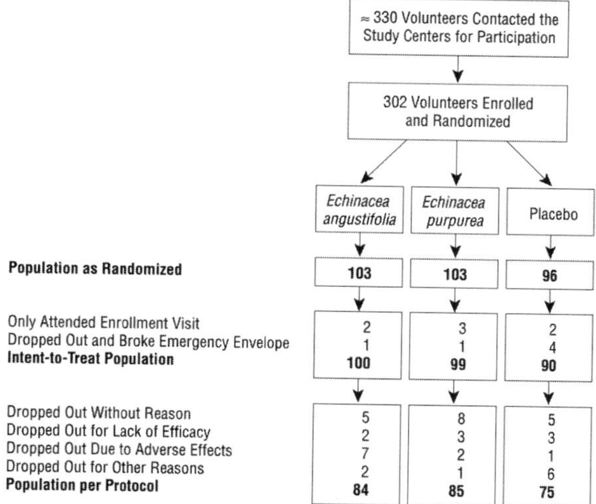

Figure 1. Trial profile.

the local study coordinator owing to a misunderstanding. These 13 volunteers were excluded from the intent-to-treat analysis, which included 289 subjects (100 in the *E angustifolia* group, 99 in the *E purpurea* group, and 90 in the placebo group; Figure 1). A further 45 participants dropped out during the trial but were included in the intent-to-treat analysis.

At baseline there were no relevant differences between the groups (Table 1). Eighty-two percent of the subjects taking *E angustifolia*, 81% of those taking *E purpurea*, and 76% of those taking placebo reported at all control visits to have taken the medication always or almost always (<3 omissions in 4 weeks; *P*=.41).

A total of 113 upper respiratory tract infections occured in 96 participants; 19 infections (17%) could only be documented retrospectively. Thirty-two percent (95% confidence interval [CI], 23%–41%) of the participants in the *E angustifolia* group had at least 1 upper respiratory tract infection compared with 29% (95% CI, 20%–38%) in the *E purpurea* group and 37% (95% CI, 27%–47%) (*P*=.55) in the placebo group. This corresponds to a relative risk (compared with placebo) of 0.87 (95% CI, 0.59–1.30) in the *E angustifolia* group and 0.80 (95% CI, 0.53–1.31) in the *E purpurea* group.

The time until occurrence of the first upper respiratory tract infection was 66 days (95% CI, 61–72 days) among participants taking *E angustifolia*, 69 days (64–74 days) in the *E purpurea* group, and 65 days (59–70 days) in the placebo group (*P*=.49). The results were very similar for the randomized (*P*=.56) and the per protocol populations (*P*=.46).

There were no significant differences between the groups in the number, severity, or duration of upper respiratory tract infections (Table 2) and quality of life. Also, there was no significant difference in the time to occurrence of infections (63 vs 60 vs 57 days, *P*=.52), white blood cell counts, or the lymphocyte subpopulations among the subgroup of participants with more than 3 infections in the previous 12 months.

More subjects in the treatment groups believed that they benefited from taking the medication (*P*=.04) and believed that they had been allocated to true treatment (*P*<.001). The proportions of subjects who correctly guessed whether they had received a true treatment or a placebo did not differ significantly between groups (*P*=.52).

Eighteen subjects in the *E angustifolia* group reported 21 adverse effects, 10 subjects in the *E purpurea* group reported 13 adverse effects, and 11 subjects in the placebo group reported 12 adverse effects (*P*=.24). None of the adverse effects were serious or required therapeutic action. Seven subjects in the *E angustifolia* group dropped out owing to adverse effects, compared with 2 subjects in the *E purpurea* group and 1 in the placebo group.

Comment

This study could not show that the investigated root extracts from *E angustifolia* and *E purpurea* have an effect over placebo in the prevention of upper respiratory tract infections in the population investigated. The proportions of participants developing an infection in the 2 treatment groups were slightly lower (corresponding to relative risk reductions of 13% for *E angustifolia* root and 20% for *E*

Table 2. Results (Intent-to-Treat Population)

	Echinacea angustifolia (n=100)	*Echinacea purpurea* (n=99)	Placebo (n=90)	*P*
Main outcome measure				
Mean (95% CI*) d to first infectious episode	66 (61-72)	69 (64-74)	65 (59-70)	.49
Secondary outcome measures				
Participants with ≥1 infection, No. (%)	32 (32)	29 (29)	33 (37)	.55
Mild infection, No. (%)	22 (69)	16 (61)	21 (64)	.85
Mean (SD) duration of infection, d	7.5 (5.0)	8.5 (5.2)	8.7 (3.6)	.29
Participants with >1 infection, No. (%)	7 (7)	4 (4.0)	6 (6.6)	.74
Believed to have had benefit, %	78	70	56	.04
Believed to have received 1 of the treatments, %	61	46	24	<.001
Correct guess whether allocated to treatment or placebo, %	61	46	50	.52
Very good or good tolerability, %	95	96	97	.79
Safety parameters				
No. of participants who reported an adverse effect	18	10	11	.24
Total No. of adverse side effects reported	21	13	12	. . .
Minor gastrointestinal symptoms	9	5	6	. . .
Headache/dizziness	9	2	1	. . .
Allergic symptoms	2	2	2	. . .
Other symptoms	1	4	3	. . .

*CI indicates confidence interval.

purpurea root) than in the placebo group, but the very large CIs indicate that this could well be chance. However, 2 of the other 3 existing randomized trials on preventative effects of echinacea products yielded very similar results (15%, *P*=.08[9] and 14%, *P*>.1[10]). The third available trial[8] showed a much larger effect (49%, *P*<.05) but suffered from severe methodological shortcomings (eg, an unclear but probably large number of randomized subjects were excluded from the analysis). The heterogeneity of the investigated products precludes a sound meta-analysis of these trials. Nonetheless, we think it is plausible to recommend that any future trials of preventive effects of echinacea products should be planned to detect effect sizes of 10% to 20% relative risk reduction. If there should be a true effect in that order of magnitude, our trial was massively undersized (a power of about 20%). This situation would have changed only slightly if we had met our original aim of recruiting 450 participants; for adequate statistical power we would have had to recruit more than 1000 participants.

The most significant result in our study was observed when we asked the participants at the end of the study to guess whether they had received 1 of the 2 true treatments or placebo. Participants in the treatment groups assumed more often that they had received a true treatment than those in the placebo group. However, the rates of participants correctly guessing whether they were in the placebo or treatment group were similar in the 3 groups. These findings are difficult to interpret. There are 2 possible explanations: (1) It might be that participants in the treatment groups truly felt more subjective benefit than those in the placebo group and, therefore, assumed more often that they had received the treatment (and the opposite in the placebo group). This would mean that the treatment was more effective than placebo on a subjective level. (2) Some participants might have found out whether the treatment they received was echinacea or placebo. Because of the characteristic taste of echinacea extracts it is almost impossible to prepare a completely indistinguishable placebo.

Unblinding is rarely discussed in clinical research.[14,15] There are no reliable procedures to quantify the degree of this problem in a trial. The mutual interactions between perceived efficacy, adverse effects, and guesses make an analysis difficult. In our trial the guesses of the participants were correct in about half of the cases (53%), wrong in about one quarter (22%), and another quarter of the participants felt unable to make a guess (25%). If one quarter of the participants made a wrong guess, it seems reasonable to expect that a similar proportion of participants made a correct guess just by chance. In consequence, unblinding due to 1 of the aforementioned reasons might have happened in about 30% of the participants. This casts further doubts on our findings. However, we think that it is a strength of our study that we tried to seriously deal with that problem instead of ignoring it.

While not reaching statistical significance, our data do suggest that the *E angustifolia* root extract might be associated with more adverse effects than the *E purpurea* root extract or placebo. Overall, tolerability was good in all 3 groups.

The fact that 45% of the participants reported trying an echinacea product at least once before participation in this study demonstrates its widespread use. Further research is therefore mandatory. However, at least in Germany, it seems unlikely that the resources needed for such research will be available. Echinacea products are prepared and marketed by many relatively small manufacturers who have neither the resources nor the know-how to sponsor and coordinate rigorous large-scale studies. The problem of standardization is also still not solved; consequently, it is very difficult to assess to what degree evidence on a specific product or even on a specific lot of one product can be extrapolated to others. Finally, as phytopharmaceuticals are generally licensed as extracts, patents for specific products are not provided unless the extract has unique features. The interest of a manufacturer to invest huge amounts of money in research whose results, in case of "success," can then easily be used by competitors is limited. In conclusion, we believe that clinical research on echinacea, at least in Germany, will remain underfunded. Unfortunately, performing rigorous trials without adequate funding is nearly impossible.

The relatively small effect sizes that can be expected, based on the available data in prevention trials, and the considerable costs of such studies raise the question of whether there would be other ways to perform clinical research on echinacea while making efficient use of the limited resources. A recent rigorous trial found that early treatment (when the patients only feel the very first symptoms of a cold) with high doses of the pressed juice of *E purpurea* herb decreased significantly the number of persons developing a "full" common cold and decreased the duration of the illness.[16] Another recent trial found similar results for a mixture of *E purpurea* herb and root.[17] This type of early treatment is widespread in self-medication and might be a more promising direction for future research.

The Center for Complementary Medicine Research is sponsored by the Bavarian Parliament. This study was partly supported by Plantapharmazie, Göttingen, Germany.

References

1. Grünwald J, Büttel K. Der europäische Markt für Phytotherapeutika. *Pharm Ind.* 1996; 58:209–214.
2. Bauer R, Wagner H. *Echinacea: Handbuch für Ärzte, Apotheker und andere Naturwissenschaftler.* Stuttgart, Germany: Wissenschaftliche Verlagsgesellschaft; 1990.
3. Bauer R, Wagner H. Echinacea species as potential immunostimulatory drugs. In: Wagner H. *Economic and Medicinal Plant Research.* London, England: Academic Press; 1991:253–321.
4. Schoenhoefer PS, Schulte-Sasse H. Sind pflanzliche Immunstimulantien wirksam und unbedenklich? *Dtsch Med Wochenschr.* 1989; 114:1804–1806.
5. Blumenthal M, Goldberg A, Gruenwald J, Hall T, Riggins CW, Rister RS, eds. *The German Commission E Monographs: Therapeutic Monographs on Medicinal Plants for Human Use.* Klein S, Rister RS, trans. Austin, Tex: American Botanical Council; 1998.
6. Melchart D, Linde K, Worku F, Bauer R, Wagner H. Immunomodulation with echinacea: a systematic review of controlled clinical trials. *Phytomedicine.* 1994;1:245–254.
7. Haustein KO. Immuntherapeutika. In: Schwabe U, Paffrath D, eds. *Arzneiverordnungsreport 1994.* Stuttgart, Germany: Fischer; 1994:245–250.
8. Forth H, Beuscher N. Beeinflussung der Häufigkeit banaler Erkältungsinfekte durch Esberitox. *Z Allgemeinmedizin.* 1981; 57:2272–2275.
9. Schmidt U, Albrecht M, Schenk N. Immunstimulans senkt Häufigkeit grippaler Infekte. *Natur Ganzheitsmedizin.* 1990; 3:277–281.
10. Schöneberger D. Einfluss der immunstimulierenden Wirkung von Presssaft aus Herba Echinaceae purpureae auf Verlauf und Schweregrad von Erkältungskrankheiten. *Forum Immunol.* 1992;2:18–22.
11. Bullinger M, Heinisch M, Ludwig M, Geier S. Skalen zur Erfassung des Wohlbefindens: Psychometrische Analysen zum "Profile of Mood States" (POMS) und zum "Psychological General Well-Being Index" (PGWB). *Z Differ Diagn Psychol.* 1990;11:53–61.
12. Bullinger M, Hasford J. Evaluating quality of life measures for German clinical trials. *Control Clin Trials.* 1991;12:915–924.
13. Day SJ, Graham DF. Sample size estimation for comparing two or more treatment groups in clinical trials. *Stat Med.* 1991;10:33–44.
14. Moscucci M, Byrne L, Weintraub M, Cox C. Blinding, unblinding, and the placebo effect: an analysis of patients' guesses of treatment assignment in a double-blind clinical trial. *Clin Pharmacol Ther.* 1987;41:259–265.
15. Byrington RP, Curb JD, Mattson ME. Assessment of double-blindness at the conclusion of the Beta-blocker Heart Attack Trial. *JAMA.* 1985;253:1733–1736.
16. Hoheisel O, Sandberg M, Bertram S, Bulitta M, Schäfer M. Echinacea treatment shortens the course of the common cold: a double-blind, placebo-controlled clinical trial. *Eur J Clin Res.* 1997;9:261–269.
17. Brinkeborn R, Shah D, Geissbühler S, Degenring FH. Echinaforce zur Behandlung von akuten Erkältungen. *Schweiz Zschr Ganzheitsmedizin.* 1998;10:26–29.

35 Marijuana Smoking vs Cannabinoids for Glaucoma Therapy

Keith Green, PhD, DSc
From the Departments of Ophthalmology, and Physiology and Endocrinology, Medical College of Georgia, Augusta.

Objective
To discuss the clinical effects, including toxicological data, of marijuana and its many constituent compounds on the eye and the remainder of the body. A perspective is given on the use of marijuana and the cannabinoids in the treatment of glaucoma.

Results
Although it is undisputed that smoking of marijuana plant material causes a fall in intraocular pressure (IOP) in 60% to 65% of users, continued use at a rate needed to control glaucomatous IOP would lead to substantial systemic toxic effects revealed as pathological changes.

Conclusions
Development of drugs based on the cannabinoid molecule or its agonists for use as topical or oral antiglaucoma medications seems to be worthy of further pursuit. Among the latter chemicals, some have no known adverse psychoactive side effects. Smoking of marijuana plant material for the reduction of elevated IOP in glaucoma is ill-advised, given its toxicological profile.

Arch Ophthalmol. 1998;116:1433–1437

Previous reviews of the ocular and toxic effects of marijuana[1–6] have provided considerable background on general human responses. Use of marijuana for medicinal purposes decreased markedly in Western civilizations during the 1930s and 1940s, due to the variable potency of these herbal preparations and the parallel development of specific medications that were more potent and targeted toward specific symptoms. This philosophical alteration in medical therapy reflected changes that occurred in all branches of medicine.[7] Only in the latter part of this century has marijuana been used as a pleasure-inducing substance during liberalization of ethics and social behavior in many cultures.[8–10] After tobacco, alcohol, and caffeine, it is probably the most widely used drug in society.

More recently, legislation has been passed by certain states (with subsequent revocation in 1 state) that has led to a resurgence of interest in the evaluation of possible medical uses of marijuana. Extensive evaluations have resulted in 1 report to the director of the National Institutes of Health,[11] and will result in another from the Institute of Medicine of the National Academy of Sciences. Furthermore, a meeting on this topic held in March 1998 at New York University School of Medicine, New York, will result in publication of a book in the spring of 1999.[12] In many areas of interest, there is little but anecdotal material on which to rely, but in the area of glaucoma, there exists a substantial literature.

Medical Effects

A number of health hazards of marijuana have been identified, but some are difficult to document completely.[9,10,13] Acute effects are increased pulse rate, orthostatic hypotension, euphoria, and conjunctival hyperemia.[14,15] Long-term clinical effects in humans include respiratory, hormonal, and pulmonary toxic effects, although effects on many other organ systems, including the brain, have been noted.[14–28] Marijuana smoking leads to emphysemalike lung changes that are caused by the products of marijuana burning (ie, cannabinoids) or through the release of tars, carcinogens, and other volatile materials, as occurs with tobacco smoke.[16,17] The latter products, however, occur in greater concentration than in tobacco smoke.[19] The cognitive effects induced by marijuana are of equal concern; these assume greater relevance with chronic, repetitive exposure, especially in the age group in which glaucoma is most prevalent.[18,20–28] These factors must be considered when potential chronic use of cannabis is considered as a treatment. This is especially true of glaucoma, where continuous use would be necessary to control this 24-hour-a-day disease, requiring as many as 2920 to 3650 marijuana cigarettes per year.

The widespread effects of the cannabinoids and marijuana on many biological systems have been attributed to direct effects on certain biochemical processes, perturbations in cell membranes, or attachment to 1 of the 2 identified cannabinoid receptors, CB1 and CB2. The CB1 receptor is located in the central nervous system, whereas CB2 receptors occur in immune system tissues, such as spleen.[29–33] Through use of cannabinoid agonists such as WIN5512-2 and methanandamide, identification of cannabinoid receptors, and evaluation of their role in reflecting the biological activity of the cannabinoids, a better and more complete picture has arisen of the effects of these compounds.[29–38]

Ocular Effects

Inhalation of marijuana smoke or smoke of cigarettes laced with Δ^9-tetrahydrocannabinol (Δ^9-THC), intravenous injection of cannabinoids, or ingestion of Δ^9-THC or marijuana ("brownies") causes conjunctival hyperemia and decreased lacrimation.[1–4,6,39–41] Ocular side effects include diplopia, impairment of accommodation, photophobia, nystagmus, and blepharospasm. The ocular effects of long-term marijuana inhalation seem to be similar.[42,43] Pupillary effects appear to differ depending somewhat on the circumstances of marijuana intake.[44,45]

Different cannabinoids reduce intraocular pressure (IOP) in about 60% to 65% of humans, and marijuana and Δ^9-THC (inhaled or taken orally) also decrease IOP in the same percentage of nonglaucomatous volunteers[4,39,41,42] and of volunteer patients with glaucoma.[4,41,46] Orthostatic hypotension and 50% decreased lacrimation occur quickly after inhalation of 2% Δ^9-THC cigarettes,[41] as noted with a synthetic THC homolog. An apparent dose-response relationship occurred between cannabinoids or marijuana and IOP when groups were evaluated. Although the peak fall in IOP was dose related, the time of maximal change was unchanged. The IOP fell, on average, by about 25% (range, –45% to +5%) after smoking 2% marijuana through a water-cooled pipe.[39] Duration of the reduction of IOP is about 3 to 4 hours, by which time the IOP approaches the presmoking level.[1–4,6,39,41] The major difficulty with marijuana smoking was to separate the reduction in IOP and the euphoric effect. These findings confirmed the physiological and pharmacological effects found in experimental animals after intravenous drug administration.[47–50]

Studies in patients with primary open-angle glaucoma (POAG) indicated a reduction of IOP in 60% to 65% of the population after marijuana smoking or Δ^9-THC ingestion.[4,39,41,46] Seven of 11 patients in 1 study showed a reduction in IOP of about 30% after smoking 2% marijuana cigarettes.[46] More quantities of oral drug or marijuana were needed compared with inhaled drug, presumably due to the poorer absorption by the former route.

About 300 volunteers (nonglaucomatous subjects or patients with POAG) overall have participated in studies to examine the acute effects of marijuana smoking or cannabinoid use (topical, oral, or intravenous). Since the largest individual group was about 40 persons, this constitutes a large number of groups and a range of conditions under which marijuana or 1 of its constituents reduced IOP.

Topical Δ^9-THC was examined in rabbits, dogs, and primates for pharmacological activity[1–6,50–55] and toxic effects[56] before being tested in humans.[57–60] The best vehicle identified for delivery of the lipophilic agent in the early 1980s[55] has been superseded by vehicles that permit internalization of lipid-soluble compounds into other materials that are themselves water soluble. This provides an excellent delivery mode of a lipophilic drug through the aqueous tear environment to the lipid corneal epithelium. Other approaches have entailed water-soluble esters of a maleate salt of a Δ^9-THC–related compound.[5] This prodrug approach offers a new modality for encouraging greater drug penetration to the site of action. The development of nonpsychoactive, cannabinoid-related drugs also has resulted in separation of IOP reduction from euphoric effects, at least in experimental animal tests,[61] and holds promise for more future developments. In humans, Δ^9-THC drops were ineffective in reducing IOP in single- or multiple-drop studies, due to the induction of ocular irritation.[59,60] This effect was revealed only in humans.

Marijuana Smoking as Treatment for Glaucoma

Use of marijuana smoking as a treatment for glaucoma is not desirable for several reasons. Although drug absorption is maximum with smoking, and the user or patient can titrate the drug to a level of euphoria indicative of a pharmacological response, this approach is poor. The pathological effects on the lung already described, exposure to carcinogens, and the other pulmonary and respiratory changes at the organ and cellular levels[16,17,19] all make smoking a nonviable mechanism. The systemic toxic effects that result in pathological changes alone seem sufficient to discourage smoking marijuana.

Primary open-angle glaucoma is a 365-day-a-year disease, and since the marijuana-induced fall in IOP lasts only 3 hours, the drug consumption conceivably needed to reduce and keep IOP at a safe level would be very high. The IOP is the only readily measurable parameter that one can use as an index of POAG and is still the major indicator of what is essentially a neuropathogenic disease.[62] No indication has been obtained or reported that those highly limited number of persons who consume marijuana cigarettes as a compassionate investigational new drug have shown any maintenance of visual function or visual fields or stabilization of optic disappearance.

Since marijuana reduces IOP for 3 to 4 hours, after which the IOP returns to baseline, control of IOP at a significantly lowered value, including maintenance of IOP at a 2-hour minimal low value, requires a marijuana cigarette to be smoked 8 or 10 times a day (by those persons in whom IOP actually decreases). This use corresponds to at least 2920 and as many as 3650 marijuana cigarettes consumed per year.[3,6] It is difficult to imagine anyone consuming that much marijuana and being a productive individual who is incorporated into society and perhaps operating machinery or driving on the highways. Similarly, the systemic end-organ effects at this level of consumption have the potential of being quite high. On the other hand, the availability of once- or twice-a-day eye drops (β-blockers such as timolol maleate, or the prostaglandin agonist latanoprost) makes IOP control a reality for many patients and provides round-the-clock IOP reduction.[62]

Glaucoma treatment requires a round-the-clock reduction in IOP, and treatments are evaluated as successful if this level of activity is achieved without progression of visual field loss or optic disc changes. There has been considerable press coverage of the use of marijuana as an antiemetic[63–66] or as treatment for glaucoma. Dangers arise from 2 considerations of the latter. First, intermittent use would lead to a lack of IOP reduction on a continued basis, thereby permitting visual function loss to proceed. Second, full use of enough smoked marijuana leads to the need, as described above, of an average of at least 3300 cigarettes per year. Advocates of the latter approach often cite using marijuana for the relief of symptoms, whereas POAG has no symptoms until too late, when vision is irreversibly lost.

The advocates of marijuana smoking for glaucoma treatment also must contend with the lack of standardization of the plant material. The 480 chemicals, including 66 cannabinoids, in marijuana vary depending on the site and circumstances of growth and certainly vary in content depending on which plant part is smoked.[67–69] This variability goes counter to the requirements of the Food and Drug Administration, Washington, DC, concerning the chemical identity and performance characteristics of specific drugs. Indeed, dronabinol (Marinol), an oral form of Δ^9-THC, is approved by the Food and Drug Administration for the treatment of chemotherapy-induced nausea and acquired immunodeficiency syndrome wasting syndrome. Further, despite attempts by individual states to change their laws, marijuana remains a schedule 1 controlled substance, and federal law prevails.

Lastly, there is an increasing movement at the federal and state levels to confine tobacco smoking to highly restricted areas to reduce smoking and the exposure of nonsmokers to second-hand smoke. In the face of this societal change, it is difficult to advocate increased smoking, particularly of marijuana, in settings where smoking is normally banned.

Cannabinoids for Glaucoma Treatment

Oral or topical cannabinoids show promise for future use in glaucoma treatment. Newer topical delivery technologies are available for these lipophilic drugs, including the formation of microemulsions and use of cyclodextrins to increase the solubility in aqueous-based solutions. This is a marked improvement over the lipid-based vehicles that were the only ones available during earlier basic and clinical studies of topical cannabinoids.[51,56,59,60,70] The development of compounds related to Δ^9-THC, such as HU211 (dexanabinol), that show a complete absence of euphoric effects while retaining IOP-reducing activity[61] is a major advance. Increasing knowledge concerning the topical cannabinoid receptors and ligands that reduce IOP in rabbit or monkey eyes will allow exploration of different structural analogs that may identify compounds efficacious as potential glaucoma medications.[70–78] Topical administration also has the advantage of permitting the use of a low mass of drug per delivery volume. Even at 5% concentration, a 30-μL drop would contain only 1.5 mg.

Oral administration of cannabinoids that lack psychoactive effects but will reduce IOP could be a significant addition to the ophthalmic armamentarium against glaucoma. The cannabinoids that exist in the plant material[67–69] or as metabolites[79,80] do not appear to be viable candidates for oral use because of the inability to separate their euphoric and IOP-reducing effects.

Because they are readily characterized from a chemical perspective, the cannabinoids and related substances represent an area of focus for future studies. Such attention would allow the development of appropriate vehicles for these chemicals into the predominantly aqueous environment of the tears. Compounds would be identified that have no euphoric effects or at least a very high ratio of IOP reduction to euphoric effects. Such chemicals would eliminate any potential abuse problems while providing drugs that would reduce IOP by unique interaction with receptors or other membrane components that could be additive to other currently available glaucoma medications. In experiments where the action of cannabinoids in causing an IOP reduction has been sought, evidence points to an influence on increasing outflow of fluid from the eye as the major component. This is true for Δ^9-THC and HU211, although the binding of each of these compounds to the cannabinoid receptor differs widely. The rapidity of onset of the responses strongly suggests that an effect is occurring that can undergo rapid adjustment rather than be related to slow alterations in trabecular meshwork glycoproteins.[81]

The perspective presented herein differs in several ways from the conclusions reached by the National Institutes of Health-assembled panel to provide a written report on medicinal use of marijuana.[11] The primary difference is the focus of research efforts, which the panel concluded should have marijuana smoking as its delivery mode, whereas my review recommends cannabinoids. The reasons for this divergence of opinion are given and, I believe, are compelling for glaucoma studies to focus on individual chemicals rather than a nonstandardized plant material.

The latter has no possibility, due to the inherent variability and the plant versatility, of reaching the standards required by the Food and Drug Administration in terms of chemical identity, purity, or characterization. A contemporary review of medicinal applications that evaluated the effect of Δ^9-THC and marijuana on a broad spectrum of medical problems indicated that THC may have a role in treating nausea associated with cancer chemotherapy and in appetite stimulation. Other uses of either material were not supported.[82]

The author has no commercial or proprietary interest in any drug or product mentioned in this article.

References

1. Green K. The ocular effects of cannabinoids. In: Zadunaisky JA, Davson H, eds. *Current Topics in Eye Research*. Orlando, Fla: Academic Press Inc; 1979;1:175–215.

2. Green K. Current status of basic and clinical marihuana research in ophthalmology. In: Leopold IH, Burns RP, eds. *Symposium on Ocular Therapy*.New York, NY: John Wiley & Sons Inc; 1979;11:37–49.

3. Green K. Marihuana and the eye: a review. *J Toxicol Cutan Ocul Toxicol*. 1982;1:3–32.

4. Green K. Marijuana effects on intraocular pressure. In: Drance SM, Neufeld AH, eds. *Glaucoma: Applied Pharmacology in Medical Treatment*. New York, NY: Grune & Stratton Inc; 1984:507–526.

5. Mechoulam R, Lander H, Srebnik M, et al. Recent advances in the use of cannabinoids as therapeutic agents. In: Agurell S, Dewey WL, Willette RE, eds. *The Cannabinoids: Chemical, Pharmacologic and Therapeutic Aspects*. Orlando, Fla: Academic Press Inc; 1984: 777–793.

6. Green K, McDonald TF. Ocular toxicology of marijuana: an update. *J Toxicol Cutan Ocul Toxicol*. 1987;6:309–334.

7. Green K. History of ophthalmic toxicology. In: Chiou GCY, ed. *Ophthalmic Toxicology*. New York, NY: Raven Press; 1992:1–16.

8. Waller CW, Nair RS, McAllister AF, Urbanek B, Turner CE. *Marihuana: An Annotated Bibliography*. Vol 2. New York, NY: MacMillan Publishing Co Inc; 1982.

9. Fehr KO, Kalant H, eds. *Adverse Health and Behavioral Consequences of Cannabis Use*. Toronto, Ontario: Addictive Research Foundation; 1983.

10. Nahas GG, ed. *Marihuana in Science and Medicine*. New York, NY: Raven Press; 1984.

11. *Workshop on the Medical Utility of Marijuana: Report to the Director*. Washington, DC: National Institutes of Health; 1997.

12. Nahas GG, Sutin KN, Agurell S, eds. *Marijuana and Medicine*. Totawa, NJ: Humana Press. In press.

13. Agurell S, Dewey WL, Willette RE, eds. *The Cannabinoids: Chemical, Pharmacologic and Therapeutic Aspects*. Orlando, Fla: Academic Press Inc; 1984.

14. Graham IDP. *Cannabis and Health*. Orlando, Fla: Academic Press Inc; 1976.

15. Dewey WL. Cannabinoid pharmacology. *Pharmacol Rev*. 1986;38:151–178.

16. Tashkin DP, Shapiro BJ, Ramanna L, Taplin GV, Lee YE, Harper CE. Chronic effects of heavy marihuana smoking on pulmonary function in healthy young males. In: Braude MC, Szara S, eds. *The Pharmacology of Marihuana*. New York, NY; Raven Press; 1976:291–295.

17. Rosenkrantz H, Fleischman RW. Effects of cannabis on lungs. In: Nahas GG, Paton WDM, eds. *Marihuana: Biological Effects*. Elmsford, NY: Pergamon Press Inc; 1979:279–299.

18. Dornbush RL, Kokkevi A. The acute effects of various cannabis substances on cognitive, perceptual, and motor performance in very long-term hashish users. In: Braude MC, Szara S, eds. *The Pharmacology of Marihuana*. New York, NY: Raven Press; 1976:421–427.

19. *Marihuana and Health*. Washington, DC: National Academy of Sciences, Institute of Medicine Report; 1982.

20. Murray JB. Marijuana's effects on human cognitive functions, psychomotor functions, and personality. *J Gen Psychol*. 1986;113:23–55.

21. Devane WA, Dysarz III FA, Johnson MR, Melvin LS, Howlett AC. Determination and characterization of a cannabinoid receptor in rat brain. *Mol Pharmacol*. 1988;34:605–613.

22. Leon-Carrion J. Mental performance in long-term heavy cannabis: a preliminary report. *Psychol Rep*. 1990;67:947–952.

23. Munro S, Thomas KL, Abu-Shaar M. Molecular characterization of a peripheral receptor for cannabinoids. *Nature*. 1993;365:61–65.

24. Howlett AC. Pharmacology of cannabinoid receptors. *Ann Rev Pharmacol Toxicol*. 1995; 35:607–634.

25. Solowij N. Do cognitive impairments recover following cessation of cannabis use? *Life Sci*. 1995;5:2119–2126.

26. Solowij N, Michie PT, Fox AM. Differential impairments of selective attention due to frequency and duration of cannabis use. *Biol Psychiatry*. 1995;37:731–739.

27. Fletcher JM, Page JB, Francis DJ, et al. Cognitive correlates of long-term cannabis use in Costa Rican men. *Arch Gen Psychiatry*. 1996; 53:1051–1057.

28. Pope HG, Yurgelun-Todd D. The residual cognitive effects of heavy marijuana use in college students. *JAMA*. 1996;275:521–527.

29. Mechoulam R, Feigenbaum JJ, Lander N, et al. Enantiomeric cannabinoids: stereospecificity of psychotropic activity. *Experientia*. 1988; 44:762–764.

30. Howlett AC, Champion TM, Wilken GH, Mechoulam R. Stereochemical effects of 11–OH-Δ^8-tetrahydrocannabinol-dimethylheptyl to inhibit adenylate cyclase and bind to the cannabinoid receptor. *Neuropharmacology*. 1990;29:161–165.

31. D'Ambra TE, Estep KG, Bell MR, et al. Conformationally restrained analogues of pravadoline: nanomolar potent, enantioselective, (aminoalkyl)indole agonists of the cannabinoid receptor. *J Med Chem*. 1992;35:124–135.

32. Compton DR, Gold LH, Ward SJ, Balster RL, Martin BR. Aminoalkylindole analogs: cannabimimetic activity of a class of compounds structurally distinct from Δ^9-tetrahydrocannabinol. *J Pharmacol Exp Ther*. 1992; 263:1118–1126.

33. Lynn AB, Herkenham M. Localization of cannabinoid receptors and nonsaturable high-density cannabinoid binding sites in peripheral tissues of the rat: implications for receptor-mediated immune modulation by cannabinoids. *J Pharmacol Exp Ther*. 1994;268:1612–1613.

34. Devane WA, Hanus L, Breuer A, et al. Isolation and structure of a brain constituent that binds to the cannabinoid receptor. *Science*. 1992; 258:1946–1959.

35. Fride E, Mechoulam R. Pharmacological activity of the cannabinoid receptor agonist, anandamide, a brain constituent. *Eur J Pharmacol*. 1993;231:313–314.

36. Kuster JE, Stevenson JI, Ward SJ, D'Ambra TE, Haycock DA. Aminoalkylindole binding in rat cerebellum: selective displacement by natural and synthetic cannabinoids. *J Pharmacol Exp Ther*. 1993;264:1351–1363.

37. Abadji V, Lin S, Taha G, et al. (R)-methanandamide: a chiral novel anandamide possessing higher potency and metabolic stability. *J Med Chem*. 1994;37:1889–1893.

38. Smith PB, Compton DR, Welch SP, Razdan RK, Mechoulam R, Martin BR. The pharmacological activity of anandamide, a putative endogenous cannabinoid in mice. *J Pharmacol Exp Ther*. 1994;270:219–227.

39. Hepler RS, Frank IM, Petrus R. Ocular effects of marijuana smoking. In: Braude MC, Szara S, eds. *The Pharmacology of Marihuana*. New York, NY: Raven Press; 1976:815–824.

40. Perez-Reyes M, Wagner D, Wall ME, Davis KH. Intravenous administration of cannabinoids on intraocular pressure. In: Braude MC, Szara S, eds. *The Pharmacology of Marihuana*. New York, NY: Raven Press; 1976:829–832.

41. Merritt JC, Crawford WJ, Alexander PC, Anduze AL, Gelbart SS. Effect of marihuana on intraocular and blood pressure in glaucoma. *Ophthalmology.* 1980;87:222–228.

42. Jones RT, Benowitz N. The 30–day trip: clinical studies of cannabis tolerance and dependence. In: Braude MC, Szara S, eds. *The Pharmacology of Marihuana.* New York, NY: Raven Press; 1976:627–642.

43. Dawson WW, Jiminez-Antillon CF, Perez JM, Zeskind JA. Marihuana and vision after ten years' use in Costa Rica. *Invest Ophthalmol.* 1977;16:689–699.

44. Hepler RS, Frank IM, Ungerleider JT. Pupillary constriction after marijuana smoking. *Am J Ophthalmol.* 1972;74:1185–1190.

45. Brown B, Adams M, Halgerstrom-Portnoy G, Jones RT, Flom MC. Pupil size after use of marijuana and alcohol. *Am J Ophthalmol.* 1977; 83:350–354.

46. Hepler RS, Petrus R. Experiences with administration of marihuana to glaucoma patients. In: Cohen S, Stillman RC, eds. *The Therapeutic Potential of Marihuana.* New York, NY: Plenum Publishing Corp; 1976:63–75.

47. Green K, Bowman KA. Effect of marihuana derivatives on intraocular pressure. In: Braude MC, Szara S, eds. *The Pharmacology of Marihuana.* New York, NY: Raven Press; 1976:803–813.

48. Green K, Symonds CM, Oliver NW, Elijah RD. Intraocular pressure following systemic administration of cannabinoids. *Curr Eye Res.* 1982–1983;2:247–253.

49. El-Sohly MA, Harland EC, Benigni DA, Waller CW. Cannabinoids in glaucoma, II: the effect of different cannabinoids on intraocular pressure of the rabbit. *Curr Eye Res.* 1984;3:841–850.

50. Waller CW, Benigni DA, Harland EC, Bedford JA, Murphy JC, El-Sohly MA. Cannabinoids in glaucoma, III: the effects of different cannabinoids on intraocular pressure in the monkey. In: Agurell S, Dewey WL, Willette RE, eds. *The Cannabinoids: Chemical, Pharmacologic and Therapeutic Aspects.* Orlando, Fla: Academic Press Inc; 1984:871–880.

51. Green K, Wynn H, Bowman K. A comparison of topical cannabinoids on intraocular pressure. *Exp Eye Res.* 1978;27:239–246.

52. Howes JF. Antiglaucoma effects of topically and orally administered cannabinoids. In: Agurell S, Dewey WL, Willette RE, eds. *The Cannabinoids: Chemical, Pharmacologic and Therapeutic Aspects.* Orlando, Fla: Academic Press Inc; 1984:881–890.

53. Merritt JC, Whitaker R, Page CJ, et al. Topical Δ^8-tetrahydrocannabinol as a potential glaucoma agent. *Glaucoma.* 1982;4:253–255.

54. Merritt JC, Peiffer RL, McKinnon SM, Stapleton SS, Goodwin T, Risco JM. Topical Δ^9-tetrahydrocannabinol on intraocular pressure in dogs. *Glaucoma.* 1981;3:13–16.

55. Green K, Bigger JF, Kim L, Bowman K. Cannabinoid penetration and chronic effects in the eye. *Exp Eye Res.* 1977;24:197–205.

56. Green K, Sobel RE, Fineberg E, Wynn HR, Bowman KA. Subchronic ocular and systemic toxicity of topically applied Δ^9-tetrahydrocannabinol. *Ann Ophthalmol.* 1981; 13:1219–1222.

57. Merritt JC, Olsen JL, Armstrong JR, McKinnon SM. Topical Δ^9-tetrahydrocannabinol in humans. *J Pharm Pharmacol.* 1981;33:40–41.

58. Merritt JC, Perry DD, Russell DN, Jones BF. Topical Δ^9-tetrahydrocannabinol and aqueous dynamics in glaucoma. *J Clin Pharmacol.* 1981;21(suppl 8–9):467S–471S.

59. Green K, Roth M. Ocular effects of topical administration of Δ^9-tetrahydrocannabinol in man. *Arch Ophthalmol.* 1982;100:265–267.

60. Jay WM, Green K. Multiple-drop study of topically applied 1% Δ^9-tetrahydrocannabinol in human eyes. *Arch Ophthalmol.* 1983; 101:591–593.

61. Beilin M, Aviv H, Friedman D, et al. HU2 11, a novel synthetic, non-psychotropic cannabinoid with ocular hypotensive activity [abstract]. *Invest Ophthalmol Vis Sci.* 1993;34(suppl):1113.

62. Sugrue MF. New approaches to antiglaucoma therapy. *J Med Chem.* 1997;40:2793–2809.

63. Lucas VS, Laszlo J. Δ^9-tetrahydrocannabinol for refractory vomiting induced by cancer chemotherapy. *JAMA.* 1980;243:1241–1243.

64. Poster DS, Penta JS, Bruno S, Macdonald JS. Δ^9-tetrahydrocannabinol in clinical oncology. *JAMA.* 1981;245:2047–2051.

65. Schwartz RH, Voth EA, Sheridan MJ. Marijuana to prevent nausea and vomiting in cancer patients: a survey of clinical oncologists. *South Med J.* 1997;90:167–172.

66. Allen T. Tetrahydrocannabinol and chemotherapy [letter]. *N Engl J Med.* 1976;294:168.

67. Turner CE, El-Sohly MA, Boeren EG. Constituents of Cannabis sativa (L), XVII: a review of the natural constituents. *J Nat Prod.* 1980;43:169–234.

68. Doorenbos NJ, Fetterman PS, Quimby MW, Turner CE. Cultivation, extraction and analysis of *Cannabis sativa* (L). *Ann N Y Acad Sci.* 1971; 191:3–14.

69. Ross SA, El-Sohly MA. Constituents of *Cannabis sativa* L, XXVIII: a review of the natural constituents: 1980–1984. *Zagazig J Pharm Sci.* 1995;4:1–10.

70. Green K, Kim K. Acute dose response of intraocular pressure to topical and oral cannabinoids. *Proc Soc Exp Biol Med.* 1977; 154:228–231.

71. Mechoulam R, Lander N, Varkony TH, et al. Stereochemical requirements for cannabinoid activity. *J Med Sci.* 1980;23:1068–1072.

72. Newell FW, Stark P, Jay WM, Schanzlin DJ. Nabilone: a pressure-reducing synthetic benzopyran in open-angle glaucoma. *Ophthalmology.* 1979;86:156–160.

73. Lemberger L. Potential therapeutic usefulness of marijuana. *Ann Rev Pharmacol Toxicol.* 1980;20:151–172.

74. Razdan RK. Structure-activity relationships in cannabinoids. *Pharmacol Rev.* 1986; 38:75–149.

75. Sugrue MF, Funk HA, Leonard Y, O'Neill-Davis L, Labelle M. The ocular hypotensive effects of synthetic cannabinoids [abstract]. *Invest Ophthalmol Vis Sci.* 1996;37(suppl):831.

76. Pate DW, Jarvinen K, Urtti A, Harho P, Jarvinen T. Arachidonylethanolamide decreases intraocular pressure in normotensive rabbits. *Curr Eye Res.* 1995;14:791–797.

77. Pate DW, Jarvinen K, Urtti A, et al. Effects of topical anandamides on intraocular pressure in normotensive rabbits. *Life Sci.* 1996; 58:1849–1860.

78. Hodges LC, Reggio PH, Green K. Evidence against cannabinoid receptor involvement in intraocular pressure: effects of cannabinoids in rabbits. *Ophthalmic Res.* 1997;29:1–5.

79. Hollister LE, Gillespie HK. Delta-8– and delta-9–tetrahydrocannabinol: comparison in man by oral and intravenous administration. *Clin Pharm Ther.* 1973;14:353–357.

80. Wall ME, Brine DR, Perez-Reyes M. Metabolism of cannabinoids in man. In: Braude MC, Szara S, eds. *The Pharmacology of Marihuana.* New York, NY: Raven Press; 1976:93–113.

81. Green K. Marijuana and intraocular pressure: possible mechanisms of action. In: Nahas GG, Sutin KN, Agurell S, eds. *Marijuana and Medicine.* Totawa, NJ: Humana Press. In press.

82. Voth EA, Schwartz RH. Medicinal applications of delta-9–tetrahydrocannabinol and marijuana. *Ann Intern Med.* 1997;126:791–798.

36 Effect of a Garlic Oil Preparation on Serum Lipoproteins and Cholesterol Metabolism

A Randomized Controlled Trial

Heiner K. Berthold, MD, PhD; Thomas Sudhop, MD; Klaus von Bergmann, MD
From the Department of Clinical Pharmacology, University of Bonn, Bonn, Germany (Drs Berthold, Sudhop, and von Bergmann).

Context
Garlic-containing drugs have been used in the treatment of hypercholesterolemia even though their efficacy is not generally established. Little is known about the mechanisms of action of the possible effects on cholesterol in humans.

Objective
To estimate the hypocholesterolemic effect of garlic oil and to investigate the possible mechanism of action.

Design
Double-blind, randomized, placebo-controlled trial.

Setting
Outpatient lipid clinic.

Patients
We investigated 25 patients (mean age, 58 years) with moderate hypercholesterolemia.

Intervention
Steam-distilled garlic oil preparation (5 mg twice a day) vs placebo each for 12 weeks with wash-out periods of 4 weeks.

Main Outcome Measures
Serum lipoprotein concentrations, cholesterol absorption, and cholesterol synthesis.

Results
Baseline lipoprotein profiles were (mean [SD]): total cholesterol, 7.53 (0.75) mmol/L (291 [29] mg/dL); low-density lipoprotein cholesterol (LDL-C), 5.35 (0.78) mmol/L (207 [30] mg/dL); high-density lipoprotein cholesterol (HDL-C), 1.50 (0.41) mmol/L (58 [16] mg/dL); and triglycerides, 1.45 (0.73) mmol/L (127 [64] mg/dL). Lipoprotein levels were virtually unchanged at the end of both treatment periods (mean difference [95% confidence interval]): total cholesterol, 0.085 (–0.201 to 0.372) mmol/L (3.3 [–7.8 to 14.4] mg/dL), *P*=.54;

LDL-C, 0.001 (–0.242 to 0.245) mmol/L (0.04 [–9.4 to 9.5] mg/dL), *P*=.99; HDL-C, 0.050 (–0.028 to 0.128) mmol/L (1.9 [–1.1 to 4.9] mg/dL), *P*=.20; triclycerides, 0.047 (–0.229 to 0.135) mmol/L (4.2 [–20.3 to 12.0]) mg/dL, *P*=.60. Cholesterol absorption (37.5% [10.5%] vs 38.3% [10.7%], *P*=.58), cholesterol synthesis (12.7 [6.5] vs 13.4 [6.6] mg/kg of body weight per day, *P*=.64), mevalonic acid excretion (192 [66] vs 187 [66] μg/d, *P*=.78), and changes in the ratio of lathosterol to cholesterol in serum (4.4% [24.3%] vs 10.6% [21.1%], *P*=.62) were not different in garlic and placebo treatment.

Conclusions

The commercial garlic oil preparation investigated had no influence on serum lipoproteins, cholesterol absorption, or cholesterol synthesis. Garlic therapy for treatment of hypercholesterolemia cannot be recommended on the basis of this study.

JAMA. 1998;279:1900–1902.

Garlic (*Allium sativum*) has been advocated as a remedy for the treatment and prevention of a number of diseases. As a pharmaceutical product, its putative cardioprotective properties, such as lipid-lowering and blood pressure-lowering, antioxidant, antiplatelet, and fibrinolytic effects,[1,2] seem interesting. Studies investigating garlic's lipid-lowering effect are sometimes flawed in design because they lack adequate description of the methods and patients studied or are overtly subjected to conflicts of interest. Meta-analyses found overall effects of between 9% and 12% reduction of total cholesterol.[3,4] However, the confidence in these data is limited by the poor quality of the underlying studies and the possibility of a publication bias in that there are fewer than expected studies reporting negative results.[5] Likewise, meta-analyses based on published reports rather than on individual patient data may be misleading,[6] implying that meta-analyses provide false-positive test results.[7] The value of meta-analyses as accurate predictors of treatment outcome as compared to prospective randomized controlled trials has been questioned.[8] Well-designed recent studies[7,9] found no lipid-lowering effects, while 3 other studies reported some efficacy.[10–12]

We hypothesized that the modest lipid-lowering effect found in meta-analyses may be further understood if more were known about the possible mechanisms of the action of garlic-containing drugs on cholesterol metabolism. We designed a double-blind, randomized, placebo-controlled, cross-over trial to investigate possible influences of a garlic preparation on serum lipoproteins and cholesterol metabolism. We used a steam-distilled garlic-oil preparation.

Methods

Patients

Patients with moderate hypercholesterolemia (total cholesterol, 6.2–9.0 mmol/L [240–348 mg/dL]; triglycerides, <3.0 mmol/L [<265 mg/dL) were recruited through the local newspaper. None of the 26 unpaid patients randomized for the study (1 later dropped out because of a scheduling conflict) had taken any lipid-lowering drugs or drugs that would interfere with lipid metabolism for 8 weeks, though some were taking antihypertensive medication, hormone replacement drugs, or thyroid hormones. After ensuring that patients who had given consent to participate were free of active liver or renal diseases, diabetes, thyroid dysfunction, a history of coronary heart disease, any pathological laboratory values in the clinical chemistry or hematological routine parameters, and alcohol or other drug abuse, they entered the study whose protocol had been approved by the ethics committee of the faculty of medicine at Bonn University and performed in accordance with Declaration of Helsinki guidelines.

Food Records

Subjects were advised to adhere to their usual diet during the study, but they were prohibited from taking additional garlic or other food supplements. Food intake was assessed at the end of 2 treatment periods, using 7-day food records that were evaluated by computerized nutrient analysis.

Study Design and Treatment

The study was a single-center, double-blind, randomized, placebo-controlled, cross-over trial. A marketed enteric coated preparation (Tegra, Hermes Arzneimittel GmbH, Munich, Germany) containing 5 mg of steam-distilled garlic oil bound to a matrix of beta cyclodextrin or matching placebos whose coating tasted like garlic, was used. The daily dosage corresponds to about 4 g to 5 g of fresh garlic cloves or 4000 units of allicin-equivalents per day.[13] The active ingredients are the stable sulfur compounds diallyl disulfide (>30%) and diallyl trisulfide (>25%), which are formed from alliin and allicin.

The patients were randomly assigned to the treatment sequences placebo-garlic or garlic-placebo in blocks of 10 for the first 20 patients and in blocks of 2 for the remaining patients. After randomization, the patients were given placebo for 4 weeks in a single-blind fashion. Thereafter, they received the garlic preparation or placebo for 12 weeks in a double-blind fashion. Then a 4-week, single-blind placebo wash-out was performed followed by the 12-week, double-blind cross-over phase. Lipoprotein concentrations from blood drawn at the beginning and end of each phase were measured enzymatically using standard laboratory procedures. High-density lipoprotein cholesterol (HDL-C) was determined after anionic precipitation of apolipoprotein B–containing lipoproteins. Low-density lipoprotein cholesterol (LDL-C) was calculated according to the method of Friedewald.[14]

Evaluation of Cholesterol Metabolism. During the last week of each 12-week treatment period, cholesterol absorption and endogenous cholesterol synthesis was measured by the double-isotope continuous feeding method as described by Lütjohann et al.[15] For this purpose the patients took 1 capsule containing [D_6]cholesterol and [D_4]sitostanol 3 times a day for 1 week. The disappearance of deuterated cholesterol and its intestinal bacterial products (coprostanol and coprostanone) relative to deuterated sitostanol were measured in fecal samples by gas chromatography–mass spectrometry. The capsules also contained unlabeled sitostanol as a nonabsorbable fecal flow and recovery marker for the measurement of fecal excretion of neutral and acidic sterols. The patients kept a 7-day dietary protocol to determine their intake of nutrients and cholesterol. Cholesterol synthesis was calculated by subtracting the amount of dietary cholesterol intake from the sum of neutral and acidic sterols excreted in feces.[16] As an additional indicator of short-term changes in endogenous cholesterol synthesis, 24-hour urinary excretion of mevalonic acid was measured by gas chromatography–mass spectrometry as described by Lindenthal et al.[17] The measurement of the cholesterol precursor lathosterol in serum was determined by gas chromatography.[18]

Statistical Analysis and Analytical Precision. Statistical analysis between lipoprotein concentrations at the end of both treatment periods was performed using *t* statistical tests for cross-over designs (in the case of triglycerides after log transformation of the data), after excluding carryover effects.[19] Correlation between the change in the primary study parameter, low-density lipoproteins (LDL), and the parameters of cholesterol metabolism was analyzed using a simple linear regression model. For all tests a significance level of $P<.05$ was defined. The study was powered at a level of greater than 95% to detect differences between treatment periods of 10% LDL-C lowering (or −0.52 mmol/L [−20 mg/dL]). Statistical analyses were performed using StatView 4.1 for the Macintosh (Abacus Concepts Inc, Berkeley, Calif) and Microsoft Excel 5.0a for the Macintosh (Microsoft Inc, Redmond, Wash). All lipoprotein measurements were performed twice on 2 separate days. The average of the 2 values was used for calculations. Within-individual coefficients of variation of the measures were 4.5% (total cholesterol), 6.2% (LDL-C), 6.8% (HDL-C), and 17.4 (triglycerides), respectively. The laboratory's precision in measurement of lipoproteins (day-to-day coefficient of variation) was 0.99% (total cholesterol), 2.64% (LDL-C), 2.22% (HDL-C), and 1.14% (triglycerides).

Results

Twenty-five subjects completed the study and 1 subject had to be excluded from the fecal balance calculations because of incomplete intake of the marker capsules in 1 test period. The baseline characteristics and the serum lipoprotein profiles of the 25 patients are listed in Table 1.

The drug was generally well tolerated. Except for garlic odor and slight abdominal discomfort in a few cases, caused by both pills, no serious adverse events occurred. Laboratory safety parameters remained in the normal range. Compliance as measured by pill count was excellent and averaged 98.4%±6.3% (mean±SD) during all phases. During active-drug treatment phase, none of the subjects had a medication intake of less than 88%.

Evaluation of the two 7-day food records showed that macronutrients, cholesterol, fiber, and alcohol were consumed similarly during both phases. Body weights remained constant during the entire course of the study (Table 2). Lipoprotein concentrations were virtually unchanged between placebo and active-drug treatment (Table 1). There was a slight increase in all lipoprotein fractions during active-drug treatment compared with placebo, none statisti-

Table 1. Subject Characteristics, Baseline Data, and Differences in Effects (in Millimoles per Liter) Between Placebo and Active Drug Treatments*

Characteristic	Baseline	Differences in Effects Between Placebo and Active Drug	P
No. of subjects (F/M)	25 (14/11)		
Age, y	58.3 (7.5)	. . .	. . .
Body mass index, kg/m²	25.3 (2.5)	. . .	. . .
Total serum cholesterol, mmol/L [mg/dL]	7.53 (0.75) [291 (29)]	. . .	. . .
LDL-cholesterol, mmol/L [mg/dL]	5.35 (0.78) [207 (30)]	0.085 (–0.201 to 0.372) [3.3 (–7.8 to 14.4)]	.54
HDL-cholesterol, mmol/L [mg/dL]	1.50 (0.41) [58 (16)]	0.001 (–0.242 to 0.245) [0.04 (–9.4 to 9.5)]	.99
Triglycerides, mmol/L [mg/dL]	1.45 (0.73) [127 (64)]	0.050 (–0.028 to 0.128) [1.9 (–1.1 to 4.9)]	.20
		0.047 (–0.229 to 0.135) [4.2 (–20.3 to 12.0)]	.60

*The baseline data represent means (SDs) of all subjects that completed the study; the treatment data represent means and 95% confidence intervals. LDL indicates low-density lipoprotein; HDL, high-density lipoprotein; and ellipses, not applicable.

Table 2. Average Daily Nutrient Intake as Assessed by 7-Day Food Records at the End of the Treatments*

	Placebo			Active Drug		
	Women	Men	All	Women	Men	All
Body weight, kg	69 (6)	80 (8)	74 (9)	70 (7)	80 (8)	74 (9)
Total energy, kJ/kg	122 (29)	151 (34)	134 (34)	126 (38)	147 (21)	134 (34)
Protein, %	15.3 (1.9)	13.5 (1.7)	14.5 (2.0)	14.3 (1.5)	14.5 (2.3)	14.4 (1.9)
Carbohydrates, %	44.0 (5.9)	44.0 (4.7)	44.0 (5.3)	46.4 (5.4)	42.5 (3.8)	44.7 (5.1)
Total fat, %	32.2 (5.1)	31.8 (5.8)	32.0 (5.3)	31.9 (3.9)	31.7 (3.9)	31.8 (3.8)
Saturated fat, %	12.6 (2.4)	12.8 (3.1)	12.7 (2.7)	13.0 (2.1)	13.2 (1.7)	13.0 (1.9)
Polyunsaturated fat, %	4.7 (1.0)	4.3 (0.6)	4.5 (0.9)	4.6 (0.9)	4.2 (0.8)	4.4 (0.9)
Alcohol, %	5.7 (5.8)	8.4 (5.1)	6.9 (5.6)	4.8 (4.8)	9.0 (5.0)	6.7 (5.2)
Fiber, g/d	26 (7)	33 (10)	29 (9)	28 (11)	31 (7)	29 (9)
Cholesterol, mg/d	342 (187)	315 (84)	330 (149)	264 (82)	337 (101)	296 (97)

*The data represent means (SDs). Macronutrients are presented as percentage of total energy intake.

cally significant. The post hoc calculated power of the study of 93.8% would have been able to detect differences in the primary study parameter of LDL-C of greater than or equal to –0.429 mmol/L (–16 mg/dL) between the 2 pills.

There were virtually no effects of garlic drug on the parameters of cholesterol metabolism (placebo vs active drug; mean [SD] values): cholesterol absorption (38.3% [10.7] vs 37.5% [10.5%], P=.58), cholesterol synthesis (13.4 [6.6] vs 12.7 [6.5] mg/kg of body weight per day, P=.64), or mevalonic acid excretion in urine (187 [66] μg/d vs 192 [66] μg/d, P=.78). Changes in the ratio of lathosterol to cholesterol were not statistically different during either treatment (garlic, 4.4% [24.3%]; baseline, 1.30 [0.42] μg/mg; placebo, 10.6% [21.1%]; baseline, 1.18 [0.35] μg/mg, P=.62). Simple linear regression analyses between changes in serum LDL-C and cholesterol absorption, cholesterol synthesis, mevalonic acid excretion, or the ratio of lathosterol to cholesterol revealed no significant correlations (cholesterol absorption, r=0.26, P=.22; cholesterol synthesis, r=0.17, P=.43; mevalonic acid excretion, r=0.11, P=.61; ratio of lathosterol to cholesterol, r=0.05, P=.81).

Comment

We evaluated the effects of a commercially available garlic preparation using a double-blind, randomized, placebo-controlled study design. No changes in serum lipoprotein levels in patients with moderate hypercholesterolemia were found. Although 2 meta-analyses and a recent study had shown small but significant effects of garlic on serum lipoprotein levels,[3,4,11] there were 2 other well-designed studies that found no influence.[7,9] Thus, the overall evidence for a positive effect of garlic on serum lipid levels is questionable.

We have addressed some new questions yet to be elucidated during treatment with garlic preparations. During trials with lipid-lowering substances, it is important to exclude changes in body weight or dietary habits, especially total calories, fat, and cholesterol content of the diet.

Earlier studies were often criticized for dosage, duration of treatment, and baseline cholesterol values. Most studies used dried garlic powder preparations in doses from 600 to 900 mg/d, the equivalent of 1.8 to 2.7 g/d of fresh garlic. Nonpowder preparations, however, seem according to the literature to have a stronger lipid-lowering effect than powder preparations, although their effects showed also a greater heterogeneity.[4] Few studies have used steam-distilled garlic oils or oil-macerated garlic.[20] These preparations contain only polysulfides and other volatile thioallyls. Based on comparisons of the content of active ingredients, the dosage of our study medication would be relatively high. The duration of treatment is assumed to be sufficient to document changes in serum lipoproteins. To circumvent the notion that garlic lowers only elevated cholesterol levels,[21] our baseline levels were high enough (cholesterol, 7.53±0.75 mmol/L [291±29 mg/dL] and LDL-C, 5.35±0.78 mmol/L [207±30 mg/dL]). Although the effects of garlic on serum lipoprotein levels have been studied extensively, very little is known about its possible mechanism of action. In vitro data in rat hepatocytes suggest that allicin and ajoene inhibit cholesterol synthesis at various steps or inhibit acetate uptake into liver cells, respectively.[22,23] Validated in vivo methods for measurement of cholesterol synthesis in humans include the sterol balance technique, the determination of mevalonic acid in 24-hour urine, and the measurement of sterol precursors in serum.[24] It has been shown that the ratio of the cholesterol precursor lathosterol to cholesterol in serum is a reliable indicator of cholesterol synthesis because it closely reflects the activity of hepatic 3-hydroxy-3-methylglutaryl coenzyme A reductase.[18] In this study an influence of garlic on cholesterol synthesis, based on determinations of 3 indicators, could be excluded. Furthermore, it could be shown that absorption of cholesterol was not affected by garlic. On the basis of these findings, it can be concluded that cholesterol metabolism at multiple metabolic sites is not influenced by garlic at least with the pharmaceutical formulation used in this study. Moreover, individual changes in the effect of garlic on LDL-C concentrations did not correlate with any of the parameters of cholesterol metabolism, so that the conjecture of possible specific effects that are overridden by counterbalancing effects seems to be excluded.

Based on a meta-analysis from 1994, the total patient experience in randomized trials amounted to only 1365 individuals until then. This is a surprisingly low number, assuming that garlic may be effective in reducing elevated lipid levels without harmful side effects. Based on the results of the present study, however, there is no evidence to recommend garlic therapy for lowering serum lipid levels.

This study was supported by a research grant from Bundesministerium für Bildung, Wissenschaft, Forschung und Technologie (01EC9402).

The kind donation of the study medication by Hermes Pharmaceuticals, Munich, is gratefully acknowledged. We would like to thank all the patients in the study. We are indebted to Anja Kerksiek, Heike Prange, Susi Volz, and Katja Willmersdorf for their excellent technical assistance and Marion Zerlett for her organizational skills.

References

1. Harenberg J, Giese C, Zimmermann R. Effect of dried garlic on blood coagulation, fibrinolysis, platelet aggregation and serum cholesterol levels in patients with hyperlipoproteinemia. *Atherosclerosis.* 1988;74:247–249.
2. Neil HAW, Silagy C. Garlic: its cardioprotective properties. *Curr Opin Lipidol.* 1994;5:6–10.
3. Warshafsky S, Kamer RS, Sivak SL. Effect of garlic on total serum cholesterol: a meta-analysis. *Ann Intern Med.* 1993;119:599–605.
4. Silagy C, Neil A. Garlic as a lipid lowering agent—a meta-analysis. *J R Coll Physicians London.* 1994;28:39–45.
5. Beaglehole R. Garlic for flavour, not cardioprotection. *Lancet.* 1996;348:186–187.
6. Stewart LA, Parma MKB. Meta-analysis of the literature or of individual patient data: is there a difference? *Lancet.* 1993;341:418–422.
7. Neil HAW, Silagy CA, Lancaster T, et al. Garlic powder in the treatment of moderate hyperlipidemia. *J R Coll Physicians London.* 1996; 30:329–334.
8. LeLorier J, Gregoire G, Benhaddad A, et al. Discrepancies between meta-analyses and subsequent large randomized, controlled trials. *N Engl J Med.* 1997;337:536–542.
9. Simons LA, Balasubramaniam S, von Konigsmark M, et al. On the effect of garlic on plasma lipids and lipoproteins in mild hypercholesterolaemia. *Atherosclerosis.* 1995; 113:219–225.
10. Jain AK, Vargas R, Gotzkowsky S, et al. Can garlic reduce levels of serum lipids? a controlled clinical study. *Am J Med.* 1993;94:632–635.
11. Adler AJ, Holub BJ. Effect of garlic and fish-oil supplementation on serum lipid and lipoprotein concentrations in hypercholesterolemic men. *Am J Clin Nutr.* 1997;65:445–450.
12. Steiner M, Khan AH, Holbert D, et al. A double-blind crossover study in moderately hypercholesterolemic men that compared the effect of aged garlic extract and placebo administration on blood lipids. *Am J Clin Nutr.* 1996; 64:866–870.
13. Winkler G, Lohmüller E, Landshuter J, et al. Schwefelhaltige Leitsubstanzen in Knoblauchpräparaten. *Dtsch Apoth Ztg.* 1992;132:2312–2317.
14. Friedewald WT, Levy RJ, Frederickson DS. Estimation of the concentration of low-density-lipoprotein cholesterol in plasma, without use of the preparative ultracentrifuge. *Clin Chem.* 1972;18:499–509.
15. Lütjohann D, Meese CO, Crouse JR, et al. Evaluation of deuterated cholesterol and deuterated sitostanol for measurement of cholesterol absorption in humans. *J Lipid Res.* 1993;34:1039–1046.

16. Czubayko F, Beumers B, Lammfuss S, et al. A simplified micro-method for quantification of fecal excretion of neutral and acidic sterols for outpatient studies in humans. *J Lipid Res.* 1991; 32:1861–1867.

17. Lindenthal B, Simatupang A, Dotti MT, et al. Urinary excretion of mevalonic acid as an indicator of cholesterol synthesis. *J Lipid Res.* 1996; 37:2193–2201.

18. Björkhem I, Miettinen TA, Reihnér E, et al. Correlation between serum levels of some cholesterol precursors and activity of HMG-CoA reductase in human liver. *J Lipid Res.* 1987; 28:1137–1143.

19. Rosner B. *Fundamentals of Biostatistics.* 4th ed. Belmont, Calif: Duxbury Press; 1995:329–336.

20. Reuter II HD. Internationales Knoblauch-symposium. *Z Phythother.* 1991;12:83–93.

21. Mader FH. Treatment of hyperlipidaemia with garlic-powder tablets. *Arzneimittelforschung.* 1990;40:1111–1116.

22. Gebhardt R, Beck H, Wagner KG. Inhibition of cholesterol biosynthesis by allicin and ajoene in rat hepatocytes and HepG2 cells. *Biochim Biophys* Acta. 1994;1213:57–62.

23. Gebhardt R. Multiple inhibitory effects of garlic on cholesterol biosynthesis in hepatocytes. *Lipids.* 1993;28:613–619.

24. Jones PJH. Regulation of cholesterol biosynthesis by diet in humans. *Am J Clin Nutr.* 1997; 66:438–446.

37 Garlic Extract Therapy in Children With Hypercholesterolemia

Brian W. McCrindle, MD, MPH, FRCPC; Elizabeth Helden, BSN, MEd; William T. Conner, MBBS, MRCP, FRCPC

From the Department of Pediatrics, University of Toronto, The Hospital for Sick Children, Toronto, Ontario, (Dr McCrindle); and the Department of Pediatrics, McMaster University, St Joseph's Hospital, Hamilton, Ontario (Ms Helden and Dr Conner).

Objective

To determine whether garlic extract therapy is efficacious and safe in children with hypercholesterolemia.

Design

Randomized, double-blind, placebo-controlled clinical trial.

Setting

Specialized pediatric lipid disorders ambulatory clinic.

Participants

Thirty pediatric patients, aged 8 to 18 years, who had familial hyperlipidemia and a minimum fasting total cholesterol level greater than 4.8 mmol/L (>185 mg/dL).

Intervention

An 8-week course of a commercially available garlic extract (Kwai [Lichtwer Pharma, Berlin, Germany], 300 mg, 3 times a day) or an identical placebo.

Main Outcome Measures

Absolute and relative changes in fasting lipid profile parameters.

Results

The groups were equivalent at baseline and compliance was similar in the 2 groups (*P*=.45). There was no significant relative attributable effect of garlic extract on fasting total cholesterol (+0.6% [95% confidence interval, –5.8% to +6.9%]) or low-density lipoprotein cholesterol (–0.5% [95% confidence interval, –8.7% to +7.6%]). The lower limits of the confidence intervals did not include –10%, the minimum relative attributable effect believed to be clinically important. Likewise, no significant effect was seen on the levels of high-density lipoprotein, triglycerides, apolipoprotein B-100,

lipoprotein(a), fibrinogen, homocysteine, or blood pressure. There was a small effect on apolipoprotein A-I (+10.0% [95% confidence interval, +1.2% to +16.5%] *P* =.03). There were no differences in adverse effects between groups.

Conclusion

Garlic extract therapy has no significant effect on cardiovascular risk factors in pediatric patients with familial hyperlipidemia.

Arch Pediatr Adolesc Med. 1998;152:1089–1094

Detection and management of hypercholesterolemia in children remains controversial.[1–3] Dietary management with reduced fat and cholesterol intake is the cornerstone of therapy in children, together with attention to other cardiovascular risk factors.[4] However, a small proportion of children with hypercholesterolemia will meet the criteria for treatment with lipid-lowering medication.[1] The standard for drug therapy in children is treatment with bile acid–binding resins, which are associated with poor acceptability, tolerance, and compliance, and achieve only modest reductions in lipid profile levels.[5] Recently, there has been some interest in alternative therapies. Garlic (*Allium sativum*) and garlic extracts have been reported to be variably effective in managing hypertension and hypercholesterolemia,[6–8] although this remains to be proven conclusively.[9,10] Given concerns about the safety of long-term pharmacologic therapy in children, there is considerable interest in assessing potential "natural" treatments. To our knowledge no data regarding use of garlic extract preparations in treating hypercholesterolemia in children have been reported.

This study determined tolerance, compliance, safety, and efficacy of therapy with a commercially available garlic extract preparation in lowering cholesterol levels in participants with hypercholesterolemia. We hypothesized that compliance would be greater than 75% during the course of an 8-week study period, that less than 5% of the patients treated with the garlic extract preparation would experience unpleasant body odor, and that a mean relative attributable reduction in low-density lipoprotein (LDL) levels of 10% would be noted.

Participants and Methods

Sample Selection

Participants were recruited from the pediatric lipid disorders clinic of St Joseph's Hospital, Hamilton, Ontario, which provides assessment and management of children with primary lipid abnormalities. Some patients who had participated in previous clinical trials in the clinic were recruited by telephone and all other patients were recruited at the time of routinely scheduled clinic visits, until the sample size (N=30) was reached. All patients recruited met the inclusion criteria. Records of the number of patients approached and the proportion giving consent were not kept. Inclusion criteria were patient age (8–18 years old), a positive family history of hypercholesterolemia or premature atherosclerotic cardiovascular disease in first-degree relatives, a minimum fasting total cholesterol level at enrollment higher than 4.8 mmol/L (>185 mg/dL), participation in a dietary counseling program, and compliance with a National Cholesterol Education Program Step II diet for at least 6 months. Exclusion criteria included the presence of secondary causes of hyperlipidemia or a history of major surgery or serious illness 3 months or less prior to enrollment. This population was chosen because most of the patients unambiguously met criteria for pharmacologic therapy.[1]

Ethics

Ethics approval was obtained from the Research Ethics Board of the St Joseph's Hospital, and all parents and/or patients gave informed consent.

Design

The study was a randomized, double-blind, placebo-controlled clinical trial. Patients were instructed to stop taking any lipid-lowering medications for at least 8 weeks before the study. The medication used in the study was formulated by an independent pharmacist. The medication consisted of 1 whole 300-mg tablet of garlic extract (Kwai, Lichtwer Pharma, Berlin, Germany) containing 0.6 mg of allicin placed in a gelatin capsule with inert filler. One bulb of Chinese-grown garlic provides the same amount of allicin as that provided by 6 tablets of garlic extract. The placebo consisted of an identical gelatin capsule filled with the same inert filler only. Participants were instructed to take 1 capsule 3 times a day for an 8-week period (the manufacturer's recommended doseage for adults is 1 to 2 tablets 3 times a day). There was no information to guide dosing in pediatric patients, and the lower limit of the recommended adult dosage was chosen arbitrarily.

Randomization Procedure

Randomization was carried out independently by one of us (B.W.M.) not involved in application of the study. Using blocks of 6, a random number generator was used to create an assignment list, which was supplied to the independent pharmacist who then assigned patients consecutively when they were enrolled and their medication dispensed. The randomization list also specified the amount of medication to dispense, which covered the 8-week treatment period and a random number of additional capsules, so that all patients would have unused medication to return at the end of the study.

Blinding

The patient nurse coordinator (E.H.) and supervising physician (W.T.C.) responsible for recruitment, application of the study, and assessment were blinded as to the group assignment and total amount of medication dispensed. The independent pharmacist was not directly involved in the care of the study subjects.

Compliance

No direct biologic measure of compliance was taken. Unused medication at the end of the study period was returned and counted by the nurse coordinator. The amount of medication taken by each patient was assumed to be the amount dispensed minus the amount returned.
Compliance was expressed as the percentage of medication assumed taken vs the percentage expected to be taken if compliance was complete throughout the study period. Compliance was also assessed from a daily logbook completed by the patient for the first week of the study, and from questionnaires completed at 4 and 8 weeks after medication was started.

Main Outcome Measures

Blood samples from patients who had fasted were assessed at baseline and at study endpoint on the following factors: total cholesterol, triglycerides, high-density lipoprotein (HDL) cholesterol (with LDL cholesterol calculated), lipoprotein(a), apolipoproteins B-100 and A-I, homocysteine, and fibrinogen. These assays were performed in a single standardized lipid research laboratory with acceptable coefficients of variation. In addition, blood pressure was assessed at both time points.

Safety Monitoring

A complete physical examination that included an assessment of height and weight was performed at baseline and at study endpoint by one of us (W.T.C.). We collected data regarding symptoms and signs with the first-week daily logbook and midpoint and endpoint questionnaires. Participants were instructed to contact study personnel immediately if important adverse effects were noted or if the patient developed serious illness, required surgery, or required other pharmacologic treatment during the study period. Serum chemistry studies and complete blood cell counts were assessed and compared at baseline and endpoint.

Sample Size

Sample size estimation was based on the assumption that a 10% relative attributable reduction in the LDL cholesterol level was the minimum treatment deemed to be clinically important to justify use of medication. This assumption was based on a report that the drug caused a 12% reduction in cholesterol levels in adults.[6] Also, the only pharmacologic therapy approved for use in children who have hyperlipidemia is treatment with the bile acid–binding resins, which results in a reduction in the LDL of 10% to 15%.[1] Hypothesized LDL level lowering was −10%±5% (mean±SD) in the garlic extract and 0%±5% in the placebo groups, for a standardized treatment effect of 2.0. With a β level of .80 and an α level of .05, the estimated sample size was 11 patients per group, increased to 15 patients to compensate for potential dropouts.

Procedures

After obtaining informed consent, eligible study participants were instructed to stop taking all lipid-lowering medication for at least 8 weeks. At their initial clinic visit, patients were assessed for the following: fasting baseline blood studies, cardiovascular risk assessment including dietary assessment by food frequency questionnaire, family history questionnaire, and results from physical examination. Patients were given instructions regarding completion of the logbook and were asked to complete midpoint and endpoint questionnaires. They were then directed to the independent pharmacist who dispensed the study medication. Patients were reminded by telephone to complete the questionnaires. At the end of the 8-week study period, patients returned to the clinic with all remaining medication and the completed questionnaires and were assessed for the following: fasting blood studies, history including dietary assessment by food frequency questionnaire, and results from physical examination.

Data Analysis

Data are reported as frequencies, medians with ranges, and means with SDs as appropriate. Characteristics at baseline were compared between groups using the Fisher exact test, χ^2 test, Kruskal-Wallis analysis of variance, and *t* test. Patient changes in height, weight, blood pressure, and blood test results were assessed with paired *t* tests for each group. Mean differences in the changes between the 2 groups were compared with a Student *t* test. Difference in mean percent compliance between the 2 groups was assessed with a Student *t* test. Differences between groups in changes in lipid profile parameters adjusted for compliance were assessed with a general linear regression model. Statistical significance was set at $P<.05$.

Results

Enrollment

Thirty patients were initially enrolled in the trial and were randomly assigned to one of two groups of 15. One patient was unable to swallow the capsules and withdrew from the study; another patient was recruited and was given the original patient's allotted medication. All enrolled patients completed all components of the study protocol, and there was no incident of unmasking of patient assignment.

Baseline Characteristics

There were 16 male and 14 female patients in the study, and mean age at enrollment was 14.0±2.3 years. All patients had a positive family history of first-degree relatives with hypercholesterolemia and premature atherosclerotic heart disease. Mean fasting lipid values at baseline were total cholesterol, 6.86±1.52 mmol/L (265±59 mg/dL); LDL, 5.33±1.45 mmol/L (206±56 mg/dL); HDL, 0.95±0.22 mmol/L (37±8 mg/dL); and triglycerides, 1.26±0.52 mmol/L (112±46 mg/dL). The mean apolipoprotein B-100 level was 1.46±0.36 g/L (146±36 mg/dL); and apolipoprotein A-I, 1.12±0.14 g/L (112±14 mg/dL). Median lipoprotein(a) level was 155 g/L (15.5 mg/dL) and ranged from 24 to 2262 g/L (2.4–226.2 mg/dL), with 9 patients (30%) having significantly elevated levels. The mean fibrinogen level was 2.48±0.51 μmol/L and the homocysteine level was 7.37±2.02 μmol/L, with all patients within the normal range. No patient had hypertension and 5 patients (17%) occasionally used tobacco products (<5 cigarettes per day). Bile acid-binding resins had been previously used in 13 patients (43%); the remaining patients had been managed with dietary therapy only. All patients were judged to be sufficiently compliant with dietary goals.

Test of Randomization

Patient characteristics at baseline were not significantly different between the 2 groups, with the exception of higher homocysteine levels in the placebo group and a greater proportion of men in the garlic extract group (Table 1).

Compliance

There were no significant differences between groups regarding compliance throughout the study period. From the logbooks completed during the first week, patients in the placebo group took a mean of 93%±12% of expected doses vs 86%±27% in the garlic extract group ($P=.34$). On the midpoint questionnaire, patients in the placebo group responded that they had taken all of their medication a median of 6.25 days of the last 7 days (range, 3.5–7 days) vs a median of 7 days (range, 0–7 days) in the garlic extract group ($P=.34$). At endpoint questionnaire, patients in the placebo group responded that they had taken all of their medication a median of 7 days of the last 7 days (range, 0–7 days) vs a median of 6 days (range, 0–7 days) in the garlic extract group ($P=.34$). From returned medication counts at the end of the study, compliance during the study period was a mean of 78%±22% of expected in the placebo group vs 72%±21% in the garlic extract group ($P=.45$). Based on compliance and body weight at baseline, mean dose taken during the study period was 0.029±0.013 mg/kg per day in the placebo group vs 0.023±0.008 mg/kg per day in the garlic extract group ($P=.13$). Compliance during the study period was not significantly related to patient age or sex, previous experience with lipid-lowering medication, or fasting lipid profile parameters at baseline.

Main Outcome Measures

There were no significant differences in the relative treatment effect of garlic extract therapy regarding any of the primary outcome variables (Table 2). The mean baseline and study endpoint values for fasting lipid profile parameters for each group are shown in Figure 1. The significant relative increase in apolipoprotein A-I is associated with a *P* value of .03, which must be viewed in light of the effect of multiple comparisons. The lower limits of the 95% confidence intervals around the relative changes in total cholesterol (–5.8%) and LDL cholesterol (–8.7%) do not meet the empirically defined minimum treatment effect of –10% to achieve clinical importance. In general linear regression modeling, there were no significant differences between

Table 1. Comparison of Baseline Characteristics*

Variable	Placebo Group (n=15)	Garlic Extract–Treated Group (n=15)	*P*
Sex, male/female	5/10	11/4	.07
Age, y	14.1 ± 2.5	13.9 ± 2.2	.83
Weight, kg	54 ± 17	59 ± 18	.45
Body mass index, kg/m²	21.1 ± 4.2	22.6 ± 5.3	.40
Blood pressure, mm Hg			
Systolic	102 ± 9	102 ± 9	.85
Diastolic	60 ± 8	63 ± 10	.38
Occasional tobacco use, No. (%) of patients	3 (20)	2 (13)	1.00
Fasting lipid profile, mmol/L (mg/dL)			
Total cholesterol	6.66 ± 1.46 (257 ± 56)	7.06 ± 1.61 (276 ± 62)	.49
LDL-C†	5.07 ± 1.38 (196 ± 53)	5.59 ± 1.52 (216 ± 59)	.34
HDL-C†	0.96 ± 0.18 (37 ± 7)	0.95 ± 0.25 (37 ± 10)	.87
Triglycerides	1.38 ± 0.61 (122 ± 54)	1.14 ± 0.38 (101 ± 34)	.22
Apolipoproteins, g/L (mg/dL)			
Apolipoprotein A-I	1.16 ± 0.13 (116 ± 13)	1.07 ± 0.13 (107 ± 13)	.08
Apolipoprotein B-100	1.43 ± 0.35 [143 ± 35]	1.49 ± 0.38 [149 ± 38]	.63
Median [range] lipoprotein(a), mg/L (mg/dL)	113 [24, 955] (11.3 [2.4, 95.5])	207 [32, 2262] (20.7 [3.2, 226.2])	.17
Fibrinogen, g/L	2.54 ± 0.47	2.43 ± 0.56	.56
Homocysteine, μmol/L	8.25 ± 2.32	6.49 ± 1.17	.02

*Unless otherwise stated values are expressed as mean±SD.
†LDL-C indicates low-density lipoprotein cholesterol; HDL-C, high-density lipoprotein cholesterol. Numbers in parentheses are 95% confidence intervals. Numbers in brackets are conventional units.

Table 2. Absolute and Relative Attributable Treatment Effects of Garlic Extract Therapy*

Variable	Absolute Effect, % (95% Confidence Interval)	Relative Effect, % (95% Confidence Interval)	*P*
Fasting lipid profile, mmol/L [mg/dL]			
Total cholesterol	+0.10 (–0.29, +0.49) [+4 (–11, +19)]	+0.6 (–5.8, +6.9)	.86
LDL-C	+0.04 (–0.35, +0.43) [+2 (–14, +17)]	–0.5 (–8.7, +7.6)	.90
HDL-C	+0.03 (–0.11, +0.17) [+1 (–4, +7)]	+9.3 (–8.2, +26.8)	.29
Triglycerides	–0.18 (–0.66, +0.30) [–16 (–58, +27)]	–7.2 (–44.6, +30.2)	.70
Apolipoprotein, g/L [mg/dL]			
Apoliprotein A-I	+0.09 (+0.01, +0.17) [+9 (+1, +17)]	+10.0 (+1.2, +16.5)	.03
Apolipoprotein B-100	+0.02 (–0.08, +0.12) [+2 (–8, +12)]	+0.8 (–7.3, +8.8)	.85
Lipoprotein(a), mg/L [mg/dL]	–71 (–138, –5) [–7.1 (–13.8, –0.5)]	–9.0 (–30.2, +12.2)	.40
Fibrinogen, g/L [mg/dL]	–0.19 (–0.64, +0.26) [+19 (–64, +26)]	–7.8 (–26.3, +10.6)	.40
Homocysteine, μmol/L	+0.67 (–0.45, +1.79)	+10.5 (–5.3, +26.4)	.19
Blood pressure, mm Hg			
Systolic	+2.1 (–7.1, +11.3)	+2.3 (–6.8, +11.4)	.61
Diastolic	0 (–6.5, +6.5)	–0.4 (–11.9, +11.1)	.94

*LDL-C indicates low-density lipoprotein cholesterol; HDL-C, high-density lipoprotein cholesterol. Numbers in parentheses are 95% confidence intervals. Numbers in brackets are conventional units.

groups in changes in primary outcome variables after controlling for compliance. In the garlic extract group, the absolute and relative changes in primary outcome variables were not significantly correlated with compliance or dose taken during the study period; thus there appeared to be no dose-response gradient.

Confounding Factors

There were no significant differences between groups regarding change in weight or body mass index (calculated as weight in kilograms divided by the square of height in meters) during the study interval. Likewise, all patients continued to follow dietary recommendations and there were no significant changes regarding dietary content. No

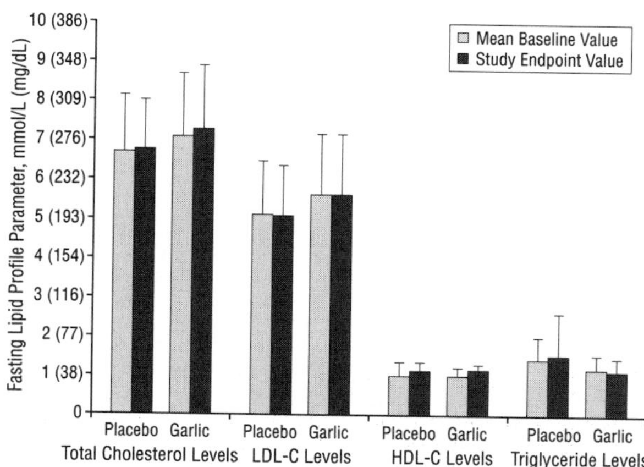

Figure 1. Changes in fasting lipid profile parameters. Height of the bars represents the mean and lines extending above bars represent 1 SD. There were no statistically significant differences in the change from baseline between placebo and garlic extract-treated groups for any fasting lipid profile parameter. LDL-C indicates low-density lipoprotein cholesterol; HDL-C, high-density lipoprotein cholesterol.

patient reported a significant change in physical activity or smoking behavior during the study period. No patient developed a noteworthy concurrent illness or was placed on any other medication.

Adverse Effects

The incidence and pattern of adverse effects was equivalent in the 2 groups. Only 1 patient in the garlic extract group experienced unpleasant body odor, but concomitantly had been working on a garlic farm during the study period. On the midpoint questionnaire, 36% of patients in the placebo group and 31% of patients in the garlic extract group reported minor adverse effects (P=1.0), the most common being headache and upset stomach. On the endpoint questionnaire, 13% of patients taking the placebo and 21% taking the garlic extract reported adverse effects (P=.66), the most common being headache. There were no significant absolute or relative attributable effects on height, weight, or blood pressure. The only significant differences in absolute attributable effect on laboratory parameters were in serum albumin level (+2.0 g/L [95% confidence interval, +0.9 to +3.0] P=.002) and hemoglobin (+5.2 g/L [95% confidence interval, +1.4 to +9.0] P=.02).

Comment

While pharmacologic lipid-lowering therapy has been shown to be effective in reducing cardiovascular morbidity and cardiovascular mortality rates and total mortality rates in adults, management of hyperlipidemia in children remains controversial.[1–3] Our study showed no significant reduction attributable to garlic extract therapy in recognized cardiovascular risk factors in children with familial hyperlipidemia, with the exception of a small increase in apolipoprotein A-I levels.

Patients are increasingly seeking alternative therapies for their illnesses, despite the fact that scientific evidence supporting the effectiveness and safety of these therapies is often lacking or conflicting. Garlic has been used for centuries to treat a wide range of ailments.[10] Recently, perhaps driven by hypotheses from dietary epidemiologic studies, there has been renewed interest in garlic and garlic preparations and their potential cardiovascular benefits. Several studies have shown improvements in lipid profile parameters,[11–15] hypertension,[15,16] platelet aggregation,[17] and plasma viscosity and fibrinolytic activity.[18] The mechanisms by which garlic or its active components might cause these effects have not been determined. Methodologic flaws of these studies and direct drug company sponsorship also weaken the strength of evidence of these studies.[6,7,9] A more recent meta-analysis was more guarded in its support of an important treatment effect related to garlic-extract therapy.[9] A recent clinical trial showed no significant lowering of cholesterol levels and no effect on LDL oxidizability, cholesterol synthesis, or LDL receptor expression.[19] In addition, to our knowledge, no study has shown any relationship between garlic extract therapy and reductions in cardiovascular morbidity and cardiovascular mortality rates or total mortality rates. Our study further supports this skepticism. Clearly, large-scale, well-designed studies are needed in this area.

Many patients may elect to adopt or persist with using garlic extract therapy despite a lack of scientific evidence supporting its effectiveness.[20] To date, reports of adverse effects related to garlic extract therapy with commercially available preparations have been limited to unpleasant body odor and mild allergic reactions.[21] No significant adverse effects that could be attributed to garlic extract therapy were noted in this study. Adverse effects on growth and development have not been studied, nor have adverse effects related to long-term use.

In summary, in a randomized, double-blind, placebo-controlled clinical trial of garlic extract therapy in hypercholesterolemic children, we found that this treatment course had no significant effect on cardiovascular risk factors.

This project was supported by the Father Sean O'Sullivan Research Centre, St Joseph's Hospital, Hamilton, Ontario.

Presented in part at the Annual Meeting of the Pediatric Academic Societies, New Orleans, La, May 1-5, 1998.

References

1. Anonymous. National Cholesterol Education Program: report of the expert panel on blood cholesterol levels in children and adolescents. *Pediatrics.* 1994;89:525–584.
2. Newman TB, Garber AM, Holtzman NA, Hulley SB. Problems with the report of the Expert Panel on blood cholesterol levels in children and adolescents. *Arch Pediatr Adolesc Med.* 1995; 149:241–247.
3. Dennison BA, Jenkins PL, Pearson TA. Challenges to implementing the current pediatric cholesterol screening guidelines into practice. *Pediatrics.* 1994;94:296–302.
4. Anonymous. Efficacy and safety of lowering dietary intake of fat and cholesterol in children with elevated low-density lipoprotein cholesterol. The Dietary Intervention Study in Children (DISC). The Writing Group for the DISC Collaborative Research Group. *JAMA.* 1995; 273:1429–1435.
5. McCrindle BW, O'Neill MB, Cullen-Dean G, Helden E. Acceptability and compliance with two forms of cholestyramine in the treatment of hypercholesterolemia in children: a randomized, crossover trial. *J Pediatr.* 1997; 130:266–273.
6. Silagy C, Neil A. Garlic as a lipid lowering agent—a meta-analysis. *J R Coll Physicians Lond.* 1994;28:39–45.
7. Warshafsky S, Kamer RS, Sivak SL. Effect of garlic on total serum cholesterol. A meta-analysis. *Ann Intern Med.* 1993;119:599–560.
8. Silagy CA, Neil HAW. A meta-analysis of the effect of garlic on blood pressure. *J Hypertension.* 1994;12:463–468.
9. Neil HA, Silagy CA, Lancaster T, et al. Garlic powder in the treatment of moderate hyperlipidaemia: a controlled trial and meta-analysis. *J R Coll Phys London.* 1996;30:329–334.
10. Kendler BS. Garlic (*Allium sativum*) and onion (*Allium cepa*): a review of their relationship to cardiovascular disease. *Prev Med.* 1987; 16:670–685.
11. Auer W, Eiber A, Hertkorn E, et al. Hypertension and hyperlipidaemia: garlic helps in mild cases. *Br J Clin Prac.* 1990;69:3–6.
12. Mader FH. Treatment of hyperlipidaemia with garlic-powder tablets: evidence from the German Association of General Practitioners' multicentric placebo-controlled double-blind study. *Arzneimittelforschung.* 1990; 40:1111–1116.
13. Jain AK, Vargas R, Gotzkowsky S, McMahon FG. Can garlic reduce levels of serum lipids? a controlled clinical study. *Am J Med.* 1993; 94:632–635.
14. Kenzelmann R, Kade F. Limitation of the deterioration of lipid parameters by a standardized garlic-ginkgo combination product. A multicenter placebo-controlled double-blind study. *Arzneimittelforschung.* 1993;43:978–981.
15. Steiner M, Khan AH, Holbert D, Lin RI. A double-blind crossover study in moderately hypercholesterolemic men that compared the effect of aged garlic extract and placebo administration on blood lipids. *Am J Clin Nutr.* 1996; 64:866–870.
16. McMahon FG, Vargas R. Can garlic lower blood pressure? a pilot study. *Pharmacotherapy.* 1993; 13:406–407.
17. Kiesewetter H, Jung F, Mrowietz C, et al. Effect of garlic therapy on thrombocyte aggregation, microcirculation, and other risk factors. *Int J Clin Pharm Ther Tox.* 1991;29:151–155.
18. Kiesewetter H, Jung F, Mrowietz C, Pindur G, Heiden M, Wenzel E. Effects of garlic on blood fluidity and fibrinolytic activity: a randomised, placebo-controlled, double-blind study. *Br J Clin Prac.* 1990;44:24–29.
19. Simons LA, Balasubramaniam S, von Konigsmark M, Parfitt A, Simons J, Peters W. On the effect of garlic on plasma lipids and lipoproteins in mild hypercholesterolaemia. *Atherosclerosis.* 1995;113:219–225.
20. Estrada CA, Young MJ. Patient preferences for novel therapy: an N-of-1 trial of garlic in the treatment for hypertension. *J Gen Int Med.* 1993;8:619–621.
21. Lautier R, Wendt V. Kontackallergie aus Alliaceae. *Dermatosen.* 1985;33:213–215.

38 A Placebo-Controlled, Double-blind, Randomized Trial of an Extract of *Ginkgo biloba* for Dementia

Pierre L. Le Bars, MD, PhD; Martin M. Katz, PhD; Nancy Berman, PhD; Turan M. Itil, MD; Alfred M. Freedman, MD; Alan F. Schatzberg, MD; for the North American EGb Study Group

From the New York Institute for Medical Research, Tarrytown (Dr Le Bars); Department of Psychiatry, Albert Einstein College of Medicine–Montefiore Medical Center, New York, NY (Dr Katz); Harbor-UCLA Medical Center, Torrance, Calif (Dr Berman); Department of Psychiatry, New York Medical College, Valhalla (Drs Itil and Freedman); and Harvard Medical Center, Boston, Mass (Dr Schatzberg). Dr Le Bars is now with the Department of Psychiatry, New York University Medical Center, New York Institute for Medical Research; Dr Itil is now with the Department of Psychiatry, New York University Medical Center; and Dr Schatzberg is now with the Department of Psychiatry and Behavioral Sciences, School of Medicine, Stanford University, Stanford, Calif. A list of investigators appears at the end of the article.

Context

EGb 761 is a particular extract of *Ginkgo biloba* used in Europe to alleviate symptoms associated with numerous cognitive disorders. Its use in dementias is based on positive results from only a few controlled clinical trials, most of which did not include standard assessments of cognition and behavior.

Objective

To assess the efficacy and safety of EGb in Alzheimer disease and multi-infarct dementia.

Design

A 52-week, randomized double-blind, placebo-controlled, parallel-group, multicenter study.

Patients

Mildly to severely demented outpatients with Alzheimer disease or multi-infarct dementia, without other significant medical conditions.

Intervention

Patients assigned randomly to treatment with EGb (120 mg/d) or placebo. Safety, compliance, and drug dispensation were monitored every 3 months with complete outcome evaluation at 12, 26, and 52 weeks.

Primary Outcome Measures

Alzheimer's Disease Assessment Scale–Cognitive subscale (ADAS-Cog), Geriatric Evaluation by Relative's Rating Instrument (GERRI), and Clinical Global Impression of Change (CGIC).

Results

From 309 patients included in an intent-to-treat analysis, 202 provided evaluable data for the 52-week end point analysis. In the intent-to-treat analysis, the EGb group had an ADAS-Cog score 1.4 points better than the placebo group (*P*=.04) and a GERRI score 0.14 points better than the placebo group (*P*=.004). The same patterns were observed with the evaluable data set in which 27% of patients treated with EGb

achieved at least a 4-point improvement on the ADAS-Cog, compared with 14% taking placebo (*P*=.005); on the GERRI, 37% were considered improved with EGb, compared with 23% taking placebo (*P*=.003). No difference was seen in the CGIC. Regarding the safety profile of EGb, no significant differences compared with placebo were observed in the number of patients reporting adverse events or in the incidence and severity of these events.

Conclusions

EGb was safe and appears capable of stabilizing and, in a substantial number of cases, improving the cognitive performance and the social functioning of demented patients for 6 months to 1 year. Although modest, the changes induced by EGb were objectively measured by the ADAS-Cog and were of sufficient magnitude to be recognized by the caregivers in the GERRI.

JAMA. 1997;278:1327–1332

The extract of *Ginkgo biloba* referred to as EGb 761 is one of the most popular plant extracts[1] used in Europe to alleviate symptoms associated with a range of cognitive disorders.[2] It has recently been approved in Germany for the treatment of dementia. The mechanism of action of EGb in the central nervous system is only partially understood, but the main effects seem to be related to its antioxidant properties, which require the synergistic action of the flavonoids, the terpenoids (ginkgolides, bilobalide), and the organic acids, principal constituents of EGb.[3] These compounds to varying degrees act as scavengers for free radicals,[2,4] which have been considered the mediators of the excessive lipid peroxidation and cell damage observed in Alzheimer disease (AD).[5–8] Although several European studies[9–13] report positive results of EGb 761 in the treatment of diverse neurological disorders, few studies using standard methods have evaluated the cognitive and behavioral effects of EGb in dementia.[13] Further, no empirical clinical trials of the extract have been conducted in the United States. Therefore, this multicenter placebo-controlled study was undertaken to assess the efficacy and safety of EGb in AD and multi-infarct dementia (MID).

Methods

Patient Population

Patients of both sexes, 45 years of age or older, with a diagnosis of uncomplicated dementia according to *Diagnostic and Statistical Manual of Mental Disorders, Third Edition, Revised (DSM-III-R)* and *International Statistical Classification of Diseases, 10th Revision (ICD-10)* criteria, either Alzheimer type (AD) or MID, were enrolled in the study. The severity of the dementia at screening was mild to moderately severe as assessed by a Mini-Mental State Examination[14] score of 9 to 26 (inclusive) and a Global Deterioration Scale score[15] of 3 to 6 (inclusive). To be eligible, patients had to have no other significant medical conditions including cardiac disease, insulin-dependent diabetes, liver disease, chronic renal insufficiency, or another psychiatric disorder as a primary diagnosis. Patients with brain mass or intracranial hemorrhage determined by computed tomography or magnetic resonance imaging were excluded.

The use of medications for preexisting conditions was not discontinued at screening, but change in regimen or prescription of new concomitant medications known to affect cognitive function was not permitted during the study. Noncompliance was monitored by pill counts and defined by a deviation of more than 20% from the study regimen.

The study protocol and the informed consent forms were approved by the institutional review boards of the Massachusetts Mental Health Center of Harvard Medical School, Boston, and New York Institute for Medical Research, Tarrytown. Written informed consent was obtained from the patients or their legal representatives and from the caregivers.

Study Design

The study used a 52-week, double-blind, fixed-dose, placebo-controlled, parallel-group randomized design and was conducted at 6 research centers in the United States. Patients underwent a 14-day single-blind placebo run-in period. Safety assessments (adverse events and vital signs), pill counts, and drug dispensation were performed at 4-, 12-, 26-, 39-, and 52-week visits. Complete assessments of primary outcome measures were required at baseline and at 12, 26, and 52 weeks. At screening and at termination, extensive medical, neurological, and psychiatric evaluations were performed, including electroencephalogram and laboratory tests (blood cell count, routine chemistry, vitamin B_{12}, folate, triiodothyronine, thyroxine, and thyrotropin). National Health Laboratories,

Cranford, NJ, was used as a central laboratory to collect and analyze all laboratory work from each site. All randomization procedures, drug packaging, storage of codes and other study materials, and study monitoring were managed by International Drug Development Corporation, Parsippany, NJ. EGb (Murdock, Springville, Utah) was supplied as a 40-mg tablet to be swallowed before each of the 3 principal daily meals, for a total daily dose of 120 mg. Patients were consecutively assigned to EGb or to placebo following a predetermined order based on separate randomization schedules for each center using balanced blocks of 10 patients. Consecutive numbers were printed on each drug study pack, and randomization codes, stored in sealed envelopes, were exclusively retained by International Drug Development Corporation independently from sponsor and investigating centers.

The EGb and the matched placebo tablets did not differ in their appearance and were film coated to ensure a similar smell and taste. EGb had the identical formulation and chemical composition as the product used in Germany (Tebonin forte, Dr. Willmar Schwabe Pharmaceuticals, Karlsruhe). The study drugs were made by a standard method and came from the same batch of Ginkgo extract. EGb is a standardized concentrated extract from the dried leaves of the *Ginkgo biloba* tree, specially produced by means of a multiple-step extraction procedure and consisting of 24% Ginkgo-flavoneglycosides and 6% terpenelactones (3.1% ginkgolides A, B, and C, 2.9% bilobalide).

Outcome Measures

The primary outcome measures assessed changes in 3 areas: (1) *Cognitive impairment* was assessed by the cognitive subscale of the Alzheimer's Disease Assessment Scale[16,17] (ADAS-Cog), a performance-based cognitive test that objectively evaluates memory, language, praxis, and orientation. The test includes 11 items with a total score ranging from 0 to 70; the higher the score, the poorer the performance. (2) *Daily living and social behavior* was assessed by the total score of the Geriatric Evaluation by Relative's Rating Instrument[18] (GERRI), a 49-item rating inventory completed by the caregiver. The total score is the grand mean of the following 3 subscale means: the GERRI-cognitive (21 items), the GERRI-social (18 items), and the GERRI-mood (10 items). The scores of each item, thus, of each subscale and of the grand mean, range from 1 to 5; the higher the score, the poorer the patient's functioning in the home environment. The questions are presented in an identical checklist at each visit and are answered by the caregiver who evaluates the patient's functioning during the 14 days prior to the assessment. The GERRI total score was found to be highly correlated with the overall symptom severity of the dementia, as assessed by the Global Deterioration Scale.[18] However, longitudinal studies of annual GERRI change scores are few[19] and its validity in this respect has yet to be rigorously tested. (3) *General psychopathology,* the changes in overall psychopathology, was assessed by the Clinical Global Impression of Change[20] (CGIC), an interview-based global rating that quantifies the clinician's judgment of the amount of change in overall impairment compared with that at the study baseline. The CGIC does not follow a structured interview and uses a 7-point ordinal scale in which 1 is an extreme score indicating that the patient improved very much, and 7 indicates extreme worsening. Secondary outcomes of the study will be presented elsewhere.

Each subject was to complete 52 weeks, but if at any time a subject showed worsening of functioning or impairment, as assessed by an increase of 1 point on the CGIC, the subject could be dropped from the study and offered admission to an uncontrolled open-label humanitarian protocol. However, the investigator was encouraged to maintain the patient in the double-blind phase for at least 6 months. The confirmatory analysis was planned on "per protocol" valid cases with missing data at the 52-week end point visit replaced by last evaluable assessments after a minimum of 20 weeks of treatment (missing data at baseline were not replaced). An analysis of efficacy on an intent-to-treat (ITT) basis[21] with last observation carried forward was formulated as a secondary analysis. However, considering the relatively low proportion of patients completing the entire study and their unequal distribution between treatment arms, the ITT analysis was selected a posteriori as the primary analysis for efficacy.

Statistical Methods

It was planned to enroll 300 patients in the study. Owing to the higher prevalence of AD compared with MID,[22,23] 70% of the total study patients were expected to have AD. However, there was no monitoring of the enrollment to control this ratio at the participating centers. The total sample size was calculated to detect a standardized treatment difference of 0.40 with a power of 80% (2-sample *t* test, α=.05, 2 sided), taking into account a predicted dropout rate of 20% during the entire course of the study. Data quality control and case classification for evaluable and ITT analyses were completed before breaking the double blind.

Prior to analysis, the distributions of the continuous variables, ie, the change scores from baseline for the ADAS-Cog and the GERRI, were tested and met the assumptions of normality. Nonparametric methods were applied for noninterval variables. The baseline Mini-Mental State Examination score was used to create a severity index for cognitive impairment.[6,24–26] Age was recoded to groups of younger than 65 years, 65 to 80 years, and older than 80 years. Paired *t* tests or median tests were performed within groups to determine if change from baseline was different from zero on the ADAS-Cog, GERRI, and CGIC.

The primary efficacy analysis used an analysis of variance model, with end point value as the dependent variable and treatment, age, and severity of cognitive impairment as factors; another model used as factors treatment, center, and severity to test for center effect. In each model, a test for interaction between factors was included. Since subjects could be removed from the study if they had a 1-point increase in the CGIC, this variable was used for testing efficacy only in the ITT analysis.

To describe the response in a manner more applicable to clinical practice, categorical variables defining positive and negative change were developed for the ADAS-Cog and the GERRI and analyzed by applying the method of cumulative logits.[27] For the ADAS-Cog, a magnitude of ±2- and ±4-point cutoffs were adopted in accord with a previous standard from the literature.[19,28–31] Because there were no guidelines for cutoff points for the GERRI, the lower and upper quartiles that bound the middle 50% of the distribution of the scores in the total population were selected (±0.2 points).

In addition to the core study on the total population, a separate analysis was performed exclusively with the AD patients. This was done for 3 reasons; first, they are a large, clinically important, well-defined, and relatively homogeneous population; second, the criteria for AD, as summarized in the *DSM-III-R* and the *ICD-10* and applied in this study, led to a high reliability of the diagnosis[32–34]; and finally, the AD subgroup of this study formed a majority of the total sample.

Results

Patient disposition during the study is summarized in Figure 1. From a total of 327 patients enrolled in the study (251 patients with AD), 309 patients were included in the ITT analysis.

Of the 18 patients not included, 15 had no data after baseline, 2 had insulin-dependent diabetes, and 1 had an unstable affective mood disorder that required multiple psychotropic drugs. The group that received EGb included

No. of Patients Screened	549	
No. of Patients Not Eligible	222	
No. of Patients Randomized	327	
	EGb	**Placebo**
Randomization	166	161
Did Not Receive Standard Intervention as Allocated	9	6
Excluded From Analysis	2	1
Followed Up		
4-wk Visit	155	154
12-wk Visit	142	141
26-wk Visit	122	122
39-wk Visit	93	75
52-wk Visit	78	59
Withdrawn (After Baseline)		
Intervention Ineffective	12	21
Caregiver Request	24	29
Unavailable for Follow-up	8	10
Adverse Event	10	4
Death	2	1
Concurrent Illness	4	5
Noncompliance With Protocol	13	14
Other	15	18
Completed Trial	78	59

Figure 1. Profile of the randomized controlled trial. Three patients were excluded from analysis because of protocol violations (2 because of diabetes mellitus and 1 because of unstable affective mood disorder).

155 patients; however, 17 of them were not compliant with the EGb regimen and an additional 15 patients did not achieve a minimum of 12 weeks of treatment. Of the 244 ITT patients reaching the 26-week visit, 202 (97 for EGb and 105 for placebo) provided evaluable data and could be included in the evaluable end point analysis.

There were 236 patients with AD in the ITT analysis, randomized to EGb (n=120) or placebo (n=116). The pattern of change in group sizes during the treatment period was similar to that in the total population.

Patient characteristics at baseline were similar between treatment groups and are summarized in Table 1. The patient characteristics for the evaluable data set were almost identical to those for the ITT group except for slightly lower values for the ADAS-Cog (17.2 and 19.9 for EGb and placebo groups, respectively).

Efficacy Analysis and ITT Analysis

Because the ITT analysis was based on last observations after baseline carried forward to end point, regardless of the actual treatment length, the average elapsed time within the study was computed for each treatment group. The EGb group had an average end point of 38.6 weeks (95% confidence interval, 35.7–41.5 weeks) compared with 34.6 weeks for the placebo group (95% confidence interval, 31.7–37.4 weeks). This difference was most

Table 1. Patient Characteristics at Baseline: Intent-to-Treat Analysis*

	All Diagnostic Groups			Alzheimer Disease		
	All	EGb Group	Placebo Group	All	EGb Group	Placebo Group
No. of subjects	309	155	154	236	120	116
No. (%) of females	166 (54)	79 (51)	87 (56)	137 (58)	65 (54)	72 (62)
Age, y	69 (10)	69 (10)	69 (10)	68 (10)	68 (10)	68 (11)
Range	45–90	47–89	45–90	45–90	47–89	45–90
Median education, y (range)	14 (0–20)	14 (1–20)	14 (0–20)	14 (0–20)	14 (1–20)	14 (0–20)
Mini-Mental State Examination score	21.1 (5.6)	21.1 (5.8)	21.2 (5.5)	21.2 (5.7)	21.1 (5.9)	21.3 (5.6)
Range	6–30	8–28	6–30	6–30	8–28	6–30
ADAS-Cog score	20.2 (15.4)	20.0 (16.0)	20.5 (14.7)	20.0 (15.8)	19.7 (16.4)	20.2 (15.2)
Range	2–64	2–64	2–63	2–64	2–64	2–63
Disease duration, y	4.2 (3.7)	4.6 (4.3)	3.9 (3.0)	4.3 (3.8)	4.6 (4.4)	4.0 (3.2)
Range	0–36	0–36	0–20	0–36	0–36	0–20

*Data are given as mean (SD), unless otherwise specified. ADAS-Cog indicates Alzheimer's Disease Assessment Scale–Cognitive subscale.

likely related to the unequal distribution of the dropout rate after the 26-week visit. Although a similar ratio of subjects withdrew from each treatment group before 26 weeks (33/155 for the EGb group and 33/154 for the placebo group), 28% (44/155) of the EGb group vs 40% (62/154) of the placebo group dropped out between 26 and 52 weeks. Consequently, 50% (78/155) of the EGb group completed the entire study compared with only 38% (59/154) of the placebo group.

The results of the ITT analysis are provided in Table 2. In this table (as well as in Table 3, for the evaluable data set), the *P* values for treatment effects in change score are the results from the analysis of variance described in the "Methods" section. Although severity of cognitive impairment was a significant factor in overall change ($P<.01$) in all analyses, no significant interaction was found between severity and treatment. Furthermore, age was not a significant factor in any analysis and no interaction was found between treatment group and center.

Regarding the ADAS-Cog, there was no significant change observed at end point for the EGb group, whereas the placebo group showed a significant worsening of 1.5 points ($P=.006$). The mean treatment difference significantly favored EGb ($P=.04$). Considering the GERRI, mild improvement was observed for the EGb group, whereas the placebo group showed significant worsening (0.08 points; $P=.02$), resulting in a statistically significant difference in favor of EGb ($P=.004$). These results are depicted graphically in Figure 2. Regarding global psychopathology, a slight worsening was observed for both treatment groups on the CGIC (departure from a score of 4, "no change"; $P<.002$), as assessed by a deviation of 0.2 points of the rating mean (59% [183/309] of the total population were considered unchanged).

When the AD subgroup was examined separately, a similar pattern of results was demonstrated across the 2 treatments; differences were significant on both the ADAS-Cog ($P=.02$) and the GERRI ($P<.001$) (Table 2).

Evaluable Population

At the 26-week time point (Table 3), a slight improvement was observed in the EGb group on the ADAS-Cog while the placebo group showed a significant worsening of 1.4 points ($P=.002$). The mean treatment difference was in favor of EGb ($P=.04$). On the GERRI, the EGb group showed a mean improvement (0.07 points) and the placebo group worsened by the same amount, resulting in a statistically significant treatment difference ($P=.04$).

For the evaluable 52-week end point analysis, the average timing of the end point was 46.6 weeks (95% confidence interval, 44.1–49.0 weeks) for the EGb group and 42.3 weeks (95% confidence interval, 39.8–44.8 weeks) for the placebo group. The difference of 4 weeks between these 2 end points followed the same pattern observed in the ITT analysis: in the EGb group, 71% (69/97) of the patients reaching 26 weeks completed the whole study compared with 51% (54/105) in the placebo group. The outcomes of the 52-week end point analysis are summarized in Table 3. There was a slight improvement for the EGb group on the ADAS-Cog, while the placebo group showed continued worsening, with an increased score from 1.4 at 26 weeks to 2.1 points at end point ($P<.001$). The mean treatment difference of –2.4 points further favored the EGb group ($P=.005$). The same course of changes were observed with the caregiver assessment. The EGb group showed significant im-

Table 2. Primary Outcome Measure Results: Intent-to-Treat Analysis*

	Mean Change From Baseline (95% CI) [n]		
	ADAS-Cog	GERRI	CGIC Rating Mean (95% CI) [n]
All diagnostic groups (N=309)			
EGb group	0.1 (–0.8 to 1.0) [136]	–0.06 (–0.13 to 0.01) [138]	4.2 (4.1 to 4.4) [155]
Placebo group	1.5 (0.4 to 2.5) [138]	0.08 (0.01 to 0.14) [132]	4.2 (4.1 to 4.3) [154]
Treatment difference	–1.4 (–2.7 to –0.0)	–0.14 (–0.23 to –0.04)	0.0 (–0.1 to 0.2)
P	.04	.004	.77
Alzheimer disease (N=236)			
EGb group	–0.2 (–1.2 to 0.8) [104]	–0.09 (–0.16 to –0.02) [104]	4.2 (4.1 to 4.4) [120]
Placebo group	1.5 (0.3 to 2.6) [103]	0.09 (0.02 to 0.17) [101]	4.2 (4.1 to 4.4) [116]
Treatment difference	–1.7 (–3.2 to –0.2)	–0.19 (–0.28 to –0.08)	0.0 (–0.2 to 0.2)
P	.02	<.001	.21

*CI indicates confidence interval; ADAS-Cog, Alzheimer's Disease Assessment Scale–Cognitive subscale; GERRI, Geriatric Evaluation by Relative's Rating Instrument; and CGIC, Clinical Global Impression of Change. The ADAS-Cog is a 70-point scale; the GERRI is a 5-point scale; and the CGIC is a 7-point ordinal scale.

Table 3. Primary Outcome Measure Results: Evaluable 26-Week Time Point and 52-Week End Point Analyses*

	ADAS-Cog, Mean (95% CI) [n]		GERRI, Mean (95% CI) [n]	
	26 wk	52 wk	26 wk	52 wk
All diagnostic groups (N=202)				
EGb group	–0.5 (–1.6 to 0.6) [95]	–0.3 (–1.3 to 0.8) [96]	–0.07 (–0.13 to 0.00) [85]	–0.09 (–0.17 to 0.02) [89]
Placebo group	1.4 (0.3 to 2.5) [102]	2.1 (0.9 to 3.4) [104]	0.07 (–0.02 to 0.16) [85]	0.10 (–0.01 to 0.19) [88]
Treatment difference	–1.9 (–3.4 to –0.3)	–2.4 (–4.0 to –0.8)	–0.14 (–0.25 to –0.02)	–0.19 (–0.31 to –0.07)
P	.04	.005	.04	.002
Alzheimer disease (N=150)				
EGb group	–0.7 (–2.0 to 0.6) [74]	–0.5 (–1.7 to 0.8) [75]	–0.08 (–0.16 to 0.01) [64]	–0.08 (–0.17 to 0.01) [67]
Placebo group	1.4 (0.2 to 2.6) [73]	2.1 (0.7 to 3.5) [75]	0.07 (0.03 to 0.17) [63]	0.12 (0.01 to 0.22) [65]
Treatment difference	–2.1 (–3.8 to –0.3)	–2.6 (–4.4 to –0.7)	–0.15 (–0.28 to –0.02)	–0.20 (–0.33 to –0.06)
P	.02	.005	.05	.004

*CI indicates confidence interval; ADAS-Cog, Alzheimer's Disease Assessment Scale–Cognitive subscale; and GERRI, Geriatric Evaluation by Relative's Rating Instrument. The ADAS-Cog is a 70-point scale; the GERRI is a 5-point scale.

provement (P=.02) while the placebo counterpart deteriorated (P=.04), resulting in a statistically significant difference of –0.19 points for the GERRI change score (P=.002).

Categorical Analysis of Positive and Negative Outcomes

To compare the number of patients showing positive or negative clinical outcomes within each treatment arm of the evaluable data set, a cumulative logit analysis was conducted using the 52-week end point on the ADAS-Cog and the GERRI classification codes described in the "Methods" section. The results are summarized in Table 4. EGb shows a higher percentage of "improvers," while the placebo shows more "decliners," leading to highly significant differences on each assessment measure. On the ADAS-Cog, 50% of the EGb patients showed an improvement by at least 2 points compared with 29% of the placebo group; this approximately 2-fold difference was still observed when the threshold to detect an improvement in cognition was set at 4 ADAS-Cog points. On the GERRI, 37% of the EGb group were considered improved and only 19% were considered worse; the placebo group demonstrated the opposite trend with 40% worsening and 23% improving.

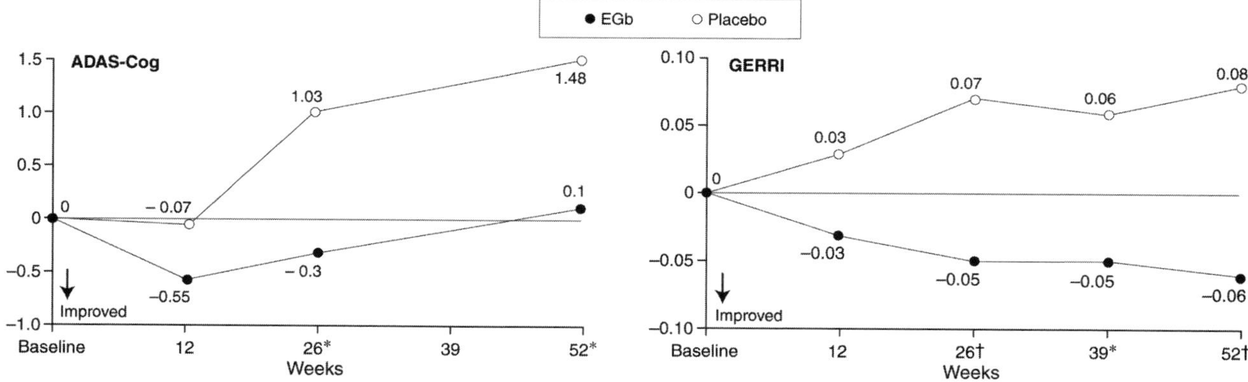

Figure 2. Mean change in the primary outcome measures for the intent-to-treat analysis. Results of Alzheimer's Disease Assessment Scale–Cognitive subscale (ADAS-Cog) and Geriatric Evaluation by Relative's Rating Instrument (GERRI) at 12-, 26-, 39-, and 52-week end points with last observation carried forward. Statistically significant differences between treatment groups are $P \leq .05$ (asterisk) and $P \leq .01$ (dagger).

Table 4. Distribution of Improvers and Decliners in the Evaluable Population*

	ADAS-Cog						GERRI			
	n	−4 or Better	−2 or Better	+2 or Worse	+4 or Worse	*P*	n	Improved	Worse	*P*
All diagnostic groups (N=202)										
EGb group	96	26 (27)	48 (50)	30 (31)	21 (22)	.005	89	33 (37)	17 (19)	.003
Placebo group	104	15 (14)	30 (29)	48 (46)	33 (32)		88	20 (23)	35 (40)	
Alzheimer disease (N=150)										
EGb group	75	22 (29)	40 (53)	23 (31)	16 (21)	.006	67	26 (39)	15 (22)	.006
Placebo group	75	10 (13)	21 (28)	35 (47)	24 (32)		65	13 (20)	27 (42)	

*Data are given as number (percent) of patients. ADAS-Cog indicates Alzheimer's Disease Assessment Scale–Cognitive subscale; GERRI, Geriatric Evaluation by Relative's Rating Instrument.

Safety

Five serious adverse events were reported during the study: 3 deaths (1 in the placebo group and 2 in the EGb group) due to acute intercurrent conditions not related to the study medication, and 1 stroke and 1 subdural hematoma (both in the placebo group) related to worsening of preexisting condition. Thirty percent (49/166) of the patients in the EGb group reported at least 1 adverse event compared with 31% (50/161) in the placebo group. When only events related to study drug were considered, 16% (27/166) of the patients in the EGb group attributed at least 1 adverse event to the study drug compared with 12% (19/161) in the placebo group. Of 188 adverse events, 97 occurred with EGb and 91 with placebo. The majority of these adverse events (167/188) were considered of mild to moderate intensity. The adverse events of severe intensity (12 for EGb, 9 for placebo) were transient and resulted in withdrawal from the trial in only 2 patients receiving EGb and 1 receiving placebo. The adverse events, regrouped in their respective anatomicophysiologic systems, were equally distributed between the 2 treatment groups with the exception of the gastrointestinal tract signs and symptoms being attributed slightly more often to EGb (18 of 29 events).

Comment

This study compared the effects of EGb with a placebo in a multicenter sample of demented patients with mild to moderately severe cognitive impairment. The results obtained from the ITT analysis and from the evaluable data demonstrated the efficacy of EGb on 2 of 3 primary outcome measures: cognitive impairment and daily living and social behavior. Although the treatment effect could not be detected by the clinician's global impression of change (CGIC), it was demonstrated through objective tests of cognitive performance (ADAS-Cog) and was of sufficient magnitude for the caregiver to recognize it in the patient's behavior (GERRI).

A concern in interpreting the study outcomes, however, relates to the substantial number of patients who withdrew after the 26-week visit. To reduce the potential bias due to the attrition of the randomization sample, the efficacy analysis was primarily based on ITT methodology. The ITT analysis, however, carries its own limitation. Dementia is inherently a deteriorating disease. By replacing missing data at end point with carried-forward values obtained early in the trial, the magnitude of the natural deterioration is underestimated; furthermore, different elapsed times in the study will tend to influence the effect size and possibly favor the group with the earliest end point. In the present sample, the EGb group included 50% of patients reaching the 52-week visit compared with only 38% of patients in the placebo group. Moreover, the average time of the end point occurred slightly earlier (4 weeks) for the placebo group. Despite these differences, apparently favorable to the placebo group, the ITT analysis showed that the EGb group maintained its baseline status (ADAS-Cog) or even improved slightly (GERRI), whereas both cognitive and social functioning worsened over time in the placebo group. These differences were observed even though 11% of the patients in the EGb group were not compliant with the drug regimen and 10% were treated with EGb for less than 12 weeks. The ITT and evaluable analyses showed EGb to be more effective, but these analyses do not completely resolve the uncertainty of the effects that may arise from nonrandom dropouts.

Of the 3 outcome measures, the CGIC failed to demonstrate a significant difference in the efficacy of the 2 treatments. Several factors may have contributed to this. First, the treatment effects may not have been large enough to allow a discrimination from placebo. Second, the CGIC appears to have low sensitivity for measurement of change in dementia over the long term. It asks the clinician to quantify the amount of change in the patient's condition compared with baseline. However, it is not a structured instrument nor is it guided by anchored criteria. Thus, its reliability suffers as the interval between the follow-up visit and the baseline evaluation increases,[35] particularly if relevant information is not systematically elicited at each follow-up visit. The problem with its sensitivity as an outcome measure in AD surfaced in the earlier tacrine studies in which only the ADAS-Cog demonstrated an advantage for tacrine over the placebo.[31] The problem was partly remedied in more recent studies by replacing the CGIC with the Clinician Interview-Based Impression rating scale.[36] The latter apparently is a more reliable and sensitive guideline-based instrument, but one not yet available when the present study was initiated.

The failure to find differences using the CGIC, however, raised the question of whether the improvements in cognition and social behavior in the EGb group, although statistically significant, were sufficiently large to be "clinically meaningful." In this respect, the categorical analysis (Table 4) of the proportions of patients whose performance improved or worsened reflects more closely how the treatment effects are manifested clinically. In clinical terms, improvement on the ADAS-Cog of 4 points may be equivalent to a 6-month delay in the progression of the disease.[17,28,31] In this study, it is noteworthy that 29% of the patients with AD treated with EGb for at least 26 weeks improved by 4 or more points compared with 13% treated with the placebo (Table 4). These ratios compare favorably with those obtained in a study of an evaluable group of patients with AD receiving a 30-week "high-dose" (160-mg) regimen of tacrine[31] (40% of the tacrine group improved by at least 4 points vs 25% of the placebo group).

The present trial, however, does not permit conclusions regarding sustained benefits, particularly if drug treatment is subsequently interrupted. In addition, this study tested a single EGb dose. It does not address whether the proportion of treatment responders will increase with higher dosages, as indicated by previous pilot studies,[37] or will remain the same but with an increase of the treatment effect. The latter finding would be more in accordance with the results obtained with 240 mg of EGb in a recent controlled trial in dementia.[13] Additional study testing multiple EGb dosages and applying a design that would distinguish a temporary stemming of the symptoms from a change in the course of the disease would be necessary to explore these important aspects.[38]

Owing to recent nosological developments[39,40] in the classification of vascular dementia (formerly MID), the frequent occurrence of mixed dementia (AD and vascular dementia), and the low clinicopathological correlation in postmortem analyses,[34] persons with MID as defined by *DSM-III-R* criteria appear to be a heterogeneous group. Moreover, no specific neuropathological criteria for the neuroimaging findings were included in the present screening framework. Thus, in view of these limitations and of the relatively small number of patients with MID, the data of the vascular subgroup were not analyzed separately. Conversely, the results of the AD subgroup have been presented since its criteria have high reliability[32,33] and it represented the majority of the study sample. However, the present findings should be considered within the limits of our study population. The number of mildly impaired vs moderately and severely impaired patients may not be representative of the AD population at large. A sizable number of mild cases may have contributed to the fairly modest changes that were observed at end point. For example, the placebo group showed only a 1.5-point worsening on the ADAS-Cog score after an average elapsed time of 35 weeks, compared with 2.0- to 2.5-point changes observed with placebo groups of previous studies.[19,30,31] A pervasive learning effect also could be suspected in view of the relatively high percentage of improvers in the placebo group. Nevertheless, considering that the baseline characteristics of the 2 treatment groups are similar and that there is no significant interaction between severity of impairment and treatment, EGb appears to stabilize and, in an additional 20% of cases (vs placebo), improve the patient's functioning for periods of 6 months to 1 year. Regarding its safety, adverse events associated with EGb were no different from those associated with placebo.

The EGb extract contains multiple compounds that are thought to act synergistically on diverse processes involved in the homeostasis of inflammation and oxidative stress, providing membrane protection[3] and, neurotransmission modulation, which may be the basis for EGb effects at the central nervous system.[2,41,42] However, further research is needed to elucidate the precise mechanism of action of EGb, to fully explore the therapeutic potential of this plant extract, and to help better understand the pathogenesis of dementia.

The 6 US investigators who participated in the data collection of this project (The North American Egb Study Group) are Myron Brazin, MD, University of Medicine and Dentistry of New Jersey/New Jersey Medical School, Denville; James Ferguson, MD, Pharmacology Research Corporation, Salt Lake City, Utah; Alfred M. Freedman, MD, New York Medical College, Valhalla; Barry Jordan, MD, Cornell University Medical College, New York, NY; Joseph Mendels, MD, Philadelphia Medical Institute, Philadelphia, Pa (now with Therapeutics PC, Wynnewood, Pa); and Alan F. Schatzberg, MD, Harvard Medical Center, Boston, Mass (now with the School of Medicine, Stanford University, Stanford, Calif).

Dr. Willmar Schwabe Pharmaceuticals provided support for this study.

The authors would like to acknowledge the patients and their families for their participation in this EGb study as well as the scientific teams of the 6 centers for their time and effort. We are indebted to J. Martorano, MD, for his invaluable advice on the manuscript. We would like to thank Neurocorp, Ltd, and its personnel: Emin Eralp, Islah Ahmed, MBBS, Meredith Lacher, MA, and Aileen Kunitz for their help in the preparation and analysis of the data.

References

1. Cott J. Natural product formulations available in Europe for psychotropic indication. *Psychopharmacol Bull.* 1995;31:745–751.

2. DeFeudis FG. In: DeFeudis FV, ed. *Ginkgo Biloba* Extract (EGb 761): *Pharmacological Activities and Clinical Applications.* Paris, France: Editions Scientifiques Elsevier; 1991:7–146.

3. Packer L, Haramaki N, Kawabata T, et al. *Ginkgo biloba* extract (EGb 761). In: Christen Y, Courtois Y, Droy-Lefaix MT, eds. *Effect of Ginkgo Biloba Extract (EGb 761) on Aging and Age-Related Disorders.* Paris, France: Editions Scientifiques Elsevier Paris; 1995:23–47.

4. Oyama Y, Fuchs PA, Katayama N, Noda K. Myricetin and quercetin, the flavonoid constituents of *Ginkgo biloba* extract, greatly reduce oxidative metabolism in both resting and Ca^{2+}-loaded brain neurons. *Brain Res.* 1994;635:125–129.

5. Richardson JS. Free radicals in the genesis of Alzheimer's disease. In: Nitsch RM, Growdon JH, Corkin S, Wurtman RJ, volume eds. *Alzheimer's Disease: Amyloid Precursor Proteins, Signal Transduction, and Neuronal Transplantation. Ann N Y Acad Sci.* 1993; 695:73–76.

6. Anderson DK, Thomas CE. Mechanisms and role of oxygen free radicals in CNS pathology. In: Racagni G, Brunello N, Langer SZ, volume eds. *Recent Advances in the Treatment of Neurodegenerative Disorders and Cognitive Dysfunction. Int Acad Biomed Drug Res.* 1994; 7:119–124.

7. Behl C, Davis JB, Lesley R, Schubert D. Hydrogen peroxide mediates amyloid β protein toxicity. *Cell.* 1994;77:817–827.

8. Benzi G, Moretti A. Are reactive oxygen species involved in Alzheimer's disease? *Neurobiol Aging.* 1995;16:661–674.

9. Warburton DM. Psycho-pharmacologie clinique de l'extrait de *Ginkgo biloba. Presse Med.* 1986; 15:1595–1604.

10. Kleijnen J, Knipschild P. *Ginkgo biloba* for cerebral insufficiency. *Br J Clin Pharmacol.* 1992; 34:352–358.

11. Letzel H, Haan J, Feil WB. Nootropics. *J Drug Dev Clin Pract.* 1996;8:77–94.

12. Hofferberth B. The efficacy of EGb 761 in patients with senile dementia of the Alzheimer type, a double-blind, placebo-controlled study on different levels of investigation. *Hum Psychopharmacol.* 1994;9:215–222.

13. Kanowski S, Herrmann WM, Stephan K, Wierich W, Hörr R. Proof of efficacy of the *Ginkgo biloba* special extract EGb 761 in outpatients suffering from mild to moderate primary degenerative dementia of the Alzheimer type or multi-infarct dementia. *Pharmacopsychiatry.* 1996;29:47–56.

14. Folstein MF, Folstein SE, McHugh PR. Mini-Mental State. *J Psychiatr Res.* 1975; 12:189–198.

15. Reisberg B, Ferris SH, de Leon MJ, et al. The Global Deterioration Scale for assessment of primary degenerative dementia. *Am J Psychiatry.* 1982;39:1136–1139.

16. Rosen WG, Mohs RC, Davis KL. A new rating scale for Alzheimer's disease. *Am J Psychiatry.* 1984;141:1356–1364.

17. Stern RG, Mohs RC, Davidson M, et al. A longitudinal study of Alzheimer's disease. *Am J Psychiatry*. 1994;151:390–396.

18. Schwartz GE. Development and validation of the Geriatric Evaluation by Relative's Rating Instrument (GERRI). *Psychol Rep.* 1983; 53:479–488.

19. Morich FJ, Bieber F, Lewis JM, et al. Nimodipine in the treatment of probable Alzheimer's disease. *Clin Drug Invest.* 1996;11:185–195.

20. US Dept of Health Education and Welfare, National Institute of Mental Health. Clinical Global Assessment Scale (CGI). In: Guy W, ed. *ECDEU Assessment Manual for Psychopharmacology.* Rockville, Md: US Dept of Health Education and Welfare, National Institute of Mental Health; 1976:218–222.

21. Gillings D, Koch G. The application of the principle of intention-to-treat to the analysis of clinical trials. *Drug Inform J.* 1991;25:411–424.

22. Jorm AF, Korten AE, Henderson AS. The prevalence of dementia. *Acta Psychiatr Scand.* 1987; 76:465–479.

23. Katzman R, Lasker B, Bernstein N. Advances in the diagnosis of dementia. In: Terry RD, ed. *Aging and the Brain.* New York, NY: Raven Press; 1988:17–62.

24. Anthony JC, LeResche L, Niaz U, Von Korff MR, Folstein MF. Limits of the 'Mini-Mental State' as a screening test for dementia and delirium among hospital patients. *Psychol Med.* 1982; 12:397–408.

25. Crum RM, Anthony JC, Bassett SS, Folstein MF. Population-based norms for the Mini-Mental State Examination by age and education level. *JAMA.* 1993;269:2386–2421.

26. Welsh K, Butters N, Hughes J, Mohs R, Heyman A. Detection of abnormal memory decline in mild cases of Alzheimer's disease using CERAD neuropsychological measures. *Arch Neurol.* 1991;48:278–281.

27. Agresti A. Tutorial on modeling ordered categorical response data. *Psychol Bull.* 1989; 105:290–301.

28. Kramer-Ginsberg E, Mohs RC, Aryan M, et al. Clinical predictors of course for Alzheimer patients in a longitudinal study: a preliminary report. *Psychopharmacol Bull.* 1988; 24:458–462.

29. Davis LK, Thal LJ, Gamzu ER, et al. A double-blind, placebo-controlled multicenter study of tacrine for Alzheimer's disease. *N Engl J Med.* 1992;327:1253–1259.

30. Farlow M, Gracon SI, Hershey LA, et al. A controlled trial of tacrine in Alzheimer's disease. *JAMA.* 1992;268:2523–2529.

31. Knapp MJ, Knopman DS, Solomon PR, et al. A 30–week randomized controlled trial of high-dose tacrine in patients with Alzheimer's disease. *JAMA.* 1994;271:985–991.

32. Morris JC, McKeel DW, Fulling K, Torack RM, Berg L. Validation of clinical diagnosis criteria for Alzheimer's disease. *Ann Neurol.* 1988; 24:17–22.

33. Baldereschi M, Amato MP, Nencini P, et al. Cross-national interrater agreement on the clinical diagnostic criteria for dementia. *Neurology.* 1994;44:239–242.

34. Victoroff J, Mack WJ, Lyness SA, Chui HC. Multicenter clinicopathological correlation in dementia. *Am J Psychiatry.* 1995; 152:1476–1484.

35. Dahlke F, Lohaus A, Gutzmann H. Reliability and clinical concepts underlying global judgments in dementia. *Psychopharmacol Bull.* 1992;28:425–432.

36. Knopman DS, Knapp MJ, Gracon SI, Davis CS. The Clinician Interview-Based Impression (CIBI): a clinician's global change rating scale in Alzheimer's disease. *Neurology.* 1994; 44:2315–2321.

37. Itil TM, Eralp E, Tsambis E, Itil KZ, Stein U. Central nervous system effects of *Ginkgo biloba*, a plant extract. *Am J Ther.* 1996;3:63–73.

38. Leber P. Observations and suggestions on antidementia drug development. *Alzheimer Dis Assoc Disord.* 1996;10(suppl 1):31–35.

39. Chui H, Victoroff JI, Margolin D, Jagust W, Shankle R, Katzman R. Criteria for the diagnosis of ischemic vascular dementia proposed by the State of California Alzheimer Disease Diagnostic and Treatment Centers (ADDTC). *Neurology.* 1992;42:473–480.

40. Lopez OL, Larumbe MR, Becker JT, et al. Reliability of NINDS-AIREN clinical criteria for the diagnosis of vascular dementia. *Neurology.* 1994;44:1240–1245.

41. Huguet F, Tarrade T. α_2-Adrenoceptor change during cerebral ageing: the effect of *Ginkgo biloba* extract. *J Pharm Pharmacol.* 1992; 44:24–27.

42. Krištofiková Z, Klaschka J. In vitro effect of *Ginkgo biloba* extract (EGb 761) on the activity of presynaptic cholinergic nerve terminals in rat hippocampus. *Dement Geriatr Cogn Disord.* 1997;8:43–48.

39 The Efficacy of *Ginkgo biloba* on Cognitive Function in Alzheimer Disease

Barry S. Oken MD; Daniel M. Storzbach PhD; Jeffrey A. Kaye MD
From the Department of Neurology (Drs Oken and Kaye) and Center for Research on Occupational and Environmental Toxicology (Dr Storzbach), Oregon Health Sciences University, and Portland Veteran Affairs Medical Center (Dr Kaye), Portland.

Objective

To determine the effect of treatment with *Ginkgo biloba* extract on objective measures of cognitive function in patients with Alzheimer disease (AD) based on formal review of the current literature.

Methods

An attempt was made to identify all English and non-English-language articles in which *G biloba* extract was given to subjects with dementia or cognitive impairment. Inclusion criteria for the meta-analysis were (1) sufficiently characterized patients such that it was clearly stated there was a diagnosis of AD by either *Diagnostic and Statistical Manual of Mental Disorders, Revised Third Edition,* or National Institute of Neurological Disorders and Stroke-Alzheimer's Disease and Related Disorders Association criteria, or there was enough clinical detail to determine this by our review; (2) clearly stated study exclusion criteria, ie, those studies that did not have stated exclusions for depression, other neurologic disease, and central nervous system-active medications were excluded; (3) use of standardized ginkgo extract in any stated dose; (4) randomized, placebo-controlled and double-blind study design; (5) at least 1 outcome measure was an objective assessment of cognitive function; and (6) sufficient statistical information to allow for meta-analysis.

Results

Of more than 50 articles identified, the overwhelming majority did not meet inclusion criteria, primarily because of lack of clear diagnoses of dementia and AD. Only 4 studies met all inclusion criteria. In total there were 212 subjects in each of the placebo and ginkgo treatment groups. Overall there was a significant effect size of 0.40 (*P*<.0001). This modest effect size translated into a 3% difference in the Alzheimer Disease Assessment Scale-cognitive subtest.

Conclusions

Based on a quantitative analysis of the literature there is a small but significant effect of 3- to 6- month treatment with 120 to 240 mg of *G biloba* extract on objective measures of

cognitive function in AD. The drug has not had significant adverse effects in formal clinical trials but there are 2 case reports of bleeding complications. In AD, there are limited and inconsistent data that preclude determining if there are effects on noncognitive behavioral and functional measures as well as on clinician's global rating scales. Further research in the area will need to determine if there are functional improvements and to determine the best dosage. Additional research will be needed to define which ingredients in the ginkgo extract are producing its effect in individuals with AD.

Arch Neurol. 1998;55:1409–1415

Ginkgo biloba is a living fossil tree having undergone little evolutionary change over almost 200 million years. While currently it is essentially extinct in the wild, it is widely cultivated for its nut as well as for its leaves. The tree has a high tolerance to urban and industrial pollution and is extremely resistant to insects, bacteria, viruses, and fungi. Extracts of the leaves have been used for 5000 years in traditional Chinese medicine for various purposes. Medicinal extracts are made from dried leaves. Studies on the biological activity of different components of the ginkgo leaf began with modern scientific methods about 20 years ago.

Currently, ginkgo extracts used for medicinal purposes are usually standardized to contain 24% ginkgo-flavone glycosides and 6% terpenoids. The terpenoids include bilobalide and the ginkgolides A, B, C, M, and J that are 20-carbon cage molecules with six 5-membered rings. The ginkgolides are antagonists of platelet-activating factor (PAF) that has numerous biological effects.[1] Besides causing platelet activation and aggregation, PAF produces proinflammatory effects (eg, increasing vascular permeability), is an extremely potent ulcerogen in the stomach, and contracts smooth muscle, including bronchial muscle. Platelet-activating factor has a direct effect on neuronal function and long-term potentiation.[2,3] An initial report[4] suggested that lissencephaly, a disorder of neural migration and dendritic branching, was associated with changes in the gene coding a PAF inactivating enzyme found in cerebral cortex, PAF acetylhydrolase. This was not confirmed in a later independent laboratory study.[5]

The other major components of ginkgo extract are the flavonoids that contribute to ginkgo's antioxidant and free radical scavenger effects.[6] Ginkgo has been found to (1) reduce cell membrane lipid peroxidation in experimental spinal cord injury similarly to methylprednisolone[7]; (2) reduce bromethalin-induced cerebral lipid peroxidation and edema[8]; (3) protect brain neurons against oxidative stress induced by peroxidation[9–11]; (4) decrease neuronal injury following ischemia or electroconvulsive shock[12]; and (5) reduce subchronic cold stress effects on receptor desensitization.[13]

Other biological effects of *G biloba* extract have been observed. It is an inhibitor of monoamine oxidase A and B.[14] Biological effects in various mammalian species have been demonstrated in many organs, such as decreasing retinal neovascularization following injury,[15] altering the immune system[16] and promoting compensation from vestibular deafferentation.[17]

Therapeutically, ginkgo may be biologically plausible to use in Alzheimer disease (AD) for several reasons. While the cause and underlying pathophysiological features of AD are unknown, prominent hypotheses as to the cause center around age-related oxidative injury.[18,19] As described earlier, the flavonoid components of ginkgo appear to be useful in animal models in preventing some types of oxidative and peroxidative neuronal injury. Another hypothesis of a cause of AD centers around an inflammatory process.[20,21] Ginkgo being a PAF antagonist has anti-inflammatory effects. Another reason for the plausibility of use of ginkgo in individuals with AD also relates to its activity as a PAF antagonist. The effect of PAF antagonism directly on brain function is fairly unexplored.[2,3]

Ginkgo has been widely used by naturopathic doctors and other alternative and complementary health care providers. Alternative or complementary medicine is widely used in North America with 34% of US adults interviewed in 1990 having used some form of alternative medicine in the past year.[22] In the United States people spend an estimated $1.5 billion per year on herbal medicines with projected annual growth of 15%.[23] Germany is one of the largest herbal users among American or western European countries with total sales in 1993 of $1.9 billion for plant-based allopathic medicines (half of these prescribed by physicians) and with 5 million prescriptions for ginkgo in 1988. Clinically, ginkgo extract is widely used in Europe for treatment of memory disorders associated with aging, including AD and vascular dementia. It is already widely used in the United States as an alternative therapy for AD despite the presence of only 1 American study.[24] Prior to the publication of that American trial, a conservative estimate at a university cognitive assessment clinic found 10% of patients using alternative medicines to improve cognitive function and an additional 29% to improve general health.[25] A less conservative estimate comes from another study[26] that found 55% of caregivers had used at least 1 alternative medicine to improve the patient's memory. Ginkgo was the major alternative treatment besides vitamins in those studies.

To help define the efficacy of *G biloba* in AD, a review of current literature and a meta-analysis of studies that met minimally acceptable scientific criteria was performed.

Methods

We attempted to identify all randomized placebo-controlled clinical trials (both English and non-English language) in which *G biloba* was administered for at least 2 months to patients with dementia or other cognitive impairment. The search for potentially relevant studies and reviews was performed through MEDLINE using the keywords "ginkgo" and "gingko [sic]." Trials referenced by articles that were found were also screened. Additionally, we had access to a listing of 60 articles with English summaries from a preliminary Cochrane Collaboration Review (http://www.cochrane.co.uk) on the use of ginkgo in dementia and related disorders. This search was done using several databases including MEDLINE, EMBASE, and PsychLit as well as references in review articles and textbooks. Additional search words included brand names for ginkgo (eg, Tanakan, Tebonin, Rokan, or Ginkoba) and a standardized extract, EGb 761.

Our goal was to evaluate only those studies that met minimally acceptable scientific standards. We therefore used the following criteria for inclusion in the quantitative review.

- Patients needed to be clearly and sufficiently characterized such that there was a clearly stated diagnosis of AD by either *Diagnostic and Statistical Manual of Mental Disorders, Revised Third Edition* or National Institute of Neurological Disorders and Stroke-Alzheimer's Disease and Related Disorders Association criteria, or there was enough clinical detail to determine this by our review.
- Studies needed to clearly state their exclusion criteria, ie, those studies that did not have stated exclusions for depression, other neurologic disease, and central nervous system-active medications were excluded. We did not exclude trials solely for the lack of neuroimaging studies on all subjects.
- The use of standardized ginkgo extract in any stated dose was required (24% or 25% ginkgo-flavone glycosides and 6% terpenoids, see above). The dose could be given by any route of administration.
- The study needed to be randomized, placebo-controlled, and double-blind. Details of the randomization procedure were not required.
- At least 1 outcome measure needed to be an objective assessment of cognitive function.

The studies that met these inclusion criteria are listed in Table 1. Studies also needed to include descriptive statistics from which effect sizes[27,28] could be computed. This only caused the exclusion of 1 article in Table 1 from the quantitative analysis.

Meta-analytic methodology was used to quantitatively assess the effects of ginkgo on objective measures of cognition for all studies that were found to meet the above-listed criteria. This statistical methodology involves computation of individual effect sizes[27,28] for each study sample which, after weighting for sample size, becomes a single case to be used in subsequent analyses. For each evaluated study we computed the effect size (g statistic) according to the methodology of Hedges and Olkin.[28]

Results

Studies Reviewed and Included

Fifty-seven articles[24,29–84] were identified, of which several were review articles. There were dozens of studies mostly in the French and German literature suggesting the efficacy of ginkgo for the treatment of memory impairment associated with aging but only a limited number were properly blinded and placebo- controlled with well-characterized subjects. Almost all reported positive effects of ginkgo. The overwhelming majority contained the diagnosis of cerebral insufficiency. However, the term *cerebral insufficiency* is vague and overinclusive with criteria that include depressed mood, fatigue, lack of motivation, dizziness, and tinnitus. Without sufficiently detailed description all articles simply using the diagnosis of cerebral insufficiency

Table 1. Studies Satisfying Inclusion Criteria*

Source, y	Diagnoses	No. of Subjects Analyzed	Study Duration wk	Dropout Rate, %	Daily Dose, mg	Ginkgo Formulation	Cognitive Outcome Measures	Other Outcome Measures
Hofferberth,[81] 1994	AD	40	12	?5	240	EGb 761	SKT, choice reaction time	SCAGS, EEG
Le Bars et al,[24] 1997	AD (*DSM-III-R*)	207	26	20	120	EGb 761	ADAS-cog	CGIC, GERRI
Kanowski et al,[86] 1996	AD (*DSM-III-R*)	125	24	30	240	EGb 761	SKT	CGI, NAB, EEG
Wesnes et al,[87] 1987	AD (dementia with appropriate medical and psychiatric exclusions)	58	12	7	120	Tanakan	10-Item battery including Benton Visual Retention Test, Digit Symbol, word list recall, and reaction time	Quality-of-life scale
Rai et al,[85] 1991	AD (dementia with appropriate medical and psychiatric exclusions)	27	24	9	120	Tanakan	MMSE, Kendrick Digit Copying and Object Learning tasks, digit recall, and classification task	EEG

*AD indicates Alzheimer disease; EGb 761, a ginko extract (Dr Willmar Schwabe Pharmaceuticals, Karlsruhe, Germany); SKT, Synrom-Kurztest; SCAGS, Sandoz Clinical Assessment Geriatric Scale; EEG, electroenephalogram; *DSM-III-R, Diagnostic and Statistical Manual of Mental Disorders, Revised Third Edition;* ADAS-Cog, Alzheimer Disease Assessment Scale-cognitive subtest; CGIC, Clinical Global Impression of Change; GERRI, Geriatric Evaluation by Relative's Rating Instrument; CGI, Clinical Global Impressions; NAB, Nurnberger Alters-Beobachtungsskala; and MMSE, Mini-Mental State Examination. The dropout rate is for 26-week data in the study by Le Bars et al.[24] The study by Rai et al[85] met criteria for inclusion other than lack of sufficient statistics for meta-analysis.

were excluded from the meta-analysis. Other potentially relevant studies were excluded for other reasons. Weitbrecht and Jansen[63] studied patients with primary degenerative dementia but did not further describe the inclusion or exclusion criteria. The patients in the study of Chartres et al[36] were receiving decreasing doses of neuroleptics and tranquilizers. There was 1 study[85] that otherwise met the inclusion criteria but could not be included in the formal meta-analysis because of a lack of sufficiently descriptive statistics. Four studies[24,81,86,87] were identified that met all criteria (Table 2). These 4 studies included patients with mild or moderate dementia severity. Although 2 of these studies[86, 24] reported additionally on patients with vascular dementia, only groups composed solely of patients diagnosed as having AD were included in the analysis.

Analysis Techniques

Of the 4 studies that met criteria, 2 reported means and SDs.[86,87] For these studies we computed the g statistic based on pooled SDs.[28] Wesnes et al[87] reported statistical analyses that aggregated their multiple cognitive measures across multiple assessments. However, we deemed it more appropriate to calculate the effect size for Wesnes et al[87] by averaging the effect sizes of their multiple cognitive measures reported for their final assessment (12 weeks). To provide more comparable treatment duration and increase total sample size, the intention-to-treat sample of Le Bars et al[24] at 26 weeks was used to calculate the study's effect size. As this study reported means and 95% confidence intervals (instead of SDs or SEs), the 95% confidence interval was used to calculate the SE, which in turn was used to calculate the SD for use in effect size calculation. Hofferberth[81] reported P values for the Mann-Whitney *U* statistic, but did not report means or SDs. The effect size for the final assessment (12 weeks) was calculated from the reported *P* value and sample sizes using the formula reported by Hedges and Olkin.[28]

The 4 studies[24,81,86,87] reported analyzable data for 212 patients treated with ginkgo and 212 with placebo. Individual group sample sizes, as shown in Table 2, ranged from 19 to 104. After appropriate weighting for sample size,[28] the mean effect size of the 4 samples was 0.41 (95% confidence interval, 0.22–0.61). This indicates that the weighted mean effect size was equivalent to a little less than half of an SD. There was significant variability in effect sizes (range, 0.1–1.1).

Adverse Effects

In a previous review,[31] no serious adverse effects were noted in any of the older studies and the incidence of significant adverse effects was similar in all placebo-treated and ginkgo-treated groups. In the studies we reviewed and the studies in our meta-analysis there were also no significant adverse effects. In all these studies doses have ranged

Table 2. Studies Satisfying Inclusion Criteria and With Sufficiently Descriptive Statistics

Source, y	Effect Size	95% Confidence Interval	No. of Subjects Taking Ginkgo	No. of Subjects Taking Placebo	P
Kanowski et al,[86] 1996	0.5156	+0.16 to +0.87	61	64	.005
Le Bars et al,[24] 1997	0.311	+0.04 to +0.59	104	103	.03
Wesnes et al,[87] 1987	0.108	−0.44 to +0.65	26	26	.69
Hofferberth,[81] 1994	1.117	+0.45 to +1.78	21	19	.001
Overall	0.413	+0.22 to +0.61	212	212	<.0001

up to 240 mg/d. Ginkgo may prolong the bleeding time and there are 2 case reports of hemorrhage in subjects who were taking ginkgo. A 33-year-old woman had been taking 120 mg of ginkgo for 2 years prior to developing bilateral subacute subdural hematomas without a known history of trauma.[88] Two simultaneously drawn bleeding times were 15 and 9.5 minutes with the upper limit for the laboratory being 9 minutes. One month after stopping ginkgo, 2 simultaneously drawn bleeding times were both 6.5 minutes. A second case report concerned a 70-year-old man who was taking aspirin daily for 3 years following coronary artery bypass surgery.[89] He developed spontaneous bleeding from the iris into the anterior chamber 1 week after beginning 80 mg/d of Ginkoba, a ginkgo extract. Another case report[90] concerned a 72-year-old who developed a small subdural hematoma several months after beginning ginkgo therapy. A final case report[91] was that of a 78-year-old who had been stable receiving warfarin for atrial fibrillation for 5 years with a prothrombin time of 16.9 seconds who presented with a left parietal intracerebral hemorrhage 2 months after beginning ginkgo therapy. These case reports are clearly of concern. However, given the large but unknown number of people taking ginkgo and the lack of such serious adverse effects reported in any of the published articles to date totaling several thousand subjects, the incidence of bleeding complications with administration of ginkgo is of unknown magnitude and significance.

Neurophysiology

Several studies on AD have included neurophysiological outcome measures. The trial by Kanowski et al[86] performed electroencephalographic frequency analysis in 36 of the subjects (17 ginkgo-treated and 19 placebo-treated subjects) enrolled at one site and found significant improvement in several electroencephalographic variables in the ginkgo group, including greater dominant posterior frequency and less theta activity. Hofferberth[81] also found a significant decrease in the theta/alpha ratio in the active group compared with the placebo group. Rai et al[85] reported a decrease in slow frequency activity in the treatment group.

Comment

Despite the widespread use of *G biloba* and more than 50 publications on its use in age-related functional and cognitive changes, there are only a handful of randomized, well-controlled studies of its use in patients with a diagnosis of AD. We identified only 1 article before 1991 that met inclusion criteria. This is consistent with the study by Kleijnen and Knipschild[30] who reviewed 40 studies through 1991 concerning the use of *G biloba* for dementia and cerebral insufficiency. Among the 40 studies, 8 were chosen to meet certain criteria for a good study (a subset of our criteria) and were discussed in more detail in a later article.[31] None of these 8 articles specifically stated that the diagnosis was AD. A single article among 8 had sufficient description such that the diagnoses were determined to be probable AD and it is included in our meta-analysis.[87] The other 7 articles and most of the clinical articles published since, especially the non–English-language articles, do not have sufficiently stringent inclusion criteria with cerebral insufficiency the most common diagnosis.

While all studies can be criticized for some aspects of design and analysis, we believe that 4 studies meet reasonable criteria for an adequate clinical trial in AD. There are some concerns regarding the performance of the studies as well as the quantitative analysis. The studies varied in length of treatment and daily dose of ginkgo (120 or 240 mg). The correct dose of ginkgo has never been formally established. While 120- and 240-mg/d doses are typical among clinical trials, animal studies have used doses of 100 mg/kg. The dose issue will need to be addressed in future studies. The dropout rate in the study of Le Bars et al[24] at 1 year was fairly high. However, to maintain comparability with the trial durations in the other studies we used the 6-month intention-to-treat data from the study of Le Bars et al.[24] The 6-month data did not have a particularly high dropout rate. The outcome measures are of variable quality with only 1 using the Alzheimer Disease Assessment Scale-cognitive subtest (ADAS-Cog).[24] However, the Syndom Kurztest is a short neuropsychological battery with high reliability that is similar to the ADAS-Cog.[92]

While the small number of trials is a limitation of this meta-analysis, the aggregate sample is fairly large. Despite the heterogeneity among study results, the similarity of effect sizes of the 2 largest studies accounting for more than 75% of the sample supports a real effect. Additionally, the fairly low effect size in the study by Wesnes et al[87] appears to be, at least in part, related to having to average the effect over their 10 outcome measures, some of which would be predicted to be insensitive to intervention. Some of the heterogeneity of effect may be related to dose with the 2 studies using a 240-mg/d dose producing greater effect sizes. Despite all the concerns, the administration of standardized *G biloba* extract appears to have a modest effect on cognitive function in AD with an effect size of about 0.4. The effect size is comparable with the donepezil trial by Rogers et al.[93] Using their ADAS-Cog placebo-treatment difference of 2.5 and 2.9 (5 and 10 mg of donepezil) and an SD of 6, estimated from their figure 1, the effect size is 0.42 and 0.48 for the doses.[93] The actual ADAS-Cog difference in the donepezil trial of 2.5 and 2.9 for the 2 doses is slightly greater than that presented in the study by Le Bars et al,[24] which also used the ADAS-Cog and observed a difference from placebo of 1.7 in their 26-week intention-to-treat data. The effect size estimate of 0.4 will be useful for design of future studies. For example, an independent samples *t* test would require about 110 subjects per group to attain a power of 90% at an effect size of 0.427. Our article does not address the issue of efficacy of ginkgo in other dementia syndromes, eg, vascular dementia, for which there is some preliminary positive results in 2 of the studies[24,88] included in our meta-analysis.

The clinical significance of this effect size of about 0.4 is less clear. Not all 4 studies[24,81,86,87] had functional, behavioral, or global change outcome measures. Since there was an insufficient number for quantitative analysis on these measures, they are briefly summarized herein. The study by Kanowski et al[86] reported a significant difference in a clinician's global rating scale but not in an activities of daily living scale. The study by Le Bars et al[24] reported no significant difference in the clinician's global rating scale, but did on the Geriatric Evaluation by Relative's Rating Instrument, their functional scale. Hofferberth[81] reported improvement in a daily function measure (the Sandoz Clinical Assessment Geriatric Scale). We need further research to determine whether there is improvement in noncognitive behavior or daily function since this is critical in evaluating the use of treatment in AD.

The component of ginkgo extract that produces its clinical effect is not known. If it turns out that the flavonoid components are producing the clinical effect, then other antioxidants may prove as effective and safer. For example, is the effect of ginkgo additive with vitamin E? Alternatively, if the terpenoid components are producing the clinical effect, then it needs to be determined which of the terpenoids is most effective (eg, ginkgolide B). This aspect of ginkgo is potentially of most interest since the unique chemical structure of the terpenoids makes it one of a limited number of good PAF antagonists. The currently available standardized extracts are only standardized to percentage of flavonoids and terpenoids. The implication of this is that the relative amounts of the ginkgolide and bilobalide components of the terpenoids or the various flavonoids may vary across preparations and even seasons.[94] The individual component chemicals in ginkgo extract, eg, ginkgolide B, are available from some manufacturers.

The enriched or special extract EGb 761 developed by Dr Willmar Schwabe Pharmaceuticals, Karlsruhe, Germany, has been used in most of the trials in Table 1. The patent for extract EGb 761 has expired so other manufacturers can use the same extraction process from the ginkgo leaf. There are no data comparing the efficacy of different formulations of ginkgo in AD, the so-called phytogenerics, even though most are standardized to 24% flavonoids and 6% terpenoids.

This article is not intended to produce specific clinical recommendations on the use of ginkgo in individuals with AD. Only additional high-quality research can address this issue. In general, physicians should inquire about alternative therapy use by patients to be aware of potential drug interactions and to ensure that the patient feels comfortable discussing alternative therapies with their nonalternative health care provider. In general, when considering alternative therapies, clinicians should ensure that patients are actually taking what is recommended. Some of the products are not pharmacy grade, do not contain known amounts of the intended drug, and may contain unknown amounts of other compounds. If considering the use of ginkgo, ensure that a standardized extract (24% flavonoids or ginkgo-flavone-glycosides and 6% terpenoids) is used. Given its mode of action on PAF and the case reports of possible hemorrhagic complications, it certainly seems prudent to be cautious in its use in patients taking anticoagulants or antiplatelet agents, or with a bleeding diathesis.

This study was supported in part by grants AG15171 (Dr Oken) and AG08017 (Dr Kaye), National Institutes of Health, Bethesda, Md.

The Cochrane Collaboration was invaluable and provided many of the reference titles along with a structured English-language summary. Dan Zajdel assisted in the preparation of the manuscript.

References

1. Koltai M, Hosford D, Guinot P, Esanu A, Braquet P. Platelet-activating factor (PAF): a review of its effects, antagonists and future clinical implications. *Drugs.* 1991; 42:9–29,174–204.

2. del Cerro S, Arai A, Lynch G. Inhibition of long-term potentiation by an antagonist of platelet-activating factor receptors. *Behav Neural Biol.* 1990;54:213–217.

3. Wieraszko A, Li G, Kornecki E, Hogan MV, Ehrlich YH. Long-term potentiation in the hippocampus induced by platelet-activating factor. *Neuron.* 1993;10:553–557.

4. Hattori M, Adachi H, Tsujimoto M, Arai H, Inoue K. Miller-Diecker lissencephaly gene encodes a subunit of brain platelet-activating factor. *Nature.* 1994;370:216–218.

5. Chong SS, Pack S, Roschke AV, Tanigami A, Carrozzo R, Smith AC. A revision of the lissencephaly and Miller-Dieker syndrome critical regions in chromosome 17p13.3. *Hum Mol Genet.* 1997;6:147–155.

6. Oyama Y, Fuchs PA, Katayama N, Noda K. Myricetin and quercetin, the flavonoid constituents of *Ginkgo biloba* extract, greatly reduce oxidative metabolism in both resting and Ca2+ loaded brain neurons. *Brain Res.* 1994;635:125–129.

7. Koc R, Akdemir H, Kurtsoy A, et al. Lipid peroxidation in experimental spinal cord injury: compensation of treatment with *ginkgo biloba*, TRH and methylprednisolone. *Res Exp Med.* 1995;195:117–123.

8. Dorman DC, Cote LM, Buck WB. Effects of an extract of gingko biloba on bromethalin-induced cerebral lipid peroxidation and edema in rats. *Am J Vet Res.* 1992;53:138–142.

9. Maitra I, Marcocci L, Droy-Lefaix MT, Packer L. Peroxyl radical scavenging activity of *ginkgo biloba* extract EGb761. *Biochem Pharmacol. 1995*;49:1649–1655.

10. Oyama Y, Chikahisa L, Ueha T, Kahemaru K, Noda K. *Ginkgo biloba* extract protects brain neurons against oxidative stress induced by hydrogen peroxide. *Brain Res.* 1996; 712:349–352.

11. Ni Y, Zhao B, Hou J, Xin W. Preventive effect of *Ginkgo biloba* extract on apoptosis in rat cerebellar neuronal cells induced by hydroxyl radicals. *Neurosci Lett.* 1996;214:115–118.

12. Birkle DL, Kurian P, Braquet P, Bazan NG. Platelet-activating factor antagonist BN52021 decreases accumulation of free polyunsaturated fatty acid in mouse brain during ischemia and electroconvulsive shock. *J Neurochem.* 1988;51:1900–1905.

13. Bolanos-Jimenez F, de Castro RM, Sarhan H, Prudhomme N, Drieu K, Fillion G. Stress-induced 5–HT1A receptor desensitization: protective effects of *ginkgo biloba* extract (EGb 761). *Fundam Clin Pharmacol.* 1995; 9:169–174.

14. White HL, Scates PW, Cooper BR. Extracts of *ginkgo biloba* leaves inhibit monoamine oxidase. *Life Sci.* 1996;58:1315–1321.

15. Baudouin C, Ettaiche M, Fredj-Reygrobellet D, Droy-Lefaix MT, Gastaud P, Lapalus P. Effects of gingko biloba extracts in a model of tractional retinal displacement. *Lens Eye Toxic Res.* 1992; 9:513–519.

16. Braquet P. Ginkgolides: *Chemistry, Biology, Pharmacology and Clinical Perspectives.* Barcelona, Spain: JR Prous Science Publishers; 1988.

17. Lacour M, Ez-Zaher L, Raymond J. Plasticity mechanisms in vestibular compensation in the cat are improved by an extract of *ginkgo biloba* (EGb 761). *Pharmacol Biochem Behav.* 1991; 40:367– 379.

18. Beal MF. Aging, energy, and oxidative stress in neurodegenerative diseases. *Ann Neurol.* 1995; 38:357–366.

19. Benzi G, Morretti A. Are reactive oxygen species involved in Alzheimer's disease? *Neurobiol Aging.* 1995;16:661–674.

20. McGeer PL, Schulzer M, McGeer EG. Arthritis and anti-inflammatory agents as possible protective factors for Alzheimer's disease. *Neurology.* 1996;47:425–432.

21. McGeer PL, McGeer EG. The inflammatory response of brain: implications for therapy of Alzheimer disease and other neurodegenerative diseases. *Brain Res Brain Res Rev.* 1995; 21:195–218.

22. Eisenberg DM, Kessler RC, Foster C, Norlock FE, Calkins DR, Delbanco TL. Unconventional medicine in the United States. *N Engl J Med.* 1993; 328:246–252.

23. Marwick C. Growing use of medicinal botanicals forces assessment by drug regulators. *JAMA.* 1995;273:607–609.

24. Le Bars PL, Katz MM, Berman N, Itil TM, Freedman AM, Schatzberg AF. A placebo-controlled, double-blind, randomized trial of an extract of *ginkgo biloba* for dementia. *JAMA.* 1997;278:1327–1332.

25. Hogan DB, Ebly EM. Complementary medicine use in a dementia clinic population. *Alzheimer Dis Assoc Disord.* 1996;10:63–67.

26. Coleman LM, Fowler LL, Williams ME. Use of unproven therapies by people with Alzheimer's disease. *J Am Geriatr Soc.* 1995;43:747–750.

27. Cohen J. Statistical Power Analysis for the Behavioral Sciences. 2nd ed. Hillsdale, NJ: *Lawrence Erlbaum Associates Publishers*; 1988.

28. Hedges LV, Olkin I. *Statistical Methods for Meta-analysis.* Orlando, Fla: Academic Press Inc; 1985.

29. Kleijnen J. *Ginkgo biloba* for intermittent claudication and cerebral insufficiency. In: Kleijnen J, ed. *Food Supplements and Their Efficacy* [dissertation]. Maastricht, the Netherlands: University of Limburg; 1991.

30. Kleijnen J, Knipschild P. *Ginkgo biloba* for cerebral insufficiency. *Br J Clin Pharmacol.* 1992; 34:352–358.

31. Kleijnen J, Knipschild P. *Ginkgo biloba. Lancet.* 1992;340:1136–1139.

32. Kleijnen J, Knipschild PG. *Ginkgo biloba.* In: Kleijnen J, Ter Riet G, Knipschild PG, eds. *Effectiviteit van alternatieve geneeswijzen: een literatuuronderzoek.* Maastricht, the Netherlands: University of Limburg; 1993:185–188.

33. Augustin P. Le tanakan en geriatrie: ètude clinique et psychomètrique chez 189 malades d'hospice. *Psychol Med.* 1976;8:123–130.

34. Bono Y, Moure P. L'insuffisance circulatoire cerebrale et son traitement par l'extrait de *ginkgo biloba. Mediterranee Med.* 1975;3:59–62.

35. Chesseboeuf L, Herard J, Trevin J. Etude comparative de deux vasoregulatours dans les hypoacousies et les syndromes vertigineux. *Med Nord Est.* 1979;3:534–539.

36. Chartres JP, Bonnan P, Martin G. Reduction de posologie de medicaments psychotropes chez des personnes agrées vivant en institution: étude a double/insu des patients prenant soit de l'extrait de *ginkgo biloba* 761 soit du placebo. *Psychol Med.* 1987;19:1365–1375.

37. Claussen CF. Mit *Ginkgo biloba* wird ihr Patienten wieder standfest: Cranio corpographie zeigt statistisch significanten Ruckgang der Vertigo- und Ataxia-symptomatik im Doppelblindversuch. *Arztliche Prax.* 1984;36:193–194.

38. Claussen CF, Kirtane MV. Randomisierte doppleblindstudie zur Wirkung von Extractum *Ginkgo biloba* bei Schwindel und Gangunsicherheit des alteren Menschen. In: Claussen CF, ed. *Presbyvertigo, Presbyataxie, Presbytinnitus: Gleichegewichts und Sinnestorungen im alter.* New York, NY: Springer-Verlag NY Inc; 1985:103–115.

39. Franco L, Cuny G, Nancy F. Etude multicentrique de l'efficacité de l'extrait de *ginkgo biloba* (EGb 761) dans le traitement des troubles mnesiques liés à l'age. *Rev Geriatr.* 1991;16:191–195.

40. Gerhardt G, Rogalla K, Jaeger J. Medikamentose Therapie von Hirnleistungsstorungen: randomisierte Vergleichstudie mit Dihydroergotoxin und Ginkgo-biloba-extrakt. *Fortschr Med.* 1990;108:384–388.

41. Grassel E. Einfluss von Ginkgo-biloba-extrakt auf die geistige Leistungsfahigkeit: Doppelblindstudie unter computerisierten Messbedingungen bei Patienten mit zerebralin Suffizienz. *Fortschr Med.* 1992;110:73–76.

42. Hamann K-F. Physikalische Therapie des vestibularen Schwindels in Verbindung mit Ginkgo-biloba Extract: eine posturographische Studie. *Therapiewoche.* 1985;35:4586–4590.

43. Haguenauer JP, Cantenot F, Koskas P, Pierart H. Traitment des troubles de l'équilibre par l'extrait de *ginkgo biloba*: étude multicentrique a double insu face au placebo. *Presse Med.* 1986;15:1569–1572.

44. Haase J, Halama P, Horr R. Wirksamkeit kurzdauernder Infusionsbehandlungen mit Ginkgo-biloba-spezialextrakt EGb761 bei Demenz vom vaskularen und Alzheimer-typ. *Z Gerontol Geriatr.* 1996;29:302–309.

45. Israel L, Dell'Accio E, Martin G, Hugonot R. Extrait de *ginkgo biloba* et exercices d'entrainement de la memoire: evaluation comparative chez des personnes agées ambulatoires. *Psychol Med.* 1987;19:1431–1439.

46. Isarel L, Ohlman T, Delomier Y, Hugonot R. Etude psychométrique de l'activité d'un extrait vegetal au cours des états d'involution senile. *Lyon Mediterranee Med.* 1977;8:1197–1199.

47. Kanowski S, Hermann WM, Stephan K, Wierich W, Horr R. Proof of efficacy of the *ginkgo biloba* special extract EGb 761 in outpatients suffering from mild to moderate primary degenerative dementia of the Alzheimer type or multi-infarct dementia. *Pharmacopsychiatry.* 1996;29:47–56.

48. Kanowski S. Ginkgo-biloba-spezialextrakt: ein Nootropikum mit nachgewiesener Wirksamkeit im indigkationsbereich Demenz. *Munch Med Wochenschr.* 1997;139:47–50.

49. Rai GS, Shovlin C, Wesnes KA. A double-blind placebo-controlled study of *ginkgo biloba* extract ("Tanakan") in elderly outpatients with mild to moderate memory impairment. *Curr Med Res Opin.* 1991;12:350–355.

50. Weiss H, Kallischnigg G. Ginkgo-biloba-extract (EGb 761): Meta-analyse von Studien zum Nachweis der therapeutischen Wirksamkeit bei Hirnleistungsstorungen bzw: peripherer arterieller Verschlusskrankheit. *Munch Med Wochenschr.* 1991;133:138–142.

51. Wesnes K, Simmons D, Rook M, Simpson P. A double-blind placebo-controlled trial of tanakan in the treatment of idiopathic cognitive impairment on the elderly. *Hum Psychopharmacol.* 1987;2:159–169.

52. Moreau P. Un nouveau stimulant circulatoire cerebral. *Nouv Presse Med.* 1975; 4:2401–2402.

53. Natali R, Rachinel J, Pouyat PM. Essai comparatif croise en O.R.L. de deux medications vasoactives. *Cah Otol Rhinol Laryngol.* 1979; 14:185–190.

54. Agnoli A. *Relazione clinica sulla specialitata "Tebonin forte."* Milan, Italy: ALSO Lab Sas; 1980.

55. Dieli G, La Mantia V, Saetta M, Costanzo E. Essai clinique a double insu de tanakan dans l'insuffisance cerebral chronique. *Lavoro Neuropshiatr.* 1981;68:1–10.

56. Schwerdfeger F. Elektronystagmographisch und klinisch dokumentierte Therapieerfahrungen mit Rokan bei Schwindelsymptomatik. *Therapiewoche.* 1981;31:8658–8667.

57. Haan J, Reckermann U, Welter FL, Sabin G, Muller E. Ginkgo-biloba-flavonglycoside: Therapiemöglichkeit der zerebralen Insuffizienz. *Med Welt.* 1982;33:1001–1005.

58. Eckmann F, Schlag H. Kontollierte Doppelblindstudie zum Wirksamkeitsnachweis von Tebonin forte bei Patienten mit zerebrovaskularer Insufficienz. *Fortschr Med.* 1982;100:31–32.

59. Eckmann F. Behandlung von Hirnleistungsstorungen mit Ginkgo-biloba Extract: Zeipunkt des Wirkungseintritts in einer Doppelblind Studie mit 60 statinaren Patienten. *Fortschr Med.* 1990;108:557–560.

60. Pidoux B, Bastien C, Niddam S. Clinical and quantitative EEG double-blind study of *ginkgo biloba* extract (GBE). *J Cereb Blood Flow Metab.* 1983;3:S556–S557.

61. Tiegeler R, Pieprzyk L. *Ginkgo biloba* bei zerebraler Insuffizienz. *Arztliche Prax.* 1984; 36:1374.

62. Gessner B, Voelp A, Klasser M. Study of the long-term action of a *ginkgo biloba* extract on vigilance and mental performance as determined by means of quantitative pharmaco-EEG and psychometric measurements. *Drug Res.* 1985;35:1459–1465.

63. Weitbrecht WV, Jansen W. Doubleblind and comparative (*ginkgo biloba* versus placebo) therapeutic study in geriatric patients with primary degenerative dementia: a preliminary evaluation. In: Agnoli J, Rapin R, Scapagnini V, Weitbrecht WV, eds. *Effects of* Ginkgo biloba *Extract on Organic Cerebral Impairment.* Montrouge, France: John Libbey Eurotext Ltd; 1985:91–99.

64. Arrigo A. Behandlung der chronischen zerebrovaskularen Insuffizienz mit Ginkgo-biloba-extrakt. *Therapiewoche.* 1986;36:5208–5218.

65. Dubreuil C. Essai therapeutique dans les surdites cochleaires aigues: étude comparative therapeutic. *Presse Med.* 1986;15:1559–1561.

66. Meyer B. Etude multicentrique des acouphenes: epidémiologie et therapeutique. *Ann Otolaryngol (Paris).* 1986;103:185–188.

67. Meyer B. Etude multicentrique randomisée a double insu face au placebo du traitment des acouphenes par l'extrait de *ginkgo biloba*. *Presse Med.* 1986;15:1562–1564.

68. Arrigo A, Cattaneo S. Clinical and psychometric evaluation of *ginkgo biloba* extract in chronic cerebro-vascular diseases. In: Agnoli J, Rapin R, Scapagnini V, Weitbrecht WV, eds. *Effects of* Ginkgo biloba *Extract on Organic Cerebral Impairment*. Montrouge, France: John Libbey Eurotext Ltd; 1985:85–89.

69. Taillandier J, Ammar A, Rabourdin JP et al. Traitement des troubles du vieillissement cerebral par l'extrait de *ginkgo biloba*: étude longitudinale multicentrique a double insu face au placebo. *Presse Med.* 1986;15:1583–1587.

70. Halama P, Bartsch G, Meng G. Hirnleistungsstorungen vaskularer Genese: randomisierte Doppelblindstudie zur Wirksamkeit von Ginkgo-biloba-extract. *Fortschr Med.* 1988; 106:408–413.

71. Halama P. *Ginkgo biloba*: Wirksamkeit eines Spezialextrakts bei Patienten mit zerebraler Insuffizienz. *Munch Med Wochenschr.* 1991; 133:190–194.

72. Halama P. Befindlichkeitsbeurteilung und Psychometrie: Testung der *Ginkgo-biloba*-wirkung bei Patienten einer neurologische Fachpraxis. *Munch Med Wochenschr.* 1991; 133:19–22.

73. Hofferberth B. Einfluss von *Ginkgo biloba* Extract auf neurophysiologische und psychometrische Messergebnisse bei Patienten mit hirnorganischem Psychosyndrom: ein Doppelblindstudie gegen Placebo. *Drug Res.* 1989;39:918–922.

74. Hofferberth B. Ginkgo-biloba-spezialextrakt bei Patienten mit hirnorganischem Psychosyndrom: Prufung der Wirksamkeit mit neurophysiologischen und psychometrischen Methoden. *Munch Med Wochenschr.* 1991;133:30–33.

75. Bruchert E, Heinrich SE, Ruf-Kohler P. Wirksamkeit von Li1370 bei alteren Patienten mit Hirnleistungsschwache: multizentrische Doppelblindstudie des fachverbandes deutscher Allgemeinarzte. *Munch Med Wochenschr.* 1991;133:9–14.

76. Vorberg G, Schenk N, Schmidt U. Wirksamkeit eines neuen Ginkgo-biloba Extraktes bei 100 Patienten mit zerebraler Insuffizienz. *Herz Gefasse.* 1989;9:936–941.

77. Schmit U, Rabinovici K, Lande S. Einfluss eines Ginkgo-spezial-extraktes auf die Befindlichkeit bei zerebraler Insuffizienz. *Munch Med Wochenschr.* 1991;133:15–18.

78. Hartmann A, Frick M. Wirkung eines Ginkgo-spezial-extraktes auf psychometrische Parameter bei Patienten mit vaskular bedingter Demenz. *Munch Med Wochenschr.* 1991; 133:23–25.

79. Maier-Hauff K. Li 1370 nach zerebraler Aneurysma-operation: Wirksamkeit bei ambulanten Patienten mit Storungen der Hirnleistungsfahigkeit. *Munch Med Wochenschr.* 1991;133:34–37.

80. Vesper J, Hansgen K-D. Efficacy of *Ginkgo biloba* in 90 outpatients with cerebral insufficiency caused by old age: results of a placebo-controlled double-blind trial. *Phytomedicine.* 1994; 1:9–16.

81. Hofferberth B. The efficacy of EGb 761 in patients with senile dementia of the Alzheimer type: a double-blind placebo-controlled study on different levels of investigation. *Hum Psychopharmacol.* 1994;9:215–222.

82. Hopfenmuller W. Nachweis der therapeutischen Wirksamkeit eines *Ginkgo biloba* Spezialextraktes: Meta-analyse von 11 klinischen Studien bei Patienten mit Hirnleistungs-storungen im Alter. *Drug Res.* 1995; 44:1005–1013.

83. Letzel H, Haan J, Feil WB. Nootropics: efficacy and tolerability of products from three active substance classes. *J Drug Dec Clin Pract.* 1996; 8:77–94.

84. Weitbrecht WV, Jansen W. Primar degenerative Demenz: Therapie mit Ginkgo-biloba: placebo-kontrollierte doppelblind and Vergleichsstudie. *Fortschr Med.* 1986;104:199–202.

85. Rai GS, Shovlin C, Wesnes KA. A double-blind placebo controlled study of *Ginkgo biloba* extract ("Tanakan") in elderly outpatients with mild to moderate memory impairment. *Curr Med Res Opin.* 1991;12:350–355.

86. Kanowski S, Herrmann WM, Stephan K, Wierich W, Horr R. Proof of efficacy of the *ginkgo biloba* special extract EGb 761 in outpatients suffering from mild to moderate primary degenerative dementia of the Alzheimer type or multi-infarct dementia. *Pharmacopsychiatry.* 1996;29:47–56.

87. Wesnes K, Simmons D, Rook M, Simpson P. A double-blind placebo-controlled trial of Tanakan in the treatment of idiopathic cognitive impairment in the elderly. *Hum Psychopharmacol.* 1987;2:159–169.

88. Rowin J, Lewis SL. Spontaneous bilateral subdural hematomas associated with chronic *ginkgo biloba* ingestion. *Neurology.* 1996; 46:1775–1776.

89. Rosenblatt M, Mindel J. Spontaneous hyphema associated with ingestion of *ginkgo biloba* extract. *N Engl J Med.* 1997;336:1108.

90. Gilbert GJ. *Ginkgo biloba*. *Neurology.* 1997; 48:1137.

91. Matthews MK. Association of *Ginkgo biloba* with intracerebral hemorrhage. *Neurology.* 1998;50:1933–1934.

92. Kim YS, Nibbelink DW. Factor structure and scoring of the SKT test battery. *J Clin Psychol.* 1993;49:61–71.

93. Rogers SL, Farlow MR, Doody RS, Mohs R, Friedhoff LT. A 24-week, double-blind placebo-controlled trial of donepezil in patients with Alzheimer's disease. *Neurology.* 1998; 50:136–145.

94. Sticher O. Quality of ginkgo preparations. *Planta Med.* 1993;59:2–11.

40 Treatment of Irritable Bowel Syndrome With Chinese Herbal Medicine

A Randomized Controlled Trial

Alan Bensoussan, MSc; Nick J. Talley, MD; Michael Hing, MBBS, FRACP; Robert Menzies, PhD; Anna Guo, PhD; Meng Ngu, PhD
From the Research Unit for Complementary Medicine, University of Western Sydney Macarthur (Mr Bensoussan), the Department of Medicine, Nepean Hospital (Dr Talley) and the Department of Behavioral Sciences (Dr Menzies). University of Sydney, Bondi Junction Endoscopy Centre (Dr Hing), Balmain Chinese Herbal Centre (Dr Guo), and Gastroenterology Unit, Concord Repatriation General Hospital (Dr Ngu), Sydney, Australia.

Context
Irritable bowel syndrome (IBS) is a common functional bowel disorder for which there is no reliable medical treatment.

Objective
To determine whether Chinese herbal medicine (CHM) is of any benefit in the treatment of IBS.

Design
Randomized, double-blind, placebo-controlled trial conducted during 1996 through 1997.

Setting
Patients were recruited through 2 teaching hospitals and 5 private practices of gastroenterologists, and received CHM in 3 Chinese herbal clinics.

Patients
A total of 116 patients who fulfilled the Rome criteria, an established standard for diagnosis of IBS.

Intervention
Patients were randomly allocated to 1 of 3 treatment groups: individualized Chinese herbal formulations (n=38), a standard Chinese herbal formulation (n=43), or placebo (n=35). Patients received 5 capsules 3 times daily for 16 weeks and were evaluated regularly by a traditional Chinese herbalist and by a gastroenterologist. Patients, gastroenterologists, and herbalists were all blinded to treatment group.

Main Outcome Measures
Change in total bowel symptom scale scores and global improvement assessed by patients and gastroenterologists and change in the degree of interference in life caused by IBS symptoms assessed by patients.

Results
Compared with patients in the placebo group, patients in the active treatment groups (standard and individualized

CHM) had significant improvement in bowel symptom scores as rated by patients (P=.03) and by gastroenterologists (P=.001), and significant global improvement as rated by patients (P=.007) and by gastroenterologists (P=.002). Patients reported that treatment significantly reduced the degree of interference with life caused by IBS symptoms (P=.03). Chinese herbal formulations individually tailored to the patient proved no more effective than standard CHM treatment. On follow-up 14 weeks after completion of treatment, only the individualized CHM treatment group maintained improvement.

Conclusion

Chinese herbal formulations appear to offer improvement in symptoms for some patients with IBS.

JAMA. 1998;280:1585–1589

Irritable bowel syndrome (IBS) is a common functional bowel disorder that accounts for a significant proportion of patients seen in gastroenterology offices[1] and is characterized by chronic or recurrent abdominal pain and disturbed defecation. Studies in the United States and Australia suggest that between 10% and 20% of the population have this disorder.[2–5] No single available treatment is reliably effective for this condition,[6,7] and patients use a variety of approaches for symptom management, including drugs, dietary modifications, and counseling.

To date, no strong scientific evidence available supports the use of Chinese herbal agents in IBS.[8] However, CHM has been used for centuries in the treatment of functional bowel disorders and is routinely used for this purpose in China. Several Chinese studies have suggested the potential effectiveness of CHM for treatment of IBS, although these have all lacked rigor in clinical trial protocol[9–13] and have had poor randomization techniques and lack of blinding.[8]

According to the fundamental principles of traditional Chinese medicine, treatment should be tailored to the individual clinical presentation of patients, even though they all may have the same medical diagnosis.[8,14,15] Furthermore, treatment needs to be modified at different stages of the patient's illness or recovery. In this study, we evaluated the effectiveness of CHM in the treatment of IBS. We compared individualized therapy against a standard Chinese herbal formulation for IBS and a placebo using a randomized, double-blind, placebo-controlled study design.

Methods

Setting and Patients

Patients were recruited from gastroenterology units in 2 teaching hospitals in Sydney, Australia, and through 5 private practices of gastroenterologists. After patient screening and subsequent review in these centers, patients' conditions were further diagnosed (according to Chinese medicine principles) and treated in 3 Chinese herbal clinics by 3 Chinese medicine practitioners.

A clinical trial notification was filed with the Therapeutic Goods Administration, Commonwealth Department of Health, Housing, Local Government and Community Services, Canberra, Australia. All herbal substances used in this trial were listed with the Australian Therapeutic Goods Administration, have been acknowledged as suitable for human consumption, and were administered within standard dosage levels. All herbs used in this trial are available over-the-counter throughout Australia. No product used in this trial was a controlled substance, animal product, or endangered species. The trial protocol was approved by the ethics committee of the University of Western Sydney Macarthur and the ethics committees of the 2 participating hospitals.

Patients between the ages of 18 and 75 years (inclusive) were screened by a gastroenterologist. Screening involved a routine clinical workup for IBS with diagnostic tests as determined appropriate by the specialist. Patients were assessed according to the Rome criteria, an established standard for diagnosis of IBS.[16,17] If diarrhea was a prominent symptom, lactose intolerance was excluded by hydrogen breath testing or during a 2-week lactose exclusion period. The inclusion and exclusion criteria are shown in Table 1. Written informed consent was obtained from all patients before entering the trial. Patients were free to withdraw from the study at any time.

Treatment Schedule

After initial gastroenterological screening (week 0), all patients entered a 2-week run-in period. A Bowel Symptom Scale (BSS) was completed at the beginning and end of the 2-week period to assess measurement reliability and to account for any degree of improvement based

Table 1. Inclusion and Exclusion Criteria

Inclusion Criteria
Age, 18-75 y inclusive
Colonic evaluation (colonoscopy or barium enema) within the previous 5 years (for 18-60 y) or within the previous 3 y (for 61-75 y)
Irritable bowel syndrome by Rome Criteria
At least 3 mo of continuous or recurrent symptoms of:
Abdominal pain or discomfort with at least some discomfort present within the last 2 wk; and ≥2 of the following on at least a quarter of occasions or days
Abdominal distention that is visible or felt by tight clothing
Pain relief with bowel action
More frequent stools with onset of pain
Looser stools with onset of pain
Mucous in stools
Feeling of incomplete evacuation
At least 1 marking on the visual analog scales for IBS symptoms to be at least 20 mm from the "not present" end of the scale
Normal liver function test and full blood cell count and urea and creatinine levels (within the last 2 wk)
Exclusion Criteria
Pregnancy or breast-feeding
Liver disease
Medications: anticholinergics, lactulose, smooth muscle relaxants, motility stimulants, and/or antidepressants. Use of these is accepted provided patient is still symptomatic for IBS, medications have been used for 3 mo, and effects of medications are stable.
Current alcoholism or drug abuse
Current psychiatric illness or dementia
Allergies to food additives
Lactose intolerance—no obvious clinical indications
Inflammatory bowel disease (ulcerative colitis, Crohn disease)
Gastric and duodenal ulcers
Cancers of the gastrointestinal tract
Celiac disease
Diabetes mellitus

simply on admission to the trial. Patients were seen on specified days by 1 of 3 herbalists during the trial period and were not permitted to change herbalist during the course of the treatment. The first consultation with the Chinese herbalist occurred at week 2, at which time the patient was randomized (by an assistant) to placebo, standard CHM, or individualized CHM treatment. The patient was reevaluated by the Chinese herbalist at 2-week intervals for 2 occasions and then at monthly intervals for 2 further occasions. Continuous treatment was administered for 16 weeks. No special instructions were given to patients regarding diet, other than to continue consumption of foods they felt comfortable with and to avoid foods known to cause them gastrointestinal tract irritation. All patients were evaluated by their gastroenterologist after 8 weeks of treatment and again at the end of the 16-week treatment period. Patients were closely monitored for any adverse effects or worsening of symptoms. Liver function tests were performed after 8 weeks of treatment. Follow-up questionnaires were sent to all patients 14 weeks after completion of the treatment period. Treatment codes were broken and revealed to patients only after completion of the follow-up questionnaires.

Randomization

Randomization was done by selection of a sealed envelope from a closed bag. Seventy sealed envelopes were prepared for each of the standard and individualized groups, and 60 envelopes were prepared for the placebo group. Patients were aware that there was a greater chance of receiving active treatment. Success in blinding was evaluated using a treatment credibility scale administered during the trial.

Herbal Preparation and Dispensing

All herbs were administered in the dried powdered form and encapsulated. A period of preparation was required before commencement of the trial to develop a suitable dispensary of 81 individual dried powdered Chinese herbs for dispensing to patients in the individualized treatment group. The standard herbal formulation was designed by Chinese herbalists and prepared by the principal supplier, Mei Yu Imports, Sydney, Australia (Table 2).[18] The placebo preparation was prepared and encapsulated by a pharmaceutical contractor and was designed to taste, smell, and look similar to a Chinese herb formula. After testing on 5 independent volunteers, the placebo was deemed indistinguishable from raw powdered Chinese herbs. All herbs and the placebo formulation were supplied in the same opaque capsules. Patients in all 3 groups were required to take 5 capsules 3 times daily.

After consulting with the Chinese herbalist, all patients were required to complete a series of questionnaires and wait 30 minutes for the preparation of their capsules. The wait time was used to avoid patients identifying whether they were receiving prepared capsules (standard or placebo) or individualized formulations that were made at the treatment center. All medication preparation occurred in a closed room by assistants who were restricted from contact with the patients. Treatment codes were held by these assistants and by the chief investigator (A.B.). A blinded primary research assistant managed all the questionnaires and was responsible for giving the capsules to the patients. All patients were treated in an equivalent fashion. Compliance was assessed by an item included in the BSS and by pill count.

Table 2. Standard Formula (Capsule Ingredients)*

Chinese Name	Pharmaceutical Name	Powdered Herb, %
Dang Shen	*Codonopsis pilosulae*, radix	7
Huo Xiang	*Agastaches seu pogostemi*, herba	4.5
Fang Feng	*Ledebouriellae sesloidis*, radix	3
Yi Yi Ren	*Coicis lachryma-jobi*, semen	7
Chai Hu	*Bupleurum chinense*	4.5
Yin Chen	*Artemesiae capillaris*, herba	13
Bai Zhu	*Atractylodis macrocephalae*, rhizoma	9
Hou Po	*Magnoliae officinalis*, cortex	4.5
Chen Pi	*Citri reticulatae*, pericarpium	3
Pao Jiang	*Zingiberis offinicinalis*, rhizoma	4.5
Qin Pi	*Fraxini*, cortex	4.5
Fu Ling	*Poriae cocos*, sclerotium (Hoelen)	4.5
Bai Zhi	*Angelicae dahuricae*, radix	2
Che Qian Zi	*Plantaginis*, semen	4.5
Huang Bai	*Phellodendri*, cortex	4.5
Zhi Gan Cao	*Glycyrrhizae uralensis*, radix	4.5
Bai Shao	*Paeoniae lactiflorae*, radix	3
Mu Xiang	*Saussureae seu vladimirae*, radix	3
Huang Lian	*Coptidis*, rhizoma	3
Wu Wei Zi	*Schisandrae*, fructus	7

*Pharmaceutical terminology from Hsu.[18]

Measurement Instruments

The BSS was used to assess change in IBS symptoms during the course of the treatment. The BSS consists of 100-mm visual analog scales related to each symptom of IBS (pain/discomfort, bloating, constipation, and diarrhea) and an overall severity scale. Patients and gastroenterologists completed this scale independently at the beginning and end of the treatment period. Patients also were monitored during the course of the trial using this scale. The BSS also included items for assessing rate of stool passage, rating the degree to which IBS symptoms interfered with life activities, and recording changes in medications usage and fiber consumption. To assess the success of patient blinding, a brief questionnaire was administered to patients after 2, 4, 10, and 16 weeks of treatment. This 4-item scale has been used to test credibility of different forms of psychological treatment[19] but also has been successfully used in acupuncture trials and shown to have good internal consistency and test-retest reliability.[20,21]

Statistical Analysis

Pearson product moment correlation was used in the analysis of reliability and validity data, and factor analysis was used to determine construct validity of the credibility scale. Outcome measures with categorical responses were analyzed using χ^2 and Fisher exact tests. For the BSS, analysis of variance was used to determine the differences among groups at baseline, end of treatment, and follow-up. All *P* values were 2-tailed, unless otherwise indicated, and the a level of significance was set at .05. Missing scale and item scores were not replaced. Data are presented according to an intention-to-treat protocol, in which patients who withdrew from the trial were recorded as having worsened (if appropriate) for categorical items only. Data for all other outcome measures are presented as per protocol analysis.

There were no reliable data that could be used to accurately predict the anticipated effect size between placebo, standard, and individualized treatment groups. We estimated that for adequate power (80%) to detect a 20% difference on the BSS scores at the α=.05 level (1-tailed test), 35 patients were needed in each group.

Results

A total of 116 subjects were recruited during an 18-month period: 35 were randomized into the placebo group, 43 into the standard group, and 38 into the individualized treatment (Figure 1). Fifteen patients withdrew during the 4-month course of the trial, and 2 patients were withdrawn from the trial for commencing a variety of relevant medications during the treatment period. Patient data on study entry are shown in Table 3. Patient groups were similar in terms of age, weight, and sex distributions. There were no significant differences among patients in the 3 groups in terms of total severity of symptoms as judged independently by both the patient and gastroenterologist, or in duration of the disease as reported by patients. Patients allocated to the placebo group had a higher mean score for constipation, while patients allocated to the standard treatment had a higher mean score for diarrhea. Compliance with study medication was high as measured by a questionnaire item and by random pill counts and did not differ between groups (95% for standard CHM, 94% for individualized CHM, and 95% for placebo). Fiber and nonstudy medication consumption did not change significantly for any group during the treatment period.

Reliability and Validity Testing

The reliability of the BSS (ie, consistency of the measure) was determined by a test-retest assessment during the run-in period prior to treatment commencing (week 0–2). Correlation between the BSS completed during the initial interview with the gastroenterologist and then 2 weeks later at the clinical treatment centers was high for total score (r=0.7; P<.01, 2-tailed) and for each individual symptom (bloating [r=0.8], pain [r=0.6], diarrhea [r=0.8], and constipation [r=0.7]).

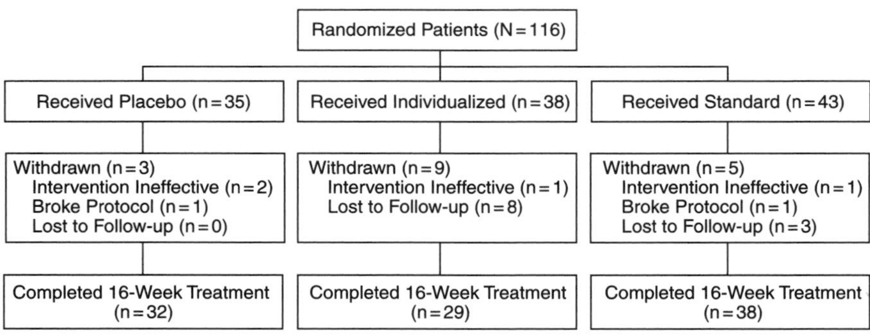

Figure 1. Patient progress through stages of the trial.

Table 3. Patient Population Characteristics Before Treatment and Mean Total Bowel Symptom Scores*

	Group, No. (SD)			
Variables	**Placebo (n=35)**	**Standard (n=43)**	**Individualized (n=38)**	***P* Values**
Characteristic				
Weight, kg	72.1 (12.8)	66.7 (16.8)	69.1 (14.4)	.29
Age, y	45.0 (13.9)	47.6 (15.1)	47.4 (13.4)	.68
Sex ratio (male:female)	0.46	0.65	0.52	.75
Baseline data				
Gastroenterologist total BSS score	182.7 (65.4)	172.2 (72.6)	166.6 (63.6)	.59
Patient total BSS score	191.2 (69.4)	189.7 (64.8)	178.5 (69.8)	.67
End of treatment				
Gastroenterologist total BSS score	147.2 (86.6) (n=30)	70.9 (63.2) (n=35)	100.4 (83.6) (n=25)	.001
Patient total BSS score	150.0 (81.6) (n=32)	106.1 (73.7) (n=38)	103.0 (74.7) (n=29)	.03
At follow-up 14 weeks after study completion				
Patient total BSS score	155.7 (84.2) (n=18)	132.6 (90.2) (n=35)	99.4 (74.8) (n=24)	.10

*Data are reported by patients and gastroenterologists at start and end of treatment period and at follow-up. BBS indicates Bowel Symptom Scale.

The credibility scale also was examined for test-retest reliability. Correlation between the first and second administration of this scale was significant (r=0.6; P<.01, 2-tailed). The correlation coefficients for each of the 4 scale items were in the range of 0.47 to 0.65. The internal consistency of the credibility scale based on interitem correlations on both occasions were uniformly high and Cronbach coefficient α (representing average interitem correlations) was .87 and .86 for the first and second occasions, respectively.

The visual analog scales within the BSS had high face validity (100-mm lines with severity marked at the extreme right and absence of symptom marked at the extreme left) and have high content validity (ie, they incorporate the key domains of interest—pain and discomfort, bloating, constipation, and diarrhea). Testing items in the scale for concurrent validity at the commencement and end of treatment showed that the gastroenterologist's assessment of the patient correlated highly with the patient's own perception of severity of symptoms. For both, Pearson correlation coefficient was in the range of r=0.63 to 0.84 for any 1 item (symptom) or for the total symptom score (P<.01 on all occasions).

Assessment of the credibility scale for construct validity through a principal components factor analysis based on the first administration revealed only 1 factor with an eigenvalue greater than 1 (2.89). This factor accounted for 72.2% of variance in this data set. All items had a high correlation with this first factor, suggesting satisfactory construct validity.

Main Outcome Measures

For all 5 main outcome measures—total mean BSS scores and global improvement as assessed by patients and gastroenterologists, and interference with life as assessed by patients—patients receiving the standard CHM formulation responded significantly better than patients in receiving placebo. Patients receiving individualized CHM treatment also responded significantly better on 4 of 5

Table 4. Perception of Improvement by Treatment Group*

Compared With Before Trial	Group, No. (%) Placebo	Standard	Individualized	*P* Value
Patient rating of response				
Improved	11 (33)	29 (76)	18 (64)	
Stayed the same	19 (57)	8 (21)	8 (29)	.007
Worsened	3 (9)	1 (3)	2 (7)	
Gastroenterologist rating of response				
Improved	9 (30)	29 (78)	15 (50)	
Stayed the same	19 (63)	7 (19)	12 (40)	.002
Worsened	2 (7)	1 (3)	3 (10)	

*Group differences calculated by using χ^2.

scores than patients receiving placebo. Overall, patients receiving individualized CHM fared slightly worse than those receiving standard CHM treatment.

At the end of treatment, there was a significant difference between the mean total BSS scores as assessed by patients, with patients in the standard CHM group and those in the individualized CHM group responding significantly better compared with placebo (Table 3). No significant differences were noted between standard and individualized CHM treatment groups.

The BSS scores completed by the gastroenterologist at the end of treatment showed a significant difference between the mean total BSS scores for patients in each group, with patients receiving standard and individualized CHM responding significantly better compared with those taking placebo (*P*=.001). A post hoc Bonferroni test demonstrated that this difference was significant for patients in the standard group (*P*=.001) but not for those in the individualized group (*P*=.08).

Patients receiving standard herbal formulations improved by 44% (according to patients) and 59% (according to gastroenterologists), in contrast to patients in the placebo group who improved 22% (according to patients) and 19% (according to gastroenterologists). Patients receiving individualized CHM improved by 42% (according to patients) and 40% (according to gastroenterologists).

There was a significant association between the treatment groups and the change in the degree to which IBS symptoms caused interference with life and activities by the end of treatment (*P*=.03). Of patients receiving the standard formulation and of those receiving individual formulations, 63% and 54%, respectively, stated that treatment resulted in IBS causing less interference in their lives and activities, compared with 37% of patients in the placebo group.

At the end of the trial, the ratings of both gastroenterologists and patients who believed that the IBS symptoms had improved, stayed the same, or worsened (Table 4) showed a significant association by treatment group (*P*=.007). Of patients receiving standard CHM and of those receiving individual CHM, 76% and 64%, respectively, stated they had improved during treatment. In contrast, only 33% of patients receiving placebo stated they had improved during treatment.

The gastroenterologists' responses also demonstrated a significant association between the treatment group and how patients felt at the end of treatment (χ^2_4=17.1; *P*=.002). Seventy-eight percent of patients receiving the standard CHM formulation, 50% of those receiving individual CHM, and 30% of those receiving placebo were judged by the gastroenterologist as having improved during treatment. There was significant correlation between patients' and gastroenterologists' assessment of global improvement and of total BSS scores at the beginning and end of the trial (all r>0.5, all significant to $P\leq.01$ level, 2-tailed).

Adverse Effects

Two patients withdrew from the trial because of discomfort associated with the treatment. One patient developed upper gastrointestinal discomfort while taking the standard CHM formulation. A second patient developed headaches (although a history of headaches existed), which gradually subsided on discontinuation of therapy. Recommencement of treatment caused gastrointestinal discomfort, and the patient was subsequently withdrawn from the study. No other major adverse effects were noted.

Liver function tests obtained after 8 weeks of treatment showed no abnormal values.

Follow-up Assessment

Results of the BSS administered to patients 14 weeks after completion of the course of treatment (but before treatment codes were revealed) demonstrated that the treatment effect weakened, with only the individualized CHM group maintaining improvement (*P*<.10) (Table 3). However, there was significant association between the treatment group and how patients felt at the 14-week follow-up (*P*=.02). Of patients who had received the standard CHM formulation and of those who had received individual CHM formulations, 63% and 75%, respectively, stated that they still felt an improvement compared with 32% of patients who received placebo.

Blinding

The success of blinding patients to treatment was tested at the beginning, end, and on 2 other occasions during the course of treatment. At 2 weeks into treatment, the overall mean on this 6-point scale was 4, indicating that patients on average viewed CHM as only moderately credible and were not a self-selected group with a bias in favor of complementary medicine. No significant difference was noted between groups at outset and at end of treatment. However, the mean credibility score decreased slightly with time for the placebo group and remained strong within the standard CHM group. Since the standard CHM treatment proved the most effective, the increased difference in credibility toward the end of the treatment may be a reflection that this group of patients was receiving the most benefit. There was a significant negative correlation between the final mean credibility score and the final patient-rated BSS score (*r*=-0.43; *P*<.01) and the final gastroenterologist-rated BSS score (*r*=-0.58; *P*<.01).

Comment

To our knowledge, this is the first clinical trial in CHM that fully adheres to the traditional Chinese diagnostic and treatment processes while using a strict and accepted methodological protocol. Our study demonstrated that CHM is effective in the management of symptoms related to IBS with, in some cases, effects lasting up to 14 weeks after completion of treatment. Patients receiving standard or individualized CHM treatment demonstrated significantly better outcomes (both clinically and statistically) than patients receiving the placebo on all 5 key outcome measures. However, patients receiving individualized CHM formulations had less improvement during treatment than patients receiving the standard formula, although this difference was not statistically significant.

The first null hypothesis that CHM treatment of IBS with a standard herbal formula is of no value is rejected. The second null hypothesis that individualized treatment of IBS according to the principles of traditional CHM is of no added value to treatment with a standard formula is partially accepted. While there were no significant differences between patients receiving standard or individualized treatment at the end of the treatment period, on follow-up, patients in the individualized treatment group had maintained more substantial improvement.

Three Chinese herbalists with contrasting Chinese medicine education backgrounds participated in this trial. In theory, their degree of education in Chinese herbalism should affect their ability to successfully tailor treatment for patients. While outcome differences between practitioners were observable for this cohort of patients, sample sizes were too small to make reliable conclusions. Furthermore, the overall differences between standard and individualized CHM may be relatively small (as both are active treatments) and require larger sample sizes. This does not, however, account for the notable improvement that was maintained in the individualized CHM group after cessation of treatment.

One plausible explanation may be that the standard CHM formulation was suitably designed to treat the complex presentations of IBS but was incapable of successfully dealing with underlying causes for most patients as viewed by Chinese medicine. The tailored formulations may have permitted the herbalists to individually address these underlying causes and deficiencies. Moreover, there may be active ingredients in the CHM formulation with properties similar to antispasmodic or anxiolytic drugs. Chinese herbal formulas are complex and viewed as a number of active ingredients working together, rather than 1 specific active substance. The standard formulation used in this study is not a sedative or anxiolytic preparation in traditional CHM terms but is a formulation considered to regulate and strengthen bowel function.

In our study, all efforts were made for the approach in the 3 treatment groups to be indistinguishable. The credibility scale was demonstrated to be a reliable and valid instrument and presents strong evidence that blinding was maintained throughout the trial. The slight decrease in credibility score seen in the placebo group toward the end of the trial was accounted for by its significant correlation with the actual treatment outcome. The authors are convinced that patients, herbalists, and gastroenterologists were all successfully blinded.

There were minimal adverse effects reported during the study. Liver function screening was included as a precaution because liver dysfunction associated with the use of Chinese herbs has been noted in other studies.[8, 22] Liver dysfunction was not expected with the type and form of herbs used in this study. In our study, liver function was reassessed after 8 weeks of treatment. We have no data on liver function after that time, and therefore cannot comment on longer-term safety of these CHM products. Raw herbs used as starting products are partly regulated in Australia.

We conclude that Chinese herbal formulations may offer symptom improvement to some patients with IBS. In this randomized, double-blinded, placebo-controlled trial CHM was shown to be effective in the management of IBS. Patients receiving the standard CHM formulation fared best during the course of treatment, while patients receiving the individualized treatments found that the benefit gained lasted beyond the treatment period. Although not all patients responded to this therapy, our findings support the consideration of further investigation of Chinese herbal medicine as a treatment option for IBS.

The study was supported by an Australian $14,000 contribution from the University of Western Sydney Macarthur, Sydney, Australia.

The authors acknowledge the financial assistance of the University of Western Sydney Macarthur, Mei Yu Imports for the contribution of all herbal materials, and Pan Laboratories, Sydney, Australia, for assistance with the design and preparation of the placebo.

This project would not have been completed without the ongoing support of gastroenterologists, nursing staff, research assistants, and Chinese herbalists. Particular thanks is given to Sungwon Chang, MStats, Kathryn Taylor, and Sue Huntley, BN; to the Gastroenterology Units of Nepean Hospital and Concord Hospital, Sydney, Australia; to herbalists Yu Long Yu and Henry Liang, MTCM; and to Gavin Barr, FRACP, Philip Barnes, MD, Chris Pokorny, FRACP, John Garvey, FRACS, Tom Borody, MD, and Laura Pearce, MBBS, Mosman Medical Centre; and to all patients who contributed their time to this study.

References

1. Drossman DA, Li Z, Andruzzi E, et al. US householder survey of functional gastrointestinal disorders. *Dig Dis Sci.* 1993;38:1569–1580.

2. Talley NJ, Zinsmeister AR, Van Dyke C, Melton III LJ. Epidemiology of colonic symptoms and the irritable bowel syndrome. *Gastroenterology.* 1991;101:927–934.

3. Heaton KW, O'Donnell LJD, Braddon FEM, et al. Irritable bowel syndrome in a British urban community. *Gastroenterology.* 1992; 102:1962–1967.

4. Jones R, Lydeard S. Irritable bowel syndrome in the general population. *BMJ.* 1992;304:87–90.

5. Talley NJ, Boyce PM, Owen BK, et al. Initial validation of a bowel symptom questionnaire and measurement of chronic gastrointestinal symptoms in Australians. *Aust N Z J Med.* 1995; 25:302–307.

6. Talley NJ, Owen BK, Boyce P, Paterson K. Psychological treatments for irritable bowel syndrome. *Am J Gastroenterol.* 1996; 91:277–283.

7. Klein KB. Controlled treatment trials in the irritable bowel syndrome. *Gastroenterology.* 1988;95:232–241.

8. Bensoussan A, Myers SP. *Towards a Safer Choice: The Practice of Traditional Chinese Medicine in Australia.* Sydney, Australia: University of Western Sydney Macarthur; 1996.

9. Yu ZX, Wang K, Li FP. Clinical trial of Chinese herbal capsule for 157 cases of irritable bowel syndrome. *Chin J Integrated Tradit West Med.* 1991;11:170–171.

10. Liu ZK. Chinese herbal medicine treatment for 120 cases of irritable bowel syndrome. *Chin J Integrated Tradit West Med.* 1990;10:615.

11. Shi ZQ. Combination treatment of Chinese and Western medicine for 30 cases of irritable bowel syndrome. *Chin J Integrated Tradit West Med.* 1989;9:241.

12. Chen DZ. Tong Xie Yao Fang with additions in treating 106 cases of irritable bowel syndrome. *Nanjing Med University J.* 1995;15:924.

13. Xu RL. Clinical realisations during the diagnosis and treatment of 55 cases of irritable bowel syndrome. *Shanxi J Tradit Chin Med.* 1995; 11:10–11.

14. Anthony HM. Some methodological problems in the assessment of complementary therapy. In: Lewith GT, Aldridge D, eds. *Clinical Research Methodology for Complementary Therapies.* London, England: Hodder & Stoughton; 1993:108–121.

15. Bensoussan A. Contemporary acupuncture research. *Am J Acupunct.* 1993;19:357–366.

16. Thompson WG, Creed F, Drossman DA, et al. Functional bowel disease and functional abdominal pain. *Gastroenterol Int.* 1992; 5:75–91.

17. Talley NJ, Nyren O, Drossman DA, et al. The irritable bowel syndrome: toward optimal design of controlled treatment trials. *Gastroenterol Int.* 1993;6:189–211.

18. Hsu H-Y. 1986 *Oriental Materia Medica.* Long Beach, Calif: Oriental Healing Arts Institute; 1986.

19. Borkovec TD, Nau SD. Credibility of analogue therapy rationales. *J Behav Ther Exp Psychiatry.* 1972;3:257–260.

20. Vincent C. Credibility assessment of trials in acupuncture. *Complementary Med Res.* 1990;4:8–11.

21. Petrie J, Hazleman B. Credibility of placebo transcutaneous nerve stimulation and acupuncture. *Clin Exp Rheumatol.* 1985;3:151–153.

22. Kane JA, Kane SP, Jain S. Hepatitis induced by traditional Chinese herbs. *Gut.* 1995; 36:146–147.

41 *Garcinia cambogia* (Hydroxycitric Acid) as a Potential Antiobesity Agent

A Randomized Controlled Trial

Steven B. Heymsfield, MD; David B. Allison, PhD; Joseph R. Vasselli, PhD; Angelo Pietrobelli, MD; Debra Greenfield, MS, RD; Christopher Nunez, MEd
From the Department of Medicine, Obesity Research Center, St Luke's–Roosevelt Hospital, Columbia University College of Physicians and Surgeons, New York, NY.

Context
Hydroxycitric acid, the active ingredient in the herbal compound *Garcinia cambogia,* competitively inhibits the extramitochondrial enzyme adenosine triphosphate–citrate (*pro*-3S)-lyase. As a citrate cleavage enzyme that may play an essential role in de novo lipogenesis inhibition, *G cambogia* is claimed to lower body weight and reduce fat mass in humans.

Objective
To evaluate the efficacy of *G cambogia* for body weight and fat mass loss in overweight human subjects.

Design
Twelve-week randomized, double-blind, placebo-controlled trial.

Setting
Outpatient weight control research unit.

Participants
Overweight men and women subjects (mean body mass index [weight in kilograms divided by the square of height in meters], approximately 32 kg/m^2).

Intervention
Subjects were randomized to receive either active herbal compound (1500 mg of hydroxycitric acid per day) or placebo, and both groups were prescribed a high-fiber, low-energy diet. The treatment period was 12 weeks. Body weight was evaluated every other week and fat mass was measured at weeks 0 and 12.

Main Outcome Measures
Body weight change and fat mass change.

Results
A total of 135 subjects were randomized to either active hydroxycitric acid (n=66) or placebo (n=69); 42 (64%) in the active hydroxycitric acid group and 42 (61%) in the placebo

group completed 12 weeks of treatment (*P*=.74). Patients in both groups lost a significant amount of weight during the 12-week treatment period (*P*<.001); however, between-group weight loss differences were not statistically significant (mean [SD], 3.2 [3.3] kg vs 4.1 [3.9] kg; *P*=.14). There were no significant differences in estimated percentage of body fat mass loss between treatment groups, and the fraction of subject weight loss as fat was not influenced by treatment group.

Conclusions

Garcinia cambogia **failed to produce significant weight loss and fat mass loss beyond that observed with placebo.**

JAMA. 1998;280:1596–1600

Excessive adiposity and its concomitant health risks are among the most common conditions managed by health care practitioners. The limited long-term effectiveness of conventional weight management, including behavioral therapy,[1] is the impetus of major efforts aimed at developing alternative pharmacologic[2] and surgical weight reduction treatment strategies.[3] A rapidly growing therapeutic area, and one widely embraced by the general public, is the use of herbal weight loss products.

An herb-derived compound, hydroxycitric acid, is now incorporated into many commercial weight loss products. Obtained from extracts of related plants native to India, mainly *Garcinia cambogia* and *Garcinia indica*, hydroxycitric acid was first identified by Watson and Lowenstein[4,5] in the late 1960s as a potent competitive inhibitor of the extramitochondrial enzyme adenosine triphosphate–citrate (*pro-3* S)-lyase. These investigators and others subsequently demonstrated both in vitro and in vivo that hydroxycitric acid in animals not only inhibited the actions of citrate cleavage enzyme and suppressed de novo fatty acid synthesis,[6] but also increased rates of hepatic glycogen synthesis,[7] suppressed food intake,[8] and decreased body weight gain.[9]

Although hydroxycitric acid appears to be a promising experimental weight control agent, studies in humans are limited and results have been contradictory[10–14] (also R. Ramos, J. Flores Saenz, F. Alarcon, unpublished data, 1996, and G. Kaats, D. Pullin, L. Parker, S. Keith, unpublished data, 1996). Supporting evidence of human hydroxycitric acid efficacy for weight control is based largely on studies with small sample sizes,[11,12] studies that failed to include a placebo-treated group,[10] and use of inaccurate measures of body lipid change.[12] Although hydroxycitric acid effectiveness remains unclear, at least [14] separate hydroxycitric acid-containing products are presently sold over-the-counter to consumers.[15] This investigation was designed to overcome limitations of earlier studies and examine the effectiveness of hydroxycitric acid for weight loss and fat mass reduction in a rigorous controlled trial.

Methods

Protocol

We tested 2 primary hypotheses in a randomized, double-blind, placebo-controlled trial: (1) *G cambogia* produces a greater reduction in body weight than placebo, and (2) *G cambogia* produces a greater reduction in total body fat mass than placebo. Advertisements were placed in local newspapers, and overweight subjects who responded and met entry criteria during a telephone screening interview were scheduled for a baseline visit. The evaluation included a physical examination, electrocardiogram, and screening blood studies. Subjects meeting entry criteria were seen within 2 weeks for randomization at treatment week 0. Subjects were assigned to placebo or active compound with equal probability through a random number generator.

The protocol with active herbal compound included *G cambogia* extract (50% hydroxycitric acid by chemical analysis), taken 3 times daily as two 500-mg caplets 30 minutes before meal ingestion. Total daily dose was *G cambogia* extract, 3000 mg, and hydroxycitric acid, 1500 mg. Placebo-treated subjects followed an identical protocol in which active compound was replaced with inert ingredients. Subjects taking active compound or placebo were provided a high-fiber, 5040-kJ/d diet plan, with 20%, 50%, and 30% of energy as fat, carbohydrate, and protein, respectively. The recommended daily food provision was divided into 3 meals with an evening snack. Subjects were asked to maintain a stable physical activity level and return for evaluation every 2 weeks for a total treatment interval of 12 weeks. Body weight was measured at each visit, and clinical information, including potential herb or weight loss adverse effects, was obtained. Biweekly pill counts and diaries were used to check patient medication compliance. Diet compliance was not quantitatively monitored during the study.

The study was approved by the institutional review board of St Luke's–Roosevelt Hospital Center, New York, NY, and all subjects gave written consent prior to participation.

Subjects

Subjects were overweight but otherwise healthy adults aged 18 to 65 years who had a body mass index (BMI, defined as weight in kilograms divided by the square of height in meters) of more than 27 kg/m^2 and at most 38 kg/m^2. Subjects were excluded if they were pregnant, had any clinically significant medical condition, were taking prescription medications or appetite suppressants on a regular basis, had a history of alcohol or other drug abuse, were allergic to any of the study products, or had dieted with weight loss in the past 6 months.

Body Composition

Body weight and height were measured to the nearest 0.1 kg and 0.5 cm using a digital scale (Weight Tronix, New York, NY) and stadiometer (Holtain, Crosswell, Wales), respectively. Total body fat mass was measured at baseline and at the 12-week visit using several different procedures.

A pencil-beam dual-energy x-ray absorptiometry (DXA) scanner (Lunar DPX, Madison, Wis) was used to estimate total body fat mass. Subjects completed the slow-mode whole body scan and fat mass estimates were provided by Lunar, Version 3.6g, software.[16] The technical error of DXA percentage fat mass estimates in our laboratory is 3.1%.[17] The remaining body fat mass measurement methods used in our laboratory for this study included underwater weighing,[18] skinfold thicknesses,[19] and bioimpedance analysis.[20]

Statistical Analysis

Based on previous research,[1] we estimated that a study that included at least 30 completed subjects in each of 2 groups would have more than 80% power at the 2-tailed a level of .05 to detect any significant differences in body weight.

The 2 study hypotheses were tested in separate sets of statistical analyses. Statistical models were used in which the outcome variable, either loss of body weight or percentage of fat mass, was set as dependent variable and assigned treatment and other covariates were set as independent variables in an intent-to-treat analysis.[21] Within the intent-to-treat analysis, missing data due to measurement failure or subject dropout were imputed by carrying the last observation forward (LOCF).[22] The baseline value of the dependent variable (ie, initial body weight or percentage of fat mass) served as a potential independent variable in each analysis. Patient age and sex also served as additional independent variables. All analyses were conducted at the 2-tailed α level of .05.

For each of the 2 dependent variables, a set of secondary analyses were conducted, including (1) evaluation of completers only; (2) imputation of all missing data with a regression procedure rather than the LOCF; (3) imputation of missing data using the EM[23] algorithm rather than the LOCF; (4) use of weight loss slopes as outcomes[24] rather than the simple baseline to final measurement change when more than 2 time points for weight were available; (5) performance of a full repeated-measures analysis of variance using all time points; and (6) performance of a multivariate analysis of covariance using all time points simultaneously in the statistical model. In no case did any of these secondary sensitivity analyses lead to different conclusions than the primary LOCF intent-to-treat analysis. We therefore report only the results of the primary intent-to-treat analysis.

At baseline, DXA readings were unavailable for several subjects who had technically poor scans or who were evaluated during a brief period in which the DXA system was undergoing repair. However, each of these subjects had 1 or more measurements of fat mass taken with the other techniques mentioned herein and summarized in earlier articles.[16–20] Estimates of total body fat mass for these subjects by DXA were inferred using single imputation plus random error models based on multiple regression analysis of all other available measurements of fat mass for that subject, as described by Graham et al.[25] Similarly, several subjects completed the entire course of treatment and received some measurement of body fat mass after treatment but not by DXA. For these subjects, estimates of total body fat mass by DXA also were imputed using the same statistical methods and the other available measurements of body fat mass.

The purported fat-mobilizing properties of hydroxycitric acid were evaluated by computing the slope of change in fat mass vs change in body weight for the 2 treatment groups. Assuming approximately a zero intercept for this relation, the anticipated regression line slopes should approach 0.7 to 0.8, the generally acknowledged fraction of weight loss as fat mass in obesity trials.[26] Promotion of fat mass loss by active hydroxycitric acid would be associated with an increased fraction of weight loss as fat mass.

Group results are expressed as mean (SD) in text and tables. Data were analyzed using the statistical programs SPSSWIN, Version 7.5, and SPSSMVA, Version 7.5 (SPSS Inc, Chicago, Ill).

Results

Baseline Characteristics

At baseline, 180 moderately overweight subjects were screened and, of those, 135 were randomized to placebo and active compound (Table 1 and Figure 1). There were 69 subjects (BMI, 31.9 [3.1] kg/m^2) in the placebo-treated group (14 men and 55 women) and 66 subjects (BMI, 31.3 [2.8] kg/m^2) in the *G cambogia*-treated group (5 men and 61 women).

Of the 69 placebo-treated subjects, 42 (61%) completed the 12-week protocol. The reasons for subject withdrawal (27 cases) are summarized in Figure 1. Of the 66 subjects randomized to active compound, 42 (64%) completed the 12 weeks of treatment. The reasons for subject withdrawal from this group (24 cases) are also summarized Figure 1. There were no significant differences in age, body weight, or BMI between subjects who withdrew from the study and those who completed the 12-week protocol. There was also no significant difference between the 2 groups in the proportion of subjects who completed the entire course of treatment (χ^2=0.11, P=.74). Among subjects completing the 12 weeks of treatment, medication compliance was 88.6% (10.9%) and 92.1% (10.0%) in the treatment and placebo groups, respectively (P=.30).

Weight Loss

Primary Analysis. The weight loss curves for placebo and treatment groups are shown in Figure 2 for subjects in the intent-to-treat analysis with LOCF. The estimated mean (SD) [median (interquartile range)] weight loss for the placebo group was 4.1 (3.9) [3.9 (4.7)] kg and for the treatment group was 3.2 (3.3) [2.6 (4.1)] kg. The weight loss within each group was significantly different from baseline (t_{134}=11.795, P<.001), although between-group weight loss differences were not statistically significant (t_{133}=1.474, P=.14). Body weight change differences remained nonsignificant after controlling for patient starting weight, sex, and age. Assumptions of the applied parametric statistical analysis such as homogeneity of variance and normality of residuals were tested and no meaningful violations were detected. Given the lack of significant findings, questions of statistical power are important. Therefore, using the observed distributions of weight change and the within-group SD thereof, we estimated that the power of the current study to detect differences between the treatment and placebo groups in terms of weight change was 89% to detect a between-group difference in weight loss as small as 2 kg at the 2-tailed α level of .05.

Secondary Analyses. In no case did any secondary analysis indicate any statistically significant effect for the active compound to produce more weight loss than placebo.

Fat Mass Loss

Primary Analysis. Results for body fat mass analysis were imputed for 9 baseline and 4 post-weight loss subjects. With the LOCF intent-to-treat analysis, the estimated mean (SD) [median (interquartile range)] percentage of body fat mass loss for the placebo group was 2.16% (2.06%) [2.20% (2.7%)] and the estimated percentage of fat mass loss for the treatment group was 1.44% (2.15%) [1.60% (1.9%)]. This difference was tested using the Welch test because the variances were significantly heterogeneous by the Levene test (P for variance heterogeneity=.03). Using the Welch test, the placebo and treatment group mean differences were not statistically significant (t_{129}=1.7, P=.08). This finding was consistent with that of the ordinary t test (t_{132}=1.78, P=.08). Using analysis of covariance with age, sex, and pretest percentage of fat mass as covariates, the percentage of fat mass differences also was nonsignificant (F_{1129}=1.57, P=.21).

Secondary Analyses. As for weight loss, all of the secondary analyses were consistent with the primary analysis. That is, in no case did analysis indicate any statistically significant effect for the active compound to produce a different percentage of body fat mass loss than the placebo.

Examination of the change in fat mass relative to change in body weight derived using least squares regression analysis for all subjects combined resulted in the relation, Δfat mass (kg)=0.77 $\times$ Δbody weight (kg) – 0.44, with r=0.89 and P<.001. The association was not changed significantly (P>.91) by adding treatment group as a second independent variable, even after adjusting for 3 additional potential covariates: initial body weight, sex, and age.

Adverse Events

No patient was removed from the study protocol for a treatment-related adverse event, and the number of reported adverse events was not significantly different between the placebo and treatment groups (eg, headache, 12

Table 1. Baseline Subject Characteristics*

Group	No. of Patients	Age, y	Weight, kg	BMI, kg/m²†	Total Body Fat Mass, %
Treatment					
Men	5	43.1 (2.8)	100.8 (11.0)	33.0 (3.7)	28.4 (2.6)
Women	61	38.2 (7.8)	82.9 (8.8)	31.1 (2.7)	41.9 (7.3)
Total	**66**	38.6 (7.7)	83.8 (10.1)	31.2 (2.8)	41.1 (7.8)
Placebo					
Men	14	40.5 (5.5)	101.7 (11.8)	32.3 (2.5)	36.6 (5.9)
Women	55	39.6 (7.6)	84.8 (10.9)	31.4 (3.2)	43.8 (4.2)
Total	**69**	39.4 (7.2)	88.2 (13.0)	31.9 (3.1)	42.0 (5.6)

*Data (except number of patients) are presented as group mean (SD).
†BMI indicates body mass index, defined as weight in kilograms divided by the square of height in meters.

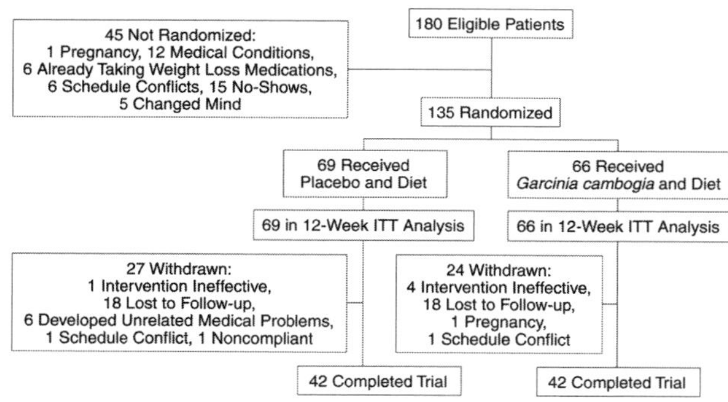

Figure 1. Study CONSORT flow diagram. ITT indicates intent-to-treat.

vs 9, respectively; upper respiratory tract symptoms, 13 vs 16, respectively; and gastrointestinal tract symptoms, 6 vs 13, respectively).

Comment

In 1883 von Lippmann isolated hydroxycitric acid, a minor constituent of sugar beets.[27] More than half a century later, in 1941, Martius and Maué[28] discovered that the (+) isomer of a racemic hydroxycitric acid mixture is attacked by the enzyme isocitrate dehydrogenase. The (–) hydroxycitric acid isomer of hydroxycitric acid was first isolated by Lewis and Neelakantan in 1964,[29] and by 1969 Watson and colleagues[5] reported the powerful inhibition by (–) hydroxycitric acid of citrate cleavage enzyme. Evidently, the additional hydroxyl group's steric position, compared with citric acid, enhances its binding affinity and competitively inhibits catalytic action by the enzyme. Citrate, entering the cytoplasm from mitochondria, cannot be cleaved to release acetyl coenzyme A, the substrate for de novo fatty acid synthesis. Despite these century-old, well-grounded observations, there has been little effort to critically test the basic assumption underlying therapeutic use of hydroxycitric acid in overweight humans: that hydroxycitric acid inhibition of lipid synthesis will significantly reduce body fat mass beyond that observed with a placebo capsule.

The present study, carried out during a 12-week evaluation period and using accepted experimental design and in vivo analytic methods, failed to support the hypothesis that hydroxycitric acid as prescribed promotes either additional weight or fat mass loss beyond that observed with placebo. Specifically, body weight and fat mass change during the 12-week study period did not differ significantly between placebo and treatment groups. These results apply to both the primary and secondary statistical analyses. Additionally, there were no observed selective fat-mobilizing effects specifically attributable to the active agent, hydroxycitric acid.

Seven earlier *G cambogia* trials have appeared in peer-reviewed literature,[11,14] as abstracts,[12,13] and in industrial publications as an open-label study[10] and randomized controlled trials.[11–14] We chose to collectively review these studies even though *G cambogia* typically was used in combination with other ingredients for the claimed purpose of enhancing weight loss.

Of the 7 studies reviewed, 5 reported significant ($P<.05$) effects of *G cambogia* alone or in combination with other ingredients on body weight or fat mass loss in overweight humans (Table 2). These earlier studies all have limitations when specifically considering *G cambogia* as a weight loss agent, including lack of placebo control or double-blinding in 1 study,[10] coadministration of *G cambogia* in combination with other potentially active ingredients in 5 studies,[10,11,13,14] use of an inaccurate body composition method (near-infrared interactance)[12] in 1 study, and failure as of yet to publish study results in peer-reviewed literature in all but 2[13,14] of the 7 studies. However, our present investigation, carried out using accepted clinical trial design procedures and applying accurate body composition methods, failed to support a specific weight loss effect of *G cambogia* administered as recommended. The present 12-week study period also exceeded in duration all previous study treatment periods, which ranged from 4 to 8 weeks.

In our present investigation we failed to detect a weight loss or fat-mobilizing effect of active herb. The question therefore arises whether there exist conditions differing from those used in the present study that might support hydroxycitric acid efficacy. The 5040-kJ/d low-fat diet recommended in our current study was intended to mimic diets commonly prescribed as a component of weight control programs. The possibility exists that the lipid synthesis–inhibiting properties of hydroxycitric acid may be more evident in subjects relapsing following a failed diet attempt, particularly if high-carbohydrate foods are ingested.[30]

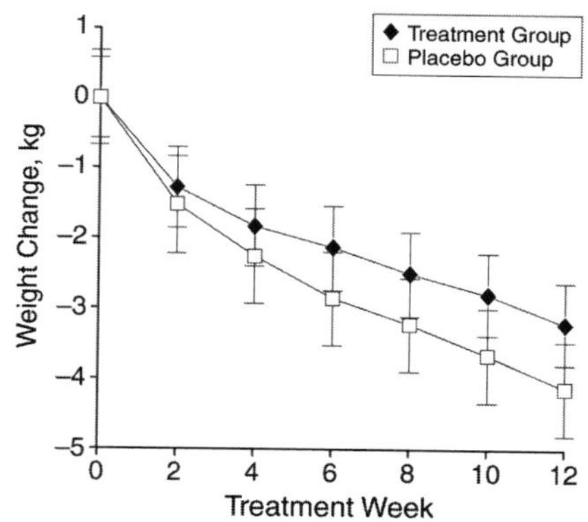

Figure 2. Weight-change curves for 2 study groups. Results are plotted for group means (±95% confidence limits) for 69 subjects in the placebo group and 66 subjects in the treatment group. Data are from last-observation-carried-forward intent-to-treat analysis.

Table 2. Summary of Previous *Garcinia cambogia* Studies*

Author(s)	Publication Type	Study Design	Study Agent(s)	Sample	Duration, wk	Major Observations
Badmaev and Majeed[10]	Industrial	Single arm, open label	GCE, 500 mg, chromium picolinate, 100 µg, 3 times per day and healthy eating/exercise	77 obese adults, with 55 completing trial	8	5.5% weight loss in women, 4.9% in men†; combined, *P*<.001 vs baseline
Conte[11]	Peer-reviewed	Randomized, double-blind, placebo controlled	*Garcinia indica* extract 500 mg, nickel chromium, 100 µg, 3 times per day and low-fat substitution diet	54 obese subjects randomized, with 39 completing trial	8	Active, 11.14 lb, vs placebo, 4.2 lb†‡
Ramos et al (unpublished data)	Abstract	Randomized, double-blind, placebo controlled	GCE, 500 mg, 3 times per day, and low-fat 4200–6300 kJ/d diet	40 obese subjects randomized, with 35 completing trial	8	Active, 4.1 (1.8) kg, vs placebo, 1.3 (0.9) kg (*P*<.05)§
Kaats et al (unpublished data)	Abstract	Randomized, double-blind, placebo controlled	GCE, 1500 mg/d, chromium picolinate, 600 µg/d, L-carnitine, 1200 mg/d, and low-fat, high-fiber diet	200 subjects randomized, with 186 completing trial	4	Active, −2.84 lb, vs placebo, −1.4 lb fat mass loss (*P*<.01)†
Thom[12]	Abstract	Randomized, double-blind, placebo controlled	Hydroxycitric acid, 1320 mg/d, in 3 divided doses, and 5040-kJ/d low-fat diet	60 subjects randomized; number completing trial not reported	8	Active, 6.4 kg, vs placebo, 3.8 kg weight loss (*P*<.001); weight loss as fat, 87% in active vs 80% in placebo group†‡
Rothacker and Waitman[13]	Abstract	Randomized, double-blind, placebo controlled	GCE, 800 mg, natural caffeine, 50 mg, and chromium polynicotinate, 40 µg, 3 times per day, and 5040-kJ/d diet	50 obese subjects randomized, with 48 completing trial	6	Active, −4.0% (3.5%) vs placebo, −3.0% (3.1%) body fat mass (*P*=.30)
Girola et al[14]	Peer-reviewed	Randomized, double-blind, placebo controlled	GCE, 55 mg, chrome, 19 mg, and chitosan, 240 mg; randomized to 1 of 3 groups, active medication twice per day, placebo twice per day, or 1 placebo and 1 active medication per day; all groups treated with hypocaloric diet	150 obese subjects; number completing trial not reported	4	Active, twice per day, −12.5% (1.2%); active, once per day, −7.9% (0.9%); twice per day placebo, −4.3% (1.0%); "overweight reduction" (*P*<.01 for all 3 vs baseline)§

*GCE indicates *Garcinia cambogia* extract.
†No SDs reported.
‡No statistical analysis reported.
§Numbers in parentheses are SD.

Another concern is related to the timing and dosage considerations of hydroxycitric acid. Sullivan and colleagues[31] showed that the effects of hydroxycitric acid in animals depend on time of administration in relation to a meal, with hydroxycitric acid maximally effective when administered 30 to 60 minutes prior to feeding. The approach used in our study and the others we reviewed suggested hydroxycitric acid ingestion about 30 minutes prior to meal intake, the lower end of the maximally effective range. A related concern is that hydroxycitric acid provided in divided doses also was found to be more effective than the same amount given as a single dose.[8] Although divided doses typically are used in weight loss protocols, human doses ranging between 750 and 1500 mg/d of hydroxycitric acid are at the extreme low end of the in vivo dose-response range established by Sullivan and colleagues.[32] Thus, in light of the many requirements for its effective use, it seems unlikely that the maximal effects of hydroxycitric acid will be realized in human weight loss studies unless treatment conditions are well defined and patient diet and medication compliance are tightly monitored.

Our study explored product safety only in the form of clinical evaluations and reported adverse events. No significant differences were observed between placebo and treatment groups in number of reported adverse events and no subjects were removed from the study for a treatment-related adverse event. Additional studies, potentially with larger subject groups, are needed to gather specific information on the long-term safety of *G cambogia.*

An important concern in all pharmacological trials, particularly those in which herbal products are evaluated, is the amount and bioavailability of the active agent. As standard procedure, we confirmed the presence and quantity of hydroxycitric acid in the supplied capsules using an independent testing laboratory. However, we did not measure hydroxycitric acid blood levels or evaluate tissue or cytosolic citrate-cleavage enzyme activity. Although the format of our experiment closely resembles current use of *G cambogia* as a weight loss product, our conclusions should not be interpreted as a failure to support the validity of the biochemical effects of hydroxycitric acid identified by earlier investigators.

In conclusion, our study evaluated the hypothesis that the active ingredient of *G cambogia,* hydroxycitric acid, has beneficial weight and fat mass loss effects. Our findings, obtained in a prospective, randomized, double-blind study, failed to detect either weight loss or fat-mobilizing effects of hydroxycitric acid beyond those of placebo. These observations, the first, to our knowledge, to appear in a peer-reviewed article using currently accepted experimental and statistical methods, do not support a role as currently prescribed for the widely used herb *G cambogia* as a facilitator of weight loss.

This study was supported by National Institutes of Health grants RR00645 and P30DK26687 and a contract with Thompson Medical Company, West Palm Beach, Fla, manufacturer of products that include *G cambogia.*

References

1. National Task Force on the Prevention and Treatment of Obesity. Long-term pharmacotherapy in the management of obesity. *JAMA.* 1996;276:1907–1915.
2. Bray GA. Use and abuse of appetite suppressant drugs in the treatment of obesity. *Ann Intern Med.* 1993;119:707–713.
3. National Institutes of Health Consensus Development Conference statements: gastrointestinal surgery for severe obesity. *Am J Clin Nutr.* 1992;55(suppl):487S–619S.
4. Watson JA, Lowenstein JM. Citrate and the conversion of carbohydrate into fat. *J Biol Chem.* 1970;245:5993–6002.
5. Watson JA, Fang M, Lowenstein JM. Tricarballylate and hydroxycitrate: substrate and inhibitor of ATP: citrate oxaloacetate lyase. *Arch Biochem Biophys.* 1969;35:209–217.
6. Lowenstein JM. Effect of (-)-hydroxycitrate on fatty acid synthesis by rat liver in vivo. *J Biol Chem.* 1971;246:629–632.
7. Sullivan AC, Triscari J, Neal Miller O. The influence of (–)-hydroxycitrate on in vivo rates of hepatic glycogenesis: lipogenesis and cholesterol-genesis. *Fed Proc.* 1974;33:656.
8. Sullivan AC, Triscari J, Hamilton JG, Neal Miller O. Effect of (-)-hydroxycitrate upon the accumulation of lipid in the rat: appetite. *Lipids.* 1973;9:129–134.
9. Nageswara Rao R, Sakeriak KK. Lipid-lowering and antiobesity effect of (–) hydroxycitric acid. *Nutr Res.* 1988;8:209–212.
10. Badmaev V, Majeed M. Open field, physician controlled, clinical evaluation of botanical weight loss formula citrin. Presented at: Nutracon 1995: Nutriceuticals, Dietary Supplements and Functional Foods; July 11–13, 1995; Las Vegas, Nev.
11. Conte AA. A non-prescription alternative on weight reduction therapy. *Am J Bariatr Med.* Summer 1993:17–19.
12. Thom E. Hydroxycitrate (HCA) in the treatment of obesity. *Int J Obes.* 1996;20(suppl 4):48.
13. Rothacker DQ, Waitman BE. Effectiveness of a *Garcinia cambogia* and natural caffeine combination in weight loss: a double-blind placebo-controlled pilot study. *Int J Obes.* 1997;21(suppl 2):53.
14. Girola M, De Bernardi M, Contos S, et al. Dose effect in lipid-lowering activity of a new dietary intetrator (chitosan, Garcinia cambogia extract, and chrome). *Acta Toxicol Ther.* 1996; 17:25–40.
15. Hobbs LS. (–)-Hydroxycitrate (HCA). In: *The New Diet Pills.* Irvine, Calif: Pragmatic Press; 1994:161–174.
16. Pietrobelli A, Formica C, Wang ZM, Heymsfield SB. Dual-energy x-ray absorptiometry body composition model: review of physical concepts. *Am J Physiol.* 1997;271:E941–E951.
17. Russel-Aulet M, Wang J, Thornton J, Pierson Jr RN. Comparison of dual photon absorptiometry system for total body bone and soft tissue measurements: dual-energy x-ray versus gadolinium 153. *J Bone Miner Res.* 1991;6:411–415.

18. Heymsfield SB, Wang ZM, Withers R. Multicomponent molecular-level models for body composition analysis. In: Roche AF, Heymsfield SB, Lohman TG, eds. *Human Body Composition.* Champaign, Ill: Human Kinetics; 1996:129–147.

19. Heymsfield SB, Tighe A, Wang ZM. Nutritional assessment by anthropometric and biochemical methods. In: Shils ME, Olson JA, Shike M, eds. *Modern Nutrition in Health and Disease.* Philadelphia, Pa: Lea & Febiger; 1992:812–841.

20. Heymsfield SB, Visser M, Gallagher D, Pierson Jr RN, Wang ZM. Techniques used in measurement of body composition: an overview with emphasis on bioelectrical impedance analysis. *Am J Clin Nutr.* 1996;64(suppl):478S–484S.

21. Committee for Proprietary Medicinal Products. *Note for Guidance on Clinical Investigation of Drugs Used in Weight Control.* London, England: The European Agency for the Evaluation of Medical Products; 1997.

22. Niklson IA, Reimitz PE, Sennef C. Factors that influence the outcome of placebo-controlled antidepressant clinical trials. *Psychopharmacol Bull.* 1997;33:41–51.

23. Dempster AP, Laird NH, Rubin DB. Maximum likelihood from incomplete data via the EM algorithm. *J R Stat Soc.* 1977;39B:1–38.

24. Burstein L, Kim KS, Delandshere G. *Multilevel Investigations of Systematically Varying Slopes: Issues, Alternatives, and Consequences.* New York, NY: Academic Press; 1989.

25. Graham JW, Hoofer SM, Picnic AM. Analysis with missing data in drug prevention research. In: Des Collins LM, Seats LA, eds. *Advances in Data Analysis for Prevention Intervention Research.* Washington, DC: US Dept of Health and Human Services; 1994:13. NIDA Research Monograph 142.

26. Webster JD, Hesp R, Garrow JS. The composition of excess weight in obese women estimated by body density, total body water and total body potassium. *Hum Nutr Clin Nutr.* 1984; 38:299–306.

27. von Lippmann EO. Uber eine neue, im Rübensaft vorkommende Säure. *Ber Dtsch Chem Ges.* 1883;16:1078–1081.

28. Martius C, Maué R. Darstellung, physiologisches Verhalten und Bedeutung der (+)-Oxycitronensäure und ihrer Isomeren. *Z Physiol Chem.* 1941;269:33–40.

29. Lewis YS, Neelakantan S. (-)-Hydroxycitric acid: the principal acid in the fruits of *Garcinia cambogia. Phytochemistry.* 1965;4:610–625.

30. Vasselli JR, Shane E, Boozer CN, Heymsfield SB. *Garcinia cambogia* extract inhibits body weight gain via increased energy expenditure (EE) in rats. *FASEB J.* 1998;12(part I):A505.

31. Sullivan AC, Hamilton JG, Neal Miller O, Wheatley VR. Inhibition of lipogenesis in rat liver by (–)-hydroxycitrate. *Arch Biochem Biophys.* 1972;150:183–190.

32. Sullivan AC, Trescari J, Hamilton JG, Neal Miller O, Wheatley VR. Effect of (–)-hydroxycitrate upon the accumulation of lipid in the rat, I: lipogenesis. *Lipids.* 1973;9:121–128.

42 Saw Palmetto Extracts for Treatment of Benign Prostatic Hyperplasia

A Systematic Review

Timothy J. Wilt, MD, MPH; Areef Ishani, MD; Gerold Stark, MD; Roderick MacDonald, MS; Joseph Lau, MD; Cynthia Mulrow, MD, MS

From the Department of Veterans Affairs Coordinating Center of the Cochrane Collaborative Review Group in Prostatic Diseases and Urologic Malignancies and Minneapolis/Veterans Integrated Service Network 13 Center for Chronic Diseases Outcomes Research, Minneapolis Veterans Affairs Medical Center, Minneapolis, Minn (Drs Wilt, Ishani, and Stark and Mr MacDonald); New England Medical Center, Boston, Mass (Dr Lau); and the Department of Veterans Affairs San Antonio Cochrane Center, San Antonio, Tex (Dr Mulrow).

Objective

To conduct a systematic review and, where possible, quantitative meta-analysis of the existing evidence regarding the therapeutic efficacy and safety of the saw palmetto plant extract, *Serenoa repens,* in men with symptomatic benign prostatic hyperplasia (BPH).

Data Sources

Studies were identified through the search of MEDLINE (1966–1997), EMBASE, Phytodok, the Cochrane Library, bibliographies of identified trials and review articles, and contact with relevant authors and drug companies.

Study Selection

Randomized trials were included if participants had symptomatic BPH, the intervention was a preparation of *S repens* alone or in combination with other phytotherapeutic agents, a control group received placebo or other pharmacological therapies for BPH, and the treatment duration was at least 30 days.

Data Extraction

Two investigators for each article (T.J.W., A.I., G.S., and R.M.) independently extracted key data on design features, subject characteristics, therapy allocation, and outcomes of the studies.

Data Synthesis

A total of 18 randomized controlled trials involving 2939 men met inclusion criteria and were analyzed. Many studies did not report results in a method that permitted meta-analysis. Treatment allocation concealment was adequate in 9 studies; 16 were double-blinded. The mean study duration was 9 weeks (range, 4–48 weeks). As compared with men receiving placebo, men treated with *S repens* had decreased urinary tract symptom scores (weighted mean difference [WMD], −1.41 points [scale range, 0–19] [95% confidence interval (CI), −2.52 to −0.30] [n=1 study]), nocturia (WMD, −0.76 times per evening [95% CI, −1.22 to −0.32] [n=10 studies]), and improvement in self-rating of urinary tract symp-

toms; risk ratio for improvement (1.72 [95% CI, 1.21–2.44] [n=6 studies]), and peak urine flow (WMD, 1.93 mL/s [95% CI, 0.72–3.14] [n=8 studies]). Compared with men receiving finasteride, men treated with *S repens* had similar improvements in urinary tract symptom scores (WMD, 0.37 International Prostate Symptom Score points [scale range, 0-35] [95% CI, −0.45 to 1.19] [n=2 studies]) and peak urine flow (WMD, −0.74 mL/s [95% CI, −1.66 to 0.18] [n=2 studies]). Adverse effects due to S repens were mild and infrequent; erectile dysfunction was more frequent with finasteride (4.9%) than with *S repens* (1.1%; *P*<.001). Withdrawal rates in men assigned to placebo, *S repens,* or finasteride were 7%, 9%, and 11%, respectively.

Conclusions

The existing literature on *S repens* for treatment of BPH is limited in terms of the short duration of studies and variability in study design, use of phytotherapeutic preparations, and reports of outcomes. However, the evidence suggests that *S repens* improves urologic symptoms and flow measures. Compared with finasteride, *S repens* produces similar improvement in urinary tract symptoms and urinary flow and was associated with fewer adverse treatment events. Further research is needed using standardized preparations of *S repens* to determine its long-term effectiveness and ability to prevent BPH complications.

JAMA. 1998;280:1604–1609

Symptomatic benign prostatic hyperplasia (BPH) is one of the most common medical conditions in older men. As many as 40% of men aged 70 years or older have lower urinary tract symptoms consistent with BPH.[1] Treatment goals in the vast majority of men are to relieve irritative (urgency, frequency, and nocturia) and obstructive (weak stream, hesitancy, intermittency, and incomplete emptying) symptoms. In the United States, treatment of BPH exceeds $2 billion in costs, accounts for 1.7 million physician office visits,[2] and results in more than 300,000 prostatectomies annually.[3] Treatment options include lifestyle modification, device and surgical therapies, and pharmaceutical and phytotherapeutic preparations.[4,5]

Phytotherapy or the use of plant extracts for treating BPH symptoms was first described in Egypt in the 15th century BC. Currently, phytotherapy is common in Europe and is increasing in the western hemisphere. The sale of all botanical medications in the United States is $1.5 billion per year and the use of phytotherapies increased nearly 70% among US adults in the past year.[6,7] Phytotherapeutic agents represent nearly half the medications dispensed for treatment of BPH in Italy, compared with 5% for α-blockers and 5% for 5 α-reductase inhibitors.[8] In Germany and Austria, phytotherapy is the first-line treatment for mild-to-moderate lower urinary tract symptoms and represents more than 90% of all drugs prescribed for the treatment of BPH.[9] In the United States, phytotherapies for BPH are readily available as nonprescription dietary supplements. Most of these compounds are unlicensed and often promoted to “maintain a healthy prostate” and as a natural and harmless treatment of BPH symptoms.

There are about 30 phytotherapeutic compounds used for the treatment of BPH.[10] The most widely used is the extract of the dried ripe fruit from the American dwarf saw palmetto plant *Serenoa repens* (also known by its botanical name *Sabal serrulata*). Berries from saw palmetto were first used by the American Indians in Florida in the early 1700s to treat testicular atrophy, erectile dysfunction, and prostate gland swelling or inflammation.[10] The medicinal value of *S repens* for relief of prostate gland swelling has been reported in medical literature since the 1800s. The mechanism of action of *S repens* is not known but may include alteration of cholesterol metabolism,[11] antiestrogenic, antiandrogenic, and anti-inflammatory effects,[12–14] and a decrease in available sex hormone-binding globulin.[15] Although *S repens* has been evaluated in several randomized trials its clinical efficacy has not been clearly demonstrated.

Our goal was to systematically review the existing evidence regarding the therapeutic efficacy and safety of the saw palmetto plant extract *S repens.* We specifically assessed whether *S repens* is more effective than placebo and as effective as other pharmacological therapies in improving symptoms and/or urodynamic measurements in men with BPH.

Methods

Inclusion Criteria

Randomized controlled trials were included if participants had symptomatic BPH; the treatment intervention was a preparation of *S repens* (*S serrulata, Sabalis serrulata, Serenoa serrulata,* Permixon, PA109, Serendar, Talso, Curbicin, Prostagutt, Prostaselect, Prostagalen,

Prostavigol, Strogen forte, and SPRO 160/120) alone or in combination with other phytotherapeutic agents; a control group received either placebo or other pharmacological therapies for BPH; and the treatment duration was at least 30 days.

Identification of Relevant Trials

We searched MEDLINE for studies from 1966 to 1997 by crossing an optimally sensitive search strategy for trials from the Cochrane Collaboration with the medical subject headings *prostatic hyperplasia, phytosterols, plant extracts, sitosterols, Serenoa repens,* or *Sabal serrulata,* including all subheadings.[16] EMBASE, (1974–July 1997), Phytodok (Munich, Germany), and the Cochrane Library, including the database of the Cochrane Prostatic Diseases and Urologic Malignancies Group and the Cochrane Field for Complementary Medicine, were searched in a similar fashion. Reference lists of all identified trials and previous reviews were searched for additional trials. Expert relevant trialists and pharmaceutical companies were asked to identify additional published or unpublished trials. There were no language restrictions.

Data Extraction and Study Appraisal

Study characteristics, demographic information, enrollment criteria, therapy allocation, adverse effects, outcomes and numbers, and reasons for dropouts were extracted independently by 2 reviewers. Missing information was sought from authors and/or sponsors. Extracted data were reviewed by the principal reviewer and discrepancies resolved by discussion.

The main outcome was the efficacy of *S repens* vs placebo or active control in improving urologic symptom scale scores or global report of urinary tract symptoms (improved vs stable or worsened). Secondary outcomes included peak and mean urine flow, residual urine volume, prostate size, and nocturia.

As a measure of overall methodological study quality, we assessed the quality of concealment of treatment allocation according to a scale developed by Schulz et al,[17] assigning 1 as poorest quality and 3 as best quality. The treatment allocation included (1) trials in which concealment was inadequate (eg, such as alternation or reference to case record numbers or to dates of birth); (2) trials in which the authors either did not report an allocation concealment approach at all or reported an approach that did not fall into one of the other categories; and (3) trials deemed to have taken adequate measures to conceal allocation (eg, central randomization; numbered or coded bottles or containers; drugs prepared by the pharmacy; serially numbered, opaque, sealed envelopes, etc, that contained elements convincing of concealment). Additionally, we assessed whether study participants and investigators were blinded to the treatment provided.

Statistical Methods

A random-effects model was used to combine data for all outcomes. For continuous variables weighted mean differences and their 95% confidence intervals (CIs) were calculated using RevMan 3.0 software.[18] For categorical variables weighted risk ratios (RRs) and 95% CIs were calculated.[19] For continuous measurements, a difference between treatment means and its correlated SE of the difference were calculated using the methods of Lau[19] and Laird and Mosteller.[20] Because studies did not report the SE of the difference between the means (*S repens* and control), analyses were carried out for 3 different assumed values of correlation (0.25, 0.50, 0.75). This approach was taken to test the sensitivity of the results to this unknown parameter. Because there were no statistically significant differences in the outcomes, according to the different correlation coefficients, we used SEMs calculated with a correlation coefficient of 0.50. χ^2 Tests were used for analysis of bivariate comparisons. To assess the percentage of patients having improvement in urologic symptoms, a modified intention-to-treat analysis was performed (ie, men who dropped out or were lost to follow-up were considered to have had worsening symptoms).[21] The denominator for the modified intention-to-treat analysis included the number randomized to treatment at baseline, and the numerator included the number completing the trial and showing improvement.

Results

The combined search strategies identified 24 reports of trials; 18 met inclusion criteria.[22–39] Reasons for exclusion included duration unknown or less than 30 days (n=2 trials)[40,41]; no clinical outcomes (examining enzyme or tissue effects (n=3)[15,42,43]; and no indication of randomization (n=1).[44] Main comparisons in the remaining studies were *S repens* alone vs placebo (n=10); *S repens* in combination with other phytotherapeutic agents vs placebo (n=3); *S repens* alone vs active control (n=2); *S repens* vs another phytotherapeutic agent and vs placebo (n=1); *S repens* in combination with other phytotherapeutic agents vs active control (n=1); and *S repens* orally vs a rectal suppository form of *S repens*, a therapeutic bioequivalence study (n=1). A total of 2939 participants were randomized in the 18 trials (1118 in trials of *S repens* alone or in combination vs placebo and 1821 in trials of *S repens* alone or in combination vs active control).

A description of the individual studies is available from the authors on request. The mean age of enrollees was 65 years (range, 40–88 years). The mean study duration was 9 weeks (range, 4–48 weeks). The percentage of men who dropped out or were lost to follow-up was 9.6% (n=283) and ranged from 4% to 15%. Treatment allocation concealment was adequate in 9 studies (50%) and 16 studies (89%) were double-blinded.

Baseline and outcome data from individual studies for urologic symptoms, nocturia, peak urine flow, and residual urine volume are available from the authors on request. These results indicate that on average, participating men had urinary tract symptoms and urinary flow measures consistent with moderate BPH. The mean (SD) baseline values for these variables did not differ by treatment group and included urologic symptom scale score (International Prostate Symptom Scale [IPSS]) in 2 studies with active control (14.4 [5.9] points; scale range, 0–35; moderate BPH symptoms, 8–19); urologic symptom scale score in 1 study with placebo (7.0 [2.8] points; scale range, 0–19, based on an addition of subscores for 6 variables: pollakiuria, nocturia, dysuria, hesitancy, urgency, and perineal heaviness); nocturia (2.5 [1.47] times per night; peak urine flow, 11.2 [3.9] mL/s; and residual urine volume, 55.8 [41.5] mL). Baseline values (SD) for mean urine flow (5.7 [2.1] mL/s) and prostate volume (43.9 [21.6] cc) also did not differ by treatment group. Symptom score results were reported in 10 studies, nocturia results in 12 studies, peak urine flow in 13 studies, and residual volume in 12 studies. Many studies did not report results in a method that permitted data to be combined in a meta-analysis.

Weighted Summary Differences in Outcomes

Urinary Tract Symptoms. Summary treatment effect sizes were determined for *S repens* alone or in combination vs placebo and vs active controls. Results from participant and physician assessment indicated that *S repens* was superior to placebo and comparable with finasteride in improving urologic symptoms. The weighted mean difference for urinary symptom scale scores for *S repens* vs placebo was –1.41 points (scale range, 0–19) (28% absolute improvement vs placebo) (95% CI, –2.52 to –0.30) (n=1 study) and vs finasteride was 0.37 IPSS points (scale range, 0–35) (37% absolute improvement from baseline for *S repens* vs 40% absolute improvement from baseline for finasteride) (95% CI, –0.45 to 1.19) (n=2 studies) (Figure 1). The weighted mean difference for the combination preparation *Sabal-Urtica* vs placebo was –3.50 IPSS points (scale range, 0–35) (17% absolute improvement vs placebo) (95% CI, –6.75 to –0.25) (n=1 study).

Participants and their physicians were both more likely to report improvement in symptoms in men treated with *S repens* than with placebo. The weighted RR for participant self-rating of improvement in urinary tract symptoms for *S repens* vs placebo was 1.72 (95% CI, 1.21–2.44) (n=6 studies) (Figure 2). The weighted RR for physician rating of improved urologic symptoms for *S repens* vs placebo was 1.72 (95% CI, 1.11–2.65) (n=3 studies). Overall, 242 (74%) of 329 men (6 studies) taking *S repens* reported an improvement of urologic symptoms compared with 168 (51%) of 330 men taking placebo (*P*<.001). Physician-assessed improvement of symptoms was reported in 165 (63%) of 262 men taking *S repens* and 101 (38%) of 262 men taking placebo (*P*<.001) (3 studies).

Serenoa repens reduced nocturia 25% (absolute difference) compared with placebo. The weighted mean difference was –0.76 times per evening vs placebo (95% CI, –1.21 to –0.32) (n=10 studies) (Figure 3). *Serenoa repens* was comparable with active controls regarding nocturia. The weighted mean difference was –0.05 (95% CI, –0.49 to 0.39) (n=1 study) vs finasteride and –0.20 (95% CI, –1.69 to 1.29) (n=1 study) vs *Pygeum africanum*.

Urinary Flow Measures and Prostate Size. *Serenoa repens* was superior to placebo and comparable with finasteride in improving peak and mean urine flow rates and residual urine volume. The weighted mean differences for peak urine flow were 1.93 mL/s vs placebo (24% absolute improvement vs placebo) (95% CI, 0.72–3.14) (n=8 studies) (Figure 4), –0.74 mL/s vs finasteride (95% CI, –1.66 to 0.18) (n=2 studies), 2.0 mL/s vs gestonorone caproate (95% CI, 1.36-2.64) (n=1 study), and 1.6 mL/s for *Sabal-Urtica* vs placebo (95% CI, –0.67 to 3.87) (n=1 study). The weighted mean differences for mean urine flow were 2.22 mL/s vs placebo (28% absolute improvement vs placebo) (95% CI, 1.17–3.27) (n=4 studies) and –0.40 mL/s vs finasteride (95% CI, 0.15–0.95) (n=1 study). For residual volume the weighted mean difference was –22.05 mL vs placebo (43% absolute decrease vs placebo) (95% CI, –40.78 to –3.32) (n=6 studies) and 5.70 mL vs finasteride (95% CI, –5.42 to 16.82) (n=1 study). *Serenoa repens* did not reduce prostate size; the weighted mean differences for prostate size were –2.14 cc (95% CI, –10.92 to 6.65) (n=2 studies) vs placebo, and 4.08 cc (95% CI, 1.42–8.18) (n=1 study) vs finasteride.

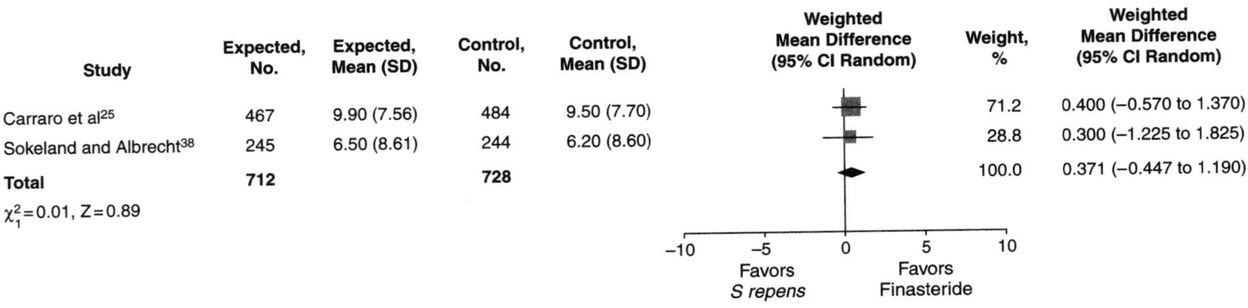

Study
Expected, No.
Expected, Mean (SD)
Control, No.
Control, Mean (SD)
Weighted Mean Difference (95% CI Random)
Weight, %
Weighted Mean Difference (95% CI Random)
Carraro et al25
467
9.90 (7.56)
484
9.50 (7.70)
71.2
0.400 (−0.570 to 1.370)
Sokeland and Albrecht38
245
6.50 (8.61)
244
6.20 (8.60)
28.8
0.300 (−1.225 to 1.825)
Total
712
728
100.0
0.371 (−0.447 to 1.190)
χ²₁=0.01, Z=0.89
−10
−5
0
5
10
Favors S repens
Favors Finasteride

Figure 1. Weighted mean differences in International Prostate Symptom Scale scores for men treated with *Serenoa repens* vs finasteride. CI indicates confidence interval.

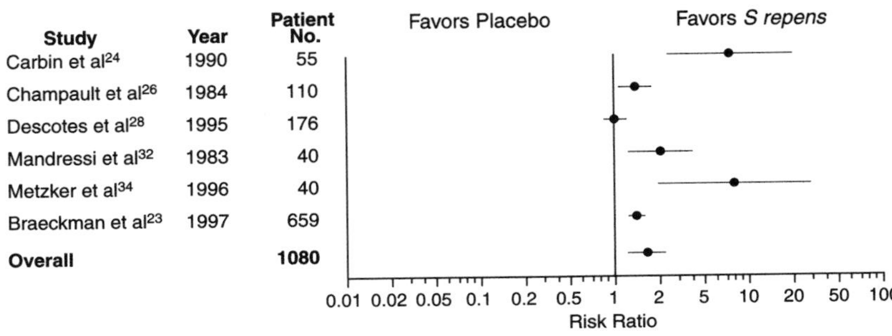

Figure 2. Weighted risk ratios for self-rating of improvement in urinary tract symptoms for men treated with *Serenoa repens* vs placebo.

Adverse Effects

Adverse effects due to *S repens* were generally mild and comparable with placebo. Withdrawal rates were *S repens*, 9.1%; placebo, 7.0%; and finasteride, 11.2% (P=.02 for *S repens* vs placebo and P=.87 vs finasteride). Erectile dysfunction was reported in 1.1% of men taking *S repens*; placebo, 0.7%; and finasteride, 4.9% (P=.58 for *S repens* vs placebo and P<.001 vs finasteride). Gastrointestinal adverse effects were reported in 1.3% of men taking *S repens*, placebo, 0.9%; and finasteride, 1.5% (P>.50 vs placebo and finasteride).

Comment

This systematic review summarizes the evidence from randomized controlled trials regarding the efficacy and safety of extracts from the saw palmetto berry *S repens* in men with lower urinary tract symptoms attributable to BPH. The available data indicate that *S repens* (alone or in combination with other phytotherapeutic agents) improves urinary tract symptoms and urinary tract flow measures. Compared with placebo, *S repens* improved urinary tract symptoms by 28%, nocturia by 25%, peak urine flow by 24%, mean urine flow by 28%, and residual urine volume by 43%. Men taking *S repens* were nearly twice as likely to report improvement in symptoms than men taking placebo. When compared with finasteride, *S repens* provided similar responses in urologic symptoms and flow measures and was associated with a lower rate of erectile dysfunction.

Participant baseline characteristics regarding age, prostate volume, peak urine flow, and symptom scale scores were comparable with previous trials and meta-analyses involving pharmacological management of BPH.[45–48] Therefore, our results are generalizable. They did not substantially change when we restricted our analysis to studies that had adequate treatment allocation concealment (level 3) or were double-blinded. Furthermore, the treatment effect sizes with regard to symptom scale scores, peak and mean urinary flow, nocturia, and residual volume are considered clinically important and similar to effects reported with other pharmacological agents.[45–48]

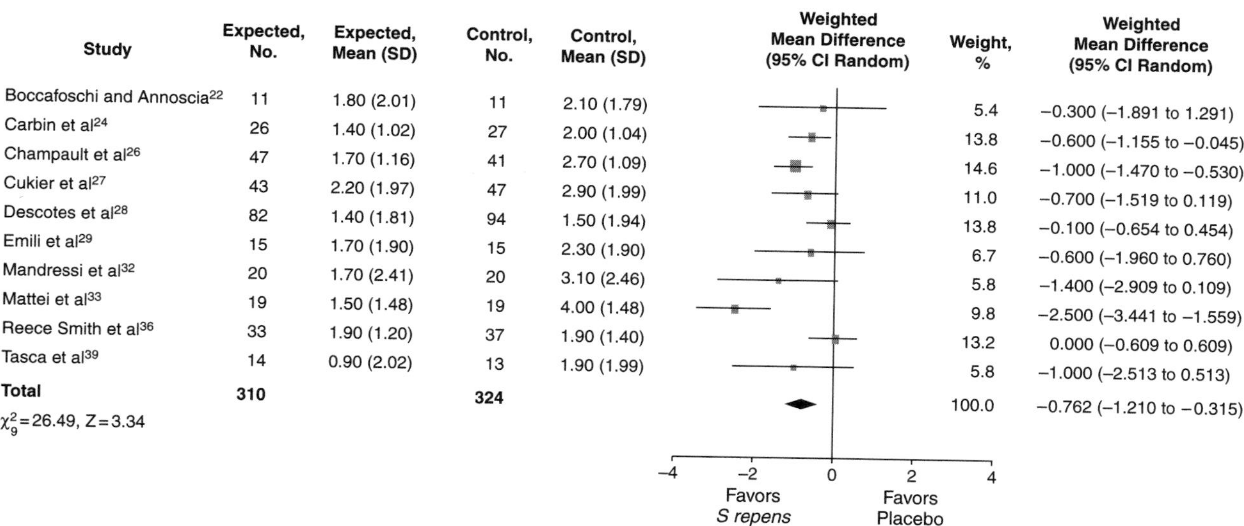

Study	Expected, No.	Expected, Mean (SD)	Control, No.	Control, Mean (SD)	Weight, %	Weighted Mean Difference (95% CI Random)
Boccafoschi and Annoscia[22]	11	1.80 (2.01)	11	2.10 (1.79)	5.4	−0.300 (−1.891 to 1.291)
Carbin et al[24]	26	1.40 (1.02)	27	2.00 (1.04)	13.8	−0.600 (−1.155 to −0.045)
Champault et al[26]	47	1.70 (1.16)	41	2.70 (1.09)	14.6	−1.000 (−1.470 to −0.530)
Cukier et al[27]	43	2.20 (1.97)	47	2.90 (1.99)	11.0	−0.700 (−1.519 to 0.119)
Descotes et al[28]	82	1.40 (1.81)	94	1.50 (1.94)	13.8	−0.100 (−0.654 to 0.454)
Emili et al[29]	15	1.70 (1.90)	15	2.30 (1.90)	6.7	−0.600 (−1.960 to 0.760)
Mandressi et al[32]	20	1.70 (2.41)	20	3.10 (2.46)	5.8	−1.400 (−2.909 to 0.109)
Mattei et al[33]	19	1.50 (1.48)	19	4.00 (1.48)	9.8	−2.500 (−3.441 to −1.559)
Reece Smith et al[36]	33	1.90 (1.20)	37	1.90 (1.40)	13.2	0.000 (−0.609 to 0.609)
Tasca et al[39]	14	0.90 (2.02)	13	1.90 (1.99)	5.8	−1.000 (−2.513 to 0.513)
Total	**310**		**324**		100.0	−0.762 (−1.210 to −0.315)

$\chi^2_9=26.49$, $Z=3.34$

Figure 3. Weighted means differences in nocturia for men treated with *Serenoa repens* vs placebo. CI indicates confidence interval.

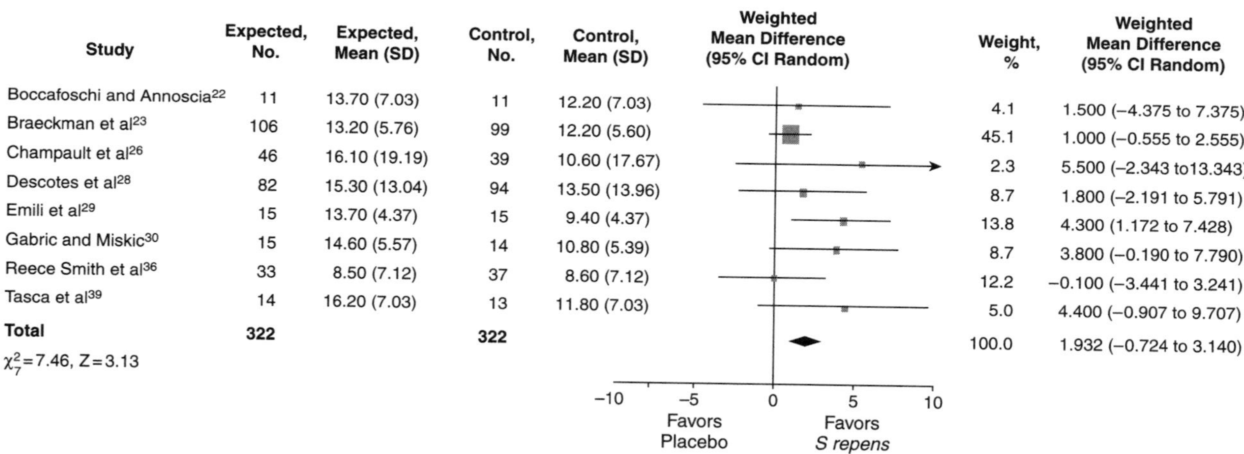

Study	Expected, No.	Expected, Mean (SD)	Control, No.	Control, Mean (SD)	Weight, %	Weighted Mean Difference (95% CI Random)
Boccafoschi and Annoscia[22]	11	13.70 (7.03)	11	12.20 (7.03)	4.1	1.500 (−4.375 to 7.375)
Braeckman et al[23]	106	13.20 (5.76)	99	12.20 (5.60)	45.1	1.000 (−0.555 to 2.555)
Champault et al[26]	46	16.10 (19.19)	39	10.60 (17.67)	2.3	5.500 (−2.343 to13.343)
Descotes et al[28]	82	15.30 (13.04)	94	13.50 (13.96)	8.7	1.800 (−2.191 to 5.791)
Emili et al[29]	15	13.70 (4.37)	15	9.40 (4.37)	13.8	4.300 (1.172 to 7.428)
Gabric and Miskic[30]	15	14.60 (5.57)	14	10.80 (5.39)	8.7	3.800 (−0.190 to 7.790)
Reece Smith et al[36]	33	8.50 (7.12)	37	8.60 (7.12)	12.2	−0.100 (−3.441 to 3.241)
Tasca et al[39]	14	16.20 (7.03)	13	11.80 (7.03)	5.0	4.400 (−0.907 to 9.707)
Total	**322**		**322**		100.0	1.932 (−0.724 to 3.140)

$\chi^2_7=7.46$, $Z=3.13$

Figure 4. Weighted mean differences in peak urinary flow rates for men treated with *Serenoa repens* vs placebo. CI indicates confidence interval.

Methodological Issues

Previous reviews of phytotherapy in the treatment of BPH were not structured systematic reviews or quantitative meta-analyses.[9,10] They included information from nonrandomized or uncontrolled studies and, therefore, may have overestimated treatment effectiveness. The number of randomized trials included in these previous studies was less than we identified. The inclusion of an EMBASE and Phytodok search identified 5 studies not listed in MEDLINE. If our search had been restricted to English-language journals, we would have missed 12 trials (67%).

Our results should be viewed with caution. Despite abstracting and analyzing 18 randomized trials that included nearly 3000 participants, many studies did not report outcomes data in a consistent fashion. Several did not report means and SDs making completion of a quantitative systematic review difficult. Funnel plot analysis for urinary tract symptoms comparing study weight with weighted mean difference revealed no publication bias.[49] Multiple attempts to contact the trialists enabled us to obtain information from additional studies.[50]

Only 3 studies reported results from standardized and validated urologic symptom scales.[25,34,38] One trial reported results from a scale that had not been standardized or validated.[23] All these studies were rated as having adequate treatment allocation concealment. Most studies were conducted prior to the development of validated urologic symptom scale scores. Results from these scales have been demonstrated to be the most valid and clinically relevant end points for assessing treatment effectiveness in men with mild to moderate symptoms of BPH.[3] Secondary outcomes were combined in only a minority of trials: mean urine flow (5 trials), peak urine flow (12 trials), residual volume (6 trials), nocturia (11 trials), and prostate size (3 trials). The treatment duration was short with only 2 studies having follow-up of at least 6 months' duration. Studies used different doses and preparations of *S repens* or were performed in combination with other phytotherapeutic compounds. The most frequently reported dosage was 160 mg of *S repens* twice per day.

Several statistical issues in combining the data in our analysis need to be mentioned. For the "self-rating of symptom improvement" outcome, there was significant heterogeneity in the treatment effects. Ideally, when significant heterogeneity of treatment effect is present, meta-regression should be explored to understand reasons for the differences. However, this was not possible here because of an insufficient number of studies and lack of standardized reporting of meaningful clinical covariates. Nonetheless, if an overall quantitative estimate is deemed to be useful, then a random-effects model that incorporates between-studies heterogeneity would be more appropriate as we have done. The random-effects model typically produces wider CIs compared with the fixed-effects model. Five of 6 studies[23,24,26,32,34] had significant treatment effects and the second largest study also had trends in the same direction, thus reducing the likelihood that the pooling produced a false-positive result.

Because of the high baseline response rate in the control groups and the wide range of the baseline rates of several studies, the choice of treatment effect metric used to combine outcomes may also affect the results. Compared with the pooled random-effects RR (RR, 1.71; 95% CI, 1.22–2.39), the pooled odds ratio (OR) is much higher (OR, 5.74; 95% CI, 2.14–15.35). The OR is frequently used to approximate the RR in the clinical trial setting. In this case, the high pooled OR creates a false impression that *S repens* is far more efficacious. We chose the more conservative metric provided by the RR in our analysis.

We were not able to determine if *S repens* prevented long-term complications of BPH, such as acute urinary retention or the need for surgical interventions. Previous studies have demonstrated that, in men with large prostates (ie, >40 cc) producing moderate to severe symptoms, finasteride is effective in relieving BPH symptoms and reducing the development of acute urinary retention and the need for surgical intervention.[45,46] However, fewer than one third of men with BPH have prostate glands more than 40 cc in size.[51] In men with "large prostates," the absolute rate of acute urinary retention or symptomatic progression requiring surgical intervention is less than 3% per year. In our review, the mean prostate volume in studies reporting prostate size was 44 cc. The available data did not allow us to determine if prostate volume was an important predictor of outcomes. Additionally, there were no reported studies comparing *S repens* with α-adrenergic blockers that met criteria. One study compared *S repens* with alfuzosin, but the duration of follow-up was only 3 weeks.[41]

The medication charges of *S repens* are less than other pharmacological therapies. A 90-day supply of saw palmetto berry (320 mg/d of *S repens*) is between $10 and $50. However, available dosages and preparations frequently vary from those used in the published trials. The pharmacy charges for a 90-day supply of finasteride or terazosin (5 mg/d) are approximately $200 and $120, respectively.[4]

Additional placebo-controlled trials are needed as well as studies that compare *S repens* with α-antagonists.[47,48] Future trials should be of sufficient size and duration to detect important differences in clinically relevant end points. At a minimum, these studies should assess and report the means and SDs at baseline and conclusion for the following variables: age, number enrolled and completing the study, standardized urologic symptom scale scores, mean and peak urine flow, voided volume, prostate size, residual urine volume, complications from BPH, need for subsequent therapy, and long-term adverse effects of *S repens*. Until then, this systematic review provides the most complete assessment regarding the efficacy and safety of *S repens* for treatment of symptomatic BPH.

In conclusion, the available evidence suggests that extracts from the saw palmetto plant, *S repens*, improve urinary tract symptoms and flow measures in men with BPH. Compared with finasteride, *S repens* produces similar improvements in urinary tract symptoms and flow measures, has fewer adverse treatment effects, and costs less. The long-term effectiveness and safety of *S repens* and its ability to prevent complications from BPH are not known.

The authors have no commercial, proprietary, or financial interest in the products or companies in this article.

This study was funded by the Department of Veterans Affairs Health Services Research and Development Service, Washington, DC.

We thank Maurizio Tiso, MS, Margaret Haugh, and Rich Crawford, MD, for their work in translating and abstracting data from the non–English-language studies.

References

1. Berry SL, Coffey DS, Walsh PC, Ewing LL. The development of human benign prostatic hyperplasia with age. *J Urol.* 1984;132:474–479.

2. Guess HA. Benign prostatic hyperplasia antecedents and natural history. *Epidemiol Rev.* 1992;14:131–153.

3. McConnell JD, Barry MJ, Bruskewitz RC. *Benign Prostatic Hyperplasia.* Rockville, Md: Agency for Health Care Policy and Research, Public Health Service, US Dept of Health and Human Services; 1994. Clinical Practice Guideline No. 8, AHCPR publication 94–0582.

4. Barry MJ. A 73-year-old man with symptomatic benign prostatic hyperplasia. *JAMA.* 1997; 278:2178–2184.

5. Oesterling JE. Benign prostatic hyperplasia. *N Engl J Med.* 1995;332:99–109.

6. *Int Med World Report.* 1998;13:8. No. 3.

7. Ernst E. Harmless herbs? a review of the recent literature. *Am J Med.* 1998;104:170–178.

8. Di Silverio F, Flammia GP, Sciarra A, et al. Plant extracts in benign prostatic hyperplasia. *Minerva Urol Nefrol.* 1993;45:143–149.

9. Buck AC. Phytotherapy for the prostate. *Br J Urol.* 1996;78:325–326.

10. Lowe FC, Ku JC. Phytotherapy in treatment of benign prostatic hyperplasia: a critical review. *Urology.* 1996;48:12–20.

11. Christensen MM, Bruskewitz RC. Clinical manifestations of benign prostatic hyperplasia and the indications for therapeutic intervention. *Urol Clin North Am.* 1990;17:509–516.

12. Dreikorn K, Richter R. Conservative nonhormonal treatment of patients with benign prostatic hyperplasia. In: Ackerman R, Schroeder FH, eds. *New Developments in Biosciences 5, Prostatic Hyperplasia.* Berlin, Germany: Walter de Gruyter & Co; 1989:109–131.

13. Marwick C. Growing use of medicinal botanicals forces assessment by drug regulators. *JAMA.* 1995;273:607–609.

14. McGuire E. *Detrusor Response to Obstruction.* Bethesda, Md: US Dept of Health and Human Services. 1987:221. NIH publication 87–2881.

15. Di Silverio F, D'Eramo G, Lubrano C, et al. Evidence that *Serenoa repens* extract displays an antiestrogenic activity in prostatic tissue of benign prostatic hypertrophy patients. *Eur Urol.* 1992;21:309–314.

16. Dickersin K, Scherer R, Lefebvre C. Identifying relevant studies for systematic reviews. *BMJ.* 1996;312:944–947.

17. Schulz KF, Chalmers I, Hayes RJ, Altman DG. Empirical evidence of bias: dimensions of methodological quality associated with estimates of treatment effects in controlled trials. *JAMA.* 1995;273:408–412.

18. *RevMan* [computer program]. Version 3.0 for Windows. Oxford, England: Update Software; 1996.

19. Lau J. *Meta-Analyst Version 0.99.* Boston, Mass: New England Medical Center; 1996.

20. Laird N, Mosteller F. Some statistical methods for combining experiment results. *Int J Technol Assess Health Care.* 1990;6:5–30.

21. Lavori PW. Clinical trials in psychiatry: should protocol deviation censor patient data? *Neuropsychopharmacology.* 1992;6:39–63.

22. Boccafoschi C, Annoscia S. Confronto fra estratto di *Serenoa repens* e placebo mediate prova clinica controllata in pazienti con adenomatosi prostatica. *Urologia.* 1983;50:1257–1268.

23. Braeckman J, Denis L, de Lavel J, et al. A double-blind, placebo-controlled study of the plant extract *Serenoa repens* in the treatment of benign hyperplasia of the prostate. *Eur J Clin Res.* 1997;9:247–259.

24. Carbin BE, Larsson B, Lindahl O. Treatment of benign prostatic hyperplasia with phytosterols. *Br J Urol.* 1990;66:639–641.

25. Carraro JC, Raynaud JP, Koch G, et al. Comparison of phytotherapy (Permixon) with finasteride in the treatment of benign prostate hyperplasia. *Prostate.* 1996;29:231–240.

26. Champault G, Patel JC, Bonnard AM. A double-blind trial of an extract of the plant *Serenoa repens* in benign prostatic hyperplasia. *Br J Clin Pharmacol.* 1984;18:461–462.

27. Cukier J, Ducassou J, Le Guillou M, et al. Permixon versus placebo: resultats d'une etude multicentrique. *C R Ther Pharmacol Clin.* 1985; 4:15–21.

28. Descotes JL, Rambeaud JJ, Deschaseaux P, Faure G. Placebo-controlled evaluation of the efficacy and tolerability of Permixon in benign prostatic hyperplasia after the exclusion of placebo responders. *Clin Drug Invest.* 1995;5:291–297.

29. Emili E, Lo Cigno M, Petrone U. Risultati clinici su un nuovo farmaco nella terapia dell'ipertofia della prostata (Permixon). *Urologia.* 1983; 50:1042–1048.

30. Gabric V, Miskic H. Behandlung des Benignen Prostata-Adenoms und der Chronischen Prostatatitis. *Therapiewoche.* 1987; 37:1775–1788.

31. Lobelenz J. Extractum *Sabal fructus* bei Benigner Prostatahyperplasie (BPH): Klinische Prufung im Stadium I und II. *Therapeutikon.* 1992;6:34–37.

32. Mandressi S, Tarallo U, Maggioni A, et al. Terapia medica dell'adenoma prostatico: confronto della efficacia dell'estratto di *Serenoa repens* (Permixon) versus l'estratto di Pigeum Africanum e placebo: Valutazione in doppio cieco. *Urologia.* 1983;50:752–758.

33. Mattei FM, Capone M, Acconcia A. Medikamentose Therapie der Benignen Prostatahyperplasie mit Einem Extrakt der Sagepalme. *TW Urol Nephrol.* 1990; 2:346–350.

34. Metzker H, Kieser M, Hölscher U. Wirksamkeit eines *Sabal-Urtica*-Kombinationspräparats bei der Behandlung der Benignen Prostatahyperplasie (BPH). *Urologe (B).* 1996; 36:292–300.

35. Pannunzio E, D'Ascenzo R, Giardinetti F, Civili P, Persichelli E. *Serenoa repens* vs gestonorone caproato nel trattamento dell'ipertofia prostatica benigna. *Urologia.* 1986;53:696–705.

36. Reece Smith H, Memon A, Smart CJ, Dewbury K. The value of Permixon in benign prostatic hypertrophy. *Br J Urol.* 1986;58:36–40.

37. Roveda S, Colombo P. Sperimentazione clinica controllata sulla bioequivalenza terapeutica e sulla tollerabilita dei prodotti a base di *Serenoa repens* in capsule da 160 mg o capsule rettali da 640 mg. *Arch Med Interna.* 1994;46:61–75.

38. Sokeland J, Albrecht J. Kombination aus Sabal und Urticaestrakt vs. finasterid bei BPH (Stad. I bis II nach Alken): Vergleich der Therapeutischen Wirksamkeit in Einer Einjahrigen Doppelblindstudie. *Urologe A.* 1997; 36:327–333.

39. Tasca A, Barulli M, Cavazzana A, Zattoni F, Artibani W, Pagano F. Trattamento della sintomatologia ostruttiva da adenoma prostatico con estratto di *Serenoa repens. Minerva Urol Nefrol.* 1985;37:87–91.

40. Comar OB, Di Rienzo A. Mepartricin versus *Serenoa repens. Riv Ital Biol Med.* 1986; 6:122–125.

41. Grasso M, Montesano A, Buonaguidi A, et al. Comparative effects of alfuzosin versus *Serenoa repens* in the treatment of symptomatic benign prostatic hyperplasia. *Arch Esp Urol.* 1995;48:97–103.

42. Strauch G, Perles P, Vergult G, et al. Comparison of finasteride (Proscar) and *Serenoa repens* (Permixon) in the inhibition of 5-alpha reductase in healthy male volunteers. *Eur Urol.* 1994;26:247–252.

43. Weisser H, Behnke B, Helpap B, Bach D, Krieg M. Enzyme activities in tissue of human benign prostatic hyperplasia after three months' treatment with the *Sabal serrulata* extract IDS 89 (Strogen) or placebo. *Eur Urol.* 1997; 31:97–101.

44. Adriazola Semino M, Lozano Ortega JL, Garcia Cobo E, et al. Tratamiento sintomatico de la hipertrofia benigna de prostata. *Arch Esp Urol.* 1992;45:211–213.

45. Boyle P, Gould AL, Roehrborn CG. Prostate volume predicts outcome of treatment of benign prostatic hyperplasia with finasteride. *Urology.* 1996;48:398–405.

46. McConnell JD, Bruskewitz R, Walsh P, et al. The effect of finasteride on the risk of acute urinary retention and the need for surgical treatment among men with benign prostatic hyperplasia. *N Engl J Med.* 1998;338:557–563.

47. Chapple CR, Wyndaele JJ, Nordling J, et al. Tamsulosin, the first prostate-selective alpha 1A-adrenoceptor antagonist: a meta-analysis of two randomized, placebo-controlled, multicentre studies in patients with benign prostatic obstruction (symptomatic BPH), European Tamsulosin Study Group. *Eur Urol.* 1996; 29:155–167.

48. Roehrborn CG, Siegel R. Safety and efficacy of doxazosin in benign prostatic hyperplasia. *Urology.* 1996;48:406–415.

49. Egger M, Davey Smith G, Schneider M, Minder C. Bias in meta-analysis detected by a simple, graphical test. *BMJ.* 1997;315:629–634.

50. Lowe F, Robertson C, Roehrborn C, Boyle P. Meta-analysis of clinical trials of Permixon. *J Urol.* 1998;159(suppl):986a.

51. Wasson JH. Finasteride to prevent morbidity from benign prostatic hyperplasia. *N Engl J Med.* 1998;338:612–613.

43 A Review of 12 Commonly Used Medicinal Herbs

Mary Ann O'Hara, MD, MSt; David Kiefer, MD; Kim Farrell, MD; Kathi Kemper, MD, MPH

From the Robert Wood Johnson Clinical Scholars Program, University of Washington Health Sciences Center (Dr O'Hara), and the University of Washington Family Medicine Network, Swedish Family Medicine Residency (Drs Kiefer and Farrell), Seattle; and the Center for Holistic Pediatric Education and Research, The Children's Hospital, Boston, Mass (Dr Kemper).

A large and increasing number of patients use medicinal herbs or seek the advice of their physician regarding their use. More than one third of Americans use herbs for health purposes, yet patients (and physicians) often lack accurate information about the safety and efficacy of herbal remedies. Burgeoning interest in medicinal herbs has increased scientific scrutiny of their therapeutic potential and safety, thereby providing physicians with data to help patients make wise decisions about their use. This article provides a review of the data on 12 of the most commonly used herbs in the United States. In addition, we provide practical information and guidelines for the judicious use of medicinal herbs.

Arch Fam Med. 1998;7:523–536

More than one third of Americans use herbs for health purposes, spending over $3.5 billion annually.[1,2] Yet patients (and physicians) often lack accurate information about the safety and efficacy of herbal remedies. Imagine the following are patients in your primary care practice. How would you advise them?

- Jane, who has chronic hepatitis C and receives medicine for both hypertension and schizophrenia, asks if she can take milk thistle to protect her liver.
- John, who has the human immunodeficiency virus, has an increasing viral load. He expresses fear of "medicine," but requests information about St John's

wort (SJW) in hopes of "naturally" curing his human immunodeficiency virus and depression.

- Sam's wife bought him valerian to help him sleep, saw palmetto for his urinary difficulties, and ginkgo to improve his memory. He is inclined to throw the herbs away but wants your opinion.
- After you inform Stephanie that she is 3 months pregnant, she asks what effects the herbs she has taken for months will have on her fetus (ginger for nausea, feverfew for headaches, and pennyroyal to induce a period).
- Your spouse has high cholesterol, your child has recurrent ear infections, and you have trouble relaxing after a hectic day at the clinic. Prompted by your patients' questions, you wonder if any herbal remedies might benefit your family.

Popular use of medicinal herbs makes it necessary for physicians to become aware of their health benefits, risks, and uncertainties so that they can educate their patients about these issues. To assist clinicians in this task, this article reviews existing data on the history, safety, and efficacy of 12 of the most commonly used and best-studied medicinal herbs (Table 1). In addition, it summarizes general information about herbal therapies, including an overview of regulatory history (Table 2), important similarities and differences between medications approved by the Food and Drug Administration (FDA) and herbal therapies (Table 3), and the nature of available data about medicinal herbs. Finally, lists of reliable introductory resources (Table 4) and guidelines for patients (Table 5) are provided.

A Historical Perspective

Plants have been used medicinally throughout history. Through the first half of this century, many herbs were considered conventional medicines and as such were included in medical curricula and formularies (eg, *United States Pharmacopoeia* and *The National Formulary*). Two important factors fostered a schism between mainstream drugs and herbal therapies in the United States: the development of a pharmaceutical industry capable of mass-producing purified chemicals, and regulatory changes by the FDA.

In 1962, thalidomide was found to be teratogenic and Congress passed an amendment to the Food and Drug Act to increase assurance of drug safety and efficacy. While successful in general, the amendment initiated a regulatory dilemma regarding herbal therapies in the United States (Table 2). No longer can substances be considered drugs based on traditional use alone. A would-be manufacturer must gain FDA approval; the profit to be made from a patented product is the motivating factor. Traditional herbal therapies cannot be patented, and therefore lack sponsors for the costly ($230 million) and lengthy (8–10 years)[3] approval process. By default, many medicinal herbs are not legally considered drugs and are not regulated as such by the FDA. The FDA suggests but cannot require that manufacturers of herbal therapies provide customers with scientific data in support of advertising claims. Furthermore, the FDA must prove that an herbal product is unsafe or ineffective before it can require the product to be removed from the market.

Herbs and FDA-Approved Medications: Similarities and Differences

Patients are often unaware of important similarities and differences between medicinal herbs and FDA-approved medications. For example, some mistakenly think of herbs as "natural" alternatives to chemicals, failing to recognize that herbs are composed of bioactive chemicals, some of which may be toxic (see Table 6 for a list of commonly used herbs with toxic effects that probably outweigh their potential benefits). Also, patients are often unaware that about 25% of modern pharmaceutical drugs have botanical origins, such as digoxin from foxglove, morphine from poppies, aspirin from willow bark, and tamoxifen from the Pacific yew tree.[4]

Unlike the FDA-approved over-the-counter and prescription medications, medicinal herbs are not required to demonstrate either safety or efficacy prior to marketing, nor are they regulated for quality. Nevertheless, herbal therapies are not necessarily less expensive than patented drugs and are rarely covered by medical insurance. In contrast to the purified, standardized, and potent FDA-approved drugs, herbs contain an array of chemicals, the relative concentration of which varies considerably depending on genetics, growing conditions, plant parts used, time of harvesting, preparation, and storage. In addition, herbs may be contaminated or misidentified at any stage from harvesting through packaging.

The Nature of Evidence About Medicinal Herbs

Most research on medicinal herbs is conducted in areas of the world where the use of medicinal herbs is mainstream, particularly in Asia and Europe. For the past 3 decades,

Table 1. Twelve Common Medicinal Herbs*

Herb *Scientific Name* **Part Used**	**Common Uses (Type of Evidence/ Recommendation)†**	**Safety‡§ǁ**	**Dose¶**	**Cost****
Chamomile *Matricaria recutita,* *Chamaemelum nobile* Flower	Mild sedative (III-C) Mild spasmolytic (III-B) Vulnerary (wound healing), (II.3-B)	GRAS†† . Rare allergic reaction and contact irritation Avoid ocular preparations	Tea as necessary Compress as necessary	$0.10 per tea bag
Echinacea *Echinacea purpurea,* *Echinacea angustifolia* Leaf, stalk, root	URI treatment (I-B) URI prevention (I-C) Vulnerary (wound healing), (III-C) Immune stimulation (III-C) Antimicrobial (HIV), (IV-C [D])	No serious side effects known Historically misidentified and contaminated Long-term use may be immunosuppressive	Not standardized Dried extract: 300–400 mg tid Tincture: 30–50 drops (1 drop=20 µL) tid	$0.25–$4 per day
Feverfew *Tanacetum parthenium* Leaf	Headache prophylaxis (I-B) Rheumatoid arthritis (I-E)	5%–15% oral or GI irritation Rebound headaches possible Avoid in pregnancy (traditional menses inducer) May potentiate platelet inhibitors	25–75 mg (1–3 leaves) bid, standardized to 0.2% parthenolide	$0.10–$0.50 per day
Garlic *Allium sativum* Cloves, root	≥9% ↓ lipids (LDL, TG), (I-B) Mild antihypertensive (I-B) Antiplatelet (II.1-B) Antioxidant (I-B) Antimicrobial (bacteria, fungus, and viruses [HIV]), (III, IV-C [D]) Cancer prevention (II.3-D) and treatment (III-D)	GRAS, including in pregnancy, lactation, and childhood No serious side effects known Mild side effects: halitosis, body odor, topical irritation, allergy (rare), GI upset May potentiate hypoglycemic and antiplatelet therapy	Fresh cloves: 0.5–1 qd Pills: 600 mg-900 mg qd, standardized to 0.6%–1.3% allicin Powder: 0.4–1.2 g	$0.04–$0.70 per day
Ginger *Zingiber officinale* Root	Antiemetic (I-B) (mildly prophylactic and therapeutic against nausea from motion, chemotherapy, pregnancy, and surgery)	GRAS, including in pregnancy, lactation, and childhood No serious side effects known May inhibit platelet aggregation GI upset (mild) Allergy (rare)	Capsules: 250–1000 mg tid-qid Tea: steep powder or fresh herb	$0.12 per dose
Ginkgo *Ginkgo biloba* Leaf	Dementia: slows cognitive deterioration (I-B) Mild effects, similar to tacrine Claudication: 50% ↑ in pain-free walking distance (II.1-B)	No serious side effects known Mild side effects: GI upset, headaches, allergic skin reactions May inhibit platelet aggregation	Use extract standardized to 6% terpenoids, 24% flavonoids 40–80 mg bid-tid	$0.30–$1.80 per day
Ginseng *Panax ginseng,* *Panax quinquefolius* Root ("Siberian ginseng" is not a true ginseng)	Endurance/adaptation enhancer —Conflicting motor results (C) —↑ Cognitive function (I-C) —Resistance to stress (III-D) —Androgenic and estrogenic (II.2-D) Enhances "quality of life" (II.1-D) Immune/endocrine stimulant (III-D)	GRAS High cost without proven benefit Avoid use with other stimulants and in patients with cardiovascular disease (potential hypertensive and chronotrope) May increase digoxin levels Mastalgia and postmenopausal bleeding (rare) Rare fatalitites attributed to contaminants	Root: 1–3g qd Pills: 100–300 mg tid, extract standardized to ≥7% ginsenosides	$0.30–$2.00 per day

the German Health Authority has systematically reviewed the evidence on about 300 herbs and formulated clinical guidelines. An English translation of the resulting *German Commission E Monographs* is due for release in 1998.[5] Although arguably the best compendium of clinical information about herbs in the world, it does not disclose the scientific basis for its conclusions. Nevertheless, such guidelines provide hypotheses to prompt quality human trials, optimally with randomized, double-blind, placebo-controlled (RDBPC) trials. Research in the United States will be bolstered by the creation of the Office of Complementary and Alternative Medicine within the National Institutes of Health, Bethesda, Md.

Table 1. Twelve Common Medicinal Herbs* *(continued)*

Herb / ***Scientific Name*** / **Part Used**	**Common Uses (Type of Evidence/ Recommendation)†**	**Safety‡§‖**	**Dose¶**	**Cost****
Goldenseal *Hydrastis canadensis* Root, rhizome	Mask illicit drugs in urine (II.3-E) Berberine constituent effects: Antidiarrheal in children (*Escherichia coli, Giardia,* and cholera), (I-B) Antiseptic, topical (III-C)	Generally well tolerated Traditional literature warns that huge (unspecified) doses can cause GI upset, hypertension, cardiac inotropy, seizures, and respiratory failure Avoid in pregnancy (uterotonic) and neonates (causes jaundice) May oppose anticoagulants	Use alternate sources of berberine, 10 mg/kg per day	$0.45–$1.25 per dose
Milk thistle *Silybum marianum* Fruit	Hepatoprotection against: —Acute hepatitis, ie, mushroom poisoning (II.3-B), drugs (III-C) —Chronic active hepatitis (I-B) —Cirrhosis (I-B, conflicting data)	No serious side effects known Rare: diarrhea, allergy	Capsules: 140 mg bid-tid, standardized to 70% silymarin IV silymarin in acute poisoning: 20-50 mg/kg per day	$0.44–$2.00 per day (oral)
St John's wort *Hypericum perforatum* Flower, leaf	Mild-moderate depression (I-B) (long-term use not yet studied) Antimicrobial (HIV), (III-C [D]) Vulnerary (III-C) Neoplastic inhibition (III-D)	Photosensitization is rare, usually in fair-skinned people taking large doses No clinical MAO-inhibition and/or related drug/food interactions Avoid use with other antidepressants	Tablets: 300 mg tid of extract standardized to 0.3% hypericin Topical	$0.17–$1.35 per day (oral)
Saw palmetto *Serenoa repens* Fruit	Benign prostatic hypertrophy (B) —↑ Flow, ↓ frequency, ↓ PVR (No. 7 II-1) —Efficacy=finasteride (I) —↓ Androgen and estrogen prostatic nuclear receptors (I) —5α reductase inhibition (IV)	Unlike finasteride, not associated with ↓ libido or changes in PSA No serious side effects or drug interactions known Mild, rare effects: GI upset, headaches, diarrhea	Tablets: 320 mg qd of extract standardized to 85%–95% fatty acids and sterols	$0.80–$1.20 per day
Valerian *Valeriana officinalis* Root	Somnogogue (sleep aid), (I-B) Spasmolytic (III-C)	GRAS Mild, rare effects: headache, palpitations, insomnia	Capsules: 400 mg qhs as necessary (≥12 years) Tea: 2–3 g=1 tsp tid Tincture: 3–5 mL tid	$0.06–$0.19 per dose

*GRAS indicates generally recognized as safe; URI, upper respiratory infection; HIV, human immunodeficiency virus; tid, three times daily; GI, gastrointestinal; bid, twice daily; LDL, low-density lipoprotein; TG, triglycerides; qd, every day; qid, four times daily; IV, intravenous; MAO, monoamine oxidase; PVR, post–void residual; PSA, prostate-specific antigen; qhs, every night. See text for more information and references.

†Adapted from study reference system of the US Preventative Services Task Force (USPSTF), 1996, 2nd edition. Type of Evidence: I indicates randomized controlled trial; II, other human study (1=placebo-controlled trial, 2=cohort or case-controlled study, 3=case series); III, animal study (vs expert opinion in USPSTF rating); IV, in vitro studies (not a category in USPSTF). Recommendation: A indicates safe and effective; B, probably safe and effective; C, probably safe, possibly effective; D, insufficient data; and E, unsafe or ineffective.

‡Data are often lacking on drug interactions and effects of long-term use.

§Content and quality of commercial products are not regulated in the United States and can vary considerably.

‖ Safety in pregnancy, lactation, and childhood is unknown (and use in these groups therefore not recommended) unless specifically indicated.

¶ Patients should use standardized preparations, which are more reliable and cost-effective.

**Range of costs for commercial products (=brands) in typical drug store.

††Generally recognized as safe as a food supplement by the FDA.

Data about the safety and efficacy of medicinal herbs are limited in a number of ways. In some cases, the best data are years old, limited to in vitro or animal studies, and/or only available in journals outside the United States. Some clinically important types of information are particularly sparse in the literature, such as the results of negative trials, drug interactions, effects in special populations (eg, children and pregnant or lactating women), and toxic reactions. In some cases, good evidence about short-term side effects comes from well-controlled human trials. However, information about the effects of long-term use is usually based on case reports rather than prospective

Table 2. Genesis of a Regulatory Dilemma: US Legislation on Herbal Remedies

Year	Act/Agency	Purpose/Details	Effects on the Status of Herbal Therapies
1906	Food and Drug Act	Outlawed misbranding and adulteration	Therapeutic herbs continue to be included in the *National Formulary* and the *United States Pharmacopoeia*
1938	Federal Food, Drug and Cosmetic Act	Required safety testing prior to marketing after new elixir killed 105 people	Most traditional remedies with history of safe use are grandfathered in under law
1962	(Kefauver-Harris) Drug Amendments	Required proof of safety and efficacy to be marketed as a drug Considered only evidence presented to expert panels, primarily by companies interested in marketing a patentable (therefore profitable) drug	Most herbs not patentable and therefore Lacked sponsor for costly approval process Never considered for approval, irrespective of efficacy or safety Reassigned status to "foods or food supplements" No longer legally considered medications No longer regulated by Food and Drug Administration (FDA) Subject to confiscation if labeled like a drug, eg, with traditional indications, doses, or cautions
. . .	FDA GRAS List	FDA maintains a list of substances generally recognized as safe (GRAS)	Includes about 250 herbs based on their use as food additives (eg, garlic and ginger)
1993	FDA Commissioner David Kessler, MD	Proposed removing herbal products from the market given booming market despite unproven safety or efficacy	More protest letters sent to Congress than about any issue since the Vietnam war, fueled by a multimillion-dollar industry campaign
1994	Dietary Supplement Health and Education Act	Shifted burden of proof to FDA (eg, that claims are misleading or an herb is unsafe) Altered restriction on labeling	Ineffective assurance of safety, efficacy, or quality Confusing guidelines about labeling: May state: effect on "structure or function of the body" or "mechanism" or "describe general well-being from consumption of the nutrient" May not state: false or misleading claims, or that the product can treat or prevent any specific disease May be accompanied by: balanced, nonpromotional literature
1997	Federal Commission on Dietary Supplements	Recommended manufacturers provide science-based evidence about product to consumers	Anticipate little effect, as lacks enforcement capability

studies. As noted earlier, traditional use has revealed serious toxic effects associated with some common medicinal herbs (see Table 6). On the other hand, the FDA categorizes about 250 herbs as "generally recognized as safe" (GRAS) for consumption based on long-term and/or widespread traditional use without significant side effects. This article reviews several herbs on the FDA GRAS list, including chamomile, garlic, ginger, ginseng, and valerian. Evidence about the safety and efficacy of these and 7 other commonly used medicinal herbs are reviewed below.

Chamomile

Matricaria recutita

Common name: German chamomile

Chamaemelum nobile (English or Roman chamomile)

Common uses: Sedative, spasmolytic, anti-inflammatory, vulnerary (wound healing)

Investigational uses: Antioxidant

Side effects: Allergy (rare)

Chamomile is a daisylike, apple-scented flower that has been used medicinally for thousands of years. Anglo-Saxons believed it was 1 of the 9 sacred herbs given to humans by the god Woden. In contemporary Germany, it is considered a cure-all. Chamomile is cultivated worldwide for use as a sedative, spasmolytic, anti-inflammatory, and vulnerary (wound-healing) agent. Few human studies have evaluated these traditional uses.

Only chamomile's vulnerary effects have been studied in a controlled human trial, with inconclusive results. A recent RDBPC trial found no difference between chamomile

Table 3. Herbs and Food and Drug Administration (FDA)–Approved Drugs: Similarities and Differences

Factor	Legal Medications (FDA-Approved)	Herbal Therapies
Mechanism	Biochemical	Biochemical
Origins	25% Plant origin	Raw plants
Efficacy	Evidence required, but not always based on well-controlled trials	Proof not required
Safety	Must be well studied, within acceptable limits, and detailed on drug label or insert	Evidence of safety not required and often unavailable Burden of proof with FDA to show herbal therapies unsafe
Dose	Established, usually by dose-response studies	Some guidelines exist, usually based on historical precedent or tradition, occasionally based on dose-response in clinical trials Standardized products are preferential and available for some herbs (eg, garlic, ginkgo, St-John's -wort, saw palmetto, and valerian) Not necessarily standardized by content of active ingredients, which are often unknown
Pharmacokinetics	Usually well characterized	Rarely known
Potency	Standardized	Varies with genetics, growing conditions, time harvested, plant part used, preparation, and storage
Proof of purity	Required	Varies greatly High potential for contamination; history of case reports
Identification	Some confusion possible with coexistence of generic and multiple trade names	Problematic, beginning with misidentification of plants at harvesting Products should be labeled with and chosen by scientific name (*genus species*, eg, *Echinacea purpurea* is the most used and studied *Echinacea* species—many of its common names are shared by other plants)
Quality control	Required	Not required Improving with self-regulation by herb industry
Cost	Wide range Elevated for patented drugs	Highly variable Extracts are the most concentrated and cost effective
Insurance coverage	Often	Rarely

and placebo in preventing mucositis in 164 patients receiving fluorouracil, half of whom used chamomile 3 times daily for 14 days).[6] However, the study was possibly too short to detect a difference, as mucositis is largely a result of immunosuppression, and therefore takes weeks to develop. In another randomized, placebo-controlled trial, radiation-induced skin reactions were less frequent and appeared later in chamomile-treated areas, but the differences were not statistically significant.[7]

Animal studies support chamomile's traditional use as a vulnerary anti-inflammatory, spasmolytic, and anxiolytic agent. The flavonoid component apigenin exhibits dose-dependent, reversible inhibition of irritant-induced skin inflammation[8] and protects against gastric ulcers induced by medications, stress, and alcohol.[9] Apigenin also binds the same receptors as benzodiazapines; it exerts anxiolytic and mild sedative effects in mice[10] and relaxes intestinal spasms.[11] In vitro, the essential oil acts as an antioxidant[12] and kills some skin pathogens (some *Staphylococcus* and *Candida* species).[13]

Chamomile is considered safe by the FDA, with no known adverse effects in pregnancy, lactation, or childhood. It caused no adverse reactions in the human trials discussed

Table 4. Introductory References

Books
Blumenthal M, Gruenwald J, Hall T, Riggins C, Rister R. *German Commission E Monographs: Medicinal Plants for Human Use.* Austin, Tex: American Botanical Council; 1998. English translation in press.
Duke JA, Emmanus PA. *The Green Pharmacy.* Emmaus, Pa: Trondal Press; 1997.
Murray M. *The Healing Power of Herbs.* 2nd ed. Rocklin, Calif: Prima Publishing; 1995.
Tyler VE. *Herbs of Choice: The Therapeutic Use of Phytomedicinals.* Binghamton, NY: Pharmaceutical Products Press; 1994.
Journals
American Botanical Council, Austin, Tex. *HerbalGram*
Facts and Comparisons, St Louis, Mo. *Lawrence Rev Nat Prod*
Online
The American Botanical Council: http://www.herbalgram.org
The Phytochemical Database: http://www.ard-grin.gov/nfrlsb/

Table 5. Medicinal Herbs: Patient Information Sheet

- Plants have been used throughout history to improve health.
- Many modern medicines came from plants. Examples include aspirin (from willow bark), morphine (from poppies), and digoxin (from foxglove. Scientists are still discovering valuable medicines in ancient plants; eg tamoxifen, which is used to treat breast cancer (from Pacific yew trees).
- Herbs used for health purposes are drugs. They are chemicals that can affect the human body in helpful or harmful ways.
- Plant products are not necessarily safe. Hemlock, for example, was used to kill Socrates. Some commonly used herbal therapies are also unsafe.
- Traditional herbal therapies are not necessarily effective. Only trials in humans comparing the herbal product with a placebo (inert substance) can determine its effectiveness, appropriate dose, and safety.
- Individual reports of benefit from any drug, including herbs, are not reliable evidence. This is because some people will feel better when treated with a medicine they believe will work, whether it does or not.
- Science is not opposed to nature, but rather is a tool to help distinguish natural products that are safe and effective from those that are not.
- Unlike medications approved by the Food and Drug Administration, herbal products
  1. Are not required to prove claims about their safety or effectiveness.
  2. Are not regulated to ensure quality control.
  3. Vary tremendously in concentration of active ingredients and other chemicals.
- If you decide to use herbs for health purposes, the following recommendations can help maximize the potential benefits and minimize the potential risks:
  1. Discuss any drugs you use, including herbal remedies, with your doctor.
  2. If you experience side effects, stop taking the herb and notify your doctor.
  3. Avoid preparations containing more than one herb.
  4. Be wary of commercial claims about herbs; seek unbiased and scientifically based sources of information. Ask your doctor or pharmacist for suggested sources.
  5. Preferentially use products that are standardized to contain a specific amount of active ingredients. Such formulations are generally more reliable, effective, and economical.
  6. Select herbal products carefully. In general, the highest quality products come from Europe or large companies in the United States with national reputations to protect. Only buy brands that list the following information on the package: the herb's common and scientific name, the name and address of the manufacturer, a batch and lot number, an expiration date, dosing guidelines, potential side effects, and details of how quality is ensured.

earlier. While chamomile's therapeutic effects and safety remain to be definitively proven in human trials, its beneficial effects seen in animals and its good safety record in widespread traditional use by humans make it an acceptable home remedy for soothing mild skin irritation, intestinal cramps, or agitated nerves. In the United States, it is commonly consumed as a tea or applied as a compress. Patients with severe allergies to ragweed should be warned about possible cross-reactivity to chamomile and other members of the aster family (eg, echinacea, feverfew, and milk thistle). It should not be taken in conjunction with other sedatives, such as benzodiazapines or alcohol.

Echinacea

Echinacea purpurea, Echinacea angustifolia,* and *Echinacea pallida

Common name: Purple coneflower

Common uses: Prevention and treatment of colds, wound healing

Investigational use: Anticancer

Side effects: Possible suppression of immunity with habitual use

Echinacea is a purple coneflower native to North America. Plains Indians valued this member of the daisy (Asteraceae) family for its medicinal properties and introduced it to European settlers. By the 1920s, this acclaimed anti-infectious and vulnerary agent was listed in the *National Formulary* and outsold all other products of one major pharmaceutical company. Its popularity dwindled after the advent of antibiotics, only to experience a resurgence in recent years. It is the most popular herb in the United States, generating more than $300 million in sales annually.[1] Three of the 9 species of *Echinacea* are used medicinally: *E purpurea, E angustifolia,* and *E pallida. Echinacea purpurea* is the most commonly used and extensively studied.

In Germany, where most studies have been conducted, echinacea is approved by the Federal Health Agency as supportive therapy for upper respiratory tract infections, urogenital infections, and wounds.[5] In the United States, echinacea is usually marketed alone or in combination with other herbs as a purported immune booster, particularly for the prevention or treatment of colds. Although 26 published controlled trials have evaluated echinacea's therapeutic effects, none is of sufficient methodologic quality to be conclusive.[14] For example, in addition to sharing the flaws of the best studies discussed later, most other controlled trials use formulations of echinacea combined with other herbs. Treatment assignment is neither random nor blind in most studies.[14]

Table 6. Common, Potentially Toxic Herbs*

Herb (Scientific Name)	Purported Use	Possible Toxic Reaction
Arnica *(Arnica montana)*	Anti-inflammatory, analgesic, antiseptic	Ingestion associated with gastrointestinal and muscle damage Safe topically, excepting rare allergic reactions
Belladonna *(Atropa belladonna),* "deadly nightshade"	Relaxant, antiulcer	Central nervous system and respiratory depression; anticholinergic
Chaparral *(Larrea tridentata)*	Anticancer	Hepatotoxic, tumor trophic
Coltsfoot *(Tussilago farfara),* "cough wort"	Antitussive, salve	Carcinogenic, hepatotoxic, genotoxic Cardiopulmonary stimulant
Comfrey *(Symphytum)*	Healing (wounds, ulcers, cancer)	Carcinogenic, hepatotoxic, genotoxic Excreted in breastmilk
Ephedra (Ma-huang) *(Ephedra sinica)*	Anorectic, stimulant, bronchodilator	Potent, highly variable α-1 and β receptor stimulation Associated with hypertensive strokes, palpitations, and nerve damage Fatalities reported
European mistletoe *(Viscum album)*	Antihypertensive, antitumor	Central nervous system and cardiac toxic reaction Gastrointestinal bleeding
Germander *(Teucrium chamaedrys)*	Anorectic	Hepatotoxic
Licorice *(Glycyrrhiza glabra)*	Expectorant, antiulcer	High or prolonged doses cause pseudoaldosteronism (saline retention and potassium depletion)
Life root *(Senecio aureus)*	Emetic Ease labor	Hepatotoxic, carcinogenic
Pennyroyal *(Hedoma pulegioides),* "squawmint," "mosquito plant"	Menstrual disorders, insect repellent	Hepatotoxic Neurotoxic Teratogenic (acetylcysteine is antidote)
Pokeroot *(Phytolacca)*	Tonic, anticancer, anti-inflammatory	Gastrointestinal, neurologic, and hematologic toxic reaction May be fatal in children
Sassafras *(Sassafras albidum)*	Stimulant, tonic, antispasmodic, anti-inflammatory	Carcinogenic
Indian snakeroot *(Rauvofilia serpentina)*	. . .	Neurotoxic reaction (sedation, depression)
Tea tree oil *(Malaleuca alternifolia)*	Antiseptic, salve	Central nervous system toxic reaction if ingested Local irritation
Yohimbe *(Pausinystalia yohimbe)*	Impotence	Cardiovascular stimulant, neurotoxic, emetic

*Select list of herbs most likely to be used by family medicine patients. Adapted from Tyler.[2, 4]

Only 2 RDBPC trials have evaluated *E purpurea's* effect on upper respiratory tract infections. In one, echinacea extract demonstrated a statistically significant decrease in symptoms and duration of "flulike" illness (n=180).[15] The effects were dose dependent; benefits were noted beginning on day 3 or 4 in patients taking 180 drops (1 drop=20 µL) of extract daily, whereas volunteers taking 90 drops per day showed no benefit. In the second RDBPC trial with 108 volunteers who had a history of recurrent URIs, prophylactic echinacea extract was associated with less frequent (14% relative risk reduction) and less severe recurrences.[16,17] In some studies, immunocompromised patients seemed to benefit the most.[14] While provocative, interpretation of the results is limited in both of the RDBPC trials by inadequate use or description of the following: diagnostic criteria, randomization process, treatment interventions, methods for assessing outcome, assurance of blinding, detail of results, and quality statistical analysis.[14]

In animal studies, echinacea affects several aspects of the immune system; components of echinacea increase the number of circulating white blood cells,[18] enhance phagocytosis,[19] stimulate cytokine production, and trigger the alternate complement pathway.[20] In vitro, echinacea displays direct bacteriostatic and antiviral activity and stimulates the production of cytokines (interferon, tumor necrosis factor, interleukin 1, and interleukin 6).[3,15] Based on its stimulation of cytokine production, echinacea is being investigated as a possible antineoplastic agent in preliminary human trials.[21]

Topical echinacea exhibits multiple vulnerary mechanisms, including the anti-infective activity noted above, stimulation of fibroblasts, and inhibition of inflammation (metabolism of arachidonate to prostaglandins).[22] In rodents, echinacea also decreases inflammation, protects against radiation-induced skin damage, and hastens wound healing.[23]

Available evidence on echinacea's therapeutic potential is incomplete, but does suggest a possible supportive role in treating infections and wounds. However, well-designed clinical trials are needed to substantiate echinacea's efficacy, clarify appropriate dosages, and confirm safety. Despite the fact that the dosage has not been standardized and that preparations are frequently adulterated, no serious side effects have been reported in more than 2.5 million prescriptions per year in Germany and more than a century of use in the United States.[24] Toxicity studies found no mutagenicity in tissue culture, and no clinical or histologic side effects in rats treated with huge doses of echinacea (5 g/kg intravenously and acutely or 8 g/kg per day orally for 1 month).[24] German guidelines discourage use of echinacea in place of antibiotics or for more than 8 weeks (one study suggests that long-term use may suppress immunity).[5]

Feverfew

Tanacetum parthenium

Common use: Migraine prophylactic
Investigational use: Antiarthritic
Side effects: Oral ulcers, rebound headaches, allergic reaction (rare)

Feverfew is a daisylike perennial found commonly in gardens and along roadsides. The name stems from the Latin *febrifugia*, "fever reducer." The first century Greek physician Dioscorides prescribed feverfew for "all hot inflammations." Also known as "featherfew," its feathery leaves are used commonly to treat arthritis and prevent migraines.[25] While feverfew did not reduce symptoms in a double-blind, placebo-controlled (DBPC) trial among patients with rheumatoid arthritis,[26] it has been shown to prevent migraines in 2 of 3 DBPC trials.

The largest and best DBPC trial was a crossover study in which feverfew use was associated with a 70% reduction in migraine frequency and severity (n=270).[27] Side effects were less frequent than with placebo. In a trial among feverfew users, subjects randomized to receive a placebo instead of continuing feverfew suffered a significant increase in the frequency and severity of headaches, nausea, and vomiting (n=20).[28] Based on these trials, Canadian health officials recently approved encapsulated feverfew leaves as an over-the-counter medication for migraine prophylaxis. However, migraines were not prevented in a subsequent randomized controlled trial (RCT) using a different formulation of feverfew (0.35%=0.5 mg of parthenolide, a suspected active ingredient).[29] This highlights the potential variability of contents and effects of different preparations of the same herb, as well as the inadequacy of standardizing herbs to a single ingredient when other bioactive constituent(s) are not well characterized.

Laboratory evidence indicates that feverfew causes vasodilation and reduces inflammation. Feverfew's constituents inhibit phagocytosis, platelet aggregation, and secretion of inflammatory mediators (arachidonic acid and serotonin).[30] Feverfew is thought to down-regulate cerebrovascular response to biogenic amines, consistent with its ability to prevent but not abort headaches, as well as the months of use needed for clinical efficacy.[25]

In summary, some feverfew preparations can prevent migraines, with efficacy that compares favorably with β-blockers and valproic acid.[31] However, side effects may limit the use of feverfew, as 5% to 15% of users develop aphthous ulcers and/or gastrointestinal (GI) tract irritation.[25] Sudden discontinuation can precipitate rebound headaches.[28] Long-term safety data are lacking. Feverfew should not be used during pregnancy (historically it has been used to induce menstrual bleeding) or in patients with coagulation problems (feverfew can alter platelet activity[30]). For patients who want to try feverfew, expert herbalists recommend a gradual dose increase up to 125 mg/d orally of encapsulated leaves (2–3 leaves) standardized to contain 0.2% parthenolide. However, according to a 1992 study, none of the commercially available North American preparations contained even half of the recommended parthenolide concentration.[32]

Garlic

Allium sativum

Common uses: Antiatherosclerosis (lipid lowering, antithrombotic, fibrinolytic, antihypertensive)
Investigational uses: Anticancer
Side effects: Sulfuric odor, contact irritation (rare)

Garlic's historic and worldwide medicinal use have made it one of the most extensively studied medicinal herbs. Nevertheless, the actual therapeutic benefits of this member of the Liliaceae family is unclear. Louis Pasteur first demonstrated garlic's antiseptic activity.[4] Both animal studies and epidemiological analyses suggest anticancer effects.[33] Most current research, popularity, and controversy relate to garlic's use as a putative antiatherosclerotic agent (via antithrombotic, antiplatelet, antihypertensive, and especially antilipidemic effects).

Mainstream medical interest in garlic's potential lipid-lowering effects was stimulated by 2 meta-analyses of RPC trials that found a 9% to 12% decrease in cholesterol in hyperlipidemic patients after at least 1 month of treatment with 600 to 900 mg/d of garlic tablets.[34,35] However, definitive conclusions were limited by methodologic flaws in the trials analyzed.

Results of subsequent better-designed RPC trials have been mixed, with most (4/7) failing to find a significant change in any lipoprotein component[36–39] These studies explicitly sought to overcome limitations of previous trials, such as by providing dietary stabilization prior to treatment and detailing methods to ensure proper control processes and laboratory standards. However, 3 of the negative trials were relatively small ($N \leq 28$), which in one case yielded a marginal power (80%) to detect the expected 9% reduction in cholesterol.[38] Three RPC trials support the positive findings of the meta-analyses, finding a 6.1% to 11.5% cholesterol reduction in the garlic-treated patients. Similar to previous studies, the lipid reduction was due to a decrease in low-density lipoprotein (LDL) ± decreased triglyceride levels.[40–43]

Of the factors that contribute to the discrepancies in data regarding garlic's antilipidemic effects, 2 are probably most important: publication bias (the preferential publication of trials with positive findings) and methodologic flaws. Both factors tend to overestimate the effect of a treatment. In contrast, excluding patients likely to benefit most (patients with severe hyperlipidemia or high-fat diets) might underestimate garlic's effect.

Blood pressure has been monitored in most recent studies of garlic's antilipidemic effects, showing a decrease (systolic and/or diastolic) in the treatment group of some, but not all, trials. Previously, a number of placebo-controlled trials that focused on the antihypertensive effects of garlic demonstrated a modest (–5% to –7%) effect.[44] Several small, nondefinitive RCTs also corroborate garlic's antiplatelet, antithrombotic, and fibrinolytic activity found in animal and in vitro studies.[45]

Dozens of trials suggest, but have not adequately proven, that garlic can decrease the risk factors for atherosclerosis, particularly hypercholesterolemia. Pending conclusive evidence from additional well-designed and adequately powered studies, it is reasonable for patients to choose to take garlic given that it is safe and generally inexpensive. Garlic is considered safe by the FDA, based on the lack of known serious adverse outcomes despite culinary and medicinal use throughout human history (including daily use by pregnant or lactating women). Malodorous breath and skin can be diminished with enteric-coated tablets or by consuming garlic with protein. Allergies and contact irritation occur rarely. Patients who decide to use garlic medicinally should be aware of a few caveats. The main purported active ingredient, allicin, is degraded by crushing, heat, and acid; thus, efficacy is optimized by consuming raw cloves or enteric-coated tablets. The usual dose is 300 mg, taken 2 to 3 times per day, standardized to at least 1.3% allicin (equivalent to approximately 3 g or 1 fresh clove daily). Finally, the quality of commercial preparations varies greatly, a problem common to many herbal therapies. In an analysis of supposedly standardized preparations, 93% were found to be so lacking in allicin that they were declared expensive placebos.[4]

Ginger

Zingiber officinale

Common uses: Antiemetic

Side effects: Heartburn, allergic reaction (rare)

Like garlic, ginger has been a popular culinary and medicinal herb for thousands of years. For 2500 years, the Chinese have used this plant as a flavoring agent and antiemetic. Ancient Greeks wrapped ginger in bread and ate it after meals as a digestive aid. Ginger is now cultivated in Asia, Africa, and the Caribbean and is used worldwide as a nausea remedy.

The characteristic odor and flavor of ginger root come from a volatile oil (1%–3% by weight) that is composed of shogaol and gingerols. In laboratory animals, the gingerols have analgesic, sedative, antipyretic, antibacterial, and GI tract motility effects.[46,47]

Ginger reduces nausea, according to some, but not all, controlled human trials. In an RDBPC crossover trial of 30 women suffering from hyperemesis gravidarum, ginger (250 mg 4 times a day) significantly decreased the severity of nausea (P=.04).[48] Two RDBPCTs report a significant decrease in perioperative nausea and vomiting in gynecological surgery patients who were given 1 g of ginger before surgery.[49,50] In one, ginger was as effective as metoclopramide in reducing the number of episodes of nausea or emesis.[44] However, in another RDBPCT, ginger was not found to be effective in preventing nausea after laparoscopic gynecologic surgery.[51] Regarding motion sickness, ginger was more effective than dimenhydrinate in one controlled trial,[52] but was not effective in another.[53] Such inconsistency of results is found in studies of conventional antiemetics as well, due in part to the difficulty in measuring symptoms such as nausea. In addition, the effect of antiemetics is often subtle and difficult to discern unless tested in a homogeneous population with a high prevalence of nausea.

It is reasonable for patients to try ginger to treat nausea, not only because data supports its efficacy, but also because it is inexpensive, readily available, and safe. Like garlic, ginger is not known to cause any serious side effects, despite worldwide culinary and medicinal use of ginger. Only 1 of the above controlled human trials noted any side effect, which, ironically, was GI tract upset. It is on the FDA's GRAS list. The usual adult dose is 250 milligrams (1/4 tsp) to 1 g of powdered root several times per day.

Ginkgo

Ginkgo biloba

Common uses: Intracerebral and peripheral vascular insufficiency (dementia and claudication)
Investigational uses: Mountain sickness
Side effects: Gastrointestinal tract disturbance, headache, contact dermatitis (each is rare/mild)

One of the oldest surviving tree species, *G biloba* has grown in China for more than 200 million years. For thousands of years, traditional Chinese medicine has used ginkgo to treat brain disorders. In the past 20 years, ginkgo has gained worldwide popularity for similar purposes, supported by evidence of its ability to promote perfusion and inhibit oxidative damage. By 1988, German physicians prescribed a standardized extract of ginkgo (Egb 761, Willmar Schwabe GmbH & Co, Karlsruhe, Germany) more than any other medication.[4] Sales in the United States soared to $240 million in 1997.[1] In Germany, where most of the research has been conducted, the federal health authorities have concluded that treatment with Egb 761 is safe and effective for peripheral and cerebral circulatory disturbances, including claudication and memory impairment.[5] Numerous European clinical trials report EGb 761's efficacy in diminishing symptoms of cerebrovascular insufficiency.[54,55]

In 1997, the first US-based trial corroborated ginkgo's efficacy in the treatment of dementia. In this year-long, RDBPC, multicenter study, EGb 761 was found to stabilize and in some cases improve cognition and social functioning in patients with mild to moderate dementia (Alzheimer disease or multi-infarct dementia).[56] In another trial, healthy geriatric patients demonstrated better cognitive function after taking EGb 761.[57]

EGb 761 improves perfusion peripherally as well as centrally. More than 15 European studies suggest a reduction of claudication symptoms in patients treated with EGb 761, including a 50% increase in pain-free walking distance.[58] Simultaneous benefits on central and peripheral perfusion are demonstrated in a randomized, placebo-controlled trial among 44 Himalayan climbers.[59] The 22 subjects treated with 160 mg/d of EGb 761 developed significantly fewer cerebral (0% vs 41.9%, $P<.002$) and respiratory symptoms (13.6% vs 81.8%, $P<.001$) of mountain sickness than climbers taking the placebo. EGb 761 also decreased vasomotor disorders of the extremities, measured by plethysmography and symptom scores.

The mechanisms of ginkgo's therapeutic effects are not fully understood. They are attributed in part to synergistic effects of its constituents, particularly the flavonoids, terpenoids, and organic acids. These act to varying degrees as scavengers of free-radicals, chemicals implicated in the pathophysiology of Alzheimer disease.[60,61] They also inhibit platelet activation factor and thereby reduce thrombosis, dilate arteries and capillaries, and block the release of chemotactic and inflammatory mediators from phagocytes.

Ginkgo's antidementia effects are similar to that of the prescription drugs donepezil and tacrine.[62,63] While statistically significant, such modest effects are of uncertain clinical benefit. However, ginkgo may have other advantages, such as improvement of peripheral vascular circulation and tolerance of altitude. In addition, ginkgo's side effects are similar to placebo vs potential hepatoxic effects with tacrine. While *G biloba* leaves may cause mild GI tract irritation, no serious adverse effects have been noted in human or animal trials, including no mutagenicity or teratogenicity.[64] In contrast, *G biloba* seeds can cause fatal neurologic and allergic reactions and are not used medicinally.[64] Patients should use the extract studied in all reported clinical trials, Egb 761. The dose is 40 mg 3 times per day or 80 mg twice per day of an extract standardized to 24% flavanoid glycoside and 6% terpenoids. Absorption is unaffected by food intake. The duration of benefit after discontinuation is unknown.[65]

Ginseng

Panax ginseng
Panax quinquefolius **(American ginseng, an endangered species)**
(*Eleutherococcus senticosus*, so-called Siberian ginseng, is *not* in the *Panax* [true ginseng] genus)
Common name: Korean ginseng
Common uses: "Tonic," performance enhancer, "adaptogen," anticancer, aphrodisiac
Investigational uses: All common uses are as of yet unproven but are under investigation
Side effects: Tachycardia, hypertension

Ginseng is one of the most popular and expensive herbs in the world. As in ancient China, ginseng is still widely believed to be a panacea; hence, its genus name *Panax*. The common name ginseng ("man-root") stems from a belief that because this root is humanoid in appearance, it can benefit all aspects of the human body. At least 6 million Americans[66] use the root of this slow-growing perennial. It is considered a tonic or adaptogen that enhances physical performance (including sexual), promotes vitality, and increases resistence to stress and aging. While in vitro and animal studies suggest that it has beneficial effects on immune and endocrine functions, evidence of its effects on humans is limited and contradictory.

One reason for lack of definitive data about ginseng's health effects is the inherent difficulty of quantifying intangible benefits such as "vitality" and "quality of life." Nevertheless, a 3-month RCT showed a significant increase in subjective "quality-of-life" scores among ginseng users (n=625).[67] Some small controlled trials report increased endurance, whereas others do not.[68] In an RDBPCT, college-aged volunteers who took 100 mg of ginseng twice daily for 12 weeks experienced a statistical improvement in the speed at which they were able to perform mathematical calculations, but did not experience improvement in motor function or other cognitive functions; no adverse effects were seen in this study.[69] To our knowledge, no studies compare ginseng's effect with that of inexpensive, widely available cognitive stimulants such as caffeine, nor has an RCT confirmed aphrodisiac effects in humans. However, ginseng was associated with a significant increase in serum hormones (testosterone, dihydroxytestosterone, follitropin, and lutropin) and in sperm numbers and motility in 46 men with oligospermia.[70] A case-control study suggests an association (but not necessarily a causal relationship) between use of ginseng and lower cancer rates (n=1987 pairs matched for age, religion, marital status, education, sex, occupation, and smoking status).[71]

In Asian cultures, ginseng is commonly consumed by pregnant women and is given to newborns in hopes of bolstering energy. A case-control study of 88 pairs of women (matched only for age and parity) found a significantly lower rate of pregnancy-induced hypertension, but a 3-fold higher incidence of gestational diabetes among ginseng consumers.[72] We do not recommend ginseng use for pregnant or lactating women or for children until safety and efficacy are proven in randomized controlled trials.

Patients who take ginseng risk paying a high price without proven benefit. Commercial preparations of ginseng cost up to $20 an ounce and vary tremendously in quality. In one analysis of 54 available ginseng products, 85% were determined "worthless," containing little or no ginseng.[73] To optimize quality and chance of efficacy, only preparations standardized to ginsenoside content should be used. Patients should be warned that *E senticosis*, marketed as "Siberian ginseng" for commercial reasons, contains no true ginseng.

Despite extensive use, adverse reactions to ginseng are rare and ginseng is on the FDA's GRAS list. However, at least 1 fatality has been attributed to contamination of a ginseng product with the potent and unpredictable herbal stimulant ephedra. While clear conclusions about the safety of ginseng cannot be drawn from the uncontrolled 1979 case series that coined the term "ginseng abuse syndrome,"[74] ginseng can act as a mild stimulant and should probably be avoided in association with other stimulants or in patients with cardiovascular disease. Rare endocrinologic effects include mastalgia and postmenopausal bleeding, both of which cease with discontinuation of ginseng.[75]

Goldenseal

Hydrastis canadensis
Common uses: Antidiarrheal and antiseptic (berberine component)
Investigational uses: Antineoplastic and anti–human immunodeficiency virus (berberine component) Side effects (large doses): Mucocutaneous irritation, GI tract upset, cardiac and uterine contractility, vasocon striction, central nervous system stimulation, neonatal jaundice (displaces bilirubin).

Cherokee Indians introduced this member of the buttercup family to European settlers. It is used topically for eye or skin irritation, and orally for infections. A recent surge in goldenseal's popularity stems from the erroneous but widespread belief that it can mask illicit drugs in urine toxicology screens. It is a also a popular but unproven cold remedy. However, one of its main bioactive constituents, berberine, is an effective antidiarrheal agent.

In one RCT, a single 400-mg dose of berberine sulfate significantly reduced stool volumes and duration of diarrhea among patients with enterotoxigenic *Escherichia coli* and *Vibrio cholerae.*[76] In another controlled trial, berberine (5 mg/kg × 6 days) was more effective than placebo and as effective as metronidazole (10 mg/kg × 6 days) in treating children with giardia.[77]

Berberine is thought to act intraluminally, as it is poorly absorbed and there is no clinical evidence for systemic anti-infective activity.[78] In vitro studies reveal possible mechanisms of berberine's antidiarrheal effects. Berberine exerts antimicrobial activity against numerous bacteria, fungi, and protozoa.[79] In addition, it blocks adhesion of bacteria to epithelial cells,[80] inhibits the intestinal secretory response of cholera and *E coli* toxins, and normalizes mucosal histology following cholera toxin damage.[81]

Despite the antidiarrheal efficacy of the chemical berberine, we do not recommend the use of the herb goldenseal for this purpose, both because of this plant's endangered status and due to the possible toxicity of its other components. For example, traditional herbal literature warns that large (unspecified) amounts of goldenseal (particularly the alkaloid hydrastine) can cause mucosal irritation, GI tract upset, uterine contractions, neonatal jaundice, hypertension, seizures, inotropic cardiac effects, and respiratory failure.[82] It may oppose heparin or coumadin anticoagulation.[83] Goldenseal should not be used by pregnant or lactating women, neonates, or patients with cardiovascular disease, epilepsy, or coagulation problems. No significant side effects have been noted in clinical or animal studies of purified berberine.

Milk Thistle

Silybum marianum
Common names: "Holy Thistle," "St Mary's Thistle"
Common uses: Hepatoprotectant, antioxidant
Investigational uses: Antihyperglycemic
Side effects: None known

For more than 2000 years, the seeds of this prickly leafed, purple-flowered plant have been used to treat liver disorders. In addition, all parts of this Kashmir native have been consumed historically as vegetables without report of toxic effects. Silymarin protects against a variety of hepatotoxic effects. Silymarin protects against a variety of hepatotoxic agents and processes in animal experiments. Evidence of its effects in humans is provocative but preliminary.

The best human data deal with silymarin's effect on cirrhosis, with conflicting results from 2 RDBPC trials.[84, 85] In the first, the 4-year mortality rate decreased by 30% in patients treated for 2 years with 140 mg of silymarin 3 times a day. Effects were greatest in alcohol-related cirrhosis. In contrast, a recent multicenter RDBPC trial in 200 patients with alcoholic cirrhosis found no differences in progression of disease or mortality after 2 years of treatment with 150 mg of silymarin 3 times per day.[85] Interestingly, glycemic control was significantly improved (lower fasting blood glucose, glycosylated hemoglobins, and insulin requirements) in a randomized, placebo-controlled trial of 60 patients taking silymarin for alcoholic cirrhosis.[86] In another RCT of patients with chronic active hepatitis, 1 week of therapy with oral silymarin (240 mg/d) resulted in decreased serum transaminases and bilirubin values.[87] European physicians routinely treat hepatotoxic mushroom poisoning with intravenous silymarin (20–50 mg/kg per day), decreasing mortality rates by more than half in several case series.[88]

In animal studies, silymarin protects liver cells against a variety of hepatotoxins, including drugs (acetaminophen, amitriptyline, and erythromycin),[89,90] toxins (a-amantin from deathcap mushrooms, alcohol, and carbon tetrachloride),[91] hemosiderin,[92] viruses, and radiation.[88] Silymarin scavenges free radicals, blocks toxin entry into cells by competing for receptor sites, inhibits inflammation, and stimulates liver regeneration. As a result, it lowers serum transaminase levels, maintains coagulation factor production, and limits necrosis.[88–91] It also prevents renal toxic reactions from cisplatin.[93]

Milk thistle warrants further investigation as a hepatoprotective and regenerative agent. No adverse effects have been reported. Diabetic patients taking silymarin should carefully monitor their blood glucose and may require reduction in standard antihyperglycemic agents to avoid hypoglycemia.[86] The common dose is a 140-mg capsule, standardized to 70% silymarin, 2 to 3 times a day. A high first-pass effect concentrates silymarin in the liver. Silymarin is poorly absorbed, so concentrated products (ie, extracts) are optimal.

St John's Wort

Hypericum perforatum
Common use: Antidepressant
Investigational uses: Anticancer, antiviral (including human immunodeficiency virus)
Side effects: Photosensitivity (rare, with large doses)

This 5-petalled yellow flower grows wild in much of the world. While reduced to 1% of its original population in the Pacific United States by ranchers who consider it a bothersome weed, in Europe it is highly valued as an antidepressant. St John's wort is by far the most common antidepressant used in Germany, where physicians prescribe it 4 times more often as fluoxetine hydrochloride.[94] Sales in the United States increased 20-fold between 1995 and 1997, from $10 million to $200 million annually.[1] St John's wort has been used for thousands of years for a myriad of conditions. It is named after St John the Baptist because it blooms around his feast day (June 24) and exudes a red color symbolic of his blood. Its scientific name derives from the Greek *hyper* and *eikon,* "to overcome an apparition," relating to ancient belief in its ability to ward off evil spirits. The vulnerary and neurologic effects of this herb were described by Galen, were repeated throughout the Middle Ages and by early American herbalists, and were recently supported by many clinical trials.

A 1996 meta-analysis of 23 randomized, controlled clinical trials of SJW concluded that it is significantly more effective than placebo in treating mild to moderate depression.[95] The 8 studies that compared *H perforatum* with low-dose tricyclics suggested equivalent efficacy, with significantly fewer side effects. The authors noted the need for further studies to determine optimal dosing, long-term side effects, efficacy in maintenance therapy, and relative safety and efficacy compared with other antidepressants.[95] In response, the Office of Complementary and Alternative Medicine of the National Institutes of Health and the National Institute of Mental Health recently allocated $4.3 million for the first clinical trial in the United States to address these issues. The 3-year multicenter trial beginning in 1998 will compare SJW with both placebo and fluoxetine hydrochloride.

The mechanism of SJW's antidepressant effects is only partially known. Some in vitro studies demonstrated monoamine oxidase inhibition, but only at concentrations unattainable in vivo.[96] Furthermore, SJW is used extensively (66 million doses in 1994 in Germany) without restriction of tyramine-containing foods and without reported side effects related to monoamine oxidase inhibition. Hypericin is the putative active ingredient. It has a high affinity for γ-aminobutyric acid, the stimulation of which is known to have antidepressant effects.[87] Other studies indicate that hypericin activates dopamine receptors but inhibits serotonin receptor expression.[97] Altered receptor regulation is consistent with the several-week lag between drug initiation and clinical efficacy, similar to other antidepressants.

In addition to SJW's antidepressant effects, evidence beyond the scope of this article supports its historical anti-inflammatory, anti-infective, and vulnerary external applications.[96] Antineoplastic and antiviral applications are experimental.

Existing data on the therapeutic effects of SJW are provocative. However, well-designed clinical trials are needed to determine long-term safety and therapeutic guidelines for use of SJW for different depressive disorders. Prior to the availability of such information, patients who choose to use SJW should use the regimen shown to be effective in the above clinical trials: 300 mg 3 times a day of an extract standardized to 0.3% hypericin. St John's wort is generally well tolerated, but can cause photosensitivity, especially in fair-skinned persons taking large doses. It should not be used during pregnancy (uterotonic) or with other psychoactive agents.

Saw Palmetto

Serenoa repens

Common uses: Benign prostatic hypertrophy (BPH), prostatitis

Side effects: Gastrointestinal tract upset, headache (each is rare and mild)

Extracts from the fruit of this short, scrubby palm have been used historically to treat urogential problems. Many modern clinical trials corroborate the ability of saw palmetto extract (SPE) to improve the signs and symptoms of BPH, for which it is a first-line treatment in much of Europe.[98]

Seven of the 8 DBPC trials that have evaluated SPE's efficacy in treating BPH demonstrate significant objective and subjective improvement in BPH symptoms in patients taking 320 mg of SPE for 1 to 3 months.[98,99] However, only 2 of these trials are randomized, and their results conflict. In the shorter randomized trial, SPE is no better than placebo in treating BPH (n=70 treated for 1 month).[100] In the larger, randomized, multicenter trial (n=176 treated for 2 months), and in the other 6 DBPC trials, SPE significantly increases urinary flow, decreases nocturia, and decreases postvoid residual.[101] Saw palmetto extract worked as well as finasteride in a randomized, 6-month study of 1098 men, with similar significant improvements in the International Prostate Symptom Score, quality of life, and peak urinary flow rate.[102] Unlike finasteride, SPE did not cause impotence, decrease libido, or alter prostate-specific antigen levels.

A mechanism of SPE's effect on BPH is demonstrated in an RDBPCT in which use of SPE for 3 months results in a significant decrease in prostatic nuclear androgen and estrogen receptors.[103] Prostate size decreased on serial ultrasounds in an open study of 505 men with BPH.[104]

Like finasteride, SPE inhibits the enzyme 5α-reductase (in vitro), blocking the conversion of testosterone to dihydroxytestosterone, a major growth stimulator of the prostate gland.[105] Saw palmetto extract also blocks the uptake of testosterone and dihydroxytestosterone by the prostate without affecting serum testosterone levels.[105] In addition, its anti-inflammatory activity (inhibition of cyclooxygenase and 5-lipoxygenase pathways) are thought to be important in decreasing the edematous component of BPH and prostatitis.[4]

These studies support the use of SPE for BPH and show that its efficacy is comparable to that of the 5α-reductase inhibitor finasteride with significantly fewer side effects. However, α1 antagonists are more effective than both SPE[106] and finasteride.[107] The usual dose of SPE is 160 mg twice daily of an extract standardized to contain 85% to 95% fatty acids and sterols. Side effects are rare (<3%) and include mild headaches and GI tract upset.[4]

Valerian

Valeriana officinalis

Common uses: Sleep-aid, anxiolytic, antispasmodic
Side effects: Headaches (rare), heart palpitations (rare), insomnia (rare)

The malodorous root of valerian, a pink-flowered perennial that grows wild in temperate areas of the Americas and Eurasia, has been a popular calming and sleep-promoting agent for centuries. German health officials have approved valerian for use as a mild sedative and sleep aid, based on several European clinical trials that demonstrate these effects.

In 2 randomized, blind, and placebo-controlled crossover trials (n=27 and n=128), valerian (400–450 mg before bedtime) resulted in significantly improved sleep quality and decreased sleep latency, with no residual sedation in the morning.[108, 109] In vitro, constituents of valerian mediate the release of γ-aminobutyric acid[110] and bind the same receptors as benzodiazepines, but with less affinity and milder clinical effects.[111] Habituation or addiction have not been reported.

In the United States, valerian is approved for use in flavoring foods and beverages such as root beer. No serious side effects have been reported. However, a small percentage of consumers experience paradoxical stimulation, including restlessness and palpitations, particularly with long-term use.[112] Some components display cytotoxic and mutagenic activity in vitro. Although these effects have not been reproduced in vivo even at high doses (1350 mg/kg), valerian probably should not be used by pregnant women. Valerian should not be taken with other sedatives or before driving or in other situations when alertness is required.

Conclusions

Physicians need to know about medicinal herbs because many patients use them and are often guided by misconceptions or inaccurate information. Whether or not physicians intend to prescribe herbal therapies, it is important that they understand the potential associated health consequences so that they can help patients make informed decisions about their use. This review aimed to familiarize clinicians with available evidence on 12 commonly used herbs, as well as to indicate areas in need of further research. Popular interest in herbal therapies is stimulating research that will help clarify issues such as the indications, effective doses, and safety of common medicinal herbs.

For patients who choose to use herbal therapies, several guidelines can help them to do so most safely and effectively (Table 5). Patients need to understand that medicinal herbs are drugs, and as such not only have potential benefits, but also the potential to interact with other drugs and to cause toxic reactions. Patients should be informed about important similarities and differences between FDA-approved drugs and herbal remedies, particularly that the herbs are not required to be proven either safe or effective prior to marketing (Table 3). Given the variable purity, potency, and quality of herbal products, they must be selected with care. In general, the best products are from Europe, where quality control regulations exist. In the United States, large stores with national reputations to protect have particular incentive to ensure quality. Finally, patients should preferably use standardized products and consult reputable sources for information about appropriate indications, contraindications, and dosing (see Tables 4 through 6).

Thanks to the following for their thoughtful comments and assistance: Lisa Butters, Maureen Brown, MD, Chris Vincent, MD, and the Swedish Medical Center Library staff.

References

1. Canedy D. Real medicine or medicine show? growth of herbal sales raises issues about value. *New York Times.* July 23, 1998:C1.

2. Tyler VE. What pharmacists should know about herbal remedies. *J Am Pharm Assoc.* 1996; 36:29–37.

3. Murray M. *The Healing Power of Herbs.* 2nd ed. Rocklin, Calif: Prima Publishing; 1995.

4. Tyler VE. *Herbs of Choice.The Therapeutic Use of Phytomedicinals.* Binghamton, NY: Haworth Press Inc; 1994.

5. Blumenthal M, Gruenwald J, Hall T, Riggins C, Rister R. *German Commission E Monographs: Medicinal Plants for Human Use.* Austin, Tex: American Botanical Council; 1998. In press.

6. Fidler P, Lorinzi C, O'Fallon J, et al. Prospective evaluation of chamomile mouthwash for the prevention of 5–FU-induced oral mucositis. *Cancer.* 1996;77:522–525.

7. Maiche A, Grohn P, Maki-Hokkonen H. Effect of chamomile cream and almond ointment on acute radiation skin reaction. *Acta Oncol.* 1991;30:395–396.

8. Gerritsen M, Carley W, Ranges G, et al. Flavonoids inhibit cytokine-induced endothelial cell adhesion protein gene expression. *Am J Pathol.* 1995;147:278–292.

9. Szelenyi I, Isaac O, Theimer K. Pharmacological experiments with compounds of chamomile: experimental studies of the ulcerprotective effect of chamomile. *Planta Med.* 1979; 35:218–227.

10. Viola H, Wasowski C, Levi de Stein M, et al. Apigenin, a component of *Matricaria recutita* flowers, is a central benzodiazopine receptor-ligand with anxiolytic effects. *Planta Med.* 1995;61:213–216.

11. Foster H, Niklas H, Lutz S. Antispasmodic effects of some medicinal plants. *Planta Med.* 1980;40:309–319.

12. Rekka E, Kourounakis A, Kourounakis P. Investigation of chamazulene on lipid peroxidation and free radical processes. *Res Commun Mol Pathol Pharmacol.* 1996;92:361–364.

13. Aggag M, Yousef R. Study of antimicrobial activity of chamomile oil. *Planta Med.* 1972; 22:140–144.

14. Melchart D, Linde K, Worku F, Bauer R, Wagner H. Immunomodulation with *Echinacea:* a systematic review of controlled clinical trials. *Phytomedicine.* 1994;1:245–254.

15. Braunig B, Dorn M, Limburg E, Knick E. Enhancement of resistance in common cold by *Echinacea purpurea. Z Phytother.* 1992; 13:7–13.

16. Hobbs C. *Echinacea:* a literature review; botany, history, chemistry, pharmacology, toxicology, and clinical uses. *HerbalGram.* 1994;30:33–47.

17. Schoneberger D. Influence of the immunostimulating effects of the pressed juice of *Echinaceae purpureae* on the duration and intensity of the common cold: results of a double-blind clinical trial. *Forum Immunol.* 1992; 2:18–22.

18. Bauer V, Jurcic K, Puhlmann J, Wagner V. Immunologic in vivo and in vitro examinations of *Echinacea* extracts. *Arzneim Forsch.* 1988; 38:276–281.

19. Roesler J, Steinmuller C, Kiderlen A, Emmendorffer A, Wagner H, Lohmann-Matthes M. Application of purified polysaccharides from cell cultures of the plant *Echinacea purpurea* to test subjects mediates activation of the phagocyte system. *Int J Immunopharmacol.* 1991;13:931–941.

20. Luettig B, Steinmuller C, Gifford G, Wagner-Matthes M. Macrophage activation by the polysaccharide arabinogalactan isolated from plant cell cultures of *Echinacea purpurea. J Natl Cancer Inst.* 1989;81:669–675.

21. Lersch C, Seuner M, Bauer A, Siemens M, Hart R, Drescher M. Nonspecific immunostimulation with low doses of cyclophosphamide (LDCY), thymostimulin, and *Echinacea purpurea* extracts (Echinacin) in patients with far-advanced colorectal cancers: preliminary results. *Cancer Invest.* 1992;10:343–348.

22. Muller-Jacki B, Breu WPA, Redl K, Greger H, Bauer R. In vitro inhibition of cyclooxygenase and 5–lipoxygenase by alkamides from *Echinacea* and *Achillea* species. *Planta Medica.* 1994;60:37–40.

23. Tubaro A, Tragni E, Del Negro P, Galli C, Della Loggia R. Anti-inflammatory activity of a polysaccharide fraction of *Echinacea angustifolia. J Pharmacol.* 1987;39:567–569.

24. Mengs U, Clare C, Poiley J. Toxicity of *Echinacea purpurea:* acute, subacute and genotoxicity studies. *Arzneim Forsch.* 1991;41:1076–1081.

25. Hobbs C. Feverfew: a review. *HerbalGram.* 1989;20:2636.

26. Patrick M, Heptinstall S, Doherty M. Feverfew in rheumatoid arthritis: a double blind, placebo controlled study. *Ann Rheum Dis.* 1989; 48:547–549.

27. Murphy J, Heptinstall S, Doherty M, Mitchell J. Randomized double-blind, placebo-controlled trial of feverfew in migraine prevention. *Lancet.* 1988;2:189–192.

28. Johnson E, Kadam N, Hylands D, Hylands P. Efficacy of feverfew as prophylactic treatment of migraine. *BMJ.* 1985;291:569–573.

29. de Weerdt C, Bootsma H, Hendricks H. Herbal medicines in migraine prevention: randomized double-blind, placebo-controlled crossover trial of a feverfew preparation.*Phytomedicine.* 1996; 3:225–230.

30. Heptinstall S, White A, Willimson L, Mitchell J. Extracts of feverfew inhibit granule secretion in blood platelets and polymorphonuclear leukocytes. *Lancet.* 1985;1:1071–1074.

31. Welch K. Drug therapy in migraine. *N Engl J Med.* 1993;329:1476–1483.

32. Heptinstall S, Awang D, Dawson B, Kindack D, Knight D, May J. Parthenolide content and bioactivity of feverfew: estimation of commercial and authenticated feverfew products. *J Pharm Phamacol.* 1992;44:391–395.

33. Dorant E, van den Brandt P, Goldbohm R, Hermus R, Sturmans F. Garlic and its significance for the prevention of cancer: a critical review. *Br J Cancer.* 1993;67:424–429.

34. Warshafshy S, Kamer R, Sivak S. Effect of garlic on total serum cholesterol. *Ann Intern Med.* 1993;1 19:599–605.

35. Silgay C, Neil A. Garlic as a lipid-lowering agent: a meta-analysis. *J R Coll Physicians London.* 1994;28:2–8.

36. Simons LA, Galaubramaniam S, von Konlgomark M, Parfitt A, Simons J, Peters W. On the effect of garlic on plasma lipids and lipoproteins in mild hypercholesterolaemia. *Atherosclerosis.* 1995;113:219–225.

37. Neil HAW, Silagy CA, Lancaster T, et al. Garlic powder in the treatment of moderate hyperlipidaemia: a controlled trial and meta-analysis. *J R Coll Physicians London.* 1996;30:329–334.

38. Isaacsohn JL, Moser M, Stein EA, et al. Garlic powder and plasma lipids and lipoproteins: a multicenter, randomized, placebo-controlled trial. *Arch Intern Med.* 1998;158:1189–1194.

39. Berthold HK, Sudhop T, von Bergman K. Effect of garlic oil preparation on serum lipoproteins and cholesterol metabolism: a randomized, controlled trial. *JAMA.* 1998;279:1900–1902.

40. Lawson D. *Human Medicinal Agents From Plants.* Springville, Utah: American Chemical Society; 1993.

41. Jain A, Vargas R, Gotzkowsky S, McMahon F. Can garlic reduce the levels of serum lipids? a controlled clinical study. *Am J Med.*1993; 94:632–635.

42. Adler AJ, Holub BJ. Effect of garlic and fish oil supplementation on serum lipid and lipoprotein concentrations in hypercholesterolemic men. *Am J Clin Nutr.* 1997;65:445–450.

43. Steiner M, Khan AH, Holbert D, Lin R. A double-blind crossover study in moderately hypercholesterolemic men that compared the effect of aged garlic extract and placebo administration on blood lipids. *Am J Clin Nutr.* 1996; 64:866–870.

44. Silagy C, Neil A. A meta-analysis of the effect of garlic on blood pressure. *J Hypertens.* 1994; 12:463–468.

45. Kleijnen J, Knipschild P, Ter Riet G. Garlic, onions and cardiovascular risk factors: a review of the evidence from human experiments with emphasis on commercially available preparations. *Br J Clin Pharmacol.* 1989;28:535–544.

46. Yamahara J, Huang Q, Li Y, Xu L, Fujimura H. Gastrointestinal motility enhancing effect of ginger and its active constituents. *Chem Pharm Bull.* 1990;38:430–431.

47. Mascolo N, Jain R, Jain S, Capasso F. Ethnopharmacologic investigations of ginger (*Zingiber officinale*). *J Ethnopharmacol.* 1989;27:129–140.

48. Fischer-Rasmussen W, Kjaer S, Dahl C, Asping U. Ginger treatment of hyperemesis gravidarum. *Eur J Obstet Gynecol Reprod Biol.* 1991;38:19–24.

49. Phillips S, Ruggier R, Hutchinson S. *Zingiber officinale* (ginger): an antiemetic for day surgery. *Anaesthesia.* 1993;48:715–717.

50. Bone M, Wilkinson D, Young J, Charlton S. The effect of ginger root on postoperative nausea and vomiting after major gynecologic surgery. *Anaesthesia.* 1990;45:669–671.

51. Arfeen Z, Owen H, Plummer J, Ilsley A, Sorby-Adams R, Doecke C. A double-blind random controlled trial of ginger for the prevention of postoperative nausea and vomiting. *Anaesth Intensive Care.* 1995;23:449–452.

52. Mowbrey D, Clayson D. Motion sickness, ginger, and psychophysics. *Lancet.* 1982; 1:656–657.

53. Stewart J, Wood M, Wood C, Mims M. Effects of ginger on motion sickness susceptibility and gastric function. *Pharmacology.* 1991; 42:111–120.

54. Hopfenmuller W. Evidence for a therapeutic effect of *Ginkgo biloba* special extract: meta-analysis of 11 clinical trials in patients with cerebrovascular insufficiency in old age. *Arzneim Forsch.* 1994;44:1005–1013.

55. Kleijnen J, Knipschild P. *Ginkgo biloba* for cerebral insufficiency. *Br J Clin Pharmacol.* 1992; 34:352–358.

56. Le Bars P, Katz M, Berman N, Turan M, Freedman A, Schatzberg A. A placebo-controlled, double-blind, randomized trial of an extract of *Ginkgo biloba* for dementia. *JAMA.* 1997;278:1327–1332.

57. Hindemarch I, Subhan Z. The pharmacological effects of *Ginkgo biloba* extract in normal healthy volunteers. *Int J Clin Pharmacol Res.* 1984;4:89–93.

58. Ernst E. *Ginkgo biloba* extract in peripheral arterial diseases: a systematic research based on controlled studies in the literature. *Fortsch Med.* 1996;114:85–87.

59. Roncin J, Schwartz F, D'Arbigny P. EGb 761 in control of acute mountain sickness and vascular reactivity to cold exposure. *Aviat Space Environ Med.* 1996;67:445–452.

60. Behl C, Davis J, Leslie R, Schubert D. Hydrogen peroxide mediates amyloid B protein toxicity. *Cell.* 1994;77:817–827.

61. Maitra I, Marcocci L, Droy-Lefais M, Packer L. Peroxyil radical scavenging activity of Ginkgo extract EGb 761. *Biochem Pharmacol.* 1995;49:1649–1655.

62. Knapp M, Knopman D, Solomon P. A 30–week randomized controlled trial of high dose tacrine in patients with Alzheimer's disease. *JAMA.* 1994;271:985–991.

63. Rogers SL, Doody RS, Mohs RC, Friedhoff LT. Donepezil improves cognition and global function in Alzheimers disease: a 15–week, double-blind, placebo-controlled study. *Arch Intern Med.* 1998;158:1021–1031.

64. Woerdenbag HJ, Van Beck TA. *Ginkgo Biloba. Adverse Effects of Herbal Drugs. Vol 3.* Berlin, Germany: Springer-Verlag; 1997.

65. Kleijnen J, Knipschild P. *Ginkgo biloba. Lancet.* 1992,340:1136–1139.

66. Lawrence Review of Natural Products. *Ginseng.* St Louis, Mo: Facts and Comparisons; 1990.

67. Marasco C, Vargas R, Salas V, Begona I. Double-blind study of a multivitamin complexes supplemented with ginseng extract. *Drugs Exp Clin Res.* 1996;22:323–329.

68. Bahrke M, Morgan W. Evaluation of the ergogenic properties of ginseng. *Sports Med.* 1994;18:229–248.

69. D'Angelo R, Grimaldi M, Caravaggi M, et al. A double-blind, placebo-controlled clinical study on the effect of a standardized ginseng extract on psychomotor performance in healthy volunteers. *J Ethnopharmacol.* 1986;16:15–22.

70. Salvati G, Genovesi G, Marcellini L, et al. Effects of *Panax ginseng C. A. Meyer saponins* on male fertility. *Panminerva Med.*1996;38:249–254.

71. Taik-Koo Y, Soo-Yong C. Preventive effect of ginseng intake against various human cancers: a case-control study on 1987 pairs. *Cancer Epidemiol Biomarkers Prev.* 1995;4:401–408.

72. Chin R. Ginseng and common pregnancy disorders. *Asia Oceanica J Obstet Gynecol.* 1991;17:379–380.

73. Castleman M. Ginseng. *Herb Q.* 1990; 48:17–24.

74. Siegel R. Ginseng abuse syndrome. *JAMA.* 1979;241:1614–1615.

75. Palmer B, Montgomery A, Monteiro J. Ginseng and mastalgia [letter]. *BMJ.* 1978;1:1284.

76. Rabbani G, Butler T, Knight J, Sanyai S, Alam K. Randomized controlled trial of berberine sulfate therapy for diarrhea due to enterotoxigenic *Escherichia coli* and *Vibrio cholerae. J Infect Dis.* 1987;155:979–984.

77. Choudhry V, Sabir M, Bhide V. Berberine in giardiasis. *Indian J Pediat.* 1972;9:143–144.

78. Bergner P. Goldenseal and the common cold. *Med Herbalism.* 1997;8:1,4–6.

79. Foster S. Goldenseal: *Hydrastis canadensis.* American Botanical Council Series. 1991:309.

80. Sun D, Courtney H, Beachey E. Berberine sulfate blocks adherence of *Streptococcus pyogenes* to epithelial cells, fibronectin, and hexadecane. *Antimicrob Agents Chemother.* 1988;32:1370–1374.

81. Sack R, Froehlich J. Berberine inhibits intestinal secretory response of *Vibrio cholera* toxins and *Escherichia coli* enterotoxins. *Infect Immun.* 1982;35:47:1–475.

82. Lawrence Review of Natural Products. *Goldenseal.* St Louis, Mo: Facts and Comparisons; 1994.

83. Newall C, Anderson L, Phillipson J. *Herbal Medicines: A Guide for Health-Care Professionals.* London, England: Pharmaceutical Press; 1996.

84. Ferenci P, Dragosics B, Dittrich H, et al. Randomized controlled trial of silymarin treatment in patients with cirrhosis of the liver. *J Hepatol.* 1989;9:105–113.

85. Pares A, Planas R, Torres M, et al. Effects of Silymarin in alcoholic cirrhosis of the liver: results of a controlled, double-blind, randomized and multicenter trial. *J Hepatol.* 1998; 28:615–621.

86. Velussi M, Cernigoi A, Viezzoli L, Dapas F, Carrau C, Zilli M. Silymarin reduces hyperinsulinemia, malondialdehyde levels and daily insulin need in cirrhotic diabetic patients. *Curr Ther Res.* 1993;53:533–545.

87. Buzzelli G, Moscarella S, Giusti A, Duchini A, Marena C, Lampertico M. A pilot study on the liver protective effect of silybin-phosphatidylchlorine complex (IdB 1016) in chronic active hepatitis. *Int J Clin Pharmacol Ther Toxicol.* 1993;31:450–460.

88. Lawrence Review of Natural Products. *Milk Thistle.* St Louis, Mo: Facts and Comparisons; 1994.

89. Muriel P, Garciapina T, Perez-Alvarez V, Mourelle M. Silymarin protects against paracetamol-induced lipid peroxidation and liver damage. *J Appl Toxicol.* 1992; 12:439–442.

90. Davila J, Lenher A, Acosta D. Protective effect of flavonoids on drug-induced hepatotoxicity in vitro. *Toxicology.* 1989;57:267–286.

91. Letteron P, Labbe G, Cegott C, et al. Mechanism for the protective effects of silymarin against carbon tetrachloride-induced lipid peroxidation and hapatotoxicity in mice. *Biochem Pharmacol.* 1990,39:2027–2034.

92. Pietrangelo A, Borella F, Casalgrandi G. Anti-oxidant activity of silybin in vivo during long term iron overload in rats. *Gastroenterology.* 1995;109:1941–1949.

93. Gaedeke J, Fels L, Bokemyere C. Cisplatin nephrotoxicity and protection by silibinin. *Nephrol Dial Transplant.* 1996;11:55–62.

94. NIH. NIH to explore St. John's wort. *Science.* 1997;278:391.

95. Linde K, Gilbert R, Murlow C, Pauls A, Weidenhammer W, Melchart D. St. John's wort for depression: an overview and meta-analysis of randomized clinical trials. *BMJ.* 1996; 313:253–257.

96. St. Johns wort (*Hypericum perforatum*): quality control, analytical and therapeutic monograph. *Am Herbal Pharmacopoeia.* 1997:1–38.

97. Muller W. Effects of *Hypericum* extract on the suppression of serotonin receptors. *J Geriatr Psychiatry Neurol.* 1994;7:S63–64.

98. Buck A. Phytotherapy for the prostate. *Br J Urol.* 1996;78:325–336.

99. Lowe F, Ku J. Phytotherapy in treatment of BPH: a critical review. *Urology.* 1996; 48:12–20.

100. Smith R, Mermon A, Smart C, et al. The value of permixon in benign prostatic hypertrophy. *Br J Urol.* 1986;58:36–40.

101. Descotes J, Rambeaud J, Deschaseaux P, Faure G. Placebo-controlled evaluation of the efficacy and tolerability of permixon in benign prostatic hyperplasia after exclusion of placebo responders. *Clin Drug Invest.* 1995;9:291–297.

102. Carraro J, Raynaud J, Koch G. Comparison of phytotherapy (Permixon) with finasteride in the treatment of BPH: a randomized international study of 1098 patients. *Prostate.* 1996;29:23:1–240.

103. Di Silverio F, D'Eramo G, Lubrano C, et al. Evidence that *Serenoa repens* extract displays an antiestrogenic activity in prostatic tissue of benign prostatic hypertrophy patients. *Eur Urol.* 1992;21:309–314.

104. Braekman J. The extract of *Serenoa repens* in the treatment of BPH: a multicenter open study. *Curr Ther Res.* 1994;55:776–785.

105. Sultan C, Terraza A, Devillier C. Inhibition of androgen metabolism and binding by a liposterolic extract of *"Serenoa repens B"* in human foreskin fibroblasts. *J Steroid Biochem.* 1984;20:515–519.

106. Grasso M, Montesano A, Buonaguidi A, et al. Comparative effects of alfuzosin versus *Serenoa repens* in the treatment of symptomatic benign prostatic hyperplasia. *Arch Esp Urol.* 1995;48:97–103.

107. Lepor H, Williford W, Barry M, et al. The efficacy of terazosin, finasteride, or both in benign prostatic hyperplasia. *N Engl J Med.* 1996;335:533–539.

108. Leatherwood P, Chauffard F, Heck E, Munoz-Box E. Aqueous extract of valerian root (*Valeriana officinalis* L.) improves sleep quality in man. *Pharmacol Biochem Behav.* 1982; 17:6541.

109. Lindahl O, Lindwell L. Double-blind study of a valerian preparation. *Pharmacol Biochem Behav.* 1989;32:1065–1066.

110. Leuschner J, Muller J, Rudmann M. Characterization of the central nervous depressant activity of a commercially available valerian root extract. *Arzneim Forsch.* 1993;43:638–641.

111. Mennini T, Bernasconi P, Bombardelli E, Morazzoni P. In vitro study of the interaction of extracts and pure compounds from *Valeriana officinalis* roots with GABA, benzodiazepine and barbiturate receptors in rat brain. *Fitoterapia.* 1993;54:291–300.

112. Hobbs C. Valerian: a literature review. *HerbalGram.* 1989;21:19–34.

44 Herbal Remedies in Psychiatric Practice

Albert H. C. Wong, MD, FRCPC; Michael Smith, MRPharmS, ND; Heather S. Boon, BScPhm, PhD

From the Clarke Institute of Psychiatry, Faculty of Medicine, University of Toronto (Dr Wong), Canadian College of Naturopathic Medicine (Mr Smith), and Faculty of Pharmacy, University of Toronto (Dr Boon), Toronto, Ontario; and Centre for Studies in Family Medicine, Department of Family Medicine, The University of Western Ontario, London (Dr Boon).

Patients' use of alternative and complementary health services has created a need for physicians to become informed about the current literature regarding these treatments. Herbal remedies may be encountered in psychiatric practice when they are used to treat psychiatric symptoms; produce changes in mood, thinking, or behavior as a side effect; or interact with psychiatric medications. English-language articles and translated abstracts or articles (where available) found on MEDLINE and sources from the alternative/complementary health field were reviewed. Each herb was assessed for its safety, side effects, drug interactions, and efficacy in treating target symptoms or diagnoses. A synopsis of the information available for each herb is presented. In many cases the quantity and quality of data were insufficient to make definitive conclusions about efficacy or safety. However, there was good evidence for the efficacy of St John's wort for the treatment of depression and for ginkgo in the treatment of memory impairment caused by dementia. More research is required for most of the herbs reviewed, but the information published to date is still of clinical interest in diagnosing, counseling, and treating patients who may be taking botanical remedies.

Arch Gen Psychiatry. 1998;55:1033–1044

It is currently estimated that alternative/complementary medicine is used by 20% to 30% of the general North American population, and use appears to be most common in patients with chronic conditions.[1,2] It is estimated that North Americans spend more than $11 billion dollars for chiropractic, naturopathic, and herbal therapies not covered by health plans each year,[1,3] and the current annual growth rate of the alternative/complementary medicine industry is estimated to be 20%.[4] Patients' growing interest in alternative/complementary medicine has created the need for accurate information that is accessible to physicians. While this review cannot be comprehensive, especially in covering remedies used in less developed countries, the botanicals commonly encountered in North America that have particular relevance to psychiatry will be discussed. The herbal remedies reviewed herein will be divided into 3 sections: (1) herbs that are commonly used to treat psychiatric symptoms (Table 1), (2) herbs that have psychotropic effects, and (3) herbs that may interact with either psychiatric illnesses or the drugs used to treat these illnesses.

Information included in this review was drawn from comprehensive MEDLINE (1986–1997) searches, frequently cited or landmark articles, sources commonly used by the alternative health care community in North America (eg, The Canadian College of Naturopathic Medicine reference library), and consensus reports from expert committees (eg, The German Commission E[5] and the European Scientific Cooperative on Phytotherapy). The efficacy of herbal interventions was rated according to criteria derived from the 1994 *Canadian Guide to Clinical Preventive Health Care* by the Canadian Task Force on the Periodic Health Examination[6] and the 1996 *Guide to Clinical Preventive Services* by the US Preventive Services Task Force.[7] This rating system was designed to provide clinically relevant guidance regarding the use of these herbs by patients. The ratings assigned to each herb, and the rating system, may be found in Table 1.

Many of the herbs discussed in this article have a variety of constituents and putative therapeutic indications. Only the information relevant to psychiatric illness, symptoms, or treatments will be considered because of space limitations. This review focuses primarily on the English-language literature. A further caveat concerns the lack of standardization, quality control, and regulation of commercial herbal products in much of the world.[8,9] The studies cited herein report results of a wide range of herbal preparations, some of which may not be applicable to other preparations of the same herb.

Herbal Remedies Commonly Used to Treat Psychiatric Symptoms

Black Cohosh

Black cohosh (*Cimicifuga racemosa* [L] Nutt) has a history of use among North American aboriginal peoples as a treatment for the hot flashes, anxiety, and dysphoria associated with menopause; as an analgesic; and to promote lactation and menses.[10] Its putative action is on the gonadotropin system, through direct estrogen ligands that suppress luteinizing hormone release, and through nonestrogen ligands that appear to decrease luteinizing hormone secretion with long-term use.[11] A variety of uncontrolled studies have demonstrated some clinical benefit in the treatment of ovarian insufficiency symptoms.[12–15]

A randomized study comparing a commercial product of *C racemosa* (Remifemin) with conventional hormonal therapy for the treatment of ovarian insufficiency symptoms showed comparable efficacy with both treatments (n=60).[16] A randomized, double-blind, placebo-controlled trial with the same product (n=80) found superior efficacy to placebo or conjugated estrogen therapy for the treatment of both physical and mental menopausal symptoms.[17] The long-term benefits of postmenopausal hormone treatment have not been compared with those of *C racemosa*. The dose of black cohosh ranges from 40 to 200 mg daily, and the onset of action is reported to be up to 2 weeks.[18]

Potential side effects include gastric upset, throbbing headaches, dysphoria, and cardiovascular depression. Caution should be exercised if the herb is taken with other hormonal therapies, since *C racemosa* likely interacts with the sex hormone system, although such interaction has not been documented. It should be avoided during pregnancy and lactation.[18,19]

German Chamomile

German chamomile (*Matricaria recutita* L) has been used for the treatment of gastrointestinal tract discomfort, peptic ulcer disease, mouth and skin irritation, pediatric colic and teething, and mild insomnia and anxiety.[18,20] The herb contains the flavonoid apigenin, which may have an affinity for the benzodiazepine receptor[21] and may also interact with the histamine system.[22] A mild hypnotic effect has been reported in mice[21] and in humans,[23–25] but no randomized or controlled clinical studies were identified. Doses commonly range from 2 to 4 g of dried flower heads 3 times daily, normally prepared as a tea.[5,18] Chamomile is also commercially available as a liquid extract (1:1, 45% ethanol), which is dosed as 1 to 4 mL 3 times daily,[18] and as a tincture (1:5, 45% ethanol), of which 3 to 10 mL is

Table 1. Herbal Remedies Commonly Used to Treat Psychiatric Symptoms*

Herb	Common Usage	Quality of Evidence Category†	Adverse Effects	Cautions/ Contraindications	Drug Interactions
Black cohosh	Menopause symptoms PMS Dysmenorrhea	I III III	GI upset (rare), headaches, CV depression	Pregnancy, lactation	Hormonal treatments (theoretical)
German chamomile	Insomnia Anxiety	III III	Allergy (rare)	Allergy to sunflower family of plants	None reported
Evening primrose	Schizophrenia ADHD Dementia	IV IV IV	None reported	Mania, epilepsy	Phenothiazines, NSAIDs, corticosteroids, β-blockers, anticoagulants
Ginkgo	"Cerebrovascular insufficiency" symptoms Dementia	I I	Headache, GI upset	Pregnancy, lactation, potential bleeding (eg, PUD)	Anticoagulants
Hops	Insomnia	III	Allergy, menstrual irregularity	Depression, pregnancy, lactation	Sedative-hypnotics, alcohol (both theoretical)
Kava	Insomnia Anxiety Seizures	III III IV	Scaling of skin on extremities	Pregnancy, lactation	Benzodiazepines, alcohol
Lemon balm	Insomnia Anxiety	IV III	None reported	Thyroid disease, pregnancy, lactation	CNS depressants, thyroid medications
Passion flower	Insomnia Anxiety	III III	Hypersensitivity vasculitis, sedation	Pregnancy, lactation	Insufficient data
Skullcap	Insomnia Anxiety Seizures	IV IV IV	Sedation, confusion, seizures	Pregnancy, lactation	Insufficient data
St John's wort	Depression	I	Photosensitivity, GI upset, sedation, anticholinergic	CV disease, pregnancy, lactation, pheochromocytoma	Drugs that interact with MAOIs
Valerian	Insomnia Anxiety	III III	Sedation	Pregnancy, lactation	CNS depressants

*PMS indicates premenstrual syndrome; GI, gastrointestinal; CV, cardiovascular; ADHD, attention deficit with hyperactivity disorder; NSAIDs, nonsteroidal anti-inflammatory drugs; PUD, peptic ulcer disease, CNS, central nervous system; and MAOIs, monoamine oxidase inhibitors.

†Quality of evidence: I, evidence from at least 2 properly randomized controlled trials; II-1, evidence from well-designed trials without randomization; II-2, evidence from well-designed cohort or case-controlled analytic studies, preferably from more than 1 center or research group; II-3, evidence obtained from multiple time series with or without the intervention; dramatic results from uncontrolled experiments could also be regarded as this type of evidence; III, opinions of respected authorities based on clinical experience, descriptive studies, or reports of expert committees; and IV, insufficient evidence to warrant conclusions about efficacy or safety.

taken 3 times daily.[18] Potential adverse reactions are rare and mainly allergic in nature.[19,23,24,26–28]

Evening Primrose

Some authors have proposed the use of evening primrose (*Oenothera biennis* L) in the treatment of schizophrenia, childhood hyperactivity, and dementia, apparently on the basis of isolated reports of prostaglandin abnormalities in schizophrenia[29] and attention-deficit/hyperactivity disorder.[30–32] There is little scientific evidence or cultural tradition to support this usage. The pharmacological constituents of interest are the essential and nonessential fatty acids: *cis*-linoleic acid, *cis*-γ-linolenic acid, oleic acid, palmitic acid, and stearic acid.[19,33,34] However, the empirical evidence for changes in fatty acid levels after oral administration is sparse,[35] and the literature on the efficacy of fatty acid administration in the treatment of schizophrenia and attention-deficit/hyperactivity disorder is contradictory.[36–38] In addition, there is currently insufficient information to recommend evening primrose in the treatment of dementia.[19,39] The majority of evening primrose oil supplements contain 8% *cis*-γ-linolenic acid, and the daily adult dose ranges from 6 to 8 g, normally given in divided doses.[19]

In general, evening primrose oil is relatively safe,[40–42] but it should be used with caution in mania[43] and epilepsy.[19,41,43] There have been cases in which evening primrose oil appears to have exacerbated epilepsy. Drugs that may interact adversely with evening primrose include phenothiazines,[37,39,44] nonsteroidal anti-inflammatory drugs, corticosteroids,[45] β-blockers,[39] and anticoagulants.[43]

Ginkgo

The ginkgo tree (*Ginkgo biloba* L) is one of the oldest deciduous tree species on earth.[46] It has been used for medicinal purposes extensively in Europe and has a minor role in traditional Chinese medicine.[47–49] Its indications are varied and include dementia, "chronic cerebrovascular insufficiency," and "cerebral trauma."[47,48] Standardized commercial preparations are widely available and usually contain the active constituents flavone glycosides (24%) and terpenoids (6%).[50,51] Most clinical studies have used specific extracts of *Ginkgo* (EGb 761 and LI 1370) that are equivalent to the commercial preparations. The dose for most indications is 40 mg of standardized extract 3 times daily,[20,48] which must be given for 1 to 3 months before the full therapeutic effects are apparent.[48,52]

There is considerable evidence that *Ginkgo* extracts can improve vascular perfusion[53–59] by modulating vessel wall tone[60–69] and can decrease thrombosis[70] through antagonism of platelet activating factor.[71–75] Ischemic sites may benefit in particular from ginkgo treatment.[76–84] The antioxidant properties that have been attributed to the flavonoid components found in ginkgo are believed to play an important role in its postulated neuroprotective and ischemia-reperfusion–protective effects.[85–91] The extract EGb 761 has been shown to have both hydroxyl radical scavenging activity and superoxide dismutase-like activity.[68,92]

Kleijnen and Knipschild[53] reviewed 40 controlled trials on the use of ginkgo in the treatment of "chronic cerebral insufficiency." Although only 8 of the studies were deemed to be of good quality, all but 1 found clinically significant improvement in symptoms, such as memory loss, concentration difficulties, fatigue, anxiety, and depressed mood. Studies investigating the use of ginkgo to augment memory or treat memory loss have produced conflicting results. Generally, some improvement is reported in patients with moderate to severe memory impairment, but no significant improvement is seen in those with mild to no memory impairment.[93–103]

There is also evidence, derived from randomized, controlled trials, that ginkgo extracts are effective in the treatment of psychopathological conditions and memory impairment caused by Alzheimer and vascular dementia.[104–107] For example, 1 multicenter, randomized, double-blind, placebo-controlled trial (N=216) assessed the use of ginkgo in the treatment of outpatients diagnosed with primary degenerative dementia of the Alzheimer type or multi-infarct dementia of mild to moderate severity (*DSM-III-R*[108] criteria). The participants were given either 120 mg of *G biloba* extract (EGb 761) or placebo twice daily. Response to treatment was defined as response to a minimum of 2 of the 3 primary outcome variables: the Clinical Global Impressions (item 2) to assess psychopathology, the Syndrom-Kurztest to assess memory and attention, and the Nurnberger Alters-Beobachtungsskala rating scale to assess the ability to perform the activities of daily life. The investigators reported that the frequency of response was significantly ($P<.005$) higher in the ginkgo-treated group, which was confirmed by intention-to-treat analyses.[104]

A recent North American multicenter, randomized, controlled trial in a similar patient population (outpatients with mild to severe Alzheimer disease or multi-infarct dementia) followed 309 patients for 52 weeks and reported similar results. Patients in this study received 40 mg of *G biloba* extract (EGb 761) or placebo 3 times daily, and the following outcome measures were used: the Alzheimer's Disease Assessment Scale–Cognitive subscale, the Geriatric Evaluation by Relative's Rating Instrument, and the Clinical Global Impression of Change. With an intention-to-treat analysis, those taking ginkgo scored significantly higher on both the Alzheimer's Disease Assessment Scale–Cognitive subscale (P=.04) and the Geriatric Evaluation by Relative's Rating Instrument (P=.005). There was no difference reported between the 2 groups in the Clinical Global Impression of Change scores. The investigators concluded that, although the changes in the ginkgo-treated groups were modest, they were of sufficient magnitude to be recognized by caregivers.[107]

Ginkgo has been used by patients in an attempt to treat impotence, including antidepressant-induced sexual dysfunction. In one open trial (N=60), patients with proved arterial erectile dysfunction who had not previously responded to papaverine ingested 60 mg of *G biloba* extract daily for 12 to 18 months. Fifty percent of the men had gained potency after 6 months of therapy; however, the role of *Ginkgo* in this recovery is difficult to determine, given the large psychological component of impotence and the fact that this trial was not blinded. There are no reports cited in the MEDLINE literature that investigated the use of ginkgo for antidepressant-induced sexual dysfunction.

There is one randomized, controlled trial showing improvement in resistant depression with ginkgo as an augmenting agent with conventional antidepressants.[109] One in vitro study reported that compounds present in both dried and fresh *Ginkgo* leaves have monoamine oxidase (MAO) (both A and B) inhibitory activity;[110] however, there is currently no evidence that *G biloba* extracts ingested in normal dosages by humans will inhibit MAO activity in the brain. Finally, there is evidence from animal studies that ginkolide B may have a neuroprotective effect in brain injury.[84,111,112]

Side effects from ginkgo appear to be relatively uncommon, but include headache, gastrointestinal tract upset, and skin allergy to the *Ginkgo* fruit.[48,49,53,61,113–115] Of these, headache is the most common, and it is best prevented by starting with a low dose and gradually titrating to the required dose. Many researchers have suggested that ginkgo theoretically may potentiate other anticoagulants or increase bleeding time; however, these effects rarely have clinically significant implications. Millions of people take ginkgo every year, yet only 2 reported cases of bleeding problems (neither a confirmed drug interaction) may be found in the literature.[116,117] Caution should still be exercised when ginkgo is taken in conjunction with anticoagulant treatment (including aspirin) or where there is a risk of bleeding (eg, peptic ulcer disease, subdural hematoma). Safety in pregnancy and lactation has not been established.

Hops

Although hops (*Humulus lupulus* L) is used by the brewing industry to produce beer, the female flowers of the plant also have a long medicinal history as a mild sedative.[25,118] Hops is also currently used as a mild hypnotic agent[18,33,119–121]; however, there are no clinical studies of its use as a single agent to treat specific symptoms or illnesses, such as insomnia or anxiety disorders. The sedating effects of hops may be mediated by one of its constituent volatile oils, 2-methyl-3-butene-2-ol,[20,121,122] but there is insufficient information to confirm this. Adverse effects include allergy and disruption of menstrual cycles.[19,25,123,124] Hops is commonly given 3 times daily and before bed in the following doses: 0.5 to 1 g of dried flowers, 0.5 to 1 mL of liquid extract (1:1, 45% ethanol), or 1 to 2 mL of tincture (1:5, 60% ethanol).[18] The use of hops should be avoided in depression, in pregnancy, and during lactation.[18,19,25] Although there are currently no documented case examples, care should be taken when hops is used with sedative-hypnotic agents and alcohol, as a potentiation of their effect may be seen.

Kava

Preparations made from the roots of kava (*Piper methysticum*, Forst) have been used extensively by the peoples of the South Pacific for both medicinal and cultural purposes.[125] Medicinally, it is reputed to have anxiolytic, anticonvulsant, sedative, and muscle relaxant properties.[125,126] While a number of pharmacologically active agents have been identified, most interest has centered on the α-pyrones commonly referred to as kavalactones. Conflicting evidence exists regarding the affinity of kava pyrones for various γ-aminobutyric acid (GABA) or benzodiazepine-binding sites.[127,128] Kavain, a kavalactone, has been shown to block the voltage-dependent sodium ion channel.[129] In animals, kava has been reported to exhibit neuroprotective effects against ischemia.[130] Anticonvulsive effects have also been noted.[131–133] Many published works regarding kava are in German, but a number of reviews are available in English.[125,134]

Kava has been reported to produce changes on the electroencephalogram similar to those seen with diazepam.[135] Several human clinical trials suggest that kava products standardized for kavalactone content (70%) may be beneficial in the management of anxiety and tension of nonpsychotic origin.[136,137] Kava appears not to adversely affect cognitive function, mental acuity, or coordination[125,138] in comparison with oxazepam, as measured by event-related potentials during cognitive testing.[139,140] Clinical trials with kava have used doses of standardized preparations that range from 100 to 200 mg of kavalactones daily in divided doses or a single dose at bedtime.[126]

Long-term administration with higher doses (eg, 400 mg of kavalactones) may result in scaling of the skin on the extremities.[125,126] It has been hypothesized that kava produces a vitamin B deficiency that results in the scaling. However, administration of nicotinamide (100 mg daily for 3 weeks) did not resolve the condition.[141] Kava may interact with benzodiazepines; there is 1 controversial case report involving alprazolam.[142] While the consumption of large amounts of alcohol has been noted to potentiate the actions of kava in mice,[143] administration of a standardized kava extract in a placebo-controlled, double-blind study showed few adverse effects.[144] The possibility exists that concomitant administration may potentiate the action of other centrally mediated agents.[126]

Lemon Balm

An aromatic member of the mint family, lemon balm (*Melissa officinalis* L) has a history of use as an anxiolytic.[25,121] Although 1 article has reported hypnotic and analgesic effects in mice,[145] there are currently no clinical studies demonstrating hypnotic or anxiolytic effects in humans, even though some authors endorse this use.[25,118,119] One study using a combination product containing valerian and lemon balm showed a sleep-promoting effect, but it is difficult to conclude what role lemon balm played in this effect.[146] Doses of lemon balm range from 1 to 4 g daily.[25] No side effects have been reported from ingestion of lemon balm; however, safety in pregnancy and lactation has not been established. Lemon balm may potentiate the effects of other central nervous system (CNS) depressants, including alcohol,[145] and may interact with thyroid medications or thyroid disease.[33,147–150]

Passion Flower

Passion flower (*Passiflora incarnata* L) is native to the Americas, where its perennial vine leaves have been used as a sedative by indigenous peoples such as the Aztecs.[19,33,151] Its current use as a sedative-hypnotic[118,119,151–153] is supported by the findings of some animal studies[153–157]; however, the active ingredients[118,151,158,159] and mechanism of action remain obscure. No clinical studies of *P incarnata* alone have been found, although one randomized, controlled trial that used a commercial preparation containing *P incarnata* in addition to valerian showed benefit in the treatment of adjustment disorder with anxious mood.[160] Passion flower is often given 3 times daily in the following doses: 0.25 to 1 g of dried herb (commonly taken as a tea); 0.5 to 1 mL of liquid extract (1:1; 25% alcohol); or 0.5 to 2.0 mL of tincture (1:8; 45% alcohol).[18,19]

Hypersensitivity vasculitits[161] and "altered consciousness"[162] have been reported with products containing passion flower. Passion flower may cause sedation, and so the usual precautions regarding operation of a motor vehicle or machinery should be observed.[153] Excessive use during pregnancy and lactation should be avoided.[19] Interactions with other psychotropic medications have not been adequately studied.

Skullcap

Members of the genus *Scutellaria* have a long history of medicinal use; the roots in traditional Chinese medicine and the aerial parts in western herbalism.[19,163] Skullcap (*Scutellaria laterifolia* L) has been used as a sedative and anticonvulsant.[119,164] The active ingredients and pharmacology are not well documented. In addition, existing studies are not necessarily applicable to preparations that patients may be taking, because different species and parts of the plant are used.[113] Skullcap is available in several dosage forms that are commonly taken 3 times daily: 1 to 2 g of dried herb or 2 to 4 mL of liquid extract (1:1; 25% alcohol).[18] Adverse reactions include giddiness, confusion, sedation, seizures,[165,166] and possibly hepatotoxic effects[166] (the hepatotoxic effect in this case was later attributed to another ingredient of the preparation[167]). Although there is insufficient information to make specific recommendations regarding safety, skullcap should be avoided in pregnancy and lactation, and may interact with other CNS drugs.[168]

St John's Wort

The use of St John's wort (*Hypericum perforatum* L) may be traced back to the texts of the ancient Greek physicians Hippocrates, Pliny, and Galen, and continued through the Classical, Renaissance, and Victorian eras.[169,170] Its contemporary usage has been as an antidepressant, for which there is more rigorous evidence than for any other herbal remedy.[171,172] The active ingredients responsible for antidepressant action have been investigated (mainly hypericin and pseudohypericin),[173–177] but the putative mechanism of action of St John's wort extracts remains controversial.

The hypericins were found to be absorbed within 2 hours, in a dose-dependent manner. These compounds are widely distributed and have a plasma half-life of 24 hours, allowing steady-state concentrations to be reached in 4 days.[175,176] It is estimated that 14% to 21% of the compounds are systemically available.[176] In vitro experiments found hypericin mainly in the cytoplasmic membrane and cytoplasm, with smaller amounts found in the nucleus.[178]

Hypericum extracts show affinity for a variety of neurotransmitter receptors, including: adenosine, $GABA_A$, $GABA_B$, serotonin $(5\text{-HT})_1$, central benzodiazepine, forskolin, inositol triphosphate, and the MAO A and B enzymes.[179] Hypericin by itself has an affinity for the N-methyl-D-aspartate receptor.[180] However, the concentrations required for in vivo activity are unlikely to be attained after oral administration, except for activity at the GABA receptors.[180] Various authors have proposed serotonin reuptake inhibition,[181,182] decreased serotonin receptor expression,[183] altered receptor regulation,[182] inhibition of benzodiazepine binding,[184] increased excretion of adrenergic metabolites,[185] and inhibition of MAO[186,187] to explain the clinically observed antidepressant effects. Although MAO inhibitor activity is an attractive explanation for the antidepressant actions of St John's wort, studies are unable to confirm that putative MAO inhibition is responsible for antidepressant effects.[187–189]

Animal studies show changes, similar to those seen with other antidepressants, on behavioral tests.[190] Changes are seen in assays of motor activity, exploratory behavior, analgesia, ketamine sleeping time, and temperature.[191 192] Rats treated for 6 months with LI 160 (a commercial hypericum extract) were found to have significantly increased numbers (50% more) of both 5-HT_{1A} and 5-HT_{2A} serotonin receptors, without changes in affinity.[193] Human studies show electroencephalographic changes with St John's wort that are different from those seen with tricyclic antidepressants: shortening of evoked potential latencies and enhancement of theta and beta-2 regions of the resting electroencephalogram in the absence of sleep changes.[194,195]

There is strong evidence of efficacy in mild to moderate depression, as reviewed by Linde et al.[171] That meta-analysis included 23 randomized trials with a total of 1757 outpatients, in which extracts of St John's wort alone (20 of 23 trials) or in combination with other herbs (3 of 23) were tested against placebo (15 trials) or antidepressant drugs (8 trials). Outcome was assessed by means of a pooled estimate of the "responder rate ratio" (response rate in the hypericum group vs the control group). St John's wort was reported to be clearly superior to placebo and comparable with conventional drug treatment, with lower side-effect and dropout rates in the hypericum group. Concerns raised in the article by Linde et al include the heterogeneity of patients, interventions, extract preparations, and diagnostic classifications among the various trials. A more recent review (but not meta-analysis) of 12 randomized trials (11 of which were included in the meta-analysis by Volz[172]) expressed similar concerns regarding the methods of the original studies, the possibility of subtherapeutic control drug dosing, and the variability of hypericum preparations. Overall, there are inadequate data regarding long-term use and efficacy in severe depression. There are concerns regarding the standardization and quality control of commercial preparations.[196,197] Clearly, more research is needed to address these shortcomings in the literature.

Many commercial St John's wort products are standardized extracts (0.3% hypericin) of which 300 to 900 mg are given daily in 3 divided doses.[171] This is approximately equivalent to 2 to 4 g of the dried herb.[19] In general, fewer adverse effects are seen with hypericum than with conventional antidepressants,[171,198] but they may include photodermatitis,[199] delayed hypersensitivity, gastrointestinal tract upset, dizziness, dry mouth, sedation, restlessness, and constipation.[19,171,200,201] There do not appear to be significant adverse effects on cardiac conduction with hypericum extracts.[202] The use of St John's wort is contraindicated in pregnancy, lactation, exposure to strong sunlight, and pheochromocytoma.[19] Because of the lack of information regarding the mechanism of action of *H perforatum* extracts, the potential for MAO inhibitor–like drug interactions cannot be excluded.[19,203]

Valerian

Valerian (*Valeriana officalis* L and *Valeriana* species) has a rich history of use throughout the world for a variety of indications, including as a sedative.[20] Research on the mechanism of action has yielded contradictory findings. Extracts of valerian have affinity for $GABA_A$ receptors,[204,205] likely because of the relatively high content of GABA itself that has been documented to be a constituent of valerian.[206,207] The amount of GABA present in aqueous extracts of valerian is sufficient to induce release of GABA in synaptosomes and may also inhibit GABA reuptake.[208,209] However, since GABA does not readily cross the blood-brain barrier, the relevance of these findings to central sedating effects is questionable. Other postulated mechanisms of action include inhibition of the catabolism of GABA by valerenolic acid and acetylvalerenolic acid[210] and affinity for the 5-HT_A receptor by another constituent of valerian, hydroxypinoresinal.[211] Adenosine receptors may also be a target of valerian extracts.[212]

Animal behavioral tests with valerian show results consistent with other hypnotic agents such as the benzodiazepines,[211 213–222] as well as contradictory reports of anticonvulsant activity[223,224] and possible antidepressant effects.[219,225] Imaging with cerebral nuclear medicine scans in rats showed CNS depressant effects.[211,226,227]

Human clinical studies of valerian confirm a mild sedative effect,[228] although the exact effects on sleep architecture, quality, and the electroencephalogram are inconsistent.[229–235] These results are based on a relatively small number of subjects and do not evaluate the efficacy of valerian as a treatment for primary or secondary insomnia. There is no evidence to suggest that valerian is superior to existing hypnotic medications or other treatments for insomnia. This review found only 1 English-language report of a subjective anxiolytic effect.[229]

The dosage for valerian ranges from 2 to 3 g of the dried root given 3 times daily or at bedtime.[211] Adverse effects include reports of hepatotoxic effects, although the offending preparations often contained a mixture of ingredients, making it difficult to draw definitive conclusions.[236–240] There is currently insufficient information to recommend valerian in pregnancy and during lactation,[241–243] although no reports of teratogenicity were found. The sedative effects of valerian may potentiate the effects of other CNS depressants,[213, 221, 244, 245] and the usual precautions taken with other sedating agents also apply to valerian.

Herbal Remedies With CNS Effects

Capsicum

Commonly encountered in the form of chili or cayenne pepper, capsicum (*Capsicum annuum* L) has been used topically for pain relief in a variety of healing traditions.[25,246] The active ingredients form a class referred to as the capsaicinoids, of which the most important is capsaicin.[247,248] Capsaicin depletes substance P, thus inhibiting substance P–mediated pain transmission.[249–252] Numerous trials have concluded that 0.075% capsaicin cream is a safe and effective treatment for painful diabetic neuropathy.[253–258] There is also some evidence that 0.025% capsaicin cream may be useful in relieving the pain of postherpetic neuralgia.[259–264] Several proprietary creams containing capsaicin (eg, Axsain and Zostrix) are available in North America. Traditionally, *Capsicum* has been ingested as a treatment for gastrointestinal tract complaints, such as colic and dyspepsia. In addition, it is thought to improve peripheral circulation in patients with cardiovascular conditions.[19] These indications have not been investigated scientifically. *Capsicum* products used internally may elevate the secretion of catecholamines,[265] thus caution with concurrent MAO inhibitor treatment is recommended.

Chaste Tree

Found in the Mediterranean and central Asia, chaste tree (Vitex *Agnus-castus* L) has been used medicinally since the times of ancient Greece and Rome to treat symptoms of premenstrual syndrome, mastodynia, menopause, hyperprolactinemia, and menstrual irregularity.[266–269] The exact mechanism of action is unclear but likely involves modulating the prolactin axis.[118,270,271] Affinity for D_1 and D_2 dopamine receptors has also been reported.[272,273] These data point to a potential interaction with other dopaminergic drugs, such as the antipsychotics and metoclopramide.[270]

Siberian Ginseng

Siberian ginseng (*Eleuthrococcus senticosus* [Rupr and Maxim] Maxim), a member of the Araliaceae family and also known as eleuthero, is native to the northern parts of China, Japan, Korea, and eastern Russia. Used in traditional Chinese medicine for more than 400 years, the roots are thought to help fatigue and stress and to improve endurance.[274,275] This type of "ginseng" must be distinguished from plants of the genus *Panax* (eg, *Panax ginseng, Panax quinquefolius)*, which are discussed below. The eleutherosides contained in Siberian ginseng are thought to mediate the antifatigue and immunostimulatory properties attributed to this plant.[19,274,276] Eleuthero should be used cautiously with sedative-hypnotic agents, as some studies report alteration of barbiturate-induced sleeping time.[18,274,277]

Herbal Remedies That May Cause Psychiatric Symptoms

Ginseng

Often confused with *E senticosus* (Siberian ginseng), *P ginseng* CA Meyer (ie, ginseng, Chinese ginseng, Korean ginseng) and *P quinquefolius* L (ie, Canadian ginseng, American ginseng) have a long list of indications, including treating stress and fatigue and improving endurance. Although many mechanisms of action have been postulated, it probably affects the hypothalamic-pituitary-adrenal axis, resulting in elevated plasma corticotropin and corticosteroid levels.[278–284] One of the most common side effects is insomnia,[285] while others include hypertension, diarrhea, restlessness, anxiety, and euphoria.[286,287] Ginseng should be used with caution in patients with hypertension and diabetes and in conjunction with centrally acting medications.[25,276] In addition, ginseng may potentiate the effect of MAO inhibitors,[45,288–290] stimulants (including caffeine), and haloperidol.[291]

Yohimbe

Yohimbe (*Pausinystalia yohimbe* [K Schum]) is a botanical medicine derived from the bark of the *P yohimbe* (K Schum) tree.[20] The active constituents are the alkaloids, notably one of the yohimbane derivatives called yohimbine.[292] Yohimbine appears to act as an α_2-adrenoceptor antagonist,[292,293] and the hydrochloride salt is used in the treatment of erectile dysfunction.[294,295] Yohimbe bark is reputed to have aphrodisiac properties and is widely sold for this purpose.[20]

When administered to humans, yohimbine causes a variety of symptoms, including anxiety, nervousness, palpitations, and restlessness, as well as signs such as elevated 3-methoxy-4-hydroxyphenylglycol and cortisol levels.[292, 296, 297] In fact, yohimbine is one of the agents commonly used to provoke panic attacks and anxiety in studies of the pathophysiology, psychopharmacology, and treatment of anxiety disorders.[298, 299] Tricyclic antidepressants, medications with central α-adrenergic blocking properties, centrally acting sympathomimetics, MAO inhibitors, and antimuscarinic agents are all known to potentiate the action of yohimbine.[292] Yohimbine also may contribute to psychotic symptoms,[296] mania,[300] and seizures,[301] but these effects are not well documented.

Clearly, yohimbine-containing products have the potential to produce psychiatric symptoms, primarily anxiety or panic, especially in patients with preexisting panic disorder.[302] While it is important to be aware of this in examining patients with anxiety who are also taking herbal remedies, many commercial products containing yohimbe bark actually have little or no yohimbine.[303]

Conclusions

We have reviewed the most common herbal products used in North America that are likely to be encountered in psychiatric practice. With the exception of St John's wort for depression and ginkgo for dementia, there is insufficient evidence to recommend the use of herbal medicines in the treatment of psychiatric illness. None of these herbal remedies is clearly superior to current conventional treatments. Because these products are widely available and often used by the general public, more clinical research is needed to establish safety and efficacy. A working knowledge of the pharmacological data and clinical literature is necessary to properly counsel, diagnose, and treat patients who may be using herbal products. The advances of modern medicine, science, and technology are greater than at any other time in history, and the rate of discovery of new knowledge and techniques is accelerating. However, the experience and healing traditions of other cultures, whether in less developed countries or in history, should not be ignored. Contemporary medical research may finally allow us to separate the traditional remedies that can effectively treat disease from those that are superstition and myth. In addition, research into the biochemical and pharmacological effects of these herbs may uncover novel treatments for psychiatric illness or yield fresh insights into basic disease mechanisms.

References

1. Eisenberg DM, Kessler RC, Foster C, Norlock FE, Calkins DR, Delbanco TL. Unconventional medicine in the United States: prevalence, costs and patterns of use. *N Engl J Med.* 1993; 328:246–252.
2. Berger E. *Canada Health Monitor Survey #9.* Toronto, Ontario: Price Waterhouse; 1993.
3. The rise of alternative medicine. *Pharm Pract.* 1997;13:50.
4. Khaliq Y. Alternative medicine: what pharmacists need to know. *Pharm Pract.* 1997; 13:44–50, 83–85.
5. Blumenthal M, Brusse WR, Goldbert A, Gruenwald J, Hall T, Riggins CW, Rister RS, eds. *The Complete German Commission E Monographs.* Austin, Tex: American Botanical Council; 1998.
6. The Canadian Task Force on the Periodic Health Examination. *The Canadian Guide to Clinical Preventive Health Care.* Ottawa, Ontario: Health Canada; 1994.
7. US Preventive Services Task Force. *Guide to Clinical Preventive Services.* 2nd ed. Baltimore, Md: Williams & Wilkins; 1996.
8. O'Neill A. Danger and safety in medicines. *Soc Sci Med.* 1994;38:497–507.
9. Mills S. Safety awareness in complementary medicine. *Complement Ther Med.* 1996; 4:48–51.
10. Brinker F. An overview of conventional, experimental and botanical treatments of non-malignant prostate conditions. *Br J Phytother.* 1993/1994;3:154–176.
11. Ducker E-M, Kopanski L, Jarry H, Wuttke W. Effects of extracts from *Cimicifuga racemosa* on gonadotropin release in menopausal women and ovariectomized rats. *Planta Med.* 1991; 57:420–424.
12. Warnecke G. Beeinflussing klimakterisch beschwerden durch ein phytotherapeutikum. *Med Welt.* 1985;36:871–874.
13. Daiber W. Menopause symptoms: success without hormones. *Arztliche Prax.* 1983; 35:1946–1947.
14. Vorberg G. Treatment of menopause symptoms. Z *Allgemeinmedizin.* 1984;60:626–629.
15. Petho A. Menopause symptoms: is it possible to switch from hormone treatment to a botanical gynecologicum? *Arztliche Prax.* 1987; 47:1551–1553.
16. Lehmann-Willenbrock E, Riedel H. Klinische und endokrinologische untersuchungen zur therapie ovarieller ausfallserscheinungen nach hysterekomie unter belassung der adnexe. *Zentralbl Gynakol.* 1988;110:611–618.
17. Stoll W. Phytotherapeutikum beeinflust atrophisches Vaginalepithel. *Therapeutikon.* 1987;1:23–31.
18. Bradley P. *British Herbal Compendium.* Bournemouth, England: British Herbal Medicine Association; 1992.
19. Newall C, Anderson L, Phillipson J. *Herbal Medicines: A Guide for Health Care Professionals.* London, England: Pharmaceutical Press; 1996:296.
20. Tyler V. *Herbs of Choice: The Therapeutic Use of Phytomedicinals.* Binghamton, NY: Pharmaceutical Products Press; 1994:209.
21. Viola H, Wasowski C, Levi de Stein M, Wolfman C, Silveira R, Dajas F, Medina JH, Paladini AC. Apigenin, a component of *Matricaria recutita* flowers, is a central benzodiazepine receptors-ligand with anxiolyic effects. *Planta Med.* 1995;61:213–216.
22. Miller T, Wittstock U, Lindequist U, Teuscher E. Effects of some components of the essential oil of chamomile, *Chamomilla recutita* on histamine release from rat mast cells. *Planta Med.* 1996;62:60–61.
23. Berry M. The chamomiles. *Pharm J.* 1995; 254:191–193.

24. Mann C, Staba EJ. The chemistry, pharmacology, and commercial formulations of chamomile. *Herbs Spices Med Plants.* 1984;1:235–280.

25. Mills S. *The Essential Book of Herbal Medicine.* 2nd ed. London, England: Penguin Books Ltd; 1991:677.

26. Paulsen E, Andersen K, Hausen B. Compositae dermatitis in a Danish dermatology department in one year. *Contact Dermatitis.* 1993;29:6–10.

27. Hausen B. The sensitizing capacity of Compositae plants, III: test results and cross reactions in Compositae-sensitive patients. *Dermatologica.* 1979;159:1–11.

28. Hausen B, Busker E, Carle R. The sensitizing capacity of Compositae plants, VII: experimental investigations with extracts of *Chamomilla recutita* (L.) Rauschert and *Anthemis cotula* L. *Planta Med.* 1984;50:229–234.

29. Vaddadi K. The use of gamma-linoleic acid and linoleic acid to differentiate between temporal lobe epilepsy and schizophrenia. *Prostaglandins Med.* 1981;27:313–323.

30. Stevens L, Zentall S, Abate M, Kuczek A, Burgess J. Omega-3 fatty acids in boys with behaviour, learning and health problems. *Physiol Behav.* 1996;59:915–920.

31. Stevens LJ, Zentall SS, Deck JL, Abate ML, Watkins BA, Lipp SR, Burgess JR. Essential fatty acid metabolism in boys with attention-deficit hyperactivity disorder. *Am J Clin Nutr.* 1995; 62:761–768.

32. Mitchell EA, Aman MG, Turbott SS, Manku M. Clinical characteristics and serum essential fatty acid levels in hyperactive children. *Clin Paediatr.* 1987;26:406–411.

33. Leung AY, Foster S. *Encyclopedia of Common Natural Ingredients Used in Food, Drugs, and Cosmetics.* 2nd ed. Toronto, Ontario: John Wiley & Sons Inc; 1996:649.

34. Briggs CJ. Evening primrose. *Rev Pharm Can.* 1986;119:249–254.

35. Manku M, Morse-Fischer N, Horrobin D. Changes in human plasma essential fatty acid levels as a result of administration of linoleic acid and gamma-linolenic acid. *Eur J Clin Nutr.* 1988;42:55–60.

36. Vaddadi K, Courtney P, Gilleard C, Manku M, Horrobin D. A double-blind trial of essential fatty acid supplementation in patients with tardive dyskinesia. *Psychiatry Res.* 1989; 27:313–323.

37. Holman C, Bell A. A trial of evening primrose oil in the treatment of chronic schizophrenia. *J Orthomol Psychiatry.* 1983;12:302–304.

38. Blackburn M. Use of efamol (oil of evening primrose) for depression and hyperactivity in children. In: Liss AR, ed. *Pathophysiology and Roles in Clinical Medicine.* New York, NY: Alan R. Liss Inc; 1990:345–349.

39. Horrobin DF. Gammalinolenic acid: an intermediate in essential fatty acid metabolism with potential as an ethical pharmaceutical and as a food. *Rev Contemp Pharmacother.* 1990;1:1–45.

40. Chenoy R, Hussain S, Tayob Y, O'Brien P, Moss M, Morse P. Effect of oral gamalinolenic acid from evening primrose oil on menopausal flushing. *BMJ.* 1994;38:501–503.

41. Joe LA, Hart LL. Evening primrose oil in rheumatoid arthritis. *Ann Pharmacother.* 1993;27:1475–1477.

42. Kleijnen J. Evening primrose oil [see comments]. *BMJ.* 1994;309:824–825.

43. Barber HJ. Evening primrose oil: a panacea? *Pharm J.* 1988;240:723–725.

44. Cant A, Shay J, Horrobin DF. The effect of maternal supplementation with linolenic and gammalinolenic acids on the fat composition and content of human milk. *J Nutr Sci Vitaminol.* 1991;37:573–579.

45. Stockley I. *Drug Interactions: A Sourcebook of Adverse Interactions, Their Mechanisms, Clinical Importance, and Management.* 3rd ed. Cambridge, England: Blackwell Scientific Press; 1994.

46. Major RT. The ginkgo, the most ancient living tree. *Science.* 1967;157:1270–1273.

47. Foster S. *Ginkgo, Ginkgo biloba.* Austin, Tex: American Botanical Council; 1990.

48. Gaby AR. *Ginkgo biloba extract:* a review. *Altern Med Rev.* 1996;1:236–242.

49. Houghton PJ. Ginkgo. *Pharm J.* 1994; 253:122–123.

50. Sticher O. *Ginkgo biloba*—analysis and dosage forms [in German]. *Pharm Unserer Zeit.* 1992; 21:253–265.

51. Sticher O. Quality of ginkgo preparations. *Planta Med.* 1993;59:2–11.

52. Kleijnen J, Knipschild P. *Ginkgo biloba* for cerebral insufficiency. *Br J Clin Pharmacol.* 1992; 34:352–358.

53. Kleijnen J, Knipschild P. *Ginkgo biloba. Lancet.* 1992;340:1136–1139.

54. Jung F, Mrowietz C, Kiesewetter H, Wenzel E. Effect of *Ginkgo biloba* on fluidity of blood and peripheral microcirculation in volunteers. *Arzneimittelforsch.* 1990;40:589–593.

55. Liberti L. Ginkgo. *Lawrence Rev Nat Products.* February 1988.

56. Le Poncin Lafitte M, Rapin J, Rapin JR. Effects of *Ginkgo biloba* on changes induced by quantitative cerebral microembolization in rats. *Arch Int Pharmacodyn Ther.* 1980;243:236–244.

57. Gaby AR. *Ginkgo biloba* extract: a review. *Alternative Med Rev.* 1996;1:236–242.

58. Krieglstein J, Beck T, Seibert A. Influence of an extract of *Ginkgo biloba* on cerebral blood flow and metabolism. *Life Sci.* 1986;39:2327–2334.

59. Tighilet B, Lacour M. Pharmacological activity of the *Ginkgo biloba* extract (EGb 761) on equilibrium function recovery in the unilateral vestibular neurectomized cat. *J Vestib Res.* 1995;5:187–200.

60. Stucker O, Pons C, Duverger JP, Drieu K. Effects of *Ginkgo biloba* extract (EGb 761) on arteriolar spasm in a rat cremaster muscle preparation. *Int J Microcirc Clin Exp.* 1996;16:98–104.

61. DeFeudis FV. Ginkgo biloba *Extract (EGb 761): Pharamacological Activities and Clinical Applications.* Paris, France: Elsevier; 1991:3–5.

62. Vilain B, DeFeudis FV, Clostre F. Effect of an extract of *Ginkgo biloba* on the isolated ileum of the guinea pig. *Gen Pharmacol.* 1982; 13:401–405.

63. Puglisi L, Salvadori S, Gabrielli G, Pasargiklian R. Pharmacology of natural compounds, I: smooth muscle relaxant activity induced by a *Ginkgo biloba* L. extract on guinea-pig trachea. *Pharmacol Res Commun*1988;20:573–589.

64. Delaflotte S, Auguet M, DeFeudis FV, Baranes J, Clostre F, Drieu K, Braquet P. Endothelium-dependent relaxations of rabbit isolated aorta produced by carbachol and by *Ginkgo biloba* extract. *Biomed Biochim Acta.* 1984;43(suppl 8–9):S212–S216.

65. Auguet M, DeFeudis FV, Clostre F. Effects of *Ginkgo biloba* on arterial smooth muscle responses to vasoactive stimuli. *Gen Pharmacol.* 1982;13:169–171.

66. Auguet M, DeFeudis FV, Clostre F, Deghenghi R. Effects of an extract of *Ginkgo biloba* on rabbit isolated aorta. *Gen Pharmacol.* 1982; 13:225–230.

67. Hellegouarch A, Baranes J, Clostre F, Drieu K, Braquet P, DeFeudis FV. Comparison of the contractile effects of an extract of *Ginkgo biloba* and some neurotransmitters on rabbit isolated vena cava. *Gen Pharmacol.* 1985;16:129–132.

68. Pincemail J, Deby C. Antiradical properties of *Ginkgo biloba* extract [in French]. *Presse Med.* 1986;15:1475–1479.

69. Robak J, Gryglewski RJ. Flavonoids are scavengers of superoxide anions. *Biochem Pharmacol.* 1988;37:837–841.

70. Smith PF, Maclennan K, Darlington CL. The neuroprotective properties of the *Ginkgo biloba* leaf: a review of the possible relationship to platelet-activating factor (PAF). *J Ethno-pharmacol.* 1996;50:131–139.

71. Braquet P. The ginkgolides: potent platelet-activating factor antagonists isolated from *Ginkgo biloba* L.: chemistry, pharmacology and clinical applications. *Drugs Future.* 1987;12:643–699.

72. Guinot P, Caffrey E, Lambe R, Darragh A. Tanakan inhibits platelet-activating-factor-induced platelet aggregation in healthy male volunteers. *Haemostasis.* 1989;19:219–223.

73. Bourgain RH, Maes L, Andries R, Braquet P. Thrombus induction by endogenic PAF-acether and its inhibition by *Ginkgo biloba* extracts in the guinea pig. *Prostaglandins.* 1986;32:142–144.

74. Bourgain RH, Andries R, Braquet P. Effect of ginkgolide PAF-acether antagonists on arterial thrombosis. *Adv Prostaglandin Thromboxane Leukot Res.* 1987;17B:815–817.

75. Belougne E, Aguejouf O, Imbault P, Azougagh Oualane F, Doutremepuich F, Droy-LeFaix MT, Doutremepuich C. Experimental thrombosis model induced by laser beam: application of aspirin and an extract of *Ginkgo biloba*: EGb 761. *Thromb Res.* 1996;82:453–458.

76. Clostre F. From the body to the cell membrane: the different levels of pharmacological action of *Ginkgo biloba* extract [in French]. *Presse Med.* 1986;15:1529–1538.

77. Rapin JR, Le Poncin Lafitte M. Cerebral glucose consumption: the effect of *Ginkgo biloba* extract [in French]. *Presse Med.* 1986;15:1494–1497.

78. Spinnewyn B, Blavet N, Clostre F. Effects of *Ginkgo biloba* extract on a cerebral ischemia model in gerbils [in French]. *Presse Med.* 1986; 15:1511–1515.

79. Spinnewyn B, Blavet N, Clostre F, Bazan N, Braquet P. Involvement of platelet-activating factor (PAF) in cerebral post-ischemic phase in Mongolian gerbils. *Prostaglandins.* 1987; 34:337–349.

80. Koc RK, Akdemir H, Kurtsoy A, Pasaoglu H, Kavuncu I, Pasaoglu A, Karakucuk I. Lipid peroxidation in experimental spinal cord injury: comparison of treatment with *Ginkgo biloba*, TRH and methylprednisolone. *Res Exp Med.* 1995;195:117–123.

81. Otamiri T, Tagesson C. *Ginkgo biloba* extract prevents mucosal damage associated with small-intestinal ischaemia. *Scand J Gastroenterol.* 1989;24:666–670.

82. Seif-El-Nasr M, El-Fattah AA. Lipid peroxide, phospholipids, glutathione levels and superoxide dismutase activity in the rat brain after ischemia: effect of *Ginkgo biloba* extract. *Pharmacol Res.* 1995;32:273–278.

83. Birkle DL, Kurian P, Braquet P, Bazan NG. Platelet-activating factor antagonist BN52021 decreases accumulation of free polyunsaturated fatty acid in mouse brain during ischemia and electroconvulsive shock. *J Neurochem.* 1988;51:1900–1905.

84. Panetta T, Marcheselli VL, Braquet P, Spinnewyn B, Bazan NG. Effects of a platelet activating factor antagonist (BN 52021) on free fatty acids, dicylglycerols, polyphosphoinositides and blood flow in the gerbil brain: inhibition of ischemia-reperfusion induced cerebral injury. *Biochem Biophys Res Commun.* 1987;149:580–587.

85. Haramaki N, Aggarwal S, Kawabata T, Droy-Lefaix MT, Packer L. Effects of natural antioxidant *Ginkgo biloba* extract (EGB 761) on myocardial ischemia-reperfusion injury. *Free Radical Biol Med.* 1994;16:789–794.

86. Oyama Y, Chikahisa L, Ueha T, Kanemaru K, Noda K. *Ginkgo biloba* extract protects brain neurons against oxidative stress induced by hydrogen peroxide. *Brain Res.* 1996;712:349–352.

87. Oyama Y, Fuchs PA, Katayama N, Noda K. Myricetin and quercetin, the flavonoid constituents of *Ginkgo biloba* extract, greatly reduce oxidative metabolism in both resting and Ca(2+)-loaded brain neurons. *Brain Res.* 1994;635:125–129.

88. Shen JG, Zhou DY. Efficiency of *Ginkgo biloba* extract (EGb 761) in antioxidant protection against myocardial ischemia and reperfusion injury. *Biochem Mol Biol Int.* 1995;35:125–134.

89. Szabo ME, Droy-Lefaix MT, Doly M, Braquet P. Free radical-mediated effects in reperfusion injury: a histologic study with superoxide dismutase and EGb 761 in rat retina. *Ophthalmic Res.* 1991;23:225–234.

90. Maitra I, Marcocci L, Droy-Lefaix MT, Packer L. Peroxyl radical scavenging activity of *Ginkgo biloba* extract EGb 761. *Biochem Pharmacol.* 1995;49:1649–1655.

91. Rong Y, Geng Z, Lau BH. *Ginkgo biloba* attenuates oxidative stress in macrophages and endothelial cells. *Free Radical Biol Med.* 1996; 20:121–127.

92. Pincemail J, Dupuis M, Nasr C, Hans P, Haag-Berrurier M, Anton R, Deby C. Superoxide anion scavenging effect and superoxide dismutase activity of *Ginkgo biloba* extract. *Experientia.* 1989;45:708–712.

93. Stoll S, Scheuer K, Pohl O, Muller WE. *Ginkgo biloba* extract (EGb 761) independently improves changes in passive avoidance learning and brain membrane fluidity in the aging mouse. *Pharmacopsychiatry.* 1996; 29:144–149.

94. Gesser B, Voelp A, Klasser M. Study of the long-term action of a *Ginkgo biloba* extract on vigilance and mental performance as determined by means of quantitative pharmaco-EEG and psychometric measurements. *Arzneimittelforschung.* 1985;35:1459–1465.

95. Rai GS, Shovlin C, Wesnes KA. A double-blind, placebo controlled study of *Ginkgo biloba* extract ("tanakan") in elderly outpatients with mild to moderate memory impairment. *Curr Med Res Opin.* 1991;12:350–355.

96. Allain H, Raoul P, Lieury A, LeCoz F, Gandon JM, d'Arbigny P. Effect of two doses of *Ginkgo biloba* extract (EGb 761) on the dual-coding test in elderly subjects. *Clin Ther.* 1993;15:549–558.

97. Hindmarch I. Activity of *Ginkgo biloba* extract on short-term memory [in French]. *Presse Med.* 1986;15:1592–1594.

98. Subhan Z, Hindmarch I. The psychopharmacological effects of *Ginkgo biloba* extract in normal healthy volunteers. *Int J Clin Pharmacol Res.* 1984;4:89–93.

99. Semlitsch HV, Anderer P, Saletu B, Binder GA, Decker KA. Cognitive psychophysiology in nootropic drug research: effects of *Ginkgo biloba* on event-related potentials (P300) in age-associated memory impaiment. *Pharmacopsychiatry.* 1995;28:134–142.

100. Warburton DM. Clinical psychopharmacology of *Ginkgo biloba* extract [in French]. *Presse Med.* 1986;15:1595–1604.

101. Winter E. Effects of an extract of *Ginkgo biloba* on learning and memory in mice. *Pharmacol Biochem Behav.* 1991;38:109–114.

102. Wesnes K, Simmons D, Rock M, Simpson P. A double-blind placebo-controlled trial of *Gingko biloba* extract in the treatment of idiopathic cognitive impairment in the elderly. *Hum Psychopharmacol.* 1987;2:159–169.

103. Gessner B, Voelp A, Klasser M. Study of the long-term action of a *Ginkgo biloba* extract on vigilance and mental performance as determined by means of quantitative pharmaco-EEG and psychometric measurements. *Arzneimittelforschung.* 1985;35:1459–1465.

104. Kanowski S, Herrmann WM, Stephan K, Wierich W, Horr R. Proof of efficacy of the *Ginkgo biloba* special extract EGb 761 in outpatients suffering from mild to moderate primary degenerative dementia of the Alzheimer type or multi-infarct dementia. *Phytomedicine.* 1997;4:3–13.

105. Hofferberth B. The efficacy of EGb 761 in patients with senile dementia of the Alzheimer type: a double-blind, placebo-controlled study on different levels of investigation. *Hum Psychopharmacol.* 1994;9:215–222.

106. Taillandier J, Ammar A, Rabourdin JP, Ribeyre JP, Pichon J, Niddam S, Pierart H. Treatment of cerebral aging disorders with *Ginkgo biloba* extract: a longitudinal multicenter double-blind drug vs placebo study [in French]. *Presse Med.* 1986;15:1583–1587.

107. Le Bars PL, Katz MM, Berman N, Turan M, Freedman AM, Schatzberg AF. A placebo-controlled, double-blind, randomized trial of an extract of *Ginkgo biloba* for dementia. *JAMA.* 1997;278:1327–1332.

108. American Psychiatric Association. *Diagnostic and Statistical Manual of Mental Disorders, Revised Third Edition.* Washington, DC: American Psychiatric Association; 1987.

109. Schubert H, Halama P. Depressive episode primarily unresponsive to therapy in elderly patients: efficacy of *Ginkgo biloba* extract (EGb 761) in combination with antidepressants. *Geriatr Forschung.* 1993;3:45–53.

110. White HL, Scates PW, Cooper BR. Extracts of *Ginkgo biloba* leaves inhibit monoamine oxidase. *Life Sci.* 1996;58:1315–1321.

111. Attella MJ, Hoffman SW, Stasio MJ, Stein DG. *Ginkgo biloba* extract facilitates recovery from penetrating brain injury in adult male rats. *Exp Neurol.* 1989;105:62–71.

112. Rodriguez de Turco EB, Droy-Lefaix MT, Bazan NG. Decreased electroconvulsive shock-induced diacylglycerols and free fatty acid accumulation in the rat brain by *Ginkgo biloba* extract (EGb 761): selective effect in hippocampus as compared with cerebral cortex. *J Neurochem.* 1993;61:1438–1444.

113. Tyler VE. *The Honest Herbal.* 3rd ed. Philadelphia, Pa: George F. Stickley Co; 1993.

114. Lepoittevin JP, Benezra C, Asakawa Y. Allergic contact dermatitis to *Ginkgo biloba* L.: relationship with urushiol. *Arch Dermatol Res.* 1989;281:227–230.

115. Mitchell JC, Maibach HI, Guin J. Leaves of *Ginkgo biloba* not allergenic for Toxicodendron-sensitive subjects. *Contact Dermatitis.* 1981;7:47–48.

116. Rowin J, Lewis SL. Spontaneous bilateral subdural hematoma associated with chronic *Gingko biloba* ingestion. *Neurology.* 1996;46:1775–1776.

117. Rosenblatt M, Mindel J. Spontaneous hyphema associated with ingestion of *Ginkgo biloba* extract. *N Engl J Med.* 1997;336:1108.

118. Weiss RF. Herbal Medicine. 6th ed. Gothenburg, Sweden: AB Arcanum; 1988:362.

119. Hoffmann D. *Holistic Herbal.* Rockport, Calif: Element Books; 1996:256.

120. Chevalier A. *The Encyclopedia of Medicinal Plants.* London, England: Readers Digest; 1996:336.

121. Bove M. *An Encyclopedia of Natural Healing for Children and Infants.* New Canaan, Conn: Keats; 1996:303.

122. Hansel R, Wohlfart R. Narcotic action of 2–methyl-3–butene-2–ol contained in the exhalation of hops. *Z Naturforschung.* 1980; 35:1096–1097.

123. O'Donovan W. Hops dermatitis. *Lancet.* 1924;2:597.

124. Newmark FM. Hops allergy and terepene sensitivity: an occupational disease. *Ann Allergy.* 1978;41:311–312.

125. Singh Y, Blumenthal M. Kava: an overview. *Herbalgram.* 1997;39:34–54.

126. Bone K. Kava: a safe herbal treatment for anxiety. *Br J Phytother.* 1993/1994;3:147–153.

127. Jussogie A, Scmiz A, Heimke C. Kavapyrone extract enriched from *Piper methysticum* as modulator of the GABA binding site in different regions of the rat brain. *Psychopharmacology.* 1994;116:469–474.

128. Davies L, Drew C, Duffield P, Johnston GA, Jamieson DD. Kava pyrones and resin: studies on GABA(A), GABA (B), and benzodiazepine binding sites in the rodent brain. *Pharmacol Toxicol.* 1992;71:120–126.

129. Glietz J, Beile A, Peters T. Kawain inhibits vetradine-activated voltage-dependent Na+ channels in synaptosomes prepared from rat cerebral cortex. *Neuropharmacology.* 1995;24:1133–1138.

130. Backhauss C, Krieglstein J. Extract of kava and its methysticin constituents protect brain tissues against ischaemic damage in rodents. *Eur J Pharmacol.* 1992;215:265–269.

131. Kretzschmar R, Meyer HJ. Comparative experiments on the anticonvulsant efficacy of *Piper methysticum* pyrone bonds [in German]. *Arch Int Pharmacodyn.* 1969;177:261–277.

132. Kretzschmar R, Meyer HJ, Teschendorf HJ, Zollner B. Antagonistic effect of natural 5,6–hydrated kava pyrones on strychnine poisoning and experimental local tetanus [in German]. *Arch Int Pharmacodyn.* 1969;182:251–268.

133. Meyer HJ, Kretzschmar R. Research on the relationship between molecular structure and pharmacological effect of aryl-substituted 4–methoxy pyrones of the kava pyrone type [in German]. *Arzneimittelforschung.* 1969; 19:617–623.

134. Hansel R. Kava-kava in modern drug research: portrait of a medicinal plant. *Q Rev Nat Med.* Winter 1996:259–274.

135. Gebner B, Cnota P. Extract of kava-kava rhizome in comparison with diazepam and placebo. *Z Phytother.* 1994;15:30–37.

136. Volz HP, Kieser M. Kava-kava extract WS 1490 versus placebo in anxiety disorders: a randomized placebo-controlled 25–week outpatient trial. *Pharmacopsychiatry.* 1997;30:1–5.

137. Lehmann E, Kinzler E, Friedemann J. Efficacy of a special kava extract (Piper methysticum) in a patients with states of anxiety, tension and excitedness of non-mental origin: a double-blind placebo-controlled study of four weeks treatment. *Phytomedicine.* 1996;3:113–119.

138. Russell P, Bakker D, Singh N. The effects of kava on alerting and speed of access of information from long-term memory. *Bull Psychonom Soc.* 1987;25:236–237.

139. Munte T, Heinze H, Matzke M, Steitz J. Effects of oxazepam and an extract of kava roots (*Piper methysticum*) on event-related potentials in a word recognition task. *Neuropsychobiology.* 1993;27:46–53.

140. Heinze HJ, Munthe TF, Stelz J, Matzke M. Pharmacopsychological effects of oxazepam and kava extract in a visual search paradigm assessed with event related potentials. *Pharmacopsychiatry.* 1994;27:224–230.

141. Ruze P. Kava-induced dermapathy. *Lancet.* 1990;335:1142–1145.

142. Almeida JC, Grimsley EW. Coma from the health food store: interaction between kava kava and alprazolam. *Annu Int Med.* 1996;125:940–941.

143. Jamieson D, Duffield P. Positive interaction to kava in mice. *Clin Exp Pharmacol Physiol.* 1990;17:509–514.

144. Herberg K. Effect of kava-special extract ws 1490 combined with ethyl alcohol on safety-relevant performance parameters. *Blutalkohol.* 1993;30:96–105.

145. Soulimani R, Fleurentin J, Mortier F, Misslin R, Derrieu G, Pelt JM. Neurotropic action of the hydroalcoholic extract of *Melissa officianalis* in the mouse. *Planta Med.* 1991;57:105–109.

146. Dressing H, Riemann D, Low M. Insomnia: are valerian/balm combinations of equal value to benzodiazepine? *Therapiewoche.* 1992; 42:726–736.

147. Brinker F. Inhibition of endocrine function by botanical agents. *J Naturopath Med.* 1990; 1:10–18.

148. Auf'mkolk M, Ingbar JC, Amir SM, Winterhoff H, Sourgens H, Hesch RD, Ingbar SH. Inhibition by certain plant extracts of the binding and adenylate cyclase stimulatory effect of bovine thyrotropin in human thyroid membranes. *Endocrinology.* 1984;115:527–534.

149. Auf'mkolk M, Kohrle J, Gumbinger H, Winterhoff H, Hesch RD. Antihormonal effects of plant extracts: iodothyronine deiodinase of rat liver is inhibited by extracts and secondary metabolites of plants. *Horm Metab Res.* 1984;16:188–192.

150. Auf'mkolk M, Ingbar J, Kubota K, Amir SM, Ingbar SH. Extracts and auto-oxidized constituents of certain plants inhibit the receptor-binding and the biological activity of Graves' immunoglobulin. *Endocrinology.* 1985; 116:1687–1693.

151. Bergner P. Passion flower. *Med Herbalism.* 1995;7:13–14, 26.

152. Flynn J. The herbal management of stress. *Aust J Med Herbalism.* 1996;8:15–18.

153. European Scientific Cooperative on Phytotherapy. *Passiflora Herba/Passiflora: ESCOP Monographs: Fascicule 4.* Exeter, England: European Scientific Cooperative on Phytotherapy; 1997:58.

154. Soulimani R, Younos C, Jarmouni S, Bousta D, Misslin R, Mortier F. Behavioural effects of *Passiflora incarnata* L. and its indole alkaloid and flavonoid derivatives and maltol in the mouse. *J Ethnopharmacol,* 1997;57:11–20.

155. Della Loggia R, Tubaro A, Redaelli C. Evaluation of the activity on the mouse CNS of several plant extracts and a combination of them [in Italian]. *Riv Neurol.* 1981;51:297–310.

156. Speroni E, Minghetti A. Neuropharmacological activity of extracts from *Passiflora incarnata. Planta Med.* 1988;54:488–491.

157. Wolfman C, Viola H, Paladini A, Dajas F, Medina JH. Possible anxiolytic effects of chrysin, a central benzodiazepine receptor ligand isolated from Passiflora coerulea. *Pharmacol Biochem Behav.* 1994;47:1–4.

158. Meier B. *Passiflora incarnata* L. —passion flower: portrait of a medicinal plant. *Q Rev Nat Med.*1985;3:191–202.

159. Aoyagi N, Kimura R, Murata T. Studies on *Passiflora incarnata* dry extract, I: isolation of maltol and pharmacological action of maltol and ethyl maltol. *Chem Pharm Bull.* 1974; 22:1008–1013.

160. Bourin M, Bougerol T, Guitton B, Broutin E. A combination of plant extracts in the treatment of outpatients with adjustment disorder with anxious mood: controlled study versus placebo. *Fundam Clin Pharmacol.* 1997;11:127–132.

161. Smith GW, Chalmers TM, Nuki G. Vasculitis associated with herbal preparation containing *Passiflora* extract. *Br J Rheumatol.* 1993; 32:87–88.

162. Solbakken AM, Rorbakken G, Gundersen T. Nature medicine as intoxicant [in Norwegian]. *Tidsskr Nor Laegeforen.* 1997;117:1140–1141.

163. Foster S, Chongxi Y. *Herbal Emissaries: Bringing Chinese Herbs to the West.* Rochester, Vt: Healing Arts Press; 1992:356.

164. Wren R. *Potter's New Encyclopedia of Botanical Drugs and Preparations.* Saffron Walden, England: CW Daniel Co; 1988:362.

165. De Smet P. Scutellaria species. In: De Smet P, Keller K, Hansel R, Chandler R, eds. *Adverse Effects of Herbal Drugs.* Heidelberg, Germany: Springer-Verlag; 1993:289–296.

166. Perharic L, Shaw D, Colbridge M, House I, Leon C, Murray V. Toxicological problems resulting from exposure to traditional remedies and food supplements. *Drug Safety.* 1994;11:284–294.

167. De Smet P. Notes added in proof. In: De Smet P, Keller K, Hansel R, Chandler R, eds. *Adverse Effects of Herbal Drugs.* Heidelberg, Germany: Springer-Verlag; 1996:229–240.

168. D'Arcy P. Adverse reactions and interactions with herbal medicines, part 2: drug interactions. *Adverse Drug React Toxicol Rev.* 1993;12:147–162.

169. Murray MT. *The Healing Power of Herbs.* Rocklin, Calif: Prima Publishing; 1992:246.

170. Upton R. St. John's wort (*Hypericum perforatum*). In: Upton R, ed. *American Herbal Pharmacopoeia and Therapeutic Compendium.* Santa Cruz, Calif: American Herbal Pharmacopoeia; 1997.

171. Linde K, Ramirez G, Mulrow CD, Pauls A, Weidenhammer W, Melchart D. St John's wort for depression: an overview and meta-analysis of randomised clinical trials [see comments]. *BMJ.* 1996;313:253–258.

172. Volz H-P. Controlled clinical trials of hypericum extracts in depressed patients: an overview. *Pharmacopsychiatry.* 1997;30:72–76.

173. Wagner H, Bladt S. Pharmaceutical quality of hypericum extracts. *J Geriatr Psychiatry Neurol.* 1994;7(suppl 1):S65–S68.

174. Kartnig T, Gobel I, Heydel B. Production of hypericin, pseudohypericin and flavonoids in cell cultures of various *Hypericum* species and their chemotypes. *Planta Med.* 1996;62:51–53.

175. Staffeldt B, Kerb R, Brockmoller J, Ploch M, Roots I. Pharmacokinetics of hypericin and pseudohypericin after oral intake of the hypericum perforatum extract LI 160 in healthy volunteers. *J Geriatr Psychiatry Neurol.* 1994;7(suppl 1):S47–S53.

176. Kerb R, Brockmoller J, Staffeldt B, Ploch M, Roots I. Single-dose and steady-state pharmacokinetics of hypericin and pseudohypericin. *Antimicrob Agents Chemother.* 1996;40:2087–2093.

177. Nahrstedt A, Butterweck V. Biologically active and other chemical constitents of the herb of *Hypericum perforatum* L. *Pharmacopsychiatry.* 1997;30:129–134.

178. Miskovsky P, Sureau F, Chinsky L, Turpin P-Y. Subcellular distribution of hypericin in human cancer cells. *Photochem Photobiol.* 1995;62:546–549.

179. Cott JM. In vitro receptor binding and enzyme inhibition by *Hypericum perforatum* extract. *Pharmacopsychiatry.* 1997;30:108–112.

180. Cott J. NCDEU update: natural product formulations available in Europe for psychotropic indications. *Psychopharmacol Bull.* 1995; 31:745–751.

181. Perovic S, Muller WE. Pharmacological profile of hypericum extract: effect on serotonin uptake by postsynaptic receptors. *Arzneimittelforschung.* 1995;45:1145–1148.

182. Muller WE, Rolli M, Schafer C, Hafner U. Effects of hypericum extract (LI 160) in biochemical models of antidepressant activity. *Pharmacopsychiatry.* 1997;30:102–107.

183. Muller WE, Rossol R. Effects of hypericum extract on the expression of serotonin receptors. *J Geriatr Psychiatry Neurol.* 1994;7(suppl 1):S63–S64.

184. Baureithel KH, Buter KB, Engesser A, Burkard W, Schaffner W. Inhibition of benzodiazepine binding in vitro by amentoflavone, a constituent of various species of 186 *Hypericum. Pharm Acta Helv.* 1997;72:153–157.

185. Von HM, Zoller M. Antidepressive effect of a *Hypericum* extract. *Drug Res.* 1984;34:918–920.

186. Suzuki O, Katsumata Y, Oya M, Bladt S, Wagner H. Inhibition of monoamine oxidase by hypericin. *Planta Med.* 1984;50:272–274.

187. Bladt S, Wagner H. Inhibition of MAO by fractions and constituents of hypericum extract. *J Geriatr Psychiatry Neurol.* 1994;7(suppl 1):S57–S59.

188. Demisch L, Holzl J, Gollnick B, Kacmarczyk P. Identification of MAO-type-A inhibitors in *Hypericum perforatum* L. (Hyperforat). *Pharmacopsychiatry*1989;22:194.

189. Thiede HM, Walper A. Inhibition of MAO and COMT by hypericum extracts and hypericin. *J Geriatr Psychiatry Neurol.* 1994;7(suppl 1):S54–S56.

190. Von SNO, Weischer ML. Experimental animal studies of the psychotropic activity of a Hypericum extract. *Drug Res.* 1987;37:10–13.

191. Ozturk Y. Testing the antidepressant effects of *Hypericum* species on animal models. *Pharmacopsychiatry.* 1997;30:125–128.

192. Butterwick V, Wall A, Lieflander-Wulf U, Winterhoff H, Nahrstedt A. Effects of the total extract and fractions of *Hypericum perforatum* in animal assays for antidepressant activity. *Pharmacopsychiatry.* 1997;30:117–124.

193. Teufel-Mayer R, Gleitz J. Effects of long-term administration of hypericum extracts on the affinity and density of the central serotoninergic 5–HT_{1A} and 5–HT_{2A} receptors. *Pharmacopsychiatry.* 1997;30:113–116.

194. Schulz H, Jobert M. Effects of hypericum extract on the sleep EEG in older volunteers. *J Geriatr Psychiatry Neurol.* 1994;7(suppl 1):S39–S43.

195. Johnson D, Ksciuk H, Woelk H, Sauerwein-Giese E, Frauendorf A. Effects of hypericum extract LI 160 compared with maprotiline on resting EEG and evoked potentials in 24 volunteers. *J Geriatr Psychiatry Neurol.* 1994; 7(suppl 1):S44–S46.

196. De Smet PA, Nolen WA. St John's wort as an antidepressant [see comments]. *BMJ.* 1996; 313:241–242.

197. Jenike MA. Editorial. *J Geriatr Psychiatry Neurol.* 1994;7(suppl 1):S1.

198. Vorbach EU, Arnoldt KH, Hubner W-D. Efficacy and tolerability of St. John's wort extract LI 160 versus imipramine in patients with severe depressive episodes according to ICD-10. *Pharmacopsychiatry*1997;30:81–85.

199. Brockmoller J, Reum T, Bauer S, Kerb R, Hubner W-D, Roots I. Hypericin and pseudohypericin: pharmacokinetics and effects on photosensitivity in humans. *Pharmacopsychiatry.* 1997;30:94–101.

200. Harrer G, Hubner WD, Podzuweit H. Effectiveness and tolerance of the hypericum extract LI 160 compared to maprotiline: a multicenter double-blind study. *J Geriatr Psychiatry Neurol.* 1994;7(suppl 1):S24–S28.

201. Woelk H, Burkard G, Grunwald J. Benefits and risks of the hypericum extract LI 160: drug monitoring study with 3250 patients. *J Geriatr Psychiatry Neurol.* 1994;7:S34–S38.

202. Czekalla J, Gastpar M, Hubner W-D, Jager D. The effect of hypericum extract on cardiac conduction as seen in the electrocardiogram compared to that of imipramine. *Pharmaco-psychiatry.* 1997;30:86–88.

203. Gillis MC, ed. *Compendium of Pharmaceuticals and Specialties.* 31st ed. Ottawa, Ontario: Canadian Pharmaceutical Association; 1998.

204. Holzl J, Godau P. Receptor binding studies with *Valeriana officinalis* on the benzodiazepine receptor. *Planta Med.* 1989;55:642.

205. Mennini T, Bernasconi P, Bombardelli E, Morazzoni P. In vitro study on the interaction of extracts and pure compounds from *Valeriana officinalis* roots with GABA, benzodiazepine and barbiturate receptors in rat brain. *Fitoterapia.* 1993;64:291–300.

206. Cavadas C, Araujo I, Cotrim MD, Amaral T, Cunha AP, Macedo T, Ribeiro CF. In vitro study on the interaction of *Valeriana officinalis* L. extracts and their amino acids on GABAA receptor in rat brain. *Arzneimittelforschung* 1995;45:753–755.

207. Bodesheim U, Holzl J. Isolation and receptor binding properties of alkaloids and lignans from *V. officinalis* L. *Pharmazie.* 1997; 52:386–391.

208. Santos MS, Ferreira F, Faro C, Pires E, Carvalho AP, Cunha AP, Macedo T. The amount of GABA present in aqueous extracts of valerian is sufficient to account for [^{3}H]GABA release in synaptosomes. *Planta Med.* 1994;60:475–476.

209. Santos MS, Ferreira F, Cunha AP, Carvalho AP, Ribeiro CF, Macedo T. Synaptosomal GABA release as influenced by valerian root extract: involvement of the GABA carrier. *Arch Int Pharmacodyn Ther.* 1994;327:220–231.

210. Riedel E, Hansel R, Ehrke G. Inhibition of GABA catabolism by valerenic acid derivatives. *Planta Med.* 1982;46:219–220.

211. *Proposals for a European Monograph on the Medicinal Use of.* Valerianae radix *(Valerian Root).* Brussels, Belgium: European Scientific Cooperative for Phytotherapy; 1990.

212. Holzl J. Baldrian: Ein mittel gegen Schlafstorungen und Nervositat. *Dtsch Apoth Zeitung.* 1996;136:751–759.

213. Hendriks H, Bos R, Woerdenbag HJ, Koster AS. Central nervous system depressant activity of valerenic acid in the mouse. *Planta Med.* 1985;1:28–31.

214. Hendricks H, Bos R, Allersma DP, Malingre TM, Koster AS. Pharmacological screening of valerenal and some other components of essential oil of *Valeriana officinalis. Planta Med.* 1981;42:62–68.

215. Veith J, Schneider G, Lemmer B, Willems M. The influence of some degradation products of valpotriates on the motor activity of light-dark synchronized mice. *Planta Med.* 1986;3:179–183.

216. Wagner H, Jurcic K, Schaette R. Comparative studies on the sedative action of *Valeriana* extracts, valpotriates and their degradation products. *Planta Med.* 1980;36:358–365.

217. Hansel R, Keller K, Rimpler H, Schneider G. Valeriana. In: *Hagers Handbuch der Parmzeutischen Praxis.*5th ed. Berlin, Germany: Springer-Verlag; 1994:1067–1095.

218. Torrent MT, Iglesias J, Adzet T. Valoracion experimental de la actividad sedante de la tinctura de *Valeriana officinalis* L. *Circ Farmaceut.* 1972;30:107–112.

219. Sakamoto T, Mitana Y, Nakajima K. Psychotropic effects of Japanese valerian root extracts. *Chem Pharm Bull.* 1992;40:758–761.

220. Hikino H, Hikino Y, Kobinata H, Aizawa A. Sedative properties of valeriana roots. *Shoyakugako Zasshi.* 1980;34:19–24.

221. Takamura K, Kawaguchi M, Nabata H. The preparation and pharmacological screening of kessoglycol derivative. *Yakugaku Zasshi.* 1975;95:1198–1204.

222. Takamura K, Nabata H, Kawaguchi M. The pharmacological action on the kessoglycol-8–monoacetate. *Yakugaku Zasshi.* 1975;95:1205–1209.

223. Leuschner J, Muller J, Rudmann M. Characterisation of the central nervous depressant activity of a commercially available valerian root extract. *Arzneimittelforschung.* 1993;43:638–641.

224. Hiller K-O, Zetler G. Neuropharmacological studies on ethanol extracts of *Valeriana officinalis* L. behavioural and anticonvulsant properties. *Phytother Res*1996;10:145–151.

225. Oshima Y, Matsuoka S, Ohizumi Y. Antidepressant principles of *Valeriana fauriei* roots. *Chem Pharm Bull.* 1995;43:169–170.

226. Kriegelstein J, Grusla D. Central depressant constituent in valerian [in German]. *Dtsch Apoth Zeitung.* 1988;40:2041–2046.

227. Grusla D, Holzl J, Kriegelstein J. Baldrianwirkungen im Gehirn der Ratte. *Dtsch Apoth Zeitung.* 1986;126:2249–2253.

228. Houghton PJ. The biological activity of valerian and related plants. *J Ethnopharmacol.* 1988;22:121–142.

229. Kohnen R, Oswald WD. The effects of valerian, propanolol, and their combination on activation, performance, and mood of healthy volunteers under social stress conditions. *Pharmacopsychiatry.* 1988;21:447–448.

230. Leathwood PD, Chauffard F, Heck E, Munoz-Box R. Aqueous extract of valerian root (*Valeriana officinalis* L.) improves sleep quality in man. *Pharmacol Biochem Behav.* 1982; 17:65–71.

231. Leathwood PD, Chauffard F. Quantifying the effects of mild sedatives. *J Psychiatr Res.* 1982;17:115–122.

232. Leathwood PD, Chauffard F, Munoz-Box R. Effect of *Valeriana officinalis* L. on subjective and objective sleep parameters. In: *Sixth European Congress on Sleep Research.* Zurich, Switzerland: Basel-Karger; 1983:402–405.

233. Braun R, Dittmar W, Hubner GE, Maurer HR. Influence of valtrate/isovaltrate on the hematopoiesis and metabolic liver activity in mice in vivo. *Plant Med.* 1984;1:1–4.

234. Balderer G, Borbely AA. Effect of valerian on human sleep. *Psychopharmacology.* 1985; 87:406–409.

235. Schulz H, Stolz C, Muller J. The effect of valerian extract on sleep polygraphy in poor sleepers: a pilot study. *Pharmacopsychiatry.* 1994; 27:147–151.

236. McGregor FB, Abernethy VE, Dahabra S, Cobden I, Hayes PC. Hepatotoxicity of herbal remedies. *BMJ.* 1989;299:1156–1157.

237. Shepherd C. Sleep disorders: liver damage warning with insomnia remedy. *BMJ.* 1993;306:1472.

238. Bos R, Woerdenbag HJ, De Smet PAGM, Scheffer JJC. *Valeriana* species. In: De Smet PAGM, Keller K, Hansel R, Chandler RF, eds. *Adverse Effects of Herbal Drugs* Berlin, Germany: Springer-Verlag; 1997:165–180.

239. Keochanthala-Bounthanh C, Haag-Berrurier M, Beck JP, Anton R. Effects of thiol compounds versus cytotoxicity of valpotriates on cultured hepatoma cells. *Plant Med.* 1990;56:190–192.

240. Keochanthala-Bounthanh C, Beck JP, Haag-Berrurier M, Anton R. Effects of two monoterpene esters, valtrate and didrovaltrate, isolated from *Valeriana wallichii,* on the ultrastructure of hepatoma cells in culture. *Phytother Res.* 1993;7:124–127.

241. Tufik S, Fujita K, Seabra MDL, Lobo LL. Effects of a prolonged administration of valepotriates in rats on the mothers and their offspring. *J Ethnopharmacol.* 1994;41:39–44.

242. Berglund F, Flodh H, Lundborg P, Prame B, Sannerstedt R. Drug use during pregnancy and lactation: a classification for drug information. *Acta Obstet Gynecol Scand Suppl.* 1984;126:1–55.

243. Committee ADE. *Medicines in Pregnancy: An Australian Categorization of Risk.* Canberra, Australia: Australian Government Publishing Service; 1989.

244. Shrivastava SC, Sisodia CS. Analgetic studies on *Vitax negundo* and *Valeriana wallichii. Ind Vet J.* 1970;47:170–175.

245. Takamura K, Kakimoto M, Kawaguchi M, Iwasaki T. Pharmacological studies on the constituents of crude drugs and plants. *J Pharm Soc Jpn.* 1973;93:599–606.

246. Govindarajan VS. Capsicum—production, technology, chemistry, and quality, I: history, botany, cultivation and primary processing. *CRC Crit Rev Food Sci Nutr.* 1985;22:109–176.

247. Cordell GA, Araujo OE. Capsaicin: identification, nomenclature, and pharmacotherapy. *Ann Pharmacother.* 1993;27:330–336.

248. Jentzsch K, Pock H, Kubelka W. Isolation of dihydrocapsaicin and homodihydrocapsaicin form *Capsicum* fruits. *Monatsch Chem.* 1968;99:661–663.

249. Locock RA. Capsicum. *Can Pharm J.* 1985; 118:517–519.

250. Skofitsch G, Donnerer J, Lembeck F. Comparison of nonivamide and capsaicin with regard to their pharmacokinetics and effects on sensory neurons. *Arzneimittelforschung.* 1984;34:154–156.

251. Szolesanyi J. Capsaicin, irritation, and desensitization. In: Green BG, Mason JR, Kare MR, eds. *Chemical Senses.* New York, NY: Marcel Dekker; 1990:14–76.

252. Lynn B. Capsaicin: actions on nociceptive C-fibres and therapeutic potential. *Pain.* 1990; 41:61–69.

253. Anonymous. Treatment of painful diabetic neuropathy with topical capsaicin: a multicentre, double-blind, vehicle-controlled study. *Arch Intern Med.* 1991;151:2225–2229.

254. Tandan R, Lewis GA, Krusinski PB, Badger GB, Fries TJ. Topical capsaicin in painful diabetic neuropathy: controlled study with long term follow-up. *Diabetes Care.* 1992;15:8–14.

255. Dailey GE. Effect of treatment with capsaicin on daily activities of patients with diabetic neuropathy. *Diabetes Care.* 1992;15:159–165.

256. Scheffler NM, Sheitel PL, Lipton MN. Treatment of painful diabetic neuropathy with capsaicin 0.075%. *J Am Podiatr Med Assoc.* 1991;81:288–293.

257. Basha KM, Whitehouse FW. Capsaicin: a therapeutic option for painful diabetic neuropathy. *Henry Ford Hosp Med J.* 1991; 39:138–140.

258. Pfeifer MA, Ross DR, Schrage JP, Gelber DA, Schumer MP, Crain GM, Markwell SJ, Jung S. A highly successful and novel model for treatment of chronic painful diabetic peripheral neuropathy. *Diabetes Care.* 1993;16:1103–1115.

259. Watson CP, Evans RJ, Watt VR. Post-herpetic neuralgia and topical capsaicin. *Pain.* 1988;35:289–297.

260. Watson CPN, Evans RJ, Watt VR, Birkett N. Post-herpetic neuralgia: 208 cases. *Pain.* 1988;35:289–297.

261. Bernstein JE, Korman NJ, Bickers DR, Dahl MV, Millikan LE. Topical capsaicin treatment of chronic postherpetic neuralgia. *J Am Acad Dermatol.* 1989;21:265–270.

262. Bernstein JE, Bickers DR, Dahl MV, Roshal JY. Treatment of chronic postherpetic neuralgia with topical capsaicin: a preliminary study. *J Am Acad Dermatol.* 1987;17:93–96.

263. Peikert A, Hentrich M, Ochs G. Topical 0.025% capsaicin in chronic post-herpetic neuralgia: efficacy, predictors of response and long-term course. *J Neurol.* 1991;238:452–456.

264. Bjerring P, Arendt-Nielsen L, Soderberg U. Argon laser induced cutaneous sensory and pain thresholds in post-herpetic neuralgia: quantitative modulation by topical capsaicin. *Acta Derm Venereol.* 1990;70:121–125.

265. Watanabe T, Kawada T, Yamamoto M, Iwgi K. Capsaicin, a pungent principle of hot red pepper, evokes catecholamine secretion from the adrenal medulla of anesthetized rats. *Biochem Biophys Res Commun.* 1987;142:259–264.

266. Du Mee C. Vitex *Agnus castus. Aust J Med Herbalism.* 1993;5:63–65.

267. Houghton P. *Agnus castus. Pharm J.* 1994; 253:720–721.

268. Bruckner C. In mitteleuropa genutze heilpflanzen mit milchsekretionsfordernder wirkung (galactagoga). *Gleditschia.* 1989;17:189–210.

269. Milewicz A, Gejdel E, Sworen H, Sienkiewicz K, Jedrzejak J, Teucher T, Schmitz H. Vitex *Agnus-castus* extract in the treatment of luteal phase defects due to latent hyperprolactinemia: results of a randomised placebo-controlled double-blind study. *Arzneimittelforschung Drug Res.* 1993;43:752–756.

270. Bohnert K-J. The use of Vitex *Agnus castus* for hyperprolactinemia. *Q Rev Nat Med.* Spring 1997:19–21.

271. Jarry H, Leonhardt S, Gorkow C, Wuttke W. In vitro prolactin but not LSH and FSH release is inhibited by compounds in extracts of *Agnus castus:* direct evidence for a dopaminergic principle by the dopamine receptor assay. *Exp Clin Endocrinol.* 1994;102:448–454.

272. Sliutz G, Speiser P, Schultz A, Spona J, Zellinger R. *Agnus castus* extracts inhibit prolactin secretion of rat pituitary cells. *Horm Metab.* 1993;25:253–255.

273. Jarry H, Leonhardt S, Wuttke W. *Agnus castus* as dopaminergous effective principle in mastoynon N. *Z Phytother.* 1991;12:77–82.

274. Farnsworth NR, Kinghorn AD, Soejarto D, Waller DP. Siberian ginseng (*Eleuthrococcus senticosus*): current status as an adaptogen. In: Wagner H, Hikino H, Farnsworth NR, eds. *Economic and Medicinal Plant Research.* Orlando, Fla: Academic Press; 1985:155–215.

275. Leung AY. *Encyclopedia of Common Natural Ingredients Used in Food, Drugs and Cosmetics.* New York, NY: John Wiley & Sons Inc; 1980.

276. Baldwin CA, Anderson LA, Phillipson JD. What pharmacists should know about ginseng. *Pharm J.* November 8, 1986:583–586.

277. Medon PJ, Ferguson PW, Watson CF. Effects of Eleutherococcus senticosus extracts on hexobarbital metabolism in vivo and in vitro. *J Ethnopharmacol.* 1984;10:235–241.

278. Chang H-M, But PP-H. *Pharmacology and Applications of Chinese Materia Medica.* Singapore, Republic of China: World Scientific Press; 1986.

279. Teegarden R. *Chinese Tonic Herbs.* New York, NY: Japan Publishing Inc; 1985:197.

280. Bensky D, Gamble A. *Chinese Herbal Medicine Materia Medica.* Seattle, Wash: Eastland Press; 1986.

281. Avakia EV, Evonuk E. Effects of panax ginseng extract on tissue glycogen and adrenal cholesterol depeletion during prolonged exercise. *Planta Med.* 1979;36:43–48.

282. Fulder SJ. Ginseng and the hypothalamic-pituitary control of stress. *Am J Chin Med.* 1981;9:112–118.

283. Wagner H, Norr H, Winterhoff H. Plant adaptogens. *Phytomedicine.* 1994;1:63–76.

284. Hiai S, Yokoyama H, Oura H. Features of ginseng saponin-induced corticosterone secretion. *Endocrinol Jpn.* 1979;26:737–740.

285. Scaglione F, Cattaneo G, Alessandria M, Cogo R. Efficacy and safety of the standardised ginseng extract G115 for potentiating vaccination against the influenza syndrome and protection against the common cold [published correction appears in *Drugs Exp Clin Res.* 1996;22:338]. *Drugs Exp Clin Res.* 1996;22:65–72.

286. Sonnenborn U, Hansel R, De Smit PAGM. *Adverse Effects of Herbal Drugs.* Berlin, Germany: Springer Verlag; 1992.

287. Siegel RK. Ginseng abuse syndrome. *JAMA.* 1979;241:1644–1645.

288. Shader RI, Greenblat DJ. Phenelzine and the dream machine: ramblings and reflections. *J Clin Psychopharmacol.* 1985;5:65.

289. Shader RI, Greenblatt DJ. Bees, ginseng and MAOIs revisited. *J Clin Psychopharmacol.* 1988;8:235.

290. Jones BD, Runikis AM. Interaction of ginseng with phenelzine. *J Psychopharmacol.* 1987;7:201–202.

291. Mitra SK, Chakraborti A, Bhattacharya SK. Neuropharmacological studies on *Panax ginseng. Indian J Exp Biol.* 1996;34:41–47.

292. De Smet PAGM, Keller K, Hansel R, Chandler R. *Adverse Effects of Herbal Drugs.* Berlin, Germany: Springer, Verlag; 1997:250.

293. Lambert GA, Lang WJ, Friedman E, Meller E, Gershon S. Pharmacological and biochemical properties of isomeric yohimbine alkaloids. *Eur J Pharmacol.* 1978;49:39–48.

294. Morales A, Condra M, Owen JA, Surridge DH, Fenemore J, Harris C. Is yohimbine effective in the treatment of organic impotence? results of a controlled trial. *J Urol.*1987;137:1168–1172.

295. Susset JG, Tessier CD, Wincze J, Bansal S, Malhotra C, Schwacha MG. Effect of yohimbine hydrochloride on erectile impotence: a double-blind study. *J Urol.* 1989;141:1360–1363.

296. Holmeberg G, Gershon S. Autonomic and psychic effects of yohimbine hydrochloride. *Psychopharmacologia.* 1961;2:93–106.

297. Charney DS, Woods SW, Goodman WK, Heninger GR. Neurobiological mechanisms of panic anxiety: biochemical and behavioural correlates of yohimbine-induced panic attacks. *Am J Psychiatry.* 1987;144:1030–1036.

298. Charney DS, Woods SW, Krystal JH, Nagy LM, Heninger GR. Noradrenergic neuronal dysregulation in panic disorder: the effects of intravenous yohimbine and clonidine in panic disorder patients. *Acta Psychiatr Scand.* 1992;86:273–282.

299. Rasmusson AM, Southwick SM, Hauger RL, Charney DS. Plasma neuropeptide Y (NPY) increases in humans in response to the alpha 2 antagonist yohimbine. *Neuropsychopharmacology.* 1998;19:95–98.

300. Price LH, Charney DS, Heninger GR. Three cases of manic symptoms following yohimbine administration. *Am J Psychiatry.* 1984;141:1267–1268.

301. Dunn RW, Corbett R. Yohimbine-induced seizures involve NMDA and GABAergic transmission. *Neuropharmacology.* 1992; 31:389–395.

302. Charney D, Heninger G, Breier A. Noradrenergic function in panic anxiety: effects of yohimbine in healthy subjects and patients with agoraphobia and panic disorder. *Arch Gen Psychiatry.* 1984;41:751–763.

303. De Smet P, Smeets O. Potential risks of health food products containing yohimbe extracts. *BMJ.* 1994;309:958.

45 Horse-Chestnut Seed Extract for Chronic Venous Insufficiency

A Criteria-Based Systematic Review

Max H. Pittler, MD; Edzard Ernst, MD, PhD, FRCP(Edin)
From the Department of Complementary Medicine, School of Postgraduate Medicine and Health Sciences, University of Exeter, Exeter, United Kingdom.

Objective

To assess the evidence for or against horse-chestnut seed extract (HCSE) as a symptomatic treatment of chronic venous insufficiency (CVI).

Data Sources

Computerized literature searches were performed in MEDLINE, EMBASE, BIOSIS, CISCOM, and the Cochrane Library (all from their respective institution to December 1996). The search terms were "horse chestnut," *"Aesculus hippocastanum,"* "escin," and *"Rosskastanie"* (German for "horse chestnut"). There were no restrictions on the language of publication.

Study Selection

Double-blind, randomized controlled trials of oral HCSE for patients with CVI were included. Identifiers were removed from all publications before assessment.

Data Extraction

Data were extracted in a standardized, predefined manner. Trial outcomes and the methodological quality of each trial were independently assessed by the 2 reviewers.

Data Synthesis

The superiority of HCSE is suggested by all placebo-controlled studies. The use of HCSE is associated with a decrease of the lower-leg volume and a reduction in leg circumference at the calf and ankle. Symptoms such as leg pain, pruritus, and a feeling of fatigue and tenseness are reduced. Five comparative trials against the reference medication indicate that HCSE and *O*-(β-hydroxyethyl)-rutosides are equally effective. One trial suggests a therapeutic equivalence of HCSE and compression therapy. Adverse effects are usually mild and infrequent.

Conclusions

These data imply that HCSE is superior to placebo and as effective as reference medications in alleviating the objective signs and subjective symptoms of CVI. Thus, HCSE represents a treatment option for CVI that is worth considering.

Arch Dermatol. 1998;134:1356–1360

With a prevalence of 10% to 15% in men and 20% to 25% in women, chronic venous insufficiency (CVI) is among the most common conditions afflicting humans.[1,2] It is more than a mere "cosmetic problem" because patients often require hospital admission and surgical treatment. At least two thirds of leg ulcers have evidence of venous disease in the affected limb.[2] The burden of suffering is high, and the economic costs for society are considerable. Although the therapy of choice is mechanical compression,[3] compliance is often poor, which renders oral drug treatment an attractive option.

Horse chestnut (*Aesculus hippocastanum*) is an herbal remedy traditionally used for CVI.[4] Horse-chestnut seed extract (HCSE), the active component of which is escin, a triterpenic saponin,[5–7] has shown enzyme-inhibiting activity.[8] The accumulation of leukocytes in CVI-affected limbs[9,10] with their subsequent activation[11] is considered an important pathophysiological mechanism of CVI. Horse-chestnut seed extract may work by preventing leukocyte activation.[8] Regardless of the postulated mechanism of action, the most important question concerns HCSE's clinical effectiveness. Our aim in this systematic review is to summarize the evidence from randomized controlled trials (RCTs) for or against the effectiveness of HCSE in the symptomatic treatment of CVI.

Trials and Methods

Computerized literature searches were performed to identify all RCTs of HCSE for CVI. Databases included MEDLINE, EMBASE, BIOSIS, CISCOM, and the Cochrane Library (on CD-ROM; available from the Cochrane Collaboration) (all from their respective institution to December 1996). The search terms used were "horse chestnut," "*Aesculus hippocastanum*," "escin," and "*Rosskastanie*" (German for "horse chestnut"). All manufacturers of HCSE preparations were asked to contribute published and unpublished material, and our own extensive files were scanned. The bibliographies of the studies thus retrieved were searched for further trials. There were no restrictions on the language of publication.

Identifiers of all publications were concealed by eliminating (by a person not involved in the review) the names of the author(s), journal, and institution before assessment. Trial outcomes and the methodological quality of each trial were independently assessed by both of us using a standard scoring system to measure the likelihood of bias[12] (Table 1). Disagreements in the evaluation of individual trials were resolved by discussion. Randomized controlled trials were included if performed on patients with CVI treated with HCSE monopreparations and if conducted double blind against placebo or the reference medication. Articles scoring below 3 (maximum, 5) points on the quality scale[12] were excluded. A meta-analysis of trial results for leg-volume assessment in placebo-controlled RCTs had initially been planned. Because of variations in devices used for assessment and insufficient reporting of data, this plan had to be abandoned.

Table 1. Scoring System to Measure the Likelihood of Bias*

1. Study described as randomized (this includes the use of words such as "random," "randomly," and "randomization")?
2. Study described as double blind?
3. Description of withdrawls and dropouts?
4. Method to generate the sequence of randomization described and appropriate (table of random numbers, computer generated, etc)?
5. Method of double blinding described and appropriate (identical placebo, active placebo, dummy, etc)?
6. Method to generate the sequence of randomization described and inappropriate (patients were allocated alternately or according to their date of birth, hospital number, etc).
7. Method of double blinding described and inappropriate (eg, comparison of tablet vs injection with no double dummy).

*Adapted from Jadad et al.[12] For questions 1 through 5, each yes answer equals 1 point, and each no answer equals 0 points. Deduct 1 point if question 6 or 7 apply.

Results

Sixteen RCTs were retrieved.[13–28] Relevant unpublished trials were not found. Three studies had to be excluded from this review, 2[13,14] because they were duplicate publications and 1[15] because it was not conducted with an HCSE monopreparation. Thirteen studies[16–28] fulfilled the inclusion-exclusion criteria. Eight of these[16–23] were placebo controlled, and 5[24–28] were controlled against reference medications. All trials scored at least 3 of 5 points on a standard scoring system to measure the likelihood of bias.[12] Two trials[16,17] scored 5 points on this scale, suggesting the superiority of the use of HCSE over placebo for the symptomatic treatment of CVI. Table 2 summarizes key data of all included trials ranked in a hierarchical order according to their methodological quality score.

The placebo-controlled RCTs suggest a decrease in lower-leg volume and a reduction in leg circumference at the calf and ankle with the use of HCSE. Edema provocation before and after the treatment period revealed protective effects against edema. A decrease of the capillary filtration rate by 22% in HCSE-treated patients was suggested.[17] The

Table 2. Double-blind Randomized Controlled Trials (RCTs) of Horse-Chestnut Seed Extract (HCSE) for Chronic Venous Insufficiency (CVI)*

Reference	Quality Score (Maximum 5)	Study Design	No. of Patients Entered/ No. of Dropouts	Medication (Dosage)	Treatment Period	Compliance Monitored/ ADRs Mentioned
Placebo-Controlled RCTs						
Rudofsky et al,[16] 1986	5	2 Parallel groups	40/1	HCSE (1 capsule twice a day)†	4 wk	Yes/Yes
Bisler et al,[17] 1986	5	Crossover	24/2	HCSE (2 capsules once a day)†	NA	NA/No
Pilz,[18] 1990	4	2 Parallel groups	30/2	HCSE (1 capsule twice a day)†	20 d	No/Yes
Diehm et al,[19] 1992	4	2 Parallel groups	40/1	HCSE (1 capsule twice a day)‡	6 wk	No/No
Friederich et al,[20] 1978	4	Crossover	118/23	HCSE (1 capsule twice a day)	20 d	No/Yes
Lohr et al,[21] 1986	3	2 Parallel groups	80/6	HCSE (1 capsule twice a day)	8 wk	No/Yes
Neiss and Böhm,[22] 1976	3	Crossover	233/7	HCSE (1 capsule twice a day)†	20 d	No/Yes
Steiner,[23] 1990	3	Crossover	20/NR	HCSE (1 capsule twice a day)†	2 wk	No/Yes
RCTs Against Reference Medications						
Kalbfleisch and Pfalzgraf,[24] 1989	4	2 Parallel groups	33/3	HCSE (1 capsule once a day), HR (500 mg/d)†	8 wk	No/No
Rehn et al,[25] 1996	4	3-Armed parallel groups	155/18	HCSE (1 capsule twice a day), HR (1000 mg/d [loading dose for 4 wk, then 500 mg/d [for 8 wk])†	12 wk	Yes/Yes
Diehm et al,[26] 1996	3	3-Armed parallel groups	240/NR	HCSE (1 capsule twice a day†); (compression therapy/ placebo)	12 wk	Yes/Yes
Erdlen,[27] 1989	3	2 Parallel groups	30/NR	HCSE (1 capsule twice a day)†§	4 wk	No/No
Erler,[28] 1991	3	2 Parallel groups	40/NR	HCSE (1 capsule twice a day), HR (2000 mg/d)‡	8 wk	No/No
Total			**1083/63‖**			

*ADRs indicate adverse drug reactions; NA, not applicable; CFC, capillary filtration coefficient; NR, not reported; and HR, O-(β-hydroxyethyl)-rutosides. Verum is equivalent to HCSE.
†Standardized to 50 mg of escin.
‡Standardized to 75 mg of escin.
§Reference medication was not defined.
‖Not all trials reported the number of withdrawals or dropouts.

prevalence of symptoms such as leg pain, pruritus, and the feeling of fatigue and tenseness was reduced. All 5 RCTs against reference medications demonstrated evidence for the effectiveness of HCSE for the treatment of CVI.

Although in 1 study,[28] HCSE was stated to be superior to *O*-(β-hydroxyethyl)-rutosides in protecting against edema, most trials suggest that both drugs are of equal value. One trial[26] suggests a therapeutic equivalence of HCSE and

Table 2. *(continued)*

Main End Point	Main Result
Placebo-Controlled RCTs	
Leg volume	Significant (*P*<.001) reduction by 44 mL (verum) compared with 34 mL (placebo)
CFC	Significant (*P*=.006) reduction by 22% (verum) compared with placebo
Leg circumference at ankle	Significant (*P*<.05) reduction of 0.8 cm (verum) compared with 0.1 cm (placebo) at ankle
Leg volume	Significant (*P*<.01) reduction of 84 mL (verum) compared with baseline, while reduction of 4 mL with placebo
CVI-related symptoms	Significant (*P*<.05) reduction of calf spasm, pain, fatigue, and tenseness on verum compared with placebo
Leg volume	Leg-volume reduction of 16.5 mL (verum) and 3.8 mL (placebo) (*P* value NR)
CVI-related symptoms	Significant (*P*<.05) reduction of edema, leg pain, and pruritus on verum compared with placebo
Leg volume	Significant (*P*=.009) reduction by 114 mL (verum) compared with 1 mL (placebo)
RCTs Against Reference Medications	
Leg circumference at ankle and calf	Reduction by 0.2 and 0.18 cm at ankle and calf, respectively (HCSE); values were not significantly different compared with HR
Leg volume	Significant (*P* value NR) reduction of 28 mL (HCSE), 58 mL (HR, 1000 mg/d), and 40 mL (HR, 1000 mg/d [loading dose for 4 wk, then 500 mg/d [for 8 wk]) compared with baseline
Logarithmically transformed leg volume	Reduction of 43.8 mL, 46.7 mL, and –9.8 mL in HCSE, compression therapy, and placebo groups, respectively; HCSE and compression vs placebo (*P*=.005); equivalence of HCSE compared with compression therapy (*P*=.001)
Minimal ankle circumference	Significant (*P* value NR) reduction by 0.4 cm (verum) compared with baseline; reduction of 0.4 cm (rutosides)
Leg circumference (calf, ankle) before and after edema provocation	Significant (*P* value NR) edema protective effects at calf and ankle with HCSE compared with baseline

compression therapy. This trial was not properly blinded, however, so its results are subject to bias.

Significant beneficial effects for patients with CVI are reported in trials that administered HCSE standardized to 100 to 150 mg of escin per day. Two studies[16,23] assessing the use of 100 mg of escin per day found a significant (*P*<.001 and *P*=.009, respectively) reduction of mean leg volumes after 2 weeks of treatment compared with placebo. The persistence of treatment effects is suggested by 1 study.[25] At the end of a 6-week follow-up, the mean leg volume was not significantly different from posttreatment values. Most studies used the classification system by Widmer and Stähelin[29] for categorizing patients and defining inclusion criteria (stage I: ankle edema without trophic changes; stage II: edema, hyperpigmented or depigmented areas, indurations; stage III: open or healed leg ulcer). Because no universally accepted classification of CVI exists to date, this seems the best available.[1] Eleven trials[16–20,23–28] used criteria of this classification system for including patients with CVI. Of the 1083 studied patients, 388 (35.8%) were categorized into CVI stages I to II. Three studies[17,20,26] included patients with stages I to III. Two trials,[21,22] comprising 29% of the studied patients, did not refer to this classification. The placebo response in trials assessing subjective variables as the main end point[20,22] ranged from 20% to 27%. Changes of objective variables during placebo use are summarized in Table 2.

Eight studies[16,18,20–23,25,26] reported on adverse drug reactions (ADRs). Gastrointestinal tract symptoms, dizziness, nausea, headache, and pruritus were reported. The reported frequency of ADRs ranged from 0.9% to 3.0%. In 3 studies,[18,21,23] the frequency of ADRs was not significantly different from that of placebo.

Comment

This criteria-based, systematic review suggests that HCSE is an effective therapy for CVI. Experts from Europe and the United States,[30,31] however, remain unconvinced of its effectiveness for this condition. Herbal medicine is clearly more accepted in German-speaking countries than in England or the United States. Thus, it is not surprising that most of the studies are published by German authors. This may be 1 reason why this treatment option has gone unappreciated by English-speaking clinicians.

Even though our search strategy was comprehensive, that some trials have been missed cannot be entirely ruled out. Trials with negative results have a tendency to remain unpublished.[32] In particular, in journals of complementary or alternative medicine, studies with positive findings may be overrepresented.[33] The results of these trials might conceivably be biased and, thus, present a false-positive picture. All trials scored at least 3 of 5 points on a scale assessing the likelihood of bias (Table 1).[12] Two studies[16,17] reporting that HCSE was superior to placebo scored the maximum of 5 points. Despite this, none of the studies were completely flawless. Thus, the uncertain quality of the original data might be another source of bias. Future trials of CVI should be executed and reported in a uniform manner to enable subsequent statistical pooling in meta-analyses. Attention must be paid to the control of patient compliance, and the assessment of venous function would require standardization.[34] Randomization and double-blinding procedures should be detailed in the published reports. Finally, carryover effects in crossover studies need to be taken into account.[25]

If, despite these caveats, HCSE is accepted as effective therapy for CVI, its mechanism of action may be of interest. The active component of HCSE is the saponin escin.[5] It has been shown in vitro to inhibit the activity of elastase and hyaluronidase, both involved in the enzymatic proteoglycan degradation, which constitutes part of the capillary endothelium and is the main component of the extravascular matrix.[8] Other studies[9,10] have shown increased levels of leukocytes in CVI-affected limbs and suggest a possible subsequent activation with the release of such enzymes.[11] An earlier study[35] found increased serum activity of proteoglycan hydrolases in patients with CVI that was reduced with the use of HCSE. Treatment with HCSE may shift the equilibrium between the degradation and synthesis of proteoglycans toward a net synthesis, thus preventing vascular leakage. This hypothesis has been supported by a study of animals[36]; using electromicroscopy, it demonstrated a marked reduction in vascular leakage after treatment with HCSE. Uncertainty exists about the effects of HCSE on venous tone. In vitro, HCSE increases the venous pressure of normal and pathologically altered veins. This is corroborated by studies of laboratory animals that demonstrate an increase in venous pressure and venous flow after HCSE administration.[6] Studies[16,17] of humans, however, have failed to replicate effects on venous capacity.

The conservative treatment of CVI comprises a variety of other modalities. Compression therapy improves venous return and is widely accepted as the treatment of choice.[37] In combination with heparin, it prevents venous stasis and reduces the risk of deep-vein thrombosis. The use of *O*-(β-hydroxyethyl)-rutosides has beneficial short-term effects by reducing edema and relieving symptoms of CVI. Its efficacy during long-term use has yet to be established, however.[38] The extract of *Ruscus aculeatus* decreases the capillary filtration rate in healthy volunteers and patients with CVI.[39] One recent review[40] concludes that combined treatment with edema protective agents and compression therapy has a better clinical benefit than either treatment alone.

Pruritus, nausea, gastrointestinal tract symptoms, headache, and dizziness were reported as ADRs to HCSE. In 3 studies,[18,21,23] the frequency of ADRs with HCSE use was not significantly different from that with placebo. In a recent observational study[41] involving more than 5000 patients with CVI, ADRs occurred in 0.6% of patients during treatment with HCSE. Gastrointestinal tract symptoms and calf spasm were reported most frequently. Adverse drug reactions are also reported from other symptomatic treatment options for CVI. Those of Ruscus extract include gastrointestinal tract symptoms and nausea, and ingesting *O*-(β-hydroxyethyl)-rutosides can cause allergic skin reactions.[42] About a third of Scottish surgeons reported[43] at least 1 case of skin necrosis or ulcers induced by compression therapy. These cumulative data imply that HCSE use is relatively safe.

Conclusions

The evidence presented here implies that HCSE is safe and effective as a symptomatic, short-term treatment of CVI. Publication bias and methodological shortcomings are important caveats. More rigorous RCTs are required to verify the usefulness of the treatment, especially for long-term use and as an adjunct to compression therapy.

References

1. Callam MJ. Epidemiology of varicose veins. *Br J Surg.* 1994;81:167–173.

2. Callam M. Prevalence of chronic leg ulceration and severe chronic venous disease in western countries. *Phlebologie.* 1992;7(suppl 1):6–12.

3. Partsch H. Compression therapy of the legs. *J Dermatol Surg Oncol.* 1991;17:799–805.

4. Bombardelli E, Morazzoni P, Griffini A. *Aesculus hippocastanum* L. *Fitoterapia.* 1996;57:483–511.

5. Lorenz D, Marek ML. Das therapeutische wirksame prinzip der rosskastanie (*Aesculus hippocastanum*). *Arzneimittelforschung.* 1960; 10:263–272.

6. Guillaume M, Padioleau F. Veinotonic effect, vascular protection, antiinflammatory and free radical scavenging properties of horse chestnut extract. *Arzneimittelforschung.* 1994; 44:25–35.

7. Schrader E, Schwankl W, Sieder CH, Christoffel V. Vergleichende untersuchung zur bioverfügbarkeit von β-aescin nach oraler einmalverabreichung zweier rosskastaniensamenextrakt enthaltender, galenisch unterschiedlicher darreichungsformen. *Pharmazie.* 1995;50:623–627.

8. Facino RM, Carini M, Stefani R, Aldini G, Saibene L. Anti-elastase and anti-hyaluronidase activities of saponins and sapogenins from *Hedera helix, Aesculus hippocastanum,* and *Ruscus aculeatus:* factors contributing to their efficacy in the treatment of venous insufficiency. *Arch Pharm* (Weinheim). 1995;328:720–724.

9. Moyses C, Cederholm-Williams SA, Michel CC. Haemoconcentration and accumulation of white cells in the feet during venous stasis. *Int J Microcir Clin Exp.* 1987;5:311–320.

10. Thomas PR, Nash GB, Dormandy JA. White cell accumulation in dependent legs of patients with venous hypertension: a possible mechanism for trophic changes in the skin. *BMJ.* 1988;296:1693–1695.

11. Sarin S, Andaz A, Shields DA, Scurr JH, Coleridge Smith PD. Neutrophil activation in venous disease. *J Vasc Surg.* 1993;17:444.

12. Jadad AR, Moore A, Carroll D, et al. Assessing the quality of reports of randomized clinical trials: is blinding necessary? *Control Clin Trials.* 1996; 17:1–12.

13. Pauschinger P. Klinisch experimentelle untersuchungen zur wirkung von roßkastaniensamenextrakt auf die transkapilläre filtration und das intravasale volumen an patienten mit chronisch venöser insuffizienz. *Phlebol Proktol.* 1987;16:57–61.

14. Steiner M. Ausmaß der ödemprotektiven wirkung von roßkastaniensamenextrakt. *Vasa.* 1991;20(suppl 33):217.

15. Dustmann HO, Godolias G, Seibel K. Verminderung des fußvolumens bei der chronischen venösen insuffizienz im stehversuch durch eine neue wirkstoffkombination. *Therapiewoche.* 1984;34:5077–5086.

16. Rudofsky G, Neiß A, Otto K, Seibel K. Ödemprotektive wirkung und klinische wirksamkeit von roßkastaniensamenextrakt im doppeltblindversuch. *Phlebol Proktol.* 1986;15:47–54.

17. Bisler H, Pfeifer R, Klüken N, Pauschinger P. Wirkung von roßkastaniensamenextrakt auf die transkapilläre filtration bei chronisch venöser insuffizienz [Effects of horse-chestnut seed extract on transcapillary filtration in chronic venous insufficiency]. *Dtsch Med Wochenschr.* 1986; 111:1321–1329.

18. Pilz E. Ödeme bei venenerkrankungen. *Med Welt.* 1990;40:1143–1144.

19. Diehm C, Vollbrecht D, Amendt K, Comberg HU. Medical edema protection: clinical benefit in patients with chronic deep vein incompetence: a placebo controlled double blind study. *Vasa.* 1992;21:188–191.

20. Friederich HC, Vogelsberg H, Neiss A. Ein beitrag zur bewertung von intern wirksamen venenpharmaka. *Z Hautkr.* 1978;53:369–374.

21. Lohr E, Garanin G, Jesau P, Fischer H. Ödempräventive therapie bei chronischer veneninsuffizienz mit ödemneigung. *MMW Munch Med Wochenschr.* 1986;128:59–81.

22. Neiss A, Böhm C. Zum Wirksamkeitsnachweis von roßkastaniensamenextrakt beim varikösen symptomenkomplex. *MMW Munch Med Wochenschr.* 1976;118:213–216.

23. Steiner M. Untersuchungen zur ödemvermindernden und ödemprotektiven wirkung von roßkastaniensamenextrakt. *Phlebol Proktol.* 1990;19:239–242.

24. Kalbfleisch W, Pfalzgraf H. Ödemprotektiva: äquipotente dosierung: roßkastaniensamenextrakt und O-β-hydroxyethylrutoside im vergleich. *Therapiewoche.* 1989;39:3703–3707.

25. Rehn D, Unkauf M, Klein P, Jost V, Lücker PW. Comparative clinical efficacy and tolerability of oxerutins and horse chestnut extract in patients with chronic venous insufficiency. *Arzneimittelforschung.* 1996;46:483–487.

26. Diehm C, Trampisch HJ, Lange S, Schmidt C. Comparison of leg compression stocking and oral horse-chestnut seed extract therapy in patients with chronic venous insufficiency. *BMJ.* 1996;347:292–294.

27. Erdlen F. Klinische wirksamkeit von venostasin retard im doppelblindversuch. *Med Welt.* 1989;40:994–996.

28. Erler M. Roßkastaniensamenextrakt bei der therapie peripherer venöser ödeme: ein klinischer therapievergleich. *Med Welt.* 1991; 42:593–596.

29. Widmer LK, Stähelin HB. *Peripheral Venous Disorders.* Bern, Switzerland: Hans Huber; 1978.

30. Kelley WN. *Textbook of Internal Medicine.* 2nd ed. Philadelphia, Pa: JB Lippincott; 1992.

31. Kappert A. *Lehrbuch und Atlas der Angiologie.* 12th ed. Bern, Switzerland: Hans Huber; 1989.

32. Easterbrook PJ, Berlin JA, Gopalan R, Matthews DR. Publication bias in clinical research. *BMJ.* 1991;337:867–872.

33. Ernst E, Pittler MH. Alternative therapy bias [letter]. *Nature.* 1997;385:480.

34. Vayssairat M, Debure C, Maurel A, Gaitz JP. Horse-chestnut seed extract for chronic venous insufficiency [letter]. *BMJ.* 1996;347:1182.

35. Kreysel HW, Nissen HP, Enghofer E. Erhöhte serumaktivität lysomaler enzyme bei varikosis. *Therapiewoche.* 1983;33:1098–1104.

36. Enghofer E, Seibel K, Hammersen F. Die antiexsudative wirkung von rosskastaniensamenextrakt. *Therapiewoche.* 1984;34:4130–4144.

37. Tooke JE, Lowe GDO. *A Textbook of Vascular Medicine.* London, England: Arnold; 1996.

38. Wadworth AN, Faulds D. Hydroxyethylrutosides. *Drugs.* 1992;44:1013–1032.

39. Rudofsky G. Beeinflussung der kapillären filtrationsrate durch phlebodril. *Phlebologie.* 1991;20:14–16.

40. Diehm C. The role of oedema protective drugs in the treatment of chronic venous insufficiency: a review of evidence based on placebo-controlled trials with regard to efficacy and tolerance. *Phlebology.* 1996;11:23–29.

41. Greeske K, Pohlmann BK. Rosskastaniensamenextrakt: ein wirksames therapieprinzip in der praxis [Horse-chestnut seed extract: an effective therapy principle in general practice: drug therapy of chronic venous insufficiency]. *Fortschr Med.* 1996; 114:196–200.

42. *Bundesverband der Pharmazeutischen Industrie.* Frankfurt, Germany: Editio Cantor; 1993.

43. Callam MJ, Ruckley CV, Dale JJ, Harper DR. Hazards of compression treatment of the leg: an estimate from Scottish surgeons. *BMJ.* 1987;295:1382.

46 Phytotherapeutic Approaches to Common Dermatologic Conditions

Donald J. Brown, ND; Alan M. Dattner, MD
From the President's Advisory Committee, Bastyr University of Natural Health Sciences, Seattle, Wash (Dr Brown); and ImmunoClarity Research Associates, New Rochelle, NY (Dr Dattner).

In this review, we discuss some common herbal preparations historically used for dermatologic conditions and recent studies that support their use. The traditional practice of topically treating dermatologic conditions with plant-derived medicines predates the cultures of ancient Egypt and remains vital today in the industrialized cultures of both the United States and Europe. Recent scientific studies lend support to some of the claims of herbal practitioners for the safety and efficacy of many herbs. The studies also elucidate, in some cases, the mechanisms by which these herbs act. With the growing interest in alternative and complementary therapies, practitioners need more information. Clinical studies and collected observations will help define specific indications for choice of herbal treatment based on both the skin disorder and the unique characteristics of the patient involved.

Arch Dermatol. 1998;134:1401–1404

A few topical herbal medicines such as *Aloe vera* are generally accepted as safe and efficacious medicines by dermatologists, primary care physicians, and research scientists. Regarding the safety and efficacy of many other herbal preparations, however, there is not such widespread agreement. Further studies and more organized systems of reporting and observation are needed to confirm or refute some interesting preliminary conclusions and to help define the place of herbal preparations in dermatologic therapeutics. The German system of regulating herbal medicines may provide the framework to further examine a prioritized list of these promising plant-derived medicines. Certain gaps exist within the German system, but the established practice of phytotherapy in that country can provide a practical basis for determining efficacy and safety.

This review of herbal approaches to common dermatologic conditions is intended to offer the dermatologist an introduction to commonly used herbal medicines in Germany and other European countries. The German system differs somewhat from ours, but the established practice of phytotherapy in that country can provide a practical basis for determining efficacy and safety.

Acne

While there have been some reports of success using tannin-containing herbs such as witch hazel and oak bark as topical astringents for acne, no controlled studies showing efficacy are available in the literature. Historically, alterative ("blood cleansing") herbs such as burdock root (*Arctium lappa*) have been recommended by traditional herbalists as an internal approach to acne, eczema, and psoriasis.[1(pp 107-108)] The underlying belief is that the skin is an organ with capabilities of elimination, which becomes diseased when the input of toxins is more than the liver, kidneys, and immune system can handle.

Dermatitis

Calendula

Calendula officinalis, also known as pot marigold or common marigold, is an aromatic plant with yellow or orange flowers that are broken up to make herbal preparations. *Calendula* flower preparations have long been considered valuable topical remedies for burns, bruises, cuts, and rashes. In European folk medicine, they were also recommended for use internally as antispasmodics, diaphoretics, antihelminthics, and for treatment of eczema.[2(pp118-120)] They are currently recommended by the German health authorities for topical treatment of minor wounds and leg ulcers.[3] Internal uses are limited to inflammatory lesions of the oral and pharyngeal mucosa.

Chemistry. Pentacyclic triterpene trihydroxyalcohols, flavonoids, and saponins have been isolated and may contribute to *Calendula*'s anti-inflammatory and wound-healing actions topically.[1(p1134)]

Mechanism of Action. Flower, flower/herb combinations, and extracts have been ascribed anti-inflammatory, wound-healing, and immunomodulatory actions.[4] *Calendula* is believed to stimulate granulation and increase glycoprotein and collagen metabolism at the wound site.

Clinical Use. *Calendula* is widely accepted as a topical treatment for diaper rash and other mild skin irritations or inflammation.

Recommended Use. Most topical use of *Calendula* flowers is in the form of an ointment or cream containing the equivalent of 2 to 5 g of the flower heads per 100 g of ointment, which is applied topically several times daily. A tea can be made for mouthwash or topical treatment by pouring 0.24 L of boiling water over 1 to 1.5 g of the flower heads and allowing it to steep for 10 minutes.[5(p1578)]

Safety. Topical as well as internal use of *Calendula* is generally safe. There have been rare reports of allergic contact dermatitis with topical use of *Calendula*.[6]

Chamomile

Chamomile (*Matricaria recutita*) is a member of the daisy family (Asteraceae) with distinctive yellow flowers with white rays. It is used for treatment of mild gastrointestinal tract conditions and as a mouthwash for irritation and inflammation of the oral mucosa. A number of topical products are also available for dermatitis and other mild irritations of the skin.

Chemistry. The flowers of chamomile contain 1% to 2% volatile oil.[2(pp322-325)] The key constituents in the volatile oil are α-bisabolol, α-bisabolol oxides A and B, and matricin. Matricin is usually converted to chamazulene during the extraction process. German chamomile products are often produced to contain an established amount of chamazulene and α-bisabolol. Chamomile flowers are also rich in flavonoids. The primary flavonoids are apigenin with smaller amounts of luteolin and quercetin.

Mechanism of Action. Chamomile extracts inhibit both cyclooxygenase and lipoxygenase in vitro.[7] Both apigenin and quercetin inhibit histamine release from antigen-stimulated human basophilic polymorphonuclear leukocytes.[8] According to a Tonelli croton oil ear assay, total chamomile extract and particularly its flavonoid fractions were very active following topical application.[9] Apigenin was found to be the most active flavonoid. A test with 9 healthy female volunteers demonstrated that skin penetration of flavonoids was excellent following topical administration.[10]

Clinical Use. Most of the studies have been completed in Germany using a chamomile cream or ointment (Kamillosan, Astra Medica, Frankfurt, Germany). In one trial with humans, chamomile was found to have an effect that was 60% as active as 0.25% hydrocortisone when applied topically.[11] In another trial, the chamomile ointment was effective in reducing dermatitis following a single application of sodium lauryl sulfate.[12] A multicenter study of patients with atopic dermatitis[13] showed that chamomile cream was "about as effective" as hydrocortisone and more effective than the other 2 topical preparations tested. Chamomile is also used for the treatment of minor wounds such as stasis ulcers in the elderly.[14]

Safety. Topical use of chamomile is extremely safe. There have been rare reports of contact dermatitis following topical application of the herb.[15]

Witch Hazel

Witch hazel (*Hamamelis virginiana*) has a long history of use in both traditional herbal medicine and allopathic medical practice for treatment of hemorrhoids, burns, cancer, tuberculosis, colds, and fever.[16] Topical preparations have also been used for symptomatic relief of itching and minor skin inflammation. Distilled witch hazel extracts available over-the-counter in the United States are virtually devoid of the tannins that are thought to be of use in the treatment of dermatitis.[5(pp151-152)]

Chemistry. Witch hazel leaves contain approximately 7% to 10% tannins, primarily gallotannins with some condensed catechins and proanthocyanidins.[2(pp245-247)]

Mechanism of Action. As is the case with other tannin-containing herbs (eg, oak bark and horse chestnut), witch hazel is a powerful astringent. Tannins are thought to be useful in dermatitis because they coagulate surface proteins of cells, leading to a reduction in permeability and secretions.[17] These precipitated proteins tend to form a protective layer on the skin.

The anti-inflammatory activity of 2 concentrations of witch hazel distillate (0.64 mg *Hamamelis* ketone/100 g and 2.56 mg *Hamamelis* ketone/100 g) were compared with 1% hydrocortisone, chamomile cream (Kamillosan), and 4 base preparations.[18] The witch hazel extract (Hametum) in a base of phosphotidyl choline was shown to reduce erythema induced by UV radiation and cellophane tape stripping in 24 healthy subjects almost as well as 1% hydrocortisone.

Clinical Use. The German Commission E monograph lists mild damage and inflammation of the skin as indications for the topical use of witch hazel.[19] A witch hazel–phosphotidyl choline product (Hametum) was slightly more effective than bufexamac ointment in a double-blind trial of 22 patients with atopic dermatitis of the lower arms.[6] In another clinical trial, 2 groups of subjects with atopic dermatitis (n=36 subjects), and contact dermatitis (n=80 subjects) were treated with witch hazel extract or a control preparation (substance not given).[20] In the atopic but not the contact dermatitis group, the witch hazel extract was somewhat superior to the control substance in reducing inflammation and itching. Anecdotal success in using the witch hazel–phosphotidyl choline cream has been reported in the management of atopic dermatitis in young children.[21]

Recommended Use. For topical use, a leaf extract supplying 5% to 10% of the drug can be applied to the affected area several times daily.

Other Herbal Approaches to Dermatitis

Licorice root (*Glycyrrhiza glabra* and *Glycyrrhiza uralensis*) is commonly used in traditional Chinese herbal medicine combinations for atopic dermatitis. A traditional formulation of 10 herbs (Zemaphyte) including licorice root has been widely studied in Great Britain for atopic dermatitis. The combination has proven successful in a long-term study of children[22] and a short-term study of adults.[23] Due to the bitter taste of the decoction made from the powdered herbs, compliance has been a problem. Concern has also been raised about mineral corticoid-like adverse effects and hepatotoxicity with long-term use.

Glycyrrhizin, a saponin of licorice root, and its derivative, glycyrrhetinic acid (GA), have been found to inhibit 11β-hydroxysteroid dehydrogenase, the enzyme that catalyzes conversion of cortisol to cortisone.[24] One study found that 2% GA combined with hydrocortisone enhanced the local effects of the hydrocortisone.[25] Because GA is already touted as a topical anti-inflammatory for dermatitis and psoriasis,[26] this may point to a potential concomitant use of GA with hydrocortisone not only to enhance local effects but also to reduce systemic adverse effects. Further studies are needed to test this hypothesis.

Interestingly, a similar effect was noted when aloe (*A vera*) gel was tested as a vehicle for hydrocortisone.[27] The combination was tested systemically and topically for acute inflammation in mice. In both tests, there was a greater anti-inflammatory effect noted with the combination than with hydrocortisone alone.

Psoriasis

While some of the topical anti-inflammatory herbal agents used to treat dermatitis may prove useful for the management of psoriasis, there are fewer data on the use of herbal medicines for this condition. Perhaps the best plant-derived product for psoriasis is capsaicin, the pungent principle in cayenne pepper. Two clinical trials have demonstrated the efficacy of 0.025% capsaicin cream (Zostrix) in the treatment of psoriasis. The first study of 44 patients with moderate and severe psoriasis vulgaris found that application of capsaicin cream led to a significant reduction in scaling and erythema over a 6-week period.[28] The second study of 197 patients with pruritic psoriasis used the same cream (applied 4 times daily) and found that scaling, thickness, erythema, and pruritis were all substantially reduced over a 6-week period.[29] In both studies, the most frequently reported adverse effect was a transient burning sensation at the site of application.

Better known for its topical use in wound healing and for the treatment of minor burns, aloe (*A vera*) has shown potential as a topical treatment for psoriasis in a study completed in Punjab, Pakistan.[30] Sixty subjects, aged 18 to 50 years, with slight to moderate chronic plaquelike psoriasis were recruited for this study. Subjects were randomized to receive either aloe extract (0.5%) in a hydrophilic cream or placebo topically applied 3 times daily for a maximum of 4 weeks. The aloe group had a significantly ($P<.001$) greater improvement (83.3%) than the placebo group (6.6%). The aloe group also showed a greater number of healed chronic plaques (82.8%) compared with the placebo group (7.9%).

Many practitioners of natural medicine believe that some people have problems with clearing toxins from the body. These practitioners advocate the use of herbs to support liver function. It is interesting to note that one study of young male patients with psoriasis indicates a strong correlation between a history of alcohol abuse and psoriasis.[31] An extract of milk thistle standardized to the flavonolignan silymarin has been advocated as a possible adjunctive approach to supporting the clearance of toxins by the liver.[32] Silymarin is approved for alcohol-related liver disease in Germany.[33] While anecdotal reports have suggested some benefit from use of milk-thistle extracts to treat psoriasis, clinical studies to support this theory are needed.

Herpes Simplex Labialis

Lemon Balm

Lemon balm (*Melissa officinalis*) is a perennial herb, originally native to the eastern Mediterranean region, that has a distinctive odor of lemon.

Chemistry. The leaves contain approximately 0.1% to 0.2% volatile oil. Among the chief constituents in the oil are citronella, citral-A, citral-B, and other monoterpenes and sesquiterpenes.[5(p1656)]

Mechanism of Action. Water extracts of the leaves have noted antiviral properties in vitro and have been shown to have a viricidal effect against herpes simplex virus type 1.[34]

Clinical Use. Two studies using a topical preparation of dried lemon balm extract 1% cream (Lomaherpan) were reported in 1994.[35] The first trial included 115 adult patients who were instructed to apply the lemon balm cream 5 times daily to the herpes lesion. Healing was complete in 96% of the patients at day 8; it was complete in 60% and 87% of the patients on days 4 and 6, respectively. Tolerance was excellent, with only 3 patients complaining of burning and paresthesia at the site of application.

The second trial reported was a randomized, placebo-controlled study of 67 subjects within 72 hours of onset of symptoms. The decline in the area of the lesion was greater and healing time was significantly faster ($P<.01$) in the lemon balm group than in the placebo group.

Plantain

Plantain (*P Lantago major*) is a common plant found on lawns, paths, and roadsides. The bruised leaves of the plant have a long history of topical use for insect bites and stings, as well as application to more serious conditions such as rattlesnake bites and tumors. One of us (A.M.D.) has observed the effectiveness of bruised leaves in reducing the itch and swelling from insect bites. A proprietary mixture (RE LEAF, ImmunoClarity Naturals) containing dried plantain leaf has also been useful in cases of insect bites and minor inflammations for which a drawing action is desired.

Clinical studies on the plant are limited to a report of its usefulness in poison ivy contact dermatitis[36] and a report of its wound-healing properties.[37] Physicians are more familiar with another product of the *Plantago* genus, the seed husk or psyllium seed, that is found in bulk laxatives (eg, Metamucil). The leaf contains mucilage that is made up of polysaccharides including mannose, galactose, dextrose, rhamnose, and levorotary arabinose.[38] These could provide an osmotic gradient to draw allergens from bites or stings and might competitively inhibit irritating lectins. Flavonoids have also been found in the leaf. Five phenylethanoids in *Plantago lanceolata* were identified, and 1 of these compounds was shown to inhibit arachidonic acid–induced mouse ear edema.[39] This observation may further explain the anti-inflammatory effects observed with plantain leaf applications. These effects are in sharp contrast to the well-known allergenic effects of plantain pollen and, to a lesser extent, plantain seed products.

Comment

Unless specifically referenced, some of the herbs mentioned herein need further study, both to document in an acceptable scientific manner their observed effects and to better define the indications for their most effective use. Redefinition of indications is especially important to integrate new laboratory and clinical data with information from alternative health approaches.

Many herbs are already being used by patients who seek care by dermatologists. Understanding their use and action helps the dermatologist integrate all elements of the patient's skin care regimen. The compilation of reports and observations of the effects of these herbs in patients with a variety of skin conditions will, along with further rigorous scientific studies, provide the basis for a more comprehensive knowledge of the usefulness of these herbs in clinical dermatologic practice.

References

1. Leung AY, Foster S. *Encyclopedia of Common Natural Ingredients Used in Food, Drugs, and Cosmetics.* New York, NY: John Wiley & Sons Inc; 1996.
2. Wichtl M. *Herbal Drugs and Phytopharmaceuticals.* Boca Raton, Fla: CRC Press Inc; 1994.
3. Committee of the Germany Federal Institute for Drugs and Medical Devices. Monograph Calendula flos. In: Blumenthal M, senior ed; Klein S, primary trans. *The Complete Germany Commission E Monographs: Therapeutic Guide to Herbal Medicines.* Austin, Tex: American Botanical Council; 1998:100.
4. ESCOP (European Scientific Cooperative on Phytotherapy) Secretariat. *Proposals for European Monographs on Calendulae flos/Flos cum erba.* Vol. 3. Bevrijdinglaan, Netherlands: ESCOP Secretariat; 1992.
5. Tyler VE. *Herbs of Choice: The Therapeutic Use of Phytomedicinals.* New York, NY: Pharmaceutical Products Press; 1994.
6. Hörmann HP, Korting HC. Evidence for the efficacy and safety of topical herbal drugs in dermatology, I: anti-inflammatory agents. *Phytomedicine.* 1994;1:161–171.
7. Ammon HPT, Kaul R. Pharmakologie der Kamille und ihrer Inhalftsstoffe. *Dtsch Apoth Ztg.* 1992;132(suppl 27):3–26.
8. Middleton E, Drzewiecki G. Effects of flavonoids and transitional metal cations on antigen-induced histamine release from human basophils. *Biochem Pharmacol.* 1982;31:1449–1453.
9. Della Loggia R. Lokale antiphlogistische Wirung der Kamillen-flavone. *Dtsch Apoth Ztg.* 1985;125(suppl 1):9–11.
10. Heilmann J, Merfort I, Hagerdorn U, Lippold BC. In vivo skin penetration studies of chamomile flavonoids. *Planta Med.* 1993; 59(suppl):A638.
11. Albring M, Albrecht H, Alcorn G, Lucker PV. The measuring of the antiinflammatory effect of a compound on the skin of volunteers. *Methods Find Exp Clin Pharmacol.* 1983;5:75–77.
12. Nissen HP, Blitz H, Kreyel HW. Prolifometrie, eine Methode zur beurteilung der therapeutischen wirksamkeit kon Kamillosan®-Slabe. *Z Hautkr.* 1988;63:184–190.
13. Aergeerts P, Albring M, Klaschka F, et al. Vergleichende pruüfung von Kamillosan Creme gegenüber Steroidalen (0.25% hydrocortison, 0.75% flucortinbutylester and nichsteroidsalen (5% bufexamac) externa in der Erhaltungstherapie von Ekzemerkrankungen. *Z Hautkr.* 1985;60:270–277.
14. Glowania HJ, Rauliin C, Swooda NI. The effect of chamomile on wound healing—a clinical double-blind study. *Z Hautkr.* 1987;62:1262–1271.
15. Mann C, Staba EJ. The chemistry, pharmacology, and commercial formulations of chamomile. In: Craker LE, Simon JE, eds. *Herbs, Spices, and Medicinal Plants: Recent Advances in Botany, Horticulture, and Pharmacology.* Vol. 1. Phoenix, Ariz: Oryx Press; 1986:235–280.
16. Witch hazel. *Rev Natur Med Prod.* St Louis, Mo: Facts and Comparisons; September 1990.
17. Laux P, Oschamann R. Witch hazel (*Hamarnelis virginiana*). *Z. Phytolther.* 1993;14:155–166.
18. Korting HC, Schäfer-Korting NM, Hart H, et al. Anti-inflammatory activity of hamamelis distillate applied topcially to the skin. *Eur J Clin Pharmacol.* 1993;44:315–318.
19. Committee of the Germany Federal Institute for Drugs and Medical Devices. Monograph *Hamamelidis folium.* In: Blumenthal, M, senior ed; Klein S, primary trans. *The Complete Germany Commission E Monographs: Therapeutic Guide to Herbal Medicines.* Austin, Tex: American Botanical Council; 1998:571–573.
20. Pfister R. Problems in the treatment and after care of chronic dermatoses: a clinical study on Hametum ointment [in German]. *Fortschr Med.* 1981;99:1264.
21. Brown DJ. *Herbal Prescriptions for Better Health.* Rocklin, Calif: Prima Publishing; 1996:291.
22. Sheehan MP, Atherton DJ. One year follow-up of children tested with Chinese medicinal herbs for atopic eczema. *Br J Dermatol.* 1994; 130:488–493.
23. Lachman Y, Banerjee P, Poulter LW, et al. Association of immunological changes with clinical efficacy in atopic eczema patients treated with traditional Chinese herbal therapy (Zemaphyte). *Int Arch Allergy Immunol.* 1996;109:243–249.
24. Whorwood CB, Sheppard MC, Stewart PM. Licorice inhibits 11β-hydroxysteroid dehydrogenase messenger ribonucleic acid levels and potentiates glucocorticoid hormone action. *Endocrinology.* 1993;132:2287–2292.
25. Teeluksingh S, Mackie ADR, Burt D, et al. Potentiation of hydrocortisone activity in skin by glycyrrhetinic acid. *Lancet.* 1990;335:1060–1063.
26. Evans FQ. The rational use of glycyrrhetinic acid in dermatology. *Br J Clin Pract.* 1958;12:269–279.
27. Davis RH, Parker WL, Murdoch DP. *Aloe vera* as a biologically active vehicle for hydrocortisone acetate. *J Am Podiatr Med Assoc.* 1991;81:1–9.
28. Bernstein JE, Parish LC, Rapaport M, et al. Effects of topically applied capsaicin on moderate and severe psoriasis vulgaris. *J Am Acad Dermatol.* 1986;15:504–507.
29. Ellis CN, Berberian B, Sulica VI, et al. A double-blind evaluation of topical capsaicin in pruritic psoriasis. *J Am Acad Dermatol.* 1993; 29:438–442.
30. Syed TA, Ahmad SA, Holt AH, et al. Management of psoriasis with *Aloe vera* extract in a hydrophilic cream: a placebo-controlled, double-blind study. *Trop Med Int Health.* 1996;1:505–509.
31. Poikolainen K, Reunala T, Karvonen J, Lauharanta J, Karkkainen P. Alcohol intake: a risk factor for psoriasis in young and middle aged men? *BMJ.* 1990;300:780–783.
32. Weber G, Galle K. The liver, a therapeutic target in dermatoses. *Med Welt.* 1983;34:108–111.
33. Leng-Peschlow E. Alcohol-related liver diseases—use of Legalon for therapy. *Pharmedicum.* 1994;2:22–27.
34. Dimitrova Z, Dimov B, Manolova N, et al. Antiherpes effect of *Melissa officinalis* L. extracts. *Acta Mirobiol Bulg.* 1993;29:65–72.
35. Wöbling RH, Leonhardt K. Local therapy of herpes simplex with dried extract of *Melissa officinalis. Phytomedicine.* 1994;1:25–31.
36. Duckett S. Plantain leaf for poison ivy. *N Engl J Med.* 1980;303:583.

37. Shipochliev T, Dimitrov A, Aleksandrova E. Anti-inflammatory action of a group of plant extracts [in Bulgarian]. *Veterinarno-Meditsinski Nauki.* 1981;18:87–94.

38. Murai M, Tamayama Y, Nishibe S. Phenylethanoids in the herb of *Plantago lanceolata* and inhibitory effect on arachidonic acid–induced mouse ear edema [letter]. *Planta Med.* 1995;61:479–480.

39. Brautigam M, Franz G. Schleimpolysaccharide aus Fpitzwegerichblattern. *Dtch Apoth Zeit.* 1985;125:58–62.

47 Randomized Trial of Aromatherapy

Successful Treatment for Alopecia Areata

Isabelle C. Hay, MRCP; Margaret Jamieson, SRN; Anthony D. Ormerod, FRCP
From the Department of Dermatology, Aberdeen Royal Infirmary, Foresterhill, Aberdeen, Scotland.

Objective
To investigate the efficacy of aromatherapy in the treatment of patients with alopecia areata.

Design
A randomized, double-blind, controlled trial of 7 months' duration, with follow-up at 3 and 7 months.

Setting
Dermatology outpatient department.

Participants
Eighty-six patients diagnosed as having alopecia areata.

Intervention
Eighty-six patients were randomized into 2 groups. The active group massaged essential oils (thyme, rosemary, lavender, and cedarwood) in a mixture of carrier oils (jojoba and grapeseed) into their scalp daily. The control group used only carrier oils for their massage, also daily.

Main Outcome Measures
Treatment success was evaluated on sequential photographs by 2 dermatologists (I.C.H. and A.D.O.) independently. Similarly, the degree of improvement was measured by 2 methods: a 6-point scale and computerized analysis of traced areas of alopecia.

Results
Nineteen (44%) of 43 patients in the active group showed improvement compared with 6 (15%) of 41 patients in the control group (*P*=.008). An alopecia scale was applied by blinded observers on sequential photographs and was shown to be reproducible with good interobserver agreement (κ=0.84). The degree of improvement on photographic assessment was significant (*P*=.05). Demographic analysis showed that the 2 groups were well matched for prognostic factors.

Conclusions

The results show aromatherapy to be a safe and effective treatment for alopecia areata. Treatment with these essential oils was significantly more effective than treatment with the carrier oil alone (P=.008 for the primary outcome measure). We also successfully applied an evidence-based method to an alternative therapy.

Arch Dermatol. 1998;134:1349–1352

With the recent resurgence of interest in alternative medicine, aromatherapy (aroma, from the Greek meaning spice) has attracted great public interest in its health-promoting or medicinal properties. With herbalism as its basis, aromatherapy involves the use of essential oils and essences derived from plants, flowers, and wood resins, which are generally massaged into the skin. These essential oils have been used to complement traditional medicine with some benefit.[1] As with other forms of alternative medicine, scientific bases for the claims made are few,[2,3] but in dermatologic studies, physiological and psychological benefits were found after treatment of psoriasis with aromatherapy.[4] Significant, consistent improvement in behavior occurred in 1 of 4 patients with dementia[5] in 10 repeated experiments. Aromatherapy is also useful in hospice care.[6]

As examples of proven therapeutic benefit, use of sandalwood oil has been shown to significantly inhibit skin papillomas in mice.[7] Tea tree oil is an effective bacteriocide[8] and fungicide, especially for *Malassezia furfur*.[9] Use of essential oils can also alter the barrier functions of the skin[10] and induce contact dermatitis.[11]

Cedarwood, lavender, thyme, and rosemary oils have hair growth-promoting properties. These oils have been anecdotally used to treat alopecia for more than 100 years. To date, there have been no controlled trials to evaluate this treatment. Our experience using aromatherapy provides anecdotal evidence that several patients have had marked improvement with this form of therapy. Our aim in this study was to test the hypothesis that pharmacologically active stimulants for hair growth are present in these oils and that use of these oils can be therapeutic in patients with alopecia.

Alopecia areata is a common condition affecting 1% of the Western world. It can cause substantial social and psychological distress and is often highly detrimental to the patient's well-being and self-esteem. In 1 study,[12] patients with alopecia areata had an increased risk of developing a psychiatric illness. An autoimmune cause is widely accepted. However, it is thought that stress can affect its course. Current conventional treatments have limited success or unacceptable toxic effects. The course of alopecia areata is unpredictable, but factors affecting prognosis are well established. A poor prognosis is indicated by the long duration of the condition (>1 year), associated autoimmune conditions (eg, thyroid disease), atopy, and family history.[13–16]

Patients, Materials, and Methods

Patients

Eighty-six patients diagnosed as having alopecia areata were invited to take part in this randomized, controlled trial. These patients were interviewed, and they completed a questionnaire. Patients with a medical history of hypertension, epilepsy, or pregnancy were excluded. Two of 86 patients were excluded because they had androgenic alopecia. Topical medication and intralesional corticosteroid therapy for the alopecia were discontinued before the trial.

Eighty-four patients were randomized into 2 groups by the aromatherapist (M.J.). All patients signed a written consent form before the trial.

The trained aromatherapist explained how to use the oils and demonstrated the technique of scalp massage. The oils were massaged into the scalp for a minimum of 2 minutes. A warm towel was then wrapped around the head to aid absorption of the oils. Patients were advised to use this technique every night.

There were 2 arms to the trial. The active group received the essential oils: *Thyme vulgaris* (2 drops, 88 mg), *Lavandula agustifolia* (3 drops, 108 mg), *Rosmarinus officinalis* (3 drops, 114 mg), and *Cedrus atlantica* (2 drops, 94 mg). These oils were mixed in a carrier oil, which was a combination of jojoba, 3 mL, and grapeseed, 20 mL, oils.

The control group received the same carrier oils without added essential oils, and the oils were identical except in smell, which could not be mimicked in the control.

Measurement and Evaluation

Initial and 3- and 7-month assessments were made by 3 methods:

1. A 4-point scale, such as that described by MacDonald Hull and Norris,[17] was used to check that the severity was similar in active and control groups, as follows: 1 indicates vellus hair or no hair; 2, sparse pigmented or nonpigmented terminal hair; 3, terminal regrowth with patches of alopecia areata; and 4, terminal regrowth in all areas.

2. A standardized professional photographic assessment of each volunteer was taken at the initial interview and after 3 and 7 months. Changes in these photographic assessments formed the primary outcome measure, with improvement as the most important factor. These changes were scored independently by 2 dermatologists (I.C.H. and A.D.O.) who were unaware of the therapy administered. Improvement in photographic assessment was graded using a numerical scale (Figure 1).

3. A further secondary outcome measure was performed. A map was traced onto transparent film wherever the alopecia occurred in patches. These tracings were then transferred onto flat acetate sheets. A computerized image analyzer was used to calculate the areas of alopecia at the initial assessment and after 3 and 7 months.

Statistical Methods

We calculated that if improvement occurred in 20% more patients with active treatment than in the control group it would require 47 active and 47 control patients to detect improvement at a 5% significance level with a power of 80%.[18] Statistical analysis was performed on an intention-to-treat basis. A pooled variance estimate Student *t* test for independent samples was used to test improvement in the patients' alopecia with the map-tracing method. The χ^2 test was used to detect improvement in the active and control groups. A Mann-Whitney *U* test, corrected for ties, was used to assess the significance of the degree of improvement in scored photographic assessment. The level of agreement of the alopecia scoring scale between 2 assessors was examined using the Cohen weighted κ statistic.

The trial was approved by the Joint Ethical Committee for the Grampian Health Board and by the University of Aberdeen, Aberdeen, Scotland.

Results

Eighty-four patients entered the trial; 28 (68%) of the patients in the control group and 35 (81%) of the patients in the active group completed the trial (Figure 2). The patients were well matched for the important demographic indicators that might affect response to therapy (Table 1). The distribution of patients by the 4-point scale was similar in both groups.

The improvement was statistically significant in all assessments undertaken. The primary outcome measure of improvement vs no improvement showed improvement with essential oils (P=.008, χ^2) (Table 2). The degree of improvement shown in the photographs was assessed by the Mann-Whitney *U* test and was significant (P=.05). The results of the alopecia scale, which scored the degree of improvement (from 1–6), are illustrated in Figure 3. The measurement of traced areas, which could be performed in only 32 patients, showed a mean ±SD reduction in area affected of 103.9 ± 140.0 cm^2 compared with −1.8 ± 155.0 cm^2 in the control group (Figure 4). This was significant, with P=.05 (Student *t* test). A relative risk of 2.6 (95% confidence limits, 1.2, 5.6) was calculated for the likelihood of improving on the active therapy. Weighted κ statistic was 0.84 for agreement between scorers on the assessment of the photographic scale, showing good interrater correlation.

This indicates that this is a reproducible method of assessment. One patient who received active treatment and had an excellent response (ie, a score of 6 on our scale) is pictured in Figure 5.

Comment

The responses were variable but showed a clear and statistically significant advantage to treatment with this standardized regimen of aromatherapy. Although the tradition of aromatherapy is to combine several oils, it seems likely that 1 of these agents has a stimulatory effect on hair growth. One male patient also had severe androgenic alopecia, which was not included in the assessment of efficacy, and within this area there was some moderate regrowth of hair and improvement in alopecia areata.

There was a higher dropout rate in the control group, which could be explained by the fact that the volunteers became discouraged with the 7-month protocol. The control oil was not odorless because the carrier oils have some smell, and patients did not know what aroma to expect. However, they may have surmised that their treatment was inactive and withdrew from the trial. The control group's relative lack of response again suggests a pharmacoactive property of the topically applied therapy as opposed to an

Scale	Description	Hair Regrowth, %
1	Worse	NA
2	No Change	NA
3	Slight but Definite Improvement	10-30
4	Marked Improvement	31-50
5	Very Good Improvement	51-80
6	Excellent Improvement	81-100

Figure 1. The scale used in the photographic assessment to measure changes in hair growth after intervention with active essential oils compared with the control. NA indicates not applicable.

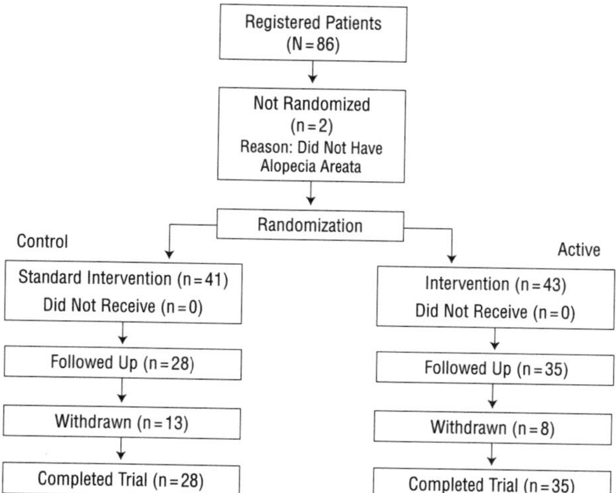

Figure 2. Flow diagram showing the randomization of patients to the active and control groups.

effect arising from the comforting, relaxing effect of massage and of the application procedure, which was the same for both groups.

Previous studies of alopecia therapies have used only subjective scales of improvement, such as those described by MacDonald Hull and Norris.[17] We found these scales less helpful because there are large intervals between the points in the alopecia scale. We validated the method of sequential photography with a standardized approach using a professional photographer's studio. Images were judged by blinded observers and showed good agreement. This proved to be the most blinded and unbiased

Table 1. Demographic and Prognostic Factors in the Active and Control Groups*

	Active Group	Control Group	Total
Age, mean ± SD, y	38.9 ± 14.6	39.3 ± 13.6	. . .
Associated conditions			
Thyroid disease	14.0	12.2	13.1
Atopy	18.6	17.1	17.9
Stress	48.8	53.7	51.2
Family history			
Alopecia areata	18.6	17.1	17.9
Autoimmune thyroid disease	18.6	24.4	21.4

*Values are expressed as percentages unless otherwise indicated. Ellipses indicate not applicable.

Table 2. Contingency Table of Improvement With Each Intervention: Active Essential Oils vs Control Carrier Oil Alone*

	Improved	Not Improved	Total
Active	19	16	**35**
Control	6	22	**28**
Total	**25**	**38**	**63**

**P* =.008 (χ^2).

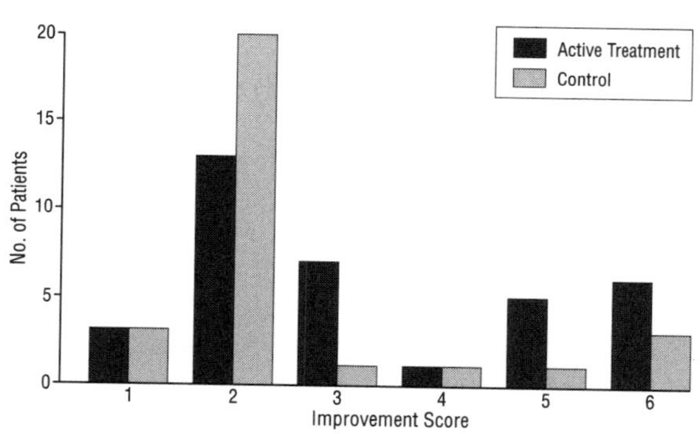

Figure 3. Results of the photographic assessment of the degree of improvement in alopecia on a 6-point scale (see Figure 1).

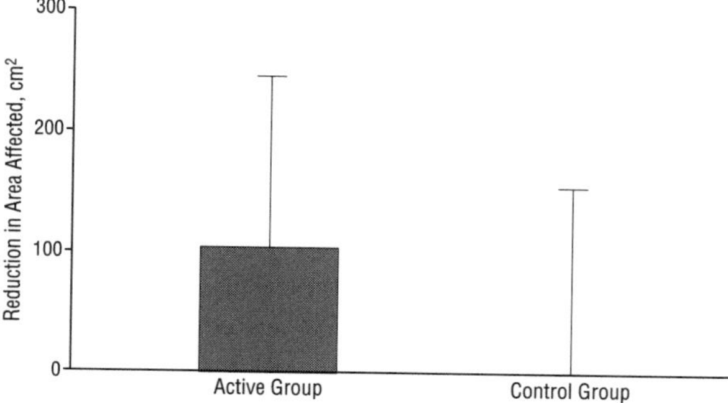

Figure 4. Results of computerized analysis of traced areas of alopecia in active and control groups. Bars indicate SD.

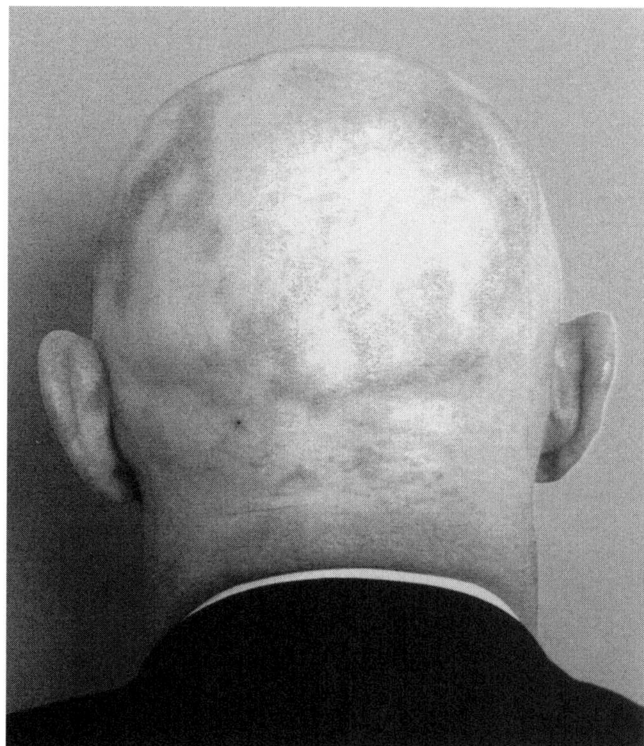
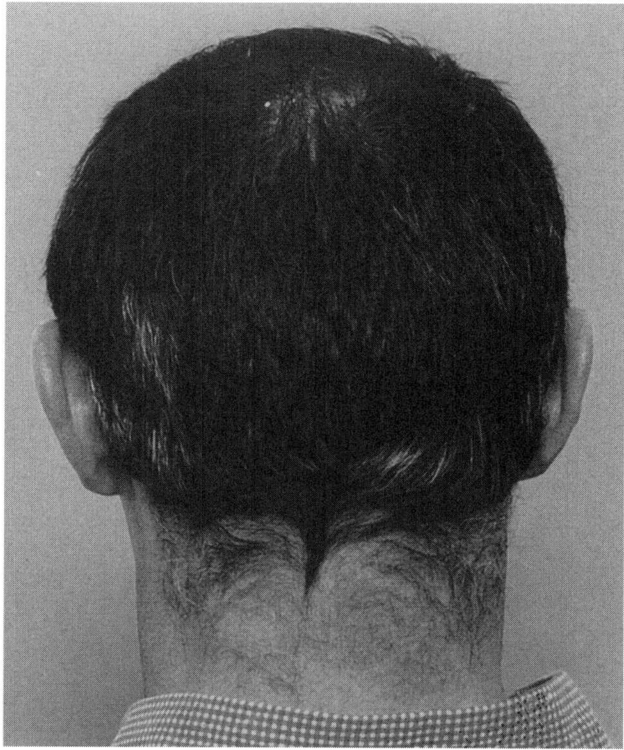

Figure 5. A patient showing an excellent response (6 on the scoring scale) to essential oil therapy.

Populations in other trials may differ in prognostic factors. Shapiro et al[20] and Gordon et al[14] found a 38% success rate in producing cosmetically acceptable regrowth in patients with alopecia using diphencyprone. A review of psoralen–UV-A therapy for alopecia areata by Taylor and Hawk[21] revealed that phototherapy was disappointing, with minimal benefit. Therefore, this aromatherapy trial, with an improvement rate of 44%, is comparable to and possibly of more benefit than trials of conventional therapies for alopecia areata. Compared with these other treatments, its safety is also greater, offering a better therapeutic ratio.

The Soroptomists International of Aberdeen, Scotland, provided financial support for the trial.

We thank Jill Mollison, BSc, for statistical advice and the members of the Aberdeen Alopecia Self Help Group for their participation.

References

1. Whitmore SM, Leake NB. Complementary therapies: an adjunct to traditional therapies. *Nurse Pract.* 1996;21:10–13.
2. Vickers A. Yes, but how do we know it's true? knowledge claims in massage and aromatherapy. *Complement Ther Nurs Midwifery.*1997; 3:63–65.
3. Martin GN. Olfactory remediation: current evidence and possible applications. *Soc Sci Med.* 1996;43:63–70.
4. Walsh D. Using aromatherapy in the management of psoriasis. *Nurs Stand.* 1996;11:53–56.
5. Brooker DJ, Snape M, Johnson E, Ward D, Payne M. Single case evaluation of the effects of aromatherapy and massage on disturbed behaviour in severe dementia. *Br J Clin Psychol.* 1997;36:287–296.
6. Welsh C. Touch with oils: a pertinent part of holistic hospice care. *Am J Hosp Palliat Care.* 1997;14:42–44.
7. Dwivedi C, Abu-Ghazaleh A. Chemopreventive effects of sandalwood oil on skin papillomas in mice. *Eur J Cancer Prev.* 1997;6:399–401.
8. Hammer KA, Carson CF, Riley TV. Susceptibility of transient and commensal skin flora to the essential oil of *Melaleuca alternifolia* (tea tree oil). *Am J Infect Control.* 1996;24:186–189.
9. Nenoff P, Haustein UF, Brandt W. Antifungal activity of the essential oil of *Melaleuca alternifolia* (tea tree oil) against pathogenic fungi in vitro. *Skin Pharmacol.* 1996;9:388–394.

10. Yamane MA, Williams AC, Barry BW. Terpene penetration enhancers in propylene glycol/water co-solvent systems: effectiveness and mechanism of action. *J Pharm Pharmacol.* 1995;47:978–989.

11. Weiss RR, James WD. Allergic contact dermatitis from aromatherapy. *Am J Contact Dermat.* 1997;8:250–251.

12. Koo YM, William VR, Shellow MD, Hallman CP, Edwards JE. Alopecia areata and increased prevalence of psychiatric disorders. *Int J Dermatol.* 1994;33:849–850.

13. van der Steen PHM, van Baar HMJ, Happle R, Boezeman JMB, Perret MJ. Prognostic factors in the treatment of alopecia areata with diphencyprone. *Am Acad Dermatol.* 1991;24:227–230.

14. Gordon PM, Aldridge RD, McVittie E, Hunter JAA. Topical diphencyprone for alopecia areata: evaluation of 48 cases after 30 months' follow up. *Br J Dermatol.* 1996;134:869–871.

15. De Prost Y, Paquez F, Touraine R. Dinitrochlorobenzene treatment of alopecia areata. *Arch Dermatol.* 1982;118:542–545.

16. Weise K, Kretzschmar L, John SM, Hamm H. Topical immunotherapy in alopecia areata: anamnestic and clinical criteria of prognostic significance. *Dermatology.* 1996;192:129–133.

17. MacDonald Hull S, Norris JF. Diphencyprone in the treatment of long standing alopecia areata. *Br J Dematol.* 1988;119:367–374.

18. Pocock SJ, Hughes MD. Estimation issues in clinical trials and overviews. *Stat Med.* 1990; 9:657–671.

19. Frattasio A, Germino M, Cargnello S, Patrone P. Side-effects during treatment with SADBE. *Contact Dermatitis.* 1997;36:118–119.

20. Shapiro J, Tan J, Ho V, Tron V. Treatment of severe alopecia areata with topical diphenulcuclopropenone and 5% minoxidil: a clinical and immunopathologic evaluation. *J Invest Dermatol.* 1995;104(suppl 5):36S.

21. Taylor CR, Hawk JLM. PUVA treatment of alopecia areata parralis, totalis and universalis: audit of ten years' experience at St. John's Institute of Dermatology. *Br J Dermatol.* 1995;133:914–918

6 Homeopathy

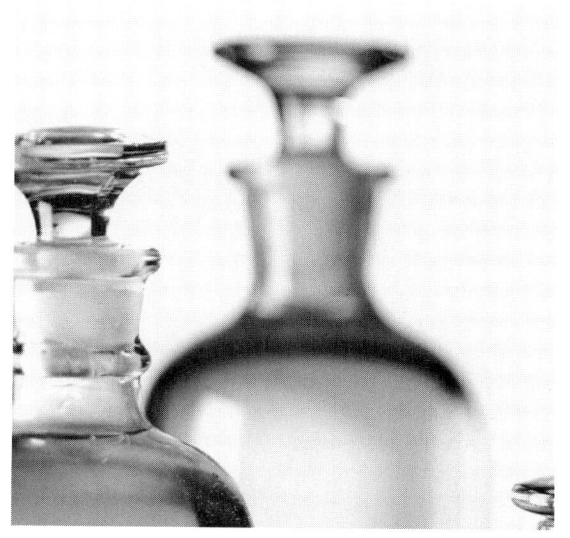

48 Patient Characteristics and Practice Patterns of Physicians Using Homeopathy

Jennifer Jacobs, MD, MPH; Edward H. Chapman, MD, DHt; Dean Crothers, MD
From the University of Washington School of Public Health and Community Medicine, Seattle (Dr Jacobs); the American Institute of Homeopathy, Alexandria, Va (Dr Chapman); and the Evergreen Center for Homeopathic Medicine, Edmonds, Wash (Dr Crothers).

Background
The use of homeopathy is growing in the United States, but little is known about practice patterns of physicians using homeopathy and the patients who seek homeopathic care.

Materials and Methods
Data for consecutive patient visits to 27 doctors of medicine and doctors of osteopathy using homeopathy in 1992 were collected and compared with the National Ambulatory Medical Care Survey of 1990.

Results
Patients seen by the homeopathic physicians were younger, more affluent, and more likely to present with long-term complaints. Physicians using homeopathic medicine surveyed spent more time with their patients, ordered fewer tests, and prescribed fewer pharmaceutical medications than physicians practicing conventional medicine.

Conclusions
While definite conclusions cannot be made based on this survey, we have documented that the use of diagnostic testing and conventional medications by physicians who use homeopathy to treat common chronic conditions is well below that of conventional primary care physicians. These findings, if associated with comparable clinical outcomes, suggest a potential for substantial cost savings. Further studies documenting outcomes, cost benefits, physician decision-making, and patient satisfaction will be required to further explore this subject.

Arch Fam Med. 1998;7:537–540

Homeopathic medicine was first developed in Germany by Samuel Hahnemann in the late 18th century. By the late 1800s, it was practiced widely in the United States, and today it is used extensively throughout the world, especially in Europe, where surveys have reported that in some countries 30% to 40% of the population has used homeopathic medicine.[1–3] Homeopathy declined in the United States in the early 20th century, but there has been increasing interest in the field in the past 10 years. In 1990, 4.8 million visits to homeopathic providers were reported in the United States and retail sales of homeopathic medicines increased from $100 million in 1988 to $250 million in 1996.[4–6] In 1997, worldwide sales of homeopathic products were estimated to be $1.15 billion.[7]

Homeopathy is based on the principle of similars, whereby highly diluted preparations of substances that can cause symptoms in healthy volunteers are used to stimulate healing in patients who have similar symptoms when ill.[8] The mechanism of action of homeopathy is not understood, and many doubt the scientific rationale of using such diluted medicines.[9] Nevertheless, a growing body of double-blind, placebo-controlled trials suggest that homeopathy may be clinically effective,[10–15] and it has been estimated that 2500 medical professionals in the United States use homeopathy to some extent in their practices.[5]

A growing number of insurers and managed care plans are offering coverage of alternative therapies ,[16–18] and it has been suggested that health care costs could be reduced by use of these therapies.[19] A survey done in France, where one third of physicians use homeopathy, found that the annual cost per person to the social security system for a homeopathic physician was 15% less than that of a conventional physician.[20] This savings was attributed to the reduction in the use of diagnostic tests and to the lower cost of homeopathic medications, which cost about one third less than conventional medicines in France.

To further our understanding of the use of alternative modalities, information is needed about patients who seek care, the problems for which care is sought, tests and treatments that are provided, and their costs. In this survey, we looked at these factors for a group of physicians using homeopathy and compared the results with similar findings from a group of physicians using conventional medicine.

Materials and Methods

In early 1992, we sent a letter requesting participation in the survey to all 102 active members of the American Institute of Homeopathy (AIH), a national organization of doctors of medicine and doctors of osteopathy who use homeopathy. Twenty-seven members agreed to participate. Physicians were asked to record data on all patient visits occurring during the week of April 6 through April 10, 1992. This survey was modeled after the National Ambulatory Medical Care Survey (NAMCS), conducted by the National Center for Health Statistics and the US Bureau of the Census. The 1990 NAMCS, which included a representative sample of general and family physicians, was used as a comparison group for the AIH physicians.[21]

Data on sequential patient visits were recorded either during or immediately after the visit on a form that was identical to that used in the 1990 NAMCS, with the addition of fields to record costs. Demographic information about the patient, payment sources, principal diagnoses, diagnostic services, medication therapy, and duration of visit was collected in both surveys.

Results

Of the 27 participating AIH physicians, 22 (81.5%) were men; the average age of the entire group was 46 years. United States geographical distribution was as follows: 7(26%), northeast; 2 (7.4%), south; (3) 11.1%, midwest; and 15 (55.5%), west. This compares with 76 (72.6%), men; 38 (37.4%), northeast; 12 (11.7%), south; 18 (17.5%), midwest; and 34 (33.5%), west of the total AIH membership of 102 physicians in 1992. Twenty-two (80%) of the 27 respondents listed their primary specialty as family practice, general practice, or homeopathic medicine. They had been practicing medicine for a median of 18 years, with an average of 11.5 years' experience using homeopathy in their practices. Twenty-four (85%) said that they used homeopathy in 75% or more of their patient visits. Demographic information about the NAMCS physicians was limited to sex (90%, men) and geographic region (18.4%, northeast; 32.3%, south; 27%, midwest; and 22.3%, west). Information about age was not collected by the NAMCS, but other sources indicate that the median age of all physicians in the United States was 44 years in 1990.[22]

A comparison of patient sex and ages showed that the AIH physicians were more likely to treat women, as well as children younger than 15 years and young to middle-aged adults, and were less likely to treat patients older than 65 years (Table 1). These physicians saw a higher percentage of white and Asian patients and a lower proportion of blacks and Hispanics.

The average percentage of new patient visits, 15%, was comparable between the 2 groups, although the AIH physicians were more likely to be seeing an old patient for

Table 1. Demographic Characteristics of Patients Seeing Physicians Using Homeopathic Medicine Compared With Physicians Using Conventional Medicine*

Characteristic	Homeopathic Medicine, % (n=1177)	Conventional Medicine, % (n=11,614)
Sex		
Female	66.2	61.0
Male	33.7	39.0
Age, y		
<15	23.9	16.6
15–24	5.2	11.6
25–44	32.6	28.5
45–64	27.8	22.8
>64	10.5	20.5
Race		
White	91.5	84.4
Black	2.9	8.5
Asian/Pacific Islander	5.5	3.0
Unspecified	0	4.0
Hispanic	2.6	5.4

*For all characteristics $P<.001$ by χ^2 test.

Table 2. Visit Type, Insurance Coverage, and Duration of Visit of Patients Seeing Physicians Using Homeopathic Medicine Compared With Physicians Using Conventional Medicine

	Homeopathic Medicine, % (n=1177)	Conventional Medicine, % (n=11,614)
Type of visit		
New patient	15.6	14.6
Old patient		
New problem	21.2	31.9
Old problem	63.2	53.5
Insurance coverage		
Self-pay	18.1	33.9
Medicare	10.4	19.0
Medicaid	3.3	12.3
Blue Cross/Blue Shield	17.5	8.6
Other commercial	37.2	20.1
HMO/prepaid plan*	6.9	13.5
Other	5.7	6.0
Duration of visit, min		
<5	2.0	11.1
6–10	7.0	33.2
11–15	17.2	32.5
>15	74.8	23.2
Mean duration, min	30.0	12.5

*HMO indicates health maintenance organization.

an old problem (Table 2). The patients seeing AIH physicians more commonly had private medical insurance, while the NAMCS patients were more likely to have Medicare or Medicaid, to belong to a health maintenance organization or other managed health care program, or to have no insurance at all. The AIH physicians spent more than twice as much time with their patients, with an average of 30 minutes per visit compared with 12.5 minutes for physicians practicing conventional medicine. This information reflects both returning and new patient visits.

While the AIH physicians spent more time with their patients, they were less likely to order diagnostic services. In the NAMCS survey, physicians ordered 1 or more diagnostic services in 68.3% of all patient visits, compared with 39.9% of visits for the AIH physicians (Table 3). The AIH physicians prescribed homeopathic medications in 79% of visits, and conventional pharmaceutical medications in 27.5% of patients visits. This compared with 68.7% of visits in the NAMCS sample where conventional medications were prescribed.

A comparison of the 10 most common diagnoses between the 2 groups indicates that the AIH physicians saw more patients for chronic illnesses (Table 4). With the exception of otitis media, which can be acute or chronic, all of the 10 most common diagnoses of the AIH patients were for chronic illnesses, such as asthma, depression, allergies, headaches, and arthritis. In contrast, there were only 3 chronic illnesses represented in the 10 most common diagnoses of the NAMCS physicians—hypertension, diabetes, and chronic sinusitis.

The average cost for a new patient visit for AIH physicians was $137 and the average time was 59.8 minutes. The average cost for a follow-up visit was $55 and the average time was 25.4 minutes. The cost of visits was not included in the NAMCS.

Comment

The results of this survey indicate that there are considerable differences in the types of patients seeking care, principal diagnoses, and the practice patterns of physicians using homeopathy when compared with physicians who practice conventional medicine. The finding that physicians using homeopathy see a younger patient population is similar to that of a 1990 survey[4] in which a larger proportion of young to middle-aged adults (the baby boomers) were found to have used unconventional therapies. The larger number of white and Asian patients is likely due to practice location, since most of the AIH survey physicians practiced in the west, where there is a larger number of Asian patients, while in the south, which was more highly represented in the NAMCS survey, there is a larger number of black and Hispanic patients. The higher percentage of patients with private medical insurance suggests that the AIH patients were in general more affluent. Conversely, the low number of

Table 3. Diagnostic Services and Medication Therapy Used by Physicians Using Homeopathic Medicine Compared With Physicians Using Conventional Medicine (Percentage of Visits)

	Homeopathic Medicine, % (n=1177)	Conventional Medicine, % (n=11,614)
Diagnostic services		
1 or more	39.9	68.3
Laboratory test(s)	9.2	19.6
Urinalysis	4.0	12.0
Chest x-ray film	0.4	3.7
Other diagnostic services	6.7	31.3
Therapy used		
Conventional medication	27.5	68.7
Homeopathic medication	79.0	NA*

*NA indicates not applicable.

Table 4. Ten Most Common Principal Diagnoses of Patients Seeking Care From Physicians Using Homeopathic Medicine Compared With Physicians Using Conventional Medicine

Homeopathic Medicine (n=1177)	Cases, %	Conventional Medicine (n=11,614)	Cases, %
Asthma	4.9	Hypertension	6.4
Depression	3.5	Upper respiratory tract infection	3.9
Otitis media	3.5	Otitis media	3.1
Allergic rhinitis	3.4	Diabetes mellitus	2.9
Headache/migraine	3.2	Acute pharyngitis	2.6
Neurotic disorders	2.9	Chronic sinusitis	2.6
Allergy (nonspecific)	2.8	Bronchitis	2.6
Dermatitis, eczema	2.6	Sprains/strains	1.7
Arthritis	2.5	Back disorders	1.4
Hypertension	2.4	Allergic rhinitis	1.4

Medicaid, Medicare, and noninsured patients seen by the homeopathic physicians suggests that interest in and access to alternative health care by low-income groups may be limited.

The AIH physicians were roughly similar to the NAMCS sample for sex and age distribution. However, major differences in geographical distribution were found, which could have affected some of the results. There was a preponderance of homeopathic physicians in the west and northeast, with a much lower proportion in the south and midwest. Whether regional differences could have affected the case mix and/or practice patterns of the physicians surveyed is unknown.

The AIH physicians were more likely to be consulted for chronic illnesses and by patients with psychological and/or functional symptoms, such as anxiety, allergies, and fatigue. These are conditions that are often difficult to treat with conventional medicine, or for which modern medicine offers mostly symptomatic relief, or treatment that does not satisfy patients. Conversely, patients with illnesses such as hypertension, diabetes mellitus, and acute injuries and infections, for which there are effective conventional treatments, were more likely to seek conventional care.

Because of the differences in the case mix, including the age and socioeconomic status of the patients and type of illnesses seen by the 2 groups, conclusions about laboratory tests, time spent, and cost per visit should be interpreted with caution. Homeopathic physicians spent more than twice as much time with their patients, which likely reflects the complexity of the homeopathic history-taking and prescribing process. Homeopathic medications are individualized to each patient, based on a wide constellation of physical, general, and mental/emotional symptoms that must be elicited at each visit.

The fewer number of diagnostic procedures and laboratory tests ordered by AIH physicians also could reflect the emphasis on history taking and physical examination to determine the diagnosis and course of treatment in homeopathic practice.[23] It is also possible that the patients seeing the AIH physicians generally were less ill and required fewer tests, or that extensive testing had already been done by another physician. The increased number of visits by old patients for old problems could also have contributed to the use of fewer tests by the AIH physicians.

As would be expected, the AIH physicians prescribed fewer conventional pharmaceutical drugs, although their use in almost 28% of patient visits suggests the complementary nature of homeopathic treatment as an adjunct to conventional treatment in many cases. In most cases, homeopathic medicines were used alone, and the cost of these medicines, as was found in the French survey, is considerably below that of standard drugs. Since visit costs were not evaluated in the NAMCS, it is difficult to make conclusions about the total cost of health care.

There are several limitations to this survey. It is unknown if the AIH members who chose to participate in the survey are representative of all members, or of the larger group of homeopathic practitioners who do not belong to this organization. It is also unknown whether patients seeing AIH members were seeing other physicians simultaneously. The NAMCS physicians recorded visits during a random week of the year, while the AIH survey was conducted in the month of April, which could lead to seasonal differences in illnesses treated. As the use of alternative modalities such as homeopathy increases, the types of patients visiting such physicians could change, affecting costs and practice patterns.

The results of this survey suggest that most patients are seen by homeopathic physicians for common, chronic complaints. While homeopathic physicians spend more time with their patients, they order fewer tests and prescribe less conventional medication. These data suggest that the cost of homeopathic care for these patients may be less than that of conventional care, although without comparable data on the actual cost of office visits, this is only speculative. Further research comparing clinical outcomes, costs, and patient satisfaction needs to be done to increase our understanding of the role of homeopathy in the health care system.

This work was done in affiliation with the American Institute of Homeopathy. Financial support was provided to the American Institute of Homeopathy by the Boiron Institute, Newton Square, Pa.

References

1. Bouchayer F. Alternative medicines: a general approach to the French situation. *Complementary Med Res.* 1990;4:4–8.
2. Wharton R, Lewith G. Complementary medicine and the general practitioner. *BMJ.* 1986; 292:1498–1500.
3. Ernst E, Kaptchuk TJ. Homeopathy revisited. *Arch Intern Med.* 1996;156:2162–2164.
4. Eisenberg DM, Kessler RC, Foster C, Norlock FE, Calkins DR, Delbanco TL. Unconventional medicine in the United States. *N Engl J Med.* 1993;328:246–252.
5. Swander H. Homeopathy: medical enigma attracts renewed attention. *Am Acad Fam Pract Rep.* 1994;21:1–2.
6. Complementary therapies: homeopathy. *Harvard Women's Health Watch.* January 1997:4.
7. Information Access Company. France leads world in homeopathy. *Marketletter.* May 1996.
8. Jonas W, Jacobs J. *Healing With Homeopathy.* New York, NY: Warner Books; 1996.
9. When to believe the unbelievable. *Nature.* 1988;333:816–818.
10. Kleijnen J, Knipschild P, ter Riet G. Clinical trials of homeopathy. *BMJ.* 1991;302:316323.
11. Reilly DT, Taylor MA, McSharry C, Aitchison T. Is homeopathy a placebo response? controlled trial of homeopathic potency, with pollen in hayfever as model. *Lancet.* 1986;2:881885.
12. Fisher P, Greenwood A, Huskisson EC, Turner P, Belon P. Effect of homeopathic treatment on fibrositis (primary fibromyalgia). *BMJ.* 1989; 299:365–366.
13. Ferley JP, Smirou D, D'Adhemar D, Balducci F. A controlled evaluation of a homeopathic preparation in the treatment of influenza-like syndromes. *Br J Clin Pharmacol.* 1989; 27:329–335.
14. Jacobs J, Jiménez LM, Gloyd SS, Gale JL, Crothers D. Treatment of acute childhood diarrhea with homeopathic medicine: a randomized clinical trial in Nicaragua. *Pediatrics.* 1994;93:719–725.
15. Reilly DT, Taylor MA, Beattie NGM, et al. Is evidence of homeopathy reproducible? *Lancet.* 1994;344:1601–1606.
16. Carton B. Health insurers embrace eye-of-newt therapy. *Wall Street Journal.* January 30, 1995:B1, B4.
17. Firshein J. Picture alternative medicine in the mainstream. *Business Health Solutions Managed Care.* April 1995:29–33.
18. Cowley G, King P, Hager M, Rosenberg D. Going mainstream. *Newsweek.* June 26, 1995:56–57.
19. Swyers MA, Silversmith L, eds. *Alternative Medicine: Expanding Medical Horizons. A Report to the National Institutes of Health on Alternative Medical Systems and Practices in the United States.* Washington, DC: US Government Printing Office; 1995:309–310.
20. *Healthcare Professionals in Private Practice in 1990.* Paris, France: National Office of Medical Insurance (CNAM); 1991. CNAM publication 61.
21. Schappert SM. *National Ambulatory Medical Care Survey: 1990 Summary.* Hyattsville, Md: National Center for Health Statistics; 1992. Advance Data From Vital and Health Statistics, No. 213.
22. American Medical Association [brochure]. *Physicians in the US: Summary Data 1980 to 1993.* Chicago, Ill: American Medical Association; 1994.
23. Vithoulkas G. *The Science of Homeopathy.* New York, NY: Grove Press; 1980.

49 A Double-blind, Controlled Clinical Trial of Homeopathy and an Analysis of Lunar Phases and Postoperative Outcome

Josef Smolle, MD; Gerhard Prause, MD; Helmut Kerl, MD
From the Departments of Dermatology (Drs Smolle and Kerl) and Anesthesiology (Dr Prause), University of Graz, Graz, Austria.

Objective

To use scientific methods to evaluate 2 claims made by practitioners of alternative medicine.

Design

A placebo-controlled, double-blind study of homeopathy in children with warts, and a cohort study of the influence of lunar phases on postoperative outcome in surgical patients.

Setting

Outpatients of a dermatology department (homeopathy study) and inpatients evaluated at an anesthesiology department (lunar phases).

Subjects

Sixty volunteers for the homeopathy study and 14,970 consecutive patients undergoing surgery under general anesthesia for the lunar phase study.

Interventions

Treatment of children with warts with individually selected homeopathic preparations (homeopathic study); surgical procedures including abdominal, vascular, cardiac, thoracic, plastic, and orthopedic operations and assessment of the lunar phase at the time of operation (lunar phase study).

Main Outcome Measures

Reduction of area occupied by warts by at least 50% within 8 weeks; death from any cause within 30 days after surgery.

Results

Nine of 30 subjects in the homeopathy group and 7 of 30 subjects in the placebo group experienced at least 50% reduction in area occupied by warts (χ^2=0.34; *P*=.56); the mortality rate was 1.20% in patients operated on during waxing moon and 1.33% in patients operated on during waning moon (χ^2=0.49; *P*=.50).

Conclusions

Statements and methods of alternative medicine—as far as they concern observable clinical phenomena—can be tested by scientific methods. When such tests yield negative results, as in the studies presented herein, the particular method or statement should be abandoned. Otherwise one would run the risk of supporting superstition and quackery.

Arch Dermatol. 1998;134:1368–1370

In recent years, methods of alternative medicine have gained increasing importance both in public opinion and among physicians. Paradoxically, the critical approach to scientific medical measures often seems to be accompanied by an approach on faith to alternative methods, even when basic data on the alternatives' clinical effectiveness and potential risks are lacking.[1]

The main reason many alternative methods are rejected by representatives of scientific medicine is that often there are few or no sound studies supporting the claims of a particular alternative method. Discussion between practitioners of scientific and alternative medicine is further hampered by the view of some representatives of alternative medicine that clinical studies are inappropriate tools to test alternative medical methods.

In this article we briefly summarize and discuss 2 studies of alternative medicine methods performed under the stringent criteria of scientific evaluation. These studies show that scientific criteria are applicable to the methods of alternative medicine; scientific methods are valuable tools for distinguishing helpful alternative medical methods from superstition and quackery.

Homeopathy in the Treatment of Common Warts

Supporters of homeopathy claim that highly diluted preparations that are chemically identical to pure water contain properties that produce beneficial effects in the treatment of various diseases. Opponents of homeopathy consider all eventual clinical benefits of homeopathic treatment to be placebo effects. In order to evaluate the efficacy of a drug beyond the placebo effect, randomized, double-blind, placebo-controlled trials should be performed. As a drawback in homeopathic trials, there is usually not a single homeopathic preparation to be tested against the placebo; rather, depending on the totality of symptoms of a patient, particular preparations are individually selected by the homeopathic physician.

We performed a double-blind, placebo-controlled study in collaboration with the Boltzmann Institute of Homeopathy, Graz, Austria.[2] In this specially designed study of children with common warts, the homeopathists prepared a list of those remedies most commonly used in treating children with warts. They arrived at a total of 12 different homeopathic preparations. For each preparation, an ordered sequence of bottles with globuli was prepared, with the true homeopathic preparation randomly alternated with pure placebo preparations. After informed written consent was obtained from appropriate subjects and their parents, the subjects were carefully examined by a homeopathic physician, and the best homeopathic preparation—as determined by the particular physician—was selected. When 1 of the 12 preselected preparations was chosen, the subject entered the study and was treated with the next bottle of the particular preparation. Neither the physician nor the subject knew whether the bottle contained the homeopathic preparation or pure placebo. When a homeopathic preparation was selected that was not in the predefined list, this patient did not enter the study. Thus, the study design guaranteed that the subject received either optimal homeopathic treatment or placebo.

The area occupied by the warts on the hands was drawn on transparent sheets and measured with a digitizer board before and after 8 weeks of treatment. Fifty percent reduction of the area involved was chosen as the primary outcome variable at the beginning of the study, and subjects demonstrating this 50% reduction qualified as *responders*.

Of the 70 subjects who signed up for the study, 3 were rejected prior to treatment (2 because the homeopathic preparation required was not on the preselected list and 1 because the subject's symptoms did not allow for a homeopathic diagnosis). Of the remaining 67 subjects, 7 withdrew from the study (3 from the placebo group and 4 from the remedy group). The reasons for withdrawal were exacerbation of warts in 2 cases (1 in each group), thrombosis of a capillary hemangioma in 1 case (placebo), and unavailability for follow-up in 4 cases (1 placebo and 3 active treatment). There were a total of 16 responders: 9 of 30 subjects in the homeopathic therapy group and 7 of 30 subjects in the placebo group (χ^2=0.34; *P*=.56). Obviously, there was no significant difference in efficacy between pure placebo and the homeopathic remedy in the context of this study.

Relationship of Lunar Phases and Postoperative Outcome

Potential influences of lunar phases on human behavior and incidence of disease have been discussed for a long time. During the last few years, several reports have been published, albeit most of them negative or inconclusive, concerning the moon's influence on suicides,[3,4] psychiatric crises,[5] car crashes,[6] and childbirths.[7] More recently, much attention has been paid in the lay press to lunar phases, particularly the full and waxing moon, as potential risk factors for postoperative complications.[8] While these claims have led to serious concern among patients and to some extent also among physicians, in a pilot study[9] no relationship between lunar phases and complications was found.

We examined the clinical records of 14,970 patients who underwent surgery under general anesthesia from 1990 to 1996 at the Department of Surgery, University of Graz, and who had had preoperative evaluation at the Department of Anesthesiology.[10] Surgical procedures included abdominal, vascular, cardiac, thoracic, plastic, and orthopedic operations. Postoperative mortality was defined as death from any cause within 30 days after surgery. Based on scientific tables of moon phases,[11] each operation was labeled as having been done at waxing, waning, or full moon. Potential relationships of lunar phases and outcome were tested by χ^2 statistics.

Of 14,970 patients, 189 (1.26%) died within 30 days after surgery. Mortality rate was 1.20% for patients operated on during waxing moon and 1.33% for patients operated on during waning moon (χ^2=0.49, *P*=.50). At full moon, mortality rate was 1.16% compared with 1.27% at other lunar phases (χ^2=0.04; *P*=.85). These data strongly indicate that postoperative mortality does not depend on lunar phases. Previous claims of a greater risk inherent in operations performed during a full or waxing moon can be disregarded as superstition, at least as far as lethal complications are concerned.

Comment

There seems to be a clear-cut difference between scientific and alternative medicine. While scientific medicine judges the truth of a given statement on observation, alternative medicine often bases its judgment solely on a philosophical model or a certain paradigm. This does not prevent scientific medicine from making errors, but it does prevent it from creating philosophical systems that have no relationship to the real world.

Supporters of alternative medical concepts often accuse representatives of scientific medicine of adhering strictly to physical facts and measurable phenomena and neglecting all other aspects of human life. Because this accusation is sometimes used to reject clinical studies like those presented herein, it should be carefully evaluated. However, we have provided 2 examples of clinical studies on aspects of alternative medicine that yielded negative results. Both studies deal with statements of alternative medicine that directly concern observable facts: homeopathists claim that children with warts will experience improvement when treated with a homeopathic remedy compared with pure water, and physicians believing in the power of lunar phases claim that the moon affects postoperative outcome. Each of these statements has proven itself subject to scientific refutation.

In conclusion, methods and statements introduced by supporters of alternative medicine should be scientifically tested whenever possible. If independent tests repeatedly support the alternative methods or statements, scientific medicine should gratefully accept this enrichment of therapeutic modalities. When, however, as here, the findings are unambiguously negative, the alternative medicine methods or statements should be abandoned.

References

1. Bühring M. *Naturheilkunde: Grundlagen, Anwendungen, Ziele*. Munich, Germany: Beck; 1997.

2. Kainz JT, Kozel G, Haidvogl M, Smolle J. Homoeopathic versus placebo therapy of children with warts on the hands: a randomized, double-blind clinical trial. *Dermatology.* 1996;193:318–320.

3. Gutierrez Garcia JM, Tusell F. Suicides and the lunar cycle. *Psychol Rep.* 1997;80:243–250.

4. Martin SJ, Kelly IW, Saklofske DH. Suicide and lunar cycles: a critical review over 28 years. *Psychol Rep.* 1992;71:787–795.

5. Gorvin JJ, Roberts MS. Lunar phases and psychiatric hospital admissions. *Psychol Rep.* 1994;75:1425–1440.

6. Kelly IW, Rotton J. Geophysical variables and behavior, XIII: comment on "lunar phase and accident injuries": the dark side of the moon and lunar research. *Percept Mot Skills.* 1983; 57:919–921.

7. Kelly IW, Martens R. Geophysical variables and behavior, LXXVIII: lunar phase and birthrate: an update. *Psychol Rep.* 1994;75:507–511.

8. Paungger J, Poppe T. *Vom richtigen Zeitpunkt: die Anwendung des Mondkalenders im täglichen Leben*. Munich, Germany: Heinrich Hugendubel Verlag; 1995.

9. Smolle J, Smolle-Juettner FM, Prause G, Ratzenhofer-Kommenda B. "Vom richtigen Zeitpunkt": Mondphasen und Operationskomplikationen. *Tagliche Praxis.* 1996; 37:309–311.

10. Smolle J, Prause G, Pierer G, et al. Mondphasen und Operationskomplikationen: eine Analyse von mehr als 14.000 Fällen. *Acta Chir Aust.* In press.

11. Meeus J. *Astronomical Tables of the Sun, Moon and Planets*. London, England: Willmann-Bell; 1983.

50 Homeopathic vs Conventional Treatment of Vertigo

A Randomized Double-blind Controlled Clinical Study

Michael Weiser, MBChB; Wolfgang Strösser, MD, MBChB; Peter Klein, MSc
From the Biologische Heilmittel Heel GmbH, Baden-Baden (Dr Weiser), Clinical Research and Pharma Consulting, Bergisch Gladbach (Dr Strösser), and Datenservice Eva Hönig GmbH, Rohrbach (Mr Klein), Germany.

Objective
To compare the efficacy and safety of a homeopathic remedy (Vertigoheel, Heel Inc, Albuquerque, NM) vs betahistine hydrochloride (active control) in the treatment of patients with vertigo of various origins in a confirmative equivalence trial.

Design
Randomized (1:1) double-blind controlled clinical trial.

Setting
Fifteen study centers (general practice) in Germany between November 1995 and November 1996.

Subjects
A total of 119 patients with vertigo of various origins (from whom 105 patients could be analyzed as intended per protocol).

Main Outcome Measures
Frequency, duration, and intensity of vertigo attacks.

Results
Both homeopathic and conventional treatments showed a clinically relevant reduction in the mean frequency, duration, and intensity of the vertigo attacks. The therapeutic equivalence of the homeopathic remedy and betahistine was established statistically.

Conclusions
Concerning the main efficacy variable, therapeutic equivalence between the homeopathic remedy and betahistine could be shown with statistical significance (confirmative analysis). Both remedies reduced the frequency, duration, and intensity of vertigo attacks during a 6-week treatment period. Also, vertigo-specific complaints were significantly reduced in both treatment groups.

Arch Otolaryngol Head Neck Surg. 1998;124:879–885

Vertigo is a common symptom with significant adverse effects on the patient's quality of life. Physicians in private practice are frequently confronted with this diagnosis, which often requires extensive investigation to determine its origin. In one study,[1] dizziness was the ninth most common symptom at initial evaluation in the outpatient setting. Vertigo may arise from lesions in the central nervous system, particularly in the nuclei of the vestibular nerve, the cerebellum, and the connections between cerebellar and vestibular nuclei. More frequently, vertigo is caused by disturbances of the vestibular nerve and vestibular cochlear system and occasionally is of vascular origin.[2] Vertigo results from abnormal processing of apparently contradicting information in the central nervous system and is often accompanied by auditory symptoms, making it more difficult for the patient to tolerate. Patients with vertigo suffer from nausea, emesis, sweating, collapse, and tinnitus. Disturbances of equilibrium, including rotational or positional vertigo, systematic imbalance, or instability, can have negative consequences on the social lives of patients and can be truly disabling.

Benign paroxysmal positional vertigo, vestibular neuritis, and Ménière disease are the primary types of vertigo, but the exact cause of vertigo often remains unknown. In many patients, a further complicating factor is that the vertigo symptoms continually change character and intensity. Positional vertigo is usually indicative of a benign vestibular disorder. The most common type is benign paroxysmal positional vertigo, which is characterized by a feeling of dizziness while lying down as well as in the sitting position. There may be dizziness from turning the head from side to side or from flexing and extending the neck. The classic finding on examination is a burst of rotary nystagmus when the patient is rapidly placed in the right- or left-ear-down position.[2] Regardless of the exact cause, it is important to reduce the frequency, intensity, and duration of vertigo attacks with an effective medication that has no adverse effects.

The following clinical trial involves a homeopathic preparation (Vertigoheel, Heel Inc, Albuquerque, NM) containing ambra grisea D6, anamirta cocculus D4, conium maculatum D3, and petroleum rectificatum D8. (Designators D6, D4, D3, and D8 denote the concentrations of the various ingredients of the homeopathic preparation.) This homeopathic remedy has been applied successfully in the treatment of vertigo in earlier studies.[3–5] The mode of action of the homeopathic remedy is not fully understood. However, its pharmacodynamic effects on acoustically evoked brainstem potentials have been investigated.[6] The present study was designed to test the therapeutic equivalence of the homeopathic remedy vs betahistine hydrochloride. Betahistine (2-pyridine) stimulates the histaminergic histamine 1 and histamine 2 receptors in the brain, which increases the cyclic adenosine monophosphate (cAMP) levels in the blood vessel walls. As a result, blood flow, especially in the brain, is increased through vasodilation. Betahistine is considered a standard treatment for patients experiencing vertigo.[7–10] Its efficacy has been determined in previous placebo-controlled studies.[11,12] Therefore, betahistine was chosen as the reference drug for this clinical trial.

Patients and Methods

Between November 1995 and November 1996, 119 patients of both sexes from 15 centers (all general practices) in Germany were considered for enrollment in the study. The main inclusion criteria were acute or chronic vertigo symptoms of various origins (including Ménière disease and vasomotor vertigo), a minimum of 3 vertigo attacks during the week before the study began, and an assessment of intensity of vertigo attacks by the patient between 2 and 4 on a 5-point rating scale (see below). The main exclusion criteria were chronic vertigo (longer than 6 months) if specifically treated during the 4 weeks before the study began; vertigo caused by psychovegetative disorders (to avoid possible noncompliance); vertigo caused by a tumor or coffee, tea, tobacco, alcohol, or drug abuse; vertigo caused by inflammation from an underlying disease; myocardial infarction within 6 months before the study began; severe metabolic disease; gastroduodenal ulcer; pheochromocytoma; or bronchial asthma. Furthermore, other concomitant vertigo or antiemetic medication, corticosteroids or antihistamines, migraine medication, psychoactive drugs, and vascular drugs were not allowed during the study (washout phase, 7 days before the study began). The study was conducted in accordance with Good Clinical Practices, consistent with the Declaration of Helsinki, and the product was manufactured in accordance with Good Manufacturing Practices, consistent with the US Food and Drug Administration's Code of Federal Regulations. The study was conducted by a contract research organization to exclude the possibility of a sponsor bias.

After being screened for eligibility, patients were randomly assigned to the homeopathic-remedy group or the betahistine group (day 1=visit 1). Randomization was performed at each center by assigning consecutive patients to the next available treatment group from a computer-generated randomization list. The study was double blind, consistent with the "double-dummy" technique[13]: because of the difference in taste between betahistine and the homeopathic remedy, corresponding placebos of the active drugs were produced that were identical in taste, as well as shape and smell. The patients in both groups took 15 drops 3 times daily of the active drug (homeopathic remedy or betahistine) plus the corresponding placebo each day for 42 consecutive days (betahistine dosage: 18 mg/d in 3 divided doses). Effectiveness and tolerability of the treatments were checked at day 3 (±1 day, visit 2), day 7 (±1 day, visit 3), and after days 14 (±2 days, visit 4), 28 (±3 days, visit 5), and 42 (±3 days, visit 6). To assess the influence of the treatment on quality of life, the patients were advised to continue normal physical activity (see below). Laboratory tests and physical examinations were conducted for each patient at the beginning (day 1) and end (day 42) of the study.

Primary Efficacy Variables

Frequency, duration, and intensity of vertigo attacks were the primary efficacy variables. These variables were assessed at visit 1 for the week before the study began (baseline) and for each study day in a diary. The mean daily duration of all vertigo attacks was assessed on a 5-point rating scale, where 0 indicates between 0 and 2 minutes; 1, between 2 and 10 minutes; 2, between 11 and 60 minutes; 3, between 1 and 6 hours; and 4, more than 6 hours. The mean daily intensity of all vertigo attacks was assessed on another 5-point rating scale, where 0 indicates no discomfort; 1, slight discomfort; 2, moderate discomfort; 3, severe discomfort; and 4, very severe discomfort. For all 3 variables, the mean daily occurrences of all vertigo attacks were assessed by the patient on an ordinal rating scale.

Secondary Efficacy Variables

Quality of Life. The quality of life was measured at visits 1 and 6 (at the last visit for patients who did not complete the study) with the validated questionnaire Medical Outcome Study-Short Form 36.[14] This questionnaire provides a comprehensive, psychometrically sound and efficient way to measure health from the patient's point of view by scoring standardized responses to standardized questions concerning physical health (physical functioning, role limitations attributed to physical problems, bodily pain, and general health) and mental health (vitality, social functioning, role limitations attributed to emotional problems, and mental health). The version translated to German and psychometrically tested was used in this study. For the questionnaires, transformed raw scores were computed according to the Medical Outcome Study-Short Form 36 manual.[14]

Severity and Impact. Severity of vertigo-specific symptoms and general impairment of daily life were assessed by means of a questionnaire that was based on the Neuro-Otologische Datenerfassung Claussen test,[3,4,6] a specific anamnestic rating scale for patients with vertigo. The questionnaire was divided into 4 parts, each containing a different set of questions. Set 1 assessed the direct vertigo symptoms, such as feeling of spinning, staggering, or elevation. Set 2 assessed the intensity of vertigo during different special exercises, such as turning the head, bending down, getting up, and laying down. Set 3 assessed vertigo-associated symptoms, such as general weakness, restrictions in hearing or seeing, headache, tinnitus, tiredness, anxiety, or insomnia. Set 4 assessed restrictions in daily life activities, such as problems while reading, going up or down stairs, using public transportation, performing housework, or walking in the dark. A total score was calculated from the scores of the individual questions and transformed to a scale of 0 (maximum number of symptoms) to 100 (no symptoms) for comparability.

Assessment of Efficacy

The patients' and investigators' global assessments of efficacy were carried out on a 5-point rating scale, where 1 indicates absolutely no complaints; 2, significant improvement; 3, slight improvement; 4, no improvement; and 5, deterioration.

The safety of the study medications was assessed by means of adverse events, clinical laboratory data (hematologic evaluations, clinical chemical evaluations, and urinalysis), and vital signs (blood pressure, pulse, body weight, and oral body temperature). Finally, the investigators and the patients assessed the global overall tolerability of the treatment at visit 6 according to the following scale: 1 indicates excellent; 2, good; 3, fair; and 4, poor.

Statistics

The sample size was calculated on the basis of the following assumptions: mean score reduction of 2 points in intensity of vertigo attacks while taking betahistine; assumed SD of score reduction, 0.8; probability of falsely rejecting the hypotheses of inferiority of homeopathic remedy, α=.05; and power of the test, $1-\beta$=0.8. The region of equivalence was stipulated at 20% (ie, a minor reduction of 0.4 score points). These assumptions mandated 50 patients per treatment group to demonstrate the equivalence of the homeopathic remedy and betahistine. Primary variables for the assessment of efficacy were the reduction of frequency, duration, and intensity of vertigo attacks, defined as the difference between the mean daily occurrences during the last study week (week 6) and the week before the study began (baseline). It was expected that the differences for the 3 variables would develop in the same direction (1-sided *t* test). The Wei-Lachin directional test[15] was performed as a simultaneous test to control the α level of .05. As a measure for effect size, the Mann-Whitney test was used (probability of superiority or inferiority of a patient in the homeopathic group compared with a patient of the betahistine group). Therefore, only ordinal information was used to assess treatment effects, reducing the possibility of biasing the treatment results because of the nonlinearity of scaling distances. The following hypotheses were stipulated in the trial protocol to show the noninferiority of the homeopathic group to the betahistine group: The treatment difference (homeopathic product minus betahistine) was equal to the lower equivalence margin for the reduction of frequency, duration, and intensity of vertigo attacks vs the alternative that the treatment difference was greater than the lower equivalence margin for at least 1 of the primary efficacy variables. Equivalence or superiority of the homeopathic remedy vs betahistine was shown if the lower limit of the 95% confidence interval (1 sided) of the Mann-Whitney statistic is larger than 0.36 (ie, moderate inferiority). The test was carried out using the validated program SmarTest.[15–17] The last-observation-carried-forward principle was used to include patients who did not complete the study (owing to cure or other reasons) in the analysis (end-point analysis). The secondary efficacy variables and the safety variables were analyzed descriptively.

Results

A total of 119 patients (59 in the homeopathic group and 60 in the betahistine group) were recruited, randomized, treated, and observed in 15 centers. The number of patients per center varied between 1 and 23. The data of 2 patients were inconsistent and not comprehensible and, therefore, were excluded from the study. Major protocol deviations (violations of inclusion or exclusion criteria, compliance, premature study termination because of patient's personal reasons, or unavailable for follow-up) led to the exclusion of 12 patients from analysis intended per protocol analysis. The per protocol analysis was chosen as the primary efficacy evaluation, because it is the more conservative analysis in equivalence trials.[18] A total of 117 patients were assessed with regard to safety. Of the 105 patients in the per protocol analysis, 9 patients (8.6%) terminated the study prematurely because of cure (homeopathic group, n=4; betahistine group, n=3) or worsening of symptoms (betahistine group, n=2). The patients in the 2 treatment groups were comparable with regard to demographic (eg, sex and age) and anamnestic (eg, abnormal findings at baseline or characterization of vertigo) data. In only a small percentage (approximately 10%) was the exact cause of vertigo known (eg, cardiovascular disease or orthostatic hypotension). In more than 70% of the patients in both treatment groups, the patients were being treated for vertigo for the first time. Patients with differential diagnoses were enrolled in the study with vestibular vertigo (rotary vertigo, positional vertigo, elevation-induced vertigo, or staggering vertigo), vasomotor vertigo (caused by circulation disturbances, eg, arteriosclerosis, hypertension, or hypotension), or both (Table 1). Whereas vestibular vertigo has a clear direction of motion (eg, rotary vertigo or elevation-induced vertigo), the vasomotor vertigo is more diffuse (eg, blurred vision or unsteadiness). The mean exposure time to treatment was 40.2 days (homeopathic remedy) vs 40.9 days (betahistine) in the per protocol analysis. In the safety population, the mean exposure times were 39.3 days (homeopathic remedy) and 37.6 days (betahistine).

Primary Efficacy Variables

The therapeutic equivalence of the homeopathic remedy and betahistine was demonstrated statistically by analyzing the primary variables. The values of the primary variables revealed no significant differences between the homeopathic group and the betahistine group before the start of treatment (baseline) and during the last study week. In all 3 primary variables, a clinically relevant reduction was found (Figure 1 and Table 2). The alternative hypothesis of noninferiority of the homeopathic remedy concerning at least 1 of the 3 vertigo criteria can therefore be accepted (Mann-Whitney statistics: $P[X<Y]=.51$ with a lower 1-sided 95% confidence limit=0.46). Concerning the frequency of vertigo attacks, a slight superiority of the homeopathic remedy in comparison to betahistine could be ascertained (Figure 1). Concerning the criteria of duration and intensity of vertigo attacks, no marked difference between the treatment groups could be ascertained. For both variables, the lower 1-sided 95% confidence limit was greater than the limit of a mean inferiority (Figure 2).

Table 1. Baseline Characteristics for Patients in the Evaluable Efficacy Sample

Parameters	Homeopathic Group (n=53)	Betahistine Group (n=52)
Sex, No. (%)		
Male	16.0 (30.2)*	13.0 (25.0)*
Female	37.0 (69.8)	39.0 (75.0)
Age, y		
Mean (SD)	50.0 (16.3)†	54.8 (15.9)†
Median (range)	49.0 (18.0-77.0)	57.0 (26.0-83.0)
Patients with abnormal findings, No. (%)‡	23.0 (39.7)	23.0 (39.0)
Patients receiving prestudy or concomitant medication, No. (%)§		
Yes	17.0 (32.1)	18.0 (34.6)
No	36.0 (67.9)	34.0 (65.4)
Characterization of vertigo, No. (%)		
Vestibular vertigo	29.0 (54.7)	35.0 (67.3)
Vasomotor vertigo‖	19.0 (35.8)	11.0 (21.2)
Both	5.0 (9.4)	6.0 (11.5)
Cause of vertigo, No. (%)		
Known	7.0 (13.2)	5.0 (9.6)
Unknown	46.0 (86.8)	47.0 (90.4)
First-time treatment of vertigo, No. (%)	39.0 (73.6)	39.0 (75.0)
Chronic or relapsed vertigo, No. (%)	14.0 (26.4)	13.0 (25.0)
Time since first occurrence of vertigo symptoms, mo, median (range)	1.3 (0.1-309.0)	1.8 (0.1-154.0)

*P=.66 by Fisher exact test.
†P=.17 by Mann-Whitney test.
‡These patients had abnormal findings (eg, problems in the musculoskeletal system or head and nape or with vascular state) at the baseline physical examination.
§Medication for treatment of abnormal findings above.
‖Vasomotor vertigo caused by circulation disturbances (eg, arteriosclerosis, hypertension, or hypotension).

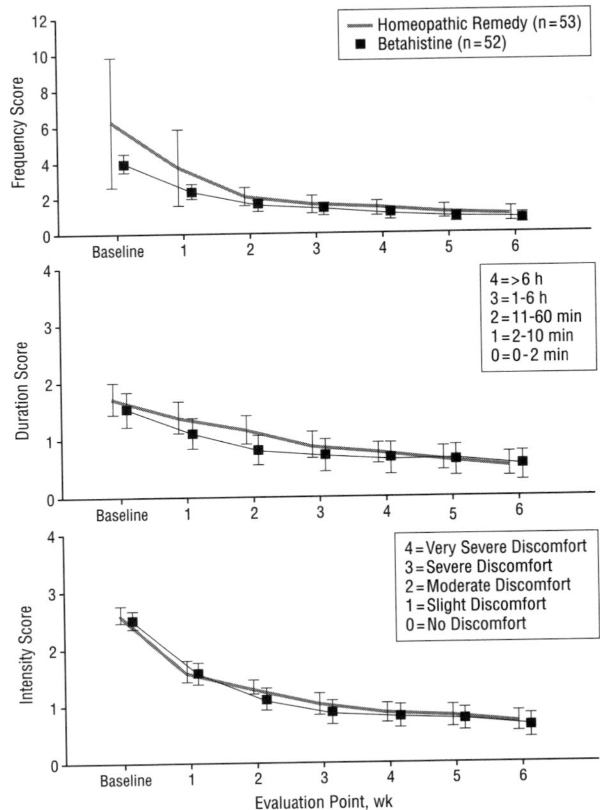

Figure 1. Mean daily frequency, duration, and intensity of vertigo attacks at baseline through week 6 are shown. Error bars indicate upper and lower 95% confidence limits.

Secondary Efficacy Variables

In all 4 categories of the vertigo-specific questionnaire, there was a significant reduction of the vertigo-specific symptoms. No marked differences were found between the 2 treatment groups (Table 3). The descriptive results for the quality-of-life questionnaire Medical Outcome Study-Short Form 36 are summarized in Table 4. Overall, in all categories of physical and mental health, an increase from baseline to visit 6 (or the last visit for patients not completing the study) can be seen. There are no striking differences between the treatment groups. The global assessment of efficacy by the investigators and the patients did not reveal striking differences between the 2 treatment groups (Mann-Whitney test, 1-sided: investigators, P=.63; patients, P=.76). A worsening of symptoms was seen in 1 (1.9%) patient (investigators' assessments) and 3 (5.8%) patients (patients' assessments) with betahistine treatment, whereas no worsening of symptoms was seen with the homeopathic treatment. In both groups, for more than 70% of the patients a significant improvement with absolutely no complaints was reported by the investigators.

Safety Variables

Fifty-seven adverse events (29 in the homeopathic group and 28 in the betahistine group) during the clinical trial were reported for 31 patients (26.5%). The causal relationship of an adverse event to the study treatment was assessed by the investigator as very probable, probable, or possible 4 times in 2 patients (homeopathic group, 3.4%) and 2 times in 1 patient (betahistine group, 1.7%). The specific adverse events were nausea, tremor of the hands

Table 2. Mean Frequency, Duration, and Intensity of Vertigo Attacks per Day in the Evaluable Efficacy Sample*

Statistics	Frequency of Vertigo Attacks† Baseline	Frequency of Vertigo Attacks† Change	Duration of Vertigo Attacks† Baseline	Duration of Vertigo Attacks† Change	Intensity of Vertigo Attacks† Baseline	Intensity of Vertigo Attacks† Change
Homeopathic group score (n=53)						
Mean (SD)	6.3 (13.1)	−5.3 (13.3)	1.7 (1.0)	−1.2 (1.2)	2.6 (0.5)	−1.9 (0.8)
Median	4.0	−3.4	2.0	−1.0	3.0	−1.9
Betahistine group score (n=52)						
Mean (SD)	4.0 (1.8)	−3.3 (2.1)	1.5 (1.1)	−1.0 (1.4)	2.5 (0.5)	−1.9 (0.8)
Median	4.0	−3.0	1.0	−1.0	2.0	−2.0
P, Mann-Whitney test	.16	...	.32	...	.30	...
P(X<Y)‡	0.42	...	0.45	...	0.45	...
95% CI‡	0.31 to 0.53	...	0.34 to 0.55	...	0.35 to 0.55	...
Single test‡						
P(X<Y)	...	0.53	...	0.51	...	0.50
90% CI, LB§	...	0.46	...	0.44	...	0.43
Simultaneous test‖						
P(X<Y)‡	...	...	...	...	...	0.51
90% CI, LB§	...	...	...	...	...	0.46

*See the "Patients and Methods" section for a description of frequency, duration, and intensity scoring. Ellipses indicate not applicable.
†Baseline measured week before treatment start; change is last 7 days of treatment minus baseline.
‡*P*(X<Y) indicates the Mann-Whitney statistic (reference measure for superiority).
§CI indicates confidence interval; LB, lower boundary.
‖Generalized multiple Mann-Whitney test (stochastic ordering).

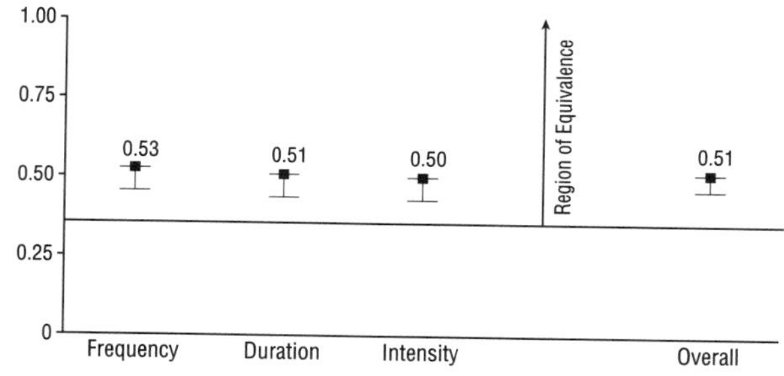

Figure 2. Equivalence or superiority in change from baseline for vertigo attacks. Data shown are Mann-Whitney statistics. Error bars indicate lower boundaries of 90% confidence intervals; solid line, upper bound of inferiority.

in the homeopathic group, and headache combined with very strong vertigo in the betahistine group. Mean relevant changes from baseline were not observed in either treatment group, neither for the clinical laboratory variables nor for the vital signs variables. There were no striking differences between the global tolerability assessments of the investigators and the patients or between the treatment groups (Mann-Whitney test, 2-sided: investigators, *P*=.46; patients, *P*=.18). For more than 90% of the patients, a good or excellent tolerability of the homeopathic remedy or betahistine was reported by the investigators.

Comment

Clinical evaluation of the efficacy of vertigo treatment is difficult. It requires the use of both objective criteria, such as frequency and duration of attacks and evidence of vestibular dysfunction, and subjective criteria, such as severity of vertigo, unsteadiness between attacks, cochlear symptoms, and vegetative symptoms. One of the main problems in the evaluation of any treatment is that the symptoms of vertigo have 2 common features: discontinuity and variability in intensity.[19,20] In the present clinical trial, all of these criteria were assessed. Subjective criteria must be given emphasis, since they reflect the patient's experience of discomfort. In this study, the homeopathic remedy proved to be as effective as betahistine in the treatment of vertigo of various origins. Concerning the associated symptoms, there was no statistically significant difference between the 2 treatment groups, whatever the population tested; this demonstrates therapeutic equivalence.

Table 3. Vertigo-Specific Questionnaire for the Evaluable Efficacy Sample*

	Set 1†			Set 2†			Set 3†			Set 4†		
Statistics‡	Baseline	Change (Visit 2)§	Change (Visit 6)§	Baseline	Change (Visit 2)§	Change (Visit 6)§	Baseline	Change (Visit 2)§	Change (Visit 6)§	Baseline	Change (Visit 2)§	Change (Visit 6)§
Homeopathic group												
Patients, No.	52.0	52.0	51.0	53.0	53.0	52.0	53.0	53.0	52.0	53.0	53.0	52.0
Score												
Mean	58.5	+7.6	+28.6	53.6	+4.6	+29.2	65.2	+3.6	+19.0	47.9	+2.4	+11.8
SD	18.2	13.2	17.2	24.2	13.1	23.6	17.2	9.8	11.3	13.5	6.8	8.9
Median	58.9	+3.6	+28.6	56.3	0.0	+25.0	67.1	+2.6	+16.5	47.4	+1.3	+11.2
Betahistine group												
Patients, No.	52.0	52.0	52.0	52.0	52.0	52.0	52.0	52.0	52.0	52.0	52.0	52.0
Score												
Mean	64.6	+8.6	+25.8	58.4	+6.1	+28.7	72.8	+5.5	+16.8	49.7	+4.8	+12.5
SD	18.2	14.6	22.8	23.8	17.5	24.9	13.8	8.5	13.5	12.8	7.4	13.2
Median	64.3	+3.6	+25.0	56.3	+3.2	+25.0	72.4	+2.6	+17.1	52.6	+3.3	+9.9
P, Mann-Whitney test	.11	...	...	.30	...	...	.04	...	...	.46	...	...
P(X<Y)	0.41	0.50	0.53	0.44	0.49	0.50	0.38	0.44	0.54	0.46	0.41	0.51
95% CI, LB	0.30	0.41	0.44	0.33	0.40	0.41	0.27	0.35	0.45	0.35	0.32	0.42
95% CI, UB	0.52	...	...	0.55	...	...	0.49	...	...	0.57	...	...

*Summary score of questionnaire transformed to a scale from 0 to 100, where 0=maximum of symptoms and 100=no symptoms. Plus signs emphasize the improvement. CI indicates confidence interval; LB, lower boundary; UB, upper boundary; and ellipses, data not applicable.
†Set 1 assessed direct vertigo symptoms; set 2, intensity of vertigo during special exercises; set 3, vertigo-associated symptoms; and set 4, restrictions in daily life activities. See the "Patients and Methods" section for further descriptions of the 4 sets.
‡*P*(X<Y) is the Mann-Whitney statistic (reference measure for superiority).
§Baseline measured week before treatment start, change (visit 2) after 3 days, and change (visit 6) after 42 days minus baseline.

All clinical trials have shortcomings. In the present study, the exact cause of vertigo was unknown in 90% of the patients. However, for more than 70% of the patients in both treatment groups, none had been treated before. In general, in this early stage of a disease, no specific differential diagnosis is given, so that one third of patients of the homeopathic group were characterized as having vasomotor vertigo. Another shortcoming of this study was the lack of a placebo control. Although there are methodological reasons for a placebo control, the ethics of not treating a serious disease like vertigo must be considered. For this study, ethical considerations outweighed the methodological ideal. Furthermore, the efficacy of betahistine in the treatment of vertigo has been demonstrated in placebo-controlled studies and is accepted as a standard treatment for patients suffering from vertigo.[11,12] Because of the taste differences between betahistine and the homeopathic remedy, a "double-dummy" design was used. This design guaranteed a high degree of blinding. Because of the lack of a placebo arm, the rate of spontaneous improvement in this trial is unknown, a common problem in clinical research. To reduce the rate of spontaneous improvement to a minimum, patients with less than 3 vertigo attacks during the week before the study began and with an intensity score lower than 2 (on a 5-point rating scale) were excluded from the study.

The patient's global impression is an important variable to assess the efficacy of antivertigo medication. Many rating scales[21] have been developed in an attempt to measure the specific influence of a disease on a patient's quality of life. A major general criticism of these instruments is that they were all developed in an attempt to provide a universal formula for evaluating the deterioration in enjoyment of life caused by a wide variety of disease processes. But some of them[22] were specifically developed to determine the deterioration in quality of life induced by a specific disease syndrome. Besides the specific vertigo questionnaire, the validated and widely used quality-of-life questionnaire Medical Outcome Study-Short Form 36 was used as a secondary variable.[14] Both treatment groups revealed slight superiorities or inferiorities for single groups of questions. But, in total, the outcome was similar. Prominent were the resultant comfort or sense of well-being of the patients; the

Table 4. Summary Scores for the Quality-of-Life Questionnaires in the Evaluable Efficacy Sample*

	Physical Health								Mental Health							
	Physical Functioning		Role Limitations Attributed to Physical Problems		Bodily Pain		General Health		Vitality		Role Limitations Attributed to Emotional Problems		Social Functioning		Mental Health	
Statistics†	**Baseline**	**Change**	**Baseline**	**Change**	**Baseline**	**Change**	**Baseline**	**Change**	**Baseline**	**Change**	**Baseline**	**Change**	**Baseline**	**Change**	**Baseline**	**Change**
Homeopathic remedy group																
Patients, No.	51.0	51.0	51.0	51.0	51.0	51.0	51.0	51.0	51.0	51.0	51.0	51.0	51.0	51.0	51.0	51.0
Summary scores																
Mean	60.8	+18.7	42.2	+27.0	65.9	+7.1	52.2	+6.6	41.7	+9.1	49.0	+30.7	64.2	+8.6	52.8	+6.4
SD	24.7	25.4	40.2	43.0	30.5	26.3	17.9	16.5	16.4	16.9	42.9	45.1	23.3	21.3	20.8	15.8
Median	60.0	+15.0	25.0	+25.0	62.0	0.0	52.0	+5.0	40.0	+10.0	66.7	0.0	62.5	0.0	48.0	+4.0
Betahistine group																
Patients, No.	51.0	51.0	50.0	50.0	51.0	51.0	51.0	50.0	51.0	51.0	50.0	50.0	51.0	51.0	51.0	51.0
Summary scores																
Mean	64.8	+16.9	43.5	+24.5	68.5	+13.9	50.7	+11.5	44.6	+11.7	57.3	+22.7	67.4	+14.2	55.9	+8.5
SD	27.1	29.5	41.0	44.2	29.2	28.8	19.0	19.7	14.4	16.1	43.2	48.3	23.9	20.8	16.6	16.1
Median	65.0	+10.0	25.0	+12.5	72.0	0.0	45.0	+10.0	40.0	+10.0	66.7	0.0	62.5	+12.5	52.0	+4.0
P, Mann-Whitney test	.31	. . .	.90	. . .	.68	. . .	.45	. . .	.23	. . .	.28	. . .	.49	. . .	.37	. . .
P(X<Y)	0.44	0.55	0.49	0.52	0.48	0.42	0.54	0.44	0.43	0.45	0.44	0.54	0.46	0.43	0.45	0.46
95% CI, LB	0.33	0.46	0.38	0.43	0.37	0.33	0.43	0.35	0.32	0.36	0.33	0.45	0.35	0.34	0.34	0.37
95% CI, UB	0.55	. . .	0.60	. . .	0.58	. . .	0.65	. . .	0.54	. . .	0.55	. . .	0.57	. . .	0.56	. . .

*Summary scores of the Medical Outcome Study-Short Form 36 questionnaires transformed to a scale of 0 to 100, with 0=lowest possible quality of life and 100=highest possible quality of life. Plus signs emphasize the improvement. Baseline measures week before treatment start; change is last 7 days of treatment minus baseline. CI, confidence interval; LB, lower boundary; UB, upper boundary; and ellipses, data not applicable.
†*P*(X<Y) indicates the Mann-Whitney statistic (reference measure for superiority).

extent to which they were able to maintain reasonable physical, emotional, and intellectual function; and the degree to which they retained their ability to participate in valued activities with family, in the workplace, and in the community.

All antivertigo medications have adverse effects, depending on their particular pharmacodynamic properties.[2] Therefore, their efficacy depends on the delicate balance between the benefits they impart in reducing the vertigo attacks and their unwanted effects. The tolerability of the homeopathic remedy and betahistine during this study was assessed as very good. Overall, it can be stated that, with the data obtained, the efficacy and safety of the homeopathic remedy in the treatment of vertigo of various origins was provable within the framework of a phase 4 clinical study.

Conclusions

The effectiveness and tolerability of a homeopathic remedy was compared with that of betahistine via a controlled double-blind study. Betahistine is considered a standard treatment for patients suffering from vertigo of various origins. Its efficacy has been reported in previous placebo-controlled studies. The study confirmed the therapeutic value of both treatments in patients suffering from vertigo of various origins as shown in the reduction of the frequency, intensity, and duration of vertigo attacks. Vertigo-specific complaints were significantly and similarly reduced in both treatment groups. The characteristics (improvement) of the quality of life, in combination with the statistically significant reduction of the vertigo attacks, are of clinical relevance. The tolerability of the homeopathic remedy and betahistine during the study was very good.

We thank W. Benik, MD, PhD, Bad Driburg, Germany; A. Bott, MD, PhD, Mannheim, Germany; G. Bretzke, MD, PhD, Zwickau, Germany; G. Buecher, MD, PhD, Ilvesheim, Germany; W. Daut, MD, PhD, Kallstadt, Germany; F. Eitner, MD, PhD, Bruehl, Germany; W. Elsel, MD, PhD, Zwickau; M. Fiebrich, MD,

Neuweiler, Germany; J. Jach-Broetzmann, MD, Mainz, Germany; D. Jost, MD, Speyer, Germany; M. Keller, MD, PhD, Donaueschingen, Germany; J. Krehbiel, MD, PhD, Roedersheim, Germany; A. Orth, MD, PhD, Speyer; F. Palm, MD, PhD, Boehl-Iggelheim, Germany; P. Schlueter, MD, PhD, Hemsbach, Germany; I. Schramm-Kempeni, MD, PhD, Neustadt, Germany; M. Schuetz, MD, PhD, Bensheim, Germany; and H.-J. Zimmermann, MD, PhD, Ingelheim, Germany for participation as clinical investigators in this study.

References

1. Kroenke K, Arrington ME, Mangelsdorff AD. The prevalence of symptoms in medical outpatients and the adequacy of therapy. *Arch Intern Med.* 1990;150:1685–1689.

2. Parker SW. Otoneurology. In: Stein JH, ed. *Internal Medicine.* 4th rev ed. St Louis, Mo: Mosby–Year Book Inc; 1994:chap 115.

3. Claussen CF. Der Schwindel und seine biologische Behandlung mit Vertigoheel: Ergebnisse von klinisch-experimentellen Untersuchungen. *Biol Med.* 1983;6:531–532.

4. Claussen CF. Die Behandlung des Syndroms des verlangsamten Hirnstamms mit Vertigoheel. *Biol Med.* 1985;14:447-470, 510–514.

5. Zenner S, Borho B, Metelmann H. Schwindel und seine Beeinflußbarkeit durch ein homöpathisches Kombinationspräparat. *Erfahrungsheilkunde.* 1991;6:423–429.

6. Claussen CF, Bergmann J, Bertora G, Claussen E. Klinisch-experimentelle Prüfung und äquilibriometrische Messungen zum Nachweis der therapeutischen Wirksamkeit eines homöpathischen Arzneimittels bestehend aus Ambra, Cocculus, Conium, und Petroleum bei der Diagnose Vertigo und Nausea. *Arzneimittelforschung.* 1984;34:1791–1798.

7. Aantaa E. Treatment of acute vestibular vertigo. *Acta Otolaryngol (Stockh).* 1991;479:44–47.

8. Elbaz P. Flunarizine and betahistine: two different therapeutic approaches in vertigo compared in a double-blind study. *Acta Octolaryngol (Stockh).* 1988;460:143–148.

9. Fraysse B, Bebear JP, Dubreuil C, Berges C, Dauman R. Betahistine dihydrochloride versus flunarizine: a double-blind study on recurrent vertigo with or without cochlear syndrome typical of Menière's disease. *Abstract Acta Otolaryngol (Stockh).* 1991;490:2–10.

10. Tran Ba Huy P, Meyrand MF. Le dichlorhydrate de bétahistine en deux prises ou en trois prises par jour. *J Fr Oto-Rhino-Laryngol.* 1992; 41(suppl 3):I-IV.

11. Canty P, Valentine J, Papworth SJ. Betahistine in peripheral vertigo: a double-blind, placebo-controlled, cross-over study of Serc® versus placebo. *J Laryngol Otol.* 1981;95:687–692.

12. Oosterveld WJ. Betahistine dihydrochloride in the treatment of vertigo of peripheral vestibular origin: a double-blind placebo controlled study. *J Laryngol Otol.* 1984;98:37–41.

13. Spilker B. *Guide to Clinical Trials.* New York, NY: Raven Press; 1990.

14. Ware JE, Kosinski M, Keller SD. *SF-36 Physical and Mental Health Summary Scales: A User's Manual.* Boston, Mass: The Health Institute, New England Medical Center; 1994.

15. Wei LJ, Lachin JM. Two-sample asymptomatically distribution-free tests for incomplete multivariate observations. *J Am Stat Assoc.* 1984;79:653–661.

16. Lachin JM. Some large-sample distribution-free estimators and tests for multivariate partially incomplete data from two populations. *Stat Med.* 1992;11:1151–1170.

17. Lachin JM. Distribution-free marginal analysis of repeated measures. *Drug Inform J.* 1996; 30:1017–1028.

18. Not Available. *Biostatistic Methodology in Clinical Trials in Applications for Marketing Authorisation for Medicinal Products.* Brussels, Belgium: European Union Committee for Proprietary Medicinal Products; 1994. Guidance note III/3630/92-EN.

19. Mizukoshi K, Watanabe I, Matsunaga T, et al. Clinical evaluation of medical treatment for Ménière's disease, using a double-blind controlled study. *Am J Otol.* 1988;9:418–422.

20. Portmann G. The old and new in Ménière's disease: over 60 years in retrospect and a look to the future. *Otolaryngol Clin North Am.* 1980;13:292–312.

21. Elinson J, Siegmann AE. *Sociomedical Health Indicators.* Farmingdale, NY: Baywood Publishing Co Inc; 1979.

22. Spilker B. *Quality-of-Life Assessment in Clinical Trials.* New York, NY: Raven Press; 1990.

51 Efficacy of Homeopathic Arnica

A Systematic Review of Placebo-Controlled Clinical Trials

E. Ernst, MD, PhD, FRCP(Edin); M. H. Pittler, MD
From the Department of Complementary Medicine, School of Postgraduate Medicine and Health Sciences, University of Exeter, Exeter, England.

Background
The efficacy of homeopathic remedies has remained controversial. The homeopathic remedy most frequently studied in placebo-controlled clinical trials is *Arnica montana.*

Objective
To systematically review the clinical efficacy of homeopathic arnica.

Materials and Methods
Computerized literature searches were performed to retrieve all placebo-controlled studies on the subject. The following databases were searched: MEDLINE, EMBASE, CISCOM, and the Cochrane Library. Data were extracted in a predefined, standardized fashion independently by both authors. There were no restrictions on the language of publications.

Results
Eight trials fulfilled all inclusion criteria. Most related to conditions associated with tissue trauma. Most of these studies were burdened with severe methodological flaws. On balance, they do not suggest that homeopathic arnica is more efficacious than placebo.

Conclusion
The claim that homeopathic arnica is efficacious beyond a placebo effect is not supported by rigorous clinical trials.

Arch Surg. 1998;133:1187–1190

Homeopathy is a system of medicine that was developed about 200 years ago and has remained highly controversial ever since.[1] Essentially it is based on the "law of similars" and on the assumption that even nonmaterial dilutions ("potentiations") can be clinically effective.[2] The law of similars claims that if a given remedy causes a certain symptom in a healthy person, the remedy should then be useful for treating that symptom in a patient who suffers from it. Homeopathic potentiations are prepared by serial dilutions and "succussions" (vigorous shaking) and often are so dilute that the likelihood of them containing a single molecule from the mother tincture is nil. Homeopaths believe that "potentizing" in this way will not reduce but rather increase the activity of the resulting remedy. It is in particular the use of highly diluted material that overtly flies in the face of science and has caused homeopathy to be regarded as placebo therapy at best and quackery at worst.

Thus, the efficacy of homeopathic remedies has always been a matter of bitter controversy.[3] Recently the issue has been addressed in various ways. A recent systematic review found most homeopathic trials to come to positive conclusions.[4] The authors, however, abstain from making a definitive conclusion as to the efficacy of homeopathic remedies. In their view, methodological problems with most clinical trials of homeopathy preclude a definitive judgement as to its efficacy.

Another approach to evaluate homeopathy is to perform a meta-analysis across all trials.[5] Even though such a meta-analysis yielded a significantly positive result, with a combined odds ratio of 2.45 favoring homeopathic remedies over placebo, the conclusions that can be drawn from such a meta-analysis are limited and several caveats have been identified. There could be indefinable bias[6] and the pooling of trials of vastly different remedies for vastly different conditions is of debatable legitimacy.[7]

A further approach is to systematically review homeopathic trials pertaining to a single disease or condition. We have chosen this method to assess homeopathy for postoperative ileus[8] and delayed-onset muscle soreness,[9] the 2 conditions most frequently submitted to controlled trials. In one case this resulted in a positive result[8] and in the other in a negative overall result[9] for homeopathy; eg, homeopathic remedies used to treat delayed-onset muscle soreness were not significantly better than placebo in alleviating symptoms. Yet again, several caveats preclude a firm conclusion.

Another approach could be to analyze homeopathic trial data by the type of remedy used; this was chosen for the present article. Its aim is to systematically review the homeopathic remedy most frequently submitted to controlled trials.

Materials and Methods

Computerized literature searches were performed to identify all placebo-controlled clinical trials of homeopathic *Arnica montana*. Databases included MEDLINE, EMBASE, CISCOM, and the Cochrane Library (all from their inception to October 1997). All 89 studies included in the above-mentioned systematic review[4] and meta-analysis[5] were also considered. One of us (E.E.) had been involved in a similar meta-analysis commissioned by the European Community.[10] This exercise included extensive handsearching of 28 specialized homeopathic journals, which resulted in the identification of more than 400 publications. The entire material was screened for this review. Furthermore, our own extensive files as well as review articles and books on homeopathy were searched for relevant publications. The bibliographies of the studies and reviews thus retrieved were searched for further trials. There were no restrictions regarding the language of publication.

Controlled clinical trials of homeopathic arnica (all potencies) vs placebo were included in this systematic review. Trials of one potency against another,[11] trials with arnica as one of several remedies with no subanalysis on a pure arnica group,[12] or studies in which arnica had been administered concomitantly with other remedies[13] were excluded. Trials not published in the peer-reviewed literature were also excluded.

All studies were read in full by both of us. Data were extracted independently in a standardized, predefined fashion (Table 1). Methodological quality of the included trials was assessed using the score according to Jadad et al[14] (Table 2). Discrepancies in the evaluation of individual trials were settled by discussion.

Results

Eight studies fulfilled all of the aforementioned inclusion criteria and were admitted to this review.[15–21] Methodological details and outcomes of these trials are summarized in Table 1. Two studies[15,17] yielded a statistically significant positive result (ie, arnica superior to placebo), 2 studies[20] had a numerically positive result (ie, no formal test statistics were applied but an advantage of the arnica

Table 1. Key Data From Placebo-Controlled Clinical Trials of Homeopathic Arnica

First Author	Condition Treated	Trial Design	Sample Size	Experimental Treatment
Hildebrandt[15]	Delayed-onset muscle soreness	Double-blind	42 Healthy women	Arnica D2 (n=6) D3 (n=6) D4 (n=6) D5 (n=6) D6 (n=6) D8 (n=6) 3 × 16 drops daily for 6 d after exercise
Kaziro[16]	Prevention of postsurgical complications	Randomized, double-blind	118 Patients after extraction of wisdom teeth	Arnica 200C twice daily for 3 days postoperatively (n=39)
Pinsent[17]	Prevention of postsurgical complications	Randomized, double-blind	59 Patients after tooth extraction	Arnica 30C 1 dose 30 min preoperatively; 3 doses each 15 min postoperatively; 1 dose every 2 h for 6 doses (n=23)
Tveiten[18]	Delayed-onset muscle soreness	Randomized, double-blind	36 Participants in the Oslo Marathon (Norway)	*Arnica montana* D30 5 pills twice daily for 5 d starting 1 d prior to race (n=20)
Gibson[19]	Acute trauma	Double-blind	20 Orthopedic patients	Arnica 30 (n=11)
Campbell[20]	Experimentally inflicted mechanical bruising	Single-blind crossover trial	13 Healthy volunteers	Arnica 10M†
Savage[21]	Experimentally inflicted mechanical bruising	Double-blind crossover trial	10 Healthy volunteers	Arnica 30C†
Livingston[22]	Stroke	Randomized double-blind	40 Patients admitted to hospital up to 7 d after acute event	Arnica "in M potency" (n=20)

*Lower creatinine kinase concentration on day 6 in group C vs placebo.
†One tablet before being bruised and 2 after, on the same day, and 2 more tablets on the next day.

groups was apparent) and 4 studies[16, 18, 19, 21] showed a significantly negative result (ie, arnica not superior to placebo). Most trials included in this review are methodologically weak. Generally speaking, the more rigorous studies[18, 22] tended to be the ones that yielded negative findings. There is no obvious common denominator to differentiate between positive and negative studies, neither in terms of potency applied nor in terms of indication. For example, one trial on delayed-onset muscle soreness had positive results[15] while another (methodologically superior) one had negative results.[18] Similarly, one study of postsurgical complications had positive results[17] and another had negative results.[16] In addition, there are no data to suggest that one potency of arnica is superior to another.

Comment

Arnica is the classic homeopathic remedy for trauma of various kinds. "The word *injury* is constantly associated with the usefulness of arnica in trauma . . . this is especially true for soft tissue damage causing bruising, bleeding, and dislocation."[22] The *Homoeopathic Pharmacy* lists as its first indication "trauma" and even recommends it as a first-aid treatment.[23] The results of this systematic review unfortunately fail to lend support to this. On balance, the trial data do not support the notion that arnica is efficacious.

There are several ways of explaining this. The evidence could be scarce and a type II error could have produced a false-negative overall picture. This is not borne out by the data presented earlier. No other homeopathic remedy has been subject to more controlled clinical trials.

The existing studies could be severely flawed and therefore produce a misleading result. The trials certainly are burdened with a multitude of methodological limitations. Small sample size and lack of test statistics are frequent and obvious ones. However, such drawbacks would be likely to create a false-positive rather than a false-negative result.

Control Treatment	Main Outcome Measures	Main Results	Comments	Jadad Score[14]
Placebo drops as per verum schedule (n=6)	Soreness intensity (rating scale) and duration, maximal isometric muscle strength, serum creatine kinase concentrations	Less decrease in muscle strength in group B vs placebo (both arms); no differences in terms of soreness intensity; shorter duration of soreness in group B (both arms) and C (left arm only) vs placebo*	No randomization; no numerical results provided (figures only); no allowance for multiple comparisons	1
Metronidazole 400 mg twice daily (n=41) Placebo twice daily for 3 d postoperatively (n=38)	Pain (visual analog scale), trismus, edema, wound healing	No difference between arnica and placebo in any outcome measure	Metronidazole was shown to be superior to placebo or arnica	2
Placebo as per verum schedule (n=36)	Pain, bleeding	Less pain with arnica, no significant difference for bleeding	41 dropouts	4
Placebo pills as per verum schedule (n=16)	Blood tests, including serum creatine kinase concentrations; soreness intensity (visual analog scale) and duration	No significant intergroup differences, but a trend for soreness and serum creatine kinase concentrations to be lower with arnica than placebo	No allowance for multiple comparisons	4
Placebo (n=9)	Pulse rate, blood pressure, respiratory rate, subjective symptoms	No significant intergroup differences	No mention of randomization, frequency and dose of medication not stated	2
Placebo	Extent of bruising, subjective symptoms	Results numerically favored arnica	Small sample size, no statistics	1
Placebo	Extent of bruising, subjective symptoms	Results numerically favored arnica	Small sample size, no statistics	2
Placebo (n=20)	3-mo mortality	No significant intergroup difference	Small baseline differences in disfavor of arnica-treated group	3

Arnica could have been applied wrongly. Homeopaths do not treat a specific condition but rather the whole human being. Thus, it is not strictly according to the teaching of Hahnemann (the "inventor" of homeopathy) to use arnica for trauma much like an allopathic drug. There are, however, exceptions to this rule, and arnica is certainly one of them. The above quotations demonstrate that arnica is used for the conditions for which it was tested in the trials reviewed here.

Therefore, the hypothesis that homeopathic arnica is, in fact, not effective beyond a placebo effect must be considered. It is not possible to "prove a negative" with these data. It is, however, possible to comment on the most likely explanation of the overall result of this systematic review.

It is concluded that the hypothesis claiming that homeopathic arnica is clinically effective beyond a placebo effect is not based on methodologically sound placebo-controlled trials.

Table 2. Scoring System to Measure the Likelihood of Bias*

Yes=1 point; no=0 points
A. Study described as randomized (this includes the use of words such as random, randomly, and randomization)?
B. Study described as double-blind?
C. Was there a description of withdrawals and dropouts?
D. Method to generate the sequence of randomization described and appropriate (table of random numbers, computer-generated, and so forth)?
E. Method of double-blinding described and appropriate (identical placebo, active placebo, or dummy)?
Deduct 1 point if:
F. Method to generate the sequence of randomization described and inappropriate (patients were allocated alternately, or according to date of birth, hospital number, and so forth).
G. Method of double-blinding described and inappropriate (comparison of tablet vs injection with no double dummy).

*Method developed by Jadad et al.[14]

References

1. Ernst E, Kaptchuk TJ. Homeopathy revisited. *Arch Intern Med*. 1996;156:2162–2164.

2. Ernst E, Hahn E.,eds. *Homeopathy: A Critical Appraisal*. Oxford, England: Butterworth-Heinemann Publishers; 1998.

3. Ernst E. The heresy of homeopathy. *Br Homeopathic J*. 1998;87:28–32.

4. Kleijnen J, Knipschild P, Ter Riet G. Clinical trials of homeopathy. *BMJ*. 1991;302:316–332.

5. Linde K, Clausius N, Ramirez G, et al. Are the clinical effects of homeopathy placebo effects? a meta-analysis of placebo-controlled trials. *Lancet*. 1997;350:834–843.

6. Vandenbrouk JP. Homeopathy trials, going nowhere. *Lancet*. 1997;350:824.

7. Langman MJS. Homeopathy trials: reasons for good ones, but are they warranted? *Lancet*. 1997;350:825.

8. Barnes J, Resch KL, Ernst E. Homeopathy for postoperative ileus: a meta-analysis. *J Clin Gastroenterol*. 1997;25:628–633.

9. Ernst E, Barnes J. Are homoeopathic remedies effective for delayed-onset muscle soreness? a systematic review of placebo-controlled trials. *Perfusion*. 1998;11:4–8.

10. Boissel JP, Ernst E, Fisher P, Fülgraff G, Garatini S, de Klerk E. Overview of data from homeopathic medicine trials. In: *European Reports*. Brussels, Belgium: EU Rep; 1996.

11. Hofmeyer GJ. Postpartum homeopathic *Arnica montana*: a potency-finding pilot study. *Br J Clin Pract*. 1990;44:619–621.

12. Lökken P, Straumsheim PA, Tveiten D, Skjelbred P, Borchgrevink CF. Effects of homeopathy on pain and other events after acute trauma. *BMJ*. 1995;310:1439–1442.

13. Bendre VV, Dharmudhikari SD. Arnica montana and hypericum in dental practice. *Hahnemannian Gleanings*. 1980;47:70–72.

14. Jadad AR, Moore RA, Carrol D, et al. Assessing the quality of reports of randomized clinical trials: is blinding necessary? *Control Clin Trials*. 1996;17:1–12.

15. Hildebrandt G, Eltze C. Über die Wirksamkeit verschiedener Potenzen von Arnica beim experimentell erzeugten Muskelkater. *Erfahrungsheilkunde*. 1984;7:430–435.

16. Kaziro GSN. Metronidazole (Flagyl) and *Arnica montana* in the prevention of postsurgical complications: a comparative placebo controlled clinical trial. *Br J Oral Maxillofac Surg*. 1984;22:42–49.

17. Pinsent RJFM, Baker GPI, Ives G, Davey RW, Jonas S. Does arnica reduce pain and bleeding after dental extraction? *Midland Homeopathy Res Group Newslett*. 1984;11:71–72.

18. Tveiten D, Bruseth S, Borchgrevink CF, Løhne K. Effect of arnica D30 on hard physical exercise: a double-blind controlled trial during the Oslo Marathon. *Tidsskr Nor Loegeforen*. 1991;111:3630–3631.

19. Gibson J, Haslam Y, Laurneson L, Newman P, Pitt R, Robins M. Double-blind trial of arnica in acute trauma patients. *Homeopathy*. 1991:41:54–55.

20. Campbell A. Two pilot controlled trials of *Arnica montana*. *Br Homeopathic J*. 1976; 65:154–158.

21. Savage RH, Roe PF. A further double blind trial to assess the benefit of *Arnica montana* in acute stroke illness. *Br Homoeopathic J*. 1978;67:211–222.

22. Livingston R. *Homeopathy, Evergreen Medicine*. Poole, England: Asher Press; 1991.

23. Kayne SB. Homeopathic Pharmacy. Edinburgh, Scotland: Churchill-Livingstone; 1997.

7 Acupuncture

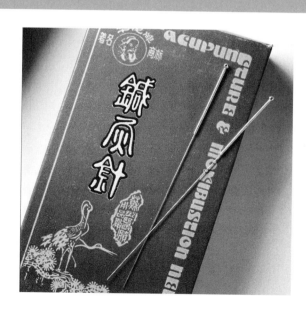

Overview

Patrick J. LaRiccia, MD
From the Department of Medicine, Presbyterian Medical Center–University of Pennsylvania Health System, and the Department of Rehabilitation Medicine, Hospital of the University of Pennsylvania–University of Pennsylvania Health System, Philadelphia.

Acupuncture is a part of traditional Chinese medicine and has been in existence for at least 2000 years. Acupuncture is based on the concepts of Yin, Yang, *Qi* (pronounced *chee*), and meridians, and is performed by piercing the skin with very fine sharp needles. The older literature on which traditional Chinese medicine is based reveals evolution of practice and concepts related to acupuncture over time.[1,2] For instance, according to ancient texts, the first acupuncture needles were made of stone, and acupuncture commonly was passed on within families or taught by apprenticeship. It is thought that acupuncture spread from China to Korea and Japan in the sixth century.[1] Use of acupuncture was documented in Europe in the 19th and 20th centuries.[1] In the United States, acupuncture is mentioned in the 1st (1892) through the 14th (1944) editions of William Osler's *The Principles and Practice of Medicine* as a treatment for acute lumbago.[1,3,4]

The central principle of acupuncture involves the concept of *Qi*, which is described as "vital energy" that courses through pathways in the body called meridians. According to acupuncture theory, when *Qi* flow through the meridians is hindered or obstructed, pain and disease can result; deficiency of *Qi* can cause fatigue. The main therapeutic goal of acupuncture is to restore the proper flow of *Qi* by stimulating acupuncture points, which are locations where the *Qi* coursing through the meridians is transported to the body surface.[5] There are 361 "regular acupuncture points," which fall on the 14 most frequently used meridians. These meridians are thought to travel essentially longitudinally along the body, but also are interconnected with each other. Most meridians are thought to have a connection to a specific visceral organ (eg, heart, lung, liver, stomach).

Performance of acupuncture involves determining which acupuncture points to stimulate. Decisions also must be made about depth and direction of needle insertion, type of needle manipulation, duration that needles are left in place, and the frequency and total number of treatments. Other considerations include whether to stimulate the acupuncture points further by application of electricity to the needles (a modern addition to acupuncture styles) or application of a heat source (traditionally provided by burning the herb *Artemisia vulgaris,* termed "moxibustion") near the acupuncture points. Different schools of thought about acupuncture (eg, traditional Chinese, Japanese, Korean, French energetics, among others) reflect various dimensions of acupuncture treatment, such as point selection, depth of insertion, and needle manipulation in different ways. For example, in mainland China, where the traditional Chinese medicine style is dominant, the depth of insertion and needle manipulation will result in a feeling of *de qi* (a temporary feeling of numbness, fullness, or heaviness). In contrast, certain Japanese acupuncture styles cause no discomfort at all.

Of the many possible applications of acupuncture, the mechanism of acupuncture analgesia has been studied most extensively. Several converging lines of evidence implicate the role of endorphins in acupuncture analgesia. For instance, although multiple opioid antagonists (eg, naloxone, naltrexone, cyclazocine) can block acupuncture analgesia,[6,7] only the L-isomer of naloxone can block the analgesic effects of acupuncture, suggesting a receptor mechanism rather than a secondary effect of naloxone such as membrane fluidization.[6,7] In animal models, microinjection of naloxone or antibodies to β-endorphin, enkephalin, or dynorphin are only successful in blocking acupuncture analgesia if the microinjections are made into areas of the nervous system where these substances are active, and animals with endorphin receptor deficiency or endorphin deficiency do less well with acupuncture analgesia.[6-10] Moreover, following acupuncture analgesia, cerebrospinal fluid endorphins increase and brain endorphins decrease. [6,11] In addition, enzyme blockers that slow endorphin breakdown enhance acupuncture analgesia,[6,12] whereas pituitary ablation and suppression techniques reduce acupuncture analgesia.[6,13] Additional research into the neurophysiology and biologic actions underlying acupuncture may help practitioners better understand the clinical benefits that have been associated with acupuncture therapy.

The following collection of articles on acupuncture research is relevant and important from multiple perspectives. From a public health perspective, these articles address prevalent medical problems that, in some cases, are not consistently responsive to standard medical care. No one will argue that neck and back pain, nicotine withdrawal, acute and chronic urticaria, postoperative pain, migraine headaches, adverse effects of medication, breech presentations, and peripheral neuropathy related to HIV infection are not part of everyday medical practice. From the perspective of adding to the body of medical knowledge, these chapters demonstrate that various types of studies can provide useful information. Specifically, this part of *Alternative Medicine: An Objective Assessment* includes 3 randomized controlled trials of acupuncture (for HIV neuropathy,[14] nicotine withdrawal,[15] and reversal of breech presentation[16]), 3 review articles on clinical applications of acupuncture (the NIH Consensus Conference Statement,[17] a systematic review of urticaria,[18] and a meta-analysis on back pain[19]), and a case study.[20]

The NIH Consensus Development Panel on Acupuncture[17] provides a broad overview of acupuncture issues and research references. Based on evaluation of randomized controlled trials, the panel identified several areas that have convincing evidence supporting acupuncture treatment, including control of postoperative nausea and vomiting, chemotherapy-induced nausea and vomiting, and postoperative dental pain. In contrast, the randomized trial of acupuncture and antidepressant medications for peripheral neuropathy related to HIV infection evaluated one specific form of acupuncture, but found that the standardized acupuncture regimen provided no clear benefit for symptom relief.[14] Likewise, the chapter on nicotine withdrawal evaluates a specific form of acupuncture treatment in a randomized, controlled, single-blinded study.[15] The meta-analysis of studies on acupuncture treatment for back pain[19] gives an excellent model for searching and synthesizing the literature of randomized controlled trials, whereas the review on urticaria[18] is informative and may stimulate more rigorously controlled research. The chapter on acupuncture in a university hospital setting presents interesting, thought-provoking information regarding the possible role of acupuncture and the dilemmas faced by a physician practicing acupuncture on an inpatient service.[20] The study on reversing breech presentation with moxibustion,[16] if replicated in other settings, may have wide public health implications.

Acupuncture is an ancient form of therapy that ultimately may prove to have many useful modern clinical applications. Publication of these chapters on acupuncture in the mainstream medical literature not only helps to address relevant clinical problems and important issues related to research methodology, but also brings acupuncture into the most open forum for evaluation and education. Such attention should serve to stimulate more research and critical evaluation of acupuncture, and should help to educate more physicians than articles in nonmainstream medical journals.

References

1. Liao SJ, Lee MHM, Ng LK. *Principles and Practice of Contemporary Acupuncture.* New York, NY: Marcel Dekker; 1994.
2. Kaptchuk TJ. *The Web That Has No Weaver: Understanding Chinese Medicine.* New York, NY: Congdon & Weed; 1983.
3. Osler WA. *The Principles and Practice of Medicine: Designed for the Use of Practitioners and Students of Medicine.* New York, NY: Appleton & Co; 1892:282.
4. Christian HA, ed. *The Osler's Principles and Practice of Medicine, 14th Edition.* New York, NY: D Appleton Century Co Inc; 1944.
5. Xinnong C, ed. *Chinese Acupuncture and Moxibustion.* Beijing, China: Foreign Languages Press; 1987:108–109.
6. Pomeranz B. Scientific basis of acupuncture. In: Stux G, Pomeranz B, eds. *Acupuncture: Textbook and Atlas.* Berlin, Germany: Springer-Verlag; 1987:1–34.
7. Cheng R, Pomeranz B. Electroacupuncture analgesia is mediated by stereospecific opiate receptors and is reversed by antagonists of type I receptors. *Life Sci.* 1979;26:631–639.
8. Han JS, Xic GX. Dynorphin: important mediator for electroacupuncture analgesia in the spinal cord of the rabbit. *Pain.* 1984;18:367–377.
9. Peets J, Pomeranz B. CXBX mice deficient in opiate receptors show poor electroacupuncture analgesia. *Nature.* 1978;273:675–676.
10. Murai M. Takeshige C, et al. Correlation between individual variations in effectiveness of acupuncture analgesia and that in contents of brain endogenous morphine-like factors [in Japanese (English summary)]. In: Takeshige C, ed. *Studies on the Mechanism of Acupuncture Analgesia Based on Animal Experiments.* Tokyo, Japan: Showa University Press; 1986.
11. Pert A, Dionne R, Ng L, Pert C, et al. Alterations in rat central nervous system endorphins following transauricular electroacupuncture. *Brain Res.* 1981;224:83–98.
12. Ehrenpreis S. Analgesic properties of enkephalinase inhibitors: animal and human studies. *Prog Clin Biol Res.* 1985;192:363–370.
13. Cheng R, Pomeranz B, Yu G. Dexamethasone partially reduces and 2% saline treatment abolishes electroacupuncture analgesia: these findings implicate pituitary endorphins. *Life Sci.* 1979;24:1481–1486.
14. Shlay JC, Chaloner K, Max MB, et al. Acupuncture and amitriptyline for pain due to HIV-related peripheral neuropathy: a randomized controlled trial. *JAMA.* 1998;280:1590–1595.
15. White AR, Resch KL, Ernst E. Randomized trial of acupuncture for nicotine withdrawal symptoms. *Arch Intern Med.* 1998;158:2251–2255.
16. Cardini F, Weixin H. Moxibustion for correction of breech presentation: a randomized controlled trial. *JAMA.* 1998;280:1580–1584.
17. NIH Consensus Development Panel on Acupuncture. Acupuncture. *JAMA.* 1998;280:1518–1524.
18. Chen CJ, Yu HS. Acupuncture treatment of urticaria. *Arch Dermatol.* 1998;134:1397–1399.
19. Ernst E, White AR. Acupuncture for back pain: a meta-analysis of randomized controlled trials. *Arch Intern Med.* 1998;158:2235–2241.
20. Nasir L. Acupuncture in a university hospital: implications for an inpatient consulting service. *Arch Fam Med.* 1998;7:593–596.

52 Acupuncture

NIH Consensus Development Panel on Acupuncture

NIH Consensus Development Conferences are convened to evaluate available scientific information and resolve safety and efficacy issues related to a biomedical technology. The resultant NIH Consensus Statements are intended to advance understanding of the technology or issue in question and to be useful to health professionals and the public.

NIH Consensus statements are prepared by a nonadvocate, nonfederal panel of experts, based on (1) presentations by investigators working in areas relevant to the consensus questions during a 2-day public session, (2) questions and statements from conference attendees during open discussion periods that are part of the public session, and (3) closed deliberations by the panel during the remainder of the second day and morning of the third. This statement is an independent report of the panel and is not a policy statement of the NIH or the federal government.

Objective

To provide clinicians, patients, and the general public with a responsible assessment of the use and effectiveness of acupuncture to treat a variety of conditions.

Participants

A nonfederal, nonadvocate, 12-member panel representing the fields of acupuncture, pain, psychology, psychiatry, physical medicine and rehabilitation, drug abuse, family practice, internal medicine, health policy, epidemiology, statistics, physiology, biophysics, and the representatives of the public. In addition, 25 experts from these same fields presented data to the panel and a conference audience of 1200. Presentations and discussions were divided into 3 phases over 2 1/2 days: (1) presentations by investigators working in areas relevant to the consensus questions during a 2-day public session; (2) questions and statements from conference attendees during open discussion periods that were part of the public session; and (3) closed deliberations by the panel during the remainder of the second day and morning of the third. The conference was organized and supported by the Office of Alternative Medicine and the Office of Medical Applications of Research, National Institutes of Health, Bethesda, Md.

Evidence

The literature, produced from January 1970 to October 1997, was searched through MEDLINE, Allied and Alternative Medicine, EMBASE, and MANTIS, as well as through a hand search of 9 journals that were not indexed by the National Library of Medicine. An extensive bibliography of 2302 references was provided to the panel and the conference audience. Expert speakers prepared abstracts of their own conference presentations with relevant citations from the literature. Scientific evidence was given precedence over clinical anecdotal experience.

Consensus Process

The panel, answering predefined questions, developed their conclusions based on the scientific evidence presented in

the open forum and scientific literature. The panel composed a draft statement, which was read in its entirety and circulated to the experts and the audience for comment. Thereafter, the panel resolved conflicting recommendations and released a revised statement at the end of the conference. The panel finalized the revisions within a few weeks after the conference. The draft statement was made available on the World Wide Web immediately following its release at the conference and was updated with the panel's final revisions within a few weeks of the conference. The statement is available at http://consensus.nih.gov.

Conclusions

Acupuncture as a therapeutic intervention is widely practiced in the United States. Although there have been many studies of its potential usefulness, many of these studies provide equivocal results because of design, sample size, and other factors. The issue is further complicated by inherent difficulties in the use of appropriate controls, such as placebos and sham acupuncture groups. However, promising results have emerged, for example, showing efficacy of acupuncture in adult postoperative and chemotherapy nausea and vomiting and in postoperative dental pain. There are other situations, such as addiction, stroke rehabilitation, headache, menstrual cramps, tennis elbow, fibromyalgia, myofascial pain, osteoarthritis, low back pain, carpal tunnel syndrome, and asthma, in which acupuncture may be useful as an adjunct treatment or an acceptable alternative or be included in a comprehensive management program. Further research is likely to uncover additional areas where acupuncture interventions will be useful.

JAMA. 1998;280:1518–1524

Acupuncture is a component of the health care system of China that can be traced back for at least 2500 years. The general theory of acupuncture is based on the premise that there are patterns of energy flow (*Qi*) through the body that are essential for health. Disruptions of this flow are believed to be responsible for disease. Acupuncture may correct imbalances of flow at identifiable points close to the skin. The practice of acupuncture to treat identifiable pathophysiological conditions in American medicine was rare until the visit of President Nixon to China in 1972. Since then, there has been an explosion of interest in the United States and Europe in the application of the technique of acupuncture to Western medicine.

Acupuncture describes a family of procedures involving stimulation of anatomical locations on the skin by a variety of techniques. There are several approaches to diagnosis and treatment in American acupuncture that incorporate medical traditions from China, Japan, Korea, and other countries. The most studied mechanism of stimulation of acupuncture points uses penetration of the skin by thin, solid, metallic needles, which are manipulated manually or by electrical stimulation. The majority of comments in this report are based on data that came from such studies. Stimulation of these areas by moxibustion, a technique that applies heat to an acupuncture point by burning a compressed, powdered, combustible substance at or near the points to be stimulated, pressure, heat, and lasers is used in acupuncture practice, but because of the paucity of studies, these techniques are more difficult to evaluate.

Acupuncture has been used by millions of American patients and performed by thousands of physicians, dentists, acupuncturists, and other clinicians for relief or prevention of pain and for a broad spectrum of health conditions. After reviewing the existing body of knowledge, the US Food and Drug Administration recently removed acupuncture needles from the category of "experimental medical devices" and now regulates them just as it does other devices, such as surgical scalpels and hypodermic syringes, under good manufacturing practices and single-use standards of sterility.

Over the years, the National Institutes of Health (NIH) has funded a variety of research projects on acupuncture, including studies on the mechanisms by which acupuncture may produce its effects, as well as clinical trials and other studies. There is also a considerable body of international literature on the risks and benefits of acupuncture, and the World Health Organization lists a variety of medical conditions that may benefit from the use of acupuncture or moxibustion. Such applications include prevention and treatment of nausea and vomiting; treatment of pain and addictions to alcohol, tobacco, and other drugs; treatment of pulmonary problems such as asthma and bronchitis; and rehabilitation from neurological damage such as that caused by stroke.

To address important issues regarding acupuncture, the NIH Office of Alternative Medicine and the NIH Office of Medical Applications of Research organized a 2½ -day conference to evaluate the scientific and medical data on the uses, risks, and benefits of acupuncture procedures for a variety of conditions. Cosponsors of the conference were the NIH's National Cancer Institute, the National Heart, Lung, and Blood Institute, the National Institute of Allergy and Infectious Diseases, the National Institute of Arthritis and Musculoskeletal and Skin Diseases, the National Institute of Dental Research, the National Institute on Drug Abuse, and the Office of Research on Women's Health of the NIH, all in Bethesda, Md. The conference brought together national and international experts in the fields of acupuncture, pain, psychology, psychiatry, physical medicine and rehabilitation, drug abuse, family practice, internal medicine, health policy, epidemiology, statistics, physiology, and biophysics, as well as representatives from the public.

After 1½ days of available presentations and audience discussion, an independent, nonfederal consensus panel weighed the scientific evidence and wrote a draft statement that was presented to the audience on the third day. The consensus statement addressed the following key questions:

1. What is the efficacy of acupuncture, compared with placebo or sham acupuncture, in the conditions for which sufficient data are available to evaluate?
2. What is the place of acupuncture in the treatment of various conditions for which sufficient data are available, in comparison or in combination with other interventions (including no intervention)?
3. What is known about the biological effects of acupuncture that helps us understand how it works?
4. What issues need to be addressed so that acupuncture can be appropriately incorporated into today's health care system?
5. What are the directions for future research?

1. What is the efficacy of acupuncture, compared with placebo or sham acupuncture, in the conditions for which sufficient data are available to evaluate?

Acupuncture is a complex intervention that may vary for different patients with similar chief complaints. The number and length of treatments and the specific points used may vary among individuals and during treatment. Given this reality, it is perhaps encouraging that there exist a number of studies of sufficient quality to assess the efficacy of acupuncture for certain conditions.

According to contemporary research standards, there is a paucity of high-quality research assessing efficacy of acupuncture compared with placebo or sham acupuncture. The vast majority of studies on acupuncture in the biomedical literature consist of case reports, case series, or intervention studies with designs inadequate to assess efficacy.

This discussion of efficacy refers to needle acupuncture (manual or electroacupuncture) because the published research is primarily on needle acupuncture and often does not encompass the full breadth of acupuncture techniques and practices. The controlled trials usually have involved only adults and did not involve long-term (ie, years) acupuncture treatment.

Efficacy of a treatment assesses the differential effect of a treatment when compared with placebo or another treatment modality using a double-blind controlled trial and a rigidly defined protocol. Articles should describe enrollment procedures, eligibility criteria, description of the clinical characteristics of the subjects, methods for diagnosis, and a description of the protocol (ie, randomization method, specific definition of treatment, and control conditions, including length of treatment and number of acupuncture sessions). Optimal trials should also use standardized outcomes and appropriate statistical analyses. This assessment of efficacy focuses on high-quality trials comparing acupuncture with sham acupuncture or placebo.

Response Rate

As with other types of interventions, some individuals are poor responders to specific acupuncture protocols. Both animal and human laboratory and clinical experience suggest that the majority of subjects respond to acupuncture, with a minority not responding. Some of the clinical research outcomes, however, suggest that a larger percentage may not respond. The reason for this paradox is unclear and may reflect the current state of the research.

Efficacy for Specific Disorders

There is clear evidence that needle acupuncture is efficacious for adult postoperative and chemotherapy nausea and vomiting and probably for the nausea of pregnancy.

Much of the research focuses on various pain problems. There is evidence of efficacy for postoperative dental pain. There are reasonable studies (although sometimes only single studies) showing relief of pain with acupuncture on diverse pain conditions such as menstrual cramps, tennis elbow, and fibromyalgia. This suggests that acupuncture may have a more general effect on pain. However, there are also studies that do not find efficacy for acupuncture in pain.

There is evidence that acupuncture does not demonstrate efficacy for cessation of smoking and may not be efficacious for some other conditions.

Although many other conditions have received some attention in the literature and, in fact, the research suggests some potential areas for the use of acupuncture, the quality or quantity of the research evidence is not sufficient to provide firm evidence of efficacy at this time.

Sham Acupuncture

A commonly used control group is sham acupuncture, using techniques that are not intended to stimulate known acupuncture points. However, there is disagreement on correct needle placement. Also, particularly in the studies on pain, sham acupuncture often seems to have either intermediate effects between the placebo and "real" acupuncture points or effects similar to those of the "real" acupuncture points. Placement of a needle in any position elicits a biological response that complicates the interpretation of studies involving sham acupuncture. Thus, there is substantial controversy over the use of sham acupuncture in control groups. This may be less of a problem in studies not involving pain.

2. What is the place of acupuncture in the treatment of various conditions for which sufficient data are available, in comparison or in combination with other interventions (including no intervention)?

Assessing the usefulness of a medical intervention in practice differs from assessing formal efficacy. In conventional practice, clinicians make decisions based on the characteristics of the patient, clinical experience, potential for harm, and information from colleagues and the medical literature. In addition, when more than 1 treatment is possible, the clinician may make the choice by taking into account the patient's preferences. Although it is often thought that there is substantial research evidence to support conventional medical practices, this is frequently not the case. This does not mean that these treatments are ineffective. The data in support of acupuncture are as strong as those for many accepted Western medical therapies.

One of the advantages of acupuncture is that the incidence of adverse effects is substantially lower than that of many drugs or other accepted medical procedures used for the same conditions. As an example, musculoskeletal conditions, such as fibromyalgia, myofascial pain, and epicondylitis (tennis elbow) are conditions for which acupuncture may be beneficial. These painful conditions are often treated with, among other things, anti-inflammatory medications (aspirin, ibuprofen) or with steroid injections. Both medical interventions have a potential for deleterious side effects but are still widely used and are considered acceptable treatments. The evidence supporting these therapies is no better than that for acupuncture.

In addition, ample clinical experience, supported by some research data, suggests that acupuncture may be a reasonable option for a number of clinical conditions. Examples are postoperative pain, myofascial pain, and low back pain. Examples of disorders for which the research evidence is less convincing but for which there are some positive clinical trials include addiction, stroke rehabilitation, carpal tunnel syndrome, osteoarthritis, and headache. Acupuncture treatment for many conditions such as asthma or addiction should be part of a comprehensive management program.

Many other conditions have been treated by acupuncture; the World Health Organization, for example, has listed more than 40 conditions for which the technique may be indicated.

3. What is known about the biological effects of acupuncture that helps us understand how it works?

Many studies in animals and humans have demonstrated that acupuncture can cause multiple biological responses. These responses can occur locally, ie, at or close to the site of application, or at a distance, mediated mainly by sensory neurons to many structures within the central nervous system. This can lead to activation of pathways affecting various physiological systems in the brain as well as in the periphery. A focus of attention has been the role of endogenous opioids in acupuncture analgesia. Considerable evidence supports the claim that opioid peptides are released during acupuncture and that the analgesic effects of acupuncture are at least partially explained by their actions. That opioid antagonists such as naloxone hydrochloride reverse the analgesic effects of acupuncture further strengthens this hypothesis. Stimulation by acupuncture may also activate the hypothalamus and the pituitary gland, resulting in a broad spectrum of systemic effects. Alteration in the secretion of neurotransmitters and neurohormones and changes in the regulation of blood flow, both centrally and peripherally, have been documented. There is also evidence of alterations in immune functions produced by acupuncture. Which of these and other physiological changes mediate clinical effects is at present unclear.

Despite considerable efforts to understand the anatomy and physiology of the "acupuncture points," the definition and characterization of these points remain controversial. Even more elusive is the scientific basis of some of the key traditional Eastern medical concepts, such as the circulation of energy flow, or *Qi*, the meridian system, and other related theories, which are difficult to reconcile with contemporary biomedical information but continue to play an important role in the evaluation of patients and the formulation of treatment in acupuncture.

Some of the biological effects of acupuncture have also been observed when "sham" acupuncture points are stimulated, highlighting the importance of defining appropriate control groups in assessing biological changes purported to be due to acupuncture. Such findings raise questions regarding the specificity of these biological changes. In addition, similar biological alterations, including the release of endogenous opioids and changes in blood pressure, have been observed after painful stimuli, vigorous exercise, and/or relaxation training; it is at present unclear to what extent acupuncture shares similar biological mechanisms.

For any therapeutic intervention, including acupuncture, the so-called nonspecific effects account for a substantial proportion of its effectiveness and thus should not be casually discounted. Many factors may profoundly determine therapeutic outcome, including the quality of the relationship between the clinician and the patient, the degree of trust, the expectations of the patient, and the compatibility of the backgrounds and belief systems of the clinician and the patient, as well as a myriad of factors that together define the therapeutic milieu.

Although much remains unknown regarding the mechanism(s) that might mediate the therapeutic effect of acupuncture, the panel is encouraged that a number of significant acupuncture-related biological changes can be identified and carefully delineated. Further research in this direction not only is important for elucidating the phenomena associated with acupuncture but also has the potential for exploring new pathways in human physiology not previously examined in a systematic manner.

4. What issues need to be addressed so that acupuncture can be appropriately incorporated into today's health care system?

The integration of acupuncture into today's health care system will be facilitated by a better understanding among providers of the language and practices of both the Eastern and Western health care communities. Acupuncture focuses on a holistic, energy-based approach to the patient rather than a disease-oriented diagnostic and treatment model.

An important factor for the integration of acupuncture into the health care system is the training and credentialing of acupuncture practitioners by the appropriate state agencies. This is necessary to allow the public and other health practitioners to identify qualified acupuncture practitioners. The acupuncture educational community has made substantial progress in this area and is encouraged to continue along this path. Educational standards have been established for training of physician and nonphysician acupuncturists. Many acupuncture educational programs are accredited by an agency that is recognized by the US Department of Education. A national credentialing agency exists for nonphysician practitioners and provides examinations for entry-level competency in the field. A nationally recognized examination for physician acupuncturists has been established.

A majority of states provide licensure or registration for acupuncture practitioners. Because some acupuncture practitioners have limited English proficiency, credentialing and licensing examinations should be provided in languages other than English when necessary. There is variation in the titles that are conferred through these processes, and the requirements to obtain licensure vary widely. The scope of practice allowed under these state requirements varies as well. Although states have the individual prerogative to set standards for licensing professions, consistency in these areas will provide greater confidence in the qualifications of acupuncture practitioners. For example, not all states recognize the same credentialing examination, thus making reciprocity difficult.

The occurrence of adverse events in the practice of acupuncture has been documented to be extremely low. However, these events have occurred on rare occasions, some of which are life threatening (eg, pneumothorax). Therefore, appropriate safeguards for the protection of patients and consumers need to be in place. Patients should be informed fully of their treatment options, expected prognoses, and relative risks, as well as informed of safety practices to minimize these risks before their receipt of acupuncture. This information must be provided in a manner that is linguistically and culturally appropriate to the patient. Use of acupuncture needles should always follow Food Drug Administration regulations, including use of sterile, single-use needles. These practices are already being performed by many acupuncture practitioners; however, these practices should be uniform. Recourse for patient grievance and professional censure are provided through credentialing and licensing procedures and are available through appropriate state jurisdictions.

It has been reported that more than 1 million Americans currently receive acupuncture each year. Continued access to qualified acupuncture professionals for appropriate conditions should be ensured. Because many individuals seek health care treatment from both acupuncturists and physicians, communication between these providers should be strengthened and improved. If a patient is under the care of an acupuncturist and a physician, both practitioners should be informed. Care should be taken to ensure that important medical problems are not overlooked. Patients and practitioners have a responsibility to facilitate this communication.

There is evidence that some patients have limited access to acupuncture services because of inability to pay. Insurance companies can decrease or remove financial barriers to access depending on their willingness to provide coverage for appropriate acupuncture services. An increasing number of insurance companies are either considering this possibility or already providing coverage for acupuncture services. Expansion of appropriate acupuncture coverage for populations served by state health insurance plans and by Medicare and Medicaid would also help remove financial barriers to access.

As acupuncture is incorporated into today's health care system and further research clarifies the role of acupuncture for various health conditions, it is expected that dissemination of this information to health care practitioners, insurance providers, policymakers, and the general public will lead to more informed decisions about the appropriate use of acupucture.

5. What are the directions for future research?

The incorporation of any new clinical intervention into accepted practice faces more scrutiny now than ever before. The demands of evidence-based medicine, outcomes research, managed care systems of health care delivery, and a plethora of therapeutic choices make the acceptance of new treatments an arduous process. The difficulties are accentuated when the treatment is based on theories unfamiliar to Western medicine and its practitioners. It is important, therefore, that the evaluation of acupuncture for the treatment of specific conditions be carried out carefully, using designs that can withstand rigorous scrutiny. To further the evaluation of the role of acupuncture in the management of various conditions, the following general areas for future research are suggested.

What Are the Demographics and Patterns of Use of Acupuncture in the United States and Other Countries?

Currently limited information on basic questions exists about who uses acupuncture, for what indications is acupuncture most commonly sought, what variations in experience and techniques used exist among acupuncture practitioners, and what differences in these patterns by geography or ethnic group exist. Descriptive epidemiologic studies can provide insight into these and other questions. This information can in turn be used to guide future research and to identify areas of greatest public health concern.

Can the Efficacy of Acupuncture for Various Conditions for Which It Is Used or for Which It Shows Promise Be Demonstrated?

Relatively few high-quality randomized controlled trials have been published on the effects of acupuncture. Such studies should be designed in a rigorous manner to allow evaluation of the effectiveness of acupuncture. Such studies should include experienced acupuncture practitioners to design and deliver appropriate interventions. Emphasis should be placed on studies that examine acupuncture as used in clinical practice and that respect the theoretical basis for acupuncture therapy.

Although randomized controlled trials provide a strong basis for inferring causality, other study designs, such as those used in clinical epidemiology or outcomes research, can also provide important insights regarding the usefulness of acupuncture for various conditions. There have been few such studies in the acupuncture literature.

Do Different Theoretical Bases for Acupuncture Result in Different Treatment Outcomes?

Competing theoretical orientations (eg, Chinese, Japanese, French) currently exist that might predict divergent therapeutic approaches (ie, the use of different acupuncture points). Research projects should be designed to assess the relative merit of these divergent approaches and to compare these systems with treatment programs using fixed acupuncture points.

To fully assess the efficacy of acupuncture, studies should be designed to examine not only fixed acupuncture points but also the Eastern medical systems that provide the foundation for acupuncture therapy, including the choice of points. In addition to assessing the effect of acupuncture in context, this would also provide the opportunity to determine if Eastern medical theories predict more effective acupuncture points.

What Areas of Public Policy Research Can Provide Guidance for the Integration of Acupuncture Into Today's Health Care System?

The incorporation of acupuncture as a treatment raises numerous questions of public policy. These include issues of access, cost-effectiveness, reimbursement by state, federal, and private payers, and training, licensure, and accreditation. These public policy issues must be founded on high-quality epidemiologic and demographic data and effective research.

Can Further Insight Into the Biological Basis for Acupuncture Be Gained?

Mechanisms that provide a Western scientific explanation for some of the effects of acupuncture are beginning to emerge. This is encouraging and may provide novel insights into neural, endocrine, and other physiological processes. Research should be supported to provide a better understanding of the mechanisms involved, and such research may lead to improvements in treatment.

Does an Organized Energetic System That Has Clinical Applications Exist in the Human Body?

Although biochemical and physiologic studies have provided insight into some of the biologic effects of acupuncture, acupuncture practice is based on a very different model of energy balance. This theory might or might not provide new insights to medical research, but it deserves further attention because of its potential for elucidating the basis for acupuncture.

Conclusions

Acupuncture as a therapeutic intervention is widely practiced in the United States. There have been many studies of its potential usefulness. However, many of these studies provide equivocal results because of design, sample size, and other factors. The issue is further complicated by inherent difficulties in the use of appropriate controls, such as creating placebo and sham acupuncture groups.

However, promising results have emerged for the use of acupuncture in treating the nausea and vomiting related to chemotherapy, adult postoperative surgery pain, and postoperative dental pain. There are other situations such as addiction, stroke rehabilitation, headache, menstrual cramps, tennis elbow, fibromyalgia, myofascial pain, osteoarthritis, low back pain, carpal tunnel syndrome, and asthma for which acupuncture may be useful as an adjunct treatment or an acceptable alternative or may be included in a comprehensive management program. Further research is likely to uncover additional areas where acupuncture interventions will be useful.

Findings from basic research have begun to elucidate the mechanisms of the action of acupuncture, including the release of opioids and other peptides in the central and peripheral nervous system, and changes in neuroendocrine function. Although much needs to be accomplished, the emergence of plausible mechanisms for the therapeutic effects of acupuncture is encouraging.

The introduction of acupuncture into the choice of treatment modalities readily available to the public is in its early stages. Issues of training, licensure, and reimbursement remain to be clarified. There is sufficient evidence, however, of its potential value to conventional medicine to encourage further studies. There is sufficient evidence of acupuncture's value to expand its use into conventional medicine and to encourage further studies of its physiology and clinical value.

Consensus Development Panel: David J. Ramsay, DM, DPhil, Panel and Conference Chairperson, President, University of Maryland, Baltimore; Marjorie A. Bowman, MD, MPA, Professor and Chair, Department of Family Practice and Community Medicine, University of Pennsylvania Health System, Philadelphia; Philip E. Greenman, DO, Associate Dean, College of Osteopathic Medicine, Michigan State University, East Lansing; Stephen P. Jiang, ACSW, Executive Director, Association of Asian Pacific Community Health Organizations, Oakland, Calif; Lawrence H. Kushi, ScD, Associate Professor, Division of Epidemiology, University of Minnesota School of Public Health, Minneapolis; Susan Leeman, PhD, Professor, Department of Pharmacology, Boston University School of Medicine, Boston, Mass; Keh-Ming Lin, MD, MPH, Professor of Psychiatry, University of California, Los Angeles, Director, Research Center on the Psychobiology of Ethnicity, Harbor-University of California, Los Angeles, Medical Center, Torrance; Daniel E. Moerman, PhD, William E. Stirton Professor of Anthropology, University of Michigan, Dearborn, Ypsilanti; Sidney H. Schnoll, MD, PhD, Chairman, Division of Substance Abuse Medicine, Professor of Internal Medicine and Psychiatry, Medical College of Virginia, Richmond; Marcellus Walker, MD, Honesdale, Pa; Christine Waternaux, PhD, Associate Professor and Chief, Biostatistics Division, Columbia University and New York State Psychiatric Institute, New York; Leonard A. Wisneski, MD, Medical Director, Bethesda Center, American WholeHealth, Bethesda, Md.

Speakers: Abass Alavi, MD, "The Role of Physiologic Imaging in the Investigation of the Effects of Pain and Acupuncture on Regional Cerebral Function"; Brian M. Berman, MD, "Overview of Clinical Trials on Acupuncture for Pain"; Stephen Birch, LicAc, PhD, "Overview of the Efficacy of Acupuncture in the Treatment of Headache and Face and Neck Pain"; Hannah V. Bradford, MAc, "Late-Breaking Data and Other News From the Clinical Research Symposium (CRS) on Acupuncture at NIH"; Xiaoding Cao, MD, PhD, "Protective Effect of Acupuncture on Immunosuppression"; Daniel C. Cherkin, PhD, "Efficacy of Acupuncture in Treating Low Back Pain: A Systematic Review of the Literature"; Patricia Culliton, MA, LAc, "Current Utilization of Acupuncture by United States Patients"; David L. Diehl, MD, "Gastrointestinal Indications"; Kevin V. Ergil, LAc, "Acupuncture Licensure, Training, and Certification in the United States"; Richard Hammerschlag, PhD, "Methodological and Ethical Issues in Acupuncture Research"; Ji-Sheng Han, MD, "Acupuncture Activates Endogenous Systems of Analgesia"; Joseph M. Helms, MD, "Acupuncture Around the World in Modern Medical Practice"; Kim A. Jobst, DM, MRCP, "Respiratory Indications"; Gary Kaplan, DO, "Efficacy of Acupuncture in the Treatment of Osteoarthritis and Musculoskeletal Pain"; Ted J. Kaptchuk, OMD, "Acupuncture: History, Context, and Long-term Perspectives"; Janet Konefal, PhD, EdD, MPH, CA, "Acupuncture and Addictions"; Lixing Lao, PhD, LAc, "Dental and Postoperative Pain"; C. David Lytle, PhD, "Safety and Regulation of Acupuncture Needles and Other Devices"; Margaret A. Naeser, PhD, LicAc, Dipl Ac, "Neurological Rehabilitation: Acupuncture and Laser Acupuncture to Treat Paralysis in Stroke and Other Paralytic Conditions and Pain in Carpal Tunnel Syndrome"; Lorenz K.Y. Ng, MD, "What Is Acupuncture?"; Andrew Parfitt, PhD, "Nausea and Vomiting"; Bruce Pomeranz, MD, PhD, "Summary of Acupuncture and Pain"; Judith C. Shlay, MD, "Neuropathic Pain"; Alan I. Trachtenberg, MD, MPH, "American Acupuncture: Primary Care, Public Health, and Policy"; Jin Yu, MD, "Induction of Ovulation With Acupuncture."

Planning Committee: Alan I. Trachtenberg, MD, MPH, Planning Committee Chairperson, Medical Officer, Office of Science Policy and Communication, National Institute on Drug Abuse, National Institutes of Health, Rockville, Md; Brian M. Berman, MD, Associate Professor of Family Medicine, Director, Center for Complementary Medicine, University of Maryland School of Medicine, Baltimore; Hannah V. Bradford, MAc, Acupuncturist, Society for Acupuncture Research, Bethesda, Md; Elsa Bray, Program Analyst, Office of Medical Applications of Research, National Institutes of Health, Bethesda; Patricia Bryant, PhD, Director Behavior, Pain, Oral Function, and Epidemiology Program, Division of Extramural Research, National Institute of Dental Research, National Institutes of Health, Bethesda; Claire M. Cassidy, PhD, Director Paradigms Found Consulting, Bethesda; Jerry Cott, PhD, Head Pharmacology Treatment Program, National Institute of Mental Health, National Institutes of Health, Rockville; George W. Counts, MD, Director Office of Research on Minority and Women's Health, National Institute of Allergy and Infectious Diseases, National Institutes of Health, Bethesda; Patricia D. Culliton, MA, LAc, Director Alternative Medicine Division, Hennepin County Medical Center, Minneapolis, Minn; Jerry M. Elliott, Program Management and Analysis Officer, Office of Medical Applications of Research, National Institutes of Health, Bethesda; John H. Ferguson, MD, Director Office of Medical Applications of Research, National Institutes of Health, Bethesda; Anita Greene, MA, Public Affairs Program Officer, Office of Alternative Medicine, National Institutes of Health, Bethesda; Debra S. Grossman, MA, Program Officer, Treatment Research Branch, Division of Clinical and Services Research, National Institute on Drug Abuse, National Institutes of Health, Rockville; William H. Hall, Director of Communications, Office of Medical Applications of Research, National Institutes of Health, Bethesda; Richard Hammerschlag, PhD, Academic Dean and Research Director, Yo San University of Traditional Chinese Medicine, Santa Monica, Calif; Freddie Ann Hoffman, MD, Deputy Director, Medicine Staff, Office of Health Affairs, US Food and Drug Administration, Rockville; Wayne B. Jonas, MD, Director, Office of Alternative Medicine, National Institutes of Health, Bethesda; Gary Kaplan, DO, President, Medical Acupuncture Research Foundation, Arlington, Va; Carol Kari, RN, LAc, MAc, President, Maryland Acupuncture Society, Member, National Alliance, Kensington; Charlotte R. Kerr, RN, MPH, MAc, Practitioner of Traditional Acupuncture, Center for Traditional Acupuncture, Columbia, Md; Thomas J. Kiresuk, PhD, Director, Center for Addiction and Alternative Medicine Research, Minneapolis; Cheryl Kitt, PhD, Program Officer Division of Convulsive Infectious and Immune Disorders, National Institute of Neurological Disorders and Stroke, National Institutes of Health, Bethesda; Janet Konefal, PhD, MPH, LAc, Associate Professor, Acupuncture Research and Training Programs, Department of Psychiatry and Behavioral Sciences, University of Miami School of Medicine, Miami, Fla; Sung J. Liao, MD, DPH, Clinical Professor of Surgical Sciences, Department of Oral and Maxillofacial Surgery, New York University College of Dentistry, Consultant Rust Institute of Rehabilitation Medicine, New York University College of Medicine, New York; Michael C. Lin, PhD, Health Scientist Administrator, Division of Heart and Vascular Diseases, National Heart, Lung, and Blood Institute, National Institutes of Health, Bethesda; C. David Lytle, PhD, Research Biophysicist, Center for Devices and Radiological Health, US Food and Drug Administration, Rockville; James D. Moran, LicAc, DAc, CAAP, CAS; President Emeritus and Doctor of Acupuncture, American Association of Oriental Medicine, The Belchertown Wellness Center, Belchertown, Mass; Richard L. Nahin, PhD, Program Officer, Extramural Affairs, Office of Alternative Medicine, National Institutes of Health, Bethesda; Lorenz K.Y. Ng, MD, RAc, Clinical Professor of Neurology, George Washington University, School of Medicine, Medical Director, Pain Management Program, National Rehabilitation Hospital, Bethesda; James Panagis, MD, Director, Orthopedics Program, Musculoskeletal Branch, National Institute of Arthritis and Musculoskeletal and Skin Diseases, National Institutes of Health, Bethesda; David J. Ramsay, DM, DPhil, Panel and Conference Chairperson, President, University of Maryland, Baltimore;

Charles R. Sherman, PhD, Deputy Director, Office of Medical Applications of Research, National Institutes of Health, Bethesda; Virginia Taggart, MPH, Health Scientist Administrator, Division of Lung Diseases, National Heart, Lung, and Blood Institute, National Institutes of Health, Bethesda; Xiao-Ming Tian, MD, RAc, Clinical Consultant on Acupuncture for the National Institutes of Health, Director, Academy of Acupuncture and Chinese Medicine, Bethesda; Claudette Varricchio, DSN, Program Director, Division of Cancer Prevention and Control, National Cancer Institute, National Institutes of Health, Rockville, Md.

Conference Sponsors: Office of Alternative Medicine, Wayne B. Jonas, MD, Director; Office of Medical Applications of Research, John H. Ferguson, MD, Director.

Conference Cosponsors: National Cancer Institute, Richard D. Klausner, MD, Director; National Heart, Lung, and Blood Institute, Claude Lenfant, MD, Director; National Institute of Allergy and Infectious Diseases, Anthony S. Fauci, MD, Director; National Institute of Arthritis and Musculoskeletal and Skin Diseases, Stephen I. Katz, MD, PhD, Director; National Institute of Dental Research, Harold C. Slavkin, DDS, Director; National Institute on Drug Abuse, Alan I. Leshner, PhD, Director; Office of Research on Women's Health, Vivian W. Pinn, MD, Director.

Bibliography

The consensus conference speakers identified the following key references in developing their presentations. A more complete bibliography prepared by the National Library of Medicine at NIH, along with the references below, was provided to the consensus panel for its consideration. The full NLM bibliography is available at: http://www.nlm.nih.gov/pubs/cbm/acupuncture.html.

Addictions

Bullock ML, Culliton PD, Olander RT. Controlled trial of acupuncture for severe recidivist alcoholism. *Lancet*. 1989;1:1435–1439.

Bullock ML, Umen AJ, Culliton PD, Olander RT. Acupuncture treatment of alcoholic recidivism: a pilot study. *Alcohol Clin Exp Res*. 1987; 11:292–295.

Clavel-Chapelon F, Paoletti C, Banhamou S. Smoking cessation rates 4 years after treatment by nicotine gum and acupuncture. *Prev Med*. 1997;26:25–28.

He D, Berg JE, Hostmark AT. Effects of acupuncture on smoking cessation or reduction for motivated smokers. *Prev Med*. 1997;26:208–214.

Konefal J, Duncan R, Clemence C. Comparison of three levels of auricular acupuncture in an outpatient substance abuse treatment program. *Altern Med J*. 1995;2:8–17.

Margolin A, Avants SK, Chang P, Kosten TR. Acupuncture for the treatment of cocaine dependence in methadone-maintained patients. *Am J Addict*. 1993;2:194–201.

White AR, Rampes H. Acupuncture in smoking cessation. In: *Cochrane Database of Systematic Reviews* [database on CD-ROM]. Oxford, England: Update Software; 1997. Updated November 24, 1996.9 The Cochrane Library; No. 2.

Gastroenterology

Cahn AM, Carayon P, Hill C, Flamant R. Acupuncture in gastroscopy. *Lancet*. 1978;1:182–183.

Chang FY, Chey WY, Ouyang A. Effect of transcutaneous nerve stimulation on esophageal function in normal subject—sevidence for a somatovisceral reflex. *Am J Chin Med*. 1996;24:185–192.

Jin HO, Zhou L, Lee KY, Chang TM, Chey WY. Inhibition of acid secretion by electrical acupuncture is mediated via β-endorphin and somatostatin. *Am J Physiol*. 1996;271:G524–G530.

Li Y, Tougas G, Chiverton SG, Hunt RH. The effect of acupuncture on gastrointestinal function and disorders. *Am J Gastroenterol*. 1992; 87:1372–1381.

General Pain

Chen XH, Han JS. All three types of opioid receptors in the spinal cord are important for 2/15 Hz electroacupuncture analgesia. *Eur J Pharmacol*. 1992;211:203–210.

Patel M, Gutzwiller F, et al. A meta-analysis of acupuncture for chronic pain. *Int J Epidemiol*. 1989;18:900–906.

Portnoy RK. Drug therapy for neuropathic pain. *Drug Ther*. 1993;23:41–53.

Shlay JC, Flaws B, Shaloner K, et al. *The Efficacy of a Standardized Acupuncture Regimen Compared to Placebo as a Treatment of Pain Caused by Peripheral Neuropathy in HIV-Infected Patients*. *JAMA*. In press.

Tang NM, Dong HW, Wang XM, Tsui ZC, Han JS. Cholecystokinin antisense RNA increases the analgesic effect induced by electroacupuncture or low dose morphine: conversion of low responder rats into high responders. *Pain*. 1997; 71:71–80.

Ter Riet G, Kleijnen J, Knipschild P. Acupuncture and chronic pain: a criteria based meta-analysis. *J Clin Epidemiol*. 1990;43:1191–1199.

Zhu CB, Li XY, Zhu YH, Xu SF. Binding sites of mu receptor increased when acupuncture analgesia was enhanced by droperidol: an autoradiographic study. *Chung Kuo Yao Li Hsueh Pao*. 1995;16:311–314.

History and Reviews

Helms JM. *Acupuncture Energetics: A Clinical Approach for Physicians*. Berkeley, Calif: Medical Acupuncture Publishers; 1996.

Hoizey D, Hoizey MJ. *A History of Chinese Medicine*. Edinburgh, Scotland: Edinburgh University Press; 1988.

Kaptchuk TJ. *The Web That Has No Weaver: Understanding Chinese Medicine*. New York, NY: Congdon & Weed; 1983.

Lao L. Acupuncture techniques and devices. *J Altern Complement Med*. 1996;2:23–25.

Liao SJ, Lee MHM, Ng NKY. *Principles and Practice of Contemporary Acupuncture*. New York, NY: Marcel Dekker Inc; 1994.

Lu GD, Needham J. *Celestial Lancets: A History and Rationale of Acupuncture and Moxa*. New York, NY: Cambridge University Press; 1980.

Lytle CD. History of the Food and Drug Administration's regulation of acupuncture devices. *J Altern Complement Med*. 1996; 2:253–256.

Mitchell BB. *Acupuncture and Oriental Medicine Laws*. Washington,DC: National Acupuncture Foundation; 1997.

Porkert M. *The Theoretical Foundations of Chinese Medicine*. Cambridge, Mass: Massachusetts Institute of Technology Press; 1974.

Stux G, Pomerantz B. *Basics of Acupuncture*. Berlin, Germany: Springer Verlag; 1995:1–250.

Unschuld PU. *Medicine in China: A History of Ideas*. Berkeley: University of California Press; 1985.

Immunology

Cheng XD, Wu GC, Jiang JW, Du LN, Cao XD. Dynamic observation on regulation of spleen lymphocyte proliferation from the traumatized rats in vitro of continued electroacupuncture. *Chin J Immunol*. 1997;13:68–70.

Du LN, Jiang JW, Wu GC, Cao XD. Effect of orphanin FQ on the immune function of traumatic rats. *Chin J Immunol*. In press.

Zhang Y, Du LN, Wu GC, Cao XD. Electroacupuncture (EA) induced attenuation of immunosuppression appearing after epidural or intrathecal injection of morphine in patients and rats. *Acupunct Electrother Res*. 1996; 21:177–186.

Miscellaneous

Medical devices: reclassification of acupuncture needles for the practice of acupuncture. *61 Federal Register*. 1996;61(236):64616–64617.

NIH Technology Assessment Workshop on Alternative Medicine. Acupuncture. *J Altern Complement Med*. 1996;2: 1–256.

Bullock ML, Pheley AM, Kiresuk TJ, Lenz SK, Culliton PD. Characteristics and complaints of patients seeking therapy at a hospital-based alternative medicine clinic. *J Altern Complement Med*. 1997;3:31–37.

Cassidy C. A survey of six acupuncture clinics: demographic and satisfaction data. In Programs and abstracts for the Proceedings of the Third Symposium of the Society for Acupuncture Research; September 16–17, 1995; Washington, DC. Pages 1–27.

Diehl DL, Kaplan G, Coulter I, Glik D, Hurwitz EL. Use of acupuncture by American physicians. *J Altern Complement Med*. 1997;3:119–126.

Musculoskeletal

Naeser MA, Hahn KK, Lieberman B. Real vs sham laser acupuncture and microamps TENS to treat carpal tunnel syndrome and worksite wrist pain: pilot study. *Lasers Surg Med Suppl*. 1996;8:7.

Nausea, Vomiting, and Postoperative Pain

Christensen PA, Noreng M, Andersen PE, Nielsen JW. Electroacupuncture and postoperative pain. *Br J Anaesth*. 1989;62:258–262.

Dundee JW, Chestnutt WN, Ghaly RG, Lynas AG. Traditional Chinese acupuncture: a potentially useful antiemetic? *BMJ*. 1986;293:583–584.

Dundee JW, Ghaly G. Local anesthesia blocks the antiemetic action of P6. *Clin Pharmacol Ther*. 1991;50:78–80.

Dundee JW, Ghaly RG, Bill KM, Chestnutt WN, Fitzpatrick KT, Lynas AG. Effect of stimulation of the P6 antiemetic point on postoperative nausea and vomiting. *Br J Anaesth*. 1989; 63:612–618.

Dundee JW, Ghaly RG, Lynch GA, Fitzpatrick KT, Abram WP. Acupuncture prophylaxis of cancer chemotherapy-induced sickness. *J R Soc Med*. 1989;82:268–271.

Dundee JW, McMillan C. Positive evidence for P6 acupuncture antiemesis. *Postgrad Med J*. 1991;67:47–52.

Lao L, Bergman S, Langenberg P, Wong RH, Berman B. Efficacy of Chinese acupuncture on postoperative oral surgery pain. *Oral Surg Med Oral Pathol Oral Radiol Endod*. 1995;79:423–428.

Martelete M, Fiori AMC. Comparative study of analgesic effect of transcutaneous nerve stimulation (TNS), electroacupuncture (EA), and meperidine in the treatment of postoperative pain. *Acupunct Electrother Res*. 1985; 10:183–193.

Sung YF, Kutner MH, Cerine FC, Frederickson EL. Comparison of the effects of acupuncture and codeine on postoperative dental pain. *Anesth Analg*. 1977;56:473–478.

Neurology

Asagai Y, Kanai H, Miura Y, Ohshiro T. Application of low reactive-level laser therapy (LLLT) in the functional training of cerebral palsy patients. *Laser Ther*.1994;6:195–202.

Han JS, Chen XH, Sun SL, et al. Effect of low- and high-frequency TENS on Met-enkephalin-Arg-Phe and dynorphin A immunoreactivity in human lumbar CSF. *Pain*. 1991;47:295–298.

Han JS, Wang Q. Mobilization of specific neuropeptides by peripheral stimulation of identified frequencies. *News Physiol Sci*. 1992;7:176–180.

Johansson K, Lindgren I, Widner H, Wiklung I, Johansson BB. Can sensory stimulation improve the functional outcome in stroke patients? *Neurology*. 1993;43:2189–2192.

Naeser MA. Acupuncture in the treatment of paralysis due to central nervous system damage. *J Altern Complement Med*. 1996;2:211–248.

Naeser MA, Alexander MP, Stlassny-Eder D, Galler V, Bachman D. Acupuncture in the treatment of paralysis in chronic and acute stroke patients: improvement correlated with specific CT scan lesion sites. *Acupunct Electrother Res*. 1994; 19:227–249.

Simpson DM, Wolfe DE. Neuromuscular complications of HIV infection and its treatment. *AIDS*. 1991;5:917–926.

Reproductive Medicine

Yang SP, He LF, Yu J. Changes in densities of hypothalamic μ opioid receptor during cupric acetate induced preovulatory LH surge in rabbit [in Chinese]. *Acta Physiol Sinica*. 1997; 49:354–358.

Yang QY, Ping SM, Yu J. Central opioid and dopamine activities in PCOS during induction of ovulation with electro-acupuncture [in Chinese]. *J Reprod Med*. 1992;1:6–19.

Yang SP, Yu J, He LF. Release of GnRH from the MBH induced by electroacupuncture in conscious female rabbits. *Acupunct Electrother Res*. 1994;19:9–27.

Yu J, Zheng HM, Ping SM. Changes in serum FSH, LH and ovarian follicular growth during electroacupuncture for induction of ovulation. *Chin J Integrated Traditional West Med*. 1995;1:13–16.

Research Methods

Birch S, Hammerschlag R. *Acupuncture Efficacy: A Compendium of Controlled Clinical Trials*. Tarrytown, NY: National Academy of Acupuncture and Oriental Medicine; 1996.

Hammerschlag R, Morris MM. Clinical trials comparing acupuncture to biomedical standard care: a criteria-based evaluation of research design and reporting. *Complement Ther Med*. 1997;5:133–140.

Kaptchuk TJ. Intentional ignorance: a history of blind assessment and placebo controls in medicine. *Bull Hist Med*. In press.

Singh BB, Berman BM. Research issues for clinical designs. *Complement Ther Med*. 1997;5:3–7.

Vincent CA. Credibility assessment in trials of acupuncture. *Complement Med Res*. 1990; 4:8–11.

Vincent CA, Lewith G. Placebo controls for acupuncture studies. *J R Soc Med*. 1995; 88:199–202.

Vincent CA, Richardson PH. The evaluation of therapeutic acupuncture: concepts and methods. *Pain*. 1986;24:1–13.

Adverse Effects

Lao L. Safety issues in acupuncture. *J Altern Complement Med*. 1996;2:27–31.

Norheim AJ, Fønnebø V. Acupuncture adverse effects are more than occasional case reports: results from questionnaires among 1135 randomly selected doctors and 197 acupuncturists. *Complement Ther Med*. 1996;4:8–13.

53 Acupuncture and Amitriptyline for Pain Due to HIV-Related Peripheral Neuropathy

A Randomized Controlled Trial

Judith C. Shlay, MD; Kathryn Chaloner, PhD; Mitchell B. Max, MD; Bob Flaws, Dipl Ac; Patricia Reichelderfer, PhD; Deborah Wentworth, MPH; Shauna Hillman, MS; Barbara Brizz, BSN, MHSEd; David L. Cohn, MD; for the Terry Beirn Community Programs for Clinical Research on AIDS

From the Denver Community Programs for Clinical Research on AIDS, Denver, Colo (Drs Shlay and Cohn); School of Statistics, University of Minnesota, St Paul (Dr Chaloner); National Institute of Dental Research (Dr Max) and National Institute of Allergy and Infectious Diseases (Dr Reichelderfer), National Institutes of Health, Bethesda, Md; Division of Biostatistics, University of Minnesota, Minneapolis (Mss Wentworth and Hillman); and Social and Scientific Systems, Inc, Rockville, Md (Ms Brizz). Mr Flaws is an acupuncturist practicing in Boulder, Colo.

Context

Peripheral neuropathy is common in persons infected with the human immunodeficiency virus (HIV) but few data on symptomatic treatment are available.

Objective

To evaluate the efficacy of a standardized acupuncture regimen (SAR) and amitriptyline hydrochloride for the relief of pain due to HIV-related peripheral neuropathy in HIV-infected patients.

Design

Randomized, placebo-controlled, multicenter clinical trial. Each site enrolled patients into 1 of the following 3 options: (1) a modified double-blind 2 × 2 factorial design of SAR, amitriptyline, or the combination compared with placebo, (2) a modified double-blind design of an SAR vs control points, or (3) a double-blind design of amitriptyline vs placebo.

Setting

Terry Beirn Community Programs for Clinical Research on AIDS (HIV primary care providers) in 10 US cities.

Patients

Patients with HIV-associated, symptomatic, lower-extremity peripheral neuropathy. Of 250 patients enrolled, 239 were in the acupuncture comparison (125 in the factorial option and 114 in the SAR option vs control points option), and 136 patients were in the amitriptyline comparison (125 in the factorial option and 11 in amitriptyline option vs placebo option).

Interventions

Standarized acupuncture regimen vs control points, amitriptyline (75 mg/d) vs placebo, or both for 14 weeks.

Main Outcome Measure

Changes in mean pain scores at 6 and 14 weeks, using a pain scale ranging from 0.0 (no pain) to 1.75 (extremely intense), recorded daily.

Results

Patients in all 4 groups showed reduction in mean pain scores at 6 and 14 weeks compared with baseline values. For both the acupuncture and amitriptyline comparisons,

changes in pain score were not significantly different between the 2 groups. At 6 weeks, the estimated difference in pain reduction for patients in the SAR group compared with those in the control points group (a negative value indicates a greater reduction for the "active" treatment) was 0.01 (95% confidence interval [CI], −0.11 to 0.12; *P*=.88) and for patients in the amitriptyline group vs those in the placebo group was −0.07 (95% CI, −0.22 to 0.08; *P*=.38). At 14 weeks, the difference for those in the SAR group compared with those in the control points group was −0.08 (95% CI, −0.21 to 0.06; *P*=.26) and for amitriptyline compared with placebo was 0.00 (95% CI, −0.18 to 0.19; *P*=.99).

Conclusions

In this study, neither acupuncture nor amitriptyline was more effective than placebo in relieving pain caused by HIV-related peripheral neuropathy.

JAMA. 1998;280:1590–1595

Peripheral neuropathies are diagnosed in 30% to 35% of patients with human immunodeficiency virus (HIV) and cause pain and dysesthesias.[1,2] Symptomatic treatment includes antidepressants, nonnarcotic and narcotic analgesics, anticonvulsants, and acupuncture.[2,3] The use of these treatments is based on anecdotal[4] information and trials in other disease conditions.[5]

We chose to examine the efficacy of 2 commonly used treatments, amitriptyline hydrochloride and acupuncture, for HIV-related peripheral neuropathy. Amitriptyline is frequently prescribed for neuropathic pain and has been shown to be an effective treatment for diabetic, hereditary, toxic, and idiopathic neuropathies.[6,7]

Although several trials that reported examining acupuncture for chronic painful conditions claim efficacy,[8,9] these studies have methodological limitations, including small sample sizes and inadequate controls for the nonspecific effects of acupuncture.[9–11] Meta-analyses of studies of acupuncture for chronic pain show a response rate of approximately 70% for acupuncture, 50% for "sham" acupuncture (needling points not considered effective), and 30% for control treatments, such as sham transcutaneous electrical nerve stimulation.[9,10,12,13]

To evaluate the effect of both a nonstandard and standard medical therapy for peripheral neuropathy, we performed a multicenter, modified double-blind, randomized, placebo-controlled study of the separate and combined efficacy of a standardized acupuncture regimen (SAR) and amitriptyline for the relief of pain caused by HIV-related peripheral neuropathy.

Methods

Study Design

We used a 2 × 2 factorial design to determine whether SAR, amitriptyline, or the combination was more effective than placebo. The SAR consisted of acupuncture points chosen by the study acupuncturists and several consultants to be effective for peripheral neuropathic pain. This regimen was compared with control points that were not "true" points defined by any standard acupuncture text[14] (Figure 1). We compared the efficacy of amitriptyline with placebo capsules of identical appearance. Enrollment in the factorial design began in May 1993, but patients at some sites were reluctant to be randomized to receive amitriptyline and some clinicians were unwilling to provide amitriptyline to their patients because it was a commonly abused drug in their communities. The study design was modified in March 1995 so that sites could choose only 1 of 3 options. Each site could (1) continue to enroll into the factorial design (factorial option), (2) enroll into a single-factor design of SAR vs control points (acupuncture option), or (3) enroll into a single-factor design of amitriptyline vs placebo (amitriptyline option) (Figure 2).

Randomization schedules were prepared using random blocks stratified by unit. Patients were randomized to treatment by the study units by telephoning the Statistical Center at the University of Minnesota, Minneapolis. The unit pharmacists were the only people unblinded to the placebo vs amitriptyline assignment, and the acupuncturists were the only people unblinded to the SAR vs control points assignments. The pain diaries and the assessments of pain relief were collected by study staff who were blinded to the treatment assignments.

Study Population

Patients were recruited from 11 units of the Terry Beirn Community Programs for Clinical Research on AIDS, an organization sponsored by the National Institutes of Health, which conducts clinical trials in primary care settings. The study was approved by each institutional review board. All participants gave written informed consent. To

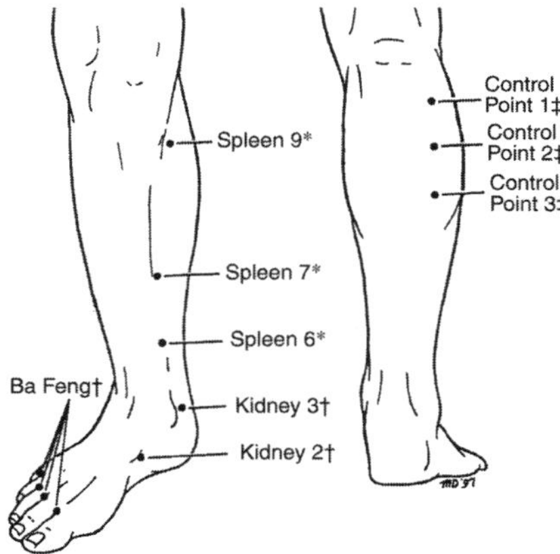

Figure 1. Standardized acupuncture regimen and control points.

be eligible, participants had to be aged 13 years or older; have documented HIV infection; have symptoms of HIV-related lower extremity peripheral neuropathy, diagnosed by a physician based on history and clinical examination; and have completed a baseline pain diary prior to randomization. Antiretroviral therapy was allowed and dosages of analgesic medication or herbal therapies used at randomization were maintained or reduced. The initiation of new treatments during the study was discouraged but allowed when necessary. Patients were excluded if they were being treated for an acute opportunistic infection or malignancy except nonsystemic Kaposi sarcoma, were pregnant, or had taken a tricyclic antidepressant or monoamine oxidase inhibitor 2 weeks before randomization.

Treatment Regimens

For the acupuncture comparison, patients were randomly assigned to receive SAR or control points twice weekly during a 6-week induction phase, followed by weekly treatment during an 8-week maintenance phase. This SAR was based on a Chinese theory that peripheral neuropathy caused by diabetes and HIV-related peripheral neuropathy have similar mechanisms. The SAR included spleen points 9, 7, and 6, with the additional supplemental points of Ba Feng (M-LE-8) for complaints of pain or numbness in the heel, Ran Gu (kidney 2) for complaints of pain or numbness in the soles, and Tai Ki (kidney 3) for complaints of pain or numbness in the heel (Figure 1).14 The control points were located on the back of the leg (Figure 1). For the SAR and control points, acupuncture needles were inserted to a specified depth. Each location was manipulated both superiorly and inferiorly. Then the needles were reinserted into the specified point. After 10 to 15 minutes, the needles were remanipulated and replaced into the original location for another 5 to 10 minutes. The depth of insertion was between 1.28 to 2.54 cm (0.5 to 1.0 in) for spleen point 9, 2.54 to 3.81 cm (1.0 to 1.5 in) for spleen point 7, and 1.5 to 3.05 cm (0.6 to 1.2 in) for spleen point 6. For the control points, insertion was less than 1.28 cm (0.5 in). Study acupuncturists received standardized training in the technique. In addition, a videotape of the acupuncture and the control treatment was provided to each of the acupuncturists in the study. To maintain blinding and to determine the need for supplemental points, the acupuncturists asked all patients a series of standard questions, irrespective of treatment arm. For those in the SAR group, spleen points 9, 7, and 6 were always used. Supplemental acupuncture points were used only if the patient answered "yes" to the corresponding question. The control points consisted of only 3 specified points.

For the amitriptyline comparison, the patients were randomized to receive a 14-week course of either amitriptyline or placebo capsules by mouth once a day. They were instructed to take them between 1 to 2 hours before bedtime. An initial daily dose of 25 mg of amitriptyline hydrochloride was increased every 2 to 3 days until a maximum dosage of 75 mg/d was reached.[15,16] The placebo capsules were identical in appearance and taste to the active capsules. Patients were followed up for the 14-week study period and for adverse event monitoring for an additonal 8 weeks after the study treatment had discontinued.

Results were monitored by the HIV Therapeutic Trials Data Safety and Monitoring Board of the National Institute of Allergy and Infectious Diseases, National Institutes of Health, Bethesda, Md. Data monitoring used the Lan–De Mets method[17] as a guideline for early stopping to account for increased type I error probability by examining the data before the designed study end.

Evaluation

Patients rated their pain in a diary once daily, choosing from the Gracely scale of 13 words that describe the intensity.18 The scale ranges from no pain (0.0), weak (0.45), mild (0.74), moderate (1.09), strong (1.36), to extremely intense (1.75). The words had been assigned magnitudes on the basis of ratio-scaling procedures that demonstrated internal consistency, reliability, and objectivity.[18] The scale has distinguished active from control interventions in experimental and clinical pain

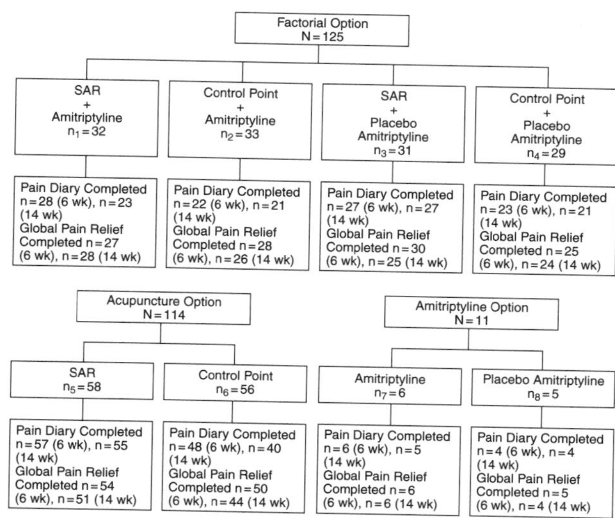

Figure 2. The standardized acupuncture regimen (SAR) vs control points (CPs) compares $n_1 + n_3 + n_5$ with $n_2 + n_4 + n_6$. The amitriptyline vs placebo compares $n_1 + n_2 + n_7 +$ with $n_3 + n_4 + n_8$.

studies.[6,18,19] At the end of both the induction and maintenance phases, patients reported their global pain relief (complete, a lot, moderate, slight, none, or worse) after they were asked the following question: "Since the beginning of the study, how would you rate the relief of pain and/or discomfort in your legs and feet?" A study physician, trained in neurologic examination, tested the patient at randomization and at 14 weeks. A neurologic summary score was computed as an average of 3 separate scores for muscle strength, sensory ability, and reflex. Each physician who performed the neurologic assessment reviewed a videotape that detailed how the examination was to be completed. The patients also completed a self-administered, 39-item, quality-of-life assessment tool.[20] The complete tool, consisting of 11 different dimensions, was administered at baseline and 14 weeks, and the dimension corresponding to physical functioning was also administered at 6 weeks. To assess the effectiveness of the blinding, all patients were asked to guess their treatment assignments at 14 weeks. Patients were monitored for grade 4 adverse events and death. Adverse experiences occurring within 8 weeks of study treatment were graded on a 5-point severity scale (grade 5 corresponding to death) according to a standardized toxicity scale. Any grade 4 or 5 event was reportable irrespective of presumed relationship to study treatment.

Statistical Analysis

Comparison of treatment groups for the primary end point of change in pain, as measured by the pain diary, used a linear model with baseline characteristics, clinical unit, and option (factorial or single factor) as covariates. If the average weekly pain score for the sixth week of treatment was present, it was used. If it was missing, the closest weekly average within the 6-week visit window of 4 to 10 weeks was used. Similarly, this was done for the 14-week end point and the visit window of 11 to 16 weeks. A linear model repeated measures analysis of the weekly pain averages was also performed, with the same explanatory variables.[21] Estimates of the difference between SAR and control points were calculated for each of the 14 weeks. The global pain relief rating was analyzed using a log-linear model, with likelihood ratio tests for differences among treatment groups, which were adjusted for option.[22]

We verified that results from the 3 treatments could be pooled by checking that the interaction term between acupuncture and amitriptyline in the factorial option and the option by treatment interaction were nonsignificant.

Secondary outcomes were the permanent discontinuation of study treatments, changes in quality of life, and changes in neurologic summary scores, which were analyzed similarly to the primary end point. All analyses were on an intent-to-treat basis. The evaluation of the blinding compared the patients' guesses of the therapy received with the treatment group. Using a log-linear model, we adjusted for option and for whether the patient reported moderate or more pain relief with the 14-week global pain relief rating.

For the original 2 × 2 factorial design, a sample size of 260 patients was calculated to provide a 90% power of detecting a mean difference between treatments of 0.20 (half the difference between "moderate" and "mild" pain) on the Gracely pain intensity scale using a type I error of .05 (2-sided). After the study design was modified, sample size requirements were estimated at 260 per group. In February 1997, the monitoring board recommended closing the study because it concluded that the results were definitive for both acupuncture and amitriptyline comparisons.

Table 1. Baseline Characteristics of Study Participants*

Characteristics	Acupuncture: SAR (n = 121)	Acupuncture: Control Points (n = 118)	Amitriptyline Hydrochloride: Active (n = 71)	Amitriptyline Hydrochloride: Placebo (n = 65)
Age, mean (SD), y	40.9 (6.8)	41.7 (8.3)	40.1 (7.1)	39.9 (5.9)
Sex, % male	88	92	94	88
Race, %				
Latino/Hispanic	12	6	11	12
Black	30	29	28	22
White	55	61	58	63
Other	3	4	3	3
Baseline pain score, mean (SD)	1.11 (0.3)	1.06 (0.4)	1.10 (0.3)	1.13 (0.3)
Karnofsky score, mean (SD)	84.5 (11.7)	84.7 (11.0)	83.7 (11.5)	83.1 (10.2)
<80, %	21	19	24	15
Disease progression history, %†	53	47	62	48
Current use of antiretrovirals, %	61	65	58	57
Current use of pain medications, %	48	46	47	54
Type of pain, %‡				
Aching/cramping	41	45	51	40
Burning/heat	35	30	28	35
Throbbing	23	22	27	12
Stabbing/sharp	36	36	35	39
Numbness/tingling	88	87	89	86
Other	24	22	30	22

*SAR indicates standardized acupuncture regimen. Values are mean percentage unless otherwise indicated.

†Defined as history of an opportunistic infection or malignancy.

‡These categories are not mutually exclusive.

Results

Study Population

From May 1993 to February 1997, 250 patients were enrolled. Of those, 239 were in the acupuncture comparison (125 in the factorial option and 114 randomized to SAR or control points), and 136 were in the amitriptyline comparison (125 from the factorial option and 11 randomized to either active or placebo amitriptyline) (Figure 2). Baseline characteristics (Table 1) were similar in the active and control groups for both comparisons.

Effects of Treatment

SAR vs Control Points. The change in pain was not significantly different between the 2 groups at either 6 or 14 weeks (Table 2). Both groups showed improvement in pain from an average intensity of "moderate" to "mild" (Figure 3). The estimated difference of the SAR group compared with the control points group was 0.01 at 6 weeks (95% confidence interval [CI], −0.11 to 0.12; *P*=.88) and −0.08 at 14 weeks (95% CI, −0.21 to 0.06; *P*=.26). At 6 weeks, the SAR group had less pain relief than patients in the control points group by 0.01 U and at 14 weeks, the SAR group had 0.08 U more relief than patients in the control points group. Repeated measures analyses of weekly pain averages during the entire 14-week period gave weekly effects, which were small and nonsignificant (*P* values ranging from .10 to .94).

There were no significant differences in the quality of life, neurologic summary score (Table 2), number of grade 4 adverse events, deaths, or discontinuations. By 14 weeks, 20% of patients randomized to the SAR group and 25% of those randomized to control points group had discontinued treatment. Three patients assigned to the SAR option and 10 assigned to the control points experienced a grade 4 adverse event (*P*=.06).

The difference in the global pain relief rating between the 2 groups was not significant at 6 weeks (*P*=.65). However, at 14 weeks, there was a nominally significant difference (*P*=.03) with a slightly higher proportion of patients in the SAR group reporting moderate or more pain relief than those in the control points group (Table 3).

Table 2. Mean Changes in Weekly Pain Diary Scores, Neurologic Score, and Quality of Life at 6 and 14 Weeks*

	Acupuncture						Amitriptyline Hydrochloride					
	SAR		Control Points				Active		Placebo			
	No.	Mean Change	No.	Mean Change	Difference (95% CI)†	P Value†	No.	Mean Change	No.	Mean Change	Difference (95% CI)‡	P Value‡
Primary Outcomes												
Pain diary, 6 wk	112	−0.21	93	−0.20	0.01 (−0.11 to 0.12)	.88	56	−0.23	54	−0.18	−0.07 (−0.22 to 0.08)	.38
Pain diary, 14 wk	105	−0.29	82	−0.19	−0.08 (−0.21 to 0.06)	.26	49	−0.26	52	−0.30	0.00 (−0.18 to 0.19)	.99
Secondary Outcomes												
Neurologic score, 14 wk	94	2.1	80	−1.4	2.2 (−1.9 to 6.3)	.30	49	0.8	49	−0.4	0.6 (−4.3 to 5.4)	.82
Quality of life												
Physical functioning, 6 wk	110	6.0	102	5.6	0.4 (−5.4 to 6.1)	.90	61	5.9	60	5.1	0.3 (−8.3 to 8.9)	.94
Physical functioning, 14 wk	97	3.4	90	1.3	3.4 (−3.3 to 10.0)	.32	52	7.1	51	0.6	6.4 (−2.7 to 15.5)	.17
Overall *P* value, 14 wk§						.64						.60

*SAR indicates standardized acupuncture regimen; CI, confidence interval.
†SAR minus control points, adjusted for unit, baseline score, and amitriptyline assignment (active, placebo, or none).
‡Active minus placebo, adjusted for unit, baseline score, and acupuncture assignment (SAR or not SAR).
§*P* value from combining 11 dimensions using method of O'Brien.[23]

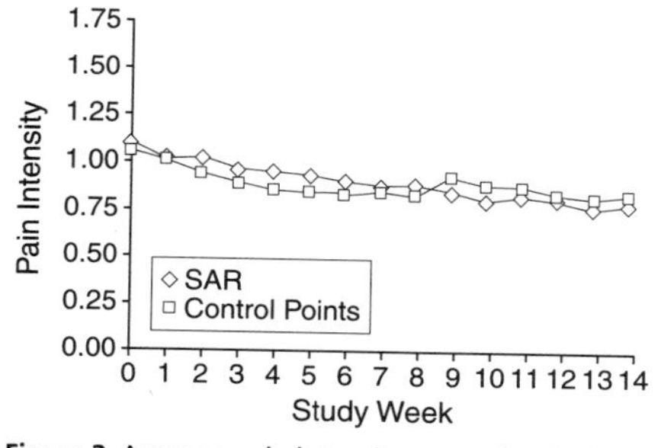

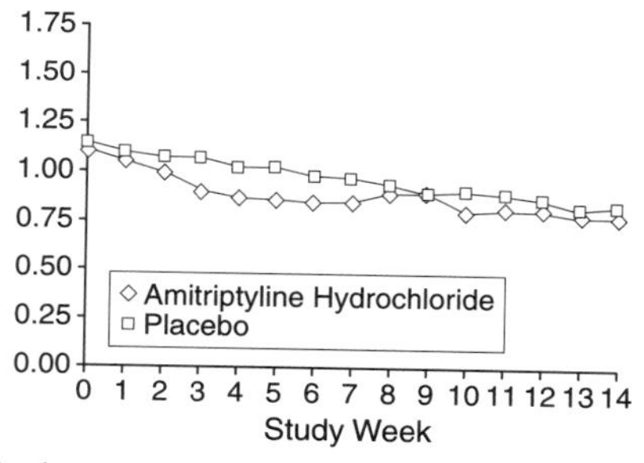

Figure 3. Average pain intensity scores for single factor options by study week. The mean weekly values of the descriptors of pain intensity are plotted. There was no statistically significant difference between the effects of the standardized acupuncture regimen (SAR) vs control points or between amitriptyline vs placebo. Pain intensity is described and rated as no pain (0.0), faint (0.04), very weak (0.36), weak (0.45), very mild (0.59), mild (0.74), moderate (1.09), barely strong (1.10), slightly intense (1.35), strong (1.36), intense (1.59), very intense (1.64), and extremely intense (1.75).[18]

However, after adjustment for multiple comparisons, the result is not significant.

Amitriptyline vs Placebo. The change in pain score at 6 and 14 weeks was not significantly different between the active and placebo groups (Table 2). As with the SAR vs control points comparison, both groups showed improvement over time (Figure 3). The estimated difference of amitriptyline compared with placebo was −0.07 at 6 weeks (95% CI, −0.22 to 0.08; *P*=.38) and 0.00 at 14 weeks (95% CI, −0.18 to 0.19; *P*=.99). That is, at 6 weeks, patients taking amitriptyline had more pain relief by 0.07 U than those taking placebo and there was no difference at 14 weeks. Repeated measures analyses of weekly pain averages indicated that the largest beneficial effect was at week 3 (*P*=.05), but after adjusting for multiple comparisons, the result was not statistically significant.

There were no statistically significant differences in quality of life, neurologic summary scores (Table 2), number of grade 4 adverse events, or deaths. Six patients assigned to the amitriptyline and 2 assigned to placebo options experienced grade 4 adverse events (*P*=.20). By 14 weeks, 35% of patients randomized to either the amitriptyline or placebo groups had discontinued drug treatment. The difference in the global pain relief rating between the 2 groups was not significant at 6 weeks (*P*=.68) or 14 weeks (*P*=.81) (Table 3).

Table 3. Global Pain Relief Rating at 6 and 14 Weeks*

	Acupuncture				Amitriptyline Hydrochloride			
	SAR		Control Points		Active		Placebo	
Global Pain Relief	**No.**	**Cumulative %**	**No.**	**Cumulative %**	**No.**	**Cumulative %**	**No.**	**Cumulative %**
6 weeks								
Complete	3	2.7	2	1.9	3	4.9	3	5.0
A lot	17	18.0	14	15.5	6	14.8	10	21.7
Moderate	37	51.4	36	50.5	22	50.8	15	46.7
Slight	29	77.5	19	68.9	14	73.8	13	68.3
None	16	91.9	22	90.3	11	91.8	11	86.7
Pain worse	9	100.0	10	100.0	5	100.0	8	100.0
No. of patients with rating	111		103		61		60	
P value†		.65				.68		
14 weeks								
Complete	8	7.8	2	2.1	1	1.7	0	0.0
A lot	19	26.5	27	30.9	12	22.4	12	22.6
Moderate	31	56.9	16	47.9	14	46.4	15	50.9
Slight	23	79.4	18	67.0	13	69.0	13	75.5
None	19	98.0	26	94.7	16	96.6	11	96.2
Pain worse	2	100.0	5	100.0	2	100.0	2	100.0
No. of patients with rating	102		94		58		53	
P value†		.03				.81		

*SAR indicates standardized acupuncture regimen.
†Likelihood ratio test for the conditional independence of relief and treatment arm; SAR vs control points comparison is adjusted for the level of the other factor (active amitriptyline, placebo amitriptyline, and no amitriptyline). Amitriptyline vs placebo comparison is adjusted for the level of the other factor (SAR, control points, or no acupuncture).

Factorial Option. The test for interaction in change of pain between the 2 factors was not significant at either 6 or 14 weeks (P=.17 and P=.31, respectively). There was no significant difference in the change in pain among the 4 groups at either 6 or 14 weeks (P=.37 and P=.64, respectively). All study groups in the factorial option showed improvement in pain.

Completeness of Data

Figure 2 shows the number of patients providing pain diary data and global pain relief ratings at 6 and 14 weeks. To examine the sensitivity of the conclusions to missing data, the analyses were repeated using 2 common methods to impute missing data. The first assumes that the patients' missing data indicated no change in their pain from baseline; the second uses the last value of the weekly pain reported to calculate the end point. Under both methods to impute the missing pain diary data, the results of the study did not reach statistical significance for either comparison at either 6 or 14 weeks.

Assessment of Treatment Blinding

For the acupuncture comparison, although the patients' guesses and the treatment assignments were not independent (P=.007, data not shown), there was a strong association between the guess and the global pain relief rating. Those reporting moderate or more relief at 14 weeks tended to guess that they received the SAR. After adjusting for option and the reported relief being moderate or more, the patients' guesses and the treatment assignments were not independent (P=.02), but the association was small. This differed in the amitriptyline comparison, in which a large proportion of patients correctly guessed the study treatment, irrespective of their level of pain relief (P<.001) (Table 4).

Comment

The main findings of this study show that treatment with this SAR had little or no effect on HIV-related peripheral neuropathy compared with the control points. Similarly, amitriptyline, as commonly used, was not significantly more effective than placebo (Table 2 and Figure 3). All treatment groups improved during the study period by the amount hypothesized in the design, suggesting that the modest decline in pain scores in all groups was either attributable to a placebo effect or patients entered the study

Table 4. Effectiveness of Participants' Blinding to Treatment Assignment*

	Acupuncture, No. (%)			Amitriptyline Hydrochloride, No. (%)	
Patient Guess	SAR	Control	Patient Guess	Active	Placebo
Moderate or more relief†					
SAR	47 (81.0)	28 (62.2)	Active	20 (74.1)	9 (33.3)
Control points	2 (3.4)	6 (13.3)	Placebo	4 (14.8)	16 (59.3)
Cannot guess	9 (15.5)	11 (24.4)	Cannot guess	3 (11.1)	2 (7.4)
Less than moderate relief†					
SAR	14 (31.8)	10 (20.4)	Active	19 (61.3)	8 (30.8)
Control points	12 (27.3)	22 (44.9)	Placebo	6 (19.4)	15 (57.7)
Cannot guess	18 (40.9)	17 (34.7)	Cannot guess	6 (19.4)	3 (11.5)
P value‡		.02			<.001

*SAR indicates standardized acupuncture regimen.
†Global pain relief rating at 14 weeks.
‡Likelihood ratio test for independence of guess and treatment adjusted for global pain relief rating at 14 weeks (moderate or more vs less than moderate).

at times of symptomatic flares and improved spontaneously thereafter.

For the acupuncture comparison, the results were strengthened by 2 methodological features of the trial. First, the sample size of approximately 120 patients per treatment group is many times larger than those in previously published trials of acupuncture,[9] and the CIs were narrow, making it unlikely that a large positive treatment effect was missed by chance. Second, the control points appeared reasonably effective in preserving the blinding (Table 4). Many of the study clinicians and, presumably, the study participants were favorably disposed toward acupuncture. If patients were able to guess their treatment better than randomly, the resulting placebo effects would be expected to bias the result in favor of this SAR,[10,12,24] thus making our finding of a similar effect even more convincing.

We cannot completely rule out the possibility that the SAR had a modest and delayed analgesic effect, in view of the nominally significant result of SAR compared with control points on the global pain relief rating at 14 weeks, although this was not seen at 6 weeks. This is unlikely, however, in view of the finding of no significant difference in the pain diary scores. Our study was designed with a sample size that provided sufficient power to detect even a small difference between the SAR and control points. The CIs at both 6 and 14 weeks rule out any clinically meaningful beneficial effects of SAR based on the primary end point of the pain diary scores.

One possible explanation for the lack of efficacy of the SAR is that we chose the wrong "active points." Consensus on the SAR was reached by 8 acupuncturists before protocol implementation. Another explanation is that the use of nonclassical points as a control provided a real effect and was not an inert control. There is evidence from animal and human studies that acupuncture at either classical or nonclassical locations may have analgesic effects[9,25,26] by mechanisms such as the release of endogenous opioids[27] or activation of other brain and spinal cord pathways that reduce pain.[28]

There is controversy over what constitutes an acceptable control group for acupuncture studies.[8,29] It is possible that the novelty of an experience like acupuncture may generate a placebo analgesic effect quite apart from specific effects produced by needling specific points.[30] Unless the study includes a "sham" acupuncture group as a control, such nonspecific effects may bias toward a result in favor of the active intervention.

The SAR chosen for this study differs from the practice of most acupuncturists, who treat patients with individualized regimens.[31] We chose to study standardized points to test the hypothesis that these specific points promote analgesia for chronic foot and leg pain[13] and because such a study is easier to blind and replicate. If the acupuncturists had used individualized treatment, the results would not be generalizable to other acupuncturists, and the treatment, if efficacious, could not be used by other practitioners. Our approach enabled us to derive a conclusion about these acupuncture points but not about individualized treatments.

Amitriptyline is used in the treatment of HIV-related peripheral neuropathy[32] but was not effective in this study. The lack of efficacy at 14 weeks was confirmed by the analysis of the secondary end points. Although the 6-week

CI did not completely rule out the beneficial effect of 0.20 that the study was designed to detect, there was no supporting evidence of beneficial effect from any of the secondary end points. In addition, another study in HIV-related peripheral neuropathy agrees with our findings.[33] The indication that the blinding was not maintained also confirms the lack of efficacy because unblinding tends to bias toward a hypothesized active intervention.[24,34]

It is possible that a higher dose of amitriptyline would have resulted in a larger treatment effect. We chose this dose based on common clinical practice and on the only 2 published prospective randomized dose-response studies of tricyclic antidepressants used for chronic pain.[15,16]

No previously controlled trials of amitriptyline in neuropathic pain have followed up patients for longer than 8 weeks.[33,35] Clinical trials of amitriptyline for neuropathies of diabetic and nondiabetic etiologies have shown larger, short-term, clinically meaningful effects.[6,7,19] Mechanisms for this include facilitation of the analgesic action of norepinephrine and serotonin released by endogenous analgesic systems[16,19] and the blockade of sodium channels in peripheral sprouts from damaged nerves.[36] Presumably, the neuropathological features of the HIV-associated distal axonal neuropathy generate painful discharges resistant to the analgesic actions of tricyclic antidepressants.[37,38]

In conclusion, this is the largest reported randomized, placebo-controlled, clinical trial of symptomatic treatment for HIV-related peripheral neuropathy. Overall, our results indicate that neither this SAR given over 14 weeks nor amitriptyline hydrochloride, 75 mg/d, was effective in relieving pain and neither therapy can be recommended for the treatment of HIV-related peripheral neuropathy. Additional clinical trials are needed because there are no effective treatments for this chronic debilitating condition.[39]

This project was supported by the National Institute of Allergy and Infectious Diseases.

We are indebted to the study participants for their cooperation and support and to other members of the Community Programs for Clinical Research on AIDS, who are as follows: Carol Anne Bosco, RN, Jill Chesnut, RN, MED, Jeffrey Cohen, MD, Marjorie Dehlinger, DNSc, Sister Mary Sarah Dolan, RN, Valerie Dratter, RN, MS, Lawrence Fox, MD, PhD, Ana Martinez, RpH, Jim Neaton, PhD, Marie Sioud, and Wendy Smith, PhD; and to Peter Jatlow, MD, for determining amitriptyline blood levels. We thank Zarina Alloo, Coleen Craig, Susan Meger, and Michelle Puplava for preparation of the manuscript. We also thank the members of the National Institute of Allergy and Infectious Diseases HIV Therapeutic Trials Data Safety and Monitoring Board, who are as follows: Baruch A. Brody, MD, Charles Carpenter, MD, David DeMets, PhD, Thomas R. Fleming, PhD, Mary A. Foulkes, MPH, PhD, Bernard Lo, MD, Julio Montaner, MD, Dianne Murphy, MD, Judith O'Fallon, PhD, James Rahal, MD, Wasima Rida, PhD, Steven Schnittman, MD, Paula Sparti, MD, Patricia N. Whitley-Williams, MD, Robert Woolson, PhD, and Abigail Zuger, MD. The following institutions and persons participated in the Community Programs for Clinical Research on AIDS: Philadelphia Fight, Philadelphia, Pa (Barbara Gallagher, Gary Seely, Regina Anthony); Denver Community Program for Clinical Research on AIDS, Denver, Colo (Michael Grodesky, Brenda Hughston, Jack Rouff); Harlem AIDS Treatment Group, New York, NY (Wafaa El-Sadr, Mary Sarah Dolan, Luis Fuentes); Community Consortium, San Francisco, Calif (Sherill Crawford, Margaret Poscher, John Nienow); Clinical Directors Network of Region II, Inc, New York, NY (Anita Vaughn, Jo Anne Staats, Margaret Granville); The Research and Education Group, Portland, Ore, (James Sampson, Doug Beers, Joyce St Arnaud); Partners in Research/New Mexico, Albuquerque (Bruce Williams, Nadine Ulibarri-Keller, Cynthia Geist); Baltimore Trials, Baltimore, Md (David Wheeler, Louise Pascal, Sandra Jones); Wayne State University, Detroit, Mich (Randa Fakhry, Rodger MacArthur, Michael Shy); North Jersey Community Research Initiative, Newark, NJ (Catherine Forrester, Norma Santos); and Washington Regional AIDS Program, Washington, DC (Douglas Ward, Barbara Standridge). In addition, the following acupuncturists participated in the study: Beverly Bakken, DOM, Dipl NCCA, Marijke S. de Vries, DOM, Andrew Fitzcharles, L Ac, Lee Forest Knowlton, L Ac, Dipl Ac, Skya Gardner-Abbate, MA, DOM, Dipl Ac, Magnolia Goh, MD, L Ac, Christopher Hudson, L Ac, Joel Kay, MD, Robert Kelly, OMD, Dipl Ac, Lixing Lao, PhD; Lorna Lee, RAc, Patricia R. Lollis, L Ac, Howard Moffet, MPH, L Ac, Joseph Odom, L Ac, Lahary Pittman, CA, CAC, Eric Serejski, M Ac, L Ac, Dipl Ac, Qing-Yao Shi, MD, L Ac, Deborah Torrance, Dipl Ac, CA, Lynsay Tunnell, DOM, Byrn Walsh, L Ac, and Wendy Whitman, L Ac.

References

1. So YT, Holtzman DM, Abrams DI, Olney RK. Peripheral neuropathy associated with AIDS. *Arch Neurol*. 1988;45:945–948.
2. Simpson DM, Tagliati M. Neurologic manifestations of HIV infection. *Ann Intern Med*. 1994; 121:769–785.
3. Armington K. Sticking it to peripheral neuropathy. *AIDS Care*. 1997;9:52–54.
4. Newshan G. HIV neuropathy treated with gabapentin. *AIDS*. 1998;12:219–221.
5. Hegarty A, Portenoy RK. Drug therapy for neuropathic pain. *Semin Neurol*. 1994; 14:213–224.
6. Max MB, Culnane M, Schafer SC, et al. Amitriptyline relieves diabetic neuropathy pain in patients with normal or depressed mood. *Neurology*. 1987;37:589–596.
7. Vrethem M, Boivie J, Arnquist H, et al. A comparison of amitriptyline and maprotiline in the treatment of painful polyneuropathy in diabetics and nondiabetics. *Clin J Pain*. 1997;13:313–323.
8. Birch S, Hammerschlag R, Berman BM. Acupuncture in the treatment of pain. *J Altern Complement Med*. 1996;2:101–124.
9. Richardson PH, Vincent CA. Acupuncture for the treatment of pain. *Pain*. 1986;24:15–40.

10. Chapman CR, Gunn CC. Acupuncture. In: Bonica JJ, ed. *The Management of Pain*. 2nd ed. Malvern, Pa: Lea & Febiger; 1990: 1805–1821.

11. Patel M, Gutzwiller F, Paccaud F, Marazzi A. A meta-analysis of acupuncture for chronic pain. *Int J Epidemiol*. 1989;18:900–906.

12. Deyo RA. Non-operative treatment. In: Frymoyer JW, ed. *The Adult Spine: Principles and Practice*. New York, NY: Raven Press; 1991:1777–1793.

13. Lewith GT, Machin D. On the evaluation of the clinical effects of acupuncture. *Pain*. 1983; 16:111–127.

14. O'Connor J, Bensky D. *Acupuncture: A Comprehensive Text*. Chicago, Ill: Eastland Press; 1981.

15. McQuay HJ, Carroll D, Glynn CJ. Dose-response for analgesic effect of amitriptyline in chronic pain. *Anaesthesia*. 1993;48:281–285.

16. Sindrup SH, Gram LH, Skjold T, et al. Concentration-response relationship in imipramine treatment of diabetic neuropathy symptoms. *Clin Pharmacol Ther*. 1990; 47:509–515.

17. Lan KKG, DeMets DL. Discrete sequential boundaries for clinical trials. *Biometrika*. 1983;70:659–663.

18. Gracely RH, McGrath P, Dubner R. Ratio scales of sensory and affective verbal pain descriptors. *Pain*. 1978;5:5–18.

19. Max MB, Lynch SA, Muir J, et al. Effects of desipramine, amitriptyline, and fluoxetine on pain in diabetic neuropathy. *N Engl J Med*. 1992; 326:1250–1256.

20. Tarlov AR, Ware JE Jr, Greenfield S, et al. The Medical Outcomes Study: an application of methods for monitoring the results of medical care. *JAMA*. 1989;262:925–930.

21. Littell RC, Milliken GA, Stroup WW, Wolfinger RD. *SAS System for Mixed Models*. Cary, NC: SAS Institute Inc; 1996.

22. Agresti A. *An Introduction to Categorial Data Analysis*. New York, NY: John Wiley & Sons Inc; 1996.

23. O'Brien PC. Procedures for comparing samples with multiple endpoints. *Biometrics*. 1984; 31:511–529.

24. Turner JA, Deyo RA, Loesor JD, et al. The importance of placebo effects in pain treatment and research. *JAMA*. 1994;271:1609–1614.

25. Lee PK, Andersen TW, Modell JH, Saga SA. Treatment of chronic pain with acupuncture. *JAMA*. 1975;232:1133–1135.

26. Gaw AC, Chang LW, Shaw LC. Efficacy of acupuncture on osteoarthritic pain. *N Engl J Med*. 1975;293:375–378.

27. Han JS, Chen XH, Sun SL, et al. Effect of low- and high-frequency TENS on Met-enkephalin-Arg-Phe and dynorphin A immunoreactivity in human lumbar CSF. *Pain*. 1991;47:295–298.

28. LeBars D, Dickerson AH, Besson JM. Diffuse noxious inhibitory controls (DNIC): effects on dorsal horn convergent neurones in the rat. *Pain*. 1979;6:283–304.

29. National Institutes of Health Consensus Conference. Acupuncture. *JAMA*. 1998; 280:1518–1524.

30. Norton GR, Goszer L, Strub H, Man SC. The effects of belief on acupuncture analgesia. *Can J Behav Sci*. 1984;16:22–29.

31. Vincent CA, Richardson PH. The evaluation of therapeutic acupuncture. *Pain*. 1986;24:1–13.

32. Fauci AS, Lane HC. Human immunodeficiency virus (HIV) disease. In: Fauci AS, Braunwald E, Isselbacher KJ, et al, eds. *Harrison's Principles of Internal Medicine*. 14th ed. New York, NY: McGraw-Hill; 1998:1790–1855.

33. Kieburtz Z, Yiannoutsos CP, Simpson D, and ACTG 242 Study Team. A double-blind, randomized clinical trial of amitriptyline and mexiletine for painful neuropathy in human immunodeficiency virus infection. *Ann Neurol*. 1997;42:429.

34. Thomson R. Side effects and placebo amplification. *Br J Psychiatry*. 1982;140:64–68.

35. Max MB. Antidepressants as analgesics. In: Fields HL, Libefkind JC, eds. *Pharmacological Approaches to the Treatment of Chronic Pain*. Vol 1. Seattle, Wash: International Association for the Study of Pain Press; 1994:229–246.

36. Jett MF, McGuirk J, Waligora D, Hunter JC. The effects of mexiletine, desipramine and fluoxetine in rat models involving central sensitization. *Pain*. 1997;69:161–169.

37. Dalakas MC, Pezeshkpour GH. Neuromuscular diseases associated with human immunodeficiency virus infection. *Ann Neurol*. 1988; 23(suppl):S28–S48.

38. Tyor WR, Wesselingh SL, Griffin JW, et al. Unifying hypothesis for the pathogenesis of HIV-associated dementia complex, vacuolar myelopathy, and sensory neuropathy. *J Acquir Immune Defic Syndr Hum Retrovirol*. 1995;9:379–388.

39. Simpson DM, Dorfman D, Olney RK, et al. Peptide T in the treatment of painful distal neuropathy associated with AIDS: results of a placebo-controlled trial. *Neurology*. 1996; 47:1254–1259.

54 Acupuncture for Back Pain

A Meta-Analysis of Randomized Controlled Trials

Edzard Ernst, MD, PhD, FRCP(Edin); Adrian R. White, MD
From the Department of Complementary Medicine, Postgraduate Medical School, University of Exeter, Exeter, England.

Background
Acupuncture is commonly used to treat back pain, but there is no published meta-analysis of trials of its effectiveness for this condition.

Objective
To perform a meta-analysis of trials of acupuncture for the treatment of back pain.

Methods
A systematic literature search was conducted to retrieve all randomized controlled trials of any form of acupuncture for any type of back pain in humans. The adequacy of the acupuncture treatment was assessed by consulting 6 experienced acupuncturists. The main outcome measure for the meta-analysis was numbers of patients whose symptoms were improved at the end of treatment.

Results
Twelve studies were included, of which 9 presented data suitable for meta-analysis. The odds ratio of improvement with acupuncture compared with control intervention was 2.30 (95% confidence interval, 1.28–4.13). For sham-controlled, evaluator-blinded studies, the odds ratio was 1.37 (95% confidence interval, 0.84–2.25).

Conclusion
Acupuncture was shown to be superior to various control interventions, although there is insufficient evidence to state whether it is superior to placebo.

Arch Intern Med. 1998;158:2235–2241

Back pain is among the most prevalent health complaints of mankind.[1] It is, therefore, associated with much individual suffering and considerable socioeconomic consequences.[2] Back pain is also the most frequent indication for using unconventional therapies.[3–5] Survey data suggest that back pain is one of the most common indications for referral to acupuncturists.[6]

Against this background, it is relevant to ask whether acupuncture can be shown to be effective. Even though several plausible mechanisms exist to explain its analgesic actions,[7] reviews of acupuncture as a treatment for painful conditions invariably conclude that the published data are insufficient to judge it as effective or ineffective.[8–12] As different pain syndromes could respond differently to acupuncture, and as no systematic review or meta-analysis of acupuncture for back pain exists, the present study was aimed at filling this gap.

Methods

Data Sources

Searches were performed for clinical trials of any form of acupuncture for back pain in 3 computerized databases: MEDLINE (1969–1996); the Cochrane Controlled Trials Register (Issue 1, 1997); and CISCOM (November 1996), a database specializing in complementary medicine including much of the "gray literature," such as unpublished studies and conference reports. Searches were performed using keywords *acupuncture, electroacupuncture,* and *backache* and text-word searches for the above terms together with *low-back pain* and *lumbago.* In addition, our files of published articles selected over the years were screened and several experts in different countries were invited to contribute published studies on the topic. The bibliographies of all articles thus retrieved together with reviews of acupuncture treatment of pain were reviewed for further references. Authors of articles published in the past 5 years (1992–1997) were contacted and asked to inform us of any other articles they were aware of. Authors of abstracts were contacted and asked to provide the full reports.

Study Selection

All articles that reported a randomized controlled trial in which dry needles were inserted into the skin and for which the process was described by the author(s) as "acupuncture" for the treatment of any type of back pain in humans were included. The basis for selecting points for needle insertion was not restricted. Articles published in the English, French, German, Spanish, Italian, or Polish language were included. Trials in which one form of acupuncture was compared with another were excluded. When more than 1 publication described a single trial, only 1 report was included.

Data Extraction

Data were extracted independently by both of us in a predefined, standardized manner. Differences were settled by discussion. For each trial, numbers of patients in experimental and control groups who were objectively rated as improved or who had returned to work were obtained. Where objective measures were not available, subjective ratings were used. Where more than 1 outcome measure was reported in this way, the least and most favorable results were extracted for separate evaluations. Where necessary, letters were sent to authors requesting these data.

Assessment of Methodological Quality

The quality of the studies was assessed by a modification of the method described by Jadad et al.[13] First, points were awarded by the investigators (E.E. and A.R.W.) in 3 categories: randomization (2 points), blinding (2 points), and description of dropouts and withdrawals (1 point). Studies were rated as "blind" if the control group received an intervention that appears likely to be indistinguishable from acupuncture (ie, sham acupuncture) and if the outcome was assessed in a blind manner, whether by a blinded observer or by the blinded subject's self-report. Second, points up to a maximum of 2 were awarded for each study according to the adequacy of the acupuncture treatment used, as assessed by blinded experts. For this purpose, an extract was prepared for each study containing only details of patients and interventions, translated into English if necessary. All means of identification were removed. Six experienced medical acupuncturists involved both in clinical practice and in teaching studied these extracts and rated the adequacy of acupuncture in each trial on a visual analog scale (VAS) that consisted of a 100-mm line. The left end of the line was labeled "complete absence of evidence that the acupuncture was adequate" and the right end was labeled "total certainty that the acupuncture was adequate." Two points were awarded for mean VAS scores of more than 66, one point for scores between 33 and 66, and zero points for scores less than 33 mm.

Data Synthesis

Meta-analyses of the data were performed using custom-written software (RevMan 3.0, Cochrane Collaboration, Oxford, England). For each trial, the total numbers of patients included in each group and the numbers whose symptoms had improved were entered into tables for comparison. Subsequently, the odds ratio (OR) for each trial was calculated, ie, the ratio of successes to failures in the genuine treatment group, divided by the same ratio in the control group. Weighting studies according to their inverse variance, the program computed a combined OR for all trials in the comparison, using the random effects model of DerSimonian and Laird.[14] Confidence intervals (CIs) were calculated from the sums of the individual variances, and were set at 95%. The primary meta-analysis combined all studies that contained data in the appropriate form. Further meta-analyses were performed to compare subsets of trials that were combined according to particular features: blinding, length of follow-up, adequacy of acupuncture, use of formula acupuncture or electrical stimulation, and number of treatment sessions.

Sensitivity Analysis

The primary meta-analysis was performed using the data that were least favorable to acupuncture. A sensitivity analysis was performed by repeating this meta-analysis using the most favorable data.

Table 1. Meta-analysis of Acupuncture for Back Pain: Trials Excluded and the Reasons for Exclusion

Source, y	Reason for Exclusion
Boas and Hatangdi,[15] 1976	Not randomized
Fox and Melzack,[19] 1976	Not randomized
Kitsenko,[27] 1976	Russian language
Laitinen,[29] 1976	Not randomized
Mendelson et al,[37, 38] 1977, 1978	Dual publication
Mazières et al,[36] 1981	Incorrect citation (no response to inquiry)
Sodipo,[42] 1981	Not randomized
Gallacchi et al,[21] 1981	Dual publication
Lehmann et al,[30] 1983	Dual publication
Lovacky et al,[33] 1987	Not randomized
Hackett et al,[24] 1988	Not needle acupuncture
Mencke et al,[40, 41] 1988	Acupuncture compared with acupuncture
Li et al,[34] 1989	Not randomized
Kitade et al,[26] 1990	Acupuncture compared with acupuncture plus D-phenylalanine
Ishimaru et al,[25] 1993	Acupuncture compared with heated-needle acupuncture
Kovacs et al,[28] 1993	Author specified "not acupuncture"

Results

Studies Identified

The search revealed 30 references for controlled trials.[15–44] Eighteen reports were excluded for the reasons given in Table 1.

Table 2 summarizes the key data from the 12 studies that were included. In 2 studies, patients were recruited after admission to hospital, either for a course of rehabilitation[30] or for management of acute back pain.[17] Patients were recruited via media advertisements in 1 study.[16] In the remaining 9 trials, patients were recruited from hospital outpatient departments. In 4 studies,[16,18,22,32] patients who were unresponsive to conventional therapy were included, and in the remaining 8 studies the included patients were described as having chronic back pain. Patients who had undergone back surgery were excluded in 2 studies[17,42] and included in 1 study;[16] 9 reports did not specify history of back surgery as a study criterion. Treatment settings were conventional health service premises in 11 studies and a dedicated acupuncture clinic in 1.[16]

In 3 studies, conventional acupuncture points were not used: Garvey et al[22] and Gunn et al[23] inserted needles into trigger points identified by tenderness, and Macdonald et al[35] placed needles superficially over trigger points. In the remaining 9 studies, recognized acupuncture points were used. In 9 studies, outcomes were measured only at the end of treatment and in 3 studies there was a follow-up period: Mendelson et al[39] and Gunn et al[23] used minimum follow-up periods of 8 and 12 weeks, respectively, and Thomas and Lundeberg[43] followed up all patients for 6 months.

Table 3 summarizes the quality ratings of all included studies. The range is wide yet the majority of studies scored 3 or more points. The expert acupuncturists held divergent opinions about the adequacy of the treatment in all studies except 1,[32] which they agreed was almost totally inadequate.

Meta-analyses

Nine studies presented data in a form suitable for inclusion in the meta-analyses. The results of the primary meta-analysis are presented in Figure 1. A total of 377 patients was included in the trials, and the overall OR was 2.30 (95% CI, 1.28–4.13). There was no significant heterogeneity between studies (χ^2_8=12.58, P>.1).

In 3 studies[16,17,23] the outcome was markedly more positive than in the remainder. These studies have no uniformity of inclusion criteria, acupuncture approach, setting, or end points that could account for the divergence. Alternative (more favorable) outcome data were available in 1 study,[17] yielding a new OR for all studies combined (Figure 1) of 2.54 (95% CI, 1.32–4.88).

Meta-analyses of Subgroups

The results of the meta-analyses of studies grouped according to design features are given in Figure 2. The OR of the 4 sham-controlled, evaluator-blinded studies[17,18,22,39] was 1.37 (95% CI, 0.84–2.25). The results were not meaningfully affected by length of follow-up, quality of acupuncture, type of acupuncture, or number of sessions. There are trends worthy of discussion but CIs of comparisons overlap, indicating that no firm conclusions can be drawn from these data.

Studies Excluded from the Meta-analysis

Three studies presented results in a form that was unsuitable for inclusion in this meta-analysis: Macdonald et al[35] concluded that acupuncture was significantly superior to control intervention, Yue[44] found a positive trend favoring acupuncture, and Gallacchi et al[21] showed no superiority of acupuncture over sham acupuncture. The total sample size of these 3 studies was 95. It seems unlikely that the omission of these studies seriously undermines the accuracy of the meta-analyses.

The funnel plot is presented in Figure 3. The studies are not evenly distributed around the combined OR, but there are too few studies to conclude whether publication bias has influenced the result of the meta-analysis.

Comment

Collectively, these data suggest that acupuncture is an effective treatment for back pain. The assessment of acupuncture for back pain is notoriously difficult for several reasons: there are many variations of acupuncture (eg, points used, method of stimulation) that are not necessarily comparable; back pain is not a distinct entity but an ill-defined category of complaints with diverse causes; acute back pain frequently disappears within days with or without treatment; concomitant treatments abound; and there is no objective, universally accepted outcome measure. The trials included in this analysis are heterogeneous in terms of study population, type of acupuncture used, outcome measure used, and length of follow-up. Thus, it is problematic to form a firm judgment.

Our search strategy was as comprehensive as possible. Yet, it is possible that some trials were not located. In particular, negative trials may not be published.[45] We also suspect that complementary medicine journals are heavily biased toward positive results.[46] Thus, systematic reviews could easily become distorted. Unfortunately, the present material gives no firm indication for or against the existence of a publication bias and we are unable confidently to exclude this source of error in our analysis.

One inclusion criterion for this analysis was randomization. We, therefore, dealt with trials of relatively high standard. The quality ratings (Table 3) show that the methodological quality was good in the majority of the studies. Only 2 trials, both published in the 1970s, were of low quality. Thus, the present meta-analysis is based largely on rigorous research, which lends weight to its findings.

All the studies recruited patients with chronic pain or who had failed to respond to conventional therapy. Only 2 studies[17,43] specifically excluded patients with previous back surgery. Thus, the majority of study participants were associated with a poor prognosis and belonged to a category that is notoriously difficult to treat. The fact that nonetheless the overall result is positive suggests that acupuncture can be helpful even for difficult cases of back pain.

In most studies, the follow-up period was inadequate. Two studies[28,43] suggest that the result measured immediately after treatment may be sustained if not improved (Figure 2). Unfortunately, this sample is too small to draw any conclusions, and the long-term effects of acupuncture on back pain remain uncertain. This, it seems, could be a fruitful area of future research.

The subgroup analyses revealed interesting trends. The OR of unblinded studies is larger than that of studies in which blinding had been introduced. This trend might indicate the importance of patient and therapist expectations in terms of clinical outcome and suggests that acupuncture (like most hands-on interventions) is associated with a powerful placebo effect.[47] In 2 studies[16,32] acupuncture was rated as inadequate, yet tended to be more effective than that judged as adequate. This seems counterintuitive at first glance but might be explained quite easily. In both cases, the descriptions of the acupuncture were minimal. Difficulty in judging the trials was reflected in the large SDs of the experts' scores (Table 3). Thus, the acupuncture technique was poorly described in these reports, but may still have been of good quality. Furthermore, it is relevant to note that both individualizing the selection of points for treatment and repeating the acupuncture more than 4 times were associated with larger effect sizes. The latter trend would be compatible with the dose-response curve of an effective therapy.

In a review of 7 acupuncture trials of acupuncture for pain, including back pain, Deyo[48] concluded that "acupuncture is little more effective than placebo therapy which mimics active treatment." Our subgroup analysis of 4 sham-controlled, evaluator-blinded studies yielded a

Table 2. Details of Randomized Sham-Controlled Trials of Acupuncture for Back Pain*

Source, y	Design	No. (Treatment, Controls)	Patients
Edelist et al,[18] 1976	RCT, pt + evaluator blind, 2 parallel arms	15, 15	LBP, no response to conventional treatment
Yue,[44] 1978	RCT, evaluator blind, 3 parallel arms	23, ?, ?	23 pts with chronic back or neck pain in experimental group
Lopacz and Gralewski,[32] 1979	RCT, nonblind, 2 parallel arms	18, 16	LBP>1 mo without root irritation
Coan et al,[16] 1980	RCT, nonblind, 2 parallel arms	25, 23	Chronic LBP
Gunn et al,[23] 1980	RCT, nonblind, 2 parallel arms	29, 27	Chronic LBP, no response to conventional treatment
Gallacchi et al,[21] 1981	RCT, nonblind, 8 parallel arms	13 to 15 in each group	Chronic "tendomyotic cervical and lumbar syndrome"
Duplan et al,[17] 1983	RCT, pt + evaluator blind, 2 parallel arms	15, 15	Acute LBP, admitted to hospital for no response to conventional treatment
Macdonald et al,[35] 1983	RCT, pt + evaluator blind, 2 parallel arms	8, 9	Chronic LBP, no response to conventional treatment
Mendelson et al,[39] 1983	RCT, pt + evaluator blind, crossover	77	Chronic LBP
Lehmann et al,[30] 1983	RCT, nonblind, 3 parallel arms	17, 18, 18	Chronic, disabling LBP
Garvey et al,[22] 1989	RCT, pt + evaluator blind, 4 parallel arms	20, 13, 14, 16	Nonradiating LBP (>4 wk), no response to conventional treatment
Thomas and Lundeberg,[43] 1994	RCT, nonblind, voluntary crossover, with untreated controls	40	Chronic "nociceptive" LBP

*Acup indicates acupuncture; RCT, randomized controlled trial; pt, patient; LBP, low back pain; EA, electroacupuncture; question mark, no sample size given for control groups; NA, not applicable; VAS, visual analog scale; SLR, straight-leg raising; and TENS, transcutaneous electrical nerve stimulation.
†End point used in the meta-analysis (not a primary end point if in parentheses).

combined OR of 1.37 (95% CI, 0.84–2.25) in favor of genuine acupuncture. Although this finding is not conclusive, it does suggest that further trials are justified to determine whether acupuncture works through specific or nonspecific effects.

It has been suggested that sham acupuncture is an unfair comparison since needling the skin can relieve pain through the process of diffuse noxious inhibitory control.[49] This effect can be minimized by needling nonmeridian, nontender points. Future studies should include both sham-control groups and other comparison groups in parallel. The optimal study in acupuncture for back pain should be randomized and fully blinded, with an adequate acupuncture technique and follow-up. It should include a sample size based on power calculation, should evaluate success with a widely accepted outcome measure, and should test acupuncture on a homogeneous subtype of back pain that has previously been suggested to respond favorably. In light of the poor reporting quality of some acupuncture trials (see above), the optimal study should, of course, detail all aspects of the method accurately.

Table 2. Details of Randomized Sham-Controlled Trials of Acupuncture for Back Pain* (continued)

Intervention (No. of Treatments)	Primary End Points	Follow-up	Result (Significance)	No. Improved in Each Group: Acup	Control
Formula EA vs sham acup (3)	Evaluator's rating of change† including pt report	None	No intergroup differences	7/15	6/15
Formula acup vs sham acup vs physiotherapy (not stated)	Pain, range of movement	None	Acup was superior to physiotherapy but not to sham	NA	NA
Formula acup + sodium chloride injection vs sham electrical stimulation (4)	Global assessment by 2 physicians†	None	Acup superior to controls (P>.05)	14/18	10/16
Individualized traditional acup vs waiting-list controls (11)	Pain score (combined pt and evaluator rating†)	10-15 wk	Pain reduction: acup, 51%; controls, 2%	19/23	5/16
Needling at muscle motor point mean 7.9) + standard physiotherapy vs physiotherapy alone	Pain and work status†	12-42 wk	Needling superior to controls (P<.01)	18/29	4/27
Formula acup vs 2 forms of sham acup vs 5 forms of laser acup (8)	VAS for pain	None	All groups improved, no intergroup differences	NA	NA
Formula acup vs sham acup (5)	Pain VAS (1) of standing 10 min,† (2) on resting†	None	Acup superior to sham for severe pain, supported by SLR changes	(1) 11/15 (2) 13/15	(1) 6/15 (2) 5/15
Superficial needling (with or without EA) vs sham TENS (10)	VAS for pain	None	Pain reduction greater after needling (P<.01)	NA	NA
Formula acup vs lidocaine injections (8)	VAS for pain (>33% relief†)	4, 12, and 16 wk	No significant difference between groups	44/77	41/77
Individualized EA (6) vs TENS (15) vs sham TENS (15); + education and exercise program	VAS for pain and disability + physician's assessment (return to work†)	Immediate and 6 mo	EA superior to TENS (P<.11); no difference between TENS and sham TENS	10/17	10/18
Trigger point needling vs vapocoolant + acupressure vs lidocaine injection lidocaine + corticosteroid injection(1)	Pt assessment of improvement†	None	Needling and acupressure yielded the best results (P>.05)	11/20	8/16
Flexible formula acup vs low-frequency EA vs high frequency EA by pt choice (average 6.8) vs waiting-list controls	Activity related to pain, mobility, verbal descriptors of pain, pt assessment of improvement†	Immediate 6 wk, 6 mo	After 6 wk all EA groups superior to untreated controls (P<.05); after 6 mo this was the only the case for low-frequency EA	17/30	4/10

If one accepts that acupuncture is an effective form of treatment for back pain, one might ask about its value compared with other forms of treatment. So far, only exercise treatments,[50] transcutaneous electrical nerve stimulation (TENS),[51] and spinal manipulation[52] have been evaluated in a systematic way. Koes et al[50] concluded that it is "uncertain whether exercise is better than other conservative treatments for back pain or whether a specific type of back pain is more effective." The review by Gadsby and Flowerdew[51] "provides some evidence to support the use of TENS." Finally, a meta-analysis of spinal manipulation found that it was of short-term benefit.[52] The last findings are so convincing that several national guidelines now recommend spinal manipulation as a first-line treatment.[53,54] It is interesting, therefore, to see that the overall OR calculated by Shekelle et al[52] for all 7 randomized control trials meta-analyzed is similar to the one emerging from this article (OR, 2.0 [95% CI, 1.48–2.77] for spinal manipulation compared with 2.30 [95% CI, 1.28–4.13] for acupuncture). This suggests equal effectiveness for both treatments. However, the usefulness of a therapy is not only determined by effectiveness—safety and costs are

Table 3. Meta-analysis of Acupuncture for Back Pain: Quality Assessment Scores of Included Studies*

Source, y	Expert Assessment Score, Mean (SD)†	Adequacy of Acupuncture‡	Quality Assessment Score: Randomization	Blinding	Dropouts	Total
Duplan et al,[17] 1983	46.5 (30.6)	1	1	2	1	5
Edelist et al,[18] 1976	49.0 (31.9)	1	1	2	1	5
Garvey et al,[22] 1989	31.3 (34.9)	1	1	2	1	5
Mendelson et al,[39] 1983	50.7 (33.1)	1	1	2	0	4
Thomas and Lundeberg,[43] 1994	69.5 (23.5)	2	1	0	1	4
Coan et al,[16] 1980	26.5 (34.2)	0	2	0	1	3
Gunn et al,[23] 1980	53.3 (33.0)	1	1	0	1	3
Gallacchi et al,[21] 1981	45.3 (37.0)	1	1	0	1	3
Lehmann et al,[30] 1983	41.5 (26.8)	1	1	0	1	3
Macdonald et al,[35] 1983	43.3 (24.1)	1	1	0	1	3
Lopacz and Gralewski,[32] 1979	9.3 (5.3)	0	1	0	0	1
Yue,[44] 1978	18.8 (35.6)	0	1	0	0	1

*In descending order of quality.

†Adequacy of acupuncture was assessed by expert panel on visual analog scale (VAS) of 0 to 100.

‡Points awarded for VAS score less than 33, zero points; VAS score of 33 to 66, 1 point; and VAS score greater than 66, 2 points.

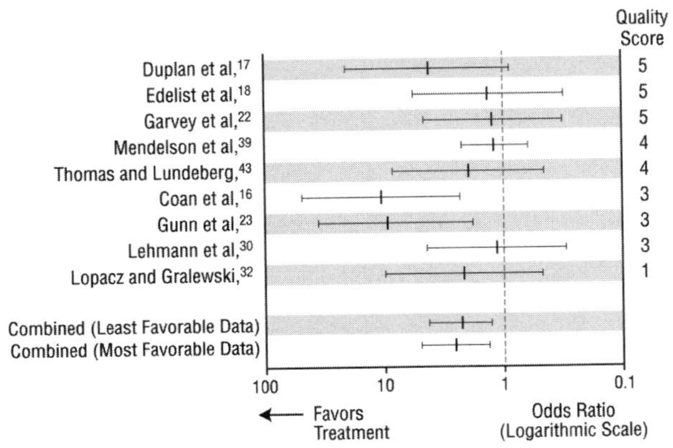

Figure 1. Meta-analysis of randomized controlled trials of acupuncture for back pain, in descending order of quality.

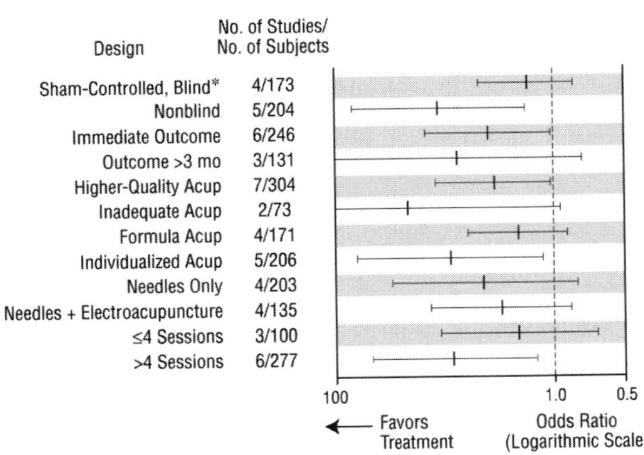

Figure 2. Meta-analyses of randomized controlled trials of acupuncture (Acup) for back pain grouped according to common design features. Asterisk indicates patient- and evaluator-blinded design.

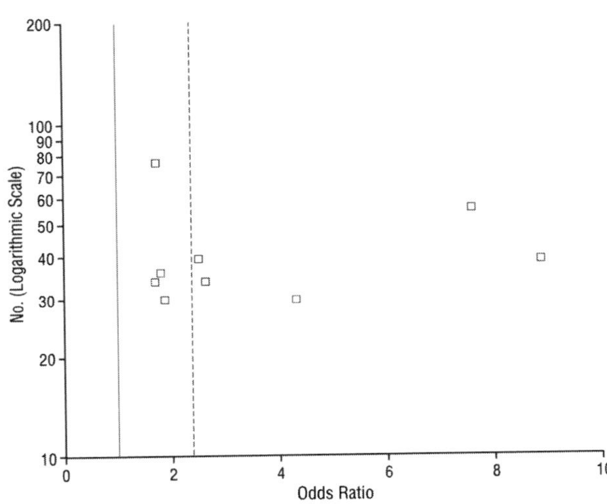

Figure 3. Funnel plot showing individual odds ratios of randomized controlled trials of acupuncture for back pain against sample size. Continuous line indicates an odds ratio of 1 (no effect); dashed line, combined odds ratios of trials.

other factors. In 2 recent surveys, we found adverse reactions of acupuncture to be considerably less frequent than those of spinal manipulation.[55] Unfortunately, no fully conclusive data about the true prevalence of adverse effects for either method exist. This, it seems, is another area of important research for the future. The costs of acupuncture may well be lower than for spinal manipulation: treatment sessions are usually shorter and often less frequent. When 1020 episodes of back pain were investigated, chiropractors had a greater mean number of visits per episode than any other profession,[56] which is supported by other data.[57] Considering the socioeconomic importance of back pain,[2] it would be relevant to establish the relative cost-effectiveness of all major treatments for this condition.

In conclusion, the combined result of all studies shows acupuncture to be superior to various control interventions. The combined results of 4 sham-controlled, evaluator-blinded studies did not show acupuncture to be superior to placebo; further studies are required to conclude with certainty whether acupuncture has specific effects in addition to its nonspecific effects.

We gratefully acknowledge V. Camp, MD, H. Dyczek, AcM, P. Marcus, MD, R. James, MD, D. Payne, MD, F. Staebler, MD, and A. Ward, MD, for help with aspects of this study.

References

1. Frymoyer JW. Back pain and sciatica. *N Engl J Med.* 1988;318:291–300.
2. Ernst E, Fialka V. Idiopathic low back pain: present impact, future directions. *Eur J Phys Med Rehabil.* 1994;4:69–72.
3. Eisenberg DM, Kessler RC, Foster C, Norlock FE, Calkins DR, Delbanco TL. Unconventional medicine in the United States. *N Engl J Med.* 1993;328:246–252.
4. Abbot NC, Ernst E. Patients' opinions about complementary medicine. *Forsch Komplementermed.* 1997;4:164–168.
5. Mintel. Complementary medicines. In: *Market Intelligence Report*. London, England: Mintel; 1997.
6. Wadlow G, Peringer E. Retrospective survey of patients of practitioners of traditional Chinese acupuncture in the UK. *Comp Ther Med.* 1996;4:1–7.
7. Han J, Terenius L. Neurochemical basis of acupuncture analgesia. *Annu Rev Pharmacol Toxicol.* 1982;22:192–220.
8. Filshie J, Morrison PJ. Acupuncture for chronic pain: a review. *Palliative Med.* 1988;2:1–14.
9. Lewith GT. How effective is acupuncture in the management of pain? *J R Coll Gen Pract.* 1984; 34:275–278.
10. Patel M, Gutzwiller F, Paccaud F, Marassi A. A meta-analysis of acupuncture for chronic pain. *Int J Epidemiol.* 1989;18:900–906.
11. Richardson PH, Vincent CA. Acupuncture for the treatment of pain: a review of evaluative research. *Pain.* 1986;24:15–40.
12. Ter Riet G, Kleijnen J, Knipschild P. Acupuncture and chronic pain: a criteria-based meta-analysis. *J Clin Epidemiol.* 1990;43:1191–1199.
13. Jadad AR, Moore RA, Carrol D, et al. Assessing the quality of reports of randomized clinical trials: is blinding necessary? *Control Clin Trials.* 1996;17:1–12.
14. DerSimonian R, Laird N. Meta-analysis in clinical trials. *Control Clin Trials.* 1986;7:177–188.
15. Boas RA, Hatangdi VS. Electrical stimulation in the relief of pain: a pilot study. *N Z Med J.* 1976;84:230–233.
16. Coan RM, Wong G, Ku SL, et al. The acupuncture treatment of low back pain: a randomized controlled study. *Am J Chin Med.* 1980;8:181–189.
17. Duplan B, Cabanel G, Piton JL, Grauer JL, Phelip X. Acupuncture et lombosciatique à la phase aiguë. *Semin Hop Paris.* 1983;59:3109–3114.
18. Edelist G, Gross AE, Langer F. Treatment of low back pain with acupuncture. *Can Anaesth Soc J.* 1976;23:303–306.
19. Fox EJ, Melzack R. Transcutaneous electrical stimulation and acupuncture: comparison of treatment for low-back pain. *Pain.* 1976; 2:141–148.
20. Gallacchi G, Muller W. Akupounktur: bringt sie etwas? *Schweiz Rundsch Med Prax.* 1983; 72:779–782.
21. Gallacchi G, Muller W, Plattner GR, Schnorrenberger CC. Akupunktur und Laserstrahlbehandlung beim Zervikal und Lumbalsyndrom. *Schweiz Med Wochenschr.* 1981;111:1360–1366.
22. Garvey TA, Marks MR, Wiesel SW. A prospective, randomized, double-blind evaluation of trigger-point injection therapy for low-back pain. *Spine.* 1989;14:962–964.
23. Gunn CC, Milbrandt WE, Little AS, Mason KE. Dry needling of muscle motor points for chronic low-back pain. *Spine.* 1980;5:279–291.
24. Hackett GI, Seddon D, Kaminski D. Electroacupuncture compared with paracetamol for acute low back pain. *Practitioner.* 1988;232:163–164.
25. Ishimaru K, Shinohara S, Kitade T, Hyodo M. Clinical efficacy of electrical heat acupuncture (first report): effect on low back pain. *Am J Acupunct.* 1993;21:13–18.
26. Kitade T, Odohara Y, Ikeuchi T. Studies on the enhanced effect of acupuncture analgesia and acupuncture anesthesia by D-phenylalanine (2nd report): schedule of administration and clinical effects in low back pain and tooth extraction. *Acupunct Electrother Res.* 1990;15:121–135.
27. Kitsenko VP. Use of acupuncture in lumbosacral radiculitis. *Zh Nevropatol Psikhiatr.* 1976; 76:872–874.
28. Kovacs FM, Abraira V, Lopez-Abente G, Pozo F. La intervencion neurroreflejoterapica en el tratamiento de la lumbalgia inespecifica: un ensayo clinico controlado, aleatorizado, a doble ciego. *Med Clin (Barc).* 1993;101:570–575.
29. Laitinen J. Acupuncture and transcutaneous electric stimulation in the treatment of chronic sacrolumbalgia and ischialgia. *Am J Chin Med.* 1976;4:169–175.
30. Lehmann TR, Russell DW, Spratt KF. The impact of patients with nonorganic physical findings on a controlled trial of transcutaneous electrical nerve stimulation and electroacupuncture. *Spine.* 1983;8:625–634.
31. Lehmann TR, Russell DW, Spratt KF, et al. Efficacy of electroacupuncture and TENS in the rehabilitation of chronic low back pain patients. *Pain.* 1986;26:277–290.
32. Lopacz S, Gralewski Z. Proba oceny winikow leczenia bolowych zespolow ledzwiowo-krzyzowych metoda igloterapii lub sugestii (Evaluation of the results of treatment of low backache by acupuncture). *Neur Neurochir Pol.* 1979;13:405–409.
33. Lovacky S, Lodin Z, Tauber O, et al. Acupuncture treatment and its effect on low back pain: correlation with beta-endorphin immunoreactivity (BEI). *Am J Acupunct.* 1987; 15:245–249.
34. Li Q, Lu S, Luo J, Liang S. An observation on the therapeutic effect of acupuncture in the treatment of sciatica. *J Traditional Chin Med.* 1989;9:90–92.
35. Macdonald AJR, Macrae KD, Master BR, Rubin A. Superficial acupuncture in the relief of chronic low back pain. *Ann R Coll Surg Engl.* 1983;65:44–46.
36. Mazières B, Frize B, Bayourthe L. Acupuncture treatment of chronic low back pain: a short-term controlled trial. *Rev Rheum.* 1981;48:447–450.

37. Mendelson G, Kidson MA, Loh ST, Scott DF, Selwood TS, Kranz H. Acupuncture analgesia for chronic low back pain. *Clin Exp Neurol.* 1978;15:182–185.

38. Mendelson G, Kranz H, Kidson MA, Loh ST, Scott DF, Selwood TS. Acupuncture for chronic back pain: patients and methods. *Clin Exp Neurol.* 1977;14:154–161.

39. Mendelson G, Selwood TS, Kranz H, Loh ST, Kidson MA, Scott DS. Acupuncture treatment of chronic back pain. *Am J Med.* 1983;74:49–55.

40. Mencke VM, Wieden TE, Hoppe M, Porschke W, Hoffmann O, Herget HF. Akupunktur des schulter-arm-syndroms und der lumbalgie-ischialgie: zwei prospektive doppelblind-studien (teil 1). *Akupunkt Theor Prax.* 1988;16:204–215.

41. Mencke VM, Wieden TE, Hoppe M, Porschke W, Hoffmann O, Herget HF. Akupunktur des schulter-arm-syndroms und der lumbalgie/ischialgie: zwei prospektive doppelblind-studien (teil 2). *Akupunkt Theor Prax.* 1988;17:5–14.

42. Sodipo JOA. Transcutaneous electrical nerve stimulation (TENS) and acupuncture: comparison of therapy for low-back pain. *Pain.* 1981;suppl 1:S277.

43. Thomas M, Lundeberg T. Importance of modes of acupuncture in the treatment of chronic nociceptive low back pain. *Acta Anaesthesiol Scand.* 1994;38:63–69.

44. Yue SJ. Acupuncture for chronic back and neck pain. *Acupunct Electrother Res.* 1978;3:323–324.

45. Dickersin K. The existence of publication bias and risk factors for its occurrence. *JAMA.* 1990;263:1385–1389.

46. Ernst E, Pittler MH. Alternative therapy bias [letter]. *Nature.* 1997;385:480.

47. Ernst E. Placebos in medicine [letter]. *Lancet.* 1995;345:65.

48. Deyo RA. Nonoperative treatment of low back disorders. In: Frymoyer JW, ed. *The Adult Spine: Principles and Practice*. New York, NY: Raven Press; 1991:chap 72.

49. LeBars D, Dickenson AH, Besson J-M. Diffuse noxious inhibitory controls (DNIC), 1: effects on dorsal horn convergent neurones in the rat. *Pain.* 1979;6:283–304.

50. Koes BW, Bouter LM, Beckerman H, van der Heijden GJMG, Knipschild PG. Physiotherapy exercises and back pain: a blinded review. *BMJ.* 1991;302:1572–1576.

51. Gadsby JG, Flowerdew MW. The effectiveness of transcutaneous electrical nerve stimulation (TENS) and acupuncture-like transcutaneous electrical nerve stimulation (ALTENS) in the treatment of patients with chronic low back pain. (Cochrane Review.) The Cochrane Library, 1997, Issue 2. Update software, Oxford, England. Updated quarterly.

52. Shekelle PG, Adams AH, Chassin MR, Hurwitz DC, Brook RH. Spinal manipulation for low-back pain. *Ann Intern Med.* 1992;117:590–597.

53. Clinical Sciences Advisory Group. *Committee Report: Back Pain*. London, England: Her Majesty's Stationery Office; 1994.

54. Royal College of General Practitioners. *National Low Back Pain Clinical Guidelines*. London, England: Royal College of General Practitioners; 1996.

55. Abbot NC, White AR, Ernst E. Complementary medicine [letter]. *Nature.* 1996;381:361.

56. Shekelle PG, Markovich M, Louie R. Comparing the costs between provider types and episodes of back pain. *Spine.* 1995;20:221–227.

57. White AR, Resch KL, Ernst E. A survey of complementary practitioners' fees, practice, and attitudes to working in the NHS. *Comp Ther Med.* 1997;5:210–214.

55 Randomized Trial of Acupuncture for Nicotine Withdrawal Symptoms

Adrian R. White, MD; Karl-Ludwig Resch, MD, PhD; Edzard Ernst, MD, PhD, FRCP(Edin)
From the Department of Complementary Medicine, Postgraduate Medical School, University of Exeter, Exeter, England. Dr Resch is now with Forschungsinstitut für Balneologie und Kurortwissenschaft, Bad Elster, Germany.

Background
Acupuncture is frequently used for smoking cessation. Positive results from uncontrolled studies have not been supported by meta-analysis of controlled trials. One possible reason for this is that the optimal acupuncture technique was not applied or that the technique was not repeated sufficiently often.

Methods
A randomized, sham-controlled trial was performed with 2 parallel treatment arms; the participant and the evaluator were unaware of which treatment was received. Seventy-six adults who wanted to stop smoking received either 100-Hz electroacupuncture with needles inserted into the appropriate point in each ear or a sham control procedure over the mastoid bone. Interventions were given on days 1, 3, and 7 of smoking cessation. Nicotine withdrawal symptoms were measured by visual analog scale scores recorded in a daily diary for 14 days; smoking cessation was confirmed objectively.

Results
There was no significant difference between the mean reduction of withdrawal symptom scores of the 2 groups from day 1 to day 14. Fifteen participants (39%) who received electroacupuncture and 16 participants (42%) who received a sham procedure were abstinent on day 14.

Conclusion
This form of electroacupuncture is no more effective than placebo in reducing nicotine withdrawal symptoms.

Arch Intern Med. 1998;158:2251–2255

Smoking is the largest single cause of preventable death in industrialized countries. A lifelong smoker's chance of reaching age 73 years is half that of a nonsmoker.[1] The government of the United Kingdom declared a target of reducing the prevalence of cigarette smoking in England from approximately 30% in 1990 to 20% by the end of the century.[2] Numerous methods are available for smoking cessation, but none is fully successful.[3] Thus, there is a need for effective programs for smoking prevention and cessation.

A population survey in 1996 suggested that 15% of respondents would use complementary therapies to give up smoking.[4] Acupuncture is a therapy frequently offered for this purpose. One possible mechanism for an effect was suggested by the finding that acupuncture released endogenous opioid peptides when it was used to treat opiate withdrawal symptoms.[5] This was supported by findings from different laboratories implying that acupuncture may reduce the withdrawal symptoms of animals that had been rendered dependent on opiates.[6,7]

Uncontrolled studies with acupuncture have reported smoking cessation rates as high as 95%.[8] However, results of a meta-analysis of controlled trials were negative,[3] which is in keeping with at least 3 possible conclusions: (1) acupuncture operates as a placebo for smoking cessation; (2) acupuncture was not applied optimally in the studies, for example, in not using electroacupuncture (EA); or (3) acupuncture may have an effect on withdrawal symptoms but not on relapse rate. This effect may be overlooked in measuring longer-term smoking cessation rates.

It was originally observed that administration of EA may have an effect on opium withdrawal symptoms.[9] Use of EA was also assumed to have an effect in tobacco addiction, but this has not been tested. We, therefore, undertook this study to investigate the hypothesis that this form of EA has a specific effect on nicotine withdrawal symptoms.

Participants and Methods

A randomized trial in which participants and evaluators were unaware of the treatment received was conducted with 2 parallel groups comparing administration of EA at genuine acupuncture points with sham stimulation at sham points.

Participants

Adults older than 21 years who smoked at least 15 cigarettes per day were recruited through media invitations. Those who had been given acupuncture previously were excluded, as were those who were pregnant, breast-feeding, or fitted with a cardiac pacemaker and those who had a known bleeding tendency. Participants were asked to make a deposit of £20, which was refunded on return of the daily symptom diary after 14 days. Signed informed consent was obtained from all participants. The study was approved by the Local Research Ethics Committee of North and East Devon Health Authority, Exeter, Devon, United Kingdom.

Predictive Baseline Variables

Baseline characteristics, including those that may predict successful smoking cessation, such as living alone or living with another smoker,[10–12] were obtained via self-completed questionnaires. The Fagerström instrument[13] was administered to assess nicotine dependency. The participants' attitude toward stopping was assessed by asking them to choose which of 5 statements most nearly matched their opinion, ranging from "I am really confident I can stop smoking now" to "I think I am going to carry on smoking."[10]

Masking and Randomization

A nurse, specially trained for the study and unaware of group allocation of participants, undertook reception duties, counseling, and measurement of outcomes. The acupuncture procedure was performed in a separate room by an acupuncturist (A.R.W.) with 14 years' clinical and teaching experience with acupuncture. The acupuncturist was not involved in counseling but maintained a neutral attitude toward all participants, with minimal verbal and nonverbal interaction.

Participants were randomly allocated to receive genuine acupuncture (group A) or a sham control procedure (group S). Group allocation was based on computer-generated block-randomization codes held in sealed opaque numbered envelopes prepared by departmental staff not involved with the study; the envelopes were opened immediately before the first intervention. Participants were informed that they would receive either low-frequency EA, which they would be aware of, or a high-frequency form, which they would "probably not feel."

Acupuncture Protocol

All participants were treated in the supine position. In group A, an acupuncture needle (7×0.2 mm, Scarborough) was placed in the point known as the "Lung" in each ear. This point lies in a depression in the center of the cavum conchae and was located by inspection. Leads from the EA apparatus (model WQ10-C, Beijing Electronic Factory, Beijing, China) were attached to the needles. The frequency of stimulation was a constant 100 Hz, and the intensity was increased to just above the threshold of sensation.

Group S members were randomized to receive either similar needles placed superficially over the center of the mastoid bone (where no acupuncture point exists) with minimum noxious stimulation or transcutaneous electrical nerve stimulation (TENS) pads fixed with adhesive tape over the mastoid bone. Leads from an inactivated version of the EA apparatus (whose indicator lights flashed without delivering any current) were attached to either needles or TENS pads. Subsequent analysis showed that there was no difference in nicotine withdrawal symptoms in these 2 subgroups of control participants. Therefore, we were satisfied that sham needling had no physiologic effects, and thus we combined outcome data from all participants in group S.

Each procedure lasted 20 minutes. The current in group A was adjusted as necessary every 5 minutes to restore the sensation; this attention was matched in group S by a routine check of the position of the wires and the "setting" of the inactive apparatus. The above procedure was repeated for each participant on days 1, 3, and 7. All participants received a brief standardized description of the reputed role of acupuncture in smoking cessation.

Credibility of Interventions

As the participants' beliefs in the intervention received are likely to affect the outcome, the credibility of the procedure was assessed by all participants immediately after the first intervention. Participants were asked to record on a Visual Analogue Scale measuring 100 mm long how confident they were that the treatment would help, whether they would recommend it to a friend, how logical it seemed, and how willing they would be to try it for a different problem. This instrument has been validated by Vincent and Lewith.[14] A fifth question was added: "How satisfactory did you find the treatment at the time?"

Outcome Measures

The primary outcome measure was the daily withdrawal symptom score. Each evening for 14 days, the participants marked a visual analog scale to indicate their responses to 6 questions: "How strong have your cravings been (ie, your desire to smoke) today?" "How irritable or frustrated have you felt?" "How moody or depressed have you been today?" "How tense or anxious have you been today?" "How much difficulty have you had in concentrating?" and "How hungry have you felt today?" An example was given of how to use a visual analog scale to score hunger. Measurement of these symptoms of nicotine withdrawal has been used previously[15] and was validated by Hughes and Hatsukami.[16]

Smoking cessation was predefined as a secondary outcome measure. It was assessed by self-reports and confirmed by expired air carbon monoxide concentration of 10 ppm or less, measured with the carbon monoxide monitor (Micro Smokerlyser, Bedfont Scientific Ltd, Kent, England).

Sample Size

In planning the trial, it was judged that a reduction in the mean withdrawal symptom scores in group A that was 20% greater than that in group S would be clinically relevant. On the basis of the results of Hughes and Hatsukami,[16] in which the SD of symptom scores was 15%, it was calculated that a sample of 24 participants would be needed to demonstrate an effect with 90% power at the 5% level of significance. It was decided to recruit 76 participants to allow for the anticipated high number of dropouts.

Statistical Analysis

Baseline variables were compared by the Student t test for continuous data and the χ^2 test for dichotomous data. Changes in mean daily nicotine withdrawal symptom scores in the 2 groups from day 1 to day 14 were compared by independent samples t test. An additional descriptive analysis consisted of changes in mean daily withdrawal scores from day 1 to day 3. Credibility scores for the different interventions were compared by the Kruskal-Wallis test. All dropouts were regarded as continuing to smoke, and the analysis was by intention-to-treat. Data were used for all days during which participants remained continuously abstinent. Statistical analysis was performed using a software program (Statistical Package for Social Sciences for Windows v6.1, SPSS Inc, Chicago, Ill).

Results

Seventy-six smokers were randomized, and the baseline characteristics of the 2 groups are shown in Table 1. The 2 groups had a similar incidence of factors that predict success in quitting, namely, 40 years or older, male, low cigarette consumption, living with spouse or partner, concern about weight gain, medical advice to stop smoking, and the presence of other smokers in the household (P>.2). Group A had made more previous attempts to stop smoking (P=.01, Mann-Whitney U test).

Fifty-two participants (68%) completed all 3 treatments. Eleven participants (29%) withdrew from group A and 13 participants (34%) withdrew from group S. Three participants stated that they withdrew because of adverse effects: 1 participant (from group S) experienced persistent fainting for the rest of the day after the first treatment;

Table 1. Baseline Characteristics of the Electroacupuncture (n=38) and Control (n=38) Groups*

Variable	Electroacupuncture Group	Sham Control Group
Age, mean ± SD, y	40.8 ± 10.9	42.5 ± 13.9
Women/men, No.	21/17	18/20
Cigarettes		
≤20	15 (40)	20 (53)
21–30	16 (42)	16 (42)
>30	7 (18)	2 (5)
No. of years smoking, mean ± SD	22.6 ± 9.5	23.8 ± 13.0
Fagerström dependency index, mean ± SD	5.5 ± 2.0	5.1 ± 1.8
Previous attempts to stop smoking, median (interquartile range)	5.0 (0–25)	3.0 (0–25)
Confidence and motivation to stop smoking, mean ± SD	3.7 ± 0.8	3.7 ± 0.8
Aged >40 y	21 (55)	22 (58)
Living alone	3 (8)	3 (8)
Other smoker in household	22 (58)	15 (40)
Advised by physician to stop	14 (37)	12 (32)
Concerned about weight gain	18 (47)	19 (50)
Consider smoking antisocial	18 (47)	13 (34)

*Values are expressed as number (percentage) unless otherwise indicated.

1 participant (from group A) had momentary pain from excessive current during adjustment in the first treatment and reacted with weeping and anorexia for several days; and 1 participant (from group S) had a headache over the mastoid areas after the first application of TENS pads. Another participant had a similar headache after application of TENS pads but did not withdraw from the study. None of the participants who withdrew stopped smoking. The remaining 21 participants who dropped out did not keep appointments and, as mentioned above, were considered to have resumed smoking.

Diaries were completed for the full 14 days by 15 participants (39%) in group A and 16 participants (42%) in group S who were still not smoking. There were no significant differences between the groups in the reductions in mean withdrawal symptom scores from day 1 to day 14 (Table 2 and Figure 1). Furthermore, there were no significant differences when the changes in scores for individual withdrawal symptoms were compared (data not presented). Diaries were completed for the first 3 days by 25 participants in group A and 24 participants in group S who stopped smoking. There were no significant differences between the groups in the reduction in mean withdrawal symptom scores from day 1 to day 3 (Table 2). At 9-month follow-up, only 3 of those quitting at 14 days were still not smoking: 1 participant from group A and 2 participants from group S.

Table 3 gives the scores for participants' responses to the 5 questions used to assess the credibility of the procedures. There was no significant difference between the credibility of the 3 procedures.

Comment

This is the first randomized trial that uses a validated measure of withdrawal symptoms to study the effect of acupuncture in smoking cessation. Its results suggest that EA does not have a specific effect in reducing nicotine withdrawal symptoms.

It has been argued that needling nonmeridian, supposedly "inactive," points on the body may release neurotransmitters and, therefore, is not an appropriate control procedure for acupuncture.[17] However, within group S, we found no difference in outcome between those who received sham acupuncture at nonmeridian points compared with those who received sham TENS. Because the latter is highly unlikely to stimulate the release of neurotransmitters, we do not believe our negative result is because of a specific effect in both arms of the study.

It could be argued that our EA technique was not optimal. Our chosen frequency was close to the 125 Hz used in the original study by Wen and Cheung.[9] There is no clinical consensus on the optimal frequency, and different investigators have used a range from 1 to 125 Hz.[9,18] Although there are suggestions that different neurotransmitters are released at different frequencies of EA,[19] it is not possible to select the precise frequency in humans to target specific transmitters. In addition, the roles of different neurotransmitters such as dopamine and the opioid peptides in nicotine withdrawal are still unknown.[20] Further trials using different frequencies of stimulation might be considered to resolve these questions.

Would these results have been different if the "Lung" point had been located by a different method, eg, by electrical resistance measurements or tenderness? Margolin et al[21] showed no difference between the "correct" and nearby "incorrect" points in the sensations or symptomatic effects resulting from stimulation; it has been argued that any benefit of acupuncture in withdrawal symptoms is likely to be caused by neurotransmitter release, and this can be triggered by stimulation anywhere within the area innervated by the vagus.[22] Based on the available evidence, we are confident that our result would not have been different if we had used a different technique to locate the point.

Was EA repeated frequently enough for any potential effect to be sustained between treatments? It could be argued that the neurotransmitter effect of acupuncture would be

Table 2. Group VAS Scores (0–100) for 6 Nicotine Withdrawal Symptoms During Smoking Cessation in Participants Receiving Electroacupuncture (Group A) or Sham Acupuncture (Group S)*

Day	Reduction in Mean VAS Score				
	Group A	Group S	Difference (A–S)	95% CI for Difference	P
	Participants Who Completed Diaries for at Least 3 Days: Group A (n = 25) and Group S (n = 24)				
2	−0.4	−6.3	5.9	−0.9 to 12.7	.08
3	4.4	−3.5	7.9	−2.1 to 17.9	.12
	Participants Who Completed Diaries for 14 Days: Group A (n = 15) and Group S (n = 16)				
2	1.2	−4.5	5.7	−1.7 to 13.1	.13
3	6.1	0.4	5.8	−5.4 to 16.9	.30
4	11.7	3.0	8.8	−6.3 to 23.8	.24
5	10.0	9.0	1.0	−14.8 to 16.9	.90
6	12.2	8.2	4.1	−12.3 to 20.4	.61
7	20.0	10.8	9.2	−8.2 to 26.5	.30
8	20.9	27.9	8.9	−7.6 to 25.4	.28
9	20.1	14.2	5.9	−11.6 to 23.4	.50
10	21.5	11.5	10.0	−7.1 to 27.1	.24
11	23.2	13.9	9.3	−8.9 to 27.4	.31
12	23.3	16.4	6.9	−11.8 to 25.6	.45
13	20.5	15.8	4.7	−14.5 to 24.0	.61
14	21.6	17.3	4.3	−20.9 to 12.3	.60

*Scores are expressed as differences from day 1; negative scores indicate symptoms worse than day 1. VAS indicates visual analog scale; CI, confidence interval.

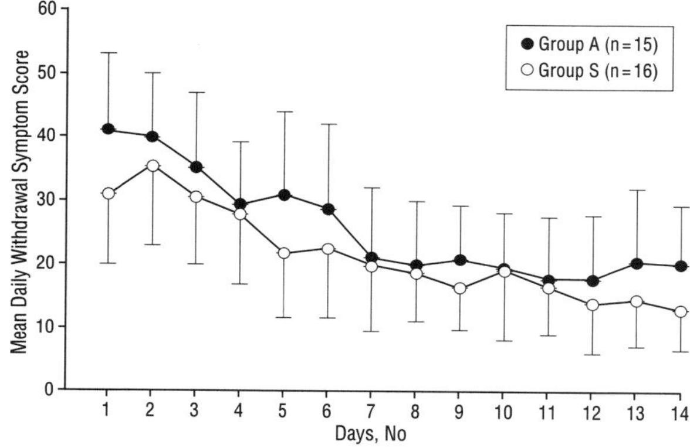

Figure 1. Mean daily nicotine withdrawal symptom scores on the visual analog scale (0–100) in participants who stopped smoking for 14 days after receiving either electroacupuncture (group A) or a sham control procedure (group S). A value of 0 can be assumed for nicotine withdrawal symptoms before participants stopped smoking (baseline). Bars indicate 95% confidence intervals.

expected to last only 4 to 8 hours and that treatment should be given 3 or 4 times every day. The need for repeated treatments would obviously limit 1 of the potential benefits of the technique, namely, its cost-effectiveness. One alternative to repeating the treatments is to maintain continuous stimulation of the auricular point with an indwelling needle or suture; trials using the latter have shown promising results, albeit at significant risk of adverse effects.[23]

Short-term (day 14) cessation rates were high in both groups (39% and 42%) and similar to those achieved with nicotine patches (eg, 36% in a study by Schneider et al[24]). The effects of acupuncture seem to be entirely nonspecific, as shown by the lack of difference between the groups. This suggests that acupuncture is a powerful placebo for this indication and thus (perhaps paradoxically) may have a place clinically as an adjunct in programs of smoking cessation. It seems to have little value in preventing relapse and would need to be used in conjunction with other methods to provide support.

We conclude that the type of acupuncture chosen for this trial is no more effective than placebo in reducing nicotine withdrawal symptoms.

Table 3. Group VAS Scores (0-100, Where 100 Is Maximum Credibility) for Participants' Assessment of the Credibility of 3 Interventions by 5 Criteria*

		Control Group		
Credibility Question	**Acupuncture Group (n=38)**	**Sham Acupuncture (n=19)**	**Sham TENS (n=19)**	***P***
Confident	76.3 (55.9–86.8)	78.9 (63.2–85.5)	73.0 (59.9–86.8)	.90
Recommend	85.5 (55.9–92.8)	89.5 (50.0–96.0)	75.0 (47.4–90.1)	.47
Logical	84.2 (55.9–92.8)	78.9 (69.7–96.0)	75.0 (44.4–94.7)	.46
Different problem	93.4 (85.5–98.7)	93.4 (80.3–97.4)	91.4 (86.9–97.4)	.78
Satisfactory	93.4 (85.5–98.0)	96.1 (81.6–98.7)	92.8 (65.5–95.1)	.33

*Values are expressed as median (interquartile range). See the "Participants and Methods" section for full descriptions of the credibility questions. VAS indicates visual analog scale; TENS, transcutaneous electrical nerve stimulation.

References

1. Phillips AN, Wannamethee SG, Walker M, Thomson A, Smith GD. Life expectancy in men who have never smoked and those who have smoked continuously: 15 year follow up of a large cohort of middle aged British men. *BMJ.* 1996;313:907–908.

2. Department of Health. *The Health of the Nation: A Strategy for Health in England.* London, England: Her Majesty's Stationery Office; 1992.

3. White AR, Rampes H. Acupuncture and smoking cessation. In: Lancaster T, Silagy C, eds. *Tobacco Addiction Module of the Cochrane Database of Systematic Reviews*[serial on CD-ROM]. Oxford, England: Update Software Ltd; 1996. Accessed December 1996.

4. *Complementary Medicines: Market Intelligence Report*. London, England: Mintel; 1997.

5. Clement-Jones V, McLoughlin L, Lowry PJ, Besser GM, Rees LH, Wen HL. Acupuncture in heroin addicts: changes in met-enkephalin and β-endorphin in blood and cerebrospinal fluid. *Lancet.* 1979;2:380–383.

6. Cheng RSS, Pomeranz B, Yu G. Electroacupuncture treatment of morphine-dependent mice reduces signs of withdrawal, without showing cross-tolerance. *Eur J Pharmacol.* 1980;68:477–481.

7. Ng LKY, Douthitt TC, Thoa NB, Albert CA. Modification of morphine-withdrawal syndrome in rats following transauricular stimulation: an experimental paradigm for auricular acupuncture. *Biol Psychiatry.* 1975;10:575–580.

8. Fuller JA. Smoking withdrawal and acupuncture. *Med J Aust.* 1982;1:28–29.

9. Wen HL, Cheung SYC. Treatment of drug addiction by acupuncture and electrical stimulation. *Asian J Med.* 1973;9:138–141.

10. Gourlay SG, Forbes A, Marriner T, Pethica D, McNeil JJ. Prospective study of factors predicting outcome of transdermal nicotine treatment in smoking cessation. *BMJ.* 1994;309:842–846.

11. DiClemente CC, Prochaska JO, Fairhurst SK, Velicer WF, Velasquez MM, Rossi JS. The process of smoking cessation: an analysis of precontemplation, contemplation and preparation stages of change. *J Consult Clin Psychol.* 1991;59:295–304.

12. Kenford SL, Fiore MC, Jorenby DE, Smith SS, Wetter D, Baker TB. Predicting smoking cessation: who will quit with and without the nicotine patch. *JAMA.* 1994;271:589–594.

13. Fagerström KO, Schneider NG. Measuring nicotine dependence: a review of the Fagerström tolerance questionnaire. *J Behav Med.* 1989; 12:159–182.

14. Vincent C, Lewith G. Placebo controls for acupuncture studies. *J R Soc Med.* 1995; 88:199–202.

15. Shiffman SM, Jarvik ME. Smoking withdrawal symptoms in two weeks of abstinence. *Psychopharmacology.* 1976;50:35–39.

16. Hughes JR, Hatsukami D. Signs and symptoms of tobacco withdrawal. *Arch Gen Psychiatry.* 1986;43:289–294.

17. Lewith G, Vincent C. Evaluation of the clinical effects of acupuncture. *Pain Forum.* 1995;4:29–39.

18. Martin GP, Waite PME. The efficacy of acupuncture as an aid to stopping smoking. *N Z Med J.* 1981;93:421–423.

19. Han JS, Chen XH, Sun SL, et al. Effect of low- and high-frequency TENS on Met-enkephalin-Arg-Phe and dynorphin A immunoreactivity in human lumbar CSF. *Pain.* 1991;47:259–298.

20. Nutt DJ. Addiction: brain mechanisms and their treatment implications. *Lancet.* 1996;347:31–36.

21. Margolin A, Avants SK, Chang P, Birch S, Kosten TR. A single-blind investigation of four auricular needle puncture configurations. *Am J Chin Med.* 1995;23:105–114.

22. McLellan AT, Grossman DS, Blaine JD, Haverkos HW. Acupuncture treatment for drug abuse: a technical review. *J Subst Abuse Treat.* 1993; 10:569–576.

23. MacHovec FJ, Man SC. Acupuncture and hypnosis compared: fifty-eight cases. *Am J Clin Hypn.* 1978;21:45–47.

24. Schneider NG, Olmstead R, Nillson F, Mody FV, Franzon M, Doan K. Efficacy of a nicotine inhaler in smoking cessation: a double-blind, placebo-controlled trial. *Addiction.* 1996; 91:1293.

56 Acupuncture Treatment of Urticaria

Chung-Jen Chen, MD; Hsin-Su Yu, MD, PhD
From the Departments of Internal Medicine (Drs Chen and Yu) and Dermatology (Dr Yu), Kaohsiung Medical College, Kaohsiung, Taiwan.

Acupuncture has long been used to treat urticaria in the Asian world. Acute urticaria can be easily and effectively treated with acupuncture. LI11 (*Quchi*), Sp10 (*Xuehai*), Sp6 (*Sanyinjiao*), and S36 (*Zusanli*) are the 4 acupuncture points most commonly prescribed. Chronic urticaria is a challenge for medical therapy. There are at least 6 kinds of acupuncture methods developed to overcome this challenge. The combination of ordinary acupuncture and auricular acupuncture has been observed to be a highly effective cure of chronic urticaria. Acupuncture point injection with thiamine hydrochloride (vitamin B_1) is also an effective treatment. However, results of these clinical observations have not been systematically confirmed for lack of a control group and the need for standard classification of urticaria. Although these observational results have clinical limitations, they do offer insight into an alternative to conventional treatment of urticaria. In the future, acupuncture or acupuncturelike techniques may provide an effective alternative for treatment of patients with urticaria, particularly those refractory to medication therapy.

Arch Dermatol. 1998;134:1397–1399

Urticaria is also known as *Fong-Tzen-Kwai* (wind-rash-patch) by the Chinese. This Chinese term *Fong* (wind) describes the onset of urticaria as appearing so fast—like wind coming so quickly.[1] Tracing back the history of traditional Chinese medicine, the description of urticaria can be found as early as 1346 years ago in a famous book of traditional Chinese medicine, entitled *Qian-Jin-Yao-Fang* (*Thousand-Ducat-Important-Prescriptions*).[2]

In traditional Chinese medicine, there are 2 diversified systems to treat urticaria. One is herbal medicine, another is acupuncture. In this article, we focus on acupuncture. The term *acupuncture* is derived from 2 Latin words—*acus* (needle) and *punctura* (puncture)—which means using needle to puncture the body (at specific acupuncture points). However, acupuncture has been applied more broadly to include not only the ordinary acupuncture (acus-punctura) but also many related methods, such as moxibustion, cupping, acupuncture point injection, and acupuncture point bleeding, among others.

Acute Urticaria

Acute urticaria is very common. It is estimated that about 15% to 23% of the population may have had this condition in the Western world.[3,4] It is also common in the Asian world. The most common cause of acute urticaria is a state of hypersensitivity to food or drugs, and it may also result from viral, bacterial, or parasitic infection.[5]

In modern medicine, most patients with acute urticaria usually can be treated successfully with antihistamines or a short course of glucocorticoids. In traditional Chinese medicine, acupuncture usually works well too.

The treatment of acute urticaria by acupuncture is easy and effective, and is performed routinely by most experienced acupuncturists. More than 90% of patients with acute urticaria experience complete relief with acupuncture therapy.[6] In acupuncture practice, the key to effective treatment for acute urticaria is to puncture the proper acupuncture points. There are 4 acupuncture points most commonly prescribed for acute urticaria: LI11 (*Quchi*), Sp10 (*Xuehai*), Sp6 (*Sanyinjiao*), and S36 (*Zusanli*)[7] (Figure 1).

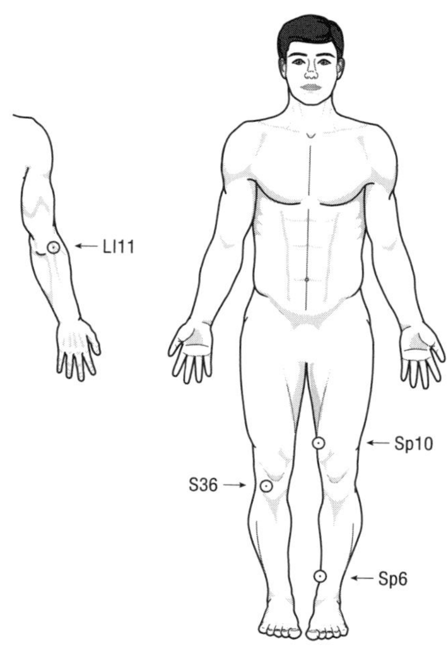

Figure 1. Illustration of 4 important acupuncture points for acute urticaria. The nomenclature of the acupuncture points is according to the recommendation of the World Health Organization.[8]

Chronic Urticaria

Chronic urticaria is defined as the occurrence of widespread wheals daily or almost daily for at least 6 weeks.[9] The causes of chronic urticaria are unknown in most cases. However, a recent study has shown that about one third of patients with chronic urticaria have circulating functional histamine-releasing autoantibodies that bind to the high-affinity IgE receptor (Fc∈ RI) or, less commonly, to IgE.[10]

Chronic urticaria can be extremely troublesome for patients. Moreover, the treatment of chronic urticaria presents a challenge for physicians. In acupuncture therapy, several strategies have been developed to treat different cases of the condition, as listed and described below.

- Ordinary acupuncture
- Combination of ordinary acupuncture and acupuncture point bleeding
- Combination of ordinary acupuncture and auricular acupuncture
- Acupuncture point injection with thiamine
- Acupuncture point injection with autologous blood
- Cupping of acupuncture point

Initially, ordinary acupuncture has been tried for the treatment of chronic urticaria. In addition to the common 4 acupuncture points described in Figure 1, other acupuncture points, such as LI4 (*Hegu*), B40 (*Weizhong*), G20 (*Fengchi*), and G31 (*Fengshi*), have been added to augment the acupuncture effect. However, only 30% to 50% of patients experience complete cure of chronic urticaria using ordinary acupuncture.[11]

Acupuncture point bleeding is 1 of the 9 classic acupuncture methods. It is believed to be able to benefit some refractory disease. Kao[12] reported that a combination of ordinary acupuncture and acupuncture point bleeding cured 83% of patients with chronic urticaria. In this report,[12] 2 acupuncture points, P3 (*Quze*) and B40 (*Weizhong*), were used for bleeding. This method definitely has improved the efficacy of acupuncture for chronic urticaria. However, not all patients, and even some acupuncturists, can tolerate the bleeding.

Subsequently, by using auricular acupuncture, which stimulates the acupuncture point of the ear, in combination with ordinary acupuncture, which stimulates several points of the body, a new combination therapy was developed. It has been reported that the combination of ordinary acupuncture with auricular acupuncture is able to cure 96% of patients with chronic urticaria.[13] In acupuncture practice, there are 4 points commonly prescribed from chronic urticaria, namely, lung, endocrine, subcortex, and shenmen (Figure 2).

Acupuncture point injection with fluid, also called "water acupuncture," is another method used in the treatment of chronic urticaria. In 1986, Tong and Song[14] reported results of a new acupuncture strategy by injecting thiamine hydrochloride (vitamin B_1) into regular acupuncture points to treat 40 cases of chronic urticaria, with disease duration of 2 to 30 years. Thirty-one patients (77.5%) were cured of chronic urticaria. During 2 years of follow-up, 4 patients (12.9%) had relapse of urticaria, and 27 patients (87.1%) were in remission.[14] This method is regarded as practical, convenient, and effective.

Lin[15] reported another type of acupuncture point injection. In his study, 38 patients with chronic urticaria were treated with autologous blood injection into acupuncture points. Another 38 patients with chronic urticaria were treated with ordinary acupuncture. The first group had a 76.3% cure rate, which was significantly ($P<.05$) higher than the 50.0% cure rate in the latter group. Although acupuncture point injection with autologus blood is effective, it is used less often than acupuncture point injection with thiamine.

Cupping therapy is an old method of acupuncture that treats disease by causing local congestion around specific areas. It was reported that the cupping on acupuncture point CV8 (*Shenque*) improved symptoms in 93.8% of patients with chronic urticaria. However, only 35.8% of patients were cured.[16] Although this method is somewhat effective, the low cure rate prevents its common use.

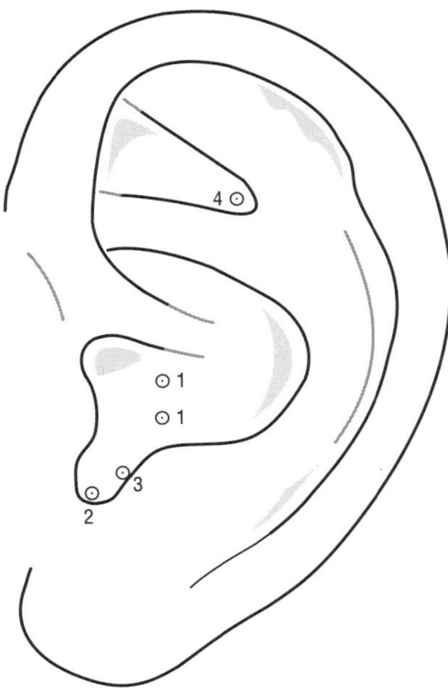

Figure 2. Illustration of 4 common points of auricular acupuncture prescribed for chronic urticaria. 1 indicates the lung point; 2, the endocrine point; 3, the subcortex point; and 4, the shenmen point.

Mechanisms of Acupuncture

Based on the above clinical observations, we can recognize that acupuncture is effective for both acute urticaria and chronic urticaria. But the effective mechanisms of acupuncture on urticaria have never been investigated directly. However, several basic studies may help us to understand its mechanisms indirectly.

It was found that adrenal production of corticosterone and cortisol in vitro was enhanced by acupuncture at acupuncture point S36 (*Zusanli*) in female rabbits.[17] Furthermore, it was found that this effect could be blocked by lesions in the ventromedian nucleus of the hypothalamus.[18] In humans, after acupuncture treatment for 15 and 45 minutes, the serum cortisol level increase was 28% and 58%, respectively, as compared with results of self-control (placebo acupuncture) studies.[19] Malizia et al[20] found that large amounts of β-endorphin and corticotropin are secreted concomitantly into peripheral blood during electroacupuncture. These above studies provide reasons to speculate that acupuncture may activate the hypothalamus-pituitary-adrenal axis and result in secretion of glucocorticoids, which suppress the immunological reaction of urticaria. However, the activation of hypothalamus-pituitary-adrenal axis may be just a part of the effective mechanisms of acupuncture on urticaria. Whether other mechanisms are also involved is not yet clear. Further studies are recommended.

Prospects for Acupuncture Treatment of Urticaria

Based on the experiences from the Asian world, acupuncture is effective for the treatment of urticaria, both the acute and chronic forms.[6,7,11–16] However, can this effect be confirmed in the Western world? Only use of the technique over a period of time and future studies will tell. However, our clinical observations do have drawbacks, such as the lack of a control group and the need for standard classification of urticaria.

Results of these clinical observations seen during the past 50 years are far from perfect. However, they provide us with an alternative way to treat patients with urticaria, especially those with chronic urticaria that is refractory to medication therapy. More attractively, several new techniques based on acupuncture theory and having acupuncturelike effects without needle insertion are being developed and assessed. These newer techniques include acupuncturelike transcutaneous electrical nerve stimulation (TENS), infrared therapy, and low-level laser therapy.[21,22]

In the future, acupuncture or acupuncturelike techniques may provide important contributions in the treatment of patients with urticaria, particularly those refractory to medication therapy.

We thank John Jun-Yang Chen, MA, June Cheng, and Yen-Cheng Chen for their help in the preparation of the manuscript.

References

1. Tsan IJ. Urticaria. In: Chin WX, ed. *Dermatology Investigation [in Chinese]*. Taipei, Taiwan: Ze-Yin Publisher; 1995:404–417.
2. Sun SM. *Qian-Jin-Yao-Fang [in Chinese]*. 3rd ed. Taipei, Taiwan: Freedom Publishers; 1982.
3. Sheldon JM, Mathews KP, Lovell RG. The vexing urticaria problem: present concepts of etiology and management. *J Allergy.* 1954; 252:525–560.
4. Swinney B. The atopic factor in urticaria. *South Med J.* 1941;34:855–858.
5. Goldstein SM. Urticaria and angioedema. In: Lawlor GJ Jr, Fischer TJ, Adelman DC, eds. *Manual of Allergy and Immunology*. 3rd ed. Boston, Mass: Little Brown & Co; 1995: 228–243.
6. Wang KD, Wang H. Acupuncture and moxibustion treatment of acute urticaria: 114 cases. *J Yunnan Coll Chin Med.* 1995;18:32.
7. Shanghai College of Traditional Medicine. *Acupuncture: A Comprehensive Text.* Seattle, Wash: Eastland Press; 1987:664–666.
8. World Health Organization. *Regional Working Group on the Standardization of Acupuncture Nomenclature*. Manila, Philippines: World Health Organization, Regional Office for the Western Pacific; 1984.
9. Greaves MW. Chronic urticaria. *N Engl J Med.* 1995;332:1767–1772.
10. Sabroe RA, Greaves MW. The pathogenesis of chronic idiopathic urticaria. *Arch Dermatol.* 1997;133:1003–1008.
11. Dai SM. *Acupuncture Reports: 2300 Cases* [in Chinese]. 4th ed. Taipei, Taiwan: Chie-Yeiblishers; 1993:118.
12. Kao FT. Acupuncture treatment of refractory urticaria: 36 cases [in Chinese]. *J Zhejiang Coll Chin Med.* 1984;19:64.
13. Kao HB. Acupuncture treatment of chronic urticaria: 48 cases [in Chinese]. *J N Chin Med.* 1983;1:36.
14. Tong YL, Song DK. Acupuncture point injection with vitamin B1 to treat chronic urticaria: clinical observation of 40 cases [in Chinese]. *J Clin Dermatol.* 1986;15:102–103.
15. Lin L. Observation on therapeutic effects of auto-hemo-injection into points on chronic urticaria [in Chinese]. *Chin Acupunct Moxibustion.* 1994;14:75–76.
16. Yang YL, Lo HC. Cupping of shenque point to treat chronic urticaria [in Chinese]. *Chin Acupunct Moxibustion.* 1993;13:51.
17. Liao YY, Seto K, Saito H, Fugita M, Kawakami M. Effects of acupuncture on adrenocortical hormone production, I: variation in ability of adrenocortical hormone production in relation to the duration of acupuncture stimulation. *Am J Chin Med.* 1979;7:367–372.
18. Liao YY, Seto K, Saito H, Kawakami M. Effect of acupuncture on adrenocortical hormone production in rabbits with a central lesion. *Am J Chin Med.* 1981;9:61–73.
19. Lee SC, Yin SJ, Lee ML, Tsai WJ, Sim CB. Effects of acupuncture on serum cortisol level and dopamine beta-hydroxylase activity in normal Chinese. *Am J Chin Med.* 1982;10:62–69.
20. Malizia E, Andreucci G, Paolucci D, Crescenzi F, Fabbri A, Fraioli F. Electroacupuncture and peripheral β-endorphin and ACTH levels. *Lancet.* 1979;2:535–536.
21. Pomeranz B. Electroacupuncture and transcutaneous electrical nerve stimulation. In: Stux G, Pomeranz B, eds. *Basics of Acupuncture.* New York, NY: Springer-Verlag; 1988:230–240.
22. Pöntinen PJ. *Low Level Laser Therapy as a Medical Treatment Modality*. Tampere, Finland: Art Upro Ltd; 1992.

57 Acupuncture in a University Hospital

Implications for an Inpatient Consulting Service

Laeth Nasir, MD
From the Department of Family Medicine, University of Nebraska Medical Center, Omaha.

This case series reviews my experience in providing acupuncture treatment to inpatients at a midwestern, tertiary care, university teaching hospital. I review 4 cases, including patients with torticollis, ileus, brain injury, and intractable migraine. The lessons learned from each of these cases are summarized, and the implications for the development of an inpatient acupuncture service are discussed.

Arch Fam Med. 1998;7:593–596

Acupuncture may have been practiced on a small scale in North America since 1876[1]; however, only recently has it become popular among large segments of the population. In China, many hospitals perform acupuncture on inpatients who have a wide range of diagnoses, in addition to carrying out traditional herbal and modern Western medical treatments. The vast majority of acupuncture in the United States is performed on an outpatient basis for chronic conditions such as pain. When acupuncture is used in the hospital, it is reported to be used primarily for the augmentation of surgical anesthesia.[2] With increasing patient and physician interest, and stronger scientific evidence of the efficacy of acupuncture, this treatment modality is being carried out more frequently in conventional medical settings. A recent National Institutes of Health Consensus Panel statement[3] addressed the increasing use of this therapeutic intervention, and reviewed the current scientific literature on the efficacy of acupuncture for many conditions. The panel's finding, that " . . . there is sufficient evidence, however, of acupuncture's value to expand its use into conventional medicine and to encourage further studies of its physiology and clinical value,"[3] has heightened interest for this treatment modality in both the lay and professional community. Recently, it was reported that at least one hospital is experimenting with providing acupuncture care to hospitalized patients for conditions such as pain relief and anxiety control[4]; however, no data exist on the use of acupuncture in a general inpatient population in the United States, in whom the average acuity and severity of illness is likely to be higher than seen in hospitalized patients in developing countries such as China.

The following case-series reviews some cases from my experience as a consultant providing acupuncture to inpatients in a midwestern, tertiary care, university teaching hospital. During the past 3 years, I have provided acupuncture treatments to 16 hospitalized patients for conditions ranging from acute pain (11 cases) to anxiety (2 cases), ileus (2 cases), and brain injury (1 case). These patients illustrate both the potential and the problems encountered in integrating this unconventional therapy into the fast-paced, highly technical world of the modern teaching hospital.

Report of Cases

Case 1

An acupuncture consultation was sought from the family medicine service for a 79-year-old woman who had presented 48 hours earlier to the emergency department with severe neck and shoulder pain and spasm. Outpatient therapy was attempted initially and failed and a medical workup failed to demonstrate any serious underlying pathologic condition to account for the pain. The patient was given progressively stronger analgesic medications to control the intense discomfort. After the failure of oral and intramuscular medications to control the pain, she received a morphine patient-controlled analgesia pump. Shortly thereafter, the patient became confused and combative. Use of the patient-controlled analgesia pump was discontinued, with gradual return of the mental status to baseline. Physical therapy was begun, the option of acupuncture was offered and refused, and a neurology consultation was obtained. Magnetic resonance angiography and imaging brain scans showed no abnormalities. Results of a lumbar puncture showed no abnormalities. A small dose of intravenous benzodiazepine was recommended but resulted in a return of the mental status changes. Physical therapy was unsuccessful owing to the intense pain experienced by the patient. The patient and her family then decided to try the acupuncture treatment. Although the patient was admittedly skeptical and apprehensive prior to the treatment, to her surprise she experienced notable reduction of her neck and shoulder pain and was able to actively move her neck through about 20° rotation and lateral flexion immediately following the acupuncture treatment, which involved the placement of needles in a finger, toe, shoulder, just inferior to the zygoma, and on her forehead. A second treatment the next day resulted in enough relief in her pain and spasm that she was able to be discharged from the hospital with a nurse providing daily follow-up and outpatient physical therapy.

One of the problems encountered in geriatric patients who are hospitalized is the high incidence of medication side effects they experience. In this case, the use of strong analgesics resulted in delirium, a condition associated with a significant mortality rate.[5] Following the principle of "do no harm" a case such as this requires creative solutions to avoid creating iatrogenic illness.

Most hospitalized patients offered acupuncture in our hospital have initially refused it or have been openly skeptical of its efficacy. They are understandably very apprehensive before the first treatment. This situation can be rather intimidating for a physician, particularly when many of the hospital staff may share some of the patients concerns; however, after treatment, most patients find that the procedure is not associated with notable discomfort. As is the case before any unfamiliar procedure, it is important to spend time building a degree of rapport with the patient prior to treatment.

Case 2

A consultation was requested from the general surgery service for a 35-year-old woman, 14 days after resection of an enterocutaneous fistula caused by Crohn's disease. The patient had a long history of Crohn's disease and had been hospitalized many times for complications of the disease. The patient initially did well postoperatively, then began complaining of increasing abdominal pain and distention that necessitated escalating doses of intravenous morphine sulfate by patient-controlled analgesia pump to achieve pain relief. The high doses of morphine resulted in an ileus that led to greater distention and discomfort. The internal medicine service was consulted, but they were unable to offer any specific solution other than to wean the patient from the morphine therapy. Any attempt to do so, however, led to an intolerable increase in discomfort. Prokinetic agents were ineffective. Total parenteral nutrition was begun. When first evaluated, the patient was alert and pain free, while receiving a morphine sulfate basal rate of 7 mg/h, with 1-mg demand doses every 15 minutes which she was using regularly. Abdominal examination revealed a healing midline abdominal incision. The abdomen was slightly distended, with absent bowel sounds, and diffuse tenderness to deep palpation.

After discussing the situation with the patient, acupuncture was begun with continuous electrical stimulation of both auricular and body points. During a 6-hour period, the basal rate of morphine sulfate was lowered to 1 mg/h, with no demand doses. The patient reported feeling "as loose as a bowl of spaghetti" and more alert. She denied pain or nausea; her vital signs were stable; and her skin was warm and dry. Orders were left with the nursing staff to page the service if the continuously stimulated needles were dislodged. A call was received about 4 hours later, at 10 PM, that the patient was experiencing pain. There had been a nursing shift change, and the information regarding the needles had not been transmitted to the nurse taking care of the patient. The needles had come unhooked from the electrical stimulating device when the patient had gotten up to go to the bathroom 2 hours before and had not been reconnected. The patient was diaphoretic, anxious, and complaining of abdominal discomfort. The basal dose of morphine sulfate was increased to 2 mg/h and the patient observed for an hour, at the end of which she reported adequate pain control. Acupuncture was discontinued for the night, with the intention of completing the weaning process the next morning. A note was left on the patient's medical record to leave the basal rate untouched if possible, but if necessary, to give the patient a very small dose of an intravenous benzodiazepine if needed for sleep.

The next morning, the patient was found to be unarousable. Apparently she had done well until about 4 AM, when she awoke with abdominal discomfort and had been given 2 mg of lorazepam (Ativan) intravenously by the surgical intern on call. Immediately, the morphine therapy was stopped, and in about 30 minutes the patient awoke with abdominal pain, diaphoresis, yawning, and midriasis. Morphine therapy was restarted, and the patient refused further acupuncture treatments.

Acupuncture has been used widely to provide detoxification for narcotic addiction.[6] In this case, tolerance to the analgesic effects of narcotics led to a vicious cycle of increasing ileus, distention, and further narcotic use. Acupuncture was initially successful in not only blocking the symptoms of narcotic withdrawal, but also in providing analgesia for the abdominal pain due to the ileus (and perhaps narcotic withdrawal). This case served to point out many weaknesses in the provision of acupuncture to our inpatient population. Clear communication among professionals is of paramount importance when many professionals simultaneously carry out many complex tasks to care for patients. Better communication and better understanding of the treatment by all involved in caring for this patient may have led to a better outcome. More education of physicians, nursing, and ancillary staff is important to ensure that the highest quality of care obtainable with this modality is achieved. Adequate manpower to provide acupuncture around the clock if necessary is another important lesson highlighted in this case, as well as the importance of providing adequate analgesia to patients to reduce anxiety and to build trust in the physician and treatment modality used.

Case 3

An acupuncture consultation was requested by a surgical specialty service for a patient who was in the intensive care unit. A 32-year-old man had suffered an apparent anoxic brain injury approximately 2 weeks earlier, and was receiving mechanical ventilation. The family had heard that acupuncture was available and had requested the consultation. Review of the patient's medical record revealed a neurology consultation that held out little, if any, hope of recovery. This was echoed in a second opinion from an independent neurologist. An ethics consultation had been obtained, and the hospital chaplaincy service was involved. Physical examination revealed the patient exhibited decorticate posturing, with no evidence of neurological activity above the brainstem. When I met with the family, they related that several years ago the patient's uncle had a transverse myelitis that had been declared irreversible by many specialists, and following a course of acupuncture, he had recovered. A long discussion took place. It was pointed out to the family that there was no evidence based on the scientific literature that this course would be effective. The family was insistent, however, and ultimately it was agreed that acupuncture would be attempted. A series of treatments was carried out over several days. There was no clinical response; however, much time was spent at the patient's bedside, and a good working relationship was developed with the family. At the end of the treatment series, they were ready to move on to recognizing the irreversibility of the patient's condition.

This case raised questions regarding the ethics of carrying out a futile treatment. It could be argued that this treatment should not be attempted, based on the lack of any evidence of its efficacy in this setting[7]; however, the same argument could be made for continuing mechanical ventilation in this case. In this situation, the futility of treatment was balanced against its possible harmfulness, wastefulness, and the family's wishes. It is possible that the lack of a trusted primary care physician may have hindered the patient's family from moving forward in the decision making regarding their loved one. Acupuncture provided an opportunity for a grieving family to develop a relationship over time with a physician accustomed to discussing end-of-life issues. Just spending unfocused "quiet time" with the patient and/or family at the bedside is a powerful tool that physicians may use too sparingly. This quiet time, during which diagnosis or therapy is carried out, is a characteristic shared by several complementary therapies, and may be as or more beneficial than is the therapy. This case reinforces the value of spending a little extra time caring for patients and families, both inside and outside of the hospital.

Case 4

An acupuncture consultation was sought by the internal medicine service for a 25-year-old woman who had been readmitted only hours after having been discharged from a 4-day hospitalization with a diagnosis of status migranosus. During that hospitalization, computed tomographic and magnetic resonance imaging studies of the brain had been performed, as well as a lumbar puncture. A neurology consultation had been obtained, and several medications were tried, including intravenous lorazepam, meperidine hydrochloride (Demerol), nalbuphine hydrochloride (Nubain), gabapentin (Neurontin), propranolol hydrochloride (Inderal), lidocaine hydrochloride nasal spray, oxygen by nasal cannula, ketorolac tromethamine (Toradol), amitryptiline hydrochloride (Elavil), dexamethasone (Decadron), and a morphine patient-controlled analgesia pump, all without relief. A psychiatric consultation was obtained. The patient's medical history was notable for recurrent severe migraine headaches since suffering from encephalitis 7 years earlier. She had been evaluated and treated for many years at 2 major regional subspecialty clinics without much change in her headache frequency or severity.

Although she voiced some skepticism that acupuncture could help her, she admitted "at this point, I would do anything to get this pain away." Within 1 hour of the treatment, she experienced resolution of her headache and was weaned from the patient-controlled analgesia pump. That night, she slept soundly, with only a mild return of the headache the next morning. The headache resolved completely following a second acupuncture treatment, and she was discharged home. She is receiving acupuncture as an outpatient and has had no recurrent headaches.

In my experience, acupuncture is often used as the treatment of last resort in the hospital. Whether it should remain as one is a question to be answered by the larger medical community through further research and multicenter studies. Its potential as a versatile and safe treatment should be balanced against concerns regarding its efficacy and cost-benefit ratio compared with other more familiar and readily available treatment modalities. Questions of acceptability to patients will likely vary according to personal preferences and health beliefs, experience with acupuncture and related treatment modalities, and the trust that they have in the judgment of their physicians.

Comment

This case-series describes some of the possible uses of acupuncture in a general inpatient population and illustrates some of the unexpected benefits and pitfalls of this procedure that may be experienced in the hospital. The cases reflect my experience in using acupuncture to treat a range of conditions. Compared with patients presenting for acupuncture in the outpatient setting, inpatients are often quite apprehensive at the prospect of receiving this therapy. This is understandable, given the unfamiliar treatments, surroundings, and severity of their illness. In contrast to the outpatient setting, where there is usually more time to build rapport and create a therapeutic alliance with the patient, physicians may often feel that they are under the gun to produce immediate results. This pressure may come from both the primary medical team and the patient, each of whom may be understandably stressed by the situation leading to the consultation.

In virtually all cases, acupuncture can be carried out without disrupting ongoing treatments. A typical treatment lasts between 10 and 20 minutes. For most inpatient indications, treatments are carried out once or twice daily. In the case of narcotic withdrawal or for postsurgical analgesia, treatment may continue for several hours.

Because of the often multifaceted problems that give rise to an acupuncture consultation, I have found that a broad range of cognitive and interpersonal skills are helpful in bridging the gap between this therapy and the highly complex hospital environment. In cases requiring follow-up, provider continuity with a generalist further promotes the transition to an outpatient setting.

As is the case with traditional consultations, any conflicting needs and expectations of patients, consultants, attending physicians, and allied health care staff need to be addressed explicitly, with clear guidelines established regarding the responsibility and end points of treatment. Further education regarding this modality for physicians and hospital staff will increase the likelihood that this treatment is used to its fullest potential for the benefit of hospitalized patients.

References

1. Helms JM. Acupuncture in the west. In: Helms JM. *Acupuncture Energetics: A Clinical Approach for Physicians.* Berkeley, Calif: Medical Acupuncture Publishers; 1995:4.

2. Mok YP. Acupuncture, analgesia and anesthesia. *Med Acupuncture.* 1996;8:4–9.

3. NIH Consens Statement Online. Available at: http://odp.od.nih.gov/consensus/statements/cdc/107/107_stmt.html. Accessed January 2, 1998.

4. Villaire M. Hospital to partner with TCM college to offer acupuncture to inpatients. *Altern Ther Health Med.* 1997;3:30.

5. Lipowski ZJ. Delerium in the elderly patient. *N Engl J Med.* 1989;320:578–582.

6. Brewington V, Smith M, Lipton D. Acupuncture as a detoxification treatment: an analysis of controlled research. *J Subst Abuse Treat.* 1994;11:289–307.

7. Savulescu J, Momeyer RW. Should informed consent be based on rational beliefs? *J Med Ethics.* 1997;23:282–288.

58 Moxibustion for Correction of Breech Presentation

A Randomized Controlled Trial

Francesco Cardini, MD; Huang Weixin, MD
From the Jiangxi Women's Hospital, Nanchang, People's Republic of China (Dr Weixin). Dr Cardini is in private practice in Verona, Italy.

Context
Traditional Chinese medicine uses moxibustion (burning herbs to stimulate acupuncture points) of acupoint BL 67 (Zhiyin, located beside the outer corner of the fifth toenail), to promote version of fetuses in breech presentation. Its effect may be through increasing fetal activity. However, no randomized controlled trial has evaluated the efficacy of this therapy.

Objective
To evaluate the efficacy and safety of moxibustion on acupoint BL 67 to increase fetal activity and correct breech presentation.

Design
Randomized, controlled, open clinical trial.

Setting
Outpatient departments of the Women's Hospital of Jiangxi Province, Nanchang, and Jiujiang Women's and Children's Hospital in the People's Republic of China.

Patients
Primigravidas in the 33rd week of gestation with normal pregnancy and an ultrasound diagnosis of breech presentation.

Interventions
The 130 subjects randomized to the intervention group received stimulation of acupoint BL 67 by *moxa* (Japanese term for *Artemisia vulgaris*) rolls for 7 days, with treatment for an additional 7 days if the fetus persisted in the breech presentation. The 130 subjects randomized to the control group received routine care but no interventions for breech presentation. Subjects with persistent breech presentation after 2 weeks of treatment could undergo external cephalic version anytime between 35 weeks' gestation and delivery.

Main Outcome Measures
Fetal movements counted by the mother during 1 hour each day for 1 week; number of cephalic presentations during the 35th week and at delivery.

Results

The intervention group experienced a mean of 48.45 fetal movements vs 35.35 in the control group (*P*<.001; 95% confidence interval [CI] for difference, 10.56–15.60). During the 35th week of gestation, 98 (75.4%) of 130 fetuses in the intervention group were cephalic vs 62 (47.7%) of 130 fetuses in the control group (*P*<.001; relative risk [RR], 1.58; 95% CI, 1.29–1.94). Despite the fact that 24 subjects in the control group and 1 subject in the intervention group underwent external cephalic version, 98 (75.4%) of the 130 fetuses in the intervention group were cephalic at birth vs 81 (62.3%) of the 130 fetuses in the control group (*P*=.02; RR, 1.21; 95% CI, 1.02–1.43).

Conclusion

Among primigravidas with breech presentation during the 33rd week of gestation, moxibustion for 1 to 2 weeks increased fetal activity during the treatment period and cephalic presentation after the treatment period and at delivery.

JAMA. 1998;280:1580–1584

In cases of breech presentation at the onset of labor, delivery is associated with additional risks: for the mother, cesarean delivery and for the neonate, physical injury. Breech presentation is common in the midtrimester pregnancy and the incidence decreases as the pregnancy approaches term because of spontaneous version.[1–4] It is reasonable to assume (although not firmly established) that fetal activity plays an important role in spontaneous version.[5–9] The incidence of breech presentation at delivery can be reduced, but not eliminated, by the use of external cephalic version (ECV).[10]

Since ancient times, traditional Chinese medicine has proposed moxibustion of acupoint BL 67 (Zhiyin) to promote version of fetuses in breech presentation. Moxibustion is a traditional Chinese method that uses the heat generated by burning herbal preparations containing *Artemisia vulgaris* (mugwort) (the Japanese name is *moxa*) to stimulate acupuncture points. Acupoint BL 67 is beside the outer corner of the fifth toenail.

At present, there are no randomized, controlled clinical trials to evaluate the efficacy of this therapy. The 2 published Chinese studies[11,12] are not randomized and are based on a mixed population of primipara and multipara subjects stimulated at varying times between the 28th and 38th weeks of pregnancy. Although both studies give encouraging results and stimulate reflection regarding possible mechanisms of action, they do not allow definitive conclusions regarding efficacy because they are not randomized, little information is provided about the population sample, and the times at which stimulation is applied are wide ranging.

Cardini et al[13] identified the stage of pregnancy at which stimulation should commence and the parity status of the groups studied as primary factors to ensure the reliability of a clinical trial concerning spontaneous or induced correction of breech presentation.

Data in the literature concerning the probability of spontaneous correction indicate that correcting breech presentation before the 32nd week is useless.[14–16] There is also a sharp differentiation between multigravidas (high likelihood of spontaneous correction of breech presentation, even between the 32nd and 35th weeks) and primigravidas or multigravidas with a previous breech presentation at term (low probability of spontaneous version after the 32nd week).[15–17]

Gottlicher and Madjaric,[15,16] by ultrasound examination of 4066 pregnant women, defined the likelihood of spontaneous correction of breech presentation from the 33rd week of pregnancy as 15.5% (95% confidence interval [CI], 2.8%–28.2%) for primigravidas and 57.5% (95% CI, 36.3%–78.7%) for multigravidas.

Westgren et al,[17] by ultrasound screening of 4600 women in the 32nd week of pregnancy, identified 310 cases (6.7%) of breech presentation, which were prospectively studied until birth. Rates of spontaneous cephalic version varied, according to whether subjects were primigravida (46%), multigravida with a previous breech presentation (32%), or multigravida with no previous breech presentation (78%). All the studies available report data relating to Western populations and we have been unable to retrieve any information regarding the spontaneous version rate from the 33rd week to term among Chinese pregnant women.

Given this background, Cardini and Marcolongo,[18] in a retrospectively controlled clinical trial, compared 23 primigravidas treated for breech presentation by moxibustion in the 32nd and 33rd week with a retrospective, untreated group at the same stage of pregnancy. The difference in prevalence of breech presentation showed borderline statistical significance (P=.05). Thus, the subgroup of primigravidas with breech presentation at the 33rd week of pregnancy seemed to be the ideal population for a randomized, controlled clinical trial.

We undertook this study to evaluate the efficacy and safety of moxibustion on acupoint BL 67 in correcting breech presentation in a population of primigravidas treated since the 33rd week of pregnancy and to evaluate the efficacy of this technique in increasing active fetal movements (AFMs).

These 2 main objectives are consistent with the hypothesis that the use of moxibustion in women whose fetuses are breech in the 33rd week of pregnancy will (1) increase fetal activity; (2) reduce the proportion of fetuses that remain in a nonvertex presentation and, hence, decrease the need for ECV; and (3) decrease the incidence of breech presentation at birth. A secondary aim of the study was to assess the efficacy of 2 different dosages of moxibustion.

Methods

This was a randomized, controlled, open clinical trial of subjects treated by moxibustion since the 33rd week of pregnancy (intervention group) vs untreated subjects (control group). Subjects with persistent breech presentation after 2 weeks' treatment (intervention group) or observation (control group) could undergo ECV. Moxibustion in the early third trimester and ECV in late pregnancy are the standard care for breech presentation in both the centers involved in the trial. Thus (and also for ethical reasons), the availability of ECV was maintained for all subjects recruited.

Subjects were included if they were primigravidas, in the 33rd week of gestation (from 32 weeks + 1 day to 33 complete weeks, based on the last menstruation date and ultrasound data), with breech presentation diagnosed by ultrasound within 24 hours of randomization, and with normal fetal biometry (biparietal diameter and abdominal circumference between the 10th and 90th percentiles). Subjects were excluded if they had pelvic defects, previous uterine surgery, uterine malformation or fibromyoma of diameter greater than 4 cm, fetal malformation, twin gestation, tocolytic therapy during pregnancy, risk of premature birth (uterine hypercontractility and/or initial shortening or dilatation of the neck, with a Bishop score ≥4), or pathological pregnancy (eg, intrauterine growth retardation, gestosis, serious infections, placenta previa, polyhydramnios, oligohydramnios) judged by the investigator to contraindicate inclusion in the study. Subjects refusing to undergo treatment were also excluded.

Study Procedures

The trial was conducted from April 1995 through August 1996 in the Women's Hospital of Jiangxi Province, Nanchang, People's Republic of China. A few subjects (23) were recruited in the nearby Jiujiang Women's and Children's Hospital, also in Jiangxi Province. The subjects were recruited during the routine management of normal pregnancies in the outpatient department. All procedures were executed by midwives (with the supervision of physicians) except ultrasound examinations and ECVs. The protocol followed the ethical standards of the Declaration of Helsinki.

Pregnant women fulfilling all criteria of the study were asked to participate. Interested subjects gave oral informed consent. Subjects had an ultrasound scan at the 33rd week. On the day of the ultrasound scan by which breech presentation was confirmed, the selected subject was randomly assigned to 1 of the 2 groups. The sample was randomly allocated by numbered envelopes (randomized in groups of 10 by the computer program PACT, Version 2.0 [Glaxo-Wellcome, London, England], in Italy). Once randomized, subjects and investigators were aware of group assignment. All subjects recruited were advised to avoid or, at least, to ask the investigators about other interventions or therapies that could contaminate the results of the trial.

All subjects were asked to return after 2 weeks for an ultrasound check on presentation. If breech presentation persisted at this time, the subject (after giving informed consent) could undergo ECV in the following weeks.

All subjects were also asked to complete 2 record forms for AFMs, 1 for each of the 2 weeks subsequent to recruitment. These 2 forms were returned at the time of the ultrasound examination. Each record form had to be completed once daily for 7 days, reporting the number of AFMs counted in 1 hour (if possible, between 5 and 8 PM) and times of starting and finishing the count.

Finally, each subject was asked to report all significant details of her pregnancy and delivery during a personal or telephone appointment after she had given birth. The following specific information was collected: date of birth, place of birth, name and address of the obstetrician normally consulted, and name and address of the obstetrician present at birth. In this way, it was possible to consult other sources of information (obstetrician normally consulted, obstetrician present at birth, patient record forms) if the subject provided incomplete or unreliable information. Because almost all the enrolled subjects gave birth in the same hospital where they had been studied, information about delivery was reliable and easy to check.

If the subject belonged to the intervention group, she was admitted to the hospital to attend an instruction session within 24 hours of randomization, alone or with her partner or the person who was actually going to help administer the treatment. Teaching the technique for applying moxibustion at home included presenting the moxibustion material (cigar-shaped rolls containing *Artemisia*), locating of acupoint BL 67, and explaining the technique for stimulation of acupoint BL 67. During the therapy the subject relaxed in the sitting or semisupine position, with the partner sitting comfortably. The therapy was executed for 30 minutes (15 minutes per side) daily for 7 days in the first 87 subjects, and twice daily in the last 43 subjects. The subjects were allowed to choose the time, ensuring no interruptions in the therapy (if possible, between 5 and 8 PM). The intensity of moxibustion was just below the individual tolerability threshold, causing hyperemia from local vasodilatation but not burn blisters.

Reasons for discontinuing stimulation and consulting the investigator (abdominal pain, other suspected adverse effects, sensation that version had occurred before completion of 7 days' treatment) were explained to the subject, together with symptoms suggesting that version had occurred (decreased pressure in the epigastrium or hypochondrium, increased pressure in the hypogastrium, pollakiuria, a "different feeling" in the abdomen). The first stimulation session was executed in the hospital and the necessary materials for the following 6 days' stimulation were dispensed, together with the AFM record forms.

Last, an examination after 1 week's treatment (visit 2) was scheduled. Visit 2 included a check on presentation and collection of the AFM record form. The presentation check was by localization of fetal heartbeats and abdominal palpation (Leopold maneuvers). Ultrasound examination was performed only in the event that the techniques described herein failed or yielded uncertain findings.[19] This was to avoid an excess of ultrasound examinations, given that an ultrasound examination was scheduled for the 35th week in all subjects. If cephalic version had not occurred, another week's treatment was advised if there were no adverse effects and the subject agreed to continue. Further *moxa* rolls were therefore dispensed to the subject with a second AFM record form. The frequency of the treatment was the same as in the first week. Visit 3 was scheduled and executed after a further week; the procedure was the same for all treated and untreated subjects as described herein (Figure 1).

Outcomes Measured

The primary outcomes were number of cephalic presentations at the 35th week and at birth and fetal motor activity. Secondary outcomes were compliance with treatment, observation of possible adverse effects in the intervention group and adverse events in both groups, number of cephalic versions after 1 and 2 weeks of treatment (ie, 34th and 35th weeks' gestation), number of cephalic versions with 2 different dosages of moxibustion (once or twice daily), number and causes of cesarean deliveries, spontaneous and induced vaginal deliveries, and Apgar score at 5 minutes.

Statistical Analysis

On the basis of the study by Cardini and Marcolongo,[18] for primigravidas it seemed possible to identify a 30% difference in the number of cephalic presentations at the 35th week and at term between the intervention and control groups, with an significance level of .05 and greater than 90% power if 60 subjects per group completed the study. Given that the reliability of the preliminary study was limited because it was based on retrospective data and that we decided to assess the efficacy of 2 different dosages of moxibustion, the number of enrolled subjects was increased to 130 per group.

Even if not attributable to 1 of the causes specified in the research protocol, discontinuation of treatment did not entail the subject's exclusion from the study. Outcomes of all subjects recruited were analyzed on the basis of intention to treat. Every possible effort was made to ascertain the reason for withdrawal.

The statistical processing was performed using Epi Info, Version 6.04 (Centers for Disease Control and Prevention, Atlanta, Ga). The χ^2 test (supplemented, where necessary, by the Fisher exact test) and the *t* test were used for comparing qualitative and continuous variables, respectively. The measurement of effects was also described in terms of relative risk (RR) with 95% confidence intervals (CIs).

Results

The total number of subjects was 260 (130 subjects per group), recruited, randomized, observed, or treated and followed up to delivery. No significant differences emerged between the intervention group and the control

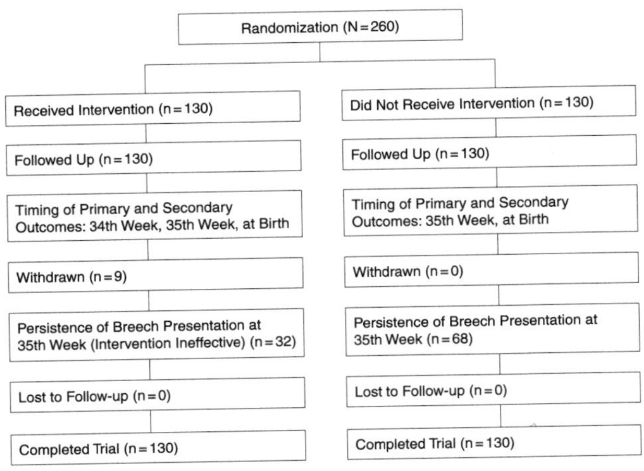

Figure 1. Profile of the randomized controlled trial.

Table 1. Comparability Between Intervention and Control Groups*

	Intervention Group (n=130)	Control Group (n=130)
Maternal age, y	25.5 (2.5)	25.2 (3.0)
Maternal height, cm	159.8 (3.9)	158.8 (3.8)
Neonatal weight, g	3234 (347)	3252 (420)
Neonatal cranial circumference, cm	34.2 (1.3)	34.3 (1.3)
Male, No. (%)	62 (47.7)	56 (43.1)
Legs straight at 33rd week, No. (%)	79 (60.8)	68 (52.3)

*Unless noted otherwise, values are expressed as mean (SD).

group (Table 1). Neither the placental localization and grading nor the amount of amniotic fluid at the 33rd week showed significant differences between the 2 groups.

The main results of the trial are summarized in Table 2. At the ultrasound check at the 35th week of gestation (2 weeks after the first visit), 98 (75.4%) of 130 fetuses in the intervention group were cephalic compared with 62 (47.7%) of 130 in the control group (*P*<.001; RR, 1.58; 95% CI, 1.29–1.94).

After 35 weeks of pregnancy, only 1 subject in the intervention group agreed to undergo ECV, but version was not obtained. Twenty-four subjects in the control group agreed to undergo ECV and in 19 subjects cephalic version was obtained. Despite this, the number of cephalic presentations at birth was still significantly different in the 2 groups: 98 (75.4%) of 130 in the intervention group compared with 81 (62.3%) of 130 in the control group (*P*=.02; RR, 1.21; 95% CI, 1.02–1.43). The results obtained excluding subjects treated with ECV are shown in Table 2.

Of the 98 cephalic versions obtained in the intervention group, 82 occurred during the first week and 16 during the second week of treatment. The cephalic or breech presentations observed at the second visit (35th week of pregnancy) remained unchanged up to term in all subjects treated and observed, except for those successfully treated with ECV.

Compliance and Adverse Effects and Events

The only intervention allowed for the subjects in the control group was ECV during the last 5 weeks of pregnancy. They were specifically questioned at the 35th week and after delivery and none reported having been treated with moxibustion or other therapies.

Among the intervention group only 1 subject failed to comply with the treatment schedule prescribed and discontinued the therapy. At the end of the first week of treatment 8 subjects withdrew from therapy, 3 on the advice of the obstetrician (for Braxton Hicks contractions, breech engagement, and maternal tachycardia and atrial sinus arrhythmia, respectively) and 5 subjects for unspecified reasons. All 9 subjects maintained the breech presentations of their fetuses to term and none of them were excluded from the statistical analysis.

The form of discomfort most frequently reported by both groups was a sense of tenderness and pressure in the epigastric region or in one of the hypochondria (epigastric crushing) attributable to the head of the breech fetus pressing against the maternal organs.

No adverse events occurred in the intervention group during treatment. After treatment, 2 premature births occurred (both at 37 weeks), 1 of which was preceded by premature rupture of the membranes (PROM). There were 4 PROMs in the intervention group.

Adverse events occurring in the control group included 3 premature births at 34, 35, and 37 weeks (the third was

Table 2. Main Results of the Trial

	No. (%)			
	Intervention Group	Control Group	*P*	RR (95% CI)*
Cephalic presentation at 35 wk	98/130 (75.4)	62/130 (47.7)	<.001	1.58 (1.29–1.94)
Cephalic presentation at birth	98/130 (75.4)	81/130 (62.3)	.02	1.21 (1.02–1.43)
Cephalic presentation at birth†	98/129 (76.0)	62/106 (58.5)	.004	1.30 (1.08–1.57)

*RR indicates relative risk; CI, confidence interval.
†Data exclude subjects treated with external cephalic version.

preceded by placental detachment with fetal distress) and 1 intrauterine fetal death (intrauterine growth retardation and oligohydramnios, spontaneous delivery at 38 weeks; growth was within normal limits at ultrasound examination at 35 weeks). The total number of PROMs in the control group was 12.

Active Fetal Movements

Regarding the efficacy of the moxibustion treatment in producing an increase in fetal motility, comparison between the 2 groups proved possible for only the first week of treatment (or observation) because all the subjects in the intervention group who achieved cephalic version in the first week of treatment filled in only the first of the 2 record forms used for the weekly AFM counts. The mean value for fetal movements recorded during a 1-hour observation period for 7 days was 48.45 for the subjects in the intervention group and 35.35 for the subjects in the control group (difference, 13.08; 95% CI, 10.56–15.60; *t* test, 10.215; *P*<.001).

Effects of 1 or 2 Moxibustion Sessions per Day

In the intervention group, the first 87 subjects received 1 stimulation per day, lasting 30 minutes, for 7 or 14 days (QD [*quaque die*] group). The last 47 subjects received 2 30-minute stimulations per day for 7 or 14 days (BID [*bis in die*] group). The 2 subgroups showed no significant differences in amount of amniotic fluid during the 33rd week, frequency of straight or bent leg position during the 33rd week, placental localization, neonatal sex, treatment compliance, or adverse effects attributable to the treatment.

At the end of the first week of treatment in the BID group, 34 (79.1%) of 43 cephalic versions were obtained compared with 48 (55.2%) of 87 in the QD group (*P*=.007; RR, 1.43; 95% CI, 1.12–1.83).

During the second week of treatment, 15 additional cephalic versions were obtained in the QD group and only 1 additional version in the BID group. Thus, the following cephalic presentation results were observed on ultrasound examination at the end of the second week of treatment: 63 (72.4%) of 87 in the QD group and 35 (81.4%) of 43 in the BID group (nonsignificant difference). The same percentages were maintained to term.

Cesarean and Vaginal Deliveries

No statistically significant differences were found in the number of cesarean deliveries performed. In the intervention group, 46 cesarean deliveries (35.4% of births) were performed, 20 of which were with cephalic presentations and 26 of which were with breech presentations. The 20 cesarean deliveries in the cephalic presentations were performed for fetopelvic disproportion (14 cases), postterm pregnancy (3 cases), or fetal distress (3 cases). The 26 cesarean deliveries in the breech presentations were performed for PROM after week 37 (10 cases), large fetus (2 cases), fetal distress (1 case), oligohydramnios (2 cases), and unspecified causes (11 cases).

In the control group, 47 cesarean deliveries (36.2%) were performed, 21 of which were with cephalic presentations and 26 of which were with breech presentations. Indications for cesarean delivery in the subjects with cephalic fetuses included fetopelvic disproportion (11 cases, 1 of which was with oligohydramnios), fetal distress (4 cases, 1 of which was in a subject with toxemia of pregnancy), sacral rotation of the occiput (2 cases), placental insufficiency (1 case), toxemia of pregnancy (1 case), PROM (1 case), and deep transverse arrest (1 case). Cesarean deliveries in the breech presentations were performed for PROM after 37 weeks (8 cases, 1 of which was with prolapse of the cord), oligohydramnios (3 cases), fetal distress (2 cases), large fetus (1 case), and unspecified causes (12 cases).

In both the intervention and control groups, cesarean delivery revealed 1 case of previously undiagnosed bicornuate uterus. In both cases, the presentation at birth was breech. Because they had been randomized, both cases were included in the statistical analysis of the data despite uterine malformations being exclusion criterion.

In regard to vaginal deliveries, the only significant difference between the 2 groups relates to the use of oxytocin, given to 7 (8.6%) of 81 subjects in the intervention group vs 25 (31.3%) of 80 in the control group (RR, 1.33 [95% CI, 1.13–1.56]; $P<.001$) before or during labor. In the intervention group, 2 vacuum-extractor and 1 forceps deliveries were performed and in the control group, 2 vacuum-extractor and 3 forceps deliveries were performed.

Apgar Scores

No neonates in the intervention group, but 7 in the control group, had Apgar scores of less than 7 at 5 minutes (Fisher exact test, $P=.006$). On grouping Apgar scores in the traditional manner, in the intervention group no neonates had Apgar scores less than 4 and 4 had scores 4 to 7; in the control group, 2 neonates had Apgar scores less than 4 and 12 had scores 4 to 7.

Comment

Moxibustion is a popular and much appreciated therapy for breech presentation in the People's Republic of China; thus, it would have been impossible to propose a "sham moxibustion" as a placebo for the control group.

Furthermore, moxibustion is a typical cheap, self-administered home therapy. This made blinding practically impossible. It was very difficult for investigators to persuade subjects to accept randomization and the consequent risk of having to do without the therapy. Consent was often obtained because of the availability of ECV later in pregnancy, but this is a much less popular and somewhat feared therapy; thus, only a few subjects, mostly belonging to the control group, opted for this solution.

Because the main results of the trial are of a qualitative type and were measured objectively (ultrasound), we believe that the lack of blinding and a placebo does not undermine the validity of the results. This is not entirely the case when considering fetal movement count, which was subjectively assessed.

The choice of sample (primigravidas at the 33rd week of gestation) appears to have been appropriate because the presentation did not change after the 35th week in any of the subjects (except for those undergoing ECV). This confirms the rarity of spontaneous fetal version (to either breech or cephalic presentation) among primigravidas after the 35th week.[16]

Two half-hour stimulations per day proved more effective in producing cephalic version than a single stimulation. On prolonging the therapy by 1 week in those cases in which cephalic version was not achieved, this difference in efficacy was partly, although not entirely, annulled. Of the 2 dosages, then, twice-daily stimulation is recommended because it did not reduce treatment compliance and had no adverse effects. Compliance with the treatment was by and large good.

In 2 cases, disorders serious enough to prompt discontinuation were observed during treatment. It was not clear whether these were adverse effects of the treatment.

No severe adverse events attributable to the treatment were observed and, in particular, there were no cases of intrauterine death or placental detachment. No cases of severe fetal anemia attributable to fetomaternal transfusion[20] were reported. The number of PROMs was similar in both groups and the number of premature births was lower in the intervention group.

Moxibustion treatment did not reduce the rate of cesarean deliveries in a population in which elective cesarean delivery is not envisaged for breech presentations. On the other hand, it is possible that the significantly higher number of breech presentations at birth in the control group may have been a factor in bringing about worse Apgar scores.

The mechanism of action of moxibustion appears to be through increased AFMs, which proved significantly stronger in the treated subjects. Although a number of studies in China[11,12,21] have investigated the neurologic path of stimulation by moxibustion and have shown evidence of its effect on maternal plasma cortisol and prostaglandins, we think that the mechanism of action of moxibustion is not entirely clear and warrants further research.

Further studies[22] are needed to establish the efficacy and safety of moxibustion at more advanced gestational ages than those considered in this trial, as well as in second pregnancies or multigravidas and populations other than Chinese. Moreover, it is not clear whether moxibustion is more or less efficacious than ECV at term for obtaining cephalic presentation given the small number of subjects (nearly all belonging to the control group) who underwent ECV. Furthermore, since moxibustion and ECV must be performed at different gestational ages, we may regard them as complementary therapies to be used in succession. As we see it, if the results of this trial are confirmed, moxibustion should be extensively used on account of its noninvasiveness, low cost, and ease of execution. In fact, it is easy to train expectant mothers (either alone or with their partners) to administer the therapy at home. Further studies are also necessary to establish whether moxibustion treatment can reduce the rate of cesarean deliveries where these are used electively for breech presentation at birth.

Additional results regarding the effects of family history, fetal sex, cranial circumference, and leg position on the likelihood of cephalic version will be presented in a subsequent article.

On the basis of the results of the trial, moxibustion, when performed in primigravidas for 1 or 2 weeks starting in the 33rd week of pregnancy, has proved to be an effective therapy for inducing a significant increase in cephalic versions within 2 weeks of the start of therapy and in cephalic presentations at birth.

The Chinese part of this research was financed by Centro di Orientamento Educativo, Milan, Italy, a nongovernmental nonprofit organization for cooperation, and by the Commission des Communauts Europtennes, Brussels, Belgium.

We particularly thank Franceseo Banfi, senior biostatician, and Roberto Scognamiglio, data manager, Glaxo Research, Verona, Italy, for statistical work; Murray Enkin, MD, FRCSC, FRCOG, Departments of Obstetrics and Gynecology, Clinical Epidemiology, and Biostatistics, McMaster University, Toronto, Ontario, and Vittorio Basevi, MD, Verona, for their precious advice regarding protocol and reporting of the results; Qiu Lunxing, MD, Nanchang, China, for his invaluable work in translation and supervision; Anthony Steele, senior lecturer in medical English at the Medicine University of Verona, Verona, Italy; and all staff directly or indirectly involved in carrying out the research.

References

1. Hickok DE, Gordon DC, Milberg JA, Williams MA, Daling JR. The frequency of breech presentation by gestational age at birth. *Am J Obstet Gynecol*. 1992;166:851–852.

2. Hill LM. Prevalence of breech presentation by gestational age. *Am J Perinatol*. 1990;7:92–93.

3. Hughey MJ. Fetal position during pregnancy. *Am J Obstet Gynecol*. 1985;153:885–886.

4. Scheer K, Nubar J. Variation of fetal presentation with gestational age. *Am J Obstet Gynecol*. 1976;125:269–270.

5. Bartlett D, Okun N. Breech presentation: a random event or an explainable phenomenon? *Dev Med Child Neurol*. 1994;36:833–838.

6. Bartlett D, Piper M, Okun N, Byrne P, Watt J. Primitive reflexes and the determination of fetal presentation at birth. *Early Hum Dev*. 1997; 48:261–273.

7. Babkin PS, Ermolenko NA. The motor adaptation syndrome in the human fetus and its dynamics in newborns. *Zh Nevrol Psikhiatr Im S S Korsakova*. 1994;94:19–21.

8. Rayl J, Gibson J, Hickok DE. A population-based case-untreated study of risk factors for breech presentation. *Am J Obstet Gynecol*. 1996; 174:28–32.

9. Sival DA. Studies on fetal motor behaviour in normal and complicated pregnancies. *Early Hum Dev*. 1993;34:13–20.

10. Hofmeyr GJ. External cephalic version facilitation at term. In: Neilson JP, Crowther CA, Hodnett ED, Hofmeyr GJ, eds. *The Cochrane Library: Pregnancy and Childbirth Module of the Cochrane Database of Systematic Reviews* [database on disk and CD-ROM]. Oxford, England: Update Software; 1998.

11. Cooperative Research Group of Moxibustion Version of Jangxi Province. Studies of version by moxibustion on Zhiyin points. In: Xiangtong Z, ed. *Research on Acupuncture, Moxibustion and Acupuncture Anesthesia*. Beijing, China: Science Press; 1980:810–819.

12. Cooperative Research Group of Moxibustion Version of Jangxi Province. Further studies on the clinical effects and the mechanism of version by moxibustion. In: *Abstracts of the Second National Symposium on Acupuncture, Moxibustion and Acupuncture Anesthesia*; August 7–10, 1984; Beijing, China.

13. Cardini F, Basevi V, Valentini A, Martellato A. Moxibustion and breech presentation: preliminary results. *Am J Chin Med*. 1991;19:105–114.

14. Boos R, Hendrik HJ, Schmidt W. Das fetale Lageverhalten in der zweiten Schwangerschaftshalfte bei Geburten aus Beckenendlage und Schadellage. *Geburtsh Frauenheilkd*. 1987;47:341–345.

15. Gottlicher S, Madjaric J. Die Lage der menschlichen Frucht im Verlauf der Schwangerschaft und die Wahrscheinlichkeit einer spontanen Drehung in die Kopflage bei Erst und Mehrgebarenden. *Geburtsh Frauenheilkd*. 1985;45:534–538.

16. Gottlicher S, Madjaric J, Morgens KL, Mittags BEL. Ein Ammenmärchen? *Geburtsh Frauenheilkd*. 1989;49:363–366.

17. Westgren M, Edvall H, Nordstrom L, Svalenius E. Spontaneous cephalic version of breech presentation in the last trimester. *Br J Obstet Gynaecol*. 1985;92:10–22.

18. Cardini F, Marcolongo A. Moxibustion for correction of breech presentation. *Am J Chin Med*. 1993;21:133–138.

19. Thorp Jr JM, Jenkins T, Watson W. Utility of Leopold maneuvers in screening formal presentation. *Obstet Gynecol*. 1991;78(3 pt 1):394–396.

20. Engel K, Gerke-Engel G, Gerhard I, Bastert G. Fetomaternal macrotransfusion after successful internal version from breech presentation by moxibustion [in German]. *Geburtsh Frauenheilkd*. 1992;52:241–243.

21. Weng J, Peng G, Yuang H, Mao S, Zhang H. The morphological investigation of the correcting abnormal fetus position by acupuncture, moxibustion and laser irradiation in the point Zhiyin. In: *Abstracts of the Second National Symposium on Acupuncture and Moxibustion and Acupuncture Anesthesia*; August 7–10, 1984; Beijing, China.

22. World Health Organization Regional Office for the Western Pacific. *Guidelines for Clinical Research on Acupuncture*. Manila, Philippines: World Health Organization Regional Publications; 1995. Western Pacific Series No. 15.

8 Manual Therapy

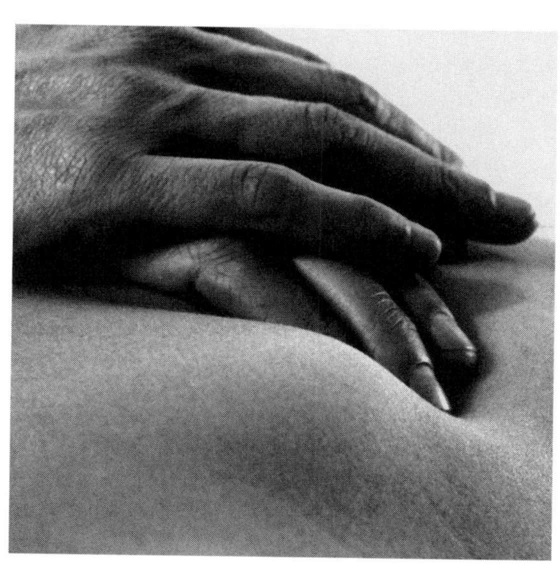

59 Chiropractic

Origins, Controversies, and Contributions

Ted J. Kaptchuk, OMD; David M. Eisenberg, MD
From the Center for Alternative Medicine Research, Department of Medicine, Beth Israel Deaconess Medical Center, Harvard Medical School, Boston, Mass.

Chiropractic is an important component of the US health care system and the largest alternative medical profession. In this overview of chiropractic, we examine its history, theory, and development; its scientific evidence; and its approach to the art of medicine. Chiropractic's position in society is contradictory, and we reveal a complex dynamic of conflict and diversity. Internally, chiropractic has a dramatic legacy of strife and factionalism. Externally, it has defended itself from vigorous opposition by conventional medicine. Despite such tensions, chiropractors have maintained a unified profession with an uninterrupted commitment to clinical care. While the core chiropractic belief that the correction of spinal abnormality is a critical health care intervention is open to debate, chiropractic's most important contribution may have to do with the patient-physician relationship.

Arch Intern Med. 1998;158:2215–2224

Chiropractic, the medical profession that specializes in manual therapy and especially spinal manipulation, is the most important example of alternative medicine in the United States and alternative medicine's greatest anomaly.

Even to call chiropractic "alternative" is problematic; in many ways, it is distinctly mainstream. Facts such as the following attest to its status and success: Chiropractic is licensed in all 50 states. An estimated 1 of 3 persons with lower back pain is treated by chiropractors.[1] In 1988 (the latest year with reliable statistics), between $2.4[2] and $4 billion[3] was spent on chiropractic care, and in 1990, 160 million office visits were made to chiropractors.[4] Since 1972, Medicare has reimbursed patients for chiropractic treatments, and these treatments are covered as well by most major insurance companies. In 1994, the Agency for Health Care Policy and Research removed much of the onus of marginality from chiropractic by declaring that spinal manipulation can alleviate low back pain.[5] In addition, the profession is growing: the number of chiropractors in the United States—now at 50,000—is expected to double by 2010 (whereas the number of physicians is expected to increase by only 16%).[6]

Despite such impressive credentials, academic medicine regards chiropractic theory as speculative at best and its claims of clinical success, at least outside of low back pain, as unsubstantiated. Only a few small hospitals permit chiropractors to treat inpatients, and to our knowledge, university-affiliated teaching centers have not yet granted chiropractors privileges to perform manipulation on patients.[7–9] Although the American Medical Association (AMA) no longer prohibits its members from consulting with chiropractors, especially since it was found guilty of conspiracy in this regard (see below), chiropractic's size and power have not translated into complete acceptance.

Contradictions and tensions exist not only between chiropractic and mainstream medicine but within chiropractic itself. Since its inception, chiropractors have disagreed about the definition of the therapy and its scope of practice. Various theories vie for dominance within the profession. A multiplicity of competing adjustment techniques also vie with each other under the rubric of chiropractic. The mode of chiropractic intervention—by means of the hands—and its unique therapeutic niche, primarily pain disorders, seem too narrow a foundation for its claim to encompass a distinct health system with autonomous licensing, credentialing, and educational institutions.

Yet, despite external conflicts and perhaps partly because of them, and despite the intraprofessional disagreements and uncertainty about its scope of practice, chiropractic has found an internal coherence that has allowed it to become an enduring presence in the United States. This integrity has to do with the profession's belief in the importance of biomechanics; the centrality of manual therapy, especially for the spine; and a clinical dynamic that provides patients with explanations, meaning, and concrete experiences that promote a strong patient-physician bond, a sense of caring, and a restored sense of well-being.

Chiropractic's Origin

Most sources date the birth of chiropractic as September 18, 1895, when Daniel David (usually called "D. D.") Palmer (1845–1913) shoved a single cervical vertebra of a deaf janitor of the Putnam Building in downtown Davenport, Iowa. A mythic aura clings to the event, partly because of its importance and because there is little agreement among witnesses about when it happened, who was there, or what actually occurred.[10] (The mythic aspect of the story may have been intentionally enhanced by selecting the date of Rosh Hashanah, the Jewish New Year, which was an occasion for revelation in 19th-century American millennialism.[11,12]) Whether fact, folklore, or both, the founding blow of chiropractic was more than a chance event or momentary inspiration. In fact, it creatively synthesized 4 previously distinct health care traditions: bonesetting, magnetic healing, orthodox science, and popular health reform.

Bonesetters

Bonesetters were a common fixture in 19th-century health care. As with the other healing crafts—midwifery, tooth-pulling, and barber-surgery—bonesetting was often part-time work and served clients who had problems that were regarded by academically trained physicians as inconsequential or beneath their dignity.[13,14] Bonesetters did much more than help mend bones. They often treated painful conditions caused by "subluxations," which meant a "joint 'put out'; and the one method of cure [is] the wrench aid, the rough movement by which it is said that the joint is 'put in' again."[15(p1)]

Palmer frequently mentioned the bonesetter's tradition, identified with it, and probably had some training in it. Palmer's innovation professionalized the craft, guaranteeing its continuation into the modern era. The upgrade extended to nomenclature; with help from a minister conversant with Greek, "bonesetting" became "chiropractic," a phrase that means "hand work."

Magnetic Healing

Although the bonesetting tradition gave chiropractic its method, "magnetic healing" provided the theory. Palmer acknowledged a special debt to magnetic healing when he wrote, "chiropractic was not evolved from medicine or any other method, except that of magnetic."[16(p111)] Derived from Anton Mesmer's (1734–1815) investigations into the supposed curative effects of animal magnetism, practitioners of magnetic healing identified the unimpeded flow of energy with health and defined illness as obstruction. For 9 years before his discovery of chiropractic, Palmer was one of a small army of healers who routinely "magnetized" their patients.[17] Palmer's major revision of traditional magnetism was to call it "innate intelligence" and to claim that its pathway was the human nervous system, especially the spinal cord. Misaligned spinal vertebrae (the redefined bonesetters' "subluxation") impinge on this beneficent flow and cause illness. By marrying magnetism to bonesetting, Palmer created a new and independent medical movement, one more capable of competing for legitimacy than either of its predecessors had been.

Orthodox Science

Neither bonesetting nor magnetic healing could be persuasively described as science. The former was clearly a folk tradition, and the latter could not shed its occult status. Chiropractic, however, could and did describe itself as science, and in the 19th century, such a label was indispensable if a medical movement hoped to emerge from a host of contending traditions. Although self-taught, Palmer saw himself as a scientist and wasted no time in adopting prevailing scientific notions of the spinal cord to chiropractic theory. An early 19th-century fascination with the spinal cord led to mainstream speculation, and by 1828, orthodox physicians began to warn about the threat posed to the organs of the body by "spinal irritation."[18] Spinal irritation in the 19th century became a catchall for a host of complaints. The theory was so well accepted that Oliver Wendell Holmes (1809–1894) could comfortably tell the 1871 graduating class of Bellevue Hospital College that he kept the phrase "spinal irritation" "on hand for patients that [*sic*] will insist on knowing the pathology of their complaints."[19(p389)] Gradually discarded by mainstream medicine and replaced by the term "neurasthenia" (and later, "depression"), spinal irritation entered into chiropractic through the subluxation terminology of bonesetters. Palmer extended the scope of spinal irritation and subluxation beyond the class of ailments that otherwise defied analysis; it was, for him, the key to understanding sickness as a whole. At the same time, the adoption of the widely accepted concept of spinal irritation lent credibility to chiropractic.

Popular Health Reform

Palmer cured the Davenport janitor of his deafness. This restoration of hearing might have been regarded as a freak occurrence were it not for a medical environment in which news of such occurrences was eagerly awaited. A well-publicized tug-of-war between "regulars" (physicians) and "irregulars" (alternative medicine practitioners) already had been sweeping the country.[20] The introduction of homeopathy, herbal medicine, "Mind Cure," Christian Science, health food, and hydropathy had prepared Americans to look for cases that, on the one hand, pointed to the limitations of mainstream medicine and, on the other, made the miraculous seem obtainable.[21] The way to perfect health was on the horizon, waiting to be grasped, described, and disseminated.

The unique union of bonesetting, magnetism, and orthodoxy was warmly received. The conflict for medical hegemony both helped and was helped by chiropractic. Palmer's invectives against the establishment of "germo-anti-toxis-vaxi-radi-electro-microbio-slush death producers"[22] resonated with the movement, as did his grandiose promises of a medicine "destined to be the grandest and greatest of this or any age"[16(p224)] because it was successful in all forms of disease. Chiropractic was the glamorous new recruit in the old war with mainstream medicine. Conventional medicine recognized the threat (see below) and had its own rhetoric ready. For example, in 1925, Morris Fishbein (1889–1976), editor of *The Journal of the American Medical Association*, wrote that chiropractors arrived on the health care scene "through the cellar . . . besmirched with dust and grime."[23(p98)]

Dissension Within the Movement

Palmer may have articulated a medical system with a single bold stroke, but neither he nor his son and successor, Bartlett Joshua Palmer (usually called "B. J.," 1882–1961), despite their best efforts, could keep it from beginning to unravel shortly thereafter.

Against the Notion of "Innate Intelligence"

Palmer's notion of innate intelligence (see the subsection on "Magnetic Healing" under "Chiropractic's Origin") was in dispute from the beginning. Many of his first disciples, destined themselves to be influential teachers of chiropractic, never adopted it. The list of those who reject the innate as "religious baggage" reads like an honor roll of chiropractic's history.[24] Willard Carver (1866–1940), who founded a core group of chiropractic teaching institutions, thought a physiological theory of nerves was sufficient.[25] John A. Howard (1876–1953), who came to chiropractic from a conventional medical background and, in 1906, founded what became the National College of Chiropractic, was thinking of innate intelligence when he warned students not to "dwindle or dwarf chiropractic by making a religion out of a technic."[26(p17)] The first chair of what became the Council for Chiropractic Accreditation, Claude O. Watkins (1909–1977), called for scientific research and the abandonment of all cultist and vitalist principles, starting with that of the innate.[27]

Today, a substantial number of chiropractors are anxious to sever all remaining ties to the vitalism of innate intelligence. For these practitioners, the notion of the innate serves only to maintain chiropractic as a fringe profession[28] and to delay its "transition into legitimate professional education, with serious scholarship, research, and service."[29(p41)]

Against the Notion of Subluxation

Palmer's followers were also quick to amend the notion of subluxation. For Palmer, the term referred to the static misalignment of a single vertebra. In the earliest chiropractic text ever published (*Modernized Chiropractic*, 1906), the meaning of subluxation was expanded to include issues of joint mobility.[30] In the late 1930s, these ideas were extended further, making spinal fixation, or restricted movement, the focus of chiropractic manipulation.[31] Some early chiropractors considered curvature of the spine and posture defects caused by muscular imbalance to be crucial and bone involvement secondary,[23] while others thought that subluxation arose from fatigue or tension in the back muscle.[32] Another group[33] maintained that subluxations were disturbances in the nerves themselves or in the muscles surrounding them, rather than defects in the bones.

Support for the original notion of subluxation was also reduced by continuous biomedical criticism that points away from, and finally discounts, bone alignment as the cause of back pain.[34] The criticism of an anatomist[35] who concluded after a series of experiments that it is nearly impossible for vertebral displacement to impinge on a spinal nerve at the intervertebral foramen has also weakened allegiance to the concept.

Many chiropractors no longer refer to simple subluxation but to a "vertebral subluxation complex," with an expanded meaning of mechanical impediments beyond bone displacement that can include mobility, posture, blood flow, muscle tone, and the condition of the nerves themselves.[36] Some want to abandon the term altogether because it "threatens to strangle the discipline."[37] Others speak of manipulable spinal lesions,[38] chiropractic lesions,[39] or vertebral blockage.[40] For D. D. Palmer, the meaning of subluxation was clear and unambiguous; today, it refers to an assortment of disturbances. Subluxation is defined less in theory than in practice: subluxation is what a chiropractor corrects. What Palmer initiated with a single thrust has evolved into an array of meanings.

The "Straight-Mixer" Schism

Serious as disagreement over the innate and subluxation was for chiropractic, it is overshadowed by the struggle for self-definition. For the Palmers, mastery over the spine meant mastery over nearly all disease. They believed that chiropractic was not the best response; it was the only response. When other practitioners suggested that they might be guilty of narrow-mindedness, B. J. Palmer denounced them as "chiropractoids" who had adulterated the "specific, pure, and unadulterated" chiropractic tradition, opening the way to "mixers."[41(p49)] B. J. Palmer's labeling of "straight" practitioners at war with "mixers" is still used today to describe an unresolved schism.

"Straights" tend to rely exclusively on spinal adjustments, to emphasize innate intelligence, and to subscribe to the notion that subluxation "is the leading cause of disease in the world today."[42(p25)] Since the 1930s, straights have been a very distinct minority in the profession.[43] Nonetheless, they have been able to transform their status as purists and heirs of the lineage into influence dramatically out of proportion to their numbers.[44]

"Mixers" tend to be more open to conventional medicine and to mainstream scientific tenets. For today's majority mixers, subluxation is one of many causes of disease.[45] This translates into a greater use of therapies other than spinal manipulation. The National Board of Chiropractic Examiners[46] indicates that most chiropractors use conventional physical therapy techniques, such as corrective exercise, ice packs, bracing, bed rest, moist heat, and massage. Nutritional supplements are the next leading nonmanipulative therapy in mixer practice, and depending on state laws, some chiropractors provide acupuncture, homeopathy, herbal remedies, and even biofeedback.[47]

Paradoxically, mixers, despite their wide range of therapeutics, tend to have a narrower and more modest claim for chiropractic's scope of practice. Also, some mixers see themselves less as traditional chiropractors and more as practitioners of a generic complementary medicine.[48] A second, larger group of mixers seeks to situate themselves in the broader mainstream health care system as specialists in musculoskeletal disorders.[49]

Spinal Manipulation: The Core Chiropractic Act

Adjusting with the hands—the signature chiropractic gesture—is the unifying activity that allows chiropractic to transcend its internal discord and create a coherent profession. Overriding disputes within the profession, the core question for all chiropractors remains unchanged and agreed on: how should the hands move the vertebrae? Beneath doctrinal disparity and clinical diversity, chiropractic has an internal cohesion that is more than a defensive reaction to a critical world. Chiropractors believe that the correction of spinal abnormality—the adjustment of vertebrae—is a critical healing act.

Obviously, vertebrae move all the time. The physical activities of daily life—exercise, turning, twisting, bending—require a normal range of motion. Greater mobility, or "mobilization," can be coaxed from the joints with the assistance of a physical therapist, for example, who can stretch the lower spine by gently moving the thigh of a person lying on his or her side. Eventually, mobilization reaches an elastic barrier of resistance, known to chiropractors as "end feel."

Chiropractic manipulation is a method of moving vertebrae beyond end feel, but not so far as to destroy the integrity of joint structure. The adjustment temporarily creates an increased range of motion. The patient feels the change and often hears a popping or cracking noise, which some attribute to a sudden liberation of synovial gases.[50]

The vertebrae can be moved by direct contact—the "short-lever" technique—or through a distant linkage, or the "long-lever" method. The latter method is used, for example, when a dynamic thrust of the thigh moves a vertebra in the lower spine. "Amplitude" refers to the depth or distance traveled by a practitioner's thrust. When joints are less accessible or when a long lever is involved, the amplitude increases. The degree of force applied is yet another variable.

Emblematic Chiropractic Adjustment

Palmer claimed to have discovered the use of spinous and transverse processes of the spine as levers and to be the first to use direct contact with a vertebra that was "out."[16(p19)] B. J. Palmer developed the "recoil adjustment," in which a practitioner quickly pushes the vertebra into motion and then, instead of maintaining pressure, relies on a fast release to generate a type of rebound. B. J. Palmer thought this maneuver allowed the body's innate intelligence to set a vertebra in its exact place. With or without recoil adjustment, the short-lever technique—touching the vertebra directly at high velocity and low amplitude, that is, by moving a small distance—with the spinal or transverse process as a fulcrum is considered the typical chiropractic maneuver.

Diversity in Manipulation

Chiropractors besides the Palmers were quick to make their own contributions, and the profession soon encompassed diverse styles, which often occasioned fresh disputes.[51] Whereas the Palmers emphasized one vertebra at a time, Carver developed methods to adjust the lumbar spine as a unit. Practitioners such as Oakley Smith and Solon Langworthy borrowed long-lever osteopathic techniques and folk methods such as Bohemian (Czech) manipulation. "Diversified technique" is the label for the largest and most eclectic collection of different methods many chiropractors use.[52]

Besides the forceful techniques, gentler methods of manipulation are common in chiropractic. The sacro-occipital technique, developed by DeJarnette in the 1930s,[53] relies on the passive weight of a patient pressing down on strategically placed padded wedges to reposition the pelvis and spine. The Logan basic technique[54] applies light thumb pressure close to the sacrotuberous ligament to move the sacrum. The activator technique[55] makes use of a small spring-loaded instrument that looks like a small plunger with a hard sponge on the tip to deliver pressure to the vertebrae. Some practitioners use tables with segmental drop pieces to allow low-force, high-velocity adjustment.[56] In total, observers of the profession have counted between 96[57] and more than 200[58] specifically chiropractic-type maneuvers. Most chiropractors draw on a variety of maneuvers on the basis of education and personal affinity, and most develop their own distinctive style.[59]

Chiropractic Battle for Acceptance

Chiropractic's cohesiveness has been forged in its battle for licensing. Chiropractors fought zealously for their current legal and professional status, suspending doctrinal wars when questions of state licensing were at stake.[60] The opposition was usually organized medicine.

From the beginning, chiropractors understood that the decisive factor for success was professional self-regulation, which would mean protection from uninformed and possibly adverse supervision and the bolstering of public confidence in the modality. State recognition was first achieved in Kansas in 1913; Louisiana granted recognition in 1974. The 60 years in between testify to the vehemence with which conventional medicine resisted.

Hostility on the part of conventional medicine usually backfired. The struggle in California serves as a case in point. Tullius Ratledge (1881–1967) led a fledgling movement to license chiropractic in the state.[61] In 1916, he was sentenced to 90 days in jail for practicing medicine without a license. As with most chiropractic arrests, the charge arose not from patient complaints but from medically instigated entrapment. Chiropractors were charged with violating the medical practice act and the controversy generated publicity on a scale the licensing attempt had never enjoyed before. California chiropractors adopted the slogan, "Go to jail for chiropractic." At the height of the controversy, 450 chiropractors were jailed in a single year.[62] Undeterred, many set up portable tables to treat fellow prisoners and visiting patients. Chiropractors forgot whether a colleague believed in the innate or subluxations or was a mixer or straight. By the time a woman chiropractor collapsed after a 10-day hunger strike in jail, public sympathy had swung to the side of chiropractic's courageous practitioners, and the medical lobby had been routed. In 1922, in a state referendum, Californians voted by an overwhelming majority to license the profession, and all chiropractors still in jail were pardoned on grounds that they had been unjustly accused.[10] Each state had its version of this battle; chiropractic emerged the winner every time.

Federal acceptance was later in coming, beginning in the 1970s when state licensing was already universal. Federal recognition consolidated state acceptance by providing coverage for chiropractic under Medicaid, Medicare, and Worker's Compensation; accepting the Council of Chiropractic Education as the official accrediting agency of chiropractic colleges; granting sick leave based on chiropractic certification for federal civil service employees; allowing federal income deductions for chiropractic care; and finally, allocating federal research money through the National Institutes of Health for chiropractic research.[45]

The final victory came with what chiropractors refer to as the "trial of the century," which again pitted them against the medical establishment. From its inception in 1847, the AMA had a clause that prohibited members from consulting with practitioners "whose practice is based on an exclusive dogma."[63(p171)] In 1957, in reaction to gains made by chiropractic, the AMA explicitly interpreted this clause to forbid consultations with chiropractors, and in 1963, the AMA's Committee on Quackery was formed primarily "to contain and eliminate chiropractic."[64(p292)]

In 1976, 5 chiropractors brought a suit against the AMA and allied conventional medical organizations. In 1987, after long and costly litigation, the US District Court in Illinois found the AMA and many of its associates, including the American College of Radiology and the American College of Surgeons, guilty of conspiracy against chiropractors and in violation of the federal antitrust laws. The permanent injunction issued against the AMA required *The Journal of the American Medical Association* to publish the court's judgment.[65] In 1990, the US Supreme Court let this decision stand without comment. The AMA, chiropractic's historic enemy, had been forced to cease and desist.

Chiropractic Health Care

Chiropractic health care is based on the endemic presence of pain, especially low back pain, in the United States. Between 70% and 80% of all adults experience low back pain at some time in their lives,[66] and in any one year, more than 50% of Americans suffer from the telltale nagging-tugging sensation.[67] So pervasive is back pain in this society that, as one authority has mused,[68] it might be abnormal not to suffer from it. Chronic pain is no less a problem, and data[69] suggest that nearly a third of the American population suffers from some sort of chronic pain.

It is no secret that low back pain and chronic pain are the Achilles' heel of biomedicine and present a need and opportunity for alternative responses. By far the largest percentage of patients—at least 80%—go to chiropractors for neuroskeletal and musculoskeletal problems.[70] Of these patients, at least 65% have back pain; most other symptoms involve the neck, extremities, and head.[71]

Patient Perceptions

Many large and methodologically sound surveys from diverse sampling populations leave little doubt that patients believe chiropractic works for them. The results show that most chiropractic patients and former patients are likely to be satisfied with the treatment they received.[72–75] Studies that compare patients' satisfaction with chiropractic with that of conventional medicine in treating low back pain demonstrate marked preference for chiropractic. A 1986 survey of members of a Washington State health maintenance organization that offers both conventional and chiropractic care compared the responses of 359 patients treated by conventional physicians with those of 348 patients treated by chiropractors. Patients treated by chiropractors for low back pain were 3 times as likely—66% to 22%—to report that they were "very satisfied" with the care they had received.[76] A Utah study (1973) reported comparable results.[77] Patients perceive chiropractic as a valuable component of their health care.

Scientific Evidence for Spinal Manipulation

Obviously, unimpeachable testimonials are not sufficient evidence of effectiveness or efficacy. Science demands controlled studies to establish legitimacy, and although the methodological problems for studying low back pain are notorious,[78] especially for nonpharmacological interventions,[79] such studies are the only basis for evaluating spinal manipulation. Fortunately, about 40 randomized controlled trials (RCTs), predominantly for low back pain, exist for spinal manipulation. Unfortunately, a substantial number of these RCTs actually concern forms of spinal manipulation that may not correspond to chiropractic treatment (eg, osteopathic manipulation, British Cyriax treatment, Australian Maitland methods, and Dutch manual therapy). Despite this additional weakness, these RCTs are the basis with which to evaluate the efficacy of spinal manipulation and, it is hoped, of chiropractic. The scientific investigation of clinical manipulation has taken 4 forms: sham-controlled RCTs, equivalency RCTs comparing manipulation with conventional treatments, systematic evaluations in the form of meta-analysis, and large-scale pragmatic RCTs.

Sham-Controlled RCTs for Low Back Pain

Since 1974, at least 11 single-blind RCTs with at least 1 arm being a sham control have been performed for spinal manipulation for low back pain. Four trials[80–83] show no difference with manipulation and sham; 3 trials[84–86] clearly show a benefit; and 3 trials[87–89] allow for the possibility of some value for manipulation, depending on what is considered the outcome, the duration of the outcome, and how outcome measures are aggregated. The methodological quality of these trials, with few exceptions, is weak (eg, high dropout rates, insufficient numbers, generalizability of treatment procedures, and outcome measures with uncertain relationships to expected changes), thus making conclusions problematic. Advocates argue that the practitioners were not properly trained and too little treatment was given, and detractors argue that there was insufficient blinding and that at least 1 of the interventions used more than manipulation.[85]

Equivalency or Comparative RCTs for Low Back Pain

At least 15 equivalency trials[90–104] for low back pain have been done in which 1 group of patients received manipulation and at least 1 other group received conventional treatment. These trials make a better case for spinal manipulation. Nine trials[90–98] show significant benefits, 4 trials[99–102] indicate no difference, 1 trial[103] is difficult to interpret, and 1[104] shows improvement in only a subgroup in the post hoc analysis. Again, problems abound. For example, which outcome and what exact time were prospectively viewed as the decisive measure are sometimes unclear. Also, a large 4-arm trial (manipulation vs physical therapy vs general practitioner vs placebo ultrasound or diathermy) is difficult to characterize because it combined patients with low back pain with those with neck pain and had both equivalency and sham comparisons. The results are nonetheless interesting: manipulation and physical therapy were significantly more beneficial than the general practitioner but did not reach statistical significance when compared with the sham trial. General practitioners' results were significantly worse than those in the sham comparisons.[105]

Equivalency trials can have problems. They often do not control for unequal belief and credibility and the comparability of physician-patient contact time, and it is sometimes questionable whether the conventional therapies in the comparison group have been adequately tested. Nonetheless, this evidence can be considered impressive. Most comparison trials show manipulation to be better, and no trial finds it to be significantly worse, than conventional treatments. As 1 researcher-scholar[44(p368)] put it, "more orthodox therapy, such as standard physical medicine or analgesics, despite being more 'scientific,' is not better."

Meta-analytic Reviews for Low Back Pain

Meta-analytic attempts to objectively summarize most of the above-mentioned spinal manipulation trials for low back pain and create a larger, more statistically valid pool of subjects on which to draw conclusions have been important in the scientific discussion of spinal manipulation. The most widely reported meta-analytic study of RCTs of manipulation for low back pain concluded that

> [S]pinal manipulation is of short-term benefit in some patients, particularly those with uncomplicated, acute low-back pain. Data are insufficient concerning the efficacy of spinal manipulation for chronic low-back pain.[106(p590)]

Another meta-analysis[107] reported similar findings. Still another systematic review that studied only the 5 trials that were clearly chiropractic manipulation (as opposed to other or imprecise forms of manual therapy) and did not mathematically aggregate the outcomes reported that[108(p487)]:

> [A]lthough the small numbers of chiropractic RCTs and the poor general methodological quality precludes [*sic*] the drawing of strong conclusions, chiropractic seems to be an effective treatment of back pain. However, more studies with a better research methodology are clearly still needed.

Pragmatic RCTs for Low Back Pain

Pragmatic RCTs compare 2 treatments under conditions in which they would be applied normally or optimally. Practitioners and patients are not blinded, and these trials generally do not control for a wide range of "nonspecific" effects. The goal is clinical decision. By far the largest and most sophisticated such pragmatic experiment took place in the United Kingdom. A total of 741 men and women with chronic low back pain at 11 matched pairs of chiropractic clinics and hospital outpatient departments were randomly assigned to either chiropractic or conventional care. The results demonstrated that

> chiropractic almost certainly confers worthwhile, long term benefit in comparison with hospital outpatient management. The benefit is seen mainly in those with chronic or severe pain."[109(p1431)]

The 3-year follow-up confirmed these findings.[110] Curiously, this study contradicts the preponderance of other RCTs in which the advantages of manipulation were more pronounced for acute pain. (Extrapolating these results to the United States is difficult because the biomedical management of low back pain in these 2 countries is radically different.)

As mentioned earlier, on the basis of these RCTs and meta-analyses, the Agency for Health Care Policy and Research in December 1994 stated[5(p34)] with guarded optimism that

> [M]anipulation can be helpful for patients with acute low back problems when used within the first month of symptoms. A trial of manipulation for patients with symptoms longer than a month is probably safe, but efficacy is unproven.

Scientific Evidence for the Benefits of Chiropractic for Neck Pain and Headache

After low back pain, neck pain and headache constitute the largest such research category, comprising at least 10 trials. Of 6 trials of neck pain,[111–116] 2 sham trials[111,112] show benefits with manipulation; 2 equivalency trials[113,114] show manipulation to be superior to conventional therapy; and in the 2 comparison trials in which manipulation is additive to conventional treatment in 1 arm, 1 trial[115] shows benefits of manipulation, and 1[116] shows no difference in treatment results. Whereas in a recent meta-analysis, it was believed that conclusions "must be made cautiously because of the small number of trials," it could still report that "there is early evidence to support the use of manual treatments in combination with other treatments for short term [neck] pain relief."[117(p1296)] Another recent meta-analysis[118] of cervical manipulation had a similar outcome. Of the headache trials, the single sham control trial[119] for migraine shows a benefit with manipulation, 2 equivalency trials[120,121] (1 for post-traumatic headache and 1 for tension headache) show a benefit with manipulation, and a third[122] (muscle-contraction headache) is difficult to interpret. Again, the systematic review hesitantly concluded that the manipulation "may be beneficial for muscle tension headaches."[118(p1755)]

Scientific Evidence for the Benefits of Manipulation for Other Conditions

The evidence for chiropractic's competence for conditions beyond pain is scarce. A few such RCTs exist and include menstrual pain,[123,124] hypertension,[125,126] and chronic obstructive lung disease.[127] Drawing any conclusions, besides that there is a need for research, is premature. This uneven balance of broad claims and scarce science is undoubtedly a source of friction between the profession and the biomedical community.

Adverse Effects of Chiropractic

The scientific value of manipulation needs to be viewed in the context of possible adverse effects. Of 138 cases of serious complications due to chiropractic, a recent review[128] found more than 8 of 10 were from cervical manipulation. Serious adverse incidences from neck rotation have included vertebrobasilar accidents with consequences such as brainstem or cerebellar infarction (or both), Wallenberg syndrome, locked-in syndrome, and such problems as spinal cord compression, vertebral fracture, tracheal rupture, diaphragm paralysis, and internal carotid hematoma.[118,129–131] Although the rate of serious complications is still debatable (because the exact denominator and numerator are unknown), estimates vary from 1 in 400,000[132] to between 3 and 6 per 10 million.[118] Some researchers[133] have advocated an informed consent procedure before patients receive cervical manipulation with thrust techniques, and others[118,134] have noted that appropriate examination procedures and specific styles of manipulation may reduce the incidence of complications. The potential for complications with lumbar spine manipulation seems less serious. The chief concern is cauda equina syndrome, and the estimated rate of occurrence has been between "one in many millions of treatments"[135] to less than 1 per 100 million manipulations.[106]

The Art of Medicine and Chiropractic's Effectiveness

It could be argued that additional evidence for chiropractic's effectiveness is still required for it to establish its scientific merits, especially for use beyond treating low back pain. Regardless of what future research will demonstrate, chiropractic will undoubtedly be an important and prominent feature of US health care. Part of its strength may lie in the domain of the art of healing and how the chiropractic profession negotiates the patient-physician relationship.

For people with chronic pain or with other refractory conditions, the chiropractic visit itself can be a source of comfort even without the addition of a demonstrable scientific component. Treatment by a chiropractor can generate a sense of understanding and meaning, an experience of comfort, an expectation of change, and a feeling of empowerment.[136] Chiropractic's combination of vitalist "innate intelligence" and simple mechanical explanation can give rich vocabulary for just those illnesses conventional medicine remains poorly equipped to address. Research indicates that for many of the illnesses chiropractic treats, precise diagnosis, assurance of recovery, and physician-patient agreement about the nature of a problem hasten recovery.[137,138]

Chiropractic finds its voice exactly where biomedicine becomes inarticulate. Too often, biomedicine fails to affirm a patient's chronic pain. Patients think their experience is brushed aside by a physician who treats it as unjustified, unfounded, or annoying, attitudes that heighten a patient's anguish and intensify suffering.[139] Chiropractors never have to put a patient's pain in the category of the "mind." They never fail to find a problem. By rooting pain in a clear physical cause, chiropractic validates the patient's experience. Even for patients with acute pain, chiropractic's assertiveness, clarity, and precision provide reassurances. As an anthropologist[140(p83)] has noted:

> [T]he chiropractor provides the patient with a structured, supportive environment and theoretical explanations designed to take the mystery out of process and problems. In essence, the chiropractor first manipulates a patient's belief structure before manipulating his or her physical structure.

Chiropractic is in no sense passive; it is, from the start, engaged. Except when contraindicated (as in patients with neoplastic disease and those with extreme osteoporosis), some form of therapy is almost always indicated. For most symptoms, there is a suitable manipulation or a designated mode of redress.

Chiropractic adjustment evokes an experience of change so palpable that the patient can often hear it in the characteristic "pop" or "crack," indicating that normal range of motion has been exceeded and a state of greater mobility and ease, however temporary, has been achieved. A perception of transformation has been audibly triggered. The chiropractic approach to healing relies on the opposite of double-blindedness; it enlists the full participation and awareness of both parties.

From the first encounter on, chiropractors generate different expectations from conventional physicians. Because conventional practitioners assume that back pain, in the absence of systemic signs, is likely to be self-limited, it is not unusual for a patient to wait weeks for an appointment with a specialist or for a radiographic diagnostic assessment. Because a chiropractor believes that back pain is both explicable and amenable to treatment, a patient can usually obtain an appointment within 24 hours of a telephone call. The message of empathy, urgency, comprehension, and support conveyed by such a rapid response is reassuring and provides a heightened sense of care and compassion.

Conclusions

Chiropractic has endured, grown, and thrived in the United States, despite internal contentiousness and external opposition. Its persistence suggests it will continue to endure as an important component of health care in the United States. In response to the countless requests for the treatment of pain, chiropractors have consistently offered the promise, assurance, and perception of relief. Chiropractic's ultimate lesson may be to reinforce the principle that the patient-physician relationship is fundamentally about words and deeds of connection and compassion. Chiropractic has managed to embody this message in the gift of the hands.

This study was supported in part by grant U24 AR43441 from the National Institutes of Health, Bethesda, Md; the John E. Fetzer Institute, Kalamazoo, Mich; the Waletzky Charitable Trust, Washington, DC; the Friends of the Beth Israel Hospital, Boston, Mass; the J. E. and Z. B. Butler Foundation, New York, NY; and the Kenneth J. Germeshausen Foundation, Boston, Mass.

We thank Harvey Blume, Janet Walzer, MEd, Debora Lane, and Marcia Rich for editorial assistance and Robb Scholten, Linda Barnes, PhD, Maria Van Rompay, and Anthony Rosner, PhD, for research assistance.

References

1. Deyo RA, Tsui-Wu YJ. Descriptive epidemiology of low-back pain and its related medical care in the United States. *Spine.* 1987;12:264–268.

2. Shekelle PG. *The Use and Costs of Chiropractic Care in the Health Insurance Experiment.* Santa Monica, Calif: RAND/Agency for Health Care Policy and Research; 1994. Publication MR-401-CCR.

3. Stano M. The chiropractic services market: a literature review. In: Scheffler R, Rossiter L, eds. *Advances in Health Economics and Health Services Research.* Greenwich, Conn: JAI Press; 1992;13:191–204.

4. DeLozier JE, Gagnon RO. *National Ambulatory Medical Care Survey: 1989 Summary.* Hyattsville, Md: National Center for Health Statistics; 1991. Advance Data From Vital and Health Statistics, No. 203.

5. Bigos S, Bowyer O, Braen B, et al. *Clinical Practice Guideline No. 14: Acute Low Back Problems in Adults.* Rockville, Md: US Dept of Health and Human Services, Agency for Health Care Policy and Research; 1994. AHCPR publication 95–0642.

6. Cooper RA, Stoflet SJ. Trends in the education and practice of alternative medicine clinicians. *Health Aff (Millwood).* 1996;15:226–238.

7. Plamondon RL. Hospital privileges survey. *Am Chiropract Assoc J Chiropract.* 1993;10:32–35.

8. Mootz RD, Meeker WC, Hawk C. Chiropractic in the health care system. In: Group Health Cooperative of Puget Sound, Seattle, Wash, Center for Health Studies, eds. *Chiropractic in the United States: Training, Practice, and Research.* Rockville, Md: US Dept of Health and Human Services, Public Health Service, Agency for Health Care Policy and Research; 1997:49–65.

9. Pelletier KR, Marie A, Krasner M, Haskell WL. Current trends in the integration and reimbursement of complementary and alternative medicine by managed care, insurance carriers, and hospital providers. *Am J Health Promot.* 1997;12:112–122.

10. Wardwell WI. *Chiropractic: History and Evolution of a New Profession.* St Louis, Mo: Mosby–Year Book; 1992.

11. Doan RA. *The Miller Heresy, Millennialism, and American Culture.* Philadelphia, Pa: Temple University Press; 1987.

12. Arasola K. *The End of Historicism: Millerite Hermeneutic of Time Prophecies in the Old Testament.* Uppsala, Sweden: Faculty of Theology, University of Uppsala; 1989.

13. Cooter R. Bones of contention? orthodox medicine and the mystery of the bone-setter's craft. In: Bynum WF, Porter R, eds. *Medical Fringe and Medical Orthodoxy, 1750–1850.* London, England: Croom Helm; 1987:158–173.

14. LeVay D. British bone-setters. *Hist Med Q.* 1971;3:13–15.

15. Paget J. Cases that bonesetters cure. *BMJ.* 1867;1:1–4.

16. Palmer DD. *Textbook of the Science, Art and Philosophy of Chiropractic.* Portland, Ore: Portland Printing; 1910.

17. Fuller RC. *Mesmerism and the American Cure of Souls.* Philadelphia: University of Pennsylvania Press; 1982.

18. Shorter E. *From Paralysis to Fatigue: A History of Psychosomatic Illness in the Modern Era.* New York, NY: Free Press; 1992.

19. Holmes OW. The young practitioner. In: *Medical Essays.* Boston, Mass: Houghton Mifflin Co; 1883:370–395.

20. Whorton JC. The first holistic revolution: alternative medicine in the nineteenth century. In: Stalker D, Glymour C, eds. *Examining Holistic Medicine.* Buffalo, NY: Prometheus; 1989: 29–48.

21. Gevitz N, ed. *Other Healers: Unorthodox Medicine in America.* Baltimore, Md: Johns Hopkins University Press; 1988.

22. Palmer DD, Palmer BJ. *The Science of Chiropractic: Its Principles and Adjustments.* Davenport, Iowa: The Palmer School of Chiropractic; 1906:10.

23. Fishbein M. *The Medical Follies.* New York, NY: Boni & Liveright; 1925.

24. Waagen G, Strang V. Origin and development of traditional chiropractic philosophy. In: Haldeman S, ed. *Principles and Practice of Chiropractic.* Norwalk, Conn: Appleton & Lange; 1992:29–43.

25. Jackson RB. Willard Carver, LL.B, D.C. 1866–1943: doctor, lawyer, Indian chief, prisoner and more. *Chiropract Hist.* 1994; 14:13–24.

26. Beideman RP. Seeking the rational alternative: the National College of Chiropractic from 1906 to 1982. *Chiropract Hist.* 1983;3:17–22.

27. Keating J, Claude O. Watkins: pioneer advocate for clinical scientific chiropractic. *Chiropract Hist.* 1987;7:11–15.

28. Winterstein JF. Is traditional "chiropractic philosophy" valid today? *Philos Constructs Chiropract Profession.* 1991;1:37–40.

29. DeBoer KF. Commentary: *eine kleine nacht* musing. *Am J Chiropract Med.* 1988;1:41.

30. Faye LJ, Wiles MR. Manual examination of the spine. In: Haldeman S, ed. *Principles and Practice of Chiropractic.* Norwalk, Conn: Appleton & Lange; 1992:301–318.

31. Gillet H. The history of motion palpation. *Eur J Chiropract.* 1983;31:196–201.

32. Heese N. Major Bernard De Jarnette: six decades of sacro occipital research, 1924–1984. *Chiropract Hist.* 1991;11:13–21.

33. Homewood AE. *The Neurodynamics of the Vertebral Subluxation.* Thornhill, Ontario: Chiropractic Publishers; 1973.

34. Goldstein M. Introduction, summary and analysis. In: *The Research Status of Spinal Manipulative Therapy.* Bethesda, Md: US Dept of Health, Education, and Welfare, Public Health Service, National Institutes of Health, National Institute of Neurological and Communicative Disorders and Stroke; 1975:3–7. Publication NIH 76–998.

35. Crelin ES. A scientific test of the chiropractic theory. *Am Scientist.* 1973;61:574–580.

36. Lantz CA. The vertebral subluxation complex, I: introduction to the model and the kinesiological component. *Chiropract Res J.* 1989;13:23–26.

37. Keating JC Jr. Science and politics and the subluxation. *Am J Chiropract Med.* 1988; 113:109–110.

38. Haldeman S. Spinal manipulation therapy: a status report. *Clin Orthop.* 1983;179:62–70.

39. Keating Jr JC. Shades of straight: diversity among the purists. *J Manipulative Physiol Ther.* 1992;15:203–209.

40. Lewit K. *Manipulative Therapy and Rehabilitation of the Locomotor System.* Woburn, Mass: Butterworth-Heinemann; 1985.

41. Moore JS. *Chiropractic in America: the History of a Medical Alternative.* Baltimore, Md: Johns Hopkins University Press; 1993:42–72.

42. Hammett RJ. Perfect practice parameters: part II. *Am J Clin Chiropract.* 1993;3:3.

43. Martin SC. Chiropractic and the social context of medical technology, 1895–1925. *Technol Cult.* 1993;34:808–834.

44. Coulehan JL. Adjustment, the hands and healing. *Cult Med Psychiatry.* 1985;9:353–382.

45. Baer HA. Divergence and convergence in two systems of manual medicine: osteopathy and chiropractic in the United States. *Med Anthropol Q.* 1987;1:176–193.

46. National Board of Chiropractic Examiners. *Job Analysis of Chiropractic.* Greeley, Colo: National Board of Chiropractic Examiners; 1993.

47. Lamm LC, Wegner E, Collard D. Chiropractic scope of practice: what the law allows—update. *J Manipulative Physiol Ther.* 1993; 18:16–20.

48. Jamison JR. Holistic health care in primary practice: chiropractic contributing to a sustainable health care system. *J Manipulative Physiol Ther.* 1992;15:604–608.

49. Cassata DM. Chiropractic clinical purpose: primary care of limited specialty. *Philos Constructs Chiropract Profession.* 1991;1:6–10.

50. Kirkaldy-Willis WH, Cassidy JD. Spinal manipulation in the treatment of low-back pain. *Can Fam Physician.* 1985;31:535–540.

51. Grice A, Vernon H. Basic principles in the performance of chiropractic adjusting: historical review, classification, and objectives. In: Haldeman S, ed. *Principles and Practice of Chiropractic.* Norwalk, Conn: Appleton & Lange; 1992:443–458.

52. Gitelman R, Fligg B. Diversified technique. In: Haldeman S,ed. *Principles and Practice of Chiropractic.* Norwalk, Conn: Appleton & Lange; 1992:483–501.

53. DeJarnette MB. *Sacro Occipital Technic.* Nebraska City, Neb: MB DeJarnette; 1984.

54. Logan VF. *Logan Basic Methods.* St Louis, Mo: Logan College of Chiropractic; 1956.

55. Smith DB, Fuhr AW, Davis BP. Skin accelerometer displacement and relative bone movement of adjacent vertebrae in response to chiropractic percussion thrusts. *J Manipulative Physiol Ther.* 1989;12:26–37.

56. Bergmann TF. Manual force, mechanically assisted articular chiropractic technique using long and/or short lever contacts. *J Manipulative Physiol Ther.* 1993;16:33–36.

57. Bergmann TF. Various forms of chiropractic technique. *Chiropract Technique.* 1993; 5:53–55.

58. Williams SE. The Mercy Conference document. *Am J Clin Chiropract.* 1993;3:1, 24.

59. Bartol KM. A model for the categorization of chiropractic treatment procedures. *Chiropract Technique.* 1991;3:78–80.

60. Wardwell WI. The cutting edge of chiropractic recognition: prosecution and legislation in Massachusetts. *Chiropract Hist.* 1982;2:54–65.

61. Keating JC Jr, Brown R, Smallie P. T. F. Ratledge, the missionary of straight chiropractic in California. *Chiropract Hist.*1991;11:27–36.

62. Reed LS. *The Healing Cults. A Study of Sectarian Medical Practices: Its Extent, Causes and Control.* Chicago, Ill: University of Chicago Press; 1932.

63. Rothstein WG. *American Physicians in the 19th Century: From Sects to Science.* Baltimore, Md: Johns Hopkins University Press; 1985.

64. Gevitz N. The chiropractors and the AMA: reflections on the history of the consultation clause. *Perspect Biol Med.* 1989;32:281–299.

65. Getzendanner S. Permanent injunction order against the AMA [special communication]. *JAMA.* 1988;259:81–82.

66. Frymoyer JW. Back pain and sciatica. *N Engl J Med.* 1988;318:291–300.

67. Sternbach RA. Survey of pain in the United States: the Nuprin Pain Report. *Clin J Pain.* 1986;2:49–53.

68. Kahanovitz N. *Diagnosis and Treatment of Low Back Pain.* New York, NY: Raven Press; 1991.

69. Bonica JJ. Preface. In: Ng LKY, ed. *New Approaches to Treatment of Chronic Pain: A Review of Multidisciplinary Pain Clinics and Pain Centers.* Washington, DC: US Dept of Health and Human Services, National Institute on Drug Abuse; 1981:vii–x.

70. Mootz RD, Shekelle PG. Content of practice. In: Group Health Cooperative of Puget Sound, Seattle, Wash, Center for Health Studies, eds. *Chiropractic in the United States: Training, Practice, and Research.* Rockville, Md: US Dept of Health and Human Services, Public Health Service, Agency for Health Care Policy and Research; 1997:67–90.

71. Hurwitz EL, Coulter ID, Adams AH, Genovese BJ, Shekelle PG. Use of chiropractic services from 1985 through 1991 in the United States and Canada. *Am J Public Health.* 1998; 88:771–775.

72. Wardwell WI. The Connecticut survey of public attitudes toward chiropractic. *J Manipulative Physiol Ther.* 1989;12:109–121.

73. Nationwide survey yields insights into the public's views of chiropractic care. *ACA J Chiropract.* 1993;30:28–31.

74. Sanchez JE. A look in the mirror: a critical and exploratory study of public perceptions of the chiropractic profession in New Jersey. *J Manipulative Physiol Ther.* 1991;14:165–176.

75. Sawyer CE, Kassak K. Patient satisfaction with chiropractic care. *J Manipulative Physiol Ther.* 1993;16:25–32.

76. Cherkin DC, MacCornack FA. Patient evaluations of low back pain care from family physicians and chiropractors. *West J Med.* 1989;150:351–355.

77. Kane RL, Olsen D, Leymaster C, Woolley FR, Fisher FK. Manipulating the patient: a comparison of the effectiveness of physician and chiropractor care. *Lancet.* 1974;1:1333–1336.

78. Bloch R. Methodology in clinical back pain trials. *Spine.* 1987;12:430–432.

79. Koes BW, Bouter LM, van der Heijden GJ. Methodological quality of randomized clinical trials on treatment efficacy in low back pain. *Spine.* 1995;20:228–235.

80. Bergquist-Ullman M, Larsson U. Acute low back pain in industry: a controlled prospective study with special reference to therapy and confounding factors. *Acta Orthop Scand.* 1977;170:1–117.

81. Sims-Williams H, Jayson MI, Young SM, Baddeley H, Collins E. Controlled trial of mobilisation and manipulation for low back pain: hospital patients. *BMJ.* 1979;2:1318–1320.

82. Godfrey CM, Morgan PP, Schatzker J. A randomized trial of manipulation for low-back pain in a medical setting. *Spine.* 1984; 9:301–304.

83. Gibson T, Grahame R, Harkness J, Woo P, Blagrave P, Hills R. Controlled comparison of short-wave diathermy treatment with osteopathic treatment in non-specific low back pain. *Lancet.* 1985;1:1258–1261.

84. Waagen GN, Haldeman S, Cook G, Lopez D, DeBoer KF. Short term trial of chiropractic adjustments for the relief of chronic low back pain. *Manual Med.* 1986;2:63–67.

85. Ongley MJ, Klein RG, Dorman TA, Eek BC, Hubert LJ. A new approach to the treatment of chronic low back pain. *Lancet.* 1987; 2:143–146.

86. Triano JJ, McGregor M, Hondras MA, Brennan PC. Manipulative therapy versus education programs in chronic low back pain. *Spine.* 1995; 20:948–955.

87. Glover JR, Morris JG, Khosla T. Back pain: a randomized clinical trial of rotational manipulation of the trunk. *Br J Ind Med.* 1974;31:59–64.

88. Sims-Williams H, Jayson MI, Young SM, Baddeley H, Collins E. Controlled trial of mobilisation and manipulation for patients with low back pain in general practice. *BMJ.* 1978; 2(6148):1338–1340.

89. Hoehler FK, Tobis JS, Buerger AA. Spinal manipulation for low back pain. *JAMA.* 1981; 245:1835–1838.

90. Evans DP, Burke MS, Lloyd KN, Roberts EE, Roberts GM. Lumbar spinal manipulation on trial, part 1: clinical assessment. *Rheumatol Rehabil.* 1978;17:46–53.

91. Rasmussen GG. Manipulation in treatment of low back pain: a randomized clinical trial. *Manual Med.* 1979;1:8–10.

92. Coxhead CE, Inskip H, Meade TW, North WR, Troup JD. Multicentre trial of physiotherapy in the management of sciatic symptoms. *Lancet.* 1981;1:1065–1068.

93. Farrell JP, Twomey LT. Acute low back pain: comparison of two conservative treatment approaches. *Med J Aust.* 1982;1:160–164.

94. Nwuga VC. Relative therapeutic efficacy of vertebral manipulation and conventional treatment in back pain management. *Am J Phys Med.* 1982;61:273–278.

95. Arkuszewski Z. The efficacy of manual treatment in low back pain: a clinical trial. *Manual Med.* 1986;2:268–271.

96. Hadler NM, Curtis P, Gillings DB, Stinnett S. A benefit of spinal manipulation as adjunctive therapy for acute low-back pain: a stratified controlled trial. *Spine.* 1987;12:702–706.

97. Postacchini F, Facchini M, Palieri P. Efficacy of various forms of conservative treatment in low back pain: a comparative study. *Neuro-Orthop.* 1988;6:28–35.

98. Hsieh CYJ, Phillips RB, Adams AH, Pope MH. Functional outcomes of low back pain: comparison of four treatment groups in a randomized controlled trial. *J Manipulative Physiol Ther.* 1992;15:4–9.

99. Doran DM, Newell DJ. Manipulation in treatment of low back pain: a multicentre study *BMJ.* 1975;2:161–164.

100. Zylbergold RS, Piper MC. Lumbar disc disease: comparative analysis of physical therapy treatments. *Arch Phys Med Rehabil.* 1981; 62:176–179.

101. Waterworth RF, Hunter IA. An open study of diflunisal, conservative and manipulative therapy in the management of acute mechanical low back pain. *N Z Med J.* 1985;98:372–375.

102. Kinalski R, Kuwik W, Pietrzak D. The comparison of the results of manual therapy versus physiotherapy methods used in treatment of patients with low back pain syndromes. *J Manual Med.* 1989;4:44–46.

103. Mathews JA, Mills SB, Jenkins VM, et al. Back pain and sciatica: controlled trials of manipulation, traction, sclerosant and epidural injections. *Br J Rheumatol.* 1987;26:416–423.

104. MacDonald RS, Bell CM. An open controlled assessment of osteopathic manipulation in nonspecific low-back pain. *Spine.* 1990; 15:364–370.

105. Koes BW, Bouter LM, van Mameren H, et al. The effectiveness of manual therapy, physiotherapy, and treatment by the general practitioner for nonspecific back and neck complaints: a randomized clinical trial. *Spine.* 1992;17:28–35.

106. Shekelle PG, Adams AH, Chassin MR, Hurwitz EL, Brook RH. Spinal manipulation for low-back pain. *Ann Intern Med.* 1992; 117:590–598.

107. Anderson R, Meeker WC, Wirick BE, Mootz RD, Kirk DH, Adams A. A meta-analysis of clinical trials of spinal manipulation. *J Manipulative Physiol Ther.* 1992;15:181–194.

108. Assendelft WJ, Koes BW, van der Heijden GJ, Bouter LM. The efficacy of chiropractic manipulation for back pain: blinded review of relevant randomized clinical trials. *J Manipulative Physiol Ther.* 1992;15:487–494.

109. Meade TW, Dyer S, Browne W, Townsend J, Frank AO. Low back pain of mechanical origin: randomised comparison of chiropractic and hospital outpatient treatment. *BMJ.* 1990;300:1431–1437.

110. Meade TW, Dyer S, Browne W, Frank AO. Randomised comparison of chiropractic and hospital outpatient management of low back pain: results from extended follow-up. *BMJ.* 1995;311:349–351.

111. Kogstad OA, Karterud S, Gudmundsen J. Cerviobrachialgia: a controlled trial with conventional therapy and manipulation [in Norwegian]. *Tidsskr Nor Laegeforen.* 1978;98:845–848.

112. Cassidy JD, Lopes AA, Yong-Hing K. The immediate effect of manipulation versus mobilization on pain and range of motion in the cervical spine: a randomized controlled trial. *J Manipulative Physiol Ther.* 1992;15:570–575.

113. Brodin H. Cervical pain and mobilization. *Manual Med.* 1982;20:90–94.

114. Vernon HT, Aker P, Burns S, Viljakaanen S, Short L. Pressure pain threshold evaluation of the effect of spinal manipulation in the treatment of chronic neck pain: a pilot study. *J Manipulative Physiol Ther.* 1990;13:13–16.

115. Howe DH, Newcombe RG, Wade MT. Manipulation of the cervical spine: a pilot study. *J R Coll Gen Pract.* 1983;33:574–579.

116. Sloop PR, Smith DS, Goldenberg E, Dore C. Manipulation for chronic neck pain: a double-blind controlled study. *Spine.* 1982;7:532–535.

117. Aker PD, Gross AR, Goldsmith CH, Peloso P. Conservative management of mechanical neck pain: systematic overview and meta-analysis. *BMJ.* 1996;313:1291–1296.

118. Hurwitz EL, Aker PD, Adams AH, Meeker WC, Shekelle PG. Manipulation and mobilization of the cervical spine: a systematic review of the literature. *Spine.* 1996;21:1746–1760.

119. Parker GB, Tupling H, Pryor DS. A controlled trial of cervical manipulation of migraine. *Aust N Z J Med.* 1978;8:589–593.

120. Jensen OK, Nielsen FF, Vosmar L. An open study comparing manual therapy with the use of cold packs in the treatment of post-traumatic headache. *Cephalalgia.* 1990;10:241–250.

121. Boline PD, Kassak K, Bronfort G, Nelson C, Anderson AV. Spinal manipulation vs. amitriptyline for the treatment of chronic tension-type headaches: a randomized clinical trial. *J Manipulative Physiol Ther.* 1995; 18:148–154.

122. Hoyt WH, Shaffer F, Bard DA, et al. Osteopathic manipulation in the treatment of muscle-contraction headache. *J Am Osteopath Assoc.* 1979;78:322–325.

123. Kokjohn K, Schmid DM, Triano JJ, Brennan PC. The effect of spinal manipulation on pain and prostaglandin levels in women with primary dysmenorrhea. *J Manipulative Physiol Ther.* 1992;15:279–285.

124. Boesler D, Warner M, Alpers A, Finnerty EP, Kilmore MA. Efficacy of high-velocity low-amplitude manipulation technique in subjects with low-back pain during menstrual cramping. *J Am Osteopath Assoc.* 1993;93:203–208.

125. Morgan JP, Dickey JL, Hunt HH, Hudgins PM. A controlled trial of spinal manipulation in the management of hypertension. *J Am Osteopath Assoc.* 1985;85:308–313.

126. Yates RG, Lamping DL, Abram NL, Wright C. Effects of chiropractic treatment for blood pressure and anxiety: a randomized, controlled trial. *J Manipulative Physiol Ther.* 1988;11:484–488.

127. Miller WD. Treatment of visceral disorders by manipulative therapy. In: Goldstein M, ed. *The Research Status of Spinal Manipulative Therapy.* Bethesda, Md: National Institutes of Health; 1975:295–302.

128. Powell FC, Hanigan WC, Olivero WC. A risk/benefit analysis of spinal manipulation for relief or lumbar or cervical pain. *Neurosurgery.* 1993;33:73–78.

129. Terrett A. Vascular accidents from cervical spine manipulation: report of 107 cases. *J Aust Chiropract Assoc.* 1987;17:15–24.

130. Lee KP, Carlini WG, McCormick GF, Albers GW. Neurologic complications following chiropractic manipulation: a survey of California neurologists. *Neurology.* 1995;45:1213–1215.

131. Krueger BR, Okazaki H. Vertebral-basilar distribution infarction following chiropractic cervical manipulation. *Mayo Clin Proc.* 1980; 55:322–332.

132. Dvorak J, Orelli F. How dangerous is manipulation of the cervical spine: case report and results of a survey. *Manual Med.* 1985;2:1–4.

133. Assendelft WJJ, Bouter LM, Knipschild PG, Bouter SM. Complications of spinal manipulation: a comprehensive review of the literature. *J Fam Pract.* 1996;42:475–480.

134. Terrett AGJ, Kleynhans AM. Cerebrovascular complications of manipulation. In: Haldeman S, ed. *Principles and Practice of Chiropractic.* Norwalk, Conn: Appleton & Lange; 1992: 579–598.

135. Haldeman S, Rubinstein SM. Cauda equina syndrome following lumbar spine manipulation. *Spine.* 1992;17:1469–1473.

136. Csordas TJ. The rhetoric of transformation in ritual healing. *Cult Med Psychiatry.* 1983; 7:333–375.

137. Thomas KB. General practice consultations: is there any point of being positive? *BMJ.* 1987;294:1200–1202.

138. Bass MJ, Buck C, Turner L, Dickie G, Pratt G, Robinson HC. The physician's actions and the outcome of illness in family practice. *J Fam Pract.* 1986;23:43–47.

139. Engelbart HJ, Vrancken MA. Chronic pain from the perspective of health: a view based on systems theory. *Soc Sci Med.* 1984; 19:1383–1392.

140. Oths K. Communication in a chiropractic clinic: how a DC treats his patient. *Cult Med Psychiatry.* 1993;18:83–113.

60 Spinal Manipulation in the Treatment of Episodic Tension-Type Headache

A Randomized Controlled Trial

Geoffrey Bove, DC, PhD; Niels Nilsson, DC, MD, PhD
From the Center for Biomechanics, Department of Anatomy and Cell Biology, Odense University, Odense, Denmark. Dr Bove is now with the Department of Anesthesia and Critical Care, Beth Israel Deaconess Medical Center and Harvard Medical School, Boston, Mass.

Context
Episodic tension-type headache is common and is often treated using manual therapies. Few data exist for the efficacy of these interventions.

Objective
To determine the effects of spinal manipulation therapy on adults with episodic tension-type headache.

Design
Randomized controlled trial lasting 19 weeks.

Setting
Outpatient facility of a National Health Service–funded chiropractic research institution in Denmark.

Participants
Volunteer sample of 26 men and 49 women aged 20 to 59 years who met the diagnostic criteria for episodic tension-type headache as defined by the International Headache Society.

Intervention
Participants were randomized into 2 groups, 1 receiving soft tissue therapy and spinal manipulation (the manipulation group), and the other receiving soft tissue therapy and a placebo laser treatment (the control group). All participants received 8 treatments over 4 weeks; all treatments were performed by the same chiropractor.

Main Outcome Measures
Daily hours of headache, pain intensity per episode, and daily analgesic use, as recorded in diaries.

Results
Based on intent-to-treat analysis, no significant differences between the manipulation and control groups were observed in any of the 3 outcome measures. However, by week 7, each group experienced significant reductions in mean daily headache hours (manipulation group, reduction from 2.8 to 1.5 hours; control group, reduction from 3.4 to 1.9 hours) and mean number of analgesics per day (manipula-

tion group, reduction from 0.66 to 0.38; control group, reduction from 0.82 to 0.59). These changes were maintained through the observation period. Headache pain intensity was unchanged for the duration of the trial.

Conclusion

As an isolated intervention, spinal manipulation does not seem to have a positive effect on episodic tension-type headache.

JAMA. 1998;280:1576–1579

Tension-type headaches (TTHs) are extremely common, affecting more than one third of the population[1] and accounting for more than two thirds of all headache episodes.[2] The pain of TTHs is usually mild to moderate and typically bilateral. Symptoms are usually described as pressing or tightening with a nonpulsating quality, and symptoms characteristic of migraine (nausea, vomiting, photophobia, and phonophobia) are absent. The International Headache Society (IHS) classifies persons with 1 to 15 and 16 or more occurrences of TTH per month as having episodic TTH (ETTH) and chronic TTH, respectively.[3] Episodic tension-type headache is by far the more common form, with a 1-year prevalence of more than 38%.[1] Because many sufferers report interference with their lifestyle, ETTH has a significant socioeconomic impact.[1]

Although ETTH is typically medically treated with nonprescription analgesics, many people with ETTH seek hands-on therapy, delivered by various groups of practitioners. Several uncontrolled studies have suggested that a combination of physical treatment methods can lessen the symptoms of TTH,[4–8] and the single randomized controlled study using IHS criteria suggested a positive treatment effect of a combination of therapies (including manipulation, heat, massage, and trigger-point therapy) for chronic TTH,[9] compared with a hands-off pharmaceutical treatment protocol. In all these studies, however, it is unclear whether the effects were due to one, all, or a combination of the treatment elements. The common element in these studies was joint manipulation, recently demonstrated to be effective in the treatment of cervicogenic headache.[10] The sole report using manipulation as an isolated treatment for TTH found a reduction in pain intensity immediately after the treatment, but the subjects were not further evaluated.[11] The goal of this randomized controlled trial was to evaluate the long-term effect of joint manipulation as an isolated intervention for ETTH.

Methods

Experimental Design

This was a randomized, controlled clinical trial with a blinded observer designed to evaluate the effect of spinal manipulative therapy in the treatment of ETTH. The trial was carried out in the outpatient facility of a National Health Service–funded independent chiropractic research institution (Nordisk Institut for Kiropraktik, Odense, Denmark). Data were interpreted by a blinded observer and analyzed at the Center for Biomechanics, Faculty of Health Science, Odense University, Odense, Denmark. All procedures were approved by the regional ethics committee (permit No. 97/12), and all subjects gave verbal and written informed consent prior to participation.

Participants

Participants were recruited from the general community by advertisements in the local newspapers. Initial eligibility screening was done over the telephone, followed by a personal interview and physical examination. Eligibility criteria for participation in this study were as follows: (1) fulfillment of IHS criteria for ETTH,[3] with more than 5 but fewer than 15 headache episodes per month; (2) age 20 to 60 years; (3) score for typical headache intensity between 25 and 85 on a visual analog scale from 0 to 100; and (4) no relative or absolute contraindications to manipulation. The selection refinements of criteria 1 and 3 were designed to better allow the possibility of seeing a change by using more typical rather than very mild or severe cases. After acceptance, a participant could be excluded for any adverse reaction to treatment or any event triggering or potentially triggering a change in headache status (eg, vehicular crash with neck injury).

Participants were informed that the purpose of the trial was to compare the relative efficacy of 2 physical treatments commonly used for ETTH. Participants were instructed to continue their normal lifestyle during the trial, including their usual pattern of medication.

Interventions

After baseline data collection and randomization (see below), participants underwent 1 of 2 treatment protocols. All participants received 8 treatments over 4 weeks, all performed by one chiropractor (Birthe Hove Madsen, DC) and each lasting approximately 15 minutes. The chiropractor routinely uses both treatment protocols in daily practice and was confident in performing both techniques. The manipulation group received joint manipulation of the cervical spine as determined by the chiropractor based on palpatory examinations and also deep friction massage (including trigger-point therapy, if indicated) of the trapezius and muscles deep to it. Specific manipulation maneuvers consisted of diversified and/or toggle-recoil techniques, depending on the level of the palpated segmental dysfunction.[12] These techniques use a high-velocity, low-amplitude thrust delivered in a specific line of drive at the palpated end point of the normal passive range of motion and are often accompanied by a clicking or cracking noise.

The control group also received deep friction massage. In addition, this group underwent the application of low-power laser light (Omega Biotherapy, London, England) to the upper cervical region. No effect, apart from placebo, can be expected from low-power laser therapy.[13]

The control group was designed to be an active control group for spinal manipulation, with the added goal of making the 2 groups more similar. A control group that receives no treatment is not ideal in procedures that use physical contact; in this study, every active intervention parameter was identical in the 2 groups except for the actual manipulation procedure. Our design allowed evaluation of the contribution of spinal manipulation, as it was the only difference between the 2 groups.

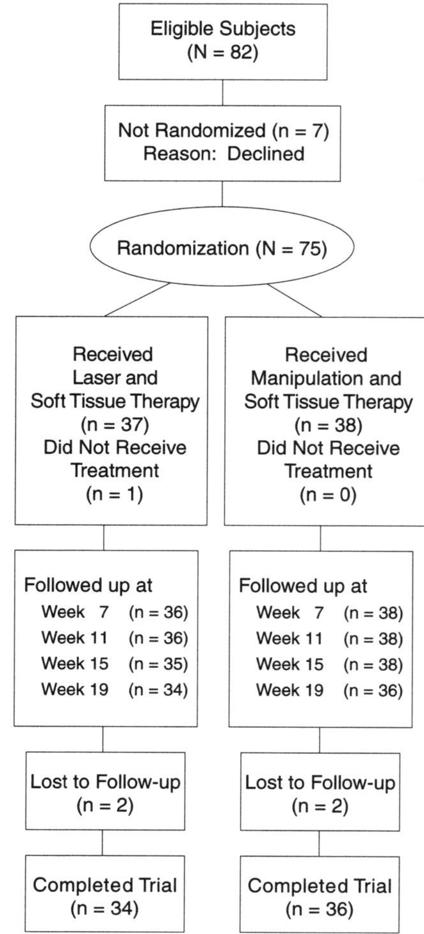

Figure 1. Progression of subjects through the trial, including withdrawal and follow-up losses.

Measurements and Procedures

The trial lasted 19 weeks. In weeks 1 and 2, data were collected to determine a baseline for the outcome variables. Before starting week 3, participants were randomized to either the manipulation group or the control group by a blinded drawing of a ticket by a secretary. In weeks 3 through 6, subjects were treated 8 times, usually twice a week. Posttreatment data were collected from headache diaries completed during weeks 7, 11, 15, and 19.

All participants were required to fill out a headache diary[14] for each of weeks 1, 2, 7, 11, 15, and 19. Recorded information included hours per day that headache was present, the intensity of the headache, and daily analgesic consumption. Additionally, to reveal any difference between the 2 physical treatment regimens in their ability to generate a placebo effect, participants scored their expected treatment outcome on a visual analog scale immediately before randomization and again immediately after the first treatment session, before a new treatment effect could have been noted.[15]

Outcome Measures

The primary outcome measures were the number of headache hours per day, mean headache intensity per headache episode, and consumption of analgesics per day. From a previous study on a similar headache population,[10] we expected most patients to stay with their preferred analgesic regimen throughout the trial period. In case of medication change, 500 mg of acetylsalicylic acid, 500 mg of paracetamol, and 200 mg of ibuprofen were regarded as equivalent doses. All data were retrieved from the diaries by assistants unaware of the treatment group assignment.

Table 1. Pretreatment Characteristics of the Study Population*

Variable	Whole Group	Control Group	Manipulation Group	*P* Value for Difference†
No. of subjects	75	37	38	. . .
Sex				
Male	26	11	15	.52
Female	49	26	23	(Fisher exact)
Age, mean (range), y	38 (20–59)	38 (20–58)	37 (22–59)	.86
Mean headache hours per day (95% CI)	3.1 (2.5–3.7)	3.4 (2.4–4.4)	2.8 (2.1–3.5)	.29
Mean headache intensity, VAS, per episode (95% CI)	38/100 (35–41/100)	37/100 (33–41/100)	37/100 (33–41/100)	.89
Mean No. of analgesics per day (95% CI)	0.74 (0.56–0.92)	0.82 (0.50–1.14)	0.66 (0.49–0.83)	.38

*CI indicates confidence interval; VAS, visual analog scale. Ellipses indicate data not applicable.
†Reported as *t* test, unless otherwise noted.

Table 2. Results of Outcome Variables During the 13-Week Follow-up Period*

Outcome Variable	Control Group	Manipulation Group	*P* Value for Difference (*t* Test)
Mean analgesics per day (95% CI)			
Week 7 (n=73)	0.59 (0.00–1.49)	0.38 (0.00–0.76)	.14
Week 11 (n=73)	0.54 (0.30–0.78)	0.41 (0.27–0.55)	.35
Week 15 (n=72)	0.60 (0.26–0.94)	0.48 (0.34–0.62)	.51
Week 19 (n=69)	0.56 (0.22–0.90)	0.48 (0.34–0.62)	.66
Mean headache hours per day (95% CI)			
Week 7 (n=74)	1.9 (0.9–2.9)	1.5 (1.1–1.9)	.33
Week 11 (n=74)	1.7 (0.9–2.5)	1.6 (1.2–2.0)	.77
Week 15 (n=73)	2.1 (1.1–3.1)	1.6 (1.2–2.0)	.30
Week 19 (n=70)	2.2 (1.2–3.2)	2.1 (1.3–2.9)	.87
Mean headache intensity (95% CI)			
Week 7 (n=74)	34 (26–38)/100	38 (30–46)/100	.43
Week 11 (n=74)	30 (26–38)/100	36 (28–44)/100	.28
Week 15 (n=73)	33 (25–41)/100	29 (23–35)/100	.41
Week 19 (n=70)	26 (20–32)/100	35 (27–43)/100	.13

*CI indicates confidence interval.

Statistical Analysis

The outcome measures were compared between pretreatment and each posttreatment period within and between the 2 treatment groups. A sample size of 84 was projected to provide a power of 90% to detect a 1-hour difference between the 2 groups in mean number of daily headache hours and a difference in headache intensity of 13/100 per episode, as scored on the visual analog scale. All tests of hypotheses and reported *P* values are 2-tailed. Statistical analysis was conducted on an intention-to-treat basis, using StatView (Abacus Concepts, Berkeley, Calif).

Results

Subjects

Participant flow and retention is summarized in Figure 1. Recruitment was conducted over a 9-month period from February through October 1997. Of the persons who responded to the advertisements and completed telephone and personal interviews, 82 fulfilled the inclusion criteria; of these, 7 did not wish to take part in the study, leaving 75 participants to enter the trial. The characteristics of the randomized participants are shown in Table 1. There were no statistically significant differences between the 2 groups with respect to age, sex, mean headache hours per day, mean headache intensity per episode, or use of analgesics. No side effects were experienced by any participant in either group.

One participant was excluded in week 5 following a neck injury due to a car crash. One participant from the placebo group was lost to follow-up at week 15 and a further 3 (manipulation group, 2; control group, 1) were lost to follow-up in week 19.

Outcomes

There was no significant difference between the 2 groups for any outcome variable before or following treatment (Table 1 and Table 2, Figure 2). However, mean headache

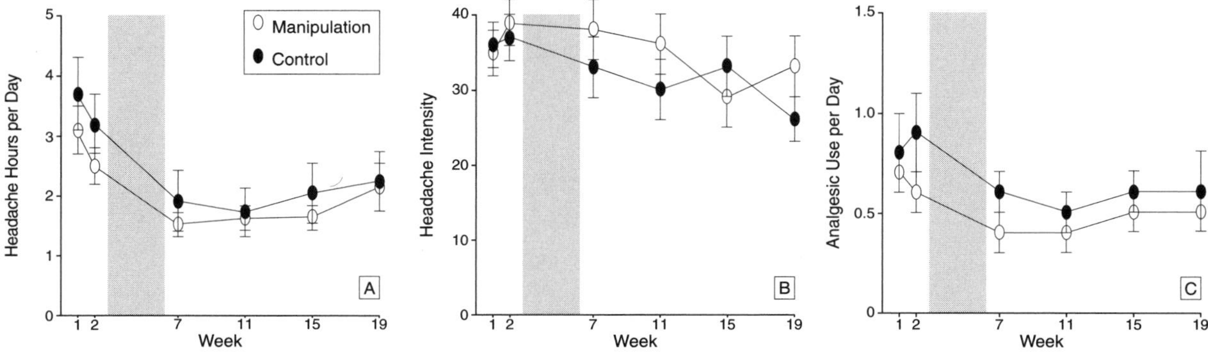

Figure 2. Results of primary outcome measures. No difference was observed between groups for any measure. Intervention in weeks 3 to 6 indicated by shaded areas. Error bars equal 1 SE.

hours per day and analgesic use within both groups showed improvement from pretreatment to week 7. The mean headache hours per day was reduced by approximately 1.5 hours by week 7 (95% confidence interval [CI], –2.4 to –0.6; Figure 2, B), and this change did not lessen significantly by the end of the trial. Headache intensity was unchanged for the duration of the trial (95% CI, –12 to 11; Figure 2, C). Analgesic consumption also lessened in both groups by week 7 (95% CI, –0.5 to –0.1; Figure 2, B). Of the 74 participants, 48 stayed with the same medication throughout the trial and 25 switched between 2 of the following: 500 mg of acetylsalicylic acid, 500 mg of paracetamol, or 200 mg of ibuprofen. One participant switched between acetylsalicylic acid and a morphine preparation; analgesic data for this person were not included in the results. Analysis of the 48 participants who continued their same medication yielded similar results (data not shown).

The expected treatment outcome was similar in both the manipulation group and the control group before (95% CI, 69–83/100 vs 68–80/100) and after (95% CI, 64–80/100 vs 69–81/100) the initial treatment. The treatment expectation did not change following the first treatment (95% CI, –2 to 10/100 vs –5 to 7/100), indicating that the 2 treatment methods had no major placebogenic differences.

Comment

This study showed that spinal manipulation did not significantly improve the outcome for ETTH. We point out that our study population was carefully selected based on accepted criteria for ETTH. In practice, ETTH and cervicogenic headache can be difficult to differentiate,[16] and often occur together.[17] Our conclusions are in stark contrast to those of an earlier and very similar study of cervicogenic headache, in which the effect of spinal manipulation was quite dramatic.[10] These data thus underline the importance of accurate diagnosis in the selection of headache patients for spinal manipulation.

The only other randomized controlled study including manipulation as a treatment for ETTH compared a hands-off pharmaceutical treatment (6 weeks of amitriptyline) with a chiropractic treatment that included personal contact, heat, massage, ergonomic advice, and spinal manipulation.[9] There was a significant decrease in overall symptoms in the chiropractic treatment group, but this effect could have been due to the higher level of personal attention given to that treatment group. Our manipulation group was comparable to that chiropractic group, and we controlled for the treatment elements of personal attention and hands-on treatment.

As always, when a controlled clinical trial fails to demonstrate a treatment effect, the question of a possible type II error (ie, overlooking a real difference) is an issue. In this trial, the number of participants was relatively small, and it is possible that a larger trial might have identified an effect in 1 or more of the outcome variables. However, the data in Table 2 and Figure 2 suggest that any such effect, statistically significant or not, would be of little clinical significance.

Support for this project came from the Nordisk Institut for Kiropraktik og Klinisk Biomekanik (Odense, Denmark), Fonden til fremme af kiropraktisk forskning og postgraduat uddannelse (Copenhagen, Denmark), the Faculty of Health Science of Odense University, and the Foundation for Chiropractic Education and Research (Boston, Mass).

The authors would like to thank Birthe Hove Madsen, DC, Andrea Bove, BSc, and Rikke Fuglsang Andersen, BSc, for their outstanding professional and technical assistance.

References

1. Schwartz BS, Stewart WF, Simon D, Lipton RB. Epidemiology of tension-type headache. *JAMA*. 1998;279:381–383.

2. Rasmussen BK, Jensen R, Schroll M, Olesen J. Epidemiology of headache in a general population: a prevalence study. *J Clin Epidemiol*. 1991;44:1147–1157.

3. Olesen J. Classification and diagnostic criteria for headache disorders, cranial neuralgias and facial pain. *Cephalgia*. 1988;8(suppl 7):1–96.

4. Droz JM, Crot F. Occipital headaches: statistical results in the treatment of vertebrogenic headache. *Ann Swiss Chiro Assoc*. 1985;8:127–136.

5. Lewit K. Ligament pain and anteflexion headache. *Eur Neurol*. 1971;5:365–378.

6. Mootz RD, Dhami MSI, Hess JA, Cook RD, Schorr DB. Chiropractic treatment of chronic episodic tension-type headache in male subjects: a case series analysis. *J Can Chiro Assoc*. 1994;38:152–159.

7. Turk Z, Ratkolb O. Mobilization of the cervical spine in chronic headaches. *Manual Med*. 1987;3:15–17.

8. Vernon H. Chiropractic manipulative therapy in the treatment of headaches. *J Manipulative Physiol Ther*. 1982;5:109–112.

9. Boline PD, Kassak K, Bronfort G, Nelson C, Anderson AV. Spinal manipulation vs amitriptyline for the treatment of chronic tension-type headaches: a randomized clinical trial. *J Manipulative Physiol Ther*. 1995;18:148–154.

10. Nilsson N, Christensen HW, Hartvigsen J. The effect of spinal manipulation in the treatment of cervicogenic headache. *J Manipulative Physiol Ther*. 1997;20:326–330.

11. Hoyt WH, Shaffer F, Bard DA, et al. Osteopathic manipulation in the treatment of muscle-contraction headache. *J Am Osteopath Assoc*.1979;78:322–325.

12. Bergmann TF, Peterson DH, Lawrence DJ. *Chiropractic Technique*. New York, New York: Churchill Livingstone; 1993.

13. Gam AN, Thorsen H, Lonnberg F. The effect of low-level laser therapy on musculoskeletal pain: a meta-analysis. *Pain*. 1993;52:63–66.

14. Nilsson N. *Cervicogenic Headache—Its Prevalence and the Effect of Spinal Manipulation*. Odense, Denmark: University of Odense; 1995.

15. Nilsson N. A randomized controlled trial of the effect of spinal manipulation in the treatment of cervicogenic headache. *J Manipulative Physiol Ther*. 1995;18:435–440.

16. Bogduk N. Headaches and cervical manipulation. *Patient Manage*. 1987;11:163–176.

17. Pfaffenrath V, Kaube H. Diagnostics of cervicogenic headache. *Funct Neurol*. 1990; 5:159–164.

9 Perspectives on Alternative Medicine

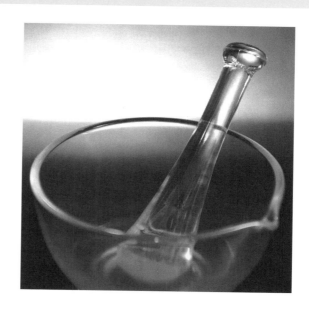

61 Alternative Medicine Meets Science

Phil B. Fontanarosa, MD; George D. Lundberg, MD
Dr Fontanarosa is Senior Editor, *JAMA*, and Dr Lundberg is Editor, *JAMA*.

JAMA. 1998;280:1618–1619

There is no alternative medicine. There is only scientifically proven, evidence-based medicine supported by solid data or unproven medicine, for which scientific evidence is lacking. Whether a therapeutic practice is "Eastern" or "Western," is unconventional or mainstream, or involves mind-body techniques or molecular genetics is largely irrelevant except for historical purposes and cultural interest. We recognize that there are vastly different types of practitioners and proponents of the various forms of alternative medicine and conventional medicine, and that there are vast differences in the skills, capabilities, and beliefs of individuals within them and the nature of their actual practices. Moreover, the economic and political forces in these fields are large and increasingly complex and have the capability for being highly contentious. Nonetheless, as believers in science and evidence, we must focus on fundamental issues—namely, the patient, the target disease or condition, the proposed or practiced treatment, and the need for convincing data on safety and therapeutic efficacy.

Despite the increasing use of alternative medicine (also termed *complementary*, *integrative*, or *unconventional* medicine) in the United States and throughout the world, most alternative therapies have not been evaluated using rigorously conducted scientific tests of efficacy based on accepted rules of evidence. The lack of properly designed and conducted randomized controlled trials is a major deficiency. For some published studies, serious concerns have been raised regarding methodological quality. A National Institutes of Health expert panel concluded that current evidence is inadequate for development of practice guidelines for alternative therapies, largely because of lack of relevant outcomes data from high-quality clinical trials.[1] However, some advocates of alternative medicine argue that many alternative therapies cannot be subjected to the standard scientific method and thus, instead must rely on anecdotes, beliefs, theories, testimonials, and opinions to support effectiveness and justify continued use.

Regardless of the origin or type of therapy, the theoretical underpinnings of its mechanism of action, or the practitioner who delivers it, the critical questions are the same. What is the therapy? What is the disease or condition for which it is being used? What is its purported benefit to the patient? What are the risks? How much does it cost? And, perhaps most important, does it work? For virtually all medical therapies and interventions, whether conventional or alternative, determination of effectiveness and recommendations for clinical application should be based on the strength of the scientific evidence using explicit criteria for grading the quality of evidence[2,3] (Table 1) and ratings for technology assessment[4] (ie, "established," "promising," "investigational," "doubtful," or "unacceptable.")

While acknowledging that many therapies used in conventional medical practice also have not been as rigorously evaluated as they should be, we agree that most alternative medicine has not been scientifically tested.[5] However, for alternative medicine therapies that are used by millions of patients every day and that generate billions of dollars in health care expenditures each year, the lack of convincing and compelling evidence on efficacy, safety, and outcomes is unacceptable and deeply troubling. We believe that physicians should become more knowledgeable about alternative medicine and increase their understanding of the possible benefits and limitations of alternative therapies. By doing so, physicians will be able to serve as more useful sources of information for their patients and advise them appropriately. As with conventional therapies, advice should be based on data and scientific information rather than anecdotal information, misperceptions, or preconceived or unfounded notions about effectiveness or lack thereof.

This theme issue of *JAMA* and the annual coordinated theme issues of the 9 American Medical Association *Archives* Journals published this month on alternative medicine represent a planned, concerted effort by the editors of these scientific journals to address some of these issues by providing physicians and other health care professionals with clinically relevant, reliable, fresh scientific information on alternative therapies. In response to our call for papers on alternative medicine,[6] we received more than 200 manuscript submissions to *JAMA* and many more manuscripts were received by the *Archives* Journals. The result, after our usual rigorous review process, is publication of more than 80 articles and editorials on alternative medicine in our 10 scientific journals, including 18 randomized trials and systematic reviews, on more than 30 different topics, and from more than 16 different countries.

Table 1. Categories for Rating Quality of Scientific Evidence for Effectiveness of an Intervention*

Quality of Evidence	
I.	Evidence obtained from at least 1 properly randomized controlled trial
II-1.	Evidence obtained from well-designed controlled trials without randomization
II-2.	Evidence obtained from well-designed cohort or case-control analytic studies, preferably from more than 1 center or research group
II-3.	Evidence obtained from multiple time series with or without the intervention. Dramatic results in uncontrolled experiments (such as the results of the introduction of penicillin treatment in the 1940s) could also be regarded as this type of evidence.
III.	Opinions of respected authorities, based on clinical experience, descriptive studies, or reports of expert committees

*Information is from Lawrence et al.[2]

This issue of *The Journal* includes 6 randomized clinical trials that evaluate the use of 6 diverse alternative medicine therapies for treatment of common clinical conditions. The results are intriguing. Bove and Nilsson[7] report that chiropractic spinal manipulation is not effective for episodic tension headache. Cardini and Weixin[8] found that moxibustion (stimulation of an acupuncture point by heat generated from burning a specific herb) is helpful for correction of breech presentation in late pregnancy. Bensoussan and colleagues[9] document that a Chinese herbal medicine formulation improves symptoms of irritable bowel syndrome. Shlay and coinvestigators[10] demonstrate that acupuncture is no more effective than amitriptyline or placebo for relieving pain due to human immunodeficiency virus–related peripheral neuropathy. Heymsfield and coworkers[11] determined that *Garcinia cambogia*, a common component of commercial weight-loss products, lacks efficacy as an antiobesity agent. In a preliminary study, Garfinkel and coworkers[12] report that a yoga-based intervention appears to hold promise for relieving some symptoms of carpal tunnel syndrome. In addition, a systematic review by Wilt and colleagues[13] suggests that saw palmetto extracts improve urologic symptoms in patients with benign prostatic hyperplasia.

Perhaps just as important as the results of their studies, these investigators demonstrate that alternative medicine therapies and interventions can and should be evaluated using explicit, focused research questions[14] along with established and accepted rigorous research methods[15] (eg, appropriate controls, effective blinding procedures, adequate power, state-of-the-art techniques for systematic reviews); incorporating measurable, objectively assessed end points (eg, blinded assessment); and reporting meaningful patient-centered outcomes.

Two other studies in this issue provide additional new information on alternative medicine. In a replication of their previous nationally representative survey,[16] Eisenberg et al[17] report that the prevalence of use of at least 1 of 16 specific alternative therapies during the previous 12 months has increased significantly (from 33.8% in 1990 to 42.1% in 1997), that the estimated number of visits to alternative medicine practitioners increased dramatically (from 427 million in 1990 to 629 million in 1997), and that only 38.5% of those who used alternative therapies discussed them with their physician. Total out-of-pocket expenditures associated with use of alternative medicine in 1997 were estimated at $27 billion. In an analysis of data from malpractice insurers from 1990 through 1996, Studdert and colleagues[18] found that claims against chiropractors, massage therapists, and acupuncturists generally occurred less frequently and usually involved less severe injury than claims against medical doctors. The authors also summarize the legal issues and principles for physicians to consider when advising or contemplating referral of patients to alternative medicine practitioners.

Taken together, the articles published in this issue of *The Journal* and in the *Archives* Journals' theme issues on alternative medicine add a substantial amount of new information and scientific data on alternative therapies to the peer-reviewed mainstream medical literature. However, given the burgeoning use of alternative medicine therapies, the increasing numbers of patients who consult both medical doctors and alternative medicine practitioners, and the increasing number of insurance companies and managed care organizations offering programs and benefits for alternative medicine,[19] the need for additional, carefully conducted, high-quality research is essential.

Priority for research funding for alternative medicine should be given to investigations of relevant clinical problems for which well-designed studies have shown encouraging results for alternative therapies, especially for conditions that are common and those for which conventional medicine has not been effective. Attention should be given to evaluation of safety and efficacy, but also to examining the effectiveness of a treatment strategy, with consideration of community practice settings, patient expectations and compliance, and cost-effectiveness.[20] Collaborative research, especially among the federally funded centers for alternative medicine research in the US and with international alternative medicine research centers, may improve efficiency in answering important research questions. We encourage high-quality, rigorous research on alternative medicine and invite authors to submit their best papers for our objective evaluation and consideration for publication.

However, until solid evidence is available that demonstrates the safety, efficacy, and effectiveness of specific alternative medicine interventions, uncritical acceptance of untested and unproven alternative medicine therapies must stop. Alternative therapies that have been shown to be of no benefit (aside from possible placebo effect) or that cause harm should be abandoned immediately. Physicians, insurance plans, medical centers and hospitals, managed care organizations, and government policymakers should base decisions regarding incorporation of and payment for alternative medicine therapies on evidence-based research and objective cost-effectiveness analyses[19] rather than on consumer interest, market demand or competition, well-publicized anecdotal reports, or political pressures from well-organized and influential interest groups.

Ultimately, answering fundamental questions about efficacy, safety, appropriate clinical applications, and meaningful outcomes for all medical therapies, including those considered alternative medicine, requires critical and objective assessment using accepted principles of scientific investigation and rigorous standards for evaluation of scientific evidence. For patients, for physicians and other health care professionals, and for alternative medicine practitioners—indeed, for all who share the goal of improving the health of individuals and of the public—there can be no alternative.

References

1. Practice and Policy Guidelines Panel, National Institutes of Health Office of Alternative Medicine. Clinical practice guidelines in complementary and alternative medicine: an analysis of opportunities and obstacles. *Arch Fam Med*. 1997;6:149–154.

2. Lawrence RS, Mickalide AD. Preventive services in clinical practice: designing the periodic health examination. *JAMA*. 1987;257:2205–2207.

3. Cook DJ, Guyatt GH, Laupacis A, et al. Clinical recommendations using levels of evidence for antithrombotic agents. *Chest*. 1995; 108(suppl):227S–230S.

4. Kalousdian S, Schneider AL, Loeb JM, et al. Technology assessment: an American Medical Association perspective. *Arch Fam Med*. 1992; 1:291–295.

5. Angell M, Kassirer JP. Alternative medicine: the risks of untested and unregulated remedies. *N Engl J Med*. 1998;339:839–841.

6. Fontanarosa PB, Lundberg GD. Complementary, alternative, unconventional, and integrative medicine: call for papers for the annual coordinated theme issues of the AMA journals. *JAMA*. 1997;278:2111–2112.

7. Bove G, Nilsson N. Spinal manipulation in the treatment of episodic tension-type headache: a randomized controlled trial. *JAMA*. 1998; 280:1576–1579.

8. Cardini F, Weixin H. Moxibustion for correction of breech presentation: a randomized controlled trial. *JAMA*. 1998;280:1580–1584.

9. Bensoussan A, Talley NJ, Hing M, et al. Treatment of irritable bowel syndrome with Chinese herbal medicine: a randomized controlled trial. *JAMA*. 1998;280:1585–1589.

10. Shlay JC, Chaloner K, Max MB, et al. Acupuncture and amitriptyline for pain due to HIV-related peripheral neuropathy: a randomized controlled trial. *JAMA*. 1998;280:1590–1595.

11. Heymsfield SB, Allison DB, Vasselli JR, et al. *Garcinia cambogia* (hydroxycitric acid) as a potential antiobesity agent: a randomized controlled trial. *JAMA*. 1998;280:1596–1600.

12. Garfinkel MS, Singhal A, Katz WA, et al. Yoga-based intervention for carpal tunnel syndrome: a randomized trial. *JAMA*. 1998; 280:1601–1603.

13. Wilt TJ, Ishani A, Stark G, et al. Saw palmetto extracts for treatment of benign prostatic hyperplasia: a systematic review. *JAMA*. 1998;280:1604–1609.

14. Vickers A, Cassileth B, Ernst E, et al. How should we research unconventional therapies? a panel report from the Conference on Complementary and Alternative Research Methodology, National Institutes of Health. *Int J Technol Assess Health Care*. 1997;13:111–121.

15. Levin JS, Glass TA, Kushi LH, et al. Quantitative methods in research on complementary and alternative medicine: a methodological manifesto. *Med Care*. 1997;35:1079–1094.

16. Eisenberg DM, Kessler RC, Foster C, et al. Unconventional medicine in the United States: prevalence, costs, and patterns of use. *N Engl J Med*. 1993;328:246–252.

17. Eisenberg DM, Davis RB, Ettner SL, et al. Trends in alternative medicine use in the United States, 1990–1997: results of a follow-up national survey. *JAMA*. 1998;280:1569–1575.

18. Studdert DM, Eisenberg DM, Miller FH, et al. Medical malpractice implications of alternative medicine. *JAMA*. 1998;280:1610–1615.

19. Pelletier KR, Marie A, Krasner M, Haskell WL. Current trends in the integration and reimbursement of complementary and alternative medicine by managed care, insurance carriers, and hospital providers. *Am J Health Promotion*. 1997;12:112–122.

20. Welch HG. Valuing clinical strategies early in their development. *Ann Intern Med*. 1992; 116:262–264.

62 "Conventional" and "Unconventional" Medicine

Can They Be Integrated?

James E. Dalen, MD, MPH
Dr Dalen is Editor, *Archives of Internal Medicine.*

Arch Intern Med. 1998;158:2179–2181

This issue of the *Archives,* as well as the 8 other specialty journals and *JAMA*, is dedicated to complementary, alternative, and integrated medicine. Complementary and alternative medicine are also termed *unconventional* medical therapy, which Eisenberg et al[1] have defined as "medical interventions that are not taught extensively at US medical schools or generally provided at US hospitals." *Conventional* medicine can then be defined as medical interventions that are taught extensively at US medical schools and generally provided at US hospitals.

Eisenberg and colleagues[1] noted that 34% (60 million) of the general public in the United States reported using 1 or more forms of unconventional medicine in 1990. The most frequently used unconventional modalities are various forms of relaxation therapy,[2,3] chiropractic,[4] acupuncture,[5,6] massage therapy,[7] and herbal/mineral/vitamin supplements.[8–10] The number of visits to unconventional providers in the United States in 1990 was greater than the number of visits to all primary care physicians. The total expenditures for unconventional therapy in 1990 amounted to $13.7 billion, $10.3 billion of which was paid out-of-pocket. In the vast majority of cases (89%), these visits to unconventional providers were not prescribed by a physician, and 72% of the patients did not discuss these visits with their physicians.[1]

What is the reason for this incredible disconnect? Patients seek unconventional medical care because they believe that it will, or does, help them. Why are conventional physicians reluctant to refer patients to unconventional therapy?

Some of the terms that are frequently used to differentiate conventional therapy from unconventional therapy are listed below:

Conventional	Unconventional
Mainstream	Alternative
Orthodox	Unorthodox
Regular	Irregular
Scientific	Unscientific
Evidence based	Not evidence based
Allopathic	Naturopathic
Western	
Modern	

Perhaps the most compelling (and most inflammatory) label is that conventional medicine is scientific and that unconventional is unscientific. It is a fact that many conventional physicians (ie, graduates of US medical schools) state that they do not refer patients to practitioners of unconventional medicine because their methods are not scientific and their qualifications are uncertain.

The definition of what is scientific in medicine obviously varies over time. I am sure that the leading conventional US physician of the 18th Century, Benjamin Rush, and his colleagues were convinced that bloodletting and purging were examples of scientific medicine. (I am not sure that George Washington agreed!)

At the present time in American medicine, scientific medicine is that which is judged to be evidence based. What is evidence-based medicine? In the 1990s, it means that a therapy has been shown to improve well-defined patient outcomes by well-designed, appropriately powered, randomized, controlled clinical trials. All drugs that have been approved by the Food and Drug Administration since the 1960s have met this standard. Conversely, many therapies introduced before the 1960s do not meet our current definition of scientific, or evidence-based, medicine.

Let us look at our current therapies for cardiovascular diseases. Cardiovascular diseases and their outcomes—myocardial infarction, stroke, pulmonary embolism, and death—are readily and reliably documented. Many of them are treated with antithrombotic agents. Three of the major antithrombotic agents that are prescribed by Western-trained physicians for millions of patients every day were introduced prior to the era of the randomized clinical trial: warfarin,[11] aspirin,[12] and heparin.[13]

What is the scientific evidence that these 3 drugs prevent myocardial infarction, stroke, pulmonary embolism, or death? The American College of Chest Physicians (ACCP) Consensus Conference on Antithrombotic Therapy was convened in 1985 to examine the available evidence and to make recommendations for antithrombotic therapy. Their recommendations were graded A, B, or C according to the rules of evidence described by Sackett[14] (Table 1). Grade A recommendations, based on the results of appropriately designed randomized clinical trials, were considered to be evidence based.

After the available evidence on the efficacy and safety of these agents was examined, it was found that only 24% of the 1986 recommendations were based on grade A evidence; ie, only 24% of their recommendations were evidence based as currently defined.[15] Of note, 55% of their recommendations were based on uncontrolled clinical observations and therefore were grade C (most evidence for the efficacy of unconventional therapies is grade C at best.) The ACCP consensus conferences helped to stimulate a flurry of appropriately designed randomized clinical trials on antithrombotic therapy from 1986 to 1998. The fifth ACCP Consensus Conference on Antithrombotic Therapy, which took place in 1998,[16] reflects the impact of these trials: 44% of the 1998 recommendations are grade A, ie, evidenced based. Nearly all the recommendations for therapies recently approved by the Food and Drug Administration (thrombolytics, ticoplidine, platelet glycoprotein II/IIIA antagonists) are grade A. However, many of the recommendations for the older, widely prescribed drugs (warfarin, heparin, and aspirin) remain grade C (not evidence based). If these therapies (eg, warfarin to prevent stroke in patients with mitral stenosis complicated by atrial fibrillation) are not evidence based as currently defined, are they unconventional therapies?

The reason that most unconventional therapies are not evidence based as currently defined is that most of them were introduced long before (in some cases centuries before) the advent of the randomized controlled clinical trial. It is also true that most therapies considered to be unconventional arose outside modern mainstream Western medicine.

Further examples of non-evidence-based therapies that are or have been widely prescribed by Western physicians for patients with cardiovascular disease are evident in the use of various procedures (which are less tightly regulated than drugs.) Coronary artery bypass grafts were first performed in 1964.[17] The efficacy of this procedure based on the early reports seemed self-evident. Therefore, the procedure was performed in hundreds of thousands of patients with coronary artery disease, even though its efficacy was not confirmed by randomized clinical trials until 1977.[18] Percutaneous transluminal coronary angioplasty followed a similar course. It was described in 1979,[19] and, as in the case of coronary artery bypass grafts, was then performed in hundreds of thousands of patients prior to the first randomized clinical trial demonstrating efficacy in 1992.[20] The procedure of bedside pulmonary artery catheterization was described in 1970,[21] and it has been performed in millions of patients without scientific evidence that it improves patient outcomes.[22] In fact, some studies have suggested that it may in fact cause harm to some patients.[23]

Table 1. Relation Between Levels of Evidence and Grades of Recommendations*

Level of Evidence	Grade of Recommendation
Level I: Large randomized trials with clear-cut results (and low risk of error)	A
Level II: Small randomized trials with uncertain results (and moderate to high risk of error)	B
Level III: Nonrandomized, contemporaneous controls	
Level IV: Nonrandomized, historical controls	C
Level V: No controls, case-series only	

*From Sackett.[14]

Table 2. Comparison of Conventional and Unconventional Therapies

	Conventional	Unconventional
Prescribed by graduates of US medical schools	Routinely	Infrequently
Date introduced	Mostly 20th Century, especially second half	Most prior to 20th Century
Scientific, evidence based as currently defined	Many	Very few
Site of origin	"Mainstream"	Out of mainstream

It is clear that many of the therapies prescribed by Western-trained physicians are not evidence based as currently defined. Does this mean that they should be defined as unconventional therapies? I believe that the reason that they are not considered to be unconventional therapies is that they were introduced from the mainstream of Western medicine. Does this mean that they should be abandoned? I think not. It means that they should be subjected to appropriately designed randomized clinical trials to establish their efficacy and safety.

Table 2 compares various characteristics of conventional medical therapies with those of unconventional therapies. The fact that unconventional therapies are infrequently prescribed by graduates of US medical schools is not surprising, since unconventional therapy is infrequently taught in US medical schools. As noted above, many, but not all, conventional therapies are evidence based, whereas very few unconventional therapies are evidence based. One of the reasons that most unconventional modalities are not evidence based is that the majority of them were introduced prior to the 20th Century; therefore, they were not subjected to randomized clinical trials.

In my opinion, the principal distinguishing characteristic of unconventional and conventional medicine therapies is their source of introduction. Conventional therapies are introduced by mainstream Western physicians and scientists, whereas most unconventional modalities are introduced by "outsiders." I agree with Goodwin and Tangum,[24] who, in this issue of the *Archives*, conclude that American academic medicine has a bias against outsiders who make therapeutic suggestions, especially when they take their message directly to the public.

Promising unconventional therapies must be subjected to the same level of scientific scrutiny that we now require for drug therapies introduced by "mainstream" medicine. As physicians whose job description requires us to help people, we cannot reject "out-of-hand" any proposed therapies just because they did not originate in modern mainstream medicine. We cannot wear blinders!

This is the challenge for integrative medicine! The leaders of integrative medicine must sort through the myriad of proposed unconventional therapies to determine which should be subjected to appropriately designed clinical trials. The best candidates for study may be those that meet at least grade C levels of evidence, as outlined by Sackett in Table 1.

If a therapy that arose from outside the mainstream of modern Western medicine can pass the same level of scrutiny that we expect of conventional therapies, it should be integrated into mainstream medicine and added to the therapeutic armamentarium of the well-trained, conventional physician. We can do no less for our patients!

We could learn from the Navajo, as described by Kim and Kwok[25] in this issue of the *Archives*. The Navajo have integrated *unconventional* Western medicine, which is provided by the Indian Health Service, into their centuries-old *conventional* health care, which is provided by native healers.

References

1. Eisenberg DM, Kessler RC, Foster C, Norlock FE, Calkins DR, Delbanco TL. Unconventional medicine in the United States. *N Engl J Med.* 1993: 328;246–252.
2. Kabat-Zinn J, Lipworth L, Burney R. The clinical use of mindfulness meditation for the self-regulation of chronic pain. *J Behav Med.* 1985;8:163–190.
3. Bernhard J, Kristeller J, Kabat-Zinn J. Effectiveness of relaxation and visualization techniques as an adjunct to phototherapy and photochemotherapy of psoriasis. *J Am Acad Dermatol.* 1988;19:572–573.
4. Kaptchuk TJ, Eisenberg DM. Chiropractic: origins, controversies, and contributions. *Arch Intern Med.* 1998;158:2215–2224.
5. White AR, Resch K-L, Ernst E. Randomized trial of acupuncture for nicotine withdrawal symptoms. *Arch Intern Med.* 1998;158:2251–2255.
6. Ernst E, White AR. Acupuncture for back pain: a meta-analysis of randomized controlled trials. *Arch Intern Med.* 1998;158:2235–2241.

7. Field T, Henteleff T, Hernandez-Reif M, et al. Children with asthma have improved pulmonary functions after massage therapy. *J Pediatr.* 1998;132:854–858.

8. Winslow LC, Kroll DJ. Herbs as medicines. *Arch Intern Med.* 1998;158:2192–2199.

9. Miller LG. Herbal medicinals: selected clinical considerations focusing on known or potential drug-herb interactions. *Arch Intern Med.* 1998;158:2200–2211.

10. Mashour NH, Lin GI, Frishman WH. Herbal medicine for the treatment of cardiovascular disease: clinical considerations. *Arch Intern Med.* 1998;158:2225–2234.

11. Murray G. Anticoagulants in venous thrombosis and the prevention of pulmonary embolism. *Surg Gynecol Obstet.* 1947;84:665–668.

12. Craven LL. Acetylsalicylic acid, possible preventive of coronary thrombosis. *Ann West Med Surg.* 1950;4:95–99.

13. Barritt DW, Jordan SC. Anticoagulant drugs in the treatment of pulmonary embolism: a controlled trial. *Lancet.* 1960;1:1309–1312.

14. Sackett DL. Rules of evidence and clinical recommendations on the use of antithrombotic agents. *Chest.* 1986;89(suppl):2S–3S.

15. First ACCP Conference on Antithrombotic Therapy. *Chest.* 1986;89(suppl):1S–106S.

16. Fifth ACCP Conference on Antithrombotic Therapy. *Chest.* In press.

17. Garrett HG, Dennis EW, DeBakey ME. Aortocoronary bypass with saphenous vein graft. *JAMA.* 1973;223:792–794.

18. Murphy ML, Hultgren HN, Detre K, Thomsen J, Takaro T. Treatment of chronic stable angina: a preliminary report of survival data of the randomized Veterans Administration Cooperative Study. *N Engl J Med.* 1977;297:621–627.

19. Grüntzig AR, Senning Å, Siegenthaler WE. Nonoperative dilation of coronary-artery stenosis: percutaneous transluminal coronary angioplasty. *N Engl J Med.* 1979;301:61–68.

20. Parisi AF, Folland ED, Hartigan P. A comparison of angioplasty with medical therapy in the treatment of single-vessel coronary artery disease. *N Engl J Med.* 1992;326:10–16.

21. Swan HJC, Ganz W, Forrester J, Marcus H, Diamond G, Chonette D. Catheterization of the heart in man with use of a flow-directed balloon-tipped catheter. *N Engl J Med.* 1970;283:447–451.

22. Dalen JE, Bone RC. Is it time to pull the pulmonary artery catheter? *JAMA.* 1996; 276:916–918.

23. Connors AF, Speroff T, Dawson NV, et al. The effectiveness of right heart catheterization in the initial care of critically ill patients. *JAMA.* 1996;276:889–897.

24. Goodwin JS, Tangum MR. Battling quackery: attitudes about micronutrient supplements in American academic medicine. *Arch Intern Med.* 1998;158:2187–2191.

25. Kim C, Kwok YS. Navajo use of native healers. *Arch Intern Med.* 1998;158:2245–2249.

63 Alternative Medicine and Dermatology

The Unconventional Issue

Kenneth A. Arndt, MD; Robert S. Stern, MD.
Dr Arndt is Editor, *Archives of Dermatology*, and Dr Stern is Coeditor.

Arch Dermatol. 1998;134:1472

This month's issue of the *Archives* and all other scientific journals of the American Medical Association are devoted to the discussion of complementary, alternative, unconventional, and integrative medicine. This topic is particularly applicable to patients with cutaneous disease and to dermatologic clinicians. It is the rare practitioner who has not seen patients who have used folk remedies, herbal medicines, acupuncture, diet, hypnosis, biofeedback, or other remedies outside of traditional allopathic medicine in pursuit of relief from, or cure of, their cutaneous disease. The high percentage of the population who use complementary therapies and the extraordinary number of visits to unconventional medical practitioners, a number that is estimated to exceed the number of visits to primary care physicians, have stimulated us to become more knowledgeable about these areas and to evaluate such practices in an effort to improve our care of patients and to integrate truly helpful remedies into patient care. The National Institutes of Health, Bethesda, Md, has established an Office of Alternative Medicine, which spends tens of millions of dollars per year on research in this area.

For this issue, we solicited manuscripts from authors around the world asking them to describe the practices in their geographic areas, to give observations about alternative medicine, and to report on the use of unconventional and "off-label" topical and systemic remedies for dermatologic problems in their geographic areas. There is a paucity of data on which to make rational decisions concerning the use of many of these alternative medications. While several articles in this issue provide new and well-evaluated information concerning traditional health care and topical therapies, the majority of articles present information, history, comments, descriptions, and opinions about this topic. All manuscripts were critically reviewed in our editorial office for their educational value and interest to those dealing with cutaneous disease, although it was not possible to evaluate many of these articles in the traditional peer-reviewed fashion. We have tried to present a wide spectrum of opinions and a comprehensive overview of the current status of unconventional medical care of dermatologic disease. Some authors see alternative approaches as offering great potential benefits to our patients. Other authors doubt the validity of alternative medicine and the evidence that supports it. In contrast to the emphasis of this month's issue on unconventional and largely unproven (according to the standards of modern science) methods of health care, next month's issue will be devoted to articles on evidence-based medicine and the application of modern statistical and scientific techniques to decision making in the care of the individual patient.

This issue provides an opportunity to learn more about diverse and unusual therapeutic methods, such as aromatherapy, horse chestnut seed extract, traditional Chinese medicines, acupuncture, spa therapy, mind-body medicine and spirituality, and phytotherapy, which are in use today, and it presents a fascinating history of these therapies as practiced in the Old World. Greater knowledge of alternative medicine and its philosophical background and practical uses should result in better care for our patients and stimulate clinical research that will allow further consideration of its appropriate use and mechanisms of action.

64 Alternative Neurology

Roger N. Rosenberg, MD
Dr Rosenburg is Editor, *Archives of Neurology.*

Arch Neurol. 1998;55:1394–1395

The largest growth industry in health care in the United States according to an article by Brody[1] in the *New York Times* is alternative medicine. It is estimated that 42% of American adults used some type of alternative care, including herbal therapy (17%), chiropractic (16%), massage therapy (14%), vitamin therapy (13%), yoga (5%), and acupuncture (2%) among other therapies. Patients with neurologic diseases and healthy individuals hoping to avoid neurologic diseases are seeking these remedies. Brody reported that among 1500 adults interviewed, 44% said they would use an alternative method if traditional medical care was not producing the desired results. Brody also says that

> Americans are voting with their feet and pocketbooks. Studies have shown that patients make more visits each year to alternative care practitioners than to primary care physicians, and most of them pay out of their own pockets for the care they receive.[1]

The types of common problems for which patients seek relief include back pain, anxiety, allergies, arthritis, depression, and insomnia.[1] Astin[2] analyzed in more depth these issues in his recent article titled "Why Patients Use Alternative Medicine." It is of considerable interest and perhaps unexpected but patients seek alternative medical therapy not because they are dissatisfied with conventional medicine. Rather, Astin found that along with being more educated and reporting poor health status, the majority of alternative medicine users appear to be doing so because these alternatives are more "congruent with their own values, beliefs, and philosophical orientations toward health and life."[2] Alternative medicine is used as a supplement to provide a "holistic" approach to life and health in addition to conventional medicine.[2]

In this issue of the *Archives*, we explore the region of alternative neurology. The response to a call for articles was vigorous and varied. Neurologic disease is difficult to treat and thereby offers room for speculative approaches and ideas. Several articles were amusing and even fanciful. They have not been included in the ARCHIVES. Seven articles with enterprising and creative ideas worthy of scientific consideration have been accepted and are presented along with 4 editorials to put them into critical perspective. Vining and colleagues[3] have reexplored the efficacy of the ketogenic diet for epilepsy. The diet has a biochemical rationale for effectiveness in patients refractory to standard antiepileptic drug therapy. Why the diet works in some patients is not known but increasing brain lipid levels and inducing acidosis are 2 issues to explore. An accompanying editorial by Roach[4] provides an important perspective on the point that if the ketogenic diet can be systematically examined, then other forms of nontraditional therapy might be elucidated. It is a paradigm that deserves additional analysis.

Naeser et al[5] offer insight into the new area of computer-assisted therapy for aphasia. Can patients who have communication deficits be aided by the vast communicative abilities of the computer and be retrained to learn and comprehend? Specific lesion sites were identified that can be appropriate for this approach. You can visualize that this is the beginning of a new era in neurologic rehabilitation. Albert[6] provides the necessary neurologic overview in his thoughtful editorial on the "Treatment of Aphasia."

Then, we come to the therapy for Alzheimer disease (AD). Many articles were submitted offering enterprising theories and therapies for this most serious of neurologic diseases. Insight into one herbal approach that may indeed have a positive effect is provided by the literature of *Ginkgo biloba*. The neurologic community is polarized on this herb or drug and considerable thought and care overall is supplied by Oken et al[7] in their review. It is an important contribution not only for its objective analysis of this agent but also on how to approach and analyze contrasting views of an emerging new neuropharmacologic agent.

Clarke et al[8] present good data indicating that patients with AD have low blood levels of folate and vitamin B_{12}, and elevated total homocysteine levels and that these changes are contributory to the causation of the disease rather than being a consequence of it. Diaz-Arrastia[9] states his view on this provocative set of findings in his editorial. Vitamins to treat patients with AD will not be the sufficient, total form of therapy but a positive response to them offers important biological clues to what needs to be done in future neurobiological research for AD.

What types of protocols need to be designed to best evaluate new alternative therapies for AD? Two enterprising articles by Karlawish and Whitehouse[10] and by Knopman and colleagues[11] examine this critical issue. Should nonplacebo-controlled trials be used in which new drugs are tested against current drugs that have some positive effect? Or should conventional placebo-controlled trials continue? They provide the fodder for debate on this point, as it will eventually apply to many degenerative neurologic diseases. Farlow[12] presents us with a balanced view on this matter in his forthright and direct editorial.

It has been an educational and scientific experience for our reviewers and editors to evaluate these articles and the issues they represent. We hope you, our readers, find them stimulating and provocative. The real objective is that they will induce new thinking and new unconventional approaches to treat the conventional, serious neurologic disorder.

References

1. Brody JE. Alternative medicine makes inroads, but watch out for the curves. *New York Times*. April 28, 1998:B9.
2. Astin JA. Why patients use alternative medicine. *JAMA*. 1998;279:1548–1553.
3. Vining EPG, Freeman JM, Ballaban-Gil K, et al, and The Ketogenic Diet Multi-Center Study Group. A multicenter study of the efficacy of the ketogenic diet. *Arch Neurol*. 1998; 55:1433–1437.
4. Roach ES. Alternative neurology: the ketogenic diet. *Arch Neurol*. 1998;55:1403–1404.
5. Naeser MA, Baker EH, Palumbo CL, et al. Lesion site patterns in severe, nonverbal aphasia to predict outcome with a computer-assisted treatment program. *Arch Neurol*. 1998; 55:1438–1448.
6. Albert ML. Treatment of aphasia. *Arch Neurol*. 1998;55:1417–1419.
7. Oken BS, Storzbach DM, Kaye JA. The efficacy of *Ginkgo biloba on* cognitive function in Alzheimer disease. *Arch Neurol*. 1998; 55:1409–1415.
8. Clarke R, Smith AD, Jobst KA, et al. Folate, vitamin B^{12}, and serum total homocysteine levels in confirmed Alzheimer disease. *Arch Neurol*. 1998;55:1449–1455.
9. Diaz-Arrastia R. Hyperhomocysteinemia: a new risk factor for Alzheimer disease? *Arch Neurol*. 1998;55:1407–1408.
10. Karlawish JHT, Whitehouse PJ. Is the placebo control obsolete in a world after donepezil and vitamin E? *Arch Neurol*. 1998;55:1420–1424.
11. Knopman D, Kahn J, Miles S. Clinical research designs for emerging treatments for Alzheimer disease: moving beyond placebo-controlled trials. *Arch Neurol*. 1998;55:1425–1429.
12. Farlow MR. New treatments in Alzheimer disease and the continued need for placebo-controlled trials. *Arch Neurol*. 1998;55:1396–1398.

"It has been estimated that consumers waste $500 million a year on medical quackery and another $500 million annually on some 'health foods' which have no beneficial effect."—John F. Kennedy, Message to Congress on Problems of the Aged, February 21, 1963[1]

65 Alternative Medicine and Surgery

Claude H. Organ, Jr, MD
Dr Organ is Editor, *Archives of Surgery.*

Arch Surg. 1998;133:1154–1155

The November 1998 issue of the *Archives of Surgery* covers the topic of alternative medicine from a surgical viewpoint. The 10 scientific journals of the American Medical Association, beginning in 1990, have published theme issues on the following topics: Caring for the Uninsured and the Underinsured (1991), Violence (1992), Molecular Medicine and Genetics (1993), Disease Prevention and Health Promotion (1994), Emerging and Reemerging Global Microbial Threats (1995), Managed Care (1996), and Quality of Care (1997).

The theme issue concept was identified to stimulate research and writing on a specific subject, emphasize a subject for our readers, change public knowledge and attitudes, influence public policy, provide timely in-depth reference sources in one place, enhance research funding for a field, and call attention to the messages and the messengers.[2]

Many terms have been used to identify alternative medicine, such as *complementary medicine*, *integrative medicine*, *unconventional approaches to improve outcomes for nontraditional modalities*, and so on. The topic becomes more penetrating when applied to the discipline of surgery: alternative surgery, alternatives to surgery, alternatives vs surgery, nonoperative management, and alternative operations. A need for definition regarding alternative medicine becomes relative, depending on several variables, and is not the same as controversial, innovative, or another point of view. Abundant evidence exists that data are not available to recommend many of these approaches. (In God we trust but everyone else must have data.) Although physicians have viewed alternative medicine with skepticism, attitudes are changing toward these nontraditional therapeutic modalities. Scientific methods to determine therapeutic outcomes and their safety are needed.

On a recent flight, I sat next to a woman obviously in severe distress with noticeable abdominal distention, pallor, weakness, and other accompanying signs of a metastatic malignancy. She was en route to Mexico to receive a miracle treatment for ovarian cancer. Physicians who had been treating her for more than 2 years had given up all hope. She exhibited a genuine belief that a miracle was possible. This experience caused me to reflect on her plight and aphorisms I heard in my early years about cancer cures (such as "people who eat a lot of raw onions do not get cancer").

The National Institutes of Health Office of Alternative Medicine, established in 1992, is being considered as a national center for complementary and alternative medicine research. The National Institutes of Health spend approximately $40 million annually for research topics involving dietary manipulation and behavioral medicine. Many types of alternative therapy are being investigated, such as relaxation, massage, imagery, spiritual healing, lifestyle diets (such as macrobiotics), herbal medicine, megavitamin therapy, imagery healing, biofeedback, hypnosis, homeopathy, acupuncture, physiological exercise, and prayer. Considerable concern has been registered regarding the amount of funding for pseudoscientific studies. Wetzel et al[3] have recently surveyed 125 US medical schools. One hundred seventeen responded (94%) and, of that group, 75 (64%) reported offering elective courses in complementary or alternative medicine. According to their study, 1 of 3 US adults use chiropractic, acupuncture, homeopathy, or other alternative therapies.

New biomedical journals devoted to the scientific evaluation of unconventional health claims have been launched: *Alternative Medicine Digest*, *Alternative Medicine Alert* (in its 16th issue), and *Alternative Medicine*. These are accompanied by an increase in dialogue, seminars, and postgraduate courses. Our shelves are increasingly occupied with books on these subjects: *Herbal Drugs and Phytopharmaceuticals, Handbook of Medicinal Mints (Aromathematics),* and *Chemistry and Application of Green Tea.*

Dating back to 1993, Eisenberg et al[4] reported that one third of the population of the United States used unconventional therapies not widely taught in medical schools. Approximately $13.7 billion was being used for unconventional therapy, of which $10.3 billion was paid out of pocket.

Scientists traditionally require an understanding of how a treatment works prior to its use. A tendency to substitute new unproven therapies for traditional medicine continues. It is our obligation to employ time-honored investigations to determine their validity. Scientists testing alternative treatments should encourage rigorous research protocols to deal with our skepticism and traditionalism.

Ebert,[5] past executive director of the American College of Surgeons, has reminded us that

> the majority of these modalities have no official approval and have not undergone legitimate clinical trials. When a surgeon writes a prescription for a particular medication, the patient's perception is that this is a proper medication that has been approved for the use for which it has been prescribed. The alternative health product market in the United States is gigantic. When a physician specifically recommends or sells a product, however, he or she is implying endorsement of a quality product.

The Complementary Care Center at the New York and Presbyterian hospitals serves as a site for research projects investigating the efficacy of hypnosis with radical prostatectomy, the effects of aromatherapy on stress reduction in coronary artery disease, the effect of meditation on patients with angina, the effectiveness of herbs on patients undergoing menopause, the development of a guided-imagery research protocol for patients with heart failure, and the effectiveness of tai chi and chi gong for patients with heart failure.[6]

Intercessory prayer is part of a clinical trial at Duke University imploring spiritual interventions for seriously ill patients. Crater, a nurse practitioner at Duke University Medical School, stated that in this randomized study when the patient's option is prayer, she triggers a chain reaction around the world: she (1) calls a group of Carmelite nuns near Baltimore who are given the name of a patient in the study, the diagnosis, etc, and the nuns pray at their next service for this patient; (2) e-mails notification to 2 groups of Buddhist monks, one in Nepal and the other outside of Paris; (3) contacts a Jewish group in Jerusalem that slips the name into the Western Wall; and (4) contacts Baptist Moravians and members of other denominations in the United States. Crater has about 100 people from 8 religious groups all praying for the patient's well-being. Other researchers at Duke have initiated a $4 million trial of St John's wort, a herb found in health food stores.[7]

Centers that study alternative medicine (pro and con) are being established nationwide. Sampson from the Stanford School of Medicine has started a journal, *The Scientific Review of Alternative Medicine*, to provide a home for clinical essays examining alternative treatments. However, Herbert, a professor of medicine and a lawyer at the Mount Sinai School of Medicine, refers to acupuncture as "quackupuncture." Herbert recently won a $2.5 million judgment against an alternative practitioner who had treated a cancer patient with hair analysis, coffee enemas, and an expensive daily regimen of 150 dietary supplements and hadn't noticed the growth of tumors. Herbert worries that an increased interest in alternative medicine is going to lead to the unwitting endorsement of health care fraud by the nation's leading medical schools.[7]

Twenty-one experienced therapeutic touch practitioners were unable to detect the investigator's "energy field." Their failure to substantiate therapeutic touch's most fundamental claim is unrefuted evidence that the claims of therapeutic touch are groundless and that further professional use is unjustified.[8] Lundberg, editor of *JAMA*, states that

> this simple statistically valid study which tested the theoretical basis for therapeutic touch [the human energy field] found that such a field does not exist. I believe that practitioners should disclose these results to patients. Third-party payers should question whether they should pay for this procedure and patients should save their money and refuse to pay for this procedure until or unless additional honest experimentation demonstrates an actual effect.[9]

In a personal communication in August 1998, Peskin, a surgical colleague of mine and member of the Editorial Board of the *Archives of Surgery*, reasoned:

> Surgeons, in general, have been slow to recognize this trend. They have been guided in their thinking by the concepts of scientific proof and long-standing tradition. They, and their consultation colleagues, have sought to provide the best surgical attention to each patient's disease, realizing that, while the overwhelming majority of these problems are correctable or curable by current techniques, there are a number of patients whose disability will persist despite all available conventional therapeusis. These are precisely the individuals who seek complementary medical care. Continuing, we are beyond the time when we can ignore the need for patients to satisfy their own desires that all that is possible has been done. It certainly is not a reflection of lack of confidence in the surgeon on the part of the patient, but more like a feeling that seems prevalent today—the desire or expectation of perfect health.

For the present Peskin advises that you

> learn all you can about these alternative techniques to help advise your patients appropriately when asked, participate in legitimate research endeavors to establish or disapprove the effectiveness of alternative treatment if you see fit, and communicate with your patients in a nonaggressive fashion when they avail themselves of these modalities. Surgeons should ask patients about their use of unconventional therapy as part of the medical record so as to improve overall care.

We agree.

I express appreciation to the contributors of this issue: E. Ernst, MD, and M. H. Pittler, MD ("Efficacy of Homeopathic Arnica: A Systematic Review of Placebo-Controlled Clinical Trials"); L. D. Britt, MD, and Frederic J. Cole, MD ("Alternative Surgery in Trauma Management"); Arthur J. Donovan, MD, Thomas V. Berne, MD, and John A. Donovan, MD ("Perforated Duodenal Ulcer: An Alternative Therapeutic Plan"); Roger S. Foster, Jr, MD, and William C. Wood, MD ("Alternative Strategies in the Management of Primary Breast Cancer"); Lars G. Svensson, MD, and Richard P. Cambria, MD ("Expanding Surgical Options Using Minimally Invasive Techniques for Cardio-aortic and Aortic Procedures"); A. James Beyer III, MD, Romano Delcore, MD, and Lawrence Y. Cheung, MD ("Nonoperative Treatment of Biliary Tract Disease"); and J. G. Rothschild, MD ("What Alternatives Has Minimally Invasive Surgery Provided the Surgeon?").

As surgeons, we are continually challenged by the dilemma of our own successes. These creative developments through research have been helpful with our number 1 goal: improved patient care. As a profession and as guardians of safe new methods for our patients, we must exercise this responsibility guided by legitimate, time-honored, clinical trials.

References

1. Kennedy JF. Message to Congress on problems of the aged. In: Strauss MB, ed. *Familiar Medical Quotations*. Boston, Mass: Little Brown & Co; 1968:126–127.
2. Lundberg GD, Wennberg JE. A *JAMA* these issue on quality of care: a new proposal and a call for action. *JAMA*. 1997;278:1615–1616.
3. Wetzel MS, Eisenberg DM, Kaptchuk TJ. Courses involving complementary and alternative medicine at US medical schools. *JAMA*. 1998;280:784–787.
4. Eisenberg DM, Kessler RC, Foster C, Norlock FE, Calkins DR, Delbanco TL. Unconventional medicine in the United States: prevalence, costs, and patterns of use. *N Engl J Med*. 1993;328:246–252.
5. Ebert PA. As I see it. *Bull Am Coll Surg*. 1998; 82:4–5.
6. McCarthy R. Science or sorcery? *Gen Surg News*. 1998;4–6.
7. Wheeler DL. From homeopathy to herbal therapy, researchers focus on alternative medicine. *Chron Higher Educ*. 1998;20–21.
8. Rosa L, Rosa E, Sarner L, Barrett S. A close look at therapeutic touch. *JAMA*. 1998; 279:1005–1010.
9. Lundberg GD. A close look at therapeutic touch [editorial]. *JAMA*. 1998;279:1064.

66 Alternative and Complementary Therapies

An Agenda for Otolaryngology

John H. Krouse, MD
From the Department of Otolaryngology–Head and Neck Surgery, University of South Florida, Tampa.

Arch Otolaryngol Head Neck Surg. 1998;124:1199–1200

Over the past decade, there has been an emergence of interest in complementary and alternative medicine among many Western nations. It has been estimated that about 30% to 40% of Americans use various alternative therapies for many illnesses.[1,2] A similar prevalence has been reported in the United Kingdom.[3] One estimate of the financial impact is that more than $13 billion is spent annually on complementary and alternative techniques in the United States alone.[4]

In 1992, the National Institutes of Health established an Office of Alternative Medicine to define the range of practice in complementary and alternative techniques and to encourage relevant outcomes studies in this area. It recognized 7 categories of alternative medicine: (1) mind-body interventions; (2) bioelectromagnetic therapies; (3) alternative systems of medical practice; (4) manual healing methods; (5) pharmacological and biological treatments; (6) herbal medicine; and (7) diet and nutrition.[5] Within these various categories are included such diverse practices as acupuncture, homeopathy, chiropractic, Eastern medicine, therapeutic touch, and chelation therapy.

Many reasons have been given to explain the rapid growth in the interest of alternative and complementary therapies. A primary factor in this growth is the desire of patients to seek options and alternatives for the treatment of chronic disease.[6] Paralleling this growing interest in complementary medicine is the increasing availability of alternative and complementary treatments,[7] permitting greater access of patients to these techniques. With a patient-physician relationship that is becoming more balanced and democratic as well,[7] patients can feel more empowered to explore options outside the field of traditional allopathic or osteopathic medicine.

Despite the wide interest of patients in the field of alternative and complementary therapies, physicians have often been neutral to them at best, and frankly hostile to them at worst. Until very recently, physicians received little or no training in alternative medicine throughout their medical school education and residency. In addition, many alternative and complementary therapies are based on belief systems and models that are foreign to Western medicine. The target conditions to be treated, the conception of the factors leading to those conditions, and the treatment methods and their outcome measures often conflict with the scientific basis of disease accepted by Western physicians.[1] Therefore, physicians frequently approach alternative and complementary therapies with skepticism and disdain.

Beyond scientific criticisms concerning the safety and efficacy of alternative medicine, other factors appear to play a role in its slow acceptance by many physicians. The traditions of Western medicine are deeply embedded in an anthropological context bounded by religion, history, culture, and the philosophy of science.[8,9] Technologies chosen for therapeutic intervention are selected based on a scientific framework influenced by these factors. There is social pressure to maintain traditional relationships, involving the influence of power bases such as governments and third-party insurers, financial influences including funding of research and reimbursement for service delivery, and public consensus.[9] Acceptance of treatment practices seen as foreign to Western thought such as alternative and complementary medicine requires a paradigm shift in the delivery of care. This paradigm shift will involve a stronger emphasis on health promotion and disease prevention through understanding the relationships among these various influences, including psychosocial, cultural, and environmental factors, as well as biological dysfunction.[10]

In the field of otolaryngology–head and neck surgery, there has been little or no research performed examining the effects of complementary and alternative therapies on the wide range of disorders of the head and neck. A thorough search of the MEDLINE database yielded only a handful of studies examining complementary treatment of disorders such as tinnitus—disorders generally considered refractory to standard medical therapies. Reports of alternative treatment of other otolaryngological problems are quite rare, and no scientific studies are generally available evaluating their safety and efficacy.

With the broad appeal of alternative and complementary therapies in the United States, it is important that otolaryngologists in both academic and community practice actively participate in the development and evaluation of alternative techniques that impact on disorders of the head and neck. To facilitate this participation, our specialty must implement an agenda ensuring its primary role in the process of blending complementary therapies with traditional otolaryngological methods. Four items are important in the implementation of this agenda:

1. The need for an open-minded approach. To allow an objective assessment of the potential benefits and risks of alternative and complementary therapies, it is first essential that otolaryngologists remain open to concepts, models, and therapies that may seem foreign or unusual to them.

2. The need for new models and heuristics. Since standard models of health and illness may not allow an accurate understanding of alternative and complementary therapies, the development of new frameworks emphasizing the importance of health promotion and disease prevention is essential in permitting the application and evaluation of these therapies.

3. The need for novel techniques and methods. Standard therapeutic modalities may not allow the smooth integration of alternative and complementary therapies, so innovative approaches to the delivery of standard otolaryngological care must be blended with creative complementary treatments to frame a new approach to practice.

4. The need for controlled scientific research. Since not all alternative and complementary therapies are equally safe and efficacious, and since skepticism concerning these techniques will remain high, controlled, prospective scientific studies are critical in demonstrating those techniques that have merit and those that should be abandoned.

It is clear that an increasing number of patients will continue to seek alternatives to traditional medical therapies, especially for conditions that are chronic in nature and those that are poorly responsive to standard medical techniques and treatments. It is essential that otolaryngologists recognize this current trend and work at its forefront to evaluate its safety and efficacy and to ensure the smooth integration of beneficial complementary and alternative therapies in standard practice. Through this method we can continue to act as responsible agents for our patients and enhance the safe and effective treatment of disorders of the head and neck.

References

1. Practice and Policy Guidelines Panel, National Institutes of Health Office of Alternative Medicine. Clinical practice guidelines in complementary and alternative medicine. *Arch Fam Med*. 1997;6:149–154.

2. Kligman E. Alternative medicine. *Iowa Med*. 1997;87:232–234.

3. Ernst E. Complementary medicine: common misconceptions. *J R Soc Med*. 1995;88:245–247.

4. Schimpff SC. Complementary medicine. *Curr Opin Oncol*. 1997;9:327–331.

5. Gordon JS. Alternative medicine and the family physician. *Am Fam Physician*. 1996; 54:2205–2212.

6. Burg MA. Women's use of complementary medicine: combining mainstream medicine with alternative practices. *J Fla Med Assoc*. 1996;83:482–488.

7. Lynoe N. Ethical and professional aspects of the practice of alternative medicine. *Scand J Soc Med*. 1992;20:217–225.

8. Hess DJ. Technology and alternative cancer therapies: an analysis of heterodoxy and constructivism. *Med Anthropol Q*. 1996;10:657–674.

9. Gursoy A. Beyond the orthodox: heresy in medicine and the social sciences from a cross-cultural perspective. *Soc Sci Med*. 1996;43:577–599.

10. Schuck JR, Chappell LT, Kindness G. Causal modeling and alternative medicine. *Altern Ther Health Med*. 1997;3:40–47.

67 Alternative Medicine—Learning From the Past, Examining the Present, Advancing to the Future

Wayne B. Jonas, MD
From the Office of Alternative Medicine, National Institutes of Health, Bethesda, Md.

JAMA. 1198;280:1616–1618

Medical practices outside the mainstream of "official" medicine have always been an important part of the public's health care. Healers and herbalists, bonesetters and barbers, shamans and spiritualists have offered the public a multiplicity of ways to address the confusion and suffering that accompany disease. A century ago in the United States there was a period of "enchantment" with unorthodox medicine. Homeopaths, herbalists, psychic and magnetic healers, and "eclectics" proliferated—most with little to no training, regulation of practice, or standards for quality of care. The prominence and configuration of these "irregulars," as they were called, has waxed and waned, depending on the perceived value of orthodox medicine, the needs of the public, and the changing values of society. The prominence of these practices subsided with the development of scientific medicine in this century and its dramatic advances in the understanding and treatment of disease.[1]

Historically, orthodox medicine fights these practices vigorously by denouncing and attacking them, restricting access to them, labeling them as antiscientific and quackery, and imposing penalties for practicing them. When these therapies persist and even rise in popularity despite this, mainstream medicine then turns more friendly, examining them, identifying similarities they have with the orthodox, and incorporating or "integrating" them into the routine practice of medicine.[2] In the past, orthodox medicine has benefited from their selective integration by abandoning ineffective therapies such as bloodletting, adopting new drugs such as digitalis, and developing more rigorous scientific methods with which to test these practices, such as blinding and randomization.[2,3]

The increasing popularity of complementary and alternative medicine (now used by more than 40% of the public) reflects changing needs and values in modern society in general.[4] This includes a rise in prevalence of chronic disease, an increase in public access to worldwide health information, reduced tolerance for paternalism, an increased sense of entitlement to a quality life, declining faith that scientific breakthroughs will have relevance for the personal treatment of disease, and an increased interest in spiritualism.[5–7] In addition, concern about the adverse effects and escalating costs of conventional health care are fueling the search for alternative approaches to the prevention and management of illness.[6,7] As the public's use of healing practices outside conventional medicine accelerates, ignorance about these practices by physicians and scientists risks broadening the communication gap between the public and the profession that serves them.[4,8]

Today, the overwhelming effort is toward attempts at "integrating" alternative practices into the mainstream. Sixty percent of medical schools have begun to teach about alternative medicine practices,[9] hospitals are creating complementary and integrated medicine programs, health suppliers are offering expanded benefits packages that include the services of alternative practitioners,[10] and biomedical research organizations are investing more substantial amounts toward the investigation of these practices. For example, the Office of Alternative Medicine at the National Institutes of Health has just become the National Center for Complementary and Alternative Medicine, with a budget of $50 million. The activities of the Office of Alternative Medicine[11] and the publication of this issue of *JAMA* illustrate that quality scientific research can be conducted and published on alternative medicine topics. It appears that complementary and alternative medicine has again "come of age" in the United States. However, the rush to embrace a new integration of alternative and conventional medicine should be approached with great caution. Alternative medicine, like conventional medicine, has pros and cons, promotes bad ideas and good ones, and promises to hold both benefits and risks. Without critical assessment of what should be integrated and what should not, we risk developing a health care system that costs more, is less safe, and fails to address the management of chronic disease in a publicly responsible manner. The potential risks and benefits of alternative medicine must be examined carefully before heading into a new but not necessarily better health care world.

Risks of Embracing Alternative Medicine

Quality of Care

The formal components of medical physician licensure usually are not required of alternative medicine practitioners. These include the content and length of time of training, testing and certification, a defined scope of practice, review and audit, and professional liability with regulatory protection and statutory authorization complete with codified disciplinary action.[12] All 50 states do provide licensure requirements for chiropractic practice, but only about half do so for acupuncture and massage therapy and fewer do for homeopathy and naturopathy. Many of these practitioners operate largely unmonitored.[13]

Quality of Products

The "natural" products used by alternative medicine practitioners also are largely unmonitored and their quality is uncontrolled. These products are available on the market as dietary supplements and may be contaminated or vary tremendously in content, quality, and safety.[14] Garlic, for example, claimed for many years to have cholesterol lowering effects, may not produce such effects if processed in certain ways.[15] Thus, even if one product is proven safe and effective, other similar products on the market may have quite different effects that preclude consistent dosing. Fifteen million Americans are taking high-dose vitamins or herbal preparations along with prescription drugs, thereby risking adverse effects from unknown interactions.[4]

Quality of Science

The use of science for understanding alternative medicine is frequently missing from such practices. Most alternative medicine systems have been largely unchanged for hundreds or thousands of years. Often they begin from the teachings of a charismatic leader that are not advanced with new observations, hypothesis-driven testing, innovation, and peer-review. Claiming that their practices are too "individual" or "holistic" to study scientifically, many alternative medicine practices hide behind anecdote, case series, or "outcomes" research.[16] To accept such views is to falsely label conventional medicine as nonholistic and reject the hard-fought gains made in the use of basic biological knowledge, the randomized, controlled clinical trial, and evidence-based medicine for health care decision making.[17]

To adopt alternative medicine without developing quality standards for its practices, products, and research is to return to a time in medicine when quackery and therapeutic confusion prevailed. Modern conventional medicine excels in the areas of quality health care and the use of science: alternative medicine must change to adopt similar standards. Conventional medicine is also the world's leader in the management of infectious, traumatic, and surgical diseases, in the study of pathology, and in biotechnology and drug development. All medical practices have the ethical obligation to retain these strengths for the benefit of patients.

Risks of Conventionalizing Alternative Medicine

Healing

Most alternative medicine systems carefully attend to the illness and suffering that accompanies all disease. The time spent with each patient by an alternative medicine practitioner usually exceeds that spent by the average conventional physician, and patients are often more satisfied with their interactions with unorthodox than orthodox medical practitioners.[18] Alternative medicine practitioners provide patients with understanding, meaning, and self-care methods for managing their condition. Empowerment, participation in the healing process, time, and personal attention are essential elements of all medicine. These elements are easily lost in the subspecialization, technology, and economics of modern medicine. Conventional medicine must develop a better language for managing illness and suffering or lose this essential message that alternative medicine provides.

Adverse Effects

In the last century, unconventional medicine increased in popularity because of the use of severe treatments such as bloodletting, purging, and toxic metals by conventional medicine.[2] The popularity of alternative medicine in this century is also driven by the perception that conventional treatments are too harsh to use for chronic and non–life-threatening disease.[6,7] Iatrogenic disease caused by conventional medicine is a major cause of death and hospitalization in the United States. While some alternative medicine practices have important toxicities, many have reduced potential for adverse effects when properly delivered.[19] Conventional medicine can learn from alternative medicine how to "gentle" its approach by focusing on the patient's inherent capacity for self-healing.[20]

Costs

Skyrocketing costs of conventional medicine also are driving the search for alternatives. Savings from managed care now are maximized and health care costs are predicted to double in the next 10 years.[21] If low-cost interventions such as lifestyle changes, diet, supplement therapy, and behavioral medicine can be delivered as substitutes for high-cost drugs and technological interventions, true cost reductions and the compression of morbidity might be achieved.[22]

If there is a single strength of alternative medicine that risks being lost in its "integration" with conventional care, it is an emphasis on self-healing as the lead approach for both improving wellness and for the treatment of disease. All the major alternative medicine systems approach illness first by trying to support and induce the self-healing processes of the person. If recovery can occur from this, the likelihood of adverse effects and the need for high-impact, high-cost interventions is reduced.[23] It is this orientation toward self-healing and health promotion (salutogenesis rather than pathogenesis) that makes alternative medicine approaches to chronic disease especially attractive.[22]

The Future of Alternative Medicine

The main "obstacles to discovery," writes Daniel Boorstin,[24] are "the illusions of knowledge." Indeed, the capacity of humans to fool themselves by making claims of truth, postulating unfounded explanations, and denying the reality of observations they cannot explain is endless. Science has emerged as one of the few truly powerful approaches for mitigating this self-delusionary capacity. The clinical experimental method, in the form of the randomized, controlled trial, examines to what extent attributions and explanations of these therapies are accurate.[25]

The goals of medicine, no matter what the label, are the same for all practices.[26] Is the current trend toward "integrated" medicine a deluded temptation that will turn out to be a nightmare of unscientific practices? Or will these newfound tools of scientific medicine be used to look deeper into the processes of healing for their utility in treating disease and alleviating suffering? In the last 50 years, powerful social forces have transformed medicine.[5] If a new evidence-based "integrated" medicine does emerge, it will likely be subject to the same forces shaping the future of medicine in general. This includes the continued takeover of medicine by managed care, a more refined ability to manipulate individual susceptibilities using nanotechnology, and the ability to track quality of care and individual patient outcomes with networks of information monitoring.[27] Research in alternative medicine will help identify what is safe and effective and will further the understanding of biology by exploring, rather than marginalizing, unorthodox medical claims and findings.[28] Alternative medicine is here to stay. It is no longer an option to ignore it or treat it as something outside the normal processes of science and medicine. The challenge is to move forward carefully, using both reason and wisdom, as we attempt to separate the pearls from the mud.

References

1. Gevitz N. *Other Healers: Unorthodox Medicine in America*. Baltimore, Md: The Johns Hopkins University Press; 1988.

2. Worton JC. The history of complementary and alternative medicine. In: Jonas WB, Levin JH, eds. *Essentials of Complementary and Alternative Medicine*. Baltimore, Md: Williams & Wilkins Inc. In press.

3. Kaptchuk TJ. Intentional ignorance: the history of blind assessment and placebo controls in medicine. *Bull Hist Med*. 1998;72:389–433.

4. Eisenberg DM, Davis RB, Ettner SL, et al. Trends in alternative medicine use in the United States, 1990–1997: results of a follow-up national survey. *JAMA*. 1998;280:1569–1575.

5. Starr P. *The Social Transformation of American Medicine*. San Francisco, Calif: Harper Collins Publishers; 1982:514.

6. Furnham A, Forey J. The attitudes, behaviors and beliefs of patients of conventional vs complementary (alternative) medicine. *J Clin Psychol*. 1994;50:458–469.

7. Astin JA. Why patients use alternative medicine: results of a national study. *JAMA*. 1998;279:1548–1553.

8. Chez IRA, Jonas WB. The challenge of complementary and alternative medicine. *Am J Obstet Gynecol*. 1997;177:1156–1161.

9. Wetzel MS, Eisenberg DM, Kaptchuk TJ. Courses involving complementary and alternative medicine at US medical schools. *JAMA*. 1998;280:784–787.

10. Pelletier KR, Marie A, Krasner M, Haskell WL. Current trends in the integration and reimbursement of complementary and alternative medicine by managed care, insurance carriers, and hospital providers. *Am J Health Promotion*. 1997;12:112–123.

11. National Institutes of Health Office of Alternative Medicine. *A Report and Plan of the Office of Alternative Medicine*. Bethesda, Md: National Institutes of Health; 1998.

12. Milbank Memorial Fund. *Enhancing the Accountability of Alternative Medicine*. New York, NY: Milbank Memorial Fund; 1998.

13. Federation of the State Medical Boards of the United States Inc. *Report on Health Care Fraud From the Special Committee on Health Care Fraud*. Austin, Tex: Federation of the State Medical Boards of the United States Inc; 1997.

14. Ernst E. Harmless herbs? *Am J Med*. 1998; 104:170–178.

15. Berthold HK, Sudhop MD, von Bergmann K. Effect of a garlic oil preparation on serum lipoproteins and cholesterol metabolism. *JAMA*. 1998;279:1900–1902.

16. Coulter HL. *The Controlled Clinical Trial*: An Analysis. Washington, DC: Center for Empirical Medicine; 1991.

17. Jonas WB. Clinical trials for chronic disease: randomized, controlled clinical trials are essential. *J Natl Inst Health Res*. 1997;9:33–39.

18. Ernst E, Resch KL, Hill S. Do complementary practitioners have a better bedside manner than physicians? *J R Soc Med*. 1997;90:118–119.

19. Jonas WB. Safety in complementary medicine. In: Ernst E, ed. *Complementary Medicine: An Objective Appraisal*. Oxford, England: Butterworth-Heinemann; 1996:126–149.

20. Antonovsky A. *Unraveling the Mystery of Health: How People Manage Stress and Stay Well*. San Francisco, Calif: Jossey-Bass; 1987.

21. Smith S, Freeland M, Heffier S, McKusick D, for the Team at HEP. The next ten years of health spending. *Health Aff (Milwood)*. 1998; 17:128–140.

22. Sobel DS. Rethinking medicine: improving health outcomes with cost-effective psychosocial interventions. *Psychosom Med*. 1995;57:234–244.

23. Jonas WB. Models of medicine and models of healing. In: Jonas WB, Levin JH, eds. *Essentials of Complementary and Alternative Medicine*. Baltimore, Md: Williams & Wilkins Inc. In press.

24. Boorstin DJ. *The Discoverers*. New York, NY: Random House Inc; 1983:xv.

25. Sackett DL, Rosenberg WM, Gray JA, Haynes RB, Richardson WS. Evidence based medicine: what it is and what it isn't [editorial]. *BMJ*. 1996;312:71–72.

26. The Hastings Center. *The Goals of Medicine: Setting New Priorities*. Briarcliff Manor, NY: The Hastings Center; 1996.

27. Institute for Alternative Futures. *The Future of Complementary and Alternative Approaches (CAAs) in US Health Care*. Alexandria, Va: Institute for Alternative Futures; 1998.

28. Jonas WB. Researching alternative medicine. *Nat Med*. 1997;3:824–827.

68 Leeches, Spiders, and Astrology: Predilections and Predictions

Tom Delbanco, MD
Boston, Mass.

JAMA. 1998;280:1560–1562

I care for a patient who is 53 and obese with high lipid levels, borderline hypertension, and a strong family history of heart disease. She loves rich foods, hates exercise, and fears synthetic compounds. Recently she has avidly embraced alternative therapies and tells me glowingly about her various healers, the herbal preparations she swallows, and homeopathic medicines that limit her colds.

She is typical of many persons in my practice. People in the United States are rushing toward alternative therapies.[1] What's going on? What does the future hold in the long-standing interplay between allopathic and alternative medicine? Drawing primarily on conversations with my patients, I offer observations and predictions that suggest we are in the midst of a fad that will pass.

Conflicting Information

Confusing both doctors and patients, contradictory results emerge every week from epidemiologic data and clinical trials. When my patient asks for advice about risk prevention, my response is halting. As I peruse newspapers and medical journals, what's judged best for managing the interplay of obesity, blood pressure, lipids, and family history in a woman feeling exceedingly well changes monthly. And for my other patients, is salt in or out this year? When is wine healthy, and when is it not? What's best for back pain? How do coronary stents, phentermine, or the interferons fare this week? When so much appears uncertain or contradictory, taking the doctor's counsel seriously is difficult.

Prediction

Rigorous investigators are just beginning to study alternative medicine. As with other new areas of inquiry, few studies have carefully examined the interactions between interventions and outcomes, and few "negative" studies have been published. As scholars compare alternative therapies with sham interventions, and control for patient expectations, their findings will add to the confusion, just as conflicting data remind us that the practice of medicine combines both art and science. Soon the questions will be: How do garlic, ginseng, ginkgo, and St John's wort look this week?

Dangers and Shaken Trust

So far, the media have primarily trumpeted success stories and testimonials about alternative medicine. In contrast, a constant barrage of news highlights dangerous medications, medical mistakes, and tragic outcomes in allopathic medicine. Ironically, scientific medicine must take partial responsibility for its own bad press, now that it has grudgingly legitimized scholarly inquiry into the prevalence and nature of medical errors. All the news about disasters and about perverse incentives tempting doctors to "withhold" care leaves public trust in allopathic medicine shaken.

Prediction

Reporters thrive on trouble and are already spreading word about dangerous herbs and quackery. As they do today with allopathic medicine, the press will soon include alternate clinicians in tales of missed tumors, substance abuse, and sexual misconduct with patients.

AIDS and Scientific Failure

Earlier in this century, scientists achieved enormous prestige following their discovery of antibiotic "miracle drugs" and the polio vaccine. But since then, the public has witnessed few miracles. Moreover, few of us, whether patient or health professional, thought we would experience an epidemic with the ferocity of AIDS that has so far stymied the biomedical community. To make matters worse, medical journals, followed quickly by terrifying paperbacks in airport bookstores, carry word of new or newly virulent killer microbes. Why can't scientists sweep away the present and future dangers posed by such organisms? Why does the "war on cancer" remain a skirmish? Public confidence in biomedical science has fallen, and alternative medicine, with its primal message of hope, is currently filling a vacuum.

Prediction

Despite the public's sense that major advances are elusive, the current infusion of dollars in the National Institutes of Health (NIH) signals society's persistent hopes and expectations for science. For those populations that can afford current therapies, the transformation of AIDS into a chronic illness is reassuring, and cardiologists and oncologists are also beginning to have some striking successes. Viagra and its descendants, new vaccines, and genetic therapies will help scientists to rebuild public trust. No comparable advances within alternative medicine will balance the scales.

Time Racing By

The inexorable shrinking of time is not a phenomenon unique to medicine. Just 20 years ago we were told computers would create so much leisure time that we would struggle to fill it. Instead we fight for time to breathe. Whoever or whatever the culprits, doctors spend fewer and fewer minutes assessing and giving counsel; many patients feel a profound sense of loss, and some are angry. They are not particularly interested in how busy we are, or in our casting blame. Alternative healers stand in sharp contrast: patients appreciate the generous amounts of time they offer.

Prediction

Economic and regulatory constraints that now overwhelm allopaths will close in on alternative practitioners, forcing them to change their habits. Soon the herbalist and homeopath will also drown in charts and forms demanding comprehensive documentation. As alternative practitioners age, they will seek larger incomes. Inexorably, time with each patient will shorten.

In contrast, allopathic doctors, particularly those in primary care, will start to reclaim time, helped by patients who both take a more active role in their care and marshal a collective will that forces payers to replenish the minutes.[2] Overall the gap in time offered patients by allopathic and alternative caregivers will diminish.

Retreat From the Din

Investment bankers leave the city and refurbish inns in the countryside. Abstract art recedes, as portraits and landscapes return. Audiences ask for music played on the "original instruments" for which it was composed. Films that celebrate the Australian Outback and the Irish village captivate viewers exhausted by the day's travails. Alternative medicine's call back to nature and the "organic" is part of this wave of nostalgia.

Prediction

Allopathic doctors will learn also to lay claim to the "organic" and "natural" arts. They will move into some of the alternative medicine turf, as they develop a new vernacular that speaks in scientific terms of allopathic medicine's ability to harness nature in the battle against disease.

Changing Behaviors

As my patient demonstrates, exercising, avoiding fattening foods, or overcoming other addictions is difficult and unpleasant. Some call it laziness; others find explanations in Freud or malfunctioning neurotransmitters. In place of taking definitive action themselves, my most honest patients confess they want something done to or for them, rather than meet the demands placed on them.

Prediction
So far, neither allopathic nor alternative clinicians have significantly improved most human conduct. Despite fervent rhetoric to the contrary, both generally do things to patients, rather than stimulate them to change behaviors. But scientists will soon develop pills that will help safely with obesity, stress, addictions, and other self-destructive behavioral phenomena. At that point, alternative medicine will have trouble competing.

Sellers Go Right to the Patient

Perhaps it is fitting that this issue of *JAMA* appears during a season celebrating the contributions of Edward Bernays, inventor of "spin" and public relations.[3] Alternative medicines sell direct to the patient, and charismatic healers extolling alternative therapies captivate the media, leaving allopaths dyspneic at the starting gate.

Prediction
The pharmaceutical industry is suddenly enjoying soaring profits from soliciting patients directly, and allopathic practitioners will learn quickly to market and peddle their wares aggressively to patients. Mobilizing charisma effectively, prominent and articulate doctors will compete with and outspend alternative healers for airtime.

Paying the Bill

The recent strong economy has lessened the sting of out-of-pocket health care payments. But if they have health insurance, patients feel it should cover most services. In contrast to payers in some western European countries, insurers in the United States are only now beginning gingerly to tread the alternative waters. Some are already beating a hasty retreat.

Prediction
Fee-for-service remains the rule for alternative practitioners. So far, chiropractors and massage therapists depend on patients coming to them and spend little time teaching family or friends to manipulate or massage at home. A volatile economy and mounting health care costs will accelerate incentives for providers to do less and for patients to stay away. How alternative therapists (and allopathic providers) will deal with rapidly shifting incentives remains an open question, but salaried health professionals, no matter what their practice persuasion, will increasingly become the norm. Then the battle for who gets paid what will begin in earnest!

Efficacy and the Placebo Effect

Focusing on quality of life, comfort, and hope, alternative practitioners have much to teach the allopath who short-changes such human needs. For such fundamental aspects of care, do we really need to put each intervention to a scientific test? If a clinician spends ample time laying on hands and addressing issues warmly and hopefully with a patient, we don't need a controlled trial demonstrating the value of such interchange. But daggers flash when alternative clinicians claim their wares are not only entirely safe but also effective beyond the placebo effect.

Prediction
Although Congress has rendered the Food and Drug Administration virtually toothless in overseeing the safety and efficacy of alternative medicines,[4] academic medicine will soon shatter claims for activity beyond placebo. Moneys spent on research by the NIH Office of Alternative Medicine are already under harsh scrutiny.[5] The fight is on. A brilliant albeit acerbic bench scientist recently asked a speaker discussing research in alternative medicine at our Medicine Grand Rounds,"Why don't we form a center at Harvard for the scientific study of astrology? After all, it's far more popular than homeopathy and massage therapy!" His point is clear: the public should not stand for spending tax revenues on studies not worth doing.

In France, touring a huge factory manufacturing homeopathic medicines, I watched technicians wearing spotless whites grind up spiders, immerse the morsels in water, dilute the slurry so that the spider molecules disappeared, and shake the fluid obsessively. For such a potion, rigorous scientific inquiry will not demonstrate physiologic impact beyond placebo, and once this is clear, alternative practices that claim such superiority will be dealt a heavy blow.

Moreover, given their safety, low cost, and efficacy, placebos and their virtues will be discussed frankly among allopathic clinicians and their patients. These powerful substances will be advertised in medical journals, but in contrast to the past, doctors will now dispense them without subterfuge or deceit.[6,7] They will simply tell their patients, "This is a placebo. We have little idea right now why it works, but it often does. Give it a try."

Fad, or Here to Stay?

Fads come and go quickly. In the past, allopathic medicine touted leeches, frozen stomachs, and thalidomide (leeches may be coming back, and thalidomide has returned, albeit with strict oversight). Today tennis is out; golf is in. Convertibles are deemed dangerous; monstrous SUVs rule the roads. Specialists look for work; primary care doctors are in demand.

Prediction

Alternative therapies, bathed invariably in optimism and hope, invoke harmony with nature and the human need for mystery. In contrast, scientific medicine focuses on trouble, dysfunction, and disorder, with practitioners discoursing on cancers "eating at the flesh" and autoimmune diseases "turning bodies against themselves." Whatever the guiding metaphors, for those long-steeped in a heritage of chicken soup, religion, copper bracelets—or penicillin—fads will have little impact.[8]

But the current explosion in alternative medicine is rooted differently. Signs of this fact are plentiful: yuppies lead the charge; messianic proselytizers harangue; profiteers follow the scent of blood; philanthropists make huge contributions; media hype drowns out the negatives; and patients spend money that might better go elsewhere. For many recent converts, the lust for alternative medicine seems to run in parallel to the appetite for cosmetic surgery designed to reclaim passing years, signaling both decadence and self-indulgence.

Well before its explosive growth in the United States, alternative medicine proliferated in western Europe. Recent conversations with doctors and patients there suggest that in some regions the bloom is fading, particularly as national health systems constrain medical costs and scrutinize the quality of care.

As my point-counterpoint suggests, the current fascination with alternative medicine will have a lasting and, on the whole, salutary impact on allopathic practice. But I predict that patients' romance with the field will diminish with time, leaving a core of true believers similar to those of the past.

What about my patient? All clinicians are learning that good care, as well as their economic survival, depends on taking into account patients' cultural heritage and habits, on respecting and addressing expectations, beliefs, and unique preferences. In that context, she is telling me to take seriously the messages alternative medicine sends, and I am ready to listen. But how can I help? In the end, whether we focus on allopathic medicine, alternative medicine, or both, she and I need to find a way to improve her lifestyle and prevent future vascular disaster. Right now, we have a long way to go.

I thank Andrew, Jill, and Suzanne Delbanco, Lisa Iezzoni, MD, and Richard Rockefeller, MD, for exceedingly helpful critique of the manuscript.

References

1. Eisenberg DM, Davis RB, Ettner SL, et al. Trends in alternative medicine use in the United States, 1990–1997: results of a follow-up national survey. *JAMA*. 1998;280:1569–1575.

2. Hart JT. Expectations of health care: promoted, managed or shared? *Health Expectations*. 1998;1:3–13.

3. Tye L. *The Father of Spin: Edward Bernays and the Birth of Public Relations*. New York, NY: Crown; 1998.

4. Delbanco TL. Bitter herbs: mainstream, magic, and menace. *Ann Intern Med*. 1994; 121:803–804.

5. Angell M, Kassirer JP. Alternative medicine—the risks of untested and unregulated remedies. *N Engl J Med*. 1998;339:839–841.

6. Brown W. Placebo as a treatment for depression. *Neuropsychopharmacology*. 1994; 10:265–269.

7. Delbanco TL. Commentary on "Placebo as a treatment for depression." *Neuropsychopharmacology*. 1994;10:279–280.

8. Gevitz N. *Other Healers: Unorthodox Medicine in America*. Baltimore, Md: Johns Hopkins University Press; 1988.

69 Factors That Shape Alternative Medicine

Daniel P. Eskinazi, DDS, PhD, LAc
From the Rosenthal Center for Complementary and Alternative Medicine, Columbia University College of Physicians and Surgeons, New York, NY.

JAMA. 1998;280:1621–1623

The lack of relevant high-quality scientific research has often been given as a reason[1,2] to explain why a large number of health care practices are termed *alternative*. However, the fact that it required congressional intervention[3,4] for the National Institutes of Health (NIH) to earmark 0.02% ($2 million) of its $10.7 billion 1992 budget to evaluate practices used by more than 35% of the US population suggests that issues beyond the scientific were involved. Nonscientific factors have played a major role in limiting scientific exploration of these areas, have discouraged potential investigators, and have dictated greater profitability elsewhere. This article examines current definitions of alternative medicine and proposes a new one, outlining those factors, sociological (academic), political, regulatory, and economic, that must be considered when exploring this field.

Definitions of Alternative Medicine

Despite increasing use of alternative medicine,[5] the creation of the NIH Office of Alternative Medicine (OAM), and increasing health insurance coverage for alternative therapies, no clear definition of alternative medicine has been established. When definitions have been proposed, they included either ad hoc lists of practices felt to be alternative[6,7] or categorical criteria that are changing rapidly[8] and, therefore, do not allow for a lasting definition of alternative medicine.

Lists of alternative medical practices are disparate[6,7] and encompass complex traditional health care systems, eg, Chinese (traditional Chinese medicine), East Indian (Ayurveda), Native American,[9,10] as well as their integrated and complementary components practiced as distinct entities (eg, medicinal herbs, acupuncture, dietary principles, and spiritual practices). These lists also include a wide variety of discrete modalities and products more difficult to categorize. Furthermore, among the proponents of practices such as hypnosis, osteopathy, and chiropractic (which have been taught in degree-granting institutions for more than a century), there is little consensus as to whether these modalities are alternative or mainstream.

Alternative medicine also has been defined as what is not taught in medical schools or not covered by insurance.[8] These definitions also have drawbacks because their reference criteria are changing rapidly and are not consistent across the country. For example, in the 75 US medical schools that offer courses in alternative medicine, the curriculum varies widely.[11] Health insurance coverage for alternative practices also varies widely among insurers and regionally. Most important, these definitions do not provide a rationale for the term *alternative medicine* to encompass such diverse practices.

Commonalities Among Traditional Health Care Systems

Comprehensive traditional health care systems and their components form much of what is generally understood in the United States as alternative medicine. Other alternative practices or products not originating in a traditional health care system also represent a substantial but less coherent grouping.

Traditional health care systems represent philosophical approaches to managing health and disease that differ substantially from those of Western biomedicine.[9,10,12–14] The question of what is common to these traditional systems has been largely overlooked, but spirituality is an integral part of each. As this trait is often directly related to the dominant religion or philosophical system of the originating culture, it is taken for granted within the context of health care. For example, the ancient Chinese health care system was influenced by several spiritual schools, in particular Taoism.[12] Ayurveda, a traditional medical system of India, reflects the traditional Hindu world view.[13] Similarly, Tibetan physicians practice Buddhist meditation as an integral part of their medical training.[14]

In many traditional medical systems, the primary explanation for biological phenomena is based on the existence of a "vital force," an elusive entity designated *Qi* in China, *Ki* in Korea and Japan, *prana* in India, and *vital force* in Western traditions (eg, homeopathy). The terms *energy* and *energy medicine* are also used with increasing frequency. However, given the scientific definition of energy, this designation is misleading, as nothing is known of the nature of this hypothetical entity.

Also common to traditional health care systems is the belief in a unity underlying all diversity, implying holism (or wholism), that nothing can be considered in isolation.[12–15] In the realm of health, these principles lead to considering the person as an indivisible whole, rather than as dissected anatomic parts. Thus, diagnoses and treatments are based primarily on concepts of organ functions, although not necessarily directly correlated to the actual organ entities or their anatomic locations. In addition, it is believed that health maintenance depends on a proper interaction with the environment. Hence, therapeutic interventions include stimuli (eg, sound, color, and taste) for any of the 5 senses, as these allow the individual to interrelate with his or her environment. Similarly, means of communication with the "invisible" environment (eg, meditation or prayer) form an important part of the therapeutic approach.[12–15]

Conceptual Differences and Commonalities Between Biomedicine and Traditional Health Care

The characteristics common to traditional (alternative) systems of health (vital force, spirituality, and holism) also seem to distinguish them from biomedicine. Biomedicine is founded in part on materialism (in contrast to the vital force explanation). Materialism in this context refers to the theory that "physical matter is the only or fundamental reality, and that all beings and processes and phenomena are manifestations or results of matter."[15] While biomedicine does not necessarily reject religion or spirituality, it does not routinely incorporate these aspects into diagnosis and treatment (unlike traditional systems). Consistent with this philosophical theory, biomedicine considers biological entities more or less as equal to the sum of their anatomic parts (a view opposite to holism) and endeavors to elucidate molecular, physiological, and pathological mechanisms believed to form the basis of biological processes. Allopathic medical treatment often logically consists of interventions chosen to interfere with identified pathological molecular processes.

As it has not been scientifically demonstrated that "physical matter is the only reality," materialism, therefore, is akin to a religion, ie, "a system of beliefs held to with ardor and faith."[15] Western allopathic medicine would, therefore, have the same fundamental quality as traditional systems of health: it reflects the dominant philosophical belief system of the society in which it developed.

Proposed Definition of Alternative Medicine

I propose that *alternative medicine* be defined as a broad set of health care practices (ie, already available to the public) that are not readily integrated into the dominant health care model, because they pose challenges to diverse societal beliefs and practices (cultural, economic, scientific, medical, and educational). This definition brings into focus factors that may play a major role in the a priori acceptance or rejection of various alternative health care practices by any society. Unlike criteria of current definitions, those of the proposed definition would not be expected to change significantly without significant societal changes.

Applications of this definition to Western society include the following: (1) *cultural*—health care systems may have developed outside mainstream American culture and may not be consonant with our cultural values; (2) *economic*—therapies similar to conventional pharmacological approaches (ie, based on the use of purified molecular species, eg, antineoplastons) can be considered alternative. These tend to be therapies that are developed by private practitioners, bypass established economic networks (eg, pharmaceutical industry, research institutions, and hospitals) and have difficulties going through the steps generally required to achieve acceptance in conventional medical practice; (3) *scientific beliefs*—there exists no scientific explanation for how some practices (for example, homeopathy and noncontact practices such as *Reiki* and *Qi gong*) could possibly work. However, the paucity of research data is most likely due to their being alternative; (4) *medical*—holistic medicine practices often focus on preventive and therapeutic enhancement of existing biological mechanisms (eg, the immune system), and do not follow the allopathic model; and (5) *educational standards*—some practices are passed on from generation to generation through oral tradition, rather than through formal training at special schools or institutions.

The proposed definition also is relevant to whether the term *alternative* or *complementary* is used. The origin of a practice may be alternative (eg, culturally or economically different), while its use can be complementary with biomedicine (or other alternative practices).

Sociological and Academic Parameters

For decades Western academia has excluded alternative medicine research and practice; this has contributed much to the paucity of data in this area. Established academic researchers have been discredited and have had difficulties when attempting to conduct alternative medicine research.[16,17] At times, explicit threats were made by mainstream medicine to individuals and institutions that would associate with alternative medicine practitioners.[18] Consequently, most alternative medicine research has been conducted outside of academia by individuals with limited research training and resources, and their investigations are often methodologically inadequate.[1,2] Conversely, those studies deemed methodologically sound may lack comparability and replication. For example, lack of funding, differences among individual investigators' resources, and personal research interests have limited replication of studies in homeopathy and acupuncture.[19,20]

This atmosphere, in which academic investigators were concerned about the impact that their interest in alternative medicine might have on their good standing and their livelihood, has been particularly unfavorable to the development of high-quality academic research. This is changing, as the creation of the OAM has helped to legitimize alternative medicine evaluation and allowed these investigators to manifest openly their interest. The result has been the creation of 13 academic centers dedicated to alternative medicine assessment at major US institutions.[21]

Political, Economic, and Regulatory Parameters

The interaction of politics and science in the arena of health care, one of the most lucrative industries in the United States, has played a significant role in recent development of alternative medicine in the United States. For example, in October 1991, the US Congress instructed the NIH to create an Office of Unconventional Medical Practices,[4] later renamed the Office of Alternative Medicine. The congressional mandate was met with a less than enthusiastic response from the NIH,[22,23] but simultaneously with high public expectations.[24] Compounding the difficulties, other key governmental agencies, in particular the Food and Drug Administration (FDA), were overlooked in the mandate, although their role was necessary and complementary to that of the OAM.

Similar to other federal programs, the activities of the OAM must comply with FDA regulations and policies. Yet, FDA regulations designed for conventional drugs and devices are not always applicable for alternative medicine products. For example, regulations are designed for conventional products that require research before becoming publicly available. Considerable economic incentives usually justify corporate sponsors of new therapies to submit to the FDA's stringent and onerous regulations.[25] Conversely, alternative medicine products are, by definition, already available, which lessens the drive for research. In addition, there is little incentive for conducting alternative medicine research, as it seldom leads to significant economic benefit. For example, research into homeopathy or medicinal plants usually does not lead to economic advantages for sponsors, because these products are not proprietary. Similarly, lack of economic incentive (due to limited markets) also led to insufficient research in the biomedical area of rare diseases and required special governmental incentives.[26]

There are several reasons, other than economic ones, that current regulatory criteria may be difficult to apply to alternative practices, in particular traditional practices from other cultures. For example, these practices follow different diagnostic classifications than biomedicine, and the complex substances (eg, botanical, animal products) they use cannot easily meet the criteria established for essentially pure drugs or even for conventional biologics. However, the FDA recently has begun addressing the issues posed by evaluation of alternative medicine products. Representatives from the FDA actively participated in the organization of 2 conferences that addressed the special considerations of acupuncture[19] and of botanical medicines.[20]

Conclusion

Nonscientific factors contribute to defining the scope of alternative medicine and the context for its evaluation. Economic promise of growing markets may lead to a focus on developing profitable alternative medicine products rather than on improving health care and also may lead away from addressing issues that have prompted the public to seek alternative medicine practices. Nonscientific and scientific factors are shaping this unusually heterogeneous and potentially fruitful field and must be taken into account for a thoughtful evaluation to yield more than incremental progress.

The author wishes to thank the following individuals for stimulating discussions and helpful comments and suggestions during the preparation of this article: Richard Hammerschlag, PhD, Judith Jacobson, PhD, Fredi Kronenberg, PhD, Carrie Lewis, Janet Mindes, PhD, David Muehsam, and Patricia Muehsam, MD. In addition, the expert assistance of Marion Brandis, RN, is gratefully acknowledged.

References

1. Chez RA, Jonas WB. The challenge of complementary and alternative medicine. *Am J Obstet Gynecol.* 1997;177:1156–1161.
2. Ernst E, ed. *Complementary Medicine: An Objective Appraisal.* Oxford, England: Butterworth Heinemann; 1996.
3. Pub L No. 102–170, Department of Labor, Health and Human Services, and Education, and Related Agencies Appropriations Act, HR 102–282 (1992):29 [Conference Report].
4. NIH Revitalization Act of 1993, HR 4 (1993):117.
5. *Enhancing Accountability of Alternative Medicine.* New York, NY: Milbank Memorial Fund; 1998.
6. Rosenthal Center for Complementary and Alternative Medicine. Information sheet: what is complementary and alternative medicine? Available at: http://cpmcnet.columbia.edu/dept/rosenthal/cancer/info/whatis.html. Accessed October 1, 1998.
7. Office of Alternative Medicine home page, core CAM presentations, slides 8–12: what is CAM? Available at: http://altmed.od.nih.gov/oam/resources/present/cam-core/. Accessed October 1, 1998.
8. Eisenberg DM, Kessler RC, Foster C, et al. Unconventional medicine in the United States: prevalence, costs, and patterns of use. *N Engl J Med.* 1993;328:245–252.
9. *Alternative Medicine: Expanding Medical Horizons: A Report to the MH on Alternative Medical Systems and Practices in The United States.* Washington, DC: National Institutes of Health, Office of Alternative Medicine; 1995.
10. Micozzi MS, ed. *Fundamentals of Complementary and Alternative Medicine.* New York, NY: Churchill Livingstone; 1996.
11. Wetzel MS, Eisenberg D, Kapchuk T. Course involving complementary medicine and alternative medicine at US medical schools. *JAMA.* 1998;280:784–787.
12. Benfield H, Korngold E. *Between Heaven and Earth: A Guide to Chinese Medicine.* New York, NY: Ballantine Books; 1991:5.
13. Wise TA. Origin and history of medicine. In: Wise TA. *The Hindu System of Medicine.* New Delhi, India: Mittal Publications; 1986:1–11.
14. Donden Y. *Health Through Balance: An Introduction to Tibetan Medicine.* Ithaca, NY: Snow Lion; 1986.
15. *Merriam-Webster's Collegiate Dictionary.* 10th ed. Springfield, Mass: Merriam-Webster, Inc; 1993.
16. Schiff M. *The Memory of Water.* London, England: Harper Collins; 1995.
17. Benveniste J. Dr Jacques Benveniste replies. *Nature.* 1988;334:291.
18. Fugh-Berman A. *Alternative Medicine: What Works.* Tucson, Ariz: Odonian Press; 1996:50–52.
19. Eskinazi D, ed. NIH Technology Assessment Workshop On Alternative Medicine: Acupuncture. *J Altern Complement Med.* 1996;2:1–256. Special issue.
20. Eskinazi D, ed. *Botanicals: A Role in US Health Care.* Larchmont, NY: Mary Ann Liebert, Inc. In press.
21. Office of Alternative Medicine home page, core CAM presentations, slide No. 42: centers. Available at: http://altmed.od.nih.gov/oam/resources/present/cam-core/. Accessed October 1, 1998.
22. *Transcripts of the Alternative Medicine Program Advisory Committee Meetings September 1994–September 1997.* Washington, DC: Alternative Medicine Program Advisory Committee; 1994–1997.
23. *Hearing Before the Subcommittee on Appropriations, United States Senate,* 103rd Cong, 2nd Sess (1993). (Special hearing).
24. Jonas W. Director designee's address. Presented at: Meeting of the Alternative Medicine Program Advisory Committee; March 21, 1995; Washington, DC.
25. Siegfried JD. The drug development and approval process. *Pharma Newsl.* January 1998.
26. Burkholtz H. *The FDA Follies.* New York, NY: Basic Books; 1994:12, 110, 114.

70 Physicians' Ethical Obligations Regarding Alternative Medicine

Jeremy Sugarman, MD, MPH, MA; Larry Burk, MD
From the Division of General Internal Medicine (Dr Sugarman), Center for the Study of Aging and Human Development (Dr Sugarman), and the Departments of Philosophy (Dr Sugarman), Radiology (Dr Burk), and Office of Integrative Medicine Education (Dr Burk), Duke University, Durham, NC.

JAMA. 1998;280:1623–1625

A substantial proportion of patients use alternative medicine, spending an estimated $13 billion each year.[1–3] Complementary and alternative medicine incorporates "all health systems, modalities, and practices other than those intrinsic to the politically dominant health system of a particular society or culture" and "includes all practices and ideas self-defined by their users as preventing or treating illness or promoting health and well-being."[4] Under this definition, the scope of professional obligations regarding alternative medicine for clinicians who provide conventional medical care is unclear. Despite the popularity of alternative medicine, conventional medicine is arguably the politically dominant health system with a somewhat circumscribed set of practices that differ from alternative therapies. However, given the strong professional obligations clinicians have toward helping patients meet health-related goals, the scope of these obligations with respect to alternative medicine deserves discussion.

Alternative medicine and conventional medicine share some important goals, which provide some support for a limited professional obligation toward alternative medicine. Nevertheless, fundamental differences in these approaches raise questions about cultural relativism. While these questions are challenging, using a principle-based analysis,[5] we describe the scope of the professional obligations of clinicians who typically practice conventional medicine toward alternative medicine. We do not directly address the full range of ethical issues, including the professional responsibilities for alternative medicine practitioners, despite the obvious implications for patients.[6] Therefore, our arguments are relevant only in those situations in which alternative medicine practitioners hold the interests of patients foremost and alternative medicine is practiced with integrity and honesty. For clarity, we use "clinician" to refer to those who provide conventional medicine and "practitioner" to those who render alternative medicine.

Comparing Modalities

Conventional modalities (such as surgery and drug therapy) rely on the scientific method whereas alternative medicine modalities (such as acupuncture and therapeutic touch) do not.[7] However, there are considerable similarities among conventional medicine and some forms of alternative medicine. For example, alternative dietary supplements may be a pill or capsule and dietary therapy is an established element of the conventional treatment of heart disease.

Similarly, while the definition of alternative medicine alone sets it apart from conventional medicine, their core health-related goals may not differ radically. Bratman[8] describes 4 values espoused by alternative medicine practitioners: "(1) Use of natural remedies rather than artificial drugs, (2) Getting to the root of problems rather than treating symptoms . . . , (3) Treating the person instead of attacking the disease, and (4) Preventing illness rather than treating it after the fact, and promoting wellness rather than the mere absence of disease." Conventional clinicians share similar values. For instance, a recent international project[9] specified 4 goals of medicine: "(1) The prevention of disease and injury and the promotion and maintenance of health," "(2) The relief of pain and suffering caused by maladies," "(3) The care and cure of those with a malady, and the care of those who cannot be cured," and "(4) The avoidance of premature death and the pursuit of peaceful death."

The concordance of these values is tangible in the current national dialogue about death and dying in which both alternative medicine and conventional medicine now hold that death is not necessarily a negative outcome and palliative care is considered an appropriate option. Both approaches also endorse attention to healing as well as curing, particularly for chronic illnesses in which a cure is often not possible. Shared health-related goals and values such as these lend some support for a limited professional obligation toward alternative medicine that is consistent with a professional obligation toward helping patients achieve these goals. Nonetheless, this obligation is certainly limited to steps that have been proven to be safe and effective, but it may be further limited by the range of practices that fall within the domain of conventional medicine.

Distinct Cultures of Healing

Despite shared values and goals, alternative medicine and conventional medicine differ in important ways. First, many alternative medicine modalities are derived from cultures other than the Western one in which conventional medicine was developed, and many of the practitioners subscribe to a different worldview.[10] Second, by definition, alternative medicine represents a different approach to healing. Third, users of alternative medicine tend to perceive these modalities, in comparison to conventional ones, in greater concordance with their views toward health care.[11] Thus, there seems to be distinct cultures of healing, which is somewhat analogous to situations that conventional medicine encounters in other cultures. For instance, what constitutes appropriate research in developing countries? Should patients be told about a diagnosis of cancer? Should advance directives be discussed with patients whose culture proscribes these discussions? How should clinicians respond to requests for female circumcision?[12] In each of these cases, just as when clinicians encounter alternative medicine, it is essential to determine an appropriate response. When is a laissez-faire approach acceptable? When is there an obligation to intervene on behalf of patients? In making such determinations, it is essential to be vigilant in ensuring that these determinations are not clouded by hegemonic concerns about social status, market share, unfamiliarity, or prejudice.

Bounds of Professional Obligations

The spectrum of possible responses to alternative medicine is quite broad, ranging from an obligation to stifle harmful practices to mere acceptance of nonharmful modalities, to encouraging the use of beneficial interventions. Obviously, none of these singular approaches is adequate or appropriate in all cases. Rather, given the diversity of modalities embraced by a broad definition of alternative medicine and medical uncertainties regarding safety and efficacy, each approach is at times correct. The patient, the illness, and the alternative modality shape the appropriate set of obligations in a particular case. This obligation is refined and justified by attending to a set of inherent ethical principles of the medical profession: respect for persons, nonmaleficence, beneficence, and justice.

Respect for Persons

The ethical obligation of respect for persons, or autonomy, finds application in now well-established expectations of shared medical decision making and informed consent. Such expectations have been endorsed not only on ethical grounds, but also on prudential grounds such as enhanced compliance. Respect for persons also helps prescribe appropriate behavior in the setting of cultural relativism.[12] A thorough respect for persons permits patients to reject unwanted interventions and to make choices that are consonant with their values.

Given the ready availability of information about alternative medicine, many patients may be quite familiar with particular modalities. While a knowledge gap between clinicians and patients regarding alternative medicine modalities may exist, it does not necessarily follow that respect for patients in making decisions regarding alternative therapies excuses conventional clinicians from playing any role whatsoever. Rather, clinicians have an obligation to discuss treatment alternatives with their patients and should be frank about their level of understanding of nonconventional interventions. Even without previous knowledge of particular modalities, clinicians can help patients focus their inquiry and thereby enhance their decision making. For instance, clinicians should ensure that patients have received information about safety (including potency, bioavailability, and drug interactions) as well as efficacy.

Respecting persons also includes making recommendations and using persuasion to help them reach accepted health-related goals. The efficacy, acceptability, and safety of conventional and alternative medicine approaches for treating a particular disorder are critical in determining the precise role in a given situation.[13] For example, it is less appropriate for professionals to exert strong influence on patients' decision making regarding alternative medicine for diseases in which there is no clearly effective conventional treatment (eg, fibromyalgia), wheras such influence is appropriate when there are known effective therapies for a life-threatening disease (eg, a treatable bacterial infection).

More difficulty arises in determining the appropriate role of clinicians when there are alternative medicine approaches for conditions in which conventional therapies have some efficacy although treatment is not completely satisfactory. For example, while conventional medicine offers both disease modifying and symptomatic treatments of rheumatoid arthritis, it would be advantageous if complementary approaches could diminish the need for the use of drugs that have deleterious adverse effects (eg, steroids). Such situations are difficult because of insufficient information regarding the safety, much less the efficacy, of using alternative medicine alone or in combination with conventional medicine. This uncertainty makes truly informed decision making difficult at best and hazardous at worst. Nevertheless, clinicians should be prepared to give patients available and appropriate information about the safety and efficacy of conventional therapies in treating their illnesses, encouraging them to seek similar, reliable information about alternative medicine.

Nonmaleficence

Not harming patients unnecessarily in the process of providing care is a well-recognized ethical principle. Although clinicians may not be prescribing or providing alternative medicine, the obligation for nonmaleficence still plays an important role. In short, it is incumbent on clinicians to elicit information about patients' use of alternative medicine modalities.[13] Such information is part of taking a comprehensive medical history since use of alternative medicine might be having some influence on patients' complaints and also may guide decisions about appropriate treatment. This is critical since some alternative medicine therapies are known to be harmful.[14] In addition, there may be harmful interactions between conventional and alternative medicine therapies. For example, conventional antidepressants act on the same neurotransmitters within the central nervous system as does St John's wort.[15] Thus, a medical history that includes information about a patient's use of alternative medicine is critical in avoiding harm.

Beneficence

Clinicians have a clear obligation to help patients achieve legitimate goals of medicine such as promoting health, prolonging meaningful life, and attenuating suffering. Accordingly, effective interventions obviously should be considered in determining a plan of care for patients. Therefore, a limited obligation does exist on the part of clinicians to make patients aware of safe and effective alternative medicine modalities. Unfortunately, although efforts now are under way to provide systematic data regarding some forms of alternative medicine, few systematic data are currently available to help clinicians and patients make important decisions in this regard.[16]

In the face of popular enthusiasm about alternative medicine, physicians may feel pressured to learn to prescribe beneficial alternative medicine modalities. While learning such interventions may be beyond the scope of clinicians' professional obligations,[17] should individual clinicians elect such training, the training itself must be adequate and appropriate. Efforts are under way to provide this sort of training.[18–20] As with conventional medicine, physicians should not adopt interventions until they have sufficient experience to use interventions safely and effectively.

Accordingly, there is room for appropriate referral and consultation with alternative medicine practitioners. This includes referral and consultation when there is both an increased likelihood that the patient will benefit from the interaction and that the practitioner is experienced as well as accredited or licensed.

Justice

A central concern of justice in health care relates to fairness. Fairness suggests that patients have fair access to alternative medicine therapies as well as conventional therapies that are known to be safe, effective, and appropriate for their conditions. Nevertheless, because little clinical research has evaluated alternative medicine, few data support claims for fair access to these therapies. This predicament, similar to that encountered in caring for children and pregnant women (groups for whom there is a relative paucity of data regarding safety and efficacy of conventional therapies to guide treatment decisions)[21] suggests the need for research efforts in this area. Given the broad use of alternative medicine, as well as the possibility that some modalities will prove to be beneficial, clinicians ought to endorse legitimate efforts aimed at the careful evaluation of conventional and alternative interventions so that they will be better positioned to help guide medical decision making.[22,23] Despite this argument, some skeptical clinicians may still object, claiming that investigating these approaches wastes scarce research dollars and encourages patients to invest their money in sources of false hope.[24] Nevertheless, if this research is conducted properly, the extent to which alternative medicine therapies meet patients' expectations will be clear. Armed with these data, harmful or useless practices could be abandoned and clinicians would be better positioned to help their patients make informed decisions to reach essential health-related goals.

References

1. Cassileth BR, Lusk EJ, Strouse TB, Bodenheimer BJ. Contemporary unorthodox treatments in cancer medicine. *Ann Intern Med.* 1984; 101:105–112.
2. Cassileth BR, Lusk EJ, Guerry D, et al. Survival and quality of life among patients receiving unproven as compared with conventional cancer therapy. *N Engl J Med.* 1991;324:1180–1185.
3. Eisenberg DM, Kessler RC, Foster C, Norlock FE, Calkins DR, Delbanco TL. Unconventional medicine in the United States: prevalence, costs, and patterns of use. *N Engl J Med.* 1993; 328:246–252.
4. Hufford DJ. Whose culture, whose body, whose healing? *Altern Ther.* 1995;1:94–95.
5. Ernst E. The ethics of complementary medicine. *J Med Ethics.* 1996;22:197–198.
6. Barrett S. "Alternative" medicine: more hype than hope. In: Humber JM, Almeder RF, eds. *Alternative Medicine and Ethics.*Totowa, NJ: Humana Press; 1998:1–42.
7. Kottow MH. Classical medicine v alternative medical practices. *J Med Ethics.* 1992;18:18–22.
8. Bratman S. Alternative medicine: how well does it live up to its own ideals? *Altern Ther.* 1997;3:127–128.
9. Callahan D. Specifying the goals of medicine. *Hastings Cent Rep.* Nov-Dec 1996;(suppl):9–14.
10. Hufford DJ. Cultural diversity, folk medicine, and alternative medicine. *Altern Ther.* 1997;3:78–80.
11. Astin JA. Why patients use alternative medicine: results of a national study. *JAMA.* 1998;279:1548–1553.
12. Macklin R. Ethical relativism in a multicultural society. *Kennedy Inst Ethics J.* 1998;8:1–22.
13. Eisenberg DM. Advising patients who seek alternative medical therapies. *Ann Intern Med.* 1997;127:61–69.
14. Ernst E. Harmless herbs? a review of the recent literature. *Am J Med.*1998;104:170–178.
15. Jenike MA. Editorial. *J Geriatr Psychiatry Neurol.* 1994;7(suppl 1):1–2.
16. Workshop on Alternative Medicine. *Alternative Medicine: Expanding Medical Horizons: A Report to the National Institutes of Health on Alternative Medical Systems and Practices in the United States.* Washington, DC: US Government Printing Office; 1995.
17. Lynöe N. Ethical and professional aspects of the practice of alternative medicine. *Scand J Soc Med.* 1992;20:217–225.
18. Daly D. Alternative medicine courses taught at United States medical schools: an ongoing list. *J Altern Complement Med.* 1997;3:405–410.
19. Milan FB, Landau C, Murphy DR, et al. Teaching residents about complementary and alternative medicine in the United States. *J Gen Intern Med.* 1998;13:562–567.
20. Von Behren D. Program in integrative medicine initiates nation's first fellowship. In: Von Behren D, ed. *Arizona Health Horizons.*Tucson: Office of Public Affairs, the University of Arizona Health Sciences Center; 1997:16–17.
21. Kahn JP, Mastroianni AC, Sugarman J. *Beyond Consent: Seeking Justice in Research.* New York, NY: Oxford University Press; 1998.
22. Mack RB. [comment]. *N C Med J.* 1998; 59:24–25.
23. Rosa L, Rosa E, Sarner L, Barrett S. A close look at therapeutic touch. *JAMA.* 1998;279:1005–1010.
24. Halperin EC. Let's abolish the Office of Alternative Medicine of the National Institutes of Health. *N C Med J.* 1998;59:21–23.

71 Beyond Complementary and Allopathic Medicine

David J. Elpern, MD
Williamstown, Mass.

Arch Dermatol. 1998;134:1473–1476

"To cure sometimes/To relieve often/To comfort always" is an ancient French proverb of great import. As medical doctors, we often forget that many of our patients' disorders cannot be fixed by drugs or procedures and that others[1] will not benefit from biopsy procedures, blood tests, or sophisticated diagnostic studies. Yet, many of us seem content to function as skilled technicians; and as the time we allot to our patients constricts, the office visit becomes a venue for interventions or the hurried writing of prescriptions, and only rarely the occasion for the dispensing of comfort and caring.

This is a personal view of why I believe that complementary and alternative medicine (CAM) is so popular in the developed countries, where, in the last century, science has made such miraculous contributions to our ability to understand and impact disease states. Despite these achievements, there are more visits to CAM practitioners in the United States than to primary care physicians. Are we playing the ostrich here?

Almost 2500 years ago, Plato wrote

> There are two types of physicians—those who are free men and those who are slaves. The slaves, to speak generally, are treated by slaves, who pay them a hurried visit, or receive them in dispensaries? A physician of this kind never gives a servant any account of his complaint, nor asks him for any; he gives him some empirical injunction with an air of finished knowledge, in the brusque fashion of a dictator, and then is off in haste to the next ailing servant. . . . The free practitioner attends free men, treats their diseases by going into things thoroughly in a scientific way, and takes the patient and his family into his confidence. Thus he learns something from the sufferers, and at the same time instructs the invalid to the best of his powers. He does not give his prescriptions until he has won the patient's support. . . . Now which of the two methods is that of the better physician or director of bodily regimen?[1]

When one listens to the hue and cry about what health maintenance organizations are doing to medical care, one smiles wryly after reading Plato's words since similar problems appear to have been present in ancient times. The public is no more satisfied with the state of affairs today than the slaves of old were with the "care" they received. Today's patients, compelled to receive the care their hurried providers dictate, often feel like slaves, deprived of choice.

I believe that the high level of interest in and utilization of so-called alternative medicine relates more to the patients' perceptions of lack of caring evinced by many medical doctors than to the inherent efficacy of CAM. To use Plato's analogies, many alternative practitioners function as free men while many medical doctors are perceived to be slaves. This is especially true for the salaried physicians of medical groups. Patients who are members of these organizations for the most part must see the practitioners in their plans and do not have the perception of free choice. Even when their physicians are highly competent and compassionate, from the patient's standpoint, choice is restricted. While there are good economic reasons for this, the resulting limitation of choice has adverse effects on physician-patient encounters. Lest private practitioners get smug, those of us who accept insurance payments function similarly, in that people with insurance are compelled for the most part to attend our offices since many types of CAM visits are not covered benefits. To some extent then, most medical doctors are perceived as slaves.

If, as for auto mechanics, what physicians are confronted with was strictly technical, then this approach would be appropriate. But, many patients have disorders that are more than just mechanical in origin, and the approaches they need are different than the ones most of us are trained to offer.

Katherine Whitehorn, speaking at a colloquium on "Conventional and Complementary Approaches to Health Care" put this particularly well:

> The only thing which every form of therapy seem[s] to have in common was a reliance, greater or less, on the springs of healing within the patient; an underground reservoir, if this is not being fanciful, that could be caused to gush forth by a very great variety of drilling equipment.[2]

What Whitehorn alludes to is the fact, known to healers of all ages and persuasions, that most patients will improve without interventions.

This thesis is hardly novel, but it bears repeating: that is, often it is the therapist who is effective, not the particular therapy. Stated differently, by far, the most versatile drug in general practice is the physician.[3] The theories behind acupuncture, homeopathy, therapeutic touch, and other alternative modalities do not make scientific sense to us; and if, indeed, these techniques are really efficacious (as they often appear to be), then the orthodox explanations accepted by their practitioners are most likely specious. Whether these modalities are any better than placebo has not been proven in most cases; but what has not been adequately studied is the power and therapeutic value of the consultation itself, of the patient-healer interaction when it is entered into with free will and is not the hurried visit of a slave to a slave.

To describe the power of the consultation, I now relate 2 recent cases of mine. In one, I lacked the power to relieve, in the other, I possessed it.

Report of Cases

The Lion in Winter

Patient 1 is a retired executive from a multinational corporation who presented with pruritus and dermatitis. His internist and I investigated his complaints without any specific findings, and the working diagnosis was xerotic eczema with excoriations. The patient is a prominent and powerful man whereas I am a small town dermatologist with no academic cachet. I had prescribed all manner of topical steroids, antihistamines, and emollients, but he did not improve. Feeling that he needed a physician with more stature than I possess, I referred him to the chief of dermatology at a prestigious medical center. This necessitated a 3-hour car trip, fighting traffic in the megalopolis, and finding parking. The big kahuna saw the patient in his impressive suite at the university medical center, spent time, and dispensed his advice with great caring and confidence. A cream, similar to but no stronger than the one this patient previously had used, was prescribed, and it was more effective than anything I had prescribed. No tests were ordered and nothing else was done. The therapy in this case was the therapist, not the medicament.

The Springs of Healing

Patient 2, a 49-year-old sales clerk, was referred to me by a podiatrist, Dr X, for evaluation of a burning sensation of the left big toe. Dr X had performed a phenol ablation of the nail 2 months prior and the patient had persistent pain ever since. She saw Dr X a number of times and went to the emergency department on 2 separate occasions. Each visit triggered more tests and ended with prescriptions for pain medications and different antibiotics. Patient 2 related to me that Dr X's anxiety and indecisiveness frightened and angered her.

Findings of the examination were normal. I listened to the patient, spent about half an hour with her, showed concern about her pain and unhappiness, and told her she was going to be fine. She returned a week later, feeling about 50% better. I reassured her again. On her next visit 2 weeks later she was wearing her shoe again; the pain was gone. She had had no new tests, no new drugs. It is now 6 months later, and the patient is free of pain. I believe her healing came from within.

These cases raise many questions. Were the therapists functioning as drugs, as therapeutic agents for these patients, by reassuring them, by displaying confidence, and implying or telling them they were going to do well? Was this the kind of anodyne these patients needed? Were the podiatrist and emergency department physicians of patient 2 acting as nocebos (countertherapeutic agents) by ordering more tests and analgesics? If there are times when the therapist is the therapy, how does one find this out and how does one dispense one's self properly? Only by considering these questions will we learn these important skills—abilities that many of our professional forefathers possessed.

My thesis is that this is how most alternative practitioners function. The oft quoted bon mot "To a man with a hammer, everything looks like a nail" describes CAM practitioners, them as well as many of us. Most of them do not comprehend that frequently they are the therapy, not their particular school of healing. In other words, the patient's faith in them and their own belief in what they are doing is powerful medicine (magic) that can work in more than half of the patients who visit them.

As we contemplate the value of complementary medicine, we focus on which therapies are scientifically valid and which ones we should include in our ever-growing palaces of medical intervention. Our administrators ask, "Should acupuncturists, massage therapists, iridologists, chiropractors, and naturopaths be practicing side-by-side with MDs, medical deities?"

A recent article by a 9-year-old girl and her mother, a registered nurse, debunked the theory that energetic fields play a role in therapeutic touch[4]; yet the value of therapeutic touch would not have surprised Francis W. Peabody, the author of the most quoted article in the medical literature. "The Care of the Patient"[5] was written in 1926 by the 46-year-old respected medical scientist who at the time was dying of stomach cancer. Peabody's seminal article has nothing to do with science, but rather with the art of medicine and this is why we revere him today. He wrote

> the application of the principles of science to the diagnosis and treatment of disease is only one limited aspect of medical practice. The practice of medicine in its broadest sense includes the whole relationship of the physician with the patient. It is an art, based to an increasing extent on the medical sciences, but comprising much that still remains outside the realm of science.[5]

He goes on to conclude with this famous passage:

> The good physician knows his patients through and through, and his knowledge is bought dearly. Time, sympathy and understanding must be lavishly dispensed, but the reward is to be found in that personal bond which forms the greatest satisfaction of the practice of medicine. One of the essential qualities of the clinician is interest in humanity, for the secret of the care of the patient is in caring for the patient.[5]

In a similar vein, Franz Ingelfinger, then editor of the *New England Journal of Medicine*, when he delivered his last major lecture at Harvard Medical School, Boston, Mass, entitled it "Arrogance" and wrote

> The physician is the person to whom patients go because they need, or think they need help. Let us assume that the physician is competent and compassionate. In spite of these virtues, there is usually little he can do physically, that is by cutting or by chemical manipulation, to eradicate the cause of the patient's distress. Epidemiologists keep pointing out . . . that physicians have done little to prolong life or to eliminate serious morbidity. The figure generally quoted is that 90% of the visits by patients to doctors are caused by conditions that are either self-limited or beyond the capabilities of medicine. In other words, if we assume that physicians do make patients feel better most of the time, it is chiefly because we can reassure the patient or give a medication that is mildly palliative. Even an operation may once in a while make a patient feel better, although it does not prolong life or eradicate the source of the problems.[6]

Strangely, when Ingelfinger wrote these words, he, like Peabody, was aware that he was dying of cancer, and this article, his farewell speech, came from the heart.

Peabody and Ingelfinger stood on the shoulders of William Osler who wrote

> Often the best part of your work will have nothing to do with powders or potions, but with the exercise of an influence of the strong upon the weak, of the righteous upon the wicked, the wise upon the foolish . . . faith is the great lever of life. Without

it man can do nothing. . . . Faith in us, faith in our drugs and methods, is the great stock-in-trade of the profession.[7]

Finally, Michael Balint, a British psychiatrist, wrote an extraordinary book in the 1950s called *The Doctor, His Patient and the Illness*.[3] One of his main theses was that often the doctor functions as a drug, as the therapeutic agent. True as this may be, we do not know the answers to the following questions: What are the pharmacokinetics of the drug physician? How to administer it? What is the proper dose? What are the the adverse effects? How often should it be given? Is it addictive? What are its withdrawal effects? These and many more questions remain unanswered. Yet, the drug doctor is among the most powerful agents we possess. This is humbling. Unless one has gotten to know the patient sufficiently well it can be dangerous to administer the drug doctor.

John Balint, Michael Balint's son, has said, "In our love affair with Science we have forgotten that the end point of medicine is to make people happy, to be co-factors in helping to improve lives."[8] It is more than just being smart, making the big diagnosis, and passing the board examinations. It is taking that diagnosis and running with it, making the patient feel better, happier; and sometimes, indeed often, there will be nothing chemical or mechanical that can be done for that patient; nothing even psychological. A patient may just need caring, comforting, and having you just be there. You may be a fabulously well-trained individual, chock full of knowledge, but this will not be called for in many cases.

Plato, Peabody, Ingelfinger, Osler, and Balint are all saying the same thing, yet separated by millennia; and our medical practices today are driven by the juggernauts of the pharmaceutical industry, the companies that make expensive equipment, insurance companies, health care organizations, and other special interest groups. So many of us have sold our birthrights when we become slave physicians seeing large numbers of patients daily and concentrating on the technical. The successes of complementary practitioners would not have surprised our forefathers and should not necessarily compel us to research what they do, as Rosa et al[4] did with therapeutic touch, but rather to ask what it is that we are not providing those who consult us. We wonder why our therapeutic power is diminished and unappreciated, as we watch patients comforted, relieved, and sometimes cured by complementary healers whose entire pharmacopoeia may be suspect.

Devoting a special issue of the *Archives* to alternative medicine is the politically correct thing to do. The public welcomes it and it shows that we are open-minded. I support my patients who see alternative practitioners, even as I withhold judgment about whether these modalities are effective in and of themselves or whether they work as placebos. I believe that if the patient is getting what is needed, then that is often therapeutic, and does it really matter who gets the credit? At the same time, I also believe that the medicine we medical doctors practice should embrace all of the old French adage: "To cure sometimes/To relieve often/To comfort always" and that most (probably all) alternative disciplines cannot provide the same percentage of cures that we can. However, by limiting our purview to cure, by becoming high-priced technicians, we have driven many patients away from our offices and delivered them into the hands of well-meaning but often ungrounded therapists, who may have little to offer besides their time and caring. Most CAM practitioners probably do not realize that it is their very belief in themselves and their particular form of magic that is more powerful than their ancient or new age therapies. In a similar vein, most conventional physicians have forgotten, or may be unaware of, the words of Plato, Peabody, Ingelfinger, Osler, and Balint.

Hundreds of millions of dollars have been spent by pharmaceutical companies to get the Food and Drug Administration's approval for new drugs to combat male pattern alopecia, onychomycosis, hypercholesterolemia, and other marketable disorders. The amount spent annually on research, development, and marketing by the drug industry is in the many billions of dollars per year. At the same time, much is made of the $10 to $20 million earmarked by the the National Institutes of Health (Bethesda, Md) for research projects approved and administered by the Office of Alternative Medicine. This is clearly inadequate, and is unlikely to generate much meaningful information. On orders of magnitude, more has been expended on toenail fungus alone. The $12 million distributed to the Office of Alternative Medicine in 1997 is a pittance when one considers that it is the entire budget allocated by the federal government for the investigation of alternative therapies from acupuncture and aroma therapy to herbs to magnets to Zen massage. And how much is spent annually in investigating why placebos are more effective in more than 50% of patients with depression[9]? The will to do these kinds of studies does not exist, because this does not generate income for large companies or specific disciplines.

I believe that medically trained physicians can dispense the best care for most patients if they subscribe to the platonic ideal of the "free practitioner" and use everything that has been proven effective in the last 2500 years, not just the latest therapeutic fads. In my opinion, an open-minded medical doctor can ensure that all who seek help get what they really need. The practitioner who knows for whom, and when, surgery, a drug, the friendship of a listening face, or the laying on of hands are indicated, who can determine when the "springs of healing" need to be plumbed will make the most effective "therapeutic marriage broker." Sadly, this type of education is not dispensed by even our most enlightened medical schools.

This area needs study, and the answers would shed light on why many CAM disciplines are effective. Faith, the placebo effect, and self-healing underlie why many patients get better with acupuncture, homeopathy, massage, the other complementary modalities, and (more important) conventional medical practices. Perhaps I am too cynical. Yet, the therapist as the therapy is a concept that needs intensive study and consideration. The proverbial MEDLINE search found precious few articles on this modality that we use daily, and often unconsciously.

Often, others say it better. In a written communication by a pastoral psychotherapist friend, William Zeckhausen (April 1998), who leads physician support groups in New Hampshire wrote to me:

> By adopting an accepting attitude, by listening, showing interest and support, and by asking questions a doctor can provide the most fundamental type of help. She is then BEING a therapist, a pastor to her patients. A group therapist wrote a book on group therapy, and said what he provides is his office and chairs for the meeting, and he then attends. This was his symbolic way of saying that he keeps his ego out of what is happening, so it can happen! So, you need to affirm what you are doing; part of which is being. This is an extraordinarily important concept for physicians who do so many things for patients technically, things which alternative practitioners cannot do; because you need to learn to appreciate the healing presence of your being with patients, as well as doing for or to them. For there is often healing in 'being with,' just as there may sometimes be 'cure' in 'doing for or to.' A physician should basically try to 'be there for' as well as 'do to' some patients. Complementary practitioners can't do all that you can. But the physician has the opportunity to do both for all who visit them (written communication, April 1998).

References

1. Plato; Bury RG, trans. *The Laws*. London, England: William Heinemann; 1926:307–309.
2. Watt J. Talking health: conventional and complementary approaches. In: *The Colloquium*. London, England: The Royal Society of Medicine; 1988
3. Balint M. *The Doctor, His Patient and the Illness*. London, England: International Universities Press; 1990.
4. Rosa L, Rosa E, Sarner L, Barrett S. A close look at therapeutic touch. *JAMA*. 1998;279:1005–1010.
5. Peabody FW. The care of the patient. *JAMA*. 1927;88:877–882.
6. Ingelfinger FJ. Arrogance. *N Engl J Med*. 1980; 303:1507–1511.
7. Cushing H. *The Life of Sir William Osler*. New York, NY: Oxford University Press Inc; 1940.
8. Balint J. Lecture presented at: Williams College; January 14, 1997; Williamstown, Mass.
9. Smith A, Traganza E, Harrison G. Studies on the effectiveness of antidepressant drugs. *Psychopharmacol Bull*. 1969 (special issue):1–53.

72 Alternative Medicine

Is It All in Your Mind?

Francisco A. Tausk, MD
From the Department of Dermatology, Johns Hopkins School of Medicine, Baltimore, Md.

Therapeutic interventions may trigger nonspecific mechanisms whose effects are not attributable to the specific properties of a given treatment. Recent investigations on the placebo effect as well as other mind-body interactions are helping us to understand some of the underlying mechanisms, as well as beginning to provide us with potentially effective adjuvant treatment strategies for a variety of human diseases.

Arch Dermatol. 1998;134:1422–1425

Alternative medicine represents practices neither incorporated into the mainstream of Western medicine nor validated by traditional scientific instruments, such as double-blind, controlled trials. Notwithstanding this vague definition, many of these medical approaches are widely used by mainstream practitioners in other parts of the world, as, for example, is the case of acupuncture or herbalist medicine in Southeast Asia; thus, the alternative label partly results from cultural variables. Some of the drugs that we prescribe in dermatology lack strong scientific proof of efficacy, and yet we do not consider ourselves alternative practitioners for using them; thus, the traditional or alternative labels may be a result of our particular training. Many alternative modalities are currently classified as "mind-body interactions," and within this category we find the placebo effect.

For the last 30 years, the US Food and Drug Administration has required that to consider the beneficial effect of a drug, it has to be significantly more effective than a placebo. It is widely accepted that the specific effect of a drug or therapeutic modality is accompanied by nonspecific effects that may influence positively or negatively the outcome of the therapy. Studies that compare a drug with an inert substance are trying to determine how much of the effect is due to the drug itself, and how much is due to the natural history of the disease, expectancy, and psychological influences such as participating in a study, or believing that the subject is being administered a medicament. The effectiveness of a drug will derive from mathematical formulas that will depend on large differences between studied groups, or small changes in a large number of participating subjects. However, some health care providers and many patients are not overly concerned with the levels of statistical significance of outcome measures. In 1990, there were more visits to alternative medicine practitioners than to all primary care physicians combined, resulting in an expenditure of $13.7 billion, and most of these patients were concealing these visits from their regular physicians.[1] Similar trends have been reported elsewhere, such as in the case of Australia, where nearly 50% of the population consults alternative practices.[2] The use of a particular therapeutic modality by large numbers of individuals does not by itself validate it, but is suggestive of some perceived benefit. Since most alternative practices are based on principles that we currently do not fully understand, without the appropriate formal scientific studies we cannot differentiate their effects from placebo (understanding placebo as a therapeutic modality that does not have any specific effect in the treatment of a given disease). The effectiveness of placebos is difficult to evaluate. Since the initial studies in the 1950s,[3] suggesting that approximately 30% of the effect of therapies is due to placebo, numerous studies have examined this phenomenon. When we analyze the results, we are confronted by the observation that there is a marked variability in the reported effectiveness of the placebo arm. This is true of studies that measure the effects of the same drug, for the same disease, with a similar study population and similar protocols. Given all the conditions being equal, we have to assume that the differences seen in placebo response are due to the way they are administered. Critical to this is the manner in which the subjects' expectations are influenced by the transmittal of unconscious cues, reinforcing their belief or disbelief in the effectiveness of a particular medical intervention. In support of this is the notion that most patients participating in studies are anxious to identify if they are in the active or placebo arm of the study. Similarly, expectancy plays an important role in the outcome resulting from a placebo. Recently, Roberts et al[4] examined medical and surgical procedures that were widely used in the past, and were later abandoned following placebo controlled studies that showed their lack of effect. These authors carefully examined the data obtained from open studies at a time when they were considered highly effective by the patients as well as their physicians. They analyzed the use of glomectomies as treatment for asthma, levamisole as an immunomodulator, photodynamic therapy and organic solvents for herpes simplex infection, and gastric freezing for ulcers. Seventy percent of the almost 7000 patients who participated in these open studies in the 1960s and early 1970s were found to have obtained good to excellent results from these modalities. This report shows that belief and expectancy of patients, and especially of their health care providers, played a critical role in determining the effectiveness of treatments later found to be nonspecific by scientific measures.

The notion that the mind can affect overall health is not new. Although for many years the nervous system, immune system, and animal/human behavior have been the subject of individual study, new lines of research are now emerging that examine the interrelation between these seemingly disparate disciplines. During the last 2 decades it has become clear that numerous neuropeptides, neurotransmitters, and neurohormones not only exert effects within the neuro-endocrine systems but are also capable of augmenting or impairing the immune response by directly binding to specific receptors on the surface of immune cells.[5,6] Thus, not only are lymphoid organs innervated by noradrenergic postganglionic sympathetic fibers[7] but also the products released from peptidergic neurons have a distant effect on cells of all tissues. For example, mediators such as substance P, calcitonin gene-related peptide, somatostatin, corticotropin, vasoactive intestinal polypeptide, neuropeptide Y, among others, have a profound effect on inflammation in the skin through their effect on local keratinocytes, mast cells, Langerhans cells, and blood vessels and local and distant lymphocytes, neutrophils, and macrophages.[8,9]

"Most of our knowledge about how the brain links body memory and emotions has been gleaned through the study of classical conditioning."[10] In this process, for example, a rat perceives a noise that is paired to an electric footpad shock, and after a few such experiences (training), the rat responds automatically to the sound in the absence of shock. The noise is the conditioned stimulus, the foot shock the unconditioned stimulus, and the rat's reaction is a conditioned reaction, which consists of readily measured behavioral and physiological changes.[10] Early evidence of this mind-body connection stemmed from Pavlov's landmark classical conditioning studies in dogs, pairing the sound of a bell to the presence of food.[11] Contemporaneously, Metalnikov and Chorine[12] reported classical conditioning of the immune system in guinea pigs. The latter studies were mostly ignored until the 1970s, when Ader et al[13] and Cohen et al[14] showed classical conditioning of immunity using cyclophosphamide and saccharin as the unconditioned and conditioned stimuli, respectively. Cyclophosphamide was paired with saccharin, and the trained animals were later exposed to saccharin alone, which evoked identical immunosuppressive effects as those produced by the cyclophosphamide. Since then, numerous studies[15–17] have shown the effect of conditioning to suppress or enhance the immune response. Classical conditioning in humans is a well-recognized phenomenon, as exemplified by anticipatory nausea in patients with cancer receiving chemotherapy[18]; however, conditioning of immunity in humans has never been shown. This may be partially explained by the need of a strong and novel conditioned stimulus that is administered isolated from other environmental cues, and the difficulty in delivering this in humans because of the critical nature of our awareness.

In the last 20 years numerous human studies have shown the influence of psychosocial factors on the immune system,[19] such as the presence of stress as a determinant in the development of the common cold following inoculation of the virus to healthy volunteers.[20] Even the evolution of neoplastic diseases has been found to be influenced by these factors. Spiegel et al[21] reported that women with metastatic breast cancer, who in addition to their standard treatment participated in a weekly session of group therapy and hypnosis, had a mean survival time that was double (36.6 months) that of a control group only receiving the standard oncological treatment (18.9 months). Fawzy et al[22] found a significant increase in survival of patients with metastatic malignant melanoma who participated in weekly psychiatric group sessions for 6 weeks, compared with those who did not. Hypnosis, as a psychological intervention, has been demonstrated to effectively modulate inflammation of the skin[23–28] and has been reported in uncontrolled or anecdotal studies to modify the clinical outcome of human disease,[29] including cutaneous disorders such as eczema,[30] urticaria,[31] warts,[32,33] and psoriasis.[34] We recently proposed the use of hypnosis as a tool to provide changes in the immune response in humans, in a manner similar to or replacing the effect of placebos, suggesting that hypnosis may allow us to bypass the natural human critical ability and simultaneously magnify the stimulus administered.[35] Hypnosis is a set of procedures during which suggestions are given for distortions of perception or memory; understanding suggestion as an idea offered to a person for uncritical acceptance.[36] In a recent randomized controlled pilot study[35] we showed the significant improvement (mean, 85%) in the psoriasis activity score index (PASI)[37] in highly hypnotizable patients with psoriasis subjected to weekly hypnosis. A sizable population of patients could benefit significantly from nonspecific treatments, not only because of their effectiveness but also because of the added benefit of limited adverse effects.

When analyzing results of clinical drug studies, we many times observe that patients on the placebo arm of the study have a positive response. In studies that show figures with all of the subjects' data, we sometimes find that a number of the placebo responders have results similar to those of the active drug, whereas others show no improvement, or what is more common, further deterioration of the disease being treated. This supports the notion that in a number of diseases, some of the placebo responders do well with nonspecific treatments. Most results of drug studies are reported as overall means of the active vs placebo arms. In this fashion, the results obtained from the placebo group are averaged between those who responded well and those who (as expected) continued to deteriorate, and only when the responder group shows impressive results do the mean values show significant improvement. However, it is difficult to examine this further, since the data of individual subjects are not readily available from pharmaceutical companies and this information is denied by the Food and Drug Administration, based on the provision in the Freedom of Information Act that exempts trade secrets and confidential commercial information from public disclosure.

More difficult than identifying the effects is understanding the underlying nature of placebos (reviewed by Kirsch[38]). Multiple explanations attempt to justify the effect of nonspecific treatments on patients. One obvious explanation lies within the natural evolution of diseases, and their waxing and waning independently of the therapeutic interventions. Many a practitioner becomes a patient's champion because he/she provided the last intervention before the symptoms improved spontaneously. Deception and self-deception or demand characteristics of the situation do not usually play a role in dermatologic studies, since the results are usually measured by a validated instrument and not self-reported. Participation in clinical trials may provide some degree of comfort, decrease in stress and anxiety, as well as patient education and contact with other patients with similar conditions, which may play a role in reduction of symptoms. The constructed belief that a result will occur, or expectancy, as well as classical conditioning play a role in defining a placebo response and are difficult to differentiate from one another in some situations.

Although we do not fully understand the power of placebos, we should begin to harness their use. Recently, Nickel[39] reported that in a large trial of a drug to reduce benign prostate hypertrophy, subjects in the placebo arm of the study, as expected, suffered an increase in prostate size; surprisingly, however, they experienced marked improvement in the symptoms as well as in the objective measurements of urinary flow. Interestingly, these patients also experienced adverse effects, and 13% of the subjects had to discontinue the placebo because of the latter. This observation, which suggests that placebos may reduce the subjective as well as objective signs and symptoms, without tissue-specific anatomical modifications makes us rethink our therapeutic goals. Would it be useful to provide symptom relief through nonspecific therapies? Can we combine specific and nonspecific treatments to augment their efficacy? If so, it is important to identify modalities that provide such treatments in an ethical manner without deceiving the patients. Hypnosis has been proposed in the past as a nondeceptive technique for the provision of placebo in psychotherapy.[40] Our current interest is directed toward assessing and understanding the potential efficacy of hypnosis, classical conditioning, and a combination of both in the provision of nonspecific therapies to patients with dermatologic diseases. However, nonspecific effects are also exploited by some practitioners to deceive patients into believing in the putative-specific effect of certain treatment modalities. It is, therefore, crucial that when evaluating the effect of traditional as well as alternative therapies we apply strict scientific methods to measure their validity.

References

1. Eisenberg DM, Kessler RC, Foster C, Norlock FE, Calkins DR, Delbanco TL. Unconventional medicine in the United States: prevalence, costs, and patterns of use. *N Engl J Med.* 1993; 328:246–252.
2. MacLennan AH, Wilson DH, Taylor AW. Prevalence and cost of alternative medicine in Australia. *Lancet.* 1996;347:569–573.
3. Beecher HK. The powerful placebo. *JAMA.* 1955;159:1602–1606.
4. Roberts AH, Kewman DG, Mercier L, Hovell M. The power of non-specific effects in healing: implications for psychosocial and biological treatments. *Clin Psychol Rev.* 1993; 12:375–391.
5. Reichlin S. Neuroendocrine-immune interactions. *N Engl J Med.* 1993;329:1246–1253.
6. Chrousos G. The hypothalamic-pituitary-adrenal axis and immune-mediated inflammation. *N Engl J Med.* 1995;332:1351–1362.
7. Madden KS, Sanders VM, Felten DL. Catecholamine influences and sympathetic neural modulation of immune responsiveness. *Ann Rev Pharmacol Toxicol.* 1995;35:417–441.
8. Tausk F, Christian E, Johansson O, Milgram S. Neurobiology of the skin. In: Fitzpatrick TB, Eisen AZ, Wolff K, Freedberg IM, Austen KF, eds. *Dermatology in General Medicine.* 4th ed. New York, NY: McGraw-Hill Book Co; 1993.
9. Asahina A, Hosoi J, Grabbe S, Granstein RD. Modulation of Langerhans cell function by epidermal nerves. *J Allergy Clin Immunol.* 1995;96:1178–1182.
10. LeDoux JE. Emotion, memory and the brain. *Scientific American.* June 1994:50–57.
11. Pavlov IP. *Conditioned Reflexes.* New York, NY: Oxford University Press Inc; 1927.
12. Metalnikov S, Chorine V. Role des reflexes conditionnels dans l'immunité. *Ann Inst Pasteur.* 1926;40:894–900.
13. Ader R, Cohen N, Felten D. Psychoneuroimmunology: interactions between the nervous system and the immune system. *Lancet.* 1995; 345:99–102.
14. Cohen N, Moynihan JA, Ader R. Pavlovian conditioning of the immune system. *Int Arch Allergy Immunol.* 1994;105:101–106.
15. Russell M, Dark KA, Cummins RW, Ellman G, Callaway E, Peeke HVS. Learned histamine release. *Science.* 1984;225:733–734.
16. MacQueen G, Marshall J, Perdue M, Siegel S, Bienenstock J. Pavlovian conditioning of rat mucosal mast cells to secrete rat mast cell protease II. *Science.* 1989;243:83–84.
17. Kelley KW, Dantzer R, Mormede P, Salmon H, Aynaud JM. Conditioned taste aversion suppresses induction of delayed-type hypersensitivity immune reactions. *Physiol Behav.* 1984; 34:189–193.
18. Stockhorst U, Klosterhalfen S, Klosterhalfen W, Winkelmann M, Steingrueber HJ. Anticipatory nausea in cancer patients receiving chemotherapy: classical conditioning, etiology and therapeutical implications. *Integr Physiol Behav Sci.* 1993;28:177–181.
19. Kiecolt-Glaser J, Glaser R. Psychoneuroimmunology and health consequences: data and shared mechanisms. *Psychosom Med.* 1995;57:269–274.
20. Cohen S, Tyrrell DA, Smith AP. Psychological stress and susceptibility to the common cold. *N Engl J Med.* 1991;325:606–612.
21. Spiegel D, Kraemer HC, Bloom J, Gottheil E. Effect of psychosocial treatment on survival of patients with metastatic breast cancer. *Lancet.* 1989;2:888–891.
22. Fawzy FI, Fawzy NW, Hyun CS, et al. Malignant melanoma: effects of an early structured psychiatric intervention, coping, and affective state on recurrence and survival 6 years later. *Arch Gen Psychiatry.* 1993;50:681–689.
23. Black S. Inhibition of immediate-type hypersensitivity response by direct suggestion under hypnosis. *BMJ.* 1963;6:925–929.
24. Black S. Shift in dose-response curve of Prausnitz-Kustner reaction by direct suggestion under hypnosis. *BMJ.* 1963;6:990–992.
25. Black S, Humphrey JH, Niven JSF. Inhibition of Mantoux reaction by direct suggestion under hypnosis. *BMJ.* 1963;6:1649–1652.

26. Zachariae R, Bjerring P, Arendt-Nielsen L. Modulation of type I immediate and type IV delayed immunoreactivity using direct suggestion and guided imagery during hypnosis. *Allergy.* 1989;44:537–542.

27. Zachariae R, Bjerring P. The effect of hypnotically induced analgesia on flare reaction of cutaneous histamine prick test. *Arch Dermatol Res.* 1990;282:539–543.

28. Wyler-Harper J, Bircher AJ, Langewitz W, Kiss A. Hypnosis and the allergic response. *Schweiz Med Wochenschr.* 1994;124(suppl):67–76.

29. Frankel FH. Hypnosis as a treatment method in psychosomatic medicine. *Int J Psychiatry Med.* 1975;6:75–85.

30. Stewart AC, Thomas SE. Hypnotherapy as a treatment for atopic dermatitis in adults and children. *Br J Dermatol.* 1995;132:778–783.

31. Shertzer CL, Lookingbill DP. Effects of relaxation therapy and hypnotizability in chronic urticaria. *Arch Dermatol.* 1987;123:913–916.

32. Surman OS, Gottlieb SK, Hackett TP, Silverberg EL. Hypnosis in the treatment of warts. *Arch Gen Psychiatry.* 1973;28:439–441.

33. Ewin DM. Hypnotherapy for warts (verruca vulgaris): 41 consecutive cases with 33 cures. *Am J Clin Hypn.* 1992;1:1–10.

34. Frankel FH, Misch RC. Hypnosis in a case of long standing psoriasis in a person with character problems. *Int J Clin Exp Hypn.* 1973;21:121–130.

35. Tausk FA, Whitmore SE. A controlled study of hypnosis in the treatment of patients with psoriasis. *Psychother Psychosom.* In press.

36. Kirsch I. APA definition and description of hypnosis: defining hypnosis for the public. *Contemp Hypn.* 1994;11:142–143.

37. Fredriksson T, Petterson U. Severe psoriasis: oral therapy with a new retinoid. *Dermatologica.* 1978;157:238–244.

38. Kirsch I. Specifying nonspecifics: psychological mechanisms of placebo effects. In: Harrington A, ed. *The Placebo Effect.* Cambridge, Mass: Harvard University Press; 1997.

39. Nickel JC. Placebo therapy in benign prostatic hyperplasia: a 25–month study. Canadian PROSPECT Study Group. *Br J Urol.* 1998; 81:383–387.

40. Kirsch I. Clinical hypnosis as a nondeceptive placebo: empirically derived techniques. *Am J Clin Hypn.* 1994;37:95–106.

73 Investigating Alternative Medicine Therapies in Randomized Controlled Trials

Arthur Margolin, PhD; S. Kelly Avants, PhD; Herbert D. Kleber, MD
From the Substance Abuse Center, Yale University School of Medicine, New Haven, Conn (Drs Margolin and Avants); and Center on Addiction and Substance Abuse at Columbia University, New York, NY (Dr Kleber).

JAMA 1998;280:1626–1628

Because alternative medicine therapies are used by a significant number of Americans[1,2] and people worldwide,[3] there is an urgent need for their efficacy to be evaluated formally. The most stringent evaluation would take place within the "gold standard" for clinical research: the randomized controlled clinical trial (RCT). However, alternative medicine comprises a large and heterogeneous group of treatments,[4] many of which are procedures that are not readily testable under blinded conditions and for which the choice of appropriate control conditions is by no means straightforward. Furthermore, alternative medicine therapies may also possess a theoretical basis, may stem from a cultural tradition that is seemingly antithetical to a quantitative, biomedical framework,[4–7] or may possess little foundational research on which to base a controlled evaluation. In this article, we discuss a number of key methodological issues that arise in the controlled evaluation of one widely used alternative medicine procedure—acupuncture for the treatment of cocaine addiction, and we offer some suggestions for how these issues may be addressed.

Basis for Undertaking a Controlled Trial

An important principle governing the justification for conducting an RCT[8] is that a condition of genuine clinical uncertainty, or "equipoise,"[9] exists among clinical experts regarding the relative benefits of the trial's treatments. However, the application of this principle entails a community of colleagues sharing basic assumptions and a common knowledge base, with consensus views founded on empirical investigations. These conditions may not be satisfied with respect to considerations of alternative medicine, which typically involve heterogeneous groups comprising incommensurate cultural and evaluative frameworks and, more often than not, a paucity of systematically derived data. Even within the biomedical community, alternative medicine generates considerable controversy.[10] The application of traditional concepts of "clinical equipoise" to alternative medicine is therefore an unsettled question, much in need of elucidation and a statement of general principles. Lacking this, investigators of an alternative medicine treatment must negotiate the justification to conduct the trial, as well as criteria for informed consent, on a case-by-case basis. Relevant to this discussion is whether the alternative medicine treatment is being compared with a conventional treatment as an alternative, as a supplement, or, where no effective conventional treatment is available, with an inactive control condition, along with whatever preliminary evidence concerning safety and efficacy is available.

Auricular acupuncture for the treatment of cocaine addiction demonstrates how a confluence of circumstances, within both Western medicine and alternative medicine, creates a context within which the evaluation of an alternative treatment can generate broad support. Among the circumstances that support a formal investigation of acupuncture for the treatment of cocaine addiction are (1) Cocaine addiction is a serious public health problem. (2) There is a lack of effective conventional treatments for the disorder. (3) There is widespread provision of acupuncture for cocaine addiction. Currently more than 300 clinics in the United States offer acupuncture as part of their addiction treatment programs.[11] (4) Preliminary studies investigating the effectiveness of acupuncture in the addictions have reported positive results.[12]

Is the Treatment to Be Evaluated Codified and Accepted?

Because alternative therapies do not possess well-established clinical practice guidelines,[7] wide variations may exist in the treatment provided for a given disorder. This raises the issue of whether the experimental treatment is regarded as representative of common practice in the field, and, if so, whether the treatment has been standardized for the trial's diagnostic category. The credibility of the study will depend in part on whether before a trial is undertaken, a consensus has been reached that the treatment being tested is the most appropriate for the target disorder. This consensus can be inferred either by expert opinion, or, where it exists, through standards of practice guidelines. In addition, like conventional treatments, alternative treatments are most cogently investigated in trials that pose well-defined questions with respect to specific diagnostic categories based on validated assessment instruments. Auricular acupuncture for treating cocaine addiction satisfies these conditions insofar as the experimental treatment is codified in the widely used protocol established by the National Acupuncture Detoxification Association and can be delivered to patients meeting *Diagnostic and Statistical Manual of Mental Disorders, Fourth Edition (DSM-IV)*[13] criteria for cocaine abuse or dependence by practitioners trained by the acupuncture association.[14]

Identification of Objective Outcomes

Similar to any treatment, alternative medicine therapies are prone to expectancy effects and other influences that may lead to biased self-reports of outcomes.[4] For this reason, and in view of the possibility of selection bias as well as the need to enhance the credibility of alternative medicine research, it is important that objective measures be included in alternative medicine studies whenever possible. For example, an RCT designed to test the efficacy of acupuncture in treating cocaine addiction could address this straightforwardly by obtaining urine toxicology screens 2 or 3 times a week. Identifying objective outcomes of other alternative medicine therapies or other target disorders may present a greater challenge.

Devising Adequate Controls

The development of control conditions for alternative medicine therapies poses a number of problems, such as the mechanism of action is usually not well understood, the treatment is typically a procedure that involves some degree of interaction between patient and treatment provider, and the development of controls for procedures is significantly more complex than for pharmacotherapies.[15] Yet, given the controversy and outright skepticism concerning alternative medicine treatments, the use of well-designed controls in their evaluation is an important factor in establishing the credibility of the trial and, therefore, the treatment being evaluated. For auricular acupuncture, controls for both needle-insertion effects and nonspecific effects, such as relaxation, may be required. Controlling for needle insertion, a "ritual" that might elicit a placebo response in drug users independent of any acupuncture-specific mechanism,[16] involves inserting needles into so-called "sham" points, which are presumed to be ineffective for the target disorder. This simple statement belies numerous complexities. Traditional Chinese medicine does not include the concept of a "placebo," and the organismic model that underlies traditional acupuncture theory does not embody a concept of an "inert" treatment.[17]

Furthermore, within a Western framework, there is no biochemical "marker" of an active auricular treatment, nor is there one that would differentiate an active from a control treatment. Hence, unknown relative levels of therapeutic activity between active and control conditions constitutes a potentially serious impediment to the interpretation of findings in acupuncture research.[18]

Key issues to consider when devising a needle insertion control include ensuring the comparability of control and active treatment with regard to any aversive effects that may affect dropout or subjective response to treatment[19] (eg, pain or discomfort caused by the treatment), and identifying a theoretical and empirical basis for regarding the control treatment as less active than the experimental treatment. In addition, there would ideally be an objective method for determining specifically where the needles are to be inserted within the hypothesized "active" and control regions. In seeking guidance on these issues, the extant literature should be approached critically. For example, in preliminary studies, we found that (1) a commonly used control in auricular acupuncture studies, insertion of needles proximate to active points, though no more painful than active sites, is probably too active to be a suitable control[20,21]; (2) needling of regions on the ear helix, in points relatively removed from the active sites and that are not indicated for the treatment of addiction, is rated least active and least preferred by patients who use cocaine compared with 3 other auricular needle configurations and, therefore, may represent a more appropriate control[22]; and (3) "active" auricular sites can be differentiated from control sites on the basis of their electrical resistance characteristics.[23] However, some commercially available "electrical point finders," used to select points for needle insertion, may be unreliable due to circuit design problems and pressure artifacts.[23] The development of adequate needle-insertion controls is an area still much in need of further research. Consideration should also be given to controlling for nonspecific effects of the treatment context that may affect the target disorder. In the case of addiction, this may include controlling for the effects of relaxation induced by sitting quietly for 40 minutes daily to receive the acupuncture treatment, because relaxation has been associated with reduced drug craving.[24,25] Control conditions should possess the nonspecific elements of the acupuncture treatment context, including credible rationale, equivalent time demands, and similar patient-staff contact. We note that standard care comparison groups do not usually contain these elements. Precisely what aspects of the experimental treatment such groups control for should be carefully considered in determining their suitability in an RCT.

Difficulties of Blinding Procedures

Blinded conditions in an RCT control for a host of potential confounds and biases,[26] and they provide conservative estimates of treatment efficacy.[27,28] However, evaluations of procedures, unlike those of pharmacotherapies, are nearly impossible to conduct under conditions in which both the patients and practitioners are blinded. Training and competency are a prerequisite to providing the treatments, and experienced practitioners will know which treatment is hypothesized to be active. Unlike pharmacotherapy studies in which the active medication and the pill placebo can be made to be identical in appearance, procedures are observably different to all of the participants in the study. Therefore, acupuncture RCTs may need to be conducted unblinded, with multiple checks on bias.

Guarding Against and Checking on Bias

Following Pocock,[26] at least 3 categories of participant bias that may be considered in RCTs of alternative medicine are treatment providers, patients, and staff. For any procedure, the interaction and ongoing relationship between the treatment provider and patient presents opportunities for the treatment provider to influence outcome, knowingly or unknowingly.[29] Several approaches to check this tendency can be implemented in RCTs of alternative medicine by imposing constraints on the patient–treatment provider interaction; monitoring these interactions by a third party; and evaluating the practitioner-patient relationship across treatment groups.[30] Various factors associated with study patients also represent a potential source of bias. In any RCT, the treatments must be described simply and factually to patients to ensure properly informed consent.[31] However, this information should be communicated in a way that minimizes expectancy effects; it should neither enhance the experimental treatment nor introduce bias against the control conditions. Treatments that are regarded as credible when administered, even if they are subsequently shown to be ineffective, can result in significant improvement in the target disorder.[32] Hence, for studies of alternative medicine, it is important to design the active and control treatments to be equivalently credible and to assess the credibility of the treatments.[33] One way to accomplish this is through multiple administrations of a treatment credibility assessment instrument, which permits for comparisons across groups of patient-perceived credibility of the assigned treatment.[34,35] In any RCT, staff bias can operate on a number of different levels and must be protected against. This may be especially important in the evaluation of controversial therapies or in treatments about which participants may be thought to have strong positive or negative opinions. The use of a primary objective outcome (eg, urine toxicity screens in addiction studies) may protect against patient bias as well as staff bias influencing primary outcomes. To preclude potential staff bias from influencing patients' self-reported change, assessment interviews should be conducted by staff members blind to treatment assignment.

Conclusions

The validity and credibility of alternative medicine investigations will be enhanced by using research designs that embody the highest standards for demonstration of efficacy: the randomized clinical trial. However, controlled evaluation of alternative medicine therapies may require its practitioners to undertake a fundamental conceptual shift from a view of patients as requiring individualized treatment that may vary at each session to one in which trial participants are regarded as members of an equivalence class, defined by the diagnosis, who all will be given a standard prescribed treatment. Although in this article we have urged the use of RCTs for evaluating alternative medicine therapies and have discussed some of the problems that arise in this endeavor, we recognize that this approach may be viewed by others as irremediably distorting the content of those treatments. This complex issue, comprising a wide range of opinions concerning the cultural relativity of methodological principles, has yet to be resolved.

Supported by grants DA08513 (Dr Margolin), DA00277 (Dr Avants) from the National Institute on Drug Abuse, National Institutes of Health, Bethesda, Md, and by grants from the Conrad N. Hilton Foundation, Los Angeles, Calif, and the Office of National Drug Control Policy, Washington, DC, for grants to Dr Kleber at the Center on Addiction and Substance Abuse, New York, NY, to support the Cocaine Alternative Treatments Study, on which this article, in part, is based.

References

1. Eisenberg D, Kessler RC, Foster C, et al. Unconventional medicine in the United States. *N Engl J Med*. 1993;328:246–252.
2. Paramore LC. Use of alternative therapies. *J Pain Symptom Manage*. 1997;13:83–89.
3. Kranz R, Rosenmund A. The motivation to use complementary medicine healing methods. *Schweiz Med Wochenschr*. 1998;128:616–622.
4. National Institutes of Health. *Alternative Medicine: Expanding Medical Horizons*. Chantilly, Va: Workshop on Alternative Medicine; 1994.
5. Cassidy CM. Social science theory and methods in the study of alternative and complementary medicine. *J Altern Complement Med*. 1995; 1:19–40.
6. Vickers A, Cassileth B, Ernst E, et al. How should we research unconventional therapies? *Int J Technol Assess Health Care*. 1997;13:111–121.
7. Woolf SH, Bell HS, Berman B, et al. Clinical practice guidelines in complementary and alternative medicine. *Arch Fam Med*. 1997;6:149–154.
8. Levine RJ. Randomized clinical trials: ethical considerations. *Principles Med Biol*. 1994;1A:37–63.
9. Freedman B. Equipoise and the ethics of clinical research. *N Engl J Med*. 1987;317:141–145.
10. Council for Scientific Medicine. In defense of scientific medicine. *Sci Rev Altern Med*. 1997;1:2.
11. Culliton P, Kiresuk T. Overview of substance abuse acupuncture treatment research. *J Altern Complement Ther*. 1996;2:149–159.
12. Brewington V, Smith M, Lipton D. Acupuncture as a detoxification treatment: an analysis of controlled research. *J Subst Abuse Treat*. 1994;11:289–307.
13. American Psychiatric Association. *Diagnostic and Statistical Manual of Mental Disorders, Fourth Edition*. Washington, DC: American Psychiatric Association; 1994.
14. Brumbaugh AG. *Transformation and Recovery: A Guide for the Design and Development of Acupuncture-Based Chemical Dependence Treatment Programs*. Santa Barbara, Calif: Stillpoint Press; 1995.
15. Cook TD, Campbell DT. *Quasi-experimentation*. Boston, Mass: Houghton Mifflin Co; 1979.
16. Liao SJ, Lee MHM, Ng LKY. *Principles and Practice of Contemporary Acupuncture*. New York, NY: Marcel Dekker; 1994.
17. Wiseman N, Ellis A. *Fundamentals of Chinese Medicine*. Brookline, Mass: Paradigm Publications; 1985.
18. Lewith GT, Machin D. On the evaluation of the clinical effects of acupuncture. *Pain*. 1983; 16:111–127.
19. Kramer MS, Shapiro SH. Scientific challenges in the application of randomized trials. *JAMA*. 1984;252:2739–2745.
20. Avants SK, Margolin A, Chang P, Kosten TR, Birch S. Acupuncture for the treatment of cocaine addiction. *J Subst Abuse Treat*. 1995;12:195–205.
21. Margolin A, Chang P, Avants SK, Kosten TR. Effects of sham and real auricular needling. *Am J Chin Med*. 1993;21:103–111.
22. Margolin A, Avants SK, Chang P, Birch S, Kosten TR. A single-blind investigation of four auricular needle puncture configurations. *Am J Chin Med*. 1995;23:105–114.
23. Margolin A, Avants SK, Birch S, Falk C, Kleber HD. Methodological investigations for a multisite trial of auricular acupuncture for cocaine addiction. *J Subst Abuse Treat*. 1996;13:471–481.
24. Margolin A, Avants SK, Kosten TR. Cue-elicited cocaine craving and autogenic relaxation. *J Subst Abuse Treat*. 1994;11:549–552.
25. Klajner F, Hartman LM, Sobell MB. Treatment of substance abuse by relaxation training. *Addict Behav*. 1984;9:41–55.
26. Pocock SJ. *Clinical Trials: A Practical Approach*. New York, NY: John Wiley & Sons Inc; 1983.
27. Colditz GA, Miller JN, Mosteller F. How study design affects outcomes in comparisons of therapy, I: medical. *Stat Med*. 1989;8:441–454.
28. Schulz KF, Chalmers I, Hayes RJ, Altman DG. Empirical evidence of bias. *JAMA*. 1995; 273:408–412.

29. Shapiro AK, Shapiro E. Patient-provider relationships and the placebo effect. In: Matarazzo JD, Weiss SM, Herd JA, Miller NE, eds. *Behavioral Health: A Handbook of Health Enhancement and Disease Prevention*. New York, NY: Wiley-Interscience; 1984:371–383.

30. Horvath AO, Greenberg LS. Development and validation of the Working Alliance Inventory. *J Consult Clin Psychol*. 1989;36:223–233.

31. Meinert CL. *Clinical Trials: Design, Conduct and Analysis*. New York, NY: Oxford University Press; 1986.

32. Roberts AH, Kewman DG, Merceir L, Hovell M. The power of nonspecific effects in healing. *Clin Psychol Rev*. 1993;13:373–391.

33. Vincent CA, Richardson PH. Placebo controls for acupuncture studies. *J R Soc Med*. 1995; 88:199–202.

34. Borkovec TD, Nau SD. Credibility of analogue therapy rationales. *J Behav Ther Exp Psychiatry*. 1972;3:257–260.

35. Vincent C. Credibility assessments in trials of acupuncture. *Complement Med Res*. 1990; 4:8–11.

74 Complementary Medicine and the Cochrane Collaboration

Jeanette Ezzo, PhD; Brian M. Berman, MD; Andrew J. Vickers, MA; Klaus Linde, MD
From the Complementary Medicine Program, School of Medicine, University of Maryland, Baltimore (Drs Ezzo and Berman); Research Council for Complementary Medicine, London, England (Mr Vickers); and Center for Complementary Medicine Research, Technical University, Munich, Germany (Dr Linde).

JAMA 1998;280:1628–1630

Every year, millions of US consumers spend billions of dollars on alternative and complementary medical treatments.[1] A similar trend exists in the United Kingdom and Australia.[2–4] As people increasingly use these treatments, questions arise from consumers, clinicians, payers, and policymakers as to the effectiveness of these interventions.

The Cochrane Complementary Medicine Field

To meet the increasing demand for evidence-based complementary medicine (CM), a CM Field, funded by the National Institutes of Health Office of Alternative Medicine, was established within the Cochrane Collaboration[5] in 1996. The goal of the Cochrane Collaboration is to produce, maintain, and disseminate systematic reviews on all topics in health care. The CM Field focuses on CM topics. Two major products of the Cochrane Collaboration are a database of systematic reviews and the Cochrane Controlled Trials Registry, the largest registry of its kind.[6] Both databases are updated quarterly with information added regularly by the CM Field.

The systematic review is a method par excellence for synthesizing evidence on a given topic, and policy agencies are increasing use of it to summarize evidence.[7] Cochrane reviews are more transparent than other reviews,[8] so that conclusions are replicable and methods are explicit. Systematic reviews are valuable even when the results are inconclusive because reviews point out where knowledge gaps exist.

Search Strategies to Retrieve Randomized Trials of CM

Since the CM Field has been functioning, a great deal of effort has focused on laying the groundwork for reviews by constructing a database of randomized controlled trials (RCTs) on CM topics. Capturing all relevant trials in MEDLINE has yielded surprising challenges. The scope of practices defined as complementary within the CM Field is broader than those captured in a MEDLINE search of the term *alternative medicine*. For example, Chinese movement therapies such as Qigong and Tai Chi are considered complementary therapies by the Field's standards, but are not accessed by a hierarchical MEDLINE search of the term *alternative medicine*. Similarly, herbal remedies may be described by MEDLINE as plant extracts rather than by any alternative medicine term. To aid MEDLINE searching, a 250-line MEDLINE search strategy has been written and is available for public use.[9]

Assessments of MEDLINE sensitivity (the proportion of RCTs identified by a MEDLINE search relative to a "gold standard" of the known number of RCTs) have demonstrated that on average, MEDLINE searches yield only half of all known trials on a given topic, with CM topics usually scoring below average (eg, 17% for homeopathy, 31% for *Ginkgo biloba*, and 58% for acupuncture).[10] The first reason for low MEDLINE sensitivity may be that articles are appearing in journals not indexed by MEDLINE. This is true for acupuncture[11] and vitamin C for the common cold.[12] Of approximately 16,000 serial medical journals worldwide, MEDLINE references about 3700 (23%).[10] Of the 695 CM journals worldwide identified by the Office of Alternative Medicine and the National Library of Medicine, MEDLINE indexes 69 (10%). Collaborations between the National Library of Medicine, the CM Field, and the Office of Alternative Medicine should soon result in increasing the number of indexed CM journals and expanding the MEDLINE thesaurus to include more CM search terms.

To retrieve studies indexed in other databases, the CM Field is searching both standard medical databases and specialized CM databases. By mid-1998, the Cochrane CM Trials Registry contained more than 3500 RCTs, with only 33% identified by a MEDLINE search for RCTs in alternative medicine and 20% not found in MEDLINE. Periodically, the CM registry uploads its trials to the Cochrane Controlled Trials Registry, making these trials available to individuals with access to the Cochrane library. The CM Field maintains the CM registry, adds new trials, assists reviewers doing CM reviews, and proactively provides references to all 40 Cochrane Collaboration reviews and protocols that have a CM component. A second reason for low MEDLINE sensitivity is that articles exist in journals that are not indexed by any electronic database. Volunteers within the CM Field are now searching by hand approximately 40 indexed and nonindexed journals in English, German, Italian, Japanese, and Spanish and are reading every article published in these journals back to their first issues to locate every RCT.

Publication Bias

A third reason for low MEDLINE sensitivity is that studies exist that have never been fully published in any journal ("gray literature").[10] Estimates from conventional medicine show that only about 50% of the RCTs that appear as conference proceedings ever materialize into published journal articles.[10] Some observations[13] estimate CM gray literature to be at least as plentiful. Complementary medicine gray literature includes expected sources, such as conference proceedings and dissertations, and unexpected sources such as US patents records.[14]

Beyond the hard-to-find trials in the gray literature lie the even harder to find studies that do not appear in print anywhere and exist only in homeopathic company data files or researchers' file drawers.[13] Gray literature plus unpublished data are collectively termed unpublished studies.[15] Publication bias is "the tendency of investigators, reviewers, and editors to differentially submit or accept manuscripts for publication based on the direction or strength of the findings."[15] To the extent that publication bias exists, systematic reviews that omit unpublished studies risk overestimating treatment effects. Bias has been demonstrated both in what investigators submit to journals[16] and what conference abstracts editors accept.[17] However, whether to include unpublished studies in reviews is still a source of debate.[15] The influence of unpublished studies in CM systematic reviews is being analyzed by the CM Field as part of a review of 164 CM systematic reviews.[9] Until the value of including CM unpublished studies can be answered more conclusively, the CM Field will continue to search for unpublished studies to help answer a frequently asked question: How much evidence exists in CM?

Examining how publication bias skews the CM evidence is important for the CM Field because some forms of publication bias may be unique to CM. One question is whether both positive and negative publication biases exist in CM. Asked another way, do CM journals tend to publish results favoring CM treatments and conventional medical journals publish results not favoring CM treatments?

Examining publication bias is not always straightforward. A study by the CM Field found that studies published in Russia and China had a disproportionately high number of statistically significant results (97% and 99%, respectively) when compared with England (75%).[18] It is not yet evident whether these high proportions are due to extreme forms of publication bias or low study quality, which overestimated treatment effects.[19,20] The CM Field is obtaining translations of these studies to examine study quality. The qualitative results will determine whether it is practical to devote efforts to the tedious task of identifying unpublished studies.

Language Bias

Moher and colleagues[21] demonstrated that the quality of studies published in French, German, Spanish, and Italian is comparable with those published in English. The present research of the CM Field will extend methodological quality knowledge into studies from Russia and China. Egger and colleagues[22] demonstrated that a language-related publication bias exists in which authors who publish in both German and English tend to report nonsignificant findings in German and significant findings in English. Preliminary observations suggest that an additional language bias may exist for CM. Regardless of whether results are significant, some CM topics are almost exclusively published initially in languages other than English. A systematic review on St John's wort for depression[23] noted that none of the trials had been originally published in English, although some were subsequently published in English. A similar experience has been reported for *Gingko biloba* for cerebral insufficiency,[24] which suggests that for certain topics in CM, there may be a language-related publication lag time—a trend not reported for conventional medicine. Trends such as this underscore the importance of the CM Field's effort to retrieve trials in languages other than English and to identify biases that may be unique to CM.

Quality Assessment of RCTs

Assessing study quality also may improve the validity of systematic reviews. The finding that low-quality studies have repeatedly yielded exaggerated treatment effects has been documented for conventional medicine[19,20] and acupuncture.[25] Yet, methodological assessments are sometimes absent from non–Cochrane Collaboration CM systematic reviews. A summary of 29 meta-analyses of mind-body techniques, for example, demonstrated that only about half assessed study quality.[26] Although assessing study quality cannot compensate for fraudulent or inaccurate reporting, it can provide additional validity-related information to guide reviewers' conclusions. For CM, quality assessments will provide needed answers to another commonly asked question: How good is the quality of CM trials?

This quality question is usually raised as an implication that CM trials reflect lower methodological quality than conventional medicine trials. To examine this notion, Cochrane Collaboration methodologists are collaborating with members of the CM Field to compare the methodological quality of CM trials with conventional medicine trials on the same diseases. Low-quality meta-analyses for analgesic interventions have been found to be associated with more positive results than high-quality meta-analyses.[27] The analysis of CM reviews is to examine whether this can be replicated in low-quality vs high-quality CM reviews, and how conclusions of low-quality vs high-quality CM reviews on the same topic differ.

Reviews Completed by the CM Field

The CM Field has completed systematic reviews on acupuncture, massage, homeopathy, and herbal medicine. Nineteen reviews are in process (Table 1),[28] and the CM Field has commented on protocols of 12 planned and completed reviews.[28]

Table 1. Titles of Cochrane Systematic Reviews Pertaining to Complementary Medicine

Reviews completed
Acupuncture for asthma
Acupuncture for nicotine addiction
Balneotherapy (spa therapy) for arthritis
Cabbage leaves to reduce breast engorgement in nursing mothers
Garlic for lower-limb atherosclerosis
Homeopathy for asthma
Hypnosis for smoking cessation
Massage for low-birth-weight infants
St John's wort for depression
Vitamin E for intermittent claudication
Vitamin C for the common cold
Reviews in progress
Acupuncture for lower back pain
Acupuncture for headache
Acupuncture for osteoarthritis
Alexander technique for asthma
Echinacea for the common cold
Evening Primrose Oil for premenstrual syndrome
Gingko biloba for dementia
Gingko biloba for intermittent claudication
Manual therapy for neck pain
Manual therapy for asthma
Marine oil supplementation for type 2 diabetes mellitus
Music therapy for dementia
Padma 28 for intermittent claudication
Pygeum africanum for benign prostatic hyperplasia
Secale cereale for benign prostatic hyperplasia
Serenoa repens for benign prostatic hyperplasia
Spinal manipulation for low back pain
Therapeutic Touch for wound healing
Yoga for epilepsy

Conclusions

Although there is no guarantee that systematic reviews will result in changing policy and practice, there is increasing evidence that policy organizations rely on systematic reviews more than they have in the past[7] and that practitioners rely on reviews as a primary information source.[29] It has also been suggested that consumers can use reviews to guide decision making.[30] Traditional literature reviews, however, have lacked explicit methods and have been susceptible to biases that generally tend to overestimate treatment effects.[7] Therefore, at a time when the public is using CM treatments in record numbers and an explicit peer-reviewed and regularly updated systematic review method exists, it is imperative to apply this method to CM. The Cochrane Collaboration provides a forum of interdisciplinary cooperation in which to produce these reviews that we hope will result in improved patient care.

We thank Victoria Hadhazy for editorial assistance.

References

1. Eisenberg DM, Kessler RC, Foster CF, et al. Unconventional medicine in the United States. *N Engl J Med.* 1993;328:246–252.

2. Fulder SJ, Munroe RE. Complementary medicine in the United Kingdom: patients, practitioners and consultations. *Lancet.* 1985;2:542–545.

3. Maddocks I. Alternative medicine. *Med J Aust.* 1985;142:547–551.

4. Maclennan AH, Wilson DH, Taylor AW. Prevalence and cost of alternative medicine in Australia. *Lancet.* 1996;347:569–573.

5. Bero L, Rennie D. The Cochrane Collaboration: preparing, maintaining and disseminating systematic reviews of the effects of health care. *JAMA.* 1995;274:1935–1938.

6. Kiley R. Medical databases on the Internet. *J R Soc Med.* 1997;90:610–611.

7. Dickersin K, Manheimer E. The Cochrane Collaboration: evaluation of health care and services using systematic reviews of the results of randomized controlled trials. *Clin Obstet Gynecol.* 1998;41:315–331.

8. Jadad AR, Cook DJ, Jones A, et al. Methodology and reports of systematic reviews and meta-analyses. *JAMA.* 1998;280:278–280.

9. The Complementary Medicine Field Module. *The Cochrane Library.* Issue 4. Oxford, England: Update Software;1998.

10. Dickersin K, Scherer L, Lefevbre C. Identifying relevant studies for systematic reviews. In: Chalmers I, Altman D, eds. *Systematic Reviews.* London, England: BMJ Press;1997:17–36.

11. Hofmans EA. Acupuncture and MEDLINE. *Lancet.* 1990;336:57.

12. Kleijnen J, Knipschild P. The comprehensiveness of MEDLINE and EMBASE computer searches. *Pharmaceutisch Weekblad.* 1992;14:316–320.

13. Knipschild P. Searching for alternatives. *Lancet.* 1993;341:1135–1136.

14. Wootton JC. US patent documents on the Internet. *J Altern Complement Med.* 1997; 2:261–269.

15. Cook DJ, Guyatt GH, Ryan G, et al. Should unpublished data be included in meta-analyses? current convictions and controversies. *JAMA.* 1993;269:2749–2753.

16. Dickersin K, Min Y, Meinert CL. Factors influencing publication of research results. *JAMA.* 1992;267:374–378.

17. Callaham ML, Wears RL, Weber EJ, Barton C, Young G. Positive-outcome bias and other limitations in the outcome of research abstracts submitted to a scientific meeting. *JAMA.* 1998;280:254–257.

18. Vickers A, Goyal N, Harland R, Rees R. Do certain countries produce only positive results? *Control Clin Trials.* 1998;19:159–166.

19. Schultz KF, Chalmers I, Hayes RJ, Altman DG. Empirical evidence of bias. *JAMA.* 1995; 273:408–412.

20. Khan KS, Daya S, Jadad A. The importance of quality of primary studies in producing unbiased systematic reviews. *Arch Intern Med.* 1996;156:661–666.

21. Moher D, Fortin R, Jadad AR, et al. Completeness of reporting of trials published in languages other than English. *Lancet.* 1996;347:363–366.

22. Egger M, Zellweger-Zahner T, Schneider M, et al. Language bias in randomized controlled trials published in English and German. *Lancet.* 1997;350:326–329.

23. Linde K, Ramirez G, Mulrow CD, Pauls A, Weidenhammer W, Melchart D. St. John's wort for depression. *BMJ.* 1996;313:253–258.

24. Kleijnen J, Knipschild P. *Ginkgo biloba* for cerebral insufficiency. *Br J Clin Pharmacol.* 1992;34:352–358.

25. ter Reit G, Kleijnen J, Knipschild P. Acupuncture and chronic pain: a criteria-based meta-analysis. *J Clin Epidemiol.* 1990;43:1191–1199.

26. Fishbain DA. Chronic pain treatments meta-analyses. Paper presented at: National Institutes of Health Technology Assessment of Integration of Behavioral and Relaxation Approaches Into the Treatment of Chronic Pain and Insomnia; October 16-18, 1995; Bethesda, Md.

27. Jadad AR, McQuay HJ. Meta-analyses to evaluate analgesic interventions. *J Clin Epidemiol.* 1996;49:235–243.

28. *The Cochrane Library.* Issue 3. Oxford, England: Update Software;1998.

29. Lehmann HP, Goodman SN. Specifications for formalizing clinical significance. *Med Decis Making.* 1995;15:424.

30. Bero LA, Jadad AR. How consumers and policy-makers can use systematic reviews for decision making. *Ann Intern Med.* 1997;127:37–42.

Index

Note: Chapter authors' names and the first page of their respective articles appear in boldface.

A

B

C

D

E

F

I

N

O

P

T

U

V

W

X

Y

Z